CONSULTATIONS IN
FELINE INTERNAL MEDICINE

◆ Section Editors

CONSULTATIONS IN FELINE INTERNAL MEDICINE

4

John R. August, B. Vet. Med., M.S.,
M.R.C.V.S., Diplomate A.C.V.I.M.

Professor of Feline Internal Medicine
Department of Small Animal Medicine and Surgery
College of Veterinary Medicine
Texas A&M University
College Station, Texas

W.B. SAUNDERS COMPANY
A Harcourt Health Sciences Company
Philadelphia London New York St. Louis Sydney Toronto

W.B. SAUNDERS COMPANY
A Harcourt Health Sciences Company

The Curtis Center
Independence Square West
Philadelphia, Pennsylvania 19106

Library of Congress Cataloging-in-Publication Data

Consultations in feline internal medicine 4 / [edited by] John R. August.

p.   cm.

Includes bibliographical references (p.   ).

ISBN 0–7216–8003–8

1. Cats—Diseases.   I. August, John R.

SF985.C66 2001

636.8′0896—dc21   00–053796

Editor-in-Chief: John Schrefer
Acquisitions Editor: Ray Kersey
Developmental Editor: Hazel Hacker
Copy Editor: Mimi McGinnis
Production Manager: Peter Faber
Illustration Specialist: Lisa Lambert
Book Designer: Sasha O'Malley
Indexer: Angela Holt

CONSULTATIONS IN FELINE INTERNAL MEDICINE   ISBN 0–7216–8003–8

Printed in the United States of America.

Last digit is the print number: 9   8   7   6   5   4   3   2   1

This book is dedicated to my daughter, Jessica

◆ Contributors

Amin Ahmadzadeh, B.Sc., Ph.D.
Postdoctoral Fellow, Center for Molecular Medicine and Infectious Diseases, Virginia-Maryland Regional College of Veterinary Medicine, Virginia Tech, Blacksburg, Virginia
Immunocontraception to Help Control Feral Cat Populations

Todd W. Axlund, D.V.M.
Assistant Professor, Department of Veterinary Surgery and Medicine; Affiliate Scientist, Scott-Ritchey Research Center, College of Veterinary Medicine, Auburn University, Auburn, Alabama
Dysautonomia Revisited

Anne Bahr, D.V.M., M.S., Diplomate A.C.V.R.
Clinical Assistant Professor, Department of Large Animal Medicine and Surgery, College of Veterinary Medicine, Texas A&M University, College Station, Texas
Diagnostic Imaging of Neoplasia

Henry J. Baker, D.V.M.
Professor and Director, Scott-Ritchey Research Center, College of Veterinary Medicine, Auburn University, Auburn, Alabama
Molecular Diagnosis of Gangliosidoses: A Model for Elimination of Inherited Diseases in Pure Breeds

Claudia J. Baldwin, D.V.M., M.S., Diplomate A.C.V.I.M.
Associate Professor of Small Animal Medicine, Department of Veterinary Clinical Sciences, College of Veterinary Medicine, Iowa State University, Ames, Iowa
Thrombocytopenia

Joseph W. Bartges, B.S., D.V.M., Ph.D., Diplomate A.C.V.I.M., Diplomate A.C.V.N.
Associate Professor of Medicine and Nutrition, Department of Small Animal Clinical Sciences, College of Veterinary Medicine; Staff Internist and Nutritionist, Veterinary Teaching Hospital, The University of Tennessee, Knoxville, Tennessee
Calcium Oxalate Urolithiasis

Catherine J. Baty, D.V.M., Ph.D., Diplomate A.C.V.I.M.
Hitchings-Elion Fellow, University of North Carolina, Chapel Hill, North Carolina
Aortic Thromboembolism

Ellen N. Behrend, V.M.D., M.S., Diplomate A.C.V.I.M.
Assistant Professor, Department of Small Animal Surgery and Medicine, College of Veterinary Medicine, Auburn University, Auburn, Alabama
Adrenocortical Disease

Linda M. Berent, V.M.D.
Graduate Student, College of Veterinary Medicine, University of Illinois, Urbana, Illinois
Use of the Polymerase Chain Reaction to Detect Hemoparasites

Sonya Bettenay, B.V.Sc.(Hons.), M.A.C.V.Sc., F.A.C.V.Sc.
Staff Dermatologist, Department of Clinical Sciences, College of Veterinary Medicine and Biomedical Sciences, Colorado State University, Fort Collins, Colorado
Photodermatitis

Stephen M. Boyle, B.Sc., M.Sc., Ph.D.
Professor of Microbiology, Department of Biomedical Sciences and Pathobiology, Virginia-Maryland Regional College of Veterinary Medicine, Virginia Tech, Blacksburg, Virginia
Immunocontraception to Help Control Feral Cat Populations

Scott A. Brown, V.M.D., Ph.D., Diplomate A.C.V.I.M.
Professor, Department of Physiology, College of Veterinary Medicine, Department of Small Animal Medicine, Veterinary Medical Teaching Hospital, College of Veterinary Medicine, University of Georgia, Athens, Georgia
Diagnosis and Treatment of Systemic Hypertension

C. A. Tony Buffington, D.V.M., Ph.D., Diplomate A.C.V.I.M.
Professor, Department of Veterinary Clinical Sciences, College of Veterinary Medicine, The Ohio State University, Columbus, Ohio
New Treatments in the Medical Management of Feline Interstitial Cystitis

Karen L. Campbell, D.V.M., M.S., Diplomate A.C.V.D., Diplomate A.C.V.I.M.
Professor and Section Head, Specialty Medicine, Department of Veterinary Clinical Medicine, University of Illinois, College of Veterinary Medicine, Urbana, Illinois
Editor, Section IV; Paraneoplastic Alopecia; Bowen's Disease (Multicentric Squamous Cell Carcinoma In Situ)

Elizabeth A. Carsten, D.V.M., Diplomate A.C.V.I.M.
Staff Internist, Southwest Veterinary Internal Medicine, Tucson, Arizona
Gastrointestinal Lymphoma and Inflammatory Bowel Disease

Sharon A. Center, Diplomate A.C.V.I.M.
Professor, Internal Medicine, Department of Clinical Sciences, College of Veterinary Medicine, Cornell University, Ithaca, New York
Idiopathic Hypercalcemia

Dennis J. Chew, D.V.M., Diplomate A.C.V.I.M.

Professor, Department of Veterinary Clinical Sciences, College of Veterinary Medicine, The Ohio State University; Attending Clinician, Ohio State University Veterinary Medical Teaching Hospital, Columbus, Ohio
Idiopathic Hypercalcemia; New Treatments in the Medical Management of Feline Interstitial Cystitis

Ruthanne Chun, D.V.M., Diplomate A.C.V.I.M.(Oncology)

Assistant Professor, Department of Clinical Sciences, College of Veterinary Medicine, Kansas State University, Manhattan, Kansas
Chemotherapeutic Challenges: Special Considerations and New Agents

Joan R. Coates, D.V.M., M.S., Diplomate A.C.V.I.M.(Neurology)

Assistant Professor, Department of Small Animal Medicine and Surgery, College of Veterinary Medicine, Texas A&M University, College Station, Texas
Editor, Section VII; Congenital Cranial and Intracranial Malformations

Kirsten L. Cooke, D.V.M., Diplomate A.C.V.I.M.

Clinical Assistant Professor, Department of Small Animal Clinical Sciences, College of Veterinary Medicine, University of Florida, Gainesville, Florida
Systemic Hypertension

Rick L. Cowell, D.V.M., M.S., Diplomate A.C.V.P.

Professor, Veterinary Clinical Pathology; Director, Clinical Pathology Laboratory, Department of Veterinary Pathobiology, College of Veterinary Medicine, Oklahoma State University, Stillwater, Oklahoma
Editor, Section VIII; Thrombocytopenia

Larry D. Cowgill, D.V.M., Ph.D., Diplomate A.C.V.I.M.

Associate Professor, Department of Medicine and Epidemiology, School of Veterinary Medicine, University of California at Davis, Davis, California
Use of Hemodialysis in Chronic Renal Failure

Paul A. Cuddon, B.V.Sc.(Hons. I), Diplomate A.C.V.I.M.(Neurology)

Associate Professor, Department of Clinical Sciences, College of Veterinary Medicine and Biomedical Sciences, Colorado State University, Fort Collins, Colorado
Diabetic Neuropathy

Curtis W. Dewey, D.V.M., M.S., Diplomate A.C.V.I.M.(Neurology), Diplomate A.C.V.S.

Assistant Professor, Department of Small Animal Medicine and Surgery, College of Veterinary Medicine, Texas A&M University, College Station, Texas
Acquired Myasthenia Gravis and Other Disorders of the Neuromuscular Junction

Stephen P. DiBartola, D.V.M., Diplomate A.C.V.I.M.

Professor of Medicine, Department of Veterinary Clinical Sciences, College of Veterinary Medicine, The Ohio State University, Columbus, Ohio
Editor, Section VI; Idiopathic Hypercalcemia

Julie M. Ducoté, D.V.M.

Neurologist, Dallas Veterinary Surgical Center, Dallas, Texas
Acquired Myasthenia Gravis and Other Disorders of the Neuromuscular Junction

Denise A. Elliott, B.V.Sc., Diplomate A.C.V.I.M.

Hills Fellow in Clinical Nutrition, Department of Molecular Biosciences, School of Veterinary Medicine, University of California at Davis, Davis, California
Use of Hemodialysis in Chronic Renal Failure

Richard H. Evans, D.V.M., M.S.

Chief of Veterinary Services, Veterinary Public Health Division, Orange County Health Care Agency, Orange, California
Feline Animal Shelter Medicine

Janet E. Foley, D.V.M., Ph.D.

Microbiologist, Department of Pathology, Microbiology, and Immunology, School of Veterinary Medicine, University of California at Davis, Davis, California
Hemobartonellosis

John V. Fondacaro, D.V.M., M.S., Diplomate A.C.V.I.M.

Internist, Ultravet Diagnostics, Mineola, New York
Problems of Diabetes Regulation With Insulin Therapy

Theresa W. Fossum, D.V.M., Ph.D., Diplomate A.C.V.S.

Professor and Chief of Surgery, Department of Small Animal Medicine and Surgery, College of Veterinary Medicine, Texas A&M University, College Station, Texas
Chylothorax

Polly Foureman, Ph.D., D.V.M.

Postdoctoral Fellow, Medical Genetics, School of Veterinary Medicine, University of Pennsylvania, Philadelphia, Pennsylvania
Molecular Diagnosis of Gangliosidoses: A Model for Elimination of Inherited Diseases in Pure Breeds

Urs Giger, P.D., Dr. Med. Vet., M.S., F.V.H., Diplomate A.C.V.I.M.

Charlotte Newton Sheppard Professor of Medicine, Chief, Section of Medical Genetics, School of Veterinary Medicine, University of Pennsylvania, Philadelphia, Pennsylvania
Hereditary Erythrocyte Disorders

Deborah S. Greco, D.V.M., Ph.D., Diplomate A.C.V.I.M.

Department of Clinical Sciences, College of Veterinary Medicine and Biomedical Sciences, Colorado State University, Fort Collins, Colorado
Editor, Section III; Oral Hypoglycemic Therapy for Type 2 Diabetes Mellitus; Problems of Diabetes Regulation With Insulin Therapy; APUDomas: Pheochromocytoma, Insulinoma, and Gastrinoma

W. Grant Guilford, B.V.Sc., Ph.D., Diplomate A.C.V.I.M.

Professor, Veterinary Internal Medicine and Clinical Nutrition, Institute of Veterinary, Animal, and Biomedical Sciences, Massey University, Palmerston North, New Zealand
The Gastrointestinal Tract and Adverse Reactions to Food

Danièlle Gunn-Moore, B.Sc., B.V.M.S., Ph.D., M.A.C.V.Sc., M.R.C.V.S.

Ralston Purina Lecturer in Feline Medicine, University of Edinburgh, Edinburgh, Scotland
Feline Spongiform Encephalopathy and Borna Disease

Jean A. Hall, D.V.M., M.S., Ph.D., Diplomate A.C.V.I.M.

Assistant Professor, Department of Biomedical Sciences, College of Veterinary Medicine, Oregon State University, Corvallis, Oregon
Clinical Approach to Chronic Diarrhea

Jeffrey O. Hall, D.V.M., Ph.D., Diplomate A.B.V.T.

Assistant Professor, Utah State University; Diagnostic Toxicologist, Utah Veterinary Diagnostic Laboratory, Logan, Utah
Lily Nephrotoxicity

David A. Harbour, B.Sc., Ph.D.

Reader, Division of Molecular and Cellular Biology, University of Bristol, Bristol, England
Feline Spongiform Encephalopathy and Borna Disease

Carolyn J. Henry, D.V.M., M.S., Diplomate A.C.V.I.M.(Oncology)

Assistant Professor of Oncology, Department of Veterinary Medicine and Surgery, College of Veterinary Medicine, University of Missouri, Columbia, Missouri
Update on Vaccine-Associated Sarcomas

Leslie Henshaw, B.S., D.V.M., Diplomate A.C.V.D.

Adjunct Faculty Member, College of Veterinary Medicine, Oklahoma State University, Stillwater; Dermatologist, Tulsa Veterinary Dermatology, Tulsa, Oklahoma
Cutaneous Xanthomas

Katherine A. Houpt, V.M.D., Ph.D., Diplomate A.C.V.B.

Professor, Department of Physiology, College of Veterinary Medicine, Cornell University, Ithaca, New York
Cognitive Dysfunction in Geriatric Cats

M. Siobhan Hughes, Ph.D.

Veterinary Sciences Division, Department of Agriculture and Rural Development, Stormont, Belfast, Northern Ireland
Nontuberculous Mycobacterial Diseases

Gilbert J. Jacobs, D.V.M., A.C.V.I.M.(Cardiology)

Professor, Department of Small Animal Medicine, College of Veterinary Medicine, University of Georgia, Athens, Georgia
Cryptococcosis: New Perspectives on Etiology, Pathogenesis, Diagnosis, and Clinical Management

Katherine M. James, D.V.M.

Veterinary Education Coordinator, Veterinary Information Network, Davis, California
Medical Management of Chronic Renal Failure

Albert E. Jergens, D.V.M., M.S., Diplomate A.C.V.I.M.

Associate Professor and Staff Internist, Department of Veterinary Clinical Sciences, College of Veterinary Medicine, Iowa State University, Ames, Iowa
Editor, Section II; Diseases of the Esophagus

Lynelle R. Johnson, D.V.M., Ph.D.

Research Assistant Professor, University of Missouri, Columbia, Missouri
Respiratory Therapeutics

Robert J. Kemppainen, D.V.M., Ph.D.

Professor, Department of Anatomy and Physiology, College of Veterinary Medicine, Auburn University, Auburn, Alabama
Adrenocortical Disease

Anke Langenbach, D.V.M.

Associate Surgeon, Surgical Referral Practice of Northern Virginia, Manassas, Virginia
Hip Dysplasia

Michael R. Lappin, D.V.M., Ph.D., Diplomate A.C.V.I.M.

Department of Clinical Sciences, College of Veterinary Medicine and Biomedical Sciences, Colorado State University, Fort Collins, Colorado
Editor, Section I; Cat Ownership by Immunosuppressed People

Dennis F. Lawler, D.V.M.

Research Veterinarian, Department of Pet Nutrition Research, Ralston Purina Company, St. Louis, Missouri
Editor, Section X

Richard A. LeCouteur, B.V.Sc., Ph.D., Diplomate A.C.V.I.M.(Neurology)

Professor, Department of Surgical and Radiological Sciences, School of Veterinary Medicine; Professor, Veterinary Medical Teaching Hospital, University of California at Davis, Davis, California
Cerebral Meningiomas: Diagnostic and Therapeutic Considerations

Carol A. Lichtensteiger, D.V.M., Ph.D., Diplomate A.C.V.P.

Clinical Assistant Professor, Laboratory of Veterinary Diagnostic Medicine, College of Veterinary Medicine, University of Illinois, Urbana, Illinois
Paraneoplastic Alopecia

Daria N. Love, D.V.Sc., Ph.D., F.R.C. Path., M.A.S.M.

Associate Professor of Veterinary Microbiology, Department of Veterinary Anatomy and Pathology, and Diagnostic Services Laboratory, University Veterinary Centre, The University of Sydney, Sydney, New South Wales, Australia
Cryptococcosis: New Perspectives on Etiology, Pathogenesis, Diagnosis, and Clinical Management; Nontuberculous Mycobacterial Diseases

Leslie A. Lyons, D.V.M., Ph.D.

Department of Population Health and Reproduction, School of Veterinary Medicine, University of California at Davis, Davis, California
Understanding the Feline Genome

Dennis W. Macy, D.V.M., M.S., Diplomate A.C.V.I.M.

Department of Clinical Sciences, College of Veterinary Medicine and Biomedical Sciences, Colorado State University, Fort Collins, Colorado
Update on Vaccine-Associated Sarcomas and Current Vaccine Recommendations

David J. Maggs, B.V.Sc.(Hons.), Diplomate A.C.V.O.

Assistant Professor of Ophthalmology, University of California at Davis, Davis, California; Formerly Visiting Assistant Professor of Ophthalmology, University of Missouri, Columbia, Missouri
Update on the Diagnosis and Management of Feline Herpesvirus-1 Infection

Richard Malik, B.V.Sc., Ph.D., F.A.C.V.Sc., M.A.S.M.

Valentine Charlton Senior Lecturer in Feline Medicine, Department of Veterinary Clinical Sciences and University Veterinary Centre, University of Sydney, Sydney, New South Wales, Australia
Cryptococcosis: New Perspectives on Etiology, Pathogenesis, Diagnosis, and Clinical Management; Nontuberculous Mycobacterial Diseases

Philip A. March, D.V.M., M.S., Diplomate A.C.V.I.M.(Neurology)

Assistant Professor of Neurology, Department of Veterinary Clinical Sciences, College of Veterinary Medicine, The Ohio State University, Columbus, Ohio
Neuronal Storage Disorders

Douglas R. Martin, Ph.D.

Postdoctoral Fellow, Scott-Ritchey Research Center, College of Veterinary Medicine, Auburn University, Auburn, Alabama
Molecular Diagnosis of Gangliosidoses: A Model for Elimination of Inherited Diseases in Pure Breeds

Kyle G. Mathews, D.V.M., M.S., Diplomate A.C.V.S.

Assistant Professor, Department of Clinical Sciences, College of Veterinary Medicine, North Carolina State University, Raleigh, North Carolina
Renal Transplantation in the Management of Chronic Renal Failure

Jennifer L. Matousek, D.V.M.

Clinical Assistant Professor, Department of Veterinary Clinical Medicine, College of Veterinary Medicine, University of Illinois, Urbana, Illinois
Paraneoplastic Alopecia

G. Neal Mauldin, B.S., D.V.M., Diplomate A.C.V.I.M.(Internal Medicine, Oncology)

Assistant Professor of Veterinary Oncology, Department of Veterinary Clinical Sciences, School of Veterinary Medicine, Louisiana State University, Baton Rouge, Louisiana
Approach to Oral Tumors

Glenna E. Mauldin, D.V.M., M.S., Diplomate A.C.V.I.M.(Oncology)

Assistant Professor of Veterinary Oncology, Department of Veterinary Clinical Sciences, School of Veterinary Medicine, Louisiana State University, Baton Rouge, Louisiana
Management of the Lymphoma Patient With Concurrent Disease

Christopher A. McReynolds, D.V.M.

Department of Clinical Sciences, College of Veterinary Medicine and Biomedical Sciences, Colorado State University, Fort Collins, Colorado
Cryptosporidiosis

James H. Meinkoth, D.V.M., M.S., Ph.D., Diplomate A.C.V.P.

Associate Professor, Clinical Pathology, Department of Veterinary Pathobiology, College of Veterinary Medicine, Oklahoma State University, Stillwater, Oklahoma
Update on Cytauxzoonosis

Michele Menard, D.V.M., M.S., Ph.D., Diplomate A.C.V.P.

Cytopathologist, Veterinary Diagnostic Imaging and Cytopathology, P.C., Clackamas, Oregon
Cytologic Evaluation of Fine-Needle Liver Biopsies

Joanne B. Messick, V.M.D., Ph.D., Diplomate A.C.V.P.

Assistant Professor, Department of Veterinary Pathobiology, College of Veterinary Medicine, University of Illinois, Urbana, Illinois
Use of the Polymerase Chain Reaction to Detect Hemoparasites

Kathryn M. Meurs, D.V.M., Ph.D., Diplomate A.C.V.I.M.(Cardiology)

Assistant Professor, Department of Veterinary Clinical Sciences, College of Veterinary Medicine, The Ohio State University, Columbus, Ohio
Hypertrophic Cardiomyopathy

Angela M. Midkiff, D.V.M.

Department of Veterinary Clinical Sciences, College of Veterinary Medicine, The Ohio State University, Columbus, Ohio
Idiopathic Hypercalcemia

Kristina G. Miles, D.V.M., M.S., Diplomate A.C.V.R.

Associate Professor, Radiology Section, Department of Veterinary Clinical Sciences, College of Veterinary Medicine, Iowa State University, Ames, Iowa
Contrast Radiography for Evaluation of the Gastrointestinal Tract

Matthew W. Miller, D.V.M., M.S., Diplomate A.C.V.I.M.(Cardiology)

Associate Professor, Department of Small Animal Medicine and Surgery, College of Veterinary Medicine, Texas A&M University; Staff Cardiologist, Texas Veterinary Medical Teaching Hospital, College Station, Texas
Editor, Section V; Echocardiography; Heartworm Disease

Samantha C. Mooney, M.A.

Research Associate, The Donaldson-Atwood Cancer Clinic, New York, New York
Management of the Lymphoma Patient With Concurrent Disease

Karen A. Moriello, D.V.M., Diplomate A.C.V.D.

Clinical Associate Professor of Dermatology, Department of Medical Sciences, School of Veterinary Medicine, University of Wisconsin, Madison, Wisconsin
What to Do for the Devoted Cat Owner Who Is Allergic to Her or His Pet

Ralf S. Mueller, Dr. Med. Vet.

Assistant Professor, Veterinary Dermatology, Department of Clinical Sciences, College of Veterinary Medicine and Biomedical Sciences, Colorado State University, Fort Collins, Colorado
Mosquito-Bite Hypersensitivity

Karen R. Muñana, D.V.M., M.S., Diplomate A.C.V.I.M.(Neurology)

Assistant Professor, Department of Clinical Sciences, College of Veterinary Medicine, North Carolina State University, Raleigh, North Carolina
Inflammatory Disorders of the Central Nervous System

Todd P. Murphy, D.V.M.

Staff Surgeon, Austin Veterinary Medical Center, Austin, Texas
Hip Dysplasia

T. Mark Neer, D.V.M.

Professor of Medicine and Section Chief, Small Animal Medicine, Teaching Hospital and Clinics, College of Veterinary Medicine, Louisiana State University, Baton Rouge, Louisiana
Splenomegaly and Lymphadenopathy

Reto Neiger, D.V.M. Med., Ph.D.

Lecturer, Royal Veterinary College, University of London, London, England
Gastric Helicobacter *Infection*

Dennis O'Brien, D.V.M., Ph.D., Diplomate A.C.V.I.M.(Neurology)

Associate Professor, Department of Veterinary Medicine and Surgery, College of Veterinary Medicine, University of Missouri, Columbia, Missouri
Dysautonomia Revisited

Marc Papageorges, D.V.M., M.S., Ph.D., Diplomate A.C.V.R.

Radiologist and President, Veterinary Diagnostic Imaging and Cytopathology, P.C., Clackamas, Oregon
Cytologic Evaluation of Fine-Needle Liver Biopsies

Manon Paradis, D.V.M., M.V.Sc., Diplomate A.C.V.D.

Professor of Dermatology, Department of Clinical Sciences, Faculté de Médecine Vétérinaire, University of Montreal, Québec, Canada
Primary Hereditary Seborrhea Oleosa

Gary J. Patronek, B.S., M.S., V.M.D., Ph.D.

Director, Tufts Center for Animals and Public Policy, Agnes Varis University Chair in Science and Society, School of Veterinary Medicine, Tufts University, North Grafton, Massachusetts
Quality of Life in Long-Term Confinement

Mark E. Peterson, D.V.M., Diplomate A.C.V.I.M.

Head, Division of Endocrinology, Bobst Hospital of the Animal Medical Center; Associate Director, Caspary Research Institute, The Animal Medical Center, New York, New York
Diagnosis of Occult Hyperthyroidism

John F. Randolph, D.V.M., Diplomate A.C.V.I.M.

Professor of Medicine, Department of Clinical Sciences, College of Veterinary Medicine, Cornell University, Ithaca, New York
Idiopathic Hypercalcemia

Kenita S. Rogers, D.V.M., M.S., Diplomate A.C.V.I.M.(Internal Medicine, Oncology)

Associate Professor of Oncology and Staff Oncologist, Department of Small Animal Medicine and Surgery, College of Veterinary Medicine, Texas A&M University, College Station, Texas
Editor, Section IX; Evaluation and Treatment of Cranial Mediastinal Masses

Wayne Shapiro, M.S., D.V.M., Diplomate A.C.V.I.M.(Internal Medicine, Oncology)

Consultant, Antech Diagnostics, Irvine, California
Myeloid and Mast Cell Leukemias

Kenneth W. Simpson, B.V.M.S., Ph.D., Diplomate A.C.V.I.M.

Assistant Professor of Medicine, Department of Clinical Sciences, College of Veterinary Medicine, Cornell University, Ithaca, New York
Gastric Helicobacter Infection

Margaret R. Slater, D.V.M., Ph.D.

Associate Professor of Epidemiology, Departments of Veterinary Anatomy and Public Health and Small Animal Medicine and Surgery, College of Veterinary Medicine, Texas A&M University, College Station, Texas
Understanding and Controlling of Feral Cat Populations

Annette Smith, D.V.M., Diplomate A.C.V.I.M.

Assistant Clinical Professor, Department of Internal Medicine/Oncology, College of Veterinary Medicine, Auburn University, Auburn, Alabama
Intranasal Neoplasia

Bruce F. Smith, V.M.D., Ph.D.

Associate Professor, Scott-Ritchey Research Center, College of Veterinary Medicine, Auburn University, Auburn, Alabama
Molecular Diagnosis of Gangliosidoses: A Model for Elimination of Inherited Diseases in Pure Breeds

Gail K. Smith, V.M.D., Ph.D.

Professor of Orthopaedic Surgery, School of Veterinary Medicine; Chairman, Department of Clinical Studies, University of Pennsylvania, Philadelphia, Pennsylvania
Hip Dysplasia

Patti S. Snyder, D.V.M., M.S., Diplomate A.C.V.I.M.

Associate Professor, Department of Small Animal Clinical Sciences, College of Veterinary Medicine, University of Florida, Gainesville, Florida
Systemic Hypertension

Donald C. Sorjonen, D.V.M., M.S., Diplomate A.C.V.I.M.(Neurology)

Professor Emeritus, Department of Veterinary Surgery and Medicine, College of Veterinary Medicine, Auburn University, Auburn, Alabama
Dysautonomia Revisited

Elizabeth Sperry, B.S.

Fourth-year Veterinary Medical Student, School of Veterinary Medicine, Tufts University, North Grafton, Massachusetts
Quality of Life in Long-Term Confinement

Alan W. Spier, D.V.M.

Resident in Cardiology, Department of Veterinary Clinical Sciences, College of Veterinary Medicine, The Ohio State University, Columbus, Ohio
Hypertrophic Cardiomyopathy

Laura B. Stokking, Ph.D., D.V.M.

Resident in Dermatology, College of Veterinary Medicine, University of Illinois, Urbana, Illinois
Bowen's Disease (Multicentric Squamous Cell Carcinoma In Situ)

Dalit Strauss-Ayali, D.V.M., M.S.

Research Associate, Koret School of Veterinary Medicine, Hebrew University of Jerusalem, Rehovot, Israel
Gastric Helicobacter Infection

Cynthia J. Stubbs, D.V.M., M.S., Diplomate A.C.V.I.M.

Internist, Cobb Veterinary Internal Medicine, Marietta, Georgia
Rickettsial Diseases

Stacey A. Sullivan, D.V.M., Diplomate A.C.V.I.M.(Neurology)

Animal Neurological Clinic, Portland, Maine
Congenital Cranial and Intracranial Malformations

Joseph Taboada, D.V.M., Diplomate A.C.V.I.M.

Professor of Small Animal Internal Medicine, Department of Veterinary Clinical Sciences; Director of Professional Instruction and Curriculum, School of Veterinary Medicine, Louisiana State University, Baton Rouge, Louisiana
Approach to the Icteric Cat

William B. Thomas, D.V.M., M.S., Diplomate A.C.V.I.M.

Associate Professor of Neurology/Neurosurgery, Department of Small Animal Clinical Sciences, College of Veterinary Medicine, University of Tennessee, Knoxville, Tennessee
Vascular Disorders

Mary Anna Thrall, B.A., D.V.M., M.S.

Professor, Department of Pathology, College of Veterinary Medicine and Biomedical Sciences; Clinical Pathologist, Veterinary Teaching Hospital, Colorado State University, Fort Collins, Colorado
Mucopolysaccharidosis

Melinda K. Van Vechten, D.V.M., Diplomate A.C.V.I.M.(Internal Medicine, Oncology)

Nuclear Medicine for Pets, Sacramento, California
Complications of Therapy for Hyperthyroidism

K. Jane Wardrop, D.V.M., M.S., Diplomate A.C.V.P.

Associate Professor, Department of Veterinary Clinical Sciences, College of Veterinary Medicine, Washington State University, Pullman, Washington
Transfusion Medicine

Wendy A. Ware, D.V.M., M.S., Diplomate A.C.V.I.M.(Cardiology)

Professor, Departments of Veterinary Clinical Sciences and Biomedical Sciences, College of Veterinary Medicine, Iowa State University; Attending Cardiologist, Iowa State University Veterinary Teaching Hospital, Ames, Iowa
Holter Monitoring

Robert J. Washabau, V.M.D., Ph.D., Diplomate A.C.V.I.M.

Associate Professor of Medicine, Department of Clinical Studies, School of Veterinary Medicine, University of Pennsylvania, Philadelphia, Pennsylvania
Update on Antiemetic Therapy

Michael D. Willard, D.V.M., M.S., Diplomate A.C.V.I.M.

Professor, Department of Small Animal Medicine and Surgery, College of Veterinary Medicine, Texas A&M University, College Station, Texas
Gastrointestinal Lymphoma and Inflammatory Bowel Disease

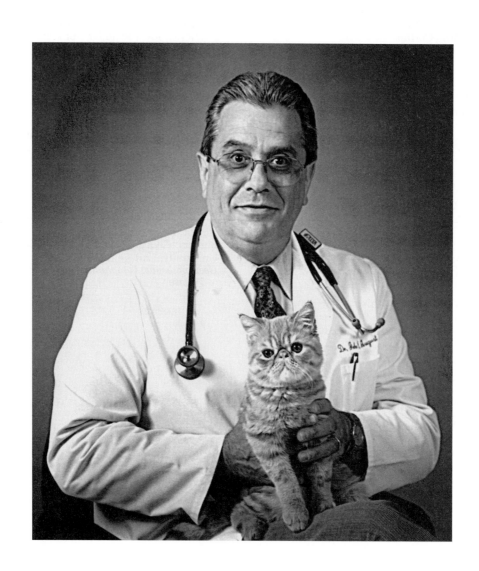

◆ Preface

In 1999, the Veterinary Medical Teaching Hospital at Texas A&M University established a feline internal medicine service to provide interested students with advanced educational opportunities, and referring practitioners and their patients with consistent access to focused medical care. The trends and forces that prompted this new venture reflect the growing stature of cats in society, their continuing evolution as true members of our families, and our increasing professional interest in their unique medical needs. The attitudes of our cat-owning clients also have changed, and most now expect us to inform them of all medical options available, however expensive or complicated.

The fourth volume of *Consultations in Feline Internal Medicine* reflects the rising expectations of the cat-owning public by addressing a fresh set of important issues affecting feline health. As the level of preventive healthcare continues to improve, more cats are becoming affected by diseases of maturity. No longer are their owners satisfied with palliative treatment; rather, more of our clients are now seeking advanced forms of treatment to provide prolonged extensions of good-quality life for their feline companions. Hence the inclusion of cutting-edge chapters in this volume on tertiary-care medicine—for example, renal transplantation, hemodialysis, the management of brain tumors, and molecular diagnosis of genetic disease in purebred cats, among many others. Paradoxically, on the other end of the spectrum, overpopulation as a result of irresponsible cat ownership continues to be a nationwide problem. For this reason, we have chosen to include several chapters on population medicine, specifically feral cat management and shelter medicine,

to help our professional colleagues address these difficult and sometimes emotion-charged issues in an informed and objective manner.

Abby and Henry, my two cats whose pictures graced the preface of the third volume, both died within the past year. Our home feels very empty without them, and I would be remiss if I did not give them a belated and posthumous thank-you for the unwavering companionship they provided me for many years.

I owe a deep debt of gratitude to the section editors and authors who worked so hard to develop this volume; they are the true unsung heroes of this project. Their names read like a Who's Who in the discipline of feline medicine and I was genuinely privileged to include them on the team. Mrs. Hazel Hacker, Senior Developmental Editor at the W.B. Saunders Company, deserves very special recognition for her contribution to the development of this book. Without Hazel's extraordinary organizational skills, attention to detail, and supportive guidance, my job would have been far more difficult, especially under the challenging circumstances that occurred during the preparation of this volume. With that said, I must give my heartfelt thanks to Dr. Michael Bevers, Dr. Cynthia Jansky, and the oncology nursing staff of St. Luke's Episcopal Hospital, Houston; you were there when we needed you.

Each volume of *Consultations in Feline Internal Medicine* complements previous volumes, and addresses carefully selected contemporary issues of clinical relevance to the progressive feline practitioner. It is my sincere hope that volume four meets your high expectations, and that you will find it to be an invaluable resource as you provide state-of-the-art care for your feline patients.

John August
College Station, Texas

◆ Contents

I
Infectious Diseases 1
Michael R. Lappin, Editor

1
Update on Vaccine-Associated Sarcomas and Current Vaccine Recommendations 3
Dennis W. Macy

2
Hemobartonellosis 12
Janet E. Foley

3
Cat Ownership by Immunosuppressed People 18
Michael R. Lappin

4
Rickettsial Diseases 28
Cynthia J. Stubbs

5
Cryptosporidiosis 34
Christopher A. McReynolds

6
Cryptococcosis: New Perspectives on Etiology, Pathogenesis, Diagnosis, and Clinical Management 39
Richard Malik, Gilbert J. Jacobs, and Daria N. Love

7
Update on the Diagnosis and Management of Feline Herpesvirus-1 Infection 51
David J. Maggs

8
Feline Spongiform Encephalopathy and Borna Disease 62
Danièlle Gunn-Moore and David A. Harbour

II
Gastrointestinal System 71
Albert E. Jergens, Editor

9
Contrast Radiography for Evaluation of the Gastrointestinal Tract 73
Kristina G. Miles

10
Approach to the Icteric Cat 87
Joseph Taboada

11
Gastric *Helicobacter* Infection 91
Kenneth W. Simpson, Dalit Strauss-Ayali, and Reto Neiger

12
Diseases of the Esophagus 99
Albert E. Jergens

13
Update on Antiemetic Therapy 107
Robert J. Washabau

14
The Gastrointestinal Tract and Adverse Reactions to Food 113
W. Grant Guilford

15
Cytologic Evaluation of Fine-Needle Liver Biopsies 118
Michele Menard and Marc Papageorges

16
Clinical Approach to Chronic Diarrhea 127
Jean A. Hall

III
Endocrine and Metabolic Diseases 137
Deborah S. Greco, Editor

17
Diabetic Neuropathy 139
Paul A. Cuddon

18
Diagnosis of Occult Hyperthyroidism 145
Mark E. Peterson

19
Complications of Therapy for Hyperthyroidism 151
Melinda K. Van Vechten

20
Adrenocortical Disease 159
Ellen N. Behrend and Robert J. Kemppainen

21

**Oral Hypoglycemic Therapy for
Type 2 Diabetes Mellitus** 169
Deborah S. Greco

22

**Problems of Diabetes Regulation With
Insulin Therapy** 175
John V. Fondacaro and
Deborah S. Greco

23

**APUDomas: Pheochromocytoma,
Insulinoma, and Gastrinoma** 181
Deborah S. Greco

IV
Dermatology 185
Karen L. Campbell, Editor

24

Mosquito-Bite Hypersensitivity 186
Ralf S. Mueller

25

Photodermatitis 190
Sonya Bettenay

26

Paraneoplastic Alopecia 196
Jennifer L. Matousek,
Karen L. Campbell, and
Carol A. Lichtensteiger

27

Primary Hereditary Seborrhea Oleosa 202
Manon Paradis

28

**Bowen's Disease (Multicentric Squamous
Cell Carcinoma In Situ)** 208
Laura B. Stokking and
Karen L. Campbell

29

Cutaneous Xanthomas 214
Leslie Henshaw

30

Nontuberculous Mycobacterial Diseases 221
Richard Malik, M. Siobhan Hughes, and
Daria N. Love

31

**What to Do for the Devoted Cat Owner
Who Is Allergic to Her or His Pet** 233
Karen A. Moriello

V
Cardiology and Respiratory
Disorders 243
Matthew W. Miller, Editor

32

Echocardiography 245
Matthew W. Miller

33

Heartworm Disease 253
Matthew W. Miller

34

Hypertrophic Cardiomyopathy 261
Kathryn M. Meurs and Alan W. Spier

35

Chylothorax 267
Theresa W. Fossum

36

Systemic Hypertension 277
Patti S. Snyder and Kirsten L. Cooke

37

Respiratory Therapeutics 283
Lynelle R. Johnson

38

Holter Monitoring 291
Wendy A. Ware

39

Aortic Thromboembolism 299
Catherine J. Baty

VI
Urinary System 307
Stephen P. DiBartola, Editor

40

Lily Nephrotoxicity 309
Jeffrey O. Hall

41

Idiopathic Hypercalcemia 311
Angela M. Midkiff, Dennis J. Chew,
John F. Randolph, Sharon A. Center,
and Stephen P. DiBartola

42

**New Treatments in the Medical
Management of Feline Interstitial Cystitis** 315
C. A. Tony Buffington and
Dennis J. Chew

43

**Renal Transplantation in the
Management of Chronic Renal Failure** 319
Kyle G. Mathews

44

**Medical Management of Chronic Renal
Failure** 328
Katherine M. James

45

**Use of Hemodialysis in Chronic Renal
Failure** 337
Denise A. Elliott and Larry D. Cowgill

46

Calcium Oxalate Urolithiasis 352
Joseph W. Bartges

47

**Diagnosis and Treatment of Systemic
Hypertension** 365
Scott A. Brown

VII
Neurology 373
Joan R. Coates, Editor

48

**Acquired Myasthenia Gravis and Other
Disorders of the Neuromuscular Junction** 374
Julie M. Ducoté and Curtis W. Dewey

49

Dysautonomia Revisited 381
Todd W. Axlund, Donald C. Sorjonen,
and Dennis O'Brien

50

**Cerebral Meningiomas: Diagnostic and
Therapeutic Considerations** 385
Richard A. LeCouteur

51

Neuronal Storage Disorders 393
Philip A. March

52

Vascular Disorders 405
William B. Thomas

53

**Congenital Cranial and Intracranial
Malformations** 413
Joan R. Coates and Stacey A. Sullivan

54

**Inflammatory Disorders of the Central
Nervous System** 425
Karen R. Muñana

VIII
Hematopoietic and Lymphatic
Systems 435
Rick L. Cowell, Editor

55

Update on Cytauxzoonosis 436
James H. Meinkoth

56

Splenomegaly and Lymphadenopathy 439
T. Mark Neer

57

Mucopolysaccharidosis 450
Mary Anna Thrall

58

Transfusion Medicine 461
K. Jane Wardrop

59

Thrombocytopenia 468
Claudia J. Baldwin and Rick L. Cowell

60

**Use of the Polymerase Chain Reaction
to Detect Hemoparasites** 479
Joanne B. Messick and
Linda M. Berent

61

Hereditary Erythrocyte Disorders 484
Urs Giger

62

Myeloid and Mast Cell Leukemias 490
Wayne Shapiro

IX
Oncology 497
Kenita S. Rogers, Editor

63

**Gastrointestinal Lymphoma and
Inflammatory Bowel Disease** 499
Elizabeth A. Carsten and
Michael D. Willard

64

**Management of the Lymphoma Patient
With Concurrent Disease** 506
Glenna E. Mauldin and
Samantha C. Mooney

65

**Chemotherapeutic Challenges: Special
Considerations and New Agents** 521
Ruthanne Chun

66

Approach to Oral Tumors 526
G. Neal Mauldin

67

Intranasal Neoplasia 529
Annette Smith

68

**Evaluation and Treatment of Cranial
Mediastinal Masses** 533
Kenita S. Rogers

69

Update on Vaccine-Associated Sarcomas 541
Carolyn J. Henry

70

Diagnostic Imaging of Neoplasia 548
Anne Bahr

X

Population Medicine 559
Dennis F. Lawler, Editor

71

**Understanding and Controlling of Feral
Cat Populations** 561
Margaret R. Slater

72

Feline Animal Shelter Medicine 571
Richard H. Evans

73

**Immunocontraception to Help Control
Feral Cat Populations** 577
Stephen M. Boyle and
Amin Ahmadzadeh

74

Cognitive Dysfunction in Geriatric Cats 583
Katherine A. Houpt

75

Hip Dysplasia 592
Anke Langenbach, Todd P. Murphy, and
Gail K. Smith

76

Understanding the Feline Genome 600
Leslie A. Lyons

77

**Molecular Diagnosis of Gangliosidoses:
A Model for Elimination of Inherited
Diseases in Pure Breeds** 615
Henry J. Baker, Bruce F. Smith,
Douglas R. Martin, and Polly Foureman

78

Quality of Life in Long-Term Confinement ... 621
Gary J. Patronek and Elizabeth Sperry

Index 635

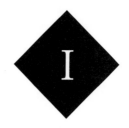

Infectious Diseases

Michael R. Lappin, Editor

◆ Update on Vaccine-Associated Sarcomas and Current
   Vaccine Recommendations 3
◆ Hemobartonellosis 12
◆ Cat Ownership by Immunosuppressed People 18
◆ Rickettsial Diseases 28
◆ Cryptosporidiosis 34
◆ Cryptococcosis: New Perspectives on Etiology,
   Pathogenesis, Diagnosis, and Clinical Management . . 39
◆ Update on the Diagnosis and Management of Feline
   Herpesvirus-1 Infections 51
◆ Spongiform Encephalopathy and Borna Disease 62

**Still-Current Information Found in *Consultations in
Feline Internal Medicine 2:***
Vaccination Against Feline Retroviruses (Chapter 5), p. 33
Diagnosis of Toxoplasmosis (Chapter 6), p. 41
Antifungal Agents (Chapter 8), p. 53
Cerebrospinal Fluid Collection and Analysis (Chapter 49),
   p. 385
Anemia: Diagnosis and Treatment (Chapter 58), p. 469
Clinical Management of Soft Tissue Sarcomas (Chapter 69),
   p. 557
Postvaccination Sarcomas (Chapter 72), p. 587
Surveillance, Prevention, and Control of Viral Diseases in
   Catteries (Chapter 75), p. 615

**Still-Current Information Found in *Consultations in
Feline Internal Medicine 3:***
Bartonella henselae: Consequences of Infection in the Cat
   (Chapter 1), p. 3
Bartonella henselae: An Important Emerging Zoonosis
   (Chapter 2), p. 7
Newer Diagnostic Testing Methodology for Infectious
   Agents (Chapter 7), p. 37
Hemobartonellosis (Chapter 59), p. 479
Clinical Perspectives on Vaccine-Associated Sarcomas
   (Chapter 67), p. 541

Elsewhere in *Consultations in Feline Internal Medicine 4:*
Approach to the Icteric Cat (Chapter 10), p. 87
Gastric *Helicobacter* Infection (Chapter 11), p. 91
Nontuberculous Mycobacterial Diseases (Chapter 30),
   p. 221
Neuronal Storage Disorders (Chapter 51), p. 393
Inflammatory Disorders of the Central Nervous System
   (Chapter 54), p. 425

Mucopolysaccharidosis (Chapter 57), p. 450

Use of the Polymerase Chain Reaction to Detect Hemoparasites (Chapter 60), p. 479

Update on Vaccine-Associated Sarcomas (Chapter 69), p. 541

Feline Animal Shelter Medicine (Chapter 72), p. 571

1

◆ Update on Vaccine-Associated Sarcomas and Current Vaccine Recommendations

Dennis W. Macy

◆ VACCINE-ASSOCIATED SARCOMAS

Epidemiologic evidence has now been published in the United States showing a strong association between the administration of inactivated feline vaccines (feline leukemia virus [FeLV] and rabies) and subsequent soft-tissue sarcoma development at sites where these vaccines have been administered.[1-5] The prevalence of soft-tissue sarcoma development at sites of vaccination has been reported as 3.6 cases in 10,000 to 1 case in 10,000 FeLV or rabies vaccines administered.[5-7] Some believe that the prevalence may be as high as 1 in 1,000 FeLV or rabies vaccines administered.[8] If these prevalence rates are to be applied to the 1991 U.S. cat population, the following projections of the number of vaccine-associated sarcomas that occurred that year can be made. In 1991, the U.S. cat population was estimated at 57 million cats.[8] Approximately 62 per cent of cats see veterinarians during any given year, and 64 per cent of the visits to veterinarians include vaccination. These data indicate that 22 million cats were vaccinated in 1991.[8] Applying the vaccine-induced tumor prevalence rate of 1 tumor per 10,000 vaccines administered, approximately 2200 cases of vaccine-associated sarcomas occurred in 1991. Using the higher estimated vaccine-associated sarcoma prevalence of 1 in 1,000 vaccinations, a total of 22,000 vaccine-associated sarcomas occurred in 1991. Because of the relatively low incidence of fibrosarcomas in cats in general (20 in 100,000), the association between vaccination and subsequent tumor development was made only after millions of doses of now-incriminated vaccines (rabies and FeLV) had been given to cats for half a decade. The number of vaccine-associated sarcomas submitted to veterinary diagnostic laboratories appears to have stabilized and has not increased during the last several years (Idexx Laboratories, Broomfield, CO, personal communication, 1998).

The national increased prevalence of feline fibrosarcomas since about 1985 paralleled the introduction and widespread use of 2 killed adjuvanted vaccines not used previously in cats in the United States.[9] Vaccine-site–associated sarcomas are believed to develop in areas of inflammation produced by these adjuvanted vaccine products, although they have been reported also with nonadjuvanted killed feline vaccines and modified-live injectable vaccines, albeit less often.[4, 5, 10–12] Killed adjuvanted rhinotracheitis/calicivirus/panleukopenia (FVRCP) vaccines were linked to soft-tissue sarcomas in several cats in Canada[13] and Australia[14] and modified-live FVRCP vaccines were linked to soft-tissue sarcomas in 3 cats in Australia.[14] Microscopically, areas of transition between inflammation and tumor development have been observed frequently in vaccine-associated sarcomas.[3, 10] The neoplasms that develop after vaccination typically are mesenchymal in origin; fibrosarcomas, malignant fibrous histiocytomas (also referred to as myofibroblastic sarcomas), osteosarcomas, chondrosarcomas, undifferentiated sarcomas, and rhabdomyosarcomas are reported most frequently.[1, 15] Vaccine-site sarcomas are histologically similar to mesenchymal tumors that arise in traumatized eyes of cats, suggesting a common pathogenesis of inflammation and wound healing in the development of tumors in these 2 syndromes.[16–18] The presence of inflammatory cells, fibroblasts, and myofibroblasts in and around vaccine-site–associated sarcomas supports this hypothesis.

A comparison of the morphologic features of vaccine-site– and nonvaccine-site–associated sarcomas found significant differences between the 2 groups of tumors.[19] Vaccine-site–associated sarcomas typically have increased amounts of necrosis, inflammatory cells (mostly lymphocytes and macrophages), and increased numbers of cycling cells as determined by the presence of mitosis when compared with nonvaccine-site sarcomas (Fig. 1–1).[19]

Hendrick[20] reported preliminary findings of an immunohistochemical study of growth factors and receptors that indicated that vaccine-associated sarcomas have a mild-to-strong positive reaction for platelet derived growth factor (PDGF) and its receptor, whereas nonvaccine-associated fibrosarcomas (NVFSA) are negative. It also was demonstrated that lymphocytes in vaccine-associated sarcomas are positive for PDGF, but lymphocytes in NVFSA and in normal lymph nodes are negative. The expression of *c-jun* also has been examined in vaccine-associated sarcomas. *C-jun* was found to be strongly positive in vaccine-associated sarcomas and not expressed in NVFSA (Fig. 1–2).

It is now believed that vaccines are not the only cause of sarcomas seen at injection sites. Virtually anything that produces local inflammation at the injection site may be responsible for injection-site sarcomas in susceptible cats, but vaccines are the only products that are given to most of the cat popu-

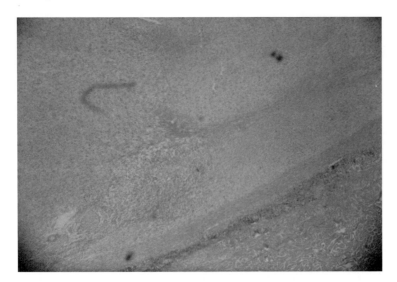

Figure 1–1. Vaccine-associated sarcoma. Note the presence of inflammation adjacent to neoplastic tissue (400×).

lation with any frequency to make a good correlation. Reports of sarcomas developing at sites of antibiotic and lufenuron administration, and the like have been reported occasionally (Kitchell B, personal communication, 1998).

Mechanisms other than inflammation also have been investigated. The potential role of viruses in the pathogenesis of vaccine-site sarcomas has been studied on a limited basis. Ellis and colleagues[21] studied whether FeLV or the feline sarcoma virus were expressed in vaccine-site–associated sarcomas in order to determine whether there might be a viral mechanism giving rise to these sarcomas. One hundred thirty vaccine-site sarcomas were evaluated using polymerase chain reaction and immunohistochemical staining, but FeLV was not detected. The possible role of the tumor suppressor gene p53 in feline sarcomas has been studied in a small number of sarcomas, and mutations in p53 were detected in only 2 of 10 fibrosarcomas studied.[22–24] More importantly, p53 not only has been shown to be increased in the tumor itself, but also in an area up to 5 cm from the tumor mass in histologically normal tissue.[24] p53 is a tumor suppressor gene, and is important in that it is up-regulated in the presence of DNA damage, and is responsible for arresting cells in G1 phase, allowing time for DNA repair, or in the case of excessive damage resulting in cellular apoptosis, preventing defective cells from further replication. The increased expression of p53 around the tumors suggests DNA damage in adjacent tissue. If p53 is defective, damaged cells will be allowed to proliferate and tumor clones to potentially develop. Abnormal p53 has been reported in some vaccine-associated sarcomas (Kanjilal S, et al, personal communication, 1999). It is suggested that vaccine-associated sarcomas may represent an example of field carcinogenesis similar to that observed in human beings with oral squamous cell carcinoma exposed to tobacco products. Further evidence of the role of this mechanism in the pathogenesis of vaccine-associated sarcomas is the finding that adjuvanted feline vaccines are mutagenic in the AL assay, whereas nonadjuvanted feline vaccines do not produce mutations and cell death (McNeil MJ, et al, personal communication, 1998). Cellular mutations are thought to be mediated by the formation of oxygen radicals associated with the inflammatory re-

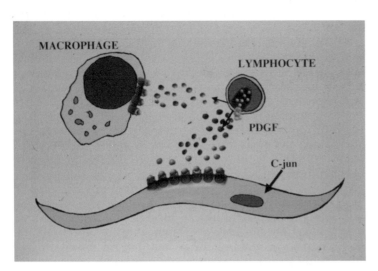

Figure 1–2. The autocrine relationship between platelet-derived growth factor (PDGF) from the macrophages and that from the receptors noted on the fibrosarcoma.

sponse to the adjuvanted vaccines. Despite other possible mechanisms, inflammation remains the most accepted hypothesis in the pathogenesis of vaccine-site–associated sarcomas.

The vaccine component thought most commonly to be associated with local postvaccinal inflammation is the adjuvant.[25] Adjuvants are used in many but not all inactivated feline vaccines. Aluminum, in the form of aluminum hydroxide or aluminum phosphate, is a common component of vaccine adjuvants and is used in some FeLV vaccines and rabies vaccines.[25] Because aluminum has been identified in postvaccinal granulomas and in some vaccine-site–associated sarcomas, it was considered a possible cause of tumor development.[3] However, aluminum may be only a marker of previous vaccination, and other vaccine components may induce inflammation or enhance the inflammatory process that results in sarcoma development in some cats. The specific role of aluminum, other adjuvants, adjuvant components, or vaccine antigens in inducing sarcomas in cats remains unknown at this time.

Although local inflammation may be induced in nearly 100 per cent of vaccinates with certain rabies and FeLV vaccines, tumors only develop in approximately 1 in 1000 of these vaccinates.[26] This fact, along with the observations that some cats develop sarcomas at every vaccine site, that some treatment failure lesions distant to the primary tumor site contain adjuvant, and that many related cats have been found to be affected with vaccine-associated sarcomas, suggests that an individual inherited susceptibility or genetic defect may play a role in the pathogenesis (Macy DW, unpublished data, 1998).

Recommendations for preventing or reducing the incidence of vaccine-associated tumors in cats are controversial. Recommendations include a change in vaccination-site location, decreased use of polyvalent vaccines, use of nonadjuvanted vaccines, avoiding the use of aluminum-based adjuvants, and not overvaccinating, among others.[27, 28]

Vaccine-site location recommendations also have been changed recently. The National Feline Vaccine-Associated Sarcoma Task Force recommends that no vaccine be given in the interscapular space, that rabies vaccine be administered subcutaneously in the distal right rear leg, that FeLV vaccine be administered subcutaneously in the distal left rear leg, and that all other vaccines be administered subcutaneously in the right shoulder region.[8, 27, 28] It appears from our research and reports by others that both intramuscular and subcutaneous administration result in local inflammation and tumor production. Subcutaneous sites are recommended for all vaccines because they will result in earlier detection of these growths if they occur. The reasoning behind these vaccine-site administration recommendations is not based so much on prevention as on earlier diagnosis and potentially a higher cure rate when treated surgically.

It would appear that the problem of vaccine-site–associated sarcomas will be with us for some time,

and the question of what to do with postvaccination lumps is a practical one. Some rabies and FeLV vaccines produce postvaccinal lumps in 100 per cent of the vaccinates, but fortunately, it has been observed that most resolve in 2 to 3 months. Very few vaccine-associated tumors occur sooner than 3 months after vaccination. Given these observations, the Vaccine-Associated Feline Sarcoma Task Force currently recommends that any vaccine-site lumps greater than 2 cm in diameter, or those that are present after 3 months from the time of vaccination, be biopsied. A biopsy will determine the magnitude of the surgery, that is, lumpectomy versus radical surgery. We do not recommend excising the mass before biopsy. Attempts at simple excision of these tumors are seldom curative and lead ultimately to local recurrence with a more difficult second surgical attempt. Even attempts at aggressive wide surgical excision are often incomplete and result in a 30 to 70 per cent failure rate.[29, 30] Treatment failure most likely is due to underestimating the extent of the primary disease. Magnetic resonance imaging or contrast-enhanced computed tomography examinations often show the magnitude of the surgery that may be needed to achieve complete removal, and are recommended when available (Fig. 1–3). The interscapular location and infiltrative nature of these tumors makes excision difficult even with partial scapulectomy, excision of epaxial muscles, and removal of dorsal cervical vertebral processes. There appears to be an advantage to refer these cases to a qualified surgeon before the second surgery is contemplated. After a second surgical intervention has been attempted, there appears to be no improvement in survival with referral to specialist surgeons. Rear-leg amputation has a higher rate of cure than surgery in the interscapular space for vaccine-site–associated sarcomas. Given the incomplete removal

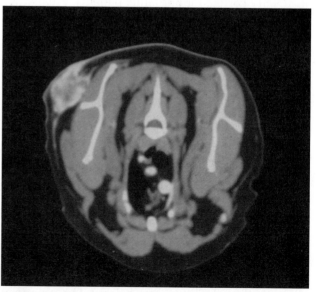

Figure 1–3. Contrast-enhanced computed tomography scan of a cat with a vaccine-associated sarcoma. Note the finger projections of the tumor.

of these tumors even with aggressive surgery, radiation often is used before or after surgery. The interim survival analysis in one study indicates a doubling of survival when radiation is combined with surgery[29] (Macy DW, unpublished data, 1998). In another study in which radiation therapy was given before surgery and complete margins were obtained, the median disease-free interval was 700 days.[31] Although the combination of surgery and radiation has increased tumor control rates in some studies, a significant number of cats still fail to respond to this combination. Several chemotherapy agents, including carboplatin, doxorubicin, cyclophosphamide, and the combination of cyclophosphamide and vincristine, have been used in cats with vaccine-associated tumor.[32] Most chemotherapeutic attempts result in partial responses, but some complete responses have been observed with these drugs. Immunomodulators have been used systemically or intralesionally, but response has been limited.[33] Although the vast majority of vaccine-site–associated sarcomas are only locally invasive, approximately 10 to 20 per cent will metastasize to the lungs or other sites.[34–36]

◆ CURRENT VACCINE RECOMMENDATIONS

Recommendations for immunization of cats should reflect current disease risk, understanding of currently available vaccines, and scientific information on immunity and disease pathogenesis, and should not be based necessarily on traditions, customs, and practices used during the 1970s. As responsible health care professionals, we must be able to evaluate our current immunization practices critically and be able to ask the same hard questions of both old and new vaccination protocols in order to pass unbiased medical judgment in determining what is medically correct for our feline patients. Finally, we must separate monetary motives from medical needs when considering annual vaccination of cats.

The current practice in preventive veterinary medicine, which has been "if it is available, give it and give it yearly" is changing. Not all cats need all available vaccines, nor do they need any of them annually. Rabies, *Microsporum canis*, feline panleukopenia (FPV), feline herpes virus-1 (FHV-1), calicivirus (FCV), FeLV, feline infectious peritonitis (FIP), *Chlamydia psittaci*, *Bordetella bronchiseptica*, and *Giardia* vaccines are available for cats. With the exception of some rabies vaccines, all feline vaccines are recommended by the manufacturer to be given annually. Are all these vaccines really necessary for every cat every year? Are there published case reports of clinical disease in vaccinated cats that miss their boosters? Do you receive all available human vaccines yearly? What is the scientific evidence that the feline immune system is that much different than that of human beings? The American Association of Feline Practitioners, at least 10 North American Colleges of Veterinary Medicine, the

American College of Veterinary Internal Medicine (oncology specialty), the U. S. Army veterinary hospitals worldwide, and veterinary virologists now endorse similar recommendations of a limited number of vaccines.[37–40] Core vaccines, those that should be administered to all cats, include FPV, FHV-1, FCV, and rabies virus. After the initial vaccination period and 1-year booster, these vaccines should be administered no more frequently than every 3 years. Vaccines considered noncore are those to be used only in some cats under special circumstances. Examples include vaccines for *B. bronchiseptica*, FIP, FeLV, *C. psittaci*, *Giardia*, and *M. canis*.

To understand the criteria for vaccine selection and booster frequency recommendations, I believe we must look at the basis of current annual vaccine labeling.[41] Other than rabies, no minimum duration of immunity data are required for veterinary vaccine licensure. Until recently, a manufacturer of U.S. veterinary vaccines could merely show protection 2 to 4 weeks after the initial vaccine series. Because the booster recommendation is *not* required to be based on scientific data, it is considered arbitrary! Manufacturers do not even have to show a rise in titer levels after boostering, let alone enhanced protection by challenge, with annual booster vaccination. This is not the case in Europe, where minimum duration of immunity data based on challenge studies must be submitted before veterinary vaccine licensure. Even with rabies vaccines, the vaccine label is not always representative of the true product. For example, a rabies vaccine that meets challenge requirements for a 3-year duration of immunity may be relabeled simply as a 1-year vaccine under current U.S. Department of Agriculture regulations. Thus a conscientious veterinarian who wanted to use a true 1-year vaccine with less adjuvant and less vaccine-site inflammation really may be using a 3-year vaccine legally relabeled as a 1-year product. The U.S. Department of Agriculture does not even require a warning label for anaphylaxis or injection-site–associated sarcoma development, despite the multiple published reports documenting these adverse events.

Because the majority of manufacturer label recommendations were determined arbitrarily, conscientious veterinarians are forced to use other criteria to establish frequency of revaccination of cats. Epidemiologic information can be very beneficial. For example, FPV is not diagnosed in the same cat twice or in cats that have ever been vaccinated, suggesting that duration of immunity after natural infection or vaccination is permanent for this agent.

Serum antibody titers are an indirect measure of protection that may be used for some diseases to determine duration of immunity.[42, 43] However, there are many limitations. For example, immunity and serum antibody responses may vary with the type of vaccine used (modified-live virus or killed). Additionally, protection against some agents may not be antibody-dependent; serum antibody titers do not necessarily reflect cellular or mucosal immunity

(FIP is a good example).[42] Serum antibody tests are not all the same; technique variation and differences between laboratories may influence interpretation of results. Finally, failure to detect antibodies against an infectious agent in a vaccinated animal does not necessarily equate to susceptibility, and should not be used as the sole basis for revaccination (rabies and rhinotracheitis are good examples).[42]

Duration of immunity studies as determined by challenge data appear to be the most believable, and unlike physicians, "we as veterinarians have the privilege of performing challenge trials." Unfortunately, challenge studies are somewhat expensive, but are not cost-prohibitive, as some vaccine manufacturers would like you to believe. The paucity of case reports of disease in previously vaccinated animals, regardless of time since last vaccinated, suggests the duration of immunity is longer than suggested by the manufacturer's label. Long-term challenge studies have been done for a small group of feline vaccines; results are discussed with each antigen that follows. Each infectious agent is unique, and so the mechanism of protection may be different. In general, those agents that produce severe systemic illness like FPV result in life-long immunity after recovery. Those agents that produce superficial infections like rhinotracheitis produce only transient immunity to infection after recovery or the development of a carrier state. In general, modified-live virus vaccines will mimic natural disease protection, so those vaccines for systemic diseases like FPV will produce lasting protection whereas those for superficial infection do not prevent infection but may reduce clinical signs associated with the infection.

Panleukopenia

FPV is caused by a parvovirus that persists through the environment. In order to prevent cat-to-cat transmission, 98 per cent of the population must be immunized.[44] This polysystemic infection is potentially deadly to the nonimmunized (especially the young), but recovery from natural infection provides life-long immunity. To my knowledge, reports of clinical FPV in vaccinated cats are lacking. Serum neutralizing antibodies were detected in serum of all 8 cats vaccinated with an inactivated FPV vaccine held in isolation for 6 years.[45] Cats vaccinated for FPV have been challenged with virulent virus at 25 months and 7.5 years; 100 per cent of the cats were protected.[46, 47] Both modified-live virus vaccine and killed vaccines provide good antibody responses. Young kittens with maternally derived FPV antibodies are resistant to challenge with virulent virus, documenting FPV serum antibodies to be protective. Because systemic humoral immune responses play a large role in protection against FPV, there is no advantage to intranasal vaccine administration.

Based on the results of these studies, annual re-vaccination recommendations for FPV appear unnecessary. It seems prudent to follow the 3-year interval recommendation for this organism.[37] However, it is doubtful that revaccination with modified-live virus FPV vaccines after the initial series increases protection against clinical disease, and the revaccination interval probably could be longer. Kittens should be vaccinated with modified-live virus or inactivated FPV every 3 to 4 weeks until 12 weeks of age and then revaccinated 1 year later. After that time, the revaccination interval should be no more than every 3 years.

Feline Herpesvirus-1

FHV-1 (viral rhinotracheitis) is the most common cause of upper respiratory disease, conjunctivitis, and keratitis in cats.[44] In general, FHV-1 results in local tissue inflammation and seldom results in systemic disease or changes in the hemogram. Naïve kittens occasionally develop lower airway inflammation and may be life-threatened. Natural FHV-1 infection results in transient and incomplete immunity in the cats. Mucosal secretory immunoglobulin A (IgA) and cell-mediated immune responses are most prominent in protecting cats against FHV-1. Infected cats may recover from clinical disease, but may remain persistently infected and shed the virus intermittently after periods of stress. Most previously infected or vaccinated cats are protected from developing severe systemic disease if re-exposed, but can be infected and shed the virus.[48] Given these characteristics of the immunity derived from natural infections, any vaccine likely will provide only short-term local immunity, but are likely to provide adequate stimulation of memory cells to prevent deep invasion of tissues and severe systemic illness.[48] Vaccinating cats previously infected with FHV-1 probably adds little additional protection. Several studies have shown FHV-1 serum neutralizing titers to be persistent after use of inactivated FHV-1 vaccines.[45, 49] In the longest study, 4 of 8 cats vaccinated with inactivated FHV-1 vaccine and held in isolation had detectable FHV-1 antibody titers 6 years later.[45] When these cats were challenged with virulent FHV-1 7.5 years after vaccination, clinical scores were 52 per cent less than those in unvaccinated control cats.[47] Similar studies have not been published for the newer modified-live virus vaccines. Modified-live virus vaccines stimulate a more lasting mucosal immunity, cell-mediated immunity, and humoral response than killed vaccines, and would be expected to provide even better protection than inactivated vaccines. Recent studies indicate that intranasal vaccines are superior to subcutaneously administered vaccines in reducing clinical disease after exposure, but have a greater incidence of local side-effects. Kittens should be vaccinated every 3 to 4 weeks until 12 weeks of age and then revaccinated 1 year later. After that time,

FHV-1 vaccines should not be administered any more frequently than every 3 years.

Feline Calicivirus

FCV induces upper respiratory disease and stomatatitis in infected cats. Disease can be severe, particularly in naïve kittens. After natural infection with FCV, immunity to reinfection is believed short, but protection against severe systemic illness is sustained.[44, 48, 49] Cats recovering from FCV-induced disease remain persistently infected and shed the virus continuously for months to years. Challenge studies in young kittens with maternally derived FCV antibodies and in immune-vaccinated cats suggests that FCV serum neutralizing titers greater than 1:16 are protective against disease after a virulent challenge.[50, 51] The role of cell-mediated or mucosal immunity in protection against disease has not been established, but both are likely to be important. After administration of inactivated FCV vaccine, serum neutralizing titers indicating protection were detected in 8 of 13 cats 5 years later.[52] In a study of cats administered inactivated FCV vaccine and then challenged with virulent FCV 7.5 years later, clinical scores were 63 per cent lower than those of unvaccinated control cats.[47] Modified-live FCV vaccines used today are likely to perform even better than the inactivated vaccine used in these studies. Because mucosal immune responses are probably important, intranasal vaccination is likely to induce more rapid protection than subcutaneous vaccination, but is likely to induce more local side-effects. Use of intranasal vaccines in combination with subcutaneous vaccines may provide better protection in the short term; however, combination protocols are unlikely to provide significantly better protection in the long-term.[53] Kittens should be vaccinated every 3 to 4 weeks until 12 weeks of age and then revaccinated 1 year later. After that time, FCV vaccines should not be administered any more frequently than every 3 years.

Chlamydia psittaci

Chlamydia psittaci infection can be subclinical or result in a moderate-to-severe conjunctivitis. Environmental conditions and poor husbandry practices appear to enhance the likelihood of clinical illness. The duration of immunity after natural infection is unknown but likely to be short. There is no correlation between circulating antibody titers and protection, and protection is likely to be associated primarily with secretary IgA mucosal immunity or cell-mediated immunity.[54] Two studies have shown significant but incomplete protection at 12 months after vaccination with an inactivated vaccine.[55, 56] *Chlamydia* vaccines do not prevent infection or eliminate shedding, but do reduce clinical signs. Because the disease is not life-threatening, is un-common, and is treated easily with inexpensive antibiotics, this vaccine is considered noncore and should be used only in catteries with a history of chlamydial disease. Veterinarians should address husbandry practices first in all cases. How frequently the vaccine should be administered is unknown. As with the other upper respiratory vaccines in cats, protection is not complete, and reduction in severity of clinical signs should be our expectation. It is likely that long-term reduction in clinical signs after exposure is associated with the presence of memory cells. Annual vaccination probably is not necessary except in catteries with sustained *Chlamydia* infections.

Bordetella bronchiseptica

Bordetella bronchiseptica is detected commonly in the airways of cats in crowded environments.[57, 58] Additionally, many cats are seropositive, proving exposure to *B. bronchiseptica*. However, most exposed cats are healthy, and significant clinical illness almost never occurs in adult cats. Occasionally, the organism has been associated with pneumonia in young kittens in stressful environments with poor sanitation. Only 1 vaccine is currently available; a modified-live intranasal product. Immunity likely is mediated by secretory IgA, and probably is short-lived as in dogs. Side-effects associated with vaccination are similar to those of the natural infection and occur in at least 2 per cent of vaccinated cats. Because clinical disease associated with *B. bronchiseptica* is mild to nonexistent in pet cats, vaccine side-effects are similar to natural infection, and clinically affected cats respond to inexpensive antibiotics, this vaccine is considered noncore. It should be administered only to cats in humane shelters or catteries where documented loss due to *Bordetella* pneumonia has occurred. If used, vaccination should be performed in conjunction with improved environmental and sanitary practices. It should be given intranasally to young kittens only.

Feline Leukemia Virus

FeLV induces a multitude of clinical syndromes in infected cats, many of which are life-threatening. The immunity after natural infection is incomplete, and some recovered cats can be reinfected with the same strain of FeLV within 3 years. Protection against natural infection is age-related; 85 per cent of cats under 12 weeks of age become persistently infected if exposed, whereas cats over 6 months of age have only a 10 to 15 per cent chance of becoming persistently infected if exposed.[59] Because the most susceptible population is the young, vaccination should be targeted at this group. Because only 10 to 15 per cent of adult cats receive any true vaccine protection beyond age-acquired immunity, and because FeLV vaccines are commonly associated with injection-site sarcomas, the risk and benefits of vaccination need to be presented to cat owners. Duration-of-immunity studies are limited, and have shown great variation between FeLV vaccine manufacturers. Some FeLV vaccines have demonstrated protection to 3 years, whereas others have shown no vaccine-related protection just 15 months after vaccine administration. (Fort Dodge Animal Health, Fort Dodge, IA, personal communication, 1996). Because antibody titers have failed to correlate reliably with FeLV vaccine protection, they should not be used in evaluating the need for revaccination of cats for FeLV.[60, 61] My research suggests the most efficacious FeLV vaccines are the most locally reactive and possibly most likely to be associated with injection-site–associated sarcoma development. These vaccines should be considered non-core and should be administered only to kittens with risk of exposure. Kittens should receive the initial vaccine series and should be revaccinated 1 year later. Additional boosters should not be given more frequently than every 3 years until more definite data on duration of immunity become available or safer vaccines are developed.

Feline Infectious Peritonitis

FIP is caused by a feline coronavirus and results in fatal disease in about 1:5,000 average client households. The duration of immunity after natural infections with feline enteric coronavirus (FECV) or the pathogenic variant (FIPV) is unknown. There is no correlation between circulating antibody titers and protection. Both secretory IgA and cell-mediated immunity are thought to provide the greatest protection against infection and clinical disease. Although cell-mediated immunity is likely to be lasting, secretory IgA protection is likely to be short-lived (1 month).[62] However, challenge studies have demonstrated some protection in cats 6 and 12 months after vaccination, which is likely to be cell-mediated.[63, 64] Studies have indicated cats must be coronavirus-negative at the time of vaccination and have a serum antibody titer less than 1:100 to receive benefit from the FIP vaccine; at least 20 to 40 per cent of the cat population has antibody titers of this magnitude. The vaccine has a 60 to 80 per cent preventive fraction at its peak protection time 2 weeks after vaccination. These findings, combined with the relatively rare incidence of disease, limits the use of this vaccine to high-risk catteries that are coronavirus-negative. It is the author's opinion that a greater decrease in mortality from FIP may be obtained through changes in husbandry practices, such as increasing the number of litter boxes and reducing crowding, rather than through routine FIP vaccination.

Microsporum canis

Mircsporum canis induces skin disease that is not life-threatening and relatively uncommon in the cat

population at large. The currently available vaccine is inactivated oil-adjuvanted, which produces significant local reactions at injection sites. This non-core vaccine is best reserved for treatment of the clinical syndrome rather than prevention. If dermatophyte vaccines were used more extensively, they probably would be linked to vaccine-site tumor development.

Giardia Species

Infection of cats with Giardia induces small bowel diarrhea that is often self-limiting or responsive to a variety of antiprotozoal drugs. Incidence varies by region, but was shown to be 2.4 per cent in one study in a presumed endemic area (north-central Colorado).[65] Administration of an inactivated, subcutaneous product resulted in lessening of clinical signs and cyst-shedding in vaccinates when compared with controls following heterogeneous challenge 1 year after vaccination. Because the product is adjuvanted, there is potential for association with vaccine-associated sarcomas. Based on incidence, availability of effective treatments, and unknown safety issues, the *Giardia* vaccine is considered non-core and should be reserved for high-risk cats or the treatment of chronic carrier cats.

Rabies

Vaccines for prevention of rabies are the only veterinary vaccines that require minimum duration of immunity studies before licensure. It should be remembered that these vaccines are tested in young, not fully developed animals and that they must protect at least 86 per cent of the vaccinates 3 years after just 1 injection.[41] Most rabies vaccines sold are inactivated products that require 2 injections to maximize immune responses. Most cases of rabies in vaccinated animals have been in those vaccinated only once. Several studies now indicate that if a pet has been vaccinated twice for rabies, you are unlikely to acquire rabies from that animal. Rabies vaccines are very effective.[66] However, they are responsible for 50 per cent of the vaccine-associated sarcomas in cats.[5] Kittens should be administered rabies vaccination according to local ordinances and revaccinated 1 year later. Then, the vaccine should not be administered more frequently than every 3 years. A canarypox-vectored rabies vaccine that must be given yearly is now available.[67] Because this vaccine does not produce chronic inflammation, it should be considered the rabies vaccine of choice for cats. More extended duration-of-immunity studies are needed to determine whether the vaccine can be administered less frequently.

REFERENCES

1. Dubielzig RR, Hawkins KL, Miller PE: Myofibroblastic sarcoma originating at the site of rabies vaccination in a cat. J Vet Diagn Invest 5:637–638, 1993.

2. Hendrick MJ, Goldschmidt MH: Do injection site reactions induce fibrosarcomas in cats? J Am Vet Med Assoc 199:968, 1991.

3. Hendrick MJ, Goldschmidt MH, Shofer F, et al: Postvaccinal sarcomas in the cat: Epidemiology and electron probe microanalytical identification of aluminum. Cancer Res 52:5391–5394, 1992.

4. Hendrick MJ, Shofer FS, Goldschmidt MH, et al: Comparison of fibrosarcomas that developed at vaccination sites and at nonvaccination sites in cats: 239 cases (1991–1992). J Am Vet Med Assoc 205:1425–1429, 1994.

5. Kass PH, Barnes WG, Spangler WL, et al: Epidemiologic evidence for a causal relation between vaccination and fibrosarcoma tumorigenesis in cats. J Am Vet Med Assoc 203:396–405, 1993.

6. Hendrick MJ, Kass PH, McGill LD, et al: Commentary: Postvaccinal sarcomas in cats. J Natl Cancer Inst 86:5, 1994.

7. Coyne MJ, Reeves NCP, Rosen DK, et al: Estimated prevalence of injection sarcomas in cats during 1992. J Am Vet Med Assoc 210:249–251, 1997.

8. Macy DW, Hendrick MJ: The potential role of inflammation in the development of postvaccinal sarcomas in cats. Vet Clin North Am Small Anim Pract 26:103–109, 1996.

9. Rhone Merieux Inc: Imrab 3 Rabies Vaccine killed virus (insert). Athens, GA. Pfizer Animal Health, personal communication, 1995.

10. Esplin DG, McGill L, Meininger A, et al: Postvaccination sarcomas in cats. J Am Vet Med Assoc 202:1245–1247, 1993.

11. Fawcett HA, Smith NP: Injection-site granuloma due to aluminum. Arch Dermatol 120:1318–1322, 1984.

12. Hendrick MJ, Dunagan C: Focal necrotizing granulomatous panniculitis associated with subcutaneous injection of rabies vaccine in cats and dogs: 10 cases (1988–1989). J Am Vet Med Assoc 198:304–305, 1991.

13. Lester S, Clemett T, Burt A: Vaccine site associated sarcomas in cats: Clinical experience and laboratory review (1982–1993). J Am Anim Hosp Assoc 32:91–95, 1996.

14. Burton G, Mason KV: Do postvaccinal sarcomas occur in Australian cats? Aust Vet J 75:102–106, 1997.

15. Hendrick MJ, Brooks JJ: Postvaccinal sarcomas in the cat: Histology and immunohistochemistry. Vet Pathol 31:126–129, 1994.

16. Dubielzig RR: Ocular sarcoma following trauma in three cats. J Am Vet Med Assoc 184:578–581, 1984.

17. Dubielzig RR, Everitt J, Shadduck JA, et al: Clinical and morphologic features of posttraumatic ocular sarcomas in cats. Vet Pathol 27:62–65, 1990.

18. Woog J, Albert DM, Gondor JR, et al: Osteosarcoma in a phthisical feline eye. Vet Pathol 20:209–214, 1983.

19. Doddy FD, Glickman LT, Glickman NW, Janovitz ED: Feline fibrosarcomas at vaccination sites and nonvaccination sites. J Comp Pathol 114:165–174, 1996.

20. Hendrick MJ: Historical review and current knowledge of risk factors involved in feline vaccine associated sarcomas. J Am Vet Med Assoc 213:1422–1423, 1998.

21. Ellis JA, Jackson ML, Bartsch RC, et al: Use of immunonohistochemistry and polymerase chain reaction for detection of coronaviruses in formalin-fixed, parathion-embedded fibrosarcomas from cats. J Am Vet Med Assoc 209:767–771, 1996.

22. Goad MEP, Lopez KM, Goad DL: Expression of tumor suppression gene and oncogenes in feline injection site-associated sarcomas. Proceedings 17th ACVIM Forum, Chicago, 1999, p. 724.

23. Mayr B, Schaffner G, Kurzbauer R, et al: Mutations in tumor suppressor gene P53 in two feline fibrosarcomas. Br Vet J 151:707–713, 1995.

24. Hershey AE, et al, personal communication, 1999.

25. Vanselow BA: The application of adjuvants to veterinary medicine. Vet Bull 57:881–896, 1987.

26. Macy DW, Bergman PJ: Postvaccinal reactions associated with three rabies and three leukemia virus vaccines in cats. Proceedings IBC Third International Symposium on Veterinary Vaccines, February 5–6, 1998, Tampa, FL.

27. AVMA/VAFSTF web site: *http://www.avma.org/vafstf/default.htm*, 1998.

28. Advisory Panel on Feline Vaccines: Feline vaccine guidelines. Feline Pract 26:14–16, 1998.

29. Hershey EA, Sorenmo K, Hendrick M, et al: Feline fibrosarcoma: Prognosis following surgical treatment: A preliminary report. Proceedings 17th Annual Veterinary Cancer Society Meeting, Chicago, December 3–6, 1997, p. 36.

30. Davidson EB, Gregory CR, Kass PH: Surgical excision of soft tissue fibrosarcomas in cats. Vet Surg 26:265–269, 1997.

31. Cronin K, Page RL, Spodnick G, et al: Radiation therapy and surgery for fibrosarcoma in 33 cats. Vet Radiol Ultrasound 39:51–56, 1998.

32. Ogilvie GK, Moore AS: Vaccine associated sarcomas in cats. *In* Managing the Veterinary Cancer Patient. Trenton, NJ, Veterinary Learning Systems, 1995.

33. Kent EM: Use of an immunostimulant as an aid in treatment and management of fibrosarcomas in three cats. Feline Pract 21:13, 1993.

34. Briscoe C, Tipscomb T, McKinney LA: Pulmonary metastasis of a feline postvaccinal fibrosarcoma. Vet Pathol 32:5, 1995.

35. Esplin DG, Campbell R: Widespread metastasis of a fibrosarcoma associated with a vaccination site in a cat. Feline Pract 23:13–16, 1995.

36. Rudmann DG, Van Alstine WG, Doddy F, et al: Pulmonary and mediastinal metastasis of a vaccination site sarcoma in a cat. Vet Pathol 33:466–469, 1996.

37. Anonymous: Guidelines for vaccination. Nashville, American Association of Feline Practitioners, 1998.

38. ACVIM Specialty Meeting minutes, May 24, 1998, San Diego.

39. David S. Rolfe, U.S. Army, personal communication, 1997.

40. Schultz RD: Current and future canine and feline vaccination programs. Vet Med 93:233–254, 1998.

41. Center for Veterinary Biologics (CVB) Ames, IA.

42. Tizard I, Ni Y: Use of serologic testing to assess immune status of companion animals. J Am Vet Med Assoc 213:54–60, 1998.

43. McCaw DL, Thompson M, Tate D, et al: Serum distemper virus and parvovirus antibody titers among dogs brought to a veterinary hospital for revaccination. J Am Vet Med Assoc 213:72–75, 1998.

44. Gaskell R, Dawson S: Feline respiratory disease. *In* Greene C (ed): Infectious Diseases of the Dog and Cat, 2nd ed. Philadelphia, WB Saunders, 1998, pp. 94–106.

45. Scott FW, Geissinger C: Duration of immunity in cats vaccinated with an inactivated feline panleukopenia, herpesvirus and calicivirus vaccine. Feline Pract 25:12–19, 1997.

46. Ackermann O, Dörr W: Prüfung der schutzdauer gege die panleukopenie der katze nach impfung mit Felidovac P. Die Blauned Hefte 66:263–267, 1983.

47. Scott FW, Geissinger CM: Long-term immunity in cats vaccinated with an inactivated trivalent vaccine. Am J Vet Res 60:652–658, 1999.

48. Scott FW: Feline respiratory viral infection. *In* Scott FW (ed): Infectious Diseases. New York, Churchill Livingstone,

49. Orr CM, Gaskell CJ: Interaction of a combined feline viral rhinotracheitis–feline calicivirus vaccine and the FVR carrier state. Vet Rec 103:200–202, 1978.

50. Povey C, Ingersoll J: Cross protection among feline caliciviruses. Infect Immunol 11:877–885, 1975.

51. Johnson RP, Povey RC: Feline calicivirus infection in kittens borne by cats persistently infected with virus. Res Vet Sci 37:114–119, 1984.

52. Tham KM, Studdert MJ: Antibody and cell mediated immune responses to feline calicivirus following inactivated vaccine and challenge. J Vet Med B 34:640–654, 1987.

53. Edinboro CH, Janowitz LK, Guptill-Yoran L, et al: A clinical trial of intranasal and subcutaneous vaccines to prevent upper respiratory infection in cats at an animal shelter. Feline Pract 27(6):7–11, 1999.

54. Mitzel JR, Strating A: Vaccination against feline pneumonitis. Am J Vet Res 38:1361–1363, 1977.

55. Kolar JR, Rude TA: Duration of immunity in cats inoculated with a commercial feline pneumonitis vaccine. Vet Med Small Anim Clin 86:1171–1173, 1981.

56. Wasmoen T, Chu HJ, Chaves L, et al: Demonstration of one year duration of immunity for an inactivated feline *Chlamydia psittaci* vaccine. Feline Pract 20:13–16, 1992.

57. Welsh R: *Bordetella bronchiseptica* infections in cats. J Am Anim Hosp Assoc 32:153–158, 1996.
58. Willoughby K, Dawson S, Jones R, et al: Isolation of *B. bronchiseptica* from kittens with pneumonia in a breeding cattery. Vet Rec 129:407, 1991.
59. Rojko J, Hardy W Jr.: Feline leukemia virus and other retroviruses. *In* Sherding R (ed): The Cat. Diseases and Clinical Management, 2nd ed. New York, Churchill Livingstone, 1994, pp. 263–432.
60. Haffer KN, Koertje WD, Derr JT, et al: Evaluation of immunosuppressive effect and efficacy of an improved potency feline leukaemia vaccine. Vaccine 8:12–16, 1990.
61. Tompkins MB, Tompkins WAF, Ogilvie GK: Immunopathogenesis of feline leukemia virus infections. Companion Anim Pract, July 1998, pp. 15–26.
62. Pedersen NC: An overview of feline enteric coronavirus and infectious peritonitis virus infections. Feline Pract 23:7–20, 1995.
63. Gerber JD, Ingersoll JD, Gast AM, et al: Protection against feline infectious peritonitis by intranasal inoculation of a temperature sensitive FIPV vaccine. Vaccine 8:536–542, 1990.
64. Fehr D, Holznagel E, Bolla S, et al: Placebo controlled evaluation of a modified live virus vaccine against infectious peritonitis: Safety and efficacy under field conditions. Vaccine 15:1101–1109, 1997.
65. Hill S, Cheney J, Taton-Allen G, et al: Prevalence of enteric zoonoses in cats. J Am Vet Med Assoc 216:687–692, 2000.
66. Greene C, Dressen D: Rabies. *In* Greene CE (ed): Infectious Diseases of the Dog and Cat, 2nd ed. Philadelphia, WB Saunders, 1998, pp. 114–126.
67. Macy DW, Chretin J: Local postvaccinal reactions of a recombinant rabies vaccine. Vet Forum, August 1999, pp. 44–49.

2

◆ Hemobartonellosis

Janet E. Foley

◆ ETIOLOGY

Haemobartonella felis (H. felis) is the causative agent of feline infectious anemia (FIA). The organism is a 0.5 μm gram-negative rod, coccus, or disc-shaped obligate epierythrocytic parasite that replicates by binary fission.[1–3] There has been significant confusion about the phylogeny and taxonomy of *H. felis*. Initially, *H. felis* was named *Eperythrozoon felis*.[4] However, *Haemobartonella* species are more tightly attached to the erythrocyte membrane, and are less commonly observed in ring forms than *Eperythrozoon* species.[1] *Eperythrozoon* species and *Haemobartonella* species were classed initially as rickettsiae on the basis of staining characteristics, obligate parasitic habit, susceptibility to tetracycline, and difficulty (or impossibility) to cultivate in vitro. Recently, analysis of the DNA sequence of the relatively conserved 16S rRNA gene has revealed that *H. felis* is only distantly related to rickettsiae (which are alpha-proteobacters). The organism should be placed in the family Mycoplasmataceae (Fig. 2–1), an evolutionarily degenerate offshoot of the low G+C gram-positive bacteria.[5–7] This classification is supported by the ultrastructure of *H. felis*; the organism has a plasma membrane but no cell wall and no internal membranous structures. As with other mycoplasmas, the cell requires cholesterol from the environment for incorporation into the plasma membrane. However, the Mycoplasma-

taceae typically are mucosal pathogens (although some species produce septicemia); *H. felis* has a cell tropism for the erythrocyte.

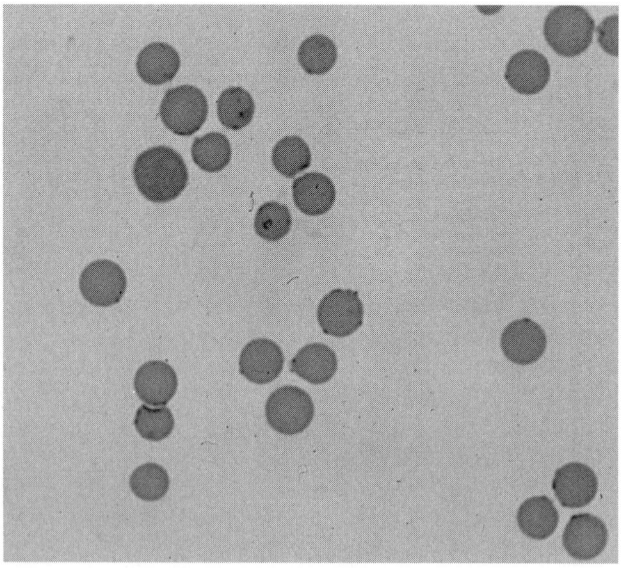

Assessment of the 16S rRNA subunit gene has revealed that there are at least 2 variants of *H. felis*, a small form (Hfsm) and large form (Hflg) that also vary in virulence. *Haemobartonella*-specific polymerase chain reaction (PCR) was designed in the 16S rRNA subunit gene for both Hfsm and Hflgs. Specific primers were predicted at position 1183 forward (GCATAATGTGTCGCAATC) and 1290 reverse (GTTTCAACTAGTACTTTCTCCC) to yield a fragment of 130 to 131 base-pairs in length. Of 20 various bacterial species, including 11 from the rickettsial and mycoplasmal clades, only *H. felis* and *Eperythrozoon suis* targets yielded 130 or 131 base-pair fragments. Sequence analysis of 16S rRNA genes indicates that the Hfsm actually is most closely related to eperythrozoa, while Hflg and other pathogenic strains from Ohio and Florida form a distinct clade within the haemobartonella, related to *Haemobartonella muris*.[5, 6] Hfsm was described previously as the California strain of *H. felis*.[6]

◆ EPIDEMIOLOGY

The epidemiology of *H. felis* infection is poorly understood, in part because the organism is difficult to detect without the only available molecular diagnostic tools. Risk factors for hemobartonellosis include age, gender, being housed indoor-outdoor, and presence of fleas. The incidence of FIA increases with age, with a peak incidence from 4 to 8 years.[8, 9] Male cats may be at greater risk for FIA.[9, 10] Infection with *H. felis* appears to be seasonal, which may relate to its association with fleas.[8, 10]

The organism can be transmitted in utero or lactationally, as well as iatrogenically by transfer of blood, by hematophagous arthropod, and orally. In utero or lactogenic infection is suggested by detection of hemobartonellosis in very young kittens.[11–14] The organism is transmitted by blood, not urine or serum,[15] which suggests that blood-sucking arthropods such as fleas might be natural vectors; one study found that significantly more cases of hemobartonellosis occurred in cats infested with fleas than in flea-free cats.[9] However, because many cases of feline hemobartonellosis were identified in Salt Lake City, Utah, in the absence of fleas, it is likely other routes of transmission occur commonly.[16] Other blood-sucking arthropods may be involved; *Haemobartonella canis* is transmitted via the brown

Figure 2–1. *Haemobartonella felis.*

dog tick *Rhipicephalus sanguineus.*[17] Experimental challenge with infectious whole blood either orally or parenterally has resulted in hemobartonellosis,[14, 15, 18] although it is difficult to envision many cats acquiring a hemoparasite naturally by ingesting infected blood from other cats. Cats have been infected iatrogenically from apparently healthy blood donors that were *H. felis* carriers.[15, 16]

◆ PATHOGENESIS AND IMMUNITY

Many aspects of the pathogenesis of FIA have not been well described. The mechanism of *H. felis* attachment to the erythrocyte is not known, but may be via pili as in *Bartonella henselae,* or some other receptor/ligand interaction. Mycoplasmas adhere to epithelial target cell receptors by means of proteins or protein conjugates, or via interaction with mycoplasmal anionic surface layers.[19] Some species of mycoplasma have electron-micrographically visible terminal organelles that are specialized for attachment to host cells, but similar structures have not been described for haemobartonellas.

Humoral and cell-mediated immune responses occur against *H. felis.* Although the organism is intimately associated with the erythrocyte membrane, the parasitism per se does not induce erythrocyte destruction. The clinical signs of hemobartonellosis are caused by the immune-mediated reactions against the organism. Hemobartonellosis is more severe in older cats than in kittens, a typical finding in diseases with an immune-mediated pathogenesis.[8, 9] Antibodies in the immunoglobulin G (IgG) class can be detected within 2 weeks after infection,[5] with the period of maximal clinical signs corresponding to the period of initial antibody production.[14] Antibody binding to *H. felis* organisms on erythrocytes initiates the complement cascade and is one trigger for splenic cleansing of parasitized erythrocytes and phagocytosis of parasitized erythrocytes by blood mononuclear cells. The reticuloendothelial system in the spleen also entraps erythrocyte–*H. felis* pairs not targeted by IgG, removing parasites from cell surfaces and returning cells to the circulation. Erythrocytes from which *H. felis* parasites have been removed may be more susceptible to osmotic lysis.[20] The increased fragility of erythrocytes in cats with active hemobartonellosis is comparable with that associated with autoimmune hemolytic anemia.[14] Acute anemia may be partially due to splenic sequestration of erythrocytes.[21] Cats with FIA typically have a positive Coombs test about 15 days after parasites appear on the cell surface.[2] *Mycoplasma pneumoniae* triggers polyclonal B-lymphocyte stimulation, resulting in production of many antibodies, including autoantibodies against erythrocytes in human beings. Other *Mycoplasma* species up-regulate B-lymphocyte and macrophage major histocompatibility complex (MHC) expression and may produce self antigens as a sequel.[22]

After a cat recovers from acute hemobartonellosis, *H. felis* organisms are sequestered in the spleen.[14, 20] Long-term immunity to *H. felis* challenge is not well understood. Earlier studies reported that cats remained chronically infected carriers.[2, 14, 23] In cats that make complete recovery, with eventual complete elimination of organisms from the spleen, it is not known whether IgG premunition may be protective and for what duration.

Splenectomy, concurrent feline leukemia virus (FeLV) or bacterial infections, and drug-induced immunosuppression have been assessed for potential to exacerbate hemobartonellosis. *H. felis* parasitemia lasted twice as long in adult splenectomized cats as in nonsplenectomized adult cats.[2] However, splenectomy performed after disease recovery resulted in a transient reappearance of organisms in the blood but no significant decrease in erythrocyte numbers.[15, 16, 24] In contrast, clinical hemobartonellosis in dogs (due to infection with *H. canis*) is virtually always observed in splenectomized dogs. Recrudescence of parasitemia in healthy carrier cats was not induced by treatment with cyclophosphamide or 6-mercaptopurine, or with experimentally induced abscesses. However, corticosteroid treatment rapidly reactivated the infection.[24]

Infection with *H. felis* leads to alterations in the immune status of the cat, resulting in immune-mediated anti-self responses, increased susceptibility to some infectious diseases such as FeLV infection, and reduced susceptibility to other infections. In unpublished studies, it was demonstrated that infection with one Hfsm isolate led to cross protection against challenge with a more virulent Hflg isolate, despite the fact the 2 agents were not serologically cross-reactive.[5] The mechanism for this cross protection is not known, but may relate to the relatively nonspecific immune modulation produced by infection with *H. felis* and other mycoplasmas. These responses potentially include up-regulation of natural killer cells and activation of macrophages by enhanced interferon gamma production.[25] Squirrel monkeys infected with *Haemobartonella* species were relatively resistant to experimental infection with *Plasmodium falciparum.*[26] Latent *Haemobartonella* infections could be activated by splenectomizing the monkeys, although 2 monkeys that did not exhibit patent hemobartonellosis after splenectomy did develop clinical disease following *P. falciparum* challenge. If the monkeys were in remission with respect to the *Haemobartonella* species infection, they were susceptible to the malaria. If *Haemobartonella* species bodies were visible on erythrocytes and had been activated recently by splenectomy, monkeys were resistant to malaria challenge.

◆ CLINICAL HEMOBARTONELLOSIS

Experimental Infections

A number of studies have reported successful experimental infection of cats by *H. felis*–infected cat blood. *Haemobartonella* bodies appear on peripheral erythrocytes 2 to 21 days after parenteral inoculation,[14-18] or 22 to 51 days after oral inoculation.[16] There were no differences between cats infected intravenously and those infected intraperitoneally with respect to date of onset of anemia, clinical signs, minimum hematocrit, or percentage of infected cells.[5] The first clinical signs (if any) occur coincidentally with visualization of the organism,[14] although cats in one study were PCR-positive in blood as early as 3 days before organisms were visible.[5] Clinical sequelae of experimental infection are typically severe, probably due to high doses of organisms in the challenge. The predominant signs included anorexia, depression, fever, anemia, dyspnea (with open-mouth breathing and cyanotic mucous membranes), hepatosplenomegaly, mesenteric lymphadenopathy, and icterus. If untreated, the mortality rate may exceed 33 per cent.[3] Less virulent strains may result in subclinical infection.[5] The primary infection lasts from 18 to 30 days.[5, 14]

After the acute severe parasitemia subsides, cats may enter a series of infection cycles consisting of periods of latency and recrudescence.[27] There may be 3 to 9 parasitemic episodes with 3 to 11 days between peaks of parasitemia.[14] During latency, there are typically far fewer *H. felis* organisms seen on erythrocytes than during acute infection. The recoveries of both erythrocyte and leukocyte numbers may be unstable, and it may require 2 to 4 months for hematologic parameters to return to normal.[14] Subsequent recrudescent attacks become increasingly less severe (in terms of per cent parasitism, reductions in hematocrit, and clinical signs) with each attack; only the first 1 or 2 attacks may be clinically apparent.[15, 23, 24] Harvey and Gaskin[24] reported that all of their experimentally infected cats became carriers, and that *H. felis* bodies were detectable approximately one-third of the time on blood smears from chronically infected cats. In another study, cyclic parasitemia was detected in 4 cats with Hfsm and 4 with Hflg.[5] Cat No. 88506, an Hfsm cat, had a recurrence of anemia and depression 7 months after acute anemia, with no clinical signs or hematologic abnormalities during the intervening period. The hematocrit during the acute attack declined from 48.6 to 31.4; during the reactivated attack, the hematocrit declined from 44.9 to 21.3. Approximately 5 per cent of erythrocytes appeared to be parasitized by *H. felis* in the later attack. Of the 7 other cats with recurrence of anemia, clinical signs and hematologic changes appeared a mean of 27 days after acute anemia. Five of these cats had visible *H. felis* organisms on erythrocytes transiently during the second attack. However, recurring cycles or recrudescence of active infection does not always occur, even in cats terminally ill with FeLV.[28]

Coinfections with *H. felis* and FeLV have been evaluated experimentally. George and Pedersen[28] inoculated an Hfsm isolate into cats with FeLV, feline immunodeficiency virus (FIV), or FeLV and FIV, and followed the course of infection by clinical pathol-

ogy and hematology. The most severely affected cats (in terms of erythrocyte reductions) were those with FeLV with or without FIV. There was no mortality as a direct result of *H. felis* infection, but 2 cats in the FeLV-only group and 1 cat with FeLV and FIV developed myeloproliferative disorders characteristic of some end-stage FeLV during weeks 6 and 7. Previously, Pedersen[23] reported that myeloproliferative disease predisposed cats to *H. felis* infection, and Kociba and coworkers[29] reported that *H. felis* infection predisposed cats to infection with FeLV viremia and aplastic anemia.

Natural Infections

Clinical and hematologic responses to *H. felis* infection are much more variable in field cases compared with experimental infections. Approximately 50 per cent of cats diagnosed with hemobartonellosis are clinically ill, whereas the other cases are detected in clinically normal cats during routine screening of blood smears. The observed clinical variability reflects agent variability, variation in host susceptibility, and possible differences in dose and route of infection. As discussed in experimental infections, Hflg isolates apparently are more pathogenic than Hfsm isolates.[5] The Hfsm isolate may have been virulent in the original case, but that cat was coinfected with FeLV, making interpretation of the relative contribution of the 2 infections difficult.

Clinical signs associated with hemobartonellosis in naturally infected cats develop gradually and include pallor, dyspnea with open-mouth breathing, weakness, and fever.[30] After primary infection, many cats become healthy carriers.[27, 31] The reservoir within the body in carrier cats is unknown, although *H. felis* organisms have been observed within splenic and pulmonary macrophages.[2]

Case reports and epidemiologic studies have demonstrated a relationship between severe FIA and stress, pregnancy, intercurrent infection, neoplasia, and FeLV infection.[9, 32] FeLV is a well-described potentiator of hemobartonellosis, but FIV is not.[30, 31, 33] In one study, 50 per cent of cats with hemobartonellosis were coinfected with FeLV.[9] In FeLV and *H. felis* coinfected cats, it may be difficult to determine which of the organisms is inducing the syndrome. An association between chronic and poorly healing abscesses and hemobartonellosis has been made.[18] Hemobartonellosis has been diagnosed in cats with chronic diarrhea, colonic impaction, pancreatitis and hepatitis, oral infections, membranous glomerulopathies, polyarthritis, and non–FeLV-associated neoplasia.[30] Cats with FIA and other concurrent disease processes usually were much sicker, with more profound and refractory anemia, than cats with FIA alone.[30]

◆ PATHOLOGY AND CLINICAL PATHOLOGY

Regenerative anemias are reported most commonly with reticulocytosis, macrocytosis, and metarubricytosis in proportion to the degree of anemia.[28, 29] In some cats with FIA, the anemia may be normocytic normochromic.[30] The hematocrit may decline to 15 per cent or lower, with hemoglobin concentrations near 12.9 g/dl.[5] Nucleated red blood cells also have been reported in cats with FIA.[5, 34–36] The nucleated erythrocytes may reflect hypoxic trauma to the bone marrow, or may be part of the normal regenerative response. Clinical signs may become apparent once the hematocrit falls below about 20 per cent at this time; about 50 per cent of cats have large numbers of parasitized erythrocytes in circulation.[14] Erythrophagocytosis by mononuclear cells is noted in peripheral blood occasionally.

Leukocyte responses in FIA are variable. Some cats develop acute leukopenia,[16, 30] possibly with toxic neutrophils[28]; others develop delayed leukopenia.[5] Some cats develop acute leukocytosis,[10, 14] others develop leukocytosis in recovery.[5]

In cats coinfected with FeLV and *H. felis*, hematologic changes may reflect both the effects of FIA and the typical myeloproliferative disease, aplastic anemia, or dyshematopoietic disorders of FeLV. Cats with naturally occurring *H. felis* and FeLV infections commonly have macrocytic hypochromic anemia[30]; experimentally coinfected cats had regenerative anemia.[28] Some FeLV- and *H. felis*–coinfected cats initially have regenerative anemia that becomes nonregenerative with the development of FeLV-associated erythroid dysplasia.[29]

Gross pathologic findings in cats with FIA are referable to anemia. The spleen may be enlarged due to reticuloendothelial and lymphoid hyperplasia as well as extramedullary hematopoiesis. Hepatomegaly and cardiomegaly may occur due to increased reticuloendothelial activity and hypoxia associated with anemia, respectively. On histopathologic examination of tissues, erythrophagocytosis by mononuclear cells in the spleen, liver, and bone marrow is seen in some cats. Hemosiderin accumulation in splenic red pulp, hepatic centrilobular necrosis, hypercellular bone marrow, and extramedullary hematopoiesis were reported in cats with FIA and FeLV.[28] Cats with chronic hemobartonellosis have been reported to have patchy atelectasis, thickening of alveolar walls, and accumulations of macrophages in alveoli,[11] as well as focal chronic pneumonia.[37]

◆ DIAGNOSIS

Microscopy

H. felis organisms are stained readily by Wright-Giemsa, other Romanowsky-type, or new methylene blue stains and appear as dark blue or gram-negative variably shaped 0.3 to 0.8 μm bodies on the surface of feline erythrocytes. There is variability in size among isolates, with Hfsm being so small that it is easily overlooked.[5, 28] The fraction of erythrocytes that is parasitized also is highly variable, and hemo-

bartonellosis may be overlooked in cats with low rates of parasitism. The fraction of parasitized erythrocytes in acutely ill cats may be as high as 95 per cent, with 10 or more *H. felis* organisms observed in pairs or chains on the surface of erythrocytes. The parasites may be confused with Howell-Jolly bodies, but these structures are at least twice as large as *H. felis* organisms and nonrefractile. Routine manual examination of blood smears for differential cell counts commonly has resulted in detection of occult hemobartonellosis in carrier cats.[30] Repeat examination over several days may facilitate detection of cases.[44]

Other stains have been proposed to increase the sensitivity of microscopy for detection of hemobartonellosis. Acridine orange, a fluorescent stain, reportedly detected *H. felis* in 15 of 57 cats tested in one study,[3] whereas only 5 were positive by Giemsa stain.[9] However, 1 cat was Giemsa-positive but not acridine orange–positive. In contrast, no increased sensitivity was observed using acridine orange in an experimental study.[5] Immunofluorescent antibody stains also have been reported.[3]

H. felis organisms appear adjacent to the erythrocyte membrane, result in invaginations of the erythrocyte, or relate to the erythrocyte by short filamentous strands. On scanning electron micrographs, a central depression of the erythrocyte in association with disc-shaped bodies is apparent.[20, 38] When the *H. felis* parasite is removed, the remaining erythrocyte membrane shows irregularities.

Culture (or Lack Thereof)

H. felis has never been cultivated in artificial media; its entire existence is intimately associated with red blood cell surfaces. Mycoplasmas in general require highly enriched media for growth. Unpublished unsuccessful culture protocols have included culture on mycoplasma media and on fresh cat blood agar.

Antibody Detection

Antibodies may be assayed by indirect fluorescent antibody assay using blood smears from experimentally infected cats,[3, 5] or enzyme-linked immunosorbent assay.[39] Substrate slides using either Hfsm or Hflg did not cross-react serologically.[5] Anti–*H. felis* IgG may be detectable by day 21 postinfection, and was reported as high as 400 by day 28.[5] These assays are not available routinely for clinicians, and the diagnostic utility has not been determined.

Polymerase Chain Reaction

Several PCRs have been used to detect *H. felis* in peripheral blood (see Chapter 60, Use of the Polymerase Chain Reaction to Detect Hemoparasites). Assays are available for both Hfsm and Hflgl.[5] In one study, the sensitivity of a *H. felis* PCR was obtained by diluting a known positive sample to endpoint of PCR detection, and determining the number of organisms represented in the last positive dilution based on the per cent parasitism per erythrocyte in the corresponding blood smear and the cat's observed total erythrocyte count.[5] Positive PCR bands were obtained on samples run with as little as 0.01 μl DNA, corresponding to 10,000 organisms. A second PCR protocol for 16S amplification of *H. felis* yielded a 1316 base-pair fragment from several *H. felis* strains and presumably the California Hflg, but did not amplify *E. suis* or Hfsm.[40] The published sensitivity was excellent, detecting from 50 to 704 organisms. A 393 base-pair specific product also was amplified by the same group,[5] which did not amplify *E. suis*. PCR apparently is more sensitive than cytology. Experimentally infected cats commonly are PCR-positive and cytology-negative.[5, 40] Cats with naturally occurring coinfections with Hfsm and Hflg have been detected by PCR; many infected cats were cytologically negative.[41] Whether determination of the *H. felis* strain infecting an individual cat will be beneficial remains to be determined. However, Hflg is detected more commonly in cats with anemia than is Hfsm.[41]

◆ TREATMENT

The treatment of choice for hemobartonellosis is the tetracyclines (tetracycline, oxytetracycline, or doxycycline). Tetracycline is prescribed commonly at 25 mg/kg orally (PO) every (q) 8 hr for 3 weeks. Oxytetracycline is convenient because it may be given less frequently, but is associated with pain on administration and local reactions at the site of injection.[30] In one study, oxytetracycline failed to clear infections even transiently.[30] In experimentally infected, anemic cats treated with tetracyclines, clinical signs resolved within 24 hours.[5] The mean hematocrit increased from 15.7 per cent pretreatment to 23.3 per cent within 24 hours. Results of PCR tests became negative by 12 hours after initiation of antibiotic therapy (oxytetracycline or doxycycline), and remained PCR-negative for the duration of antibiotic treatment. After discontinuation of antibiotics, PCR tests became positive again in 3 days in 1 cat treated with tetracycline, in 14 days in 1 cat treated with doxycycline, and in 5 days in the cat treated with oxytetracycline. The organism was detectable cytologically on some sample dates. Doxycycline was not more effective than tetracycline with respect to clinical response. In another study, cats recovered clinically and became PCR-negative shortly after treatment with doxycycline, but were PCR-positive again 84 days later.[42] The pharmacologic mechanism of tetracycline is protein synthesis inhibition, and thus it is likely static. Despite this, cats frequently respond to tetracycline within 12 hours, suggesting

that at the peak of infection, many of the *H. felis* bodies seen in blood are new and that the erythrophagocytic action in the spleen is highly effective.

Some cases of FIA are refractory to tetracycline.[11] As with mycoplasmas, *H. felis* is resistant to antibiotics with activity against cell-wall synthesis or integrity. Older recommended alternative treatments for FIA include thiacetarsamide (0.11 to 0.22 ml/kg intravenously [IV] on days 1 and 3),[23] chlorpromazine (4 to 7 mg/kg [IM] on day 1, and 2 to 3 mg/kg PO daily for days 2 to 9),[23] chloramphenicol (25 mg/kg q 12 hr PO for 21 days),[23] and a combination of spiramycin, metronidazole, and chloramphenicol. Chloramphenicol at 15 to 20 mg/kg PO, with oxytetracycline was not 100 per cent effective.[43] It also has been suggested that enrofloxacin (which is bactericidal by means of inhibition of DNA supercoiling and replication) might be as, or more, effective than tetracycline.[36] Very preliminary results in our laboratory demonstrated that enrofloxacin improved clinical signs of hemobartonellosis and increased the hematocrit, but the drug was less effective than tetracycline at eliminating *H. felis* DNA.

In addition to antibiotic therapy, supportive therapy often is necessary. Glucocorticoids (e.g., prednisolone at 1 to 2 mg/kg PO daily for the first 7 to 14 days) may be used to lessen immune-mediated erythrophagocytosis. If FIA and primary immune-mediated anemia are on the differential diagnosis list, it is reasonable to combine tetracycline and glucocorticoids in the initial treatment plan. Blood transfusion is frequently necessary, but transfused cells are very susceptible to parasitism, and we have given as many as 3 transfusions in 1 cat in a 12-hour period to maintain a hematocrit greater than 15 per cent. An alternative to transfusion is Oxyglobin (Biopure, Cambridge, MA), a polymerized bovine hemoglobin product licensed for use in anemic dogs, because it is cell-free. Some cats with hemobartonellosis have been supplemented with iron, but this is not indicated in most cats because the disease is a hemolytic anemia, not a blood-loss anemia.[12, 44]

◆ PREVENTION AND CONTROL

Because the route of transmission is unknown, definitive recommendations are difficult. However, flea control should be instituted owing to the epidemiologic association with hemobartonellosis. Cats should be housed indoors to avoid concurrent infections or conditions that might potentiate FIA.

REFERENCES

1. Kreier J, Ristic M: The biology of hemotrophic bacteria. Annu Rev Microbiol 35:325–338, 1981.
2. Maede Y: Sequestration and phagocytosis of *Haemobartonella felis* in the spleen. Am J Vet Res 40:691–695, 1979.
3. Small E, Ristic M: Haemobartonellosis. Vet Clin North Am Small Anim Pract 1:225–230, 1971.

4. Clark R: *Eperythrozoon felis* (sp. no.) in a cat. J South Afr Vet Assoc 13:15–16, 1942.
5. Foley J, Harrus S, Poland A, et al: Molecular, clinical, and pathological comparison of two distinct strains of *Hemobartonella felis* in domestic cats. Am J Vet Res 59:1581–1588, 1998.
6. Rikihisa Y, Kawahara M, Wen B, et al: Western immunoblot analysis of *Haemobartonella muris* and comparison of 16S rRNA gene sequences of *H. muris, H. felis,* and *Eperythrozoon suis*. J Clin Microbiol 35:823–829, 1997.
7. Weisburg WG, Tully JG, Rose DL, et al: A phylogenetic analysis of the mycoplasmas: Basis for their classification. J Bacteriol 171:6455–6467, 1989.
8. Hayes H, Priester W: Feline infectious anemia: risk by age, sex, and breed; prior disease; seasonal occurrence; mortality. J Small Anim Pract 14:797–804, 1973.
9. Nash A, Bobade P: *Haemobartonella felis* infection in cats from the Glasgow area. Vet Rec 119:373–375, 1986.
10. Flint J, Roepke M, Jensen R: Feline infectious anemia. I. Clinical aspects. Am J Vet Res 19:164–168, 1958.
11. Cretillat S: Feline haemobartonellosis. Fel Pract 14:22–27, 1984.
12. Fisher E: Anemia in a litter of Siamese kittens. J Small Anim Pract 24:215–219, 1983.
13. Harbutt P: A clinical appraisal of feline infectious anemia and its transmission under natural conditions. Austr Vet J 39:402–404, 1963.
14. Harvey J, Gaskin J: Experimental feline haemobartonellosis. J Am Anim Hosp Assoc 13:28–38, 1977.
15. Splitter E, Castro E, Kanawyer W: Feline infectious anemia. Vet Med Small Anim Clin 51:17–22, 1956.
16. Flint J, Roepke M, Jensen R: Feline infectious anemia. II. Experimental cases. Am J Vet Res 20:33–40, 1959.
17. Lester S, Hume J, Phipps B: *Haemobartonella canis* infection following splenectomy and transfusion. Can Vet J 36:444–445, 1995.
18. Flint JC, Moss J: Infectious anemia in cats. J Am Vet Med Assoc 122:45–48, 1953.
19. Rosendal S: Mycoplasma. *In* Gyles C, Thoen C, (eds): Pathogenesis of Bacterial Infections in Animals. Iowa State University Press, Ames, 1993, pp. 297–311.
20. Maede Y, Sonoda M: Studies on feline haemobartonellosis. III. Scanning electron microscopy of *Haemobartonella felis*. Jpn J Vet Sci 37:209–211, 1975.
21. Maede Y, Hata R: Studies on feline haemobartonellosis. II. The mechanism of anemia produced by infection with *Haemobartonella felis*. Jpn J Vet Sci 37:49–54, 1975.
22. Stuart PM, Cassell GH, Woodward JG: Induction of class II MHC antigen expression in macrophages by *Mycoplasma* species. J Immunol 142:3392–3399, 1989.
23. Pedersen N: Feline Infectious Diseases. Goleta, CA, American Veterinary Publisher, 1988.
24. Harvey J, Gaskin J: Feline haemobartonellosis: Attempts to induce relapses of clinical disease in chronically infected cats. J Am Anim Hosp Assoc 14:453–456, 1978.
25. Lai WC, Bennett M, Pakes SP, et al: Resistance to *Mycoplasma pulmonis* mediated by activated natural killer cells. J Infect Dis 161:1269–1275, 1990.
26. Contamin H, Michel JC: Haemobartonellosis in squirrel monkeys *(Saimiri sciureus)*: Antagonism between *Haemobartonella* sp. and experimental *Plasmodium falciparum* malaria. Exp Parasitol 91:297–305, 1999.
27. Small E, Ristic M: Hemobartonellosis. *In* Holzworth J (ed): Diseases of the Cat. Medicine and Surgery. Philadelphia, WB Saunders, 1987, pp. 301–308.
28. George J, Pedersen N: Haemobartonellosis in cats infected with feline leukemia virus, feline immunodeficiency virus, or both. Am J Vet Res (submitted).
29. Kociba GJ, Weiser M, Olsen R: Enhanced susceptibility to feline leukemia virus in cats with *Hemobartonella felis* infection. Leuk Rev Internat 1:88–89, 1983.
30. Bobade P, Nash A, Rogerson P: Feline hemobartonellosis: Clinical, haematological and pathological studies in natural infections and the relationship to infection with feline leukemia virus. Vet Rec 122:32–36, 1988.
31. Grindem C, Corbett W, Tompkins M: Risk factors for *Haemobartonella felis* infection in cats. J Am Vet Med Assoc 196:96–99, 1990.
32. Priester W, Hayes H: Feline leukemia after feline infectious anemia. J Natl Cancer Inst 51:289–291, 1973.
33. Cotter S, Hardy W, Essex M: Association of feline leukemia virus with lymphosarcoma and other disorders in the cat. J Am Vet Med Assoc 166:449–454, 1975.
34. Schalm O: Feline infectious anemia. Fel Pract 2:26–30, 1972.
35. VanSteenhouse JJ, Taboada J, Dorfmann M: *Hemobartonella felis* infection with atypical hematological abnormalities. J Am Anim Hosp Assoc 31:165–169, 1995.
36. VanSteenhouse J, Taboada J, Millard J: Feline hemobartonellosis. Compend Contin Educ Pract Vet 15:535–545, 1993.
37. Schwartzman R, Besch E: Feline infectious anemia. Vet Med Small Anim Clin 53:494–500, 1958.
38. Jain N, Keeton K: Scanning electron microscopic features of *Haemobartonella felis*. Am J Vet Res 34:697–700, 1973.
39. Turner C, Bloxham P, Cox F, Turner C: Unreliable diagnosis of *Haemobartonella felis*. Vet Rec 119:534–535, 1986.
40. Messick JB, Berent LM, Cooper SK: Development and evaluation of a PCR-based assay for detection of *Haemobartonella felis* in cats and differentiation of *H. felis* from related bacteria by restriction fragment length polymorphism analysis. J Clin Microbiol 36:462–466, 1998.
41. Jensen WA, Lappin MR, Reagan W, Kamkar S: Prevalence of *Haemobartonella felis* infection in cats. Am J Vet Res (In review).
42. Berent LM, Messick JB, Cooper SK: Detection of *Haemobartonella felis* in cats with experimentally induced acute and chronic infections, using a polymerase chain reaction assay. Am J Vet Res 59:1215–1220, 1998.
43. Stevenson M: Treatment for *Haemobartonella felis* in cats (Letter). Vet Rec 140:512, 1997.
44. Wilkinson G: Two further cases of feline infectious anemia. Vet Rec 77:453–454, 1965.

3
◆ Cat Ownership by Immunosuppressed People

Michael R. Lappin

Zoonotic diseases are those common to, shared by, or transmitted naturally between human beings and other vertebrate animals.[1] Zoonotic agents are transferred to human beings by direct contact with the infected cat; indirect contact with secretions from the cat; contact with contaminated vehicles like water, food, or fomites; or shared vectors. Several current reviews of cat-associated zoonoses are available.[2–5]

There are many causes of immunodeficiency in human beings. Notable causes include the human immunodeficiency virus (HIV), chemotherapy for cancer, immunosuppressive therapy for immune-mediated diseases or organ transplantation, and age-associated immunodeficiencies (very young or very old). Most zoonotic agents will infect anyone regardless of their immune status, but the severity of clinical illness often is more severe in the immunosuppressed. When immunodeficiency is detected in a family, it is often recommended that pets be removed from the household.[6, 7] Although cats can harbor many different zoonotic agents, human beings are unlikely to acquire infectious diseases from healthy, adult, parasite-free, indoor cats.[2, 3, 6, 8, 9] It is well recognized that pet ownership results in increased happiness and decreased depression, and any decision concerning cat ownership should factor in benefits as well as potential risks.[8, 10]

There are multiple infectious agents of cats capable of zoonotic transfer; some of the most common or important are listed by route of transmission in Tables 3–1 to 3–4. In immunosuppressed human beings, most concern is given to the enteric agents *Cryptosporidium* species, *Toxoplasma gondii*, *Salmonella* species, *Campylobacter* species, and *Giardia*, and infectious agents transmitted by bites and scratches, particularly *Bartonella* species and *Capnocytophaga canimorsus*. *Helicobacter* species, *Chlamydia psittaci*, *Bordetella bronchiseptica*, *Ehrlichia* species, and *Rickettsia felis* are emerging zoonoses potentially associated with cats. The following is a brief discussion of these agents. Recommendations for avoiding zoonotic transfer of infection from cats to human beings are included.

◆ SELECT ENTERIC ZOONOSES
Campylobacteriosis

Campylobacter jejuni, *Campylobacter coli*, and *Campylobacter upsalensis* infections in human beings and cats can be subclinical or result in an-

orexia, vomiting, and large-bowel diarrhea.[11, 12] Human beings usually are infected by ingesting contaminated food or water. Infection of human beings has been linked to cats in several reports.[13–16] In previous studies, up to 60 per cent of the pets from crowded environments were infected with *Campylobacter* species.[1, 12] However, in a recent study from north central Colorado, only 0 percent of cats from a shelter and 1.6 per cent of client-owned cats with or without diarrhea were culture-positive.[17] The incidence of campylobacteriosis in cats may be decreasing due to improved husbandry. Neutrophils and spirochetes may be detected on rectal cytology of affected cats, and may lead to a presumptive diagnosis of campylobacteriosis; definitive diagnosis is based on culture of feces. Several antibiotics including erythromycin, chloramphenicol, enrofloxacin, and second-generation cephalosporins are effective for treatment.

Cryptosporidiosis

Cryptosporidium parvum is a coccidian that can cause severe gastrointestinal tract disease in infected cats and human beings, (see Chapter 5, Cryptosporidiosis). Oocysts of *C. parvum* are passed sporulated and so are immediately infectious. Ingestion of as few as 1 oocyst can result in clinical illness in human beings. Many infected individuals require hospitalization for administration of intravenous fluid therapy; some people with AIDS are never cured. There are many examples of how common cryptosporidiosis is in human beings. Approximately 300,000 people in Milwaukee developed cryptosporidiosis when a water-purification system malfunctioned,[18] approximately 10 to 20 per cent of AIDS patients are infected with *C. parvum* at some time during their lives,[19] and the organism commonly causes diarrhea outbreaks in daycare centers.[20]

An enzyme-linked immunosorbent assay (ELISA) for detection of *C. parvum* immunoglobulin G (IgG) was developed and applied to serum of cats to estimate the seroprevalence of exposure.[21] *C. parvum* antibodies were detected in serum of 15.3 per cent of cats in Colorado and 8.3 per cent of cats in the United States.[21, 22] *C. parvum* oocysts have been documented in feces of many domestic cats with or without diarrhea in the United States, Japan, Scotland, Australia, and Spain.[17, 21, 23–31] Oocysts or antigens of *C. parvum* were detected in feces of 5.4 per cent of cats tested in north-central Colorado.[17]

Table 3–1. Common Enteric Zoonoses Associated With Contact With Cats or Their Excrement

Organism	Incubation	Relative Risk
Bacterial		
Campylobacter jejuni	Immediately infectious	Rare
Escherichia coli	Immediately infectious	Rare
Helicobacter species	Immediately infectious	Extremely rare
Salmonella species	Immediately infectious	Rare
Yersinia enterocolitica	Immediately infectious	Extremely rare
Parasitic—Amoeba		
Entamoeba histolytica	Immediately infectious (cysts)	Extremely rare
Parasitic—Cestodes		
Echinococcus multilocularis	Immediately infectious (cysts)	Extremely rare; regional
Parasitic—Coccidia		
Cryptosporidium parvum	Immediately infectious (oocysts)	Common
Toxoplasma gondii	Infectious after 1- to 5-day incubation—oocyst exposure from environment	Common
Parasitic—Flagellate		
Giardia species*	Immediately infectious (cysts)	Common
Parasitic—Helminths		
Ancylostoma braziliense	Larva infectious after > 3-day incubation—skin penetration	Common; regional
A. tubaeforme	from larva in environment	
Uncinaria stenocephala		
Strongyloides stercoralis	Larva immediately infectious	Rare
Toxocara cati	Larvated ova infectious after 1- to 3-week incubation—exposure from environment	Common; regional

*Trophozoites are likely to be minimally zoonotic.

Table 3–2. Common Feline Bite-, Scratch-, or Exudate-Contact–Associated Zoonoses

Organism	Clinical Syndrome	Relative Risk
Bacterial		
Bartonella species	Cat—subclinical	Common
	Human being—lymphadenopathy, fever, malaise, bacillary angiomatosis, bacillary peliosis	
Capnocytophaga canimorsus	Cat—subclinical	Rare
	Human being—bacteremia	
Francisella tularensis	Cat—septicemia, pneumonia	Extremely rare
	Human being—ulceroglandular, glandular, oculoglandular, pneumonic, or typhoidal (depending on route of infection)	
ʟ-Form bacteria	Cat—chronic draining tracts, polyarthritis	Extremely rare
	Human being—chronic draining tracts, polyarthritis	
Yersinia pestis	Cat—bubonic, bacteremic, or pneumonic	Rare; regional
	Human being—bubonic, bacteremic, or pneumonic	
Fungal		
Dermatophytes	Cat—superficial dermatologic disease	Common
	Human being—superficial dermatologic disease	
Sporothrix schenkii	Cat—chronic draining cutaneous tracts	Extremely rare
	Human being—chronic draining cutaneous tracts	
Viral		
Rabies	Cat—progressive CNS disease	Rare
	Human being—progressive CNS disease	

Abbreviation: CNS, central nervous system.

Table 3–3. Common Zoonoses Associated With Direct Contact With Respiratory or Ocular Secretions of Cats

Organism	Clinical Signs	Relative Risk
Bordetella bronchiseptica	Cat—upper respiratory; rarely, pneumonia Human being—pneumonia in immunosuppressed	Extremely rare
Chlamydia psittaci	Cat—conjunctivitis, mild upper respiratory Human being—conjunctivitis, bacteremia	Extremely rare
Francisella tularensis	Cat—septicemia, pneumonia Human being—ulceroglandular, oculoglandular, glandular, pneumonic, or typhoidal (depending on route of inoculation)	Extremely rare
Streptococcus group A	Cat—subclinical, transient carrier Human being—strep throat, septicemia	Extremely rare
Yersinia pestis	Cat—bubonic, bacteremic, or pneumonic Human being—bubonic, bacteremic, or pneumonic	Extremely rare and regional

Although it usually is undetermined where people acquire *C. parvum* infection, contaminated water is the most likely source.[32] However, cryptosporidiosis has been documented in people and cats in the same environment, suggesting that the potential for zoonotic transfer exists.[33–36] Oocysts are infectious when passed in feces, so the potential for direct zoonotic transfer exists. A feline genotype that varies considerably from human and cattle genotypes was identified.[37] The feline genotype was documented in an infected human being[38] and in an infected cow,[39] suggesting that the genotype can infect other mammals. Only 2 feline *C. parvum* cross-infection studies have been performed, but the genotypes were not determined. In one study, a feline isolate failed to cross-infect mice, rats, guinea pigs, or dogs.[40] In another study, a feline isolate cross-infected lambs.[41] In a study of HIV-infected people with cryptosporidiosis, there was no statistical association with cat ownership, suggesting that cat contact is an uncommon way to acquire cryptosporidiosis.[42] Although cats commonly are infected with *Cryptosporidium* species[17] and can shed oocysts for extended periods of time,[40, 43] only small numbers of oocysts per gram of feces are shed, and cats are very fastidious.[24] These facts may explain the lack of association between cats and human cryptosporidiosis.

Because it is impossible to determine zoonotic strains of *C. parvum* by microscopic examination, it seems prudent to assume feces from all cats infected with *C. parvum* to be a potential human health risk. Feces from all cats with diarrhea and all cats in the homes of immunosuppressed individuals should be evaluated for *C. parvum*. Infected cats generally do not shed large numbers of *Cryptosporidium* oocysts, and the oocysts are very small, which can result in false-negative fetal flotation results. Acid-fast staining of a thin fecal smear, immunofluorescent antibody staining of feces, or fecal antigen ELISA will aid in the identification of the extremely small (approximately 5 μm) oocysts.[44] The source from which cats acquire cryptosporidiosis is unknown, but because rodents commonly are infected,[45] infection may be acquired by carnivorism. It is possible that administration of paromomycin or tylosin can lessen oocyst shedding from infected cats, but data are limited.[29, 30] Fecal examination should be performed 2 weeks after cessation of treatment to assess for the presence of oocysts.

Giardiasis

Giardia is a flagellate with worldwide distribution that has been associated with diarrhea in cats and people. Mammalian isolates are all classified currently as *Giardia lamblia*. Prevalence in cats varies by the region; 3.9 per cent and 1.9 per cent of client-owned cats with or without diarrhea, respectively, were infected in a study performed in north central Colorado.[17] The organism is passed in feces as a

Table 3–4. Common Canine and Feline Urinary and Genital Tract Zoonoses

Organism	Clinical Signs	Relative Risk
Bacterial		
Leptospira species	Cat—fever, malaise, inflammatory urinary tract or hepatic disease, uveitis, CNS disease Human being—fever, malaise, inflammatory urinary tract or hepatic disease, uveitis, CNS disease	Extremely rare
Rickettsial		
Coxiella burnetii	Cat—subclinical, abortion, or stillbirth Human being—fever, pneumonitis, lymphadenopathy, myalgia, arthritis	Unknown

Abbreviation: CNS, central nervous system.

motile trophozoite or as cysts. Trophozoites usually are found only in diarrheic stool and are inactivated by gastric secretions, thus they are unlikely to be involved with zoonotic transmission. *Giardia* cysts are immediately infectious when passed in stool, so there is potential for direct zoonotic transfer.

Evaluation of human and feline *Giardia* species isolates by isoenzyme electrophoresis suggests that cats could serve as a reservoir for human infections.[46] However, cross-infection potential of *Giardia* species isolates has not been studied extensively using isolates from cats. In one study, *Giardia* species from human beings were inoculated into cats and the cats were relatively resistant to infection.[47] To date, there have been no documented cases of direct zoonotic transfer from a cat to a human being; however, it is difficult to determine the source of individual infections.

Because it is impossible to determine zoonotic strains of *Giardia* species by microscopic examination, it seems prudent to assume feces from all cats infected with *Giardia* species to be a potential human health risk. *Giardia* is a common enteric pathogen and can be detected in feces of cats with and without diarrhea. These findings emphasize that fecal examination should be performed on all cats at least yearly, and that treatment with anti-*Giardia* drugs should be administered if infection is documented. Many parasitologists feel that zinc sulfate centrifugation is the optimum procedure for demonstration of *Giardia* cysts. Use of repeated fecal examinations or fecal antigen testing may improve sensitivity of organism detection. The drugs currently used most frequently for the treatment of giardiasis in cats include metronidazole and fenbendazole. Fecal examination should be performed 2 weeks after cessation of treatment to assess for presence of cysts. Vaccination against *Giardia* could be considered in cats with recurrent infection.[48] Risk of giardiasis should be factored against risk of vaccine-associated disease. Anecdotal information suggests that vaccination may have a therapeutic effect in cats with chronic giardiasis.

Helicobacteriosis

Helicobacter species are gastric spiral organisms associated with disease in a number of animals including human beings. The prevalence of *Helicobacter*-like organisms in gastric tissues ranges from 41 to 100 per cent of healthy cats and 57 to 100 per cent of vomiting cats.[49] *Helicobacter felis, H. pametensis, H. pylori,* and "*H. heilmannii*" infections of cats have been documented.[49, 50] The principal pathogen in human beings is *H. pylori,* which has been isolated from a colony of research cats but not stray cats. The failure to find *H. pylori* in naturally exposed cats suggests that it is a reverse zoonosis.[51] There is some evidence that cats can be associated with helicobacteriosis in human beings. A genetically identical "*H. heilmannii*" was identified in an infected person and his cat.[52] An association was made with cat contact in one study of farm workers with helicobacteriosis.[53] However, in 3 other studies, including one of veterinarians, there was no epidemiologic association of cat contact with human helicobacteriosis.[54–56] Based on these reports, it appears that human beings are unlikely to acquire *Helicobacter* species infection from contact with cats.

Salmonellosis

There are more than 2000 variants of *Salmonella enteritidis.*[5] The bacterium is infectious when passed in feces, and so can be a direct zoonosis. However, it appears that most infections of human beings occur from indirect contact with contaminated water or food. Salmonellosis is severe in immunosuppressed human beings and is considered an AIDS-defining illness.[9] Many *Salmonella*-infected cats are clinically normal. Approximately 50 per cent of clinically affected cats have gastroenteritis; others are presented with abortion, stillbirth, neonatal death, or signs of bacteremia.[57–59] Neutropenia and neutrophils on rectal cytology are common findings in acute salmonellosis. Song-bird fever is a clinical syndrome noted in some cats after the ingestion of infected birds.[57] The incidence of salmonellosis varies by region and husbandry. It was reported that *Salmonella* was cultured from 1 to 18 per cent of cats.[60] However, the incidence in cats in crowded environments may be decreasing owing to improved husbandry and changes in feeding practices (less raw food). *Salmonella* species were cultured from the stool of 0.8 per cent of client-owned cats and 1.3 per cent of shelter-source cats in a recent study in north-central Colorado.[17] Cats with suspected salmonellosis should have stool or blood cultured to make a definitive diagnosis. Prevention of salmonellosis in human beings and cats is based on sanitation and control of exposure to feces. Because salmonellosis can be acquired by carnivorism, cats should not be allowed to hunt and should not be fed undercooked meats, particularly chicken products. Several antibiotics including quinolones can control clinical signs of salmonellosis. Only parenteral antibiotics should be given to cats with salmonellosis to lessen risk of antimicrobial resistance. Several cats have been reported with multiple antibiotic–resistant *Salmonella* infections.[61–63]

Toxoplasmosis

Cats are the only known definitive host for the coccidian *T. gondii,* and so are solely responsible for passage of oocysts into the environment.[64] Oocysts require 1 to 5 days in the environment to sporulate and become infectious. Once sporulated, oocysts survive for months to years in soil or contaminated water. Most other mammals serve as intermediate hosts for the organism and maintain the organism in tissues as tachyzoites or bradyzoites in tissue cysts. Approximately 30 to 40 per cent of adult human beings in the world have *T. gondii* serum antibodies, suggesting previous or current infection.[65] Infection of human beings occurs most frequently by ingestion of sporulated oocysts in the environment or by ingestion of tissue cysts in undercooked meats. Thus, prevention of toxoplasmosis in people can be achieved by avoiding those 2 life stages.

In immunocompetent human beings, clinical disease generally is mild after primary infection. Primary *T. gondii* infection is recognized rarely because the predominant clinical signs of self-limiting fever, malaise, and lymphadenopathy are nonspecific and shared with other infections. For example, toxoplasmosis has been confused with infectious mononucleosis. Clinical toxoplasmosis can be severe in immunosuppressed individuals, including the fetus, people with AIDS, and human patients treated with immunosuppressive agents for the treatment of cancer and to prevent organ transplant rejection. As T-helper cell counts decline in people with AIDS, bradyzoites in tissue cysts replicate rapidly, resulting in toxoplasmic encephalitis. Infection of a previously naïve mother during gestation commonly results in stillbirth, central nervous system disease, and ocular disease in the fetus. Thus, *T. gondii* is a very important zoonotic disease.

T. gondii infection of human beings by ingestion of oocysts has been documented several times. Clinical toxoplasmosis developed in a group of people after a common exposure in a riding stable,[66] in a group of soldiers drinking contaminated water in Panama,[67] and from an oocyst-contaminated municipal water supply.[68] However, although it cannot be stated definitively that a person will not acquire toxoplasmosis from her or his personal cat, it is extremely unlikely. Cats generally acquire *T. gondii* infection by carnivorism. After primary infection by ingestion of tissue cysts, cats shed oocysts for approximately 7 to 10 days. Thus, an individual cat will be passing oocysts into the human environment for only a small fraction of its entire life span. Because of this short oocyst-shedding period, *T. gondii* oocysts are found rarely in fecal studies. For example, the seroprevalence of *T. gondii* infection in 206 cats with and without diarrhea in north-central Colorado was 23.6 per cent, but none of the cats were shedding *T. gondii* oocysts in feces.[17] Most cats are fastidious and do not leave feces on their fur for the required 1- to 5-day oocyst-sporulation period. Oocysts were not detected on the fur of experimentally inoculated cats 7 days after they were shedding millions of oocysts in feces.[69] These findings suggest that touching individual cats is an unlikely way to acquire toxoplasmosis; this hypothesis also is supported by epidemiologic studies. In general, veterinary healthcare providers are no more likely than the general population to be seropositive for *T. gon-*

dii infection. Because oocysts are passed unsporulated and noninfectious, working with fresh feline feces (<1 day old) is not a risk for veterinary healthcare personnel. People with HIV infection who owned cats were not more likely to acquire toxoplasmosis during their illness than people with HIV infection who did not have cat contact.[70]

It is difficult to induce repeat oocyst shedding in cats previously infected with *T. gondii*. Superinfection with *Isospora* led to oocyst shedding in some *T. gondii*–infected cats.[64] Prednisolone administered at 10 to 80 mg/kg orally (PO) or methylprednisolone administered at 10 to 80 mg/kg intramuscularly (IM) induced oocyst shedding in some cats with chronic toxoplasmosis.[64] However, administration of methyprednisolone acetate administered at the more appropriate clinical dose of 5 mg/kg weekly for 4 to 6 weeks to cats infected with *T. gondii* for 14 weeks or 14 months failed to induce oocyst shedding.[71] *T. gondii*–infected cats infected with feline immunodeficiency virus (FIV) followed by feline leukemia virus (FeLV) developed immunodeficiency-associated syndromes (unpublished data), but repeat *T. gondii* oocyst shedding did not occur. Inoculation of cats with FIV or FeLV infections with *T. gondii* results in oocyst-shedding periods and number of oocysts shed similar to those for cats without FIV or FeLV infections.[64, 72] The intestinal immunity to *T. gondii* in cats is not permanent; 4 of 9 cats inoculated 6 years after primary inoculation shed oocysts even though each had high serum antibody titers.[69] In another study, *T. gondii*–infected cats with and without FIV infection failed to repeat oocyst shedding when inoculated with *T. gondii* 16 months after primary inoculation.[72] Thus, cats that are exposed frequently to *T. gondii* probably do not shed large numbers of oocysts after the first infection.

There is no serologic assay that accurately predicts when a cat shed *T. gondii* oocysts in the past, and most cats that are shedding oocysts are seronegative.[73] Most seropositive cats have completed the oocyst shedding period and are unlikely to repeat shedding; most seronegative cats would shed the organism if infected. *Because human beings are not commonly infected with* T. gondii *from contact with individual cats, and because serologic test results cannot predict the oocyst shedding status of seropositive cats accurately, testing healthy cats for toxoplasmosis is of no clinical use.*[8, 73] Fecal examination is an adequate procedure to determine when cats are actively shedding oocysts, but cannot predict when a cat has shed oocysts in the past. If owners are concerned that they may have toxoplasmosis, they should see their doctor for testing.

T. gondii infection can be avoided. Water collected from the environment should be boiled or filtered before drinking. Care should be taken to wash hands carefully after working with soil or to wear gloves. Produce from the garden should be washed carefully before ingestion. The children's sandbox should be covered when not in use. A litterbox liner should be used, and the litterbox should be cleaned daily by someone other than the immunosuppressed or pregnant person. Scalding water should be used to clean the litterbox because sporulated oocysts are extremely resistant to most disinfectants. Oocysts measuring 10×12 μm in a cat fecal sample could be *T. gondii. Hammondia hammondi* and *Besnoitia darlingi* are morphologically similar coccidians passed by cats, but are not human pathogens.[64] Feces should be collected and disposed of daily until the oocyst shedding period is complete; administration of clindamycin, sulfonamides, or pyrimethamine can reduce levels of oocyst shedding. Ingestion of *T. gondii* in tissues can result in human toxoplasmosis. Meats (particularly pork in the United States) should be cooked to medium-well to inactivate tissue cysts. Gloves should be worn when handling raw meats (including field dressing) for cooking, or hands should be cleansed thoroughly afterward. Freezing meat at $-12°C$ for several days will kill most tissue cysts. Ingestion of raw goat's milk also can result in human toxoplasmosis.

◆ SELECT BITE- AND SCRATCH-ASSOCIATED ZOONOSES

Capnocytophaga Species, *Mycoplasma felis,* and *Pasteurella* Species

Animal bites result in over 300,000 emergency room visits annually in the United States.[74] In immunocompetent individuals, the majority of the aerobic and anaerobic bacteria associated with bite or scratch wounds lead only to local infection. However, 28 to 80 per cent of cat bites become infected, and uncommon severe sequelae including meningitis, endocarditis, septic arthritis, and septic shock can occur.[74] Immunocompromised humans beings, or human beings exposed to *Pasteurella* species or *C. canimorsus* (formerly known as DF-2) more consistently develop systemic clinical illness.[75, 76] In particular, splenectomy results in increased risk. Local cellulitis is noted initially, followed by evidence of deeper tissue infection. Bacteremia and the associated clinical signs of fever, malaise, and weakness are common, and death can occur from either of these 2 genera. *Pasteurella multocida* from a cat was cultured from the lungs of a man with AIDS who had had only passive contact with the cat.[77] *Mycoplasma* species infection of people associated with cat bites, 1 with cellulitis and 1 with septic arthritis, has been reported at least twice.[78, 79] Diagnosis of bacterial infections is confirmed by culture. Treatment includes local wound drainage and systemic antibiotic therapy. Penicillin derivatives are very effective against most *Pasteurella* infections. Penicillins and cephalosporins are effective against *Capnocytophaga* in vitro. Bites and scratches should be avoided if possible, wounds should be irrigated voluminously with sterile saline solution and scrubbed, and immunosuppressed individuals should seek immediate medical attention for antimicrobial treatment.

Bartonellosis

Cats are infected with *Bartonella henselae* (previously *Rochalimaea*), *Bartonella clarridgeiae*, and *Bartonella koehlerae*.[80–82] *B. henselae* and *B. clarridgeiae*[83] have been isolated from human beings with cat-scratch disease; *B. henselae* causes bacillary angiomatosis and bacillary peliosis in immunosuppressed people. Both the type I and the type II variants of *B. henselae* can be detected in infected cats and human beings.[84, 85]

Cat-scratch disease is characterized in human beings by lymphadenopathy, fever, malaise, weight loss, ophthalmic disease, myalgia, headache, conjunctivitis, skin eruptions, and arthralgia. The incubation period is approximately 3 weeks. The syndrome may take several months to resolve completely, and resolution may or may not be aided by use of antimicrobial therapy. It is estimated that there are at least 25,000 cases of cat-scratch disease diagnosed annually in the United States, resulting in at least $12.5 million in healthcare costs.

Cats are reservoirs for *Bartonella* species, and infection of cats is extremely common. Most cases of cat-scratch disease in human beings are associated with kitten contact. The seroprevalence of *Bartonella* species in cats in the United States is as high as 54.6 to 81 per cent in some geographic areas.[86, 87] *B. henselae* has been cultured from the blood of many naturally exposed cats; cats infected with the organism by inoculation intradermally, subcutaneously, intravenously, or intramuscularly; and cats infected by fleas.[87–92] Experimental infections induced by intravenous, intramuscular, or intradermal inoculation have resulted in fever, lymphadenopathy, and neurologic diseases in some cats.[91, 92] Uveal tract inflammation and other clinical signs of disease including gingivitis and lymphadenopathy have been reported in some naturally infected cats.[93–95]

Bartonella species infection is most common in flea-infested cats from catteries,[96] and so when an immunosuppressed person wishes to adopt a new cat, an adult animal without history of flea infestation is the safest. New cats entering the environment of an immunosuppressed family should be isolated from the immunosuppressed family member while being screened for *Bartonella* species infection. Blood culture is the optimum test to prove the presence of current *Bartonella* species infection, but bacteremia can be intermittent and so false-negative results occur occasionally. Polymerase chain reaction can be used to document the presence of *Bartonella* species DNA, but results are false-negative occasionally, and positive results do not necessarily indicate that the organism is alive. Seropositive and seronegative cats can be bacteremic, which limits the diagnostic utility of serologic testing.

Bacteremia can be limited by administration of doxycycline, tetracycline, erythromycin, amoxicillin-clavulanate, or enrofloxacin, but does not cure infection in all cats.[88, 89, 97] Accordingly, whether to administer antibiotics to bacteremic cats is controversial. However, if an immunosuppressed family member is present in the household, it seems prudent to treat the infected cat. The cat should be isolated from the immunosuppressed individual until follow-up cultures or polymerase chain reaction is performed no sooner than 3 weeks after treatment. Flea control should be maintained continually.

◆ SELECT EMERGING ZOONOSES

Bordetellosis

B. bronchiseptica is a primary pathogen in dogs that is one of the causes of infectious tracheobronchitis. Many cats, particularly those in crowded environments, have serologic evidence of exposure to *B. bronchiseptica* or are culture-positive.[98, 99] In one study, *B. bronchiseptica* was isolated from 82 of 740 cats sampled.[99] The organism appears to be host-adapted in cats, with significant clinical disease almost never occurring. In the rare clinically affected cat, fever, mucopurulent nasal discharge, and cough are the most common clinical signs.[100, 101] By 1998, 39 cases of *B. bronchiseptica* infection in people had been reported, many of whom were immunodeficient.[102–104] An association with cats has been reported only once in an HIV- and *B. bronchiseptica*–coinfected person.[104] Based on these studies, it appears that *B. bronchiseptica* infection of human beings resulting from contact with cats is extremely unlikely. A vaccine is available to aid in the prevention of bordetellosis in cats. However, owing to the low risk of transmission of feline bordetellosis to human beings, there appears to be no use for the vaccine to prevent zoonoses. However, in households with immunosuppressed family members, a diagnostic work-up should be considered for cats with suspected bacterial respiratory disease. *B. bronchiseptica* is cultured easily. Doxycycline, amoxicillin-clavulanate, and quinolones are effective in controlling clinical signs of disease, but treated cats can be culture-positive for months.

Chlamydiosis

C. psittaci is a differential diagnosis for conjunctivitis and potentially rhinitis in cats. Conjunctivitis in human beings may occur after direct contact with ocular discharges from infected cats.[105, 106] A human Chlamydia species isolate that was inoculated into cats resulted in conjunctivitis and persistent infection, suggesting that the isolate was originally from a cat.[107] Chlamydia of feline origin have been associated indirectly with atypical pneumonia in an apparently immunocompetent 48-year-old man,[108] malaise and cough in an immunosuppressed woman,[109] and endocarditis and glomerulonephritis in a 40-year-old woman.[110] Care should be taken to avoid direct conjunctival contact with discharges

from the respiratory or ocular secretions of cats, especially by immunosuppressed persons. Tetracycline derivatives administered topically or orally are effective for the treatment of infected cats.

Ehrlichiosis

Ehrlichia species infection has been documented in multiple cats around the world[111, 112] (see Chapter 4, Rickettsial Diseases). To date, morulae have been detected in mononuclear cells and neutrophils. Only 1 feline *Ehrlichia* isolate has been sequenced and analyzed genetically.[113] This Swedish feline isolate was genetically identical to the human granulocytic *Ehrlichia* in Sweden and the United States. *Ehrlichia risticii* infects cats and *Ehrlichia chaffeensis* infects dogs, indicating that pets may be potential reservoirs for infection of vectors. However, it is unlikely that direct zoonotic transfer occurs. Tick control should be maintained to avoid shared vector transfer of infection.

Rickettsia felis

A clinical disease syndrome similar to Rocky Mountain spotted fever in human beings is caused by *Rickettsia prowazekii* (louse-borne or epidemic typhus). In some regions, opossums serve as a reservoir, and the organism is transmitted by *Ctenocephalides felis*. *R. felis* was discovered in a person with clinical signs referable to typhus. To date, *R. felis* has been isolated from *C. felis* collected in California, Florida, Georgia, Louisiana, New York, North Carolina, Oklahoma, Texas, and Tennessee.[114] The organism is passed transtadially and transovarially in fleas. Experimentally inoculated cats become seropositive, but are infected subclinically. It is unknown whether cats can be a reservoir for fleas or are clinically affected. However, it seems prudent to maintain flea control to lessen potential for human exposure.

◆ RECOMMENDATIONS

Because human beings are not likely to acquire an infectious disease from direct cat contact, and because cat ownership has many positive benefits, there appear to be few reasons for immunosuppressed people to relinquish their cats or to avoid cat ownership. Veterinarians should familiarize themselves with zoonotic issues and actively discuss the health risks and benefits of pet ownership with immunosuppressed clients, so that logical decisions concerning ownership and management of individual animals may be made (Table 3–5).

The safest new cat to adopt into a household with an immunosuppressed family member is a clinically normal, adult cat from a private family. Cats with

Table 3–5. Recommendations for Avoidance of Zoonotic Agents of Cats

Keep house cats indoors
Feed only processed foods
Cover children's sandboxes
Clean the litterbox daily
Clean the litterbox periodically with scalding water
Do not allow immunosuppressed individuals to clean the litterbox
Wash hands or wear gloves when gardening
Cook meat for human consumption to 80°C for 15 min minimum
Wash hands or wear gloves when handling meat
If immunosuppressed and adopting a new cat, avoid kittens from crowded environments with a history of diarrhea and ectoparasites
Administer routine anthelmintic to kittens at 6, 8, and 10 wk of age
Perform suggested work-up for enteric zoonoses
   Fecal flotation for oocysts, cysts, and ova
   Rectal cytology to observe for white blood cells and spirochetes
   Fecal wet mount to evaluate for trophozoites
   Cryptosporidium screening by IFA, ELISA or acid-fast stain
   Fecal culture
Administer periodic anthelmintics and taeniacides, particularly in cats allowed outdoors
Use heartworm preventives that aid in control of helminths
Control ectoparasites
Control potential transport hosts like flies, cockroaches, fleas, and rodents in the household
Seek veterinary care for respiratory, gastrointestinal, dermatologic, and genitourinary problems
Test new cats (or cats with ectoparasites) for *Bartonella* species infection by PCR or culture and serology

Abbreviations: ELISA, enzyme-linked immunosorbent assay; IFA, immunofluorescent antibody; PCR, polymerase chain reaction.

ectoparasites should be avoided because of increased risk of *Bartonella* species infection and the shared-vector zoonoses. Until the cat is evaluated by a veterinarian, it should be isolated from the immunosuppressed family member. Housing the cat indoors will lessen the potential for exposure to potentially zoonotic agents.

A thorough physical examination should be performed on all cats at least yearly. Because enteric zoonoses may be present in cats with and without diarrhea, fecal flotation for oocysts, cysts, and eggs, *Cryptosporidium* species examination by immunofluorescent antibody or antigen testing, and fecal culture for enteric bacteria, are all logical screening procedures. Each new cat and previously owned cats allowed outdoors also should be screened for bartonellosis yearly. Blood collected aseptically should be placed in an ethylenediaminetetraacetic acid (EDTA) tube for *Bartonella* species culture or polymerase chain reaction (see the section on bartonellosis). Serum is submitted at the same time for *Bartonella* species antibody testing. Direct contact with individual cats is an uncommon way to acquire toxoplasmosis, and there is no indication for evaluating healthy cats serologically. The cat should be treated with a drug that kills hookworms and roundworms. Fenbendazole is a good choice given at 50 mg/kg, PO, every (q) 24 hr for 3 days because it also

may be effective for the treatment of giardiasis. Flea and tick control should be instituted or maintained. Fecal material produced in the home environment should be removed daily, preferably by someone other than the immunosuppressed individual. Litterbox liners should be used, or the litterbox should be cleaned at least once weekly with scalding water. The cat should be maintained in the home environment and fed only commercially processed pet food. The owner should not allow the cat to share utensils and should avoid being licked. Care should be taken to control possible transport hosts like flies, cockroaches, and rodents in the cat's environment.

REFERENCES

1. Evans RH: Public health and important zoonoses in feline populations. *In* August JR (ed): Consultations in Feline Internal Medicine, vol. 3. Philadelphia, WB Saunders, 1997, pp. 611–629.
2. Lappin MR: Feline zoonoses. *In* Kirk RW, Bonagura JD (eds): Current Veterinary Therapy XI: Small Animal Practice. Philadelphia, WB Saunders, 1992, pp. 284–291.
3. Greene CE: Immunocompromised people and pets. *In* Greene CE (ed): Infectious Diseases of the Dog and Cat, 2nd ed. Philadelphia, WB Saunders, 1998, pp. 710–717.
4. Patronek G: Free-roaming and feral cats—Their impact on wildlife and human beings. J Am Vet Med Assoc 212:218–226, 1998.
5. Tan J: Human zoonotic infections transmitted by dogs and cats. Arch Intern Med 157:1933–1943, 1997.
6. Burton B: Pets and PWAs: Claims of health risk exaggerated. AIDS Patient Care, February 1989, pp. 34–37.
7. Spencer L: Study explores health risks and the human animal bond. J Am Vet Med Assoc 201:1669, 1992.
8. Angulo FJ, Glaser CA, Juranek DD, et al: Caring for pets of immunocompromised persons. J Am Vet Med Assoc 205:1711–1718, 1994.
9. Glaser CA, Angulo F J, Rooney JA: Animal associated opportunistic infections among persons infected with the human immunodeficiency virus. Clin Infect Dis 18:14–24, 1994.
10. Carmack B: The role of companion animals for persons with AIDS/HIV: Holistic Nurs Pract 5:24–31, 1991.
11. Fox JG, Maxwell KO, Taylor NS, et al: "*Campylobacter upsaliensis*" isolated from cats as identified by DNA relatedness and biochemical features. J Clin Microbiol 27:2376–2378, 1989.
12. Fox JG: Campylobacter infections. *In* Greene CE (ed): Infectious Diseases of the Dog and Cat, 2nd ed. Philadelphia, WB Saunders, 1998, pp. 226–229.
13. Holt PE: The role of dogs and cats in the epidemiology of human campylobacter enterocolitis. J Small Anim Pract 22:681–685, 1981.
14. Hopkins RS, Olmsted R, Istre GR: Endemic *Campylobacter jejuni* infection in Colorado: Identified risk factors. Am J Public Health 74:249–250, 1984.
15. Deming MS, Tauxe RV, Blake PA, et al: *Campylobacter* enteritis at a university: Transmission from eating chickens and from cats. Am J Epidemiol 126:526–534, 1987.
16. Gurgan T, Diker KS: Abortion associated with *Campylobacter upsaliensis*. J Clin Microbiol 32:3093–3094, 1994.
17. Hill S, Lappin MR, Cheney J, et al: Prevalence of enteric zoonotic agents in cats. J Am Vet Med Assoc 216:687–692, 2000.
18. MacKenzie WR, Hoxie NJ, Proctor ME, et al: A massive outbreak in Milwaukee of cryptosporidium infection transmitted through the public water supply. N Engl J Med 331:161–167, 1994.
19. Beneson AS: Cryptosporidiosis. *In* Control of Communica-

ble Diseases in Man, 15th ed. American Public Health Association, 1990; pp. 112–114.

20. Diers J, McCallister GL: Occurrence of *Cryptosporidium* in home daycare centers in west-central Ohio. J Parasitol 75:637–638, 1989.

21. Lappin MR, Ungar B, Brown-Hahn B, et al: Enzyme-linked immunosorbent assay for the detection of *Cryptosporidium* spp. IgG in the serum of cats. J Parasitol 83:957–960, 1997.

22. McReynolds C, Lappin MR, McReynolds L, et al: Regional seroprevalence of *Cryptosporidium parvum* IgG specific antibodies of cats in the United States. Vet Parasitol 80:187–195, 1998.

23. Arai H, Fukuda Y, Hara T, et al: Prevalence of *Cryptosporidium* infection among domestic cats in the Tokyo metropolitan district, Japan. Jpn J Med Sci 43:7–14, 1990.

24. Uga S, Matsumura T, Ishibashi K, et al: Cryptosporidiosis in dogs and cats in Hyogo Prefecture, Japan. Jpn J Parasitol 38:139–143, 1989.

25. Goodwin MA, Barsanti JA: Intractable diarrhea associated with intestinal cryptosporidiosis in a domestic cat also infected with feline leukemia virus. J Am Anim Hosp Assoc 26:365–368, 1990.

26. Mtambo MMA, Nash AS, Blewett DA, et al: *Cryptosporidium* infection in cats: Prevalence of infection in domestic and feral cats in the Glasgow area. Vet Rec 129:502–504, 1991.

27. Lent SF, Burkhardt JE, Bolka D: Coincident enteric cryptosporidiosis and lymphosarcoma in a cat with diarrhea. J Am Anim Hosp Assoc 29:492–496, 1993.

28. Nash AS, Mtambo MMA, Gibbs HA: *Cryptosporidium* infection in farm cats in the Glasgow area. Vet Rec 133:576–577, 1993.

29. Barr SC, Jamrosz GF, Hornbuckle WE, et al: Use of paromomycin for treatment of cryptosporidiosis in a cat. J Am Vet Med Assoc 205:1742–1743, 1994.

30. Lappin MR, Dowers K, Edsell, D, et al: Cryptosporidiosis and inflammatory bowel disease in a cat. Fel Pract 3:10–13, 1997.

31. Sargent KD, Morgan UM, Elliot A, et al: Morphological and genetic characterisation of *Cryptosporidium* oocysts from domestic cats. Vet Parasitol 77:221–227, 1998.

32. Juranek DD: Cryptosporidiosis: Sources of infection and guidelines for prevention. Clin Infect Dis 21:S57–S61, 1995.

33. Egger M, Nguyen X, Schaad UB, et al: Intestinal cryptosporidiosis acquired from a cat. Infection 18:177–178, 1990.

34. Bennett M, Baxby D, Blundell N, et al: Cryptosporidiosis in the domestic cat. Vet Rec 116:73–74, 1985.

35. Edelman MJ, Oldfield EC: Severe cryptosporidiosis in an immunocompetent host. Arch Intern Med 148:1873–1874, 1988.

36. Koch KL, Shandey TV, Weinstein GS, et al: Cryptosporidiosis in·a patient with hemophilia, common variable hypogammaglobulinemia, and the acquired immunodeficiency syndrome. Ann Intern Med 99:337–340, 1983.

37. Morgan UM, Constantine CC, Forbes DA, Thompson RC: Differentiation between human and animal isolates of *Cryptosporidium parvum* using rDNA sequencing and direct PCR analysis. J Parasitol 83:825–830, 1997.

38. Pieniazek NJ, Bornay-Llinares FJ, Slemenda SB et al: New *Cryptosporidium* genotypes in HIV-infected persons. Emerg Infect Dis 5:444–449, 1999.

39. Bornay-Llinares FJ, da Silva AJ, Moura INS , et al: Identification of *Cryptosporidium felis* in a cow by morphologic and molecular methods. Appl Environ Microbiol 65:1455–1458, 1999.

40. Asahi H, Koyama T, Arai H, et al: Biological nature of *Cryptosporidium* sp. isolated from a cat. Parasitol Res 77:237–240, 1991.

41. Mtambo MMA, Wright E, Nash AS, Blewett DA: Infectivity of a *Cryptosporidium* species isolated from a domestic cat *(Felis domestica)* in lambs and mice. Res Vet Sci 60:61–63, 1996.

42. Glaser CA, Safrin S, Reingold A, et al: Association between *Cryptosporidium* infection and animal exposure in HIV-infected individuals. J Acquir Immun Defic Syndr Hum Retrovirol 17:79–82, 1998.

43. McReynolds CA, Lappin MR: *Cryptosporidium parvum* oocyst shedding and serum antibody responses in experimentally infected cats. J Vet Intern Med 13:256, 1999.

44. Mtambo MMA, Nash AS, Blewett DA, et al: Comparison of staining and concentration techniques for detection of *Cryptosporidium* oocysts in cat faecal specimens. Vet Parasitol 45:49–57, 1992.

45. Chalmers RM, Sturdee AP, Bull SA, et al: The prevalence of *Cryptosporidium parvum* and *C. muris* in *Mus domesticus, Apodemus sylvaticus,* and *Clethrionomys glareolus* in an agricultural system. Parasitol Res 83:478–482, 1997.

46. Meloni BP, Lymbery AJ, Thompson RCA: Isoenzyme electrophoresis of 30 isolates of *Giardia* from humans and felines. Am J Trop Med Hyg 38:65–73, 1988.

47. Kirkpatrick CE, Green GA: Susceptibility of domestic cats to infections with *Giardia lamblia* cysts and trophozoites from human sources. J Clin Microbiol 21:678–680, 1985.

48. Olson ME, Morck DW, Ceri H: The efficacy of a *Giardia lamblia* vaccine in kittens. Can J Vet Res 60:249–256, 1996.

49. Simpson K, Neiger R, DeNovo R, et al: The relationship of *Helicobacter* spp. infection to gastric disease in dogs and cats. J Vet Intern Med 14:223–227, 2000.

50. Neiger R, Simpson KW: *Helicobacter* infection in dogs and cats: Facts and fiction. J Vet Intern Med 14:125–133, 2000.

51. El-Zaatari FAK, Woo JS, Badr A, et al: Failure to isolate *Helicobacter pylori* from stray cats indicated that *H. pylori* in cats may be an anthroponosis—An animal infection with a human pathogen. J Med Microbiol 46:372–376, 1997.

52. Dieterich C, Wiesel P, Neiger R, et al: Presence of multiple "*Helicobacter heilmannii*" strains in an individual suffering from ulcers and his two cats. J Clin Microbiol 36:1366–1370, 1998.

53. Thomas DR, Salmon RL, Meadows D, et al: Incidence of *Helicobacter pylori* in farmworkers and the role of zoonotic spread [Abstract]. Gut 37(Suppl 1):A24, 1995.

54. Ansorg R, von Heinnegg EH, Von Recklinghausen G: Cat owners' risk of acquiring a *Helicobacter pylori* infection. Zentralbl Bakteriol 283:122–126, 1995.

55. Webb PM, Knight T, Elder J, et al: Is *Helicobacter pylori* transmitted from cats to humans? Helicobacter 1:79–81, 1996.

56. Neiger R, Schmassmann A, Seidel KE: Antibodies against *Helicobacter pylori* and *Helicobacter felis* in veterinarians [Abstract]. Gastroenterol Int 11:127, 1998.

57. Scott FW: Salmonella implicated as cause of song bird fever. Feline Health Topics 3:5, 1988.

58. Dow SW, Jones RL, Henik RA, et al: Clinical features of salmonellosis in cats: Six cases (1981–1986). J Am Vet Med Assoc 194:1464–1466, 1989.

59. Foley JE, Orgad U, Hirsh DC, et al: Outbreak of fatal salmonellosis in cats following use of a high-titer modified-live panleukopenia virus vaccine. J Am Vet Med Assoc 214:67–70, 1999.

60. Greene CE: Salmonellosis. *In* Greene CE (ed): Infectious Diseases of the Dog and Cat, 2nd ed. Philadelphia, WB Saunders, 1998, pp. 235–240.

61. Low JC, Tennant B, Munro D: Multiresistant *Salmonella typhimurium* DT104 in cats. Lancet 348:1391–1392, 1996.

62. Wall PG, Davis S, Threlfall EJ, et al: Chronic carriage of multidrug resistant *Salmonella typhimurium* in a cat. J Small Anim Pract 36:279–281, 1995.

63. Wall PG, Threllfall EJ, Ward LR, et al: Multiresistant *Salmonella typhimurium* DT104 in cats: A public health risk. Lancet 348:471–472, 1996.

64. Dubey JP, Lappin MR: Toxoplasmosis and neosporosis. *In* Greene CE (ed): Infectious Diseases of the Dog and Cat, 2nd ed. Philadelphia, WB Saunders, 1998, pp. 493–503.

65. Dubey JP, Beattie CP: Toxoplasmosis of Animals and Man. Boca Raton, FL, CRC, 1988, pp. 1–220.

66. Teutsch SM, Juranek DD, Sulzer A, et al: Epidemic toxoplasmosis associated with infected cats. N Engl J Med 300:695–699, 1979.

67. Benenson MW, Takafuji ET, Lemon SM, et al. Oocyst-transmitted toxoplasmosis associated with ingestion of contaminated water. N Engl J Med 307:666–669, 1982.

68. Aramini JJ, Stephen C, Dubey JP, et al: Potential contamination of drinking water with *Toxoplasma gondii* oocysts. Epidemiol Infect 122:305–315, 1999.
69. Dubey JP: Duration of immunity to shedding *Toxoplasma gondii* oocysts by cats. J Parasitol 81:410–415, 1995.
70. Wallace MR, Rossetti RJ, Olson PE: Cats and toxoplasmosis risk in HIV-infected adults. JAMA 269:76–77, 1993.
71. Lappin MR, Dawe DL, Lindl PA, et al: The effect of glucocorticoid administration on oocyst shedding, serology, and cell mediated immune responses of cats with recent or chronic toxoplasmosis. J Am Anim Hosp Assoc 27:625–632, 1992.
72. Lappin MR, George JW, Pedersen NC, et al: Primary and secondary *Toxoplasma gondii* infection in normal and feline immunodeficiency virus infected cats. J Parasitol 82:733–742, 1996.
73. Lappin MR: Feline toxoplasmosis: Interpretation of diagnostic test results. Semin Vet Med Surg 11:154–160, 1996.
74. Talan DA, Citron DM, Abrahamian FM, et al: Bacteriologic analysis of infected dog and cat bites. N Engl J Med 340:84–92, 1999.
75. Carpenter PD, Heppner BT, Gnann JW: DF-2 bacteremia following cat bites. Report of two cases. Am J Med 82:621, 1987.
76. Valtonen M, Lauhio A, Carlson P, et al: *Capnocytophaga canimorsus* septicemia: Fifth report of a cat-associated infection and five other cases. Eur J Clin Microbiol Infect Dis 14:520–523, 1995.
77. Drabick JJ, Gasser RA, Saunders NB, et al: *Pasteurella multocida* pneumonia in a man with AIDS and nontraumatic feline exposure. Chest 103:7–11, 1993.
78. Bonilla HF, Chenoworth CE, Tully JG, et al: *Mycoplasma felis* septic arthritis in a patient with hypogammaglobulinemia. Clin Infect Dis 24:222–225, 1997.
79. McCabe SJ, Murray JF, Ruhnke HL, Rachlis A: Mycoplasma infection of the hand acquired from a cat. J Hand Surg [Am] 12:1085–1088, 1987.
80. Regnery RL, Anderson BE, Clarridge JE III, et al: Characterization of a novel *Rochalimaea species, R. henselae* sp. nov., isolated from blood of a febrile, human immunodeficiency virus–positive patient. J Clin Microbiol 30:265–274, 1992.
81. Clarridge JE, Raich TJ, Pirwani D, et al: Strategy to detect and identify *Bartonella* species in routine clinical laboratory yields *Bartonella henselae* from human immunodeficiency virus–positive patient and unique *Bartonella* strain from his cat. J Clin Microbiol 33:2107–2113, 1995.
82. Dehio C, Sander A: *Bartonella* as emerging pathogens. Trends Microbiol 7:226–228, 1999.
83. Kordick DL, Hilyard EJ, Hadfield TL, et al: *Bartonella clarridgeiae*, a newly recognized zoonotic pathogen causing inoculation papules, fever, and lymphadenopathy (cat scratch disease). J Clin Microbiol 35:1813–1818, 1997.
84. Heller R, Artois M, Xemar V, et al: Prevalence of *Bartonella henselae* and *Bartonella clarridgeiae* in stray cats. J Clin Microbiol 35:1327–1331, 1997.
85. Bergmans AMC, Schellekens JFP, van Embden JDA, et al: Predominance of two *Bartonella henselae* variants among cat-scratch disease patients in the Netherlands. J Clin Microbiol 34:254–260, 1996.
86. Jameson PH, Greene CE, Regnery RL, et al: Prevalence of *Bartonella henselae* antibodies in pet cats throughout regions of North America. J Infect Dis 172:1145–1149, 1995.
87. Chomel BB, Abbott RC, Kasten RW, et al: *Bartonella henselae* prevalence in domestic cats in California: Risk factors and association between bacteremia and antibody titers. J Clin Microbiol 33:2445–2450, 1995.
88. Regnery RL, Rooney JA, Johnson AM, et al: Experimentally induced *Bartonella henselae* infections followed by challenge exposure and antimicrobial therapy in cats. Am J Vet Res 57:1714–1719, 1996.
89. Greene CE, McDermott M, Jameson PH, et al: *Bartonella henselae* infection in cats: Evaluation during primary infection, treatment, and rechallenge infection. J Clin Microbiol 34:1682–1685, 1996.
90. Chomel BB, Kasten RW, Floyd-Hawkins K, et al: Experimental transmission of *Bartonella henselae* by the cat flea. J Clin Microbiol 34:1952–1956, 1996.
91. Kordick DL, Breitschwerdt EB: Relapsing bacteremia after blood transmission of *Bartonella henselae* to cats. Am J Vet Res 58:492–497, 1997.
92. Guptill L, Slater L, Ching-Ching W, et al: Experimental infection of young specific pathogen-free cats with *Bartonella henselae*. J Infect Dis 176:206–216, 1997.
93. Lappin MR, Black JC: *Bartonella* spp. associated uveitis in a cat. J Am Vet Med Assoc 214;1205–1207, 1999.
94. Ueno J, Hohdatsu T, Muramatsu Y, et al: Does coinfection of *Bartonella henselae* and FIV induce clinical disorders in cats? Microbiol Immunol 40:617–620, 1996.
95. Lappin MR, Jensen W, Kordick DL, et al: *Bartonella* spp. antibodies and DNA in aqueous humor of cats. J Fel Med Surg 2:61–68, 2000.
96. Foley JE, Chomel B, Kikuchi Y, et al: Seroprevalence of *Bartonella henselae* in cattery cats: Association with cattery hygiene and flea infestation. Vet Q 20:1–5, 1998.
97. Kordick DL, Papich MG, Breitschwerdt EB: Efficacy of enrofloxacin or doxycycline for treatment of *Bartonella henselae* or *Bartonella clarridgeiae* infection in cats. Antimicrob Agents Chemother 41:2448–2455, 1997.
98. Hoskins JD, Williams J, Roy AF, et al: Isolation and characterization of *Bordetella bronchiseptica* from cats in southern Louisiana. Vet Immunol Immunopathol 65:173–176, 1998.
99. Binns SH, Dawson S, Speakman AJ, et al: Prevalence and risk factors for feline *Bordetella bronchiseptica* infection. Vet Rec 144:575–580, 1999.
100. Coutts AJ, Dawson S, Binns S, et al: Studies on natural transmission of *Bordetella bronchiseptica* in cats. Vet Microbiol 48:19–27, 1996.
101. Welsh RD: *Bordetella bronchiseptica* infections in cats. J Am Anim Hosp Assoc 32:153–158, 1996.
102. Stefanelli P, Mastrantonio P, Hausman SZ, et al: Molecular characterization of two *Bordetella bronchiseptica* strains isolated from children with coughs. J Clin Microbiol 35:1550–1555, 1997.
103. Gomez L, Grazziutti M, Sumoza D, et al: Bacterial pneumonia due to *Bordetella bronchiseptica* in a patient with acute leukemia. Clin Infect Dis 26:1002–1003, 1998.
104. Dworkin MS, Sullivan PS, Buskin SE, et al: *Bordetella bronchiseptica* infection in human immunodeficiency virus–infected patients. Clin Infect Dis 28:1095–1099, 1999.
105. Bialasiewicz AA, Jahn GJ: Ocular findings in *Chlamydia psittaci*–induced keratoconjunctivitis in the human. Fortschr Ophthalmol 83:629–631, 1986.
106. Schmeer N, Jahn GJ, Bialasiewicz AA, et al: The cat as a possible source for *Chlamydia psittaci*–induced keratoconjunctivitis in the human. Tierarztl Prax 15:201–204, 1987.
107. Ostler HB, Schacter J, Dawson R: Acute follicular conjunctivitis of epizootic origin. Arch Ophthalmol 82:587–591, 1969.
108. Cotton MM, Partridge MR: Infection with feline *Chlamydia psittaci*. Thorax 53:75–76, 1998.
109. Griffins PD, Lechler RI, Treharne JD: Unusual chlamydial infection in a human renal allograft recipient. BMJ 277:1264–1265, 1978.
110. Regan RJ, Dathan JRE, Treharne JD: Infective endocarditis with glomerulonephritis associated with cat chlamydia *(C. psittaci)* infection. Br Heart J 42:349–352, 1979.
111. Lappin MR: Feline ehrlichiosis. *In* Greene CE (ed): Infectious Diseases of the Dog and Cat, 2nd ed. Philadelphia, WB Saunders, 1998, pp. 149–154.
112. Stubbs CJ, Holland CJ, Reif JS, et al: Feline ehrlichiosis: Literature review and serologic survey. Compend Contin Educ Pract Vet (in press).
113. Bjoersdorff A, Svendenius L, Owens JH, et al: Feline granulocytic ehrlichiosis—A report of a new clinical entity and characterisation of the new infectious agent. J Small Anim Pract 40:20–24, 1999.
114. Higgins JA, Radulovic S, Schriefer ME, et al: *Rickettsia felis*: A new species of pathogenic rickettsia isolated from cat fleas. J Clin Microbiol 34:671–674, 1996.

4

◆ Rickettsial Diseases

Cynthia J. Stubbs

◆ EHRLICHIOSIS

Etiologic Agent

Ehrlichia species, members of the family Rickettsiaceae, are gram-negative, obligate intracellular microorganisms. Charpentier and Groulade[1] documented the first naturally occurring case of ehrlichiosis in a cat in France in 1986. Since that time, feline ehrlichiosis has been documented around the world. Most recently, a granulocytic *Ehrlichia* species causing clinical disease in a cat was isolated and genetically characterized in Sweden.[2]

Morulae, which are intracytoplasmic inclusions formed by clusters of the rickettsia, can be found in mononuclear cells, neutrophils, and eosinophils transiently during acute illness (Fig. 4–1). In one study, electron microscopic assessment of these *Ehrlichia*-like bodies in cats revealed organisms from 0.54 to 1.3 μm, intermediate in size between *Ehrlichia canis* and *Ehrlichia sennetsu*.[3] *Ehrlichia* species morulae found in mononuclear cells include *E. canis, E. chaffeensis, E. sennetsu, E. risticii, E. bovis,* and *E. muris*.[3–5] Other *Ehrlichia* species, such as *E. equi, E. ewingii, E. phagocytophila*, and an unidentified agent that causes human granulocytic ehrlichiosis, have morulae that are found in neutrophils, and occasionally in eosinophils.[4] The granulocytic species isolated in Sweden is identical to the agent that causes human, canine, and equine granulocytic ehrlichiosis.[2] Because *Ehrlichia* species morulae have been detected in feline neutrophils, eosinophils, and mononuclear cells,[1–3, 6–11] it is likely that more than 1 *Ehrlichia* species is involved in feline ehrlichiosis.

Cats can be infected experimentally with *E. risticii*, the causative agent of Potomac horse fever.[12] Experimental infection of specific-pathogen–free cats with *E. equi*, which causes equine ehrlichiosis, also has been performed.[13] *E. canis* is presumed to infect only members of the family Canidae.[4] However, to our knowledge, experimental infections of cats with *E. canis* or other ehrlichial species have not been attempted. It is possible that one of these ehrlichial species, or a previously unidentified ehrlichial species, may be involved in the mononuclear cell infection in cats.

The distribution of feline ehrlichiosis appears to be worldwide. Internationally, antibodies that react with *Ehrlichia* species antigens have been detected in serum of cats from Sweden,[2, 14] Africa,[15] France,[1, 6] and the United States.[11, 12, 16, 17] In separate reports, seropositive cats were detected in Maryland,[12] Colorado,[11] Virginia,[16] and California.[17] In an unpublished U.S. seroprevalence study of 599 cats (Lappin MR, Holland C, Thrall M, et al: Prevalence of *Ehrlichia* spp. antibodies in serum of cats in the United States, unpublished data, 1999), antibodies to *E. canis* and/or *E. risticii* were detected in 29.2 per cent; positive cats were identified throughout the United States. Of these cats, 4.4 per cent were seropositive for *E. canis* alone, 28.5 per cent were seropositive for *E. risticii* alone, and 3 per cent were seropositive for both *Ehrlichia* species (Lappin MR, Holland C, Thrall M, et al: Prevalence of *Ehrlichia* spp. antibodies in serum of cats in the United States, unpublished data, 1999).

Pathogenesis

Because histopathologic results from naturally infected or experimentally infected cats with ehrlichiosis have not been reported, the pathogenesis of the disease is unknown. Based on clinical and laboratory findings, it appears likely to be similar to that of acute *E. canis* infection of dogs.

Transmission

The route of transmission of *Ehrlichia* species to cats currently is unknown. Ticks have been incriminated in the transmission of most *Ehrlichia* species.[4] Naturally infected cats in reports from Kenya were infested with *Haemaphysalalis leachi*,[3, 9] and the

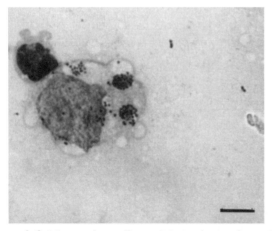

Figure 4–1. Mononuclear cell containing a cluster of organisms consistent with *Ehrlichia* species. Wright-Giemsa stain. (From Bouloy RP, Lappin MR, Holland CH, et al: Clinical ehrlichiosis in a cat. J Am Vet Med Assoc 204:1475–1478, 1994.)

naturally infected cat in Sweden was infested with *Ixodes ricinus*,[2] suggesting that feline ehrlichiosis might be a tick-borne disease.

Some naturally infected cats had flea infestations.[17] However, based on results of one study, it seems unlikely that the *Ehrlichia* species inducing antibody production in cats is transmitted by fleas (Lappin MR, Holland C, Thrall M, et el: Prevalence of *Ehrlichia* spp. antibodies in serum of cats in the United States, unpublished data, 1999). Results from that study showed that the presence of *Ehrlichia* species antibodies was not correlated statistically with the presence of *Bartonella* species antibodies, a genus thought to be transmitted by fleas.[18]

Coxiella burnetii, another rickettsial species, can be transmitted to cats by ingestion of infected rodents.[19] *E. muris* was isolated from mice, and it was proposed that cats could be infected by an *Ehrlichia* species by ingesting infected rodents or by exposure to arthropods that feed on rodents.[5, 20] However, the presence of *Ehrlichia* species antibodies in feline sera was not correlated statistically with the presence of *Toxoplasma gondii* antibodies (Lappin MR, Holland C, Thrall M, et al: Prevalence of *Ehrlichia* spp. antibodies in serum of cats in the United States, unpublished data, 1999). Because *T. gondii* infection in cats usually is acquired by ingestion of infected rodents,[21] it seems unlikely that cats are exposed to *Ehrlichia* species from contact with rodents.

Ehrlichia species infections of dogs can be transmitted by blood transfusions; therefore, this route of transmission also may occur in cats.[4] Because ehrlichial infection of cats appears to be common based on serologic studies, it may be prudent to screen blood donor cats for presence of antibodies.

Clinical Signs

Currently, there are 31 well-documented cases of feline ehrlichiosis reported worldwide.[1-3, 6-11, 17, 22] An epidemiologic study identified several other clinical associations.[23] Clinical signs of feline ehrlichiosis are diverse and similar to those associated with acute canine ehrlichiosis (Table 4–1). The most common clinical sign reported to date is fever. Anorexia, weight loss, and attitude changes consisting of lethargy, depression, general malaise, or irritable disposition also are common. Vomiting or diarrhea are more common in seropositive cats than in seronegative animals. Pain manifested as generalized hyperesthesia, lameness, or arthralgia also is common. Other clinical signs reported less frequently include pale mucous membranes, dehydration, gingivitis, polyuria, polydipsia, and tachypnea.

Laboratory Abnormalities

The most frequent hematologic change reported in cases of feline ehrlichiosis is anemia. When the anemia is characterized, most cases are nonregenerative. *Ehrlichia*-infected cats with regenerative anemia also were infected with *Hemobartonella felis*.[1, 7] Thrombocytopenia has been reported in multiple cats. Neutrophilic leukocytosis, general leukocytosis, lymphocytosis, monocytosis, leukopenia, neutropenia, and lymphopenia all have been associated with feline ehrlichiosis.

Hyperglobulinemia is a common abnormality. The hyperglobulinemia was polyclonal in the 1 cat from which a protein electrophoresis was available.[6] *Ehrlichia*-seropositive cats are 6.6 times more likely than *Ehrlichia*-seronegative cats to have monoclonal gammopathy.[23] Biochemical profile abnormalities reported less frequently include elevated blood urea nitrogen, elevated creatinine, hyperbilirubinemia, hypoalbuminemia, hyperglycemia, hypokalemia, and elevated creatine phosphokinase activity.

Diagnosis

Definitive diagnosis of feline ehrlichiosis is made by demonstration of morulae located in the cytoplasm of blood leukocytes, or identification after amplification by polymerase chain reaction (PCR). However, in most ehrlichial infections of other species, morulae usually are detectable only transiently in the acute phase of illness.[4] Thus, even though many cats are seropositive for *Ehrlichia* species antibodies, only a few cases of clinical feline ehrlichiosis have been diagnosed based on detection of morulae.

Owing to the difficulty in finding morulae, a presumptive diagnosis of ehrlichiosis is based on the combination of appropriate clinical signs, exclusion of other causes of disease, detection of serum *Ehrlichia* species antibodies, and response to antirickettsial drugs.[23] In several different reports[1–3, 6–11, 17, 22, 23] (Lappin MR, Holland C, Thrall M, et al: Prevalence of *Ehrlichia* spp. antibodies in serum of cats in the United States, unpublished data, 1999), immunofluorescent antibody (IFA) tests were adapted for use with cat serum and applied to samples from naturally infected, clinically ill cats, and healthy cats. Seroreactivity with *E. canis* and *E. risticii* morulae has been assessed most frequently. In general, there is minimal cross-reactivity between antibodies against *Ehrlichia* species and other infectious agents such as *Rickettsia rickettsii*. The granulocytic ehrlichial agent isolated in Sweden did not cross-react with *E. canis*.[2] However, antibodies against some *Ehrlichia* species commonly cross-react with other members of the genus.[4] For example, *E. chaffeensis, E. canis*, and *E. ewingii* infections commonly induce cross-reacting antibodies. Results of IFA testing can not be used to confirm the *Ehrlichia* species infecting individual cats.

Because positive serologic results can occur in healthy cats as well as in clinically ill cats, a diagnosis of ehrlichiosis should not be made based on serologic results alone. A 4-fold rise in the acute and convalescent titers also may correlate with recent or

Table 4–1. Clinical Findings for Cats With Suspected Ehrlichiosis and Morulae Morphologically Consistent With *Ehrlichia* Species

Signalment	Clinical Findings	Laboratory Findings	Diagnosis	Treatment/ Response	Reference
10-yr-old, FS, DSH (United States)	Fever, anorexia, hyperesthesia	Nonregenerative anemia, hyperglobulinemia	Morulae in mononuclear cells, *Ehrlichia canis* and *Ehrlichia risticii*–seropositive	Doxycycline/ excellent	12
10-yr-old, M, DSH (Kenya)	Fever, anorexia, dyspnea, splenomegaly, pale mucous membranes	Nonregenerative anemia, hyperglobulinemia, interstitial lung disease	Morulae in mononuclear cells, rarely in neutrophils	Tetracycline/ excellent	9
4-yr-old, M, DSH, (Kenya)	Fever, anorexia, splenomegaly, pale mucous membranes	Nonregenerative anemia	Morulae in mononuclear cells, rarely in neutrophils	Imidocarb/excellent	9
2-yr-old, F, DSH (Kenya)	Fever, anorexia, dyspnea, splenomegaly, lymphadenomegaly, pale mucous membranes	Nonregenerative anemia, neutropenia, interstitial lung disease	Morulae in mononuclear cells, rarely in neutrophils	Imidocarb/excellent	9
Adult lioness (Kenya)	Lethargy, emaciation, lymphadenomegaly	Neutrophilic leukocytosis	Morulae in mononuclear cells	Not treated	10
6-yr-old, MC, DSH (France)	Fever, anorexia, pale mucous membranes, depression	Regenerative anemia, *Haemobartonella felis*, leukocytosis, lymphocytosis, monocytosis, hyperbilirubinemia	Morulae in mononuclear cells	Tetracycline/ euthanasia	2
11-yr-old, FS, DSH (France)	Fever, weight loss, anorexia, depression, joint pain	Nonregenerative anemia, leukopenia, hypoalbuminemia, hyperglobulinemia	Morulae in lymphocytes, *E. canis*–seropositive	Doxycycline/ glucocorticoids/ euthanasia	6
9-yr-old, MC, DSH (France)	Anorexia, gingivitis, pale mucous membranes, polyuria, polydipsia, weight loss	Anemia, FeLV-positive, FIV-positive, hyperglobulinemia	Morulae in lymphocytes, *E. canis*–seropositive	Euthanasia	6
14-yr-old, MC, DSH (France)	Dyspnea, pale mucous membranes, polyuria, polydipsia, weight loss	Pleural effusion, hyperglobulinemia	Morulae in lymphocytes, *E. canis*–seropositive	Euthanasia/ lymphosarcoma	6
5-yr-old, MC, DSH (France)	Fever, lethargy, anorexia, weight loss, pale mucous membranes	Regenerative anemia, *Haemobartonella felis*, thrombocytopenia, monocytosis	Morulae in mononuclear cells	Doxycycline/ glucocorticoids	7
1-yr-old, MC, DSH (Sweden)	Fever, lethargy, anorexia, tachypnea, depression	Neutrophilia, lymphopenia	Morulae in neutrophils, PCR-positive	Doxycycline	11

Abbreviations: DSH, domestic shorthair; F, female; FeLV, feline leukemia virus; FIV, feline immunodeficiency virus; FS, female, spayed; M, male; MC, male, castrated; PCR, polymerase chain reaction.

From Stubbs CJ, Holland CJ, Reif JS, et al: Feline ehrlichiosis: A literature review and serologic survey of 344 cats in the United States. Compend Contin Educ Pract Vet 22:307–318, 2000.

active infection. The cat in Sweden was negative for antibodies against 5 different *Ehrlichia* species, including *E. canis* and *E. risticii*, when tested at presentation, but seroconverted on day 15. At that time, antibodies against the Swedish *Ehrlichia* species, *E. equi*, and *E. phagocytophila* were detected; seropositivity was maintained throughout the follow-up period (8.5 months).[2] To date, no consistent pattern of titer duration has been noted in cats with ehrlichiosis. Similar to dogs,[24] it appears that clearance of serum antibodies to *Ehrlichia* species is prolonged in some cats. One report proposed that this long clearance time was due to incomplete elimination of the organisms after treatment.[17] All 5 cats in that report ultimately became seronegative after doxycycline was administered at 10 mg/kg for 42 days.[17]

As it becomes more readily available, PCR likely will prove valuable in the diagnosis of feline ehrlichiosis and for helping determine the *Ehrlichia* species that infect cats, as in the feline case from Sweden.[2] However, PCR may not be positive in all infected cats. PCR tests using *E. risticii*–specific primers have been applied to blood from 5 *E. risticii*–seropositive cats from California that responded to treatment; each of these cats tested negative by PCR.[17]

Therapy

Clinical improvement has been documented in affected cats after administration of tetracycline, doxycycline, or imidocarb. Tetracycline, administered orally (PO) every (q) 12 hr for 7 days (dose not given), clinically resolved infection in 1 cat.[3] Doxycycline, dosed at 5 mg/kg PO q 12 hr for 21 days, was used successfully to treat 3 cats with ehrlichiosis.[11] This same drug regimen was used in 5 cats that later had to be retreated at a higher dose and for a longer duration (10 mg/kg q 12 hr for 42 days) owing to recurring leukopenia and thrombocytopenia.[17] Doxycycline, dosed at 10 mg/kg intravenously once, followed by 10 mg/kg orally for 20 days, resolved clinical signs of ehrlichiosis in 1 cat.[2] Imidocarb dipropionate given at 5 mg/kg intramuscularly and repeated after 14 days resulted in resolution of clinical disease in 2 cats.[3] Doxycycline (5 mg/kg PO q 12 hr for 4 to 6 weeks) appears to be an appropriate drug regimen for treating feline ehrlichiosis. Three cats with *Ehrlichia* species morulae were euthanatized owing to treatment failures or concurrent disease.[1, 6]

Public Health Aspects

Public health risks associated with the *Ehrlichia* species infecting cats are poorly defined. The cat in the Swedish report was infected with an *Ehrlichia* species that was identical to the agent that causes human granulocytic ehrlichiosis.[2] Whether cats may

serve as a reservoir for this ehrlichial agent, as well as develop clinical illness, needs to be determined. *E. chaffeensis*, the etiologic agent of human monocytic ehrlichiosis, can be harbored by dogs and cross-reacts serologically with *E. canis*.[25, 26] Cats are not known to be infected by *E. canis* but commonly have *E. canis* antibodies; thus, it is possible that cats also might be infected by *E. chaffeensis*.

◆ COXIELLA BURNETII

Etiologic Agent

C. burnetii, the cause of Q fever, was first linked to an acute febrile illness in employees of a meat-packing plant in Australia in 1935.[27] The organism has an affinity for the urogenital tract of many animals, in particular, cattle, sheep, goats, and cats.[28] The agent is rod-shaped, 0.25 μm in width, and ranges from 0.5 to 1.25 μm in length. *C. burnetii* is maintained in nature in ticks and reservoir hosts. Over 40 ticks can host the organism. In the vertebrate host, the organism lives intracellularly and is found within vacuoles of infected cells. A small-cell variant and a large-cell, spore-forming variant exist in nature. Once sporulated, the organism can withstand extreme environmental conditions including heat and drying, and remains viable in soil for many years.[29] The organism also is resistant to most disinfectants. *C. burnetii* has worldwide distribution; the northeastern region of North America appears to be an endemic area.[28] Seroprevalence studies performed in dogs and cats suggest that exposure may be common. In one group of shelter cats in Southern California, the seroprevalence was 20 per cent.[30]

Pathogenesis

Carrier animals shed *C. burnetii* in urine, milk, placental tissues, amniotic fluid, and feces.[29] During parturition, large numbers of *C. burnetii* organisms are shed in amniotic fluid and the placenta, potentiating zoonotic spread. Mammals are infected directly by inhalation or ingestion of infected particles. The organism also can be transmitted indirectly by tick bites. Once *C. burnetii* enters the body, replication occurs locally at the site of infection followed by systemic bacteremia. The organism has a predilection for replication in the vascular endothelium and the epithelium of the respiratory tract, renal tubules, and serosa.[29] *C. burnetii* enters cells passively and multiplies within the vacuoles in the cytoplasm, causing destruction of the cell.

Clinical Findings

Transient low-grade fever, lethargy, and anorexia last for about 3 days in cats inoculated experimentally with *C. burnetii*. The organism also has been implicated as a cause of feline abortion and neonatal mortality.[19] Although the true incidence of clinical illness from *C. burnetii* infection in naturally exposed cats is unknown, it is thought to be insignificant.

Diagnosis

Definitive diagnosis of coxiellosis in cats and human beings can be made by documentation of increasing antibody titers in serum samples taken 4 weeks apart. The organism also can be demonstrated by laboratory animal inoculation, fluorescent antibody staining of tissue samples, and PCR. Because healthy cats may have a positive titer to *C. burnetii*, a 4-fold rise in immunoglobulin G (IgG) titer is needed to confirm active infection.[30]

Pathologic Findings

Granulomatous hepatitis, myocarditis, nephritis, and diffuse granulomatous pneumonia are histologic findings in *C. burnetii*–infected kittens.

Therapy

Because clinical disease due to *C. burnetii* usually is not recognized, treatment is rarely indicated. Based on results in human beings, antirickettsial drugs including tetracycline, doxycycline, and chloramphenicol likely would be effective choices.

Public Health Aspects

Clinical signs of *C. burnetii* infection in human beings (Q fever) can be significant; infection has been associated with parturient cats.[28, 31, 32] Based on limited seroprevalence studies, infected cats may represent an important reservoir of *C. burnetii* in urban areas.[33] Clinical signs in human beings occur 2 to 6 weeks after exposure. Acute clinical syndromes may be mild and self-limiting and include fever, malaise, headache, interstitial pneumonitis, myalgia, and arthralgia.[29] Many people recover spontaneously from acute infection, but a small number of patients do not clear the organism. Chronic manifestations of Q fever include hepatitis and valvular endocarditis, which can develop years after primary infection.[19] Q fever always should be considered as a possible cause of culture-negative endocarditis in human patients; serologic testing is required to document infection.[29]

Methods to prevent infection should be taken by persons attending parturient or aborting cats, including veterinarians, breeders, researchers, and animal-shelter workers. Gloves and masks should be worn while working with these animals. If clinical signs consistent with acute Q fever develop within 2 to 6 weeks of working with a parturient or aborting cat, medical attention should be sought. Limited studies suggest investigational vaccines are effective, and may be indicated for workers with a high occupational risk of exposure once the products are approved for general use.[29]

◆ *RICKETTSIA FELIS*

Etiologic Agent and Pathogenesis

Murine typhus is a mild febrile illness in human beings caused by *Rickettsia typhi*, maintained in rats and opossums, and transmitted by the rat flea, *Xenopsylla cheopis*.[34] *Rickettsia felis* (previously called the ELB agent) is a closely related organism isolated originally from the cat flea, *Ctenocephalides felis*. This organism also has been isolated from human beings with murine typhus, opossums, and cats.[34–36] Murine typhus reached a peak in the United States during the 1930s and 1940s.[36] However, several endemic areas of disease still exist, including suburban regions of southern California and south-central Texas.

R. felis is an obligate intracellular bacterium, found in the cytoplasm of infected eukaryotic cells. In one study, *R. felis* antibodies were detected in 8 per cent of febrile cats in the northeastern United States.[35] It was estimated recently that up to 285,000 cats could be infected nationwide.[34] Little is known of the pathogenesis of this disease in cats, but the organism can be recovered from blood, urine, and other tissues of cats 14 days postinfection.[37]

Clinical Findings

Cats inoculated intradermally with *R. felis* exhibited no clinical signs and harbored the organism for only a few weeks, as demonstrated by PCR.[38] Although *R. felis* antibodies have been detected in febrile cats, it is unknown whether infection results in disease.

Diagnosis

Serologic testing using complement fixation (CF) and IFA tests have been utilized in cats that are in close association with human cases of murine typhus. A CF titer of 1:8 or higher and/or an IFA titer of 1:32 or higher was considered evidence of infection.[37] The use of PCR technology has aided in the identification of the organism.[35] However, these tests are not available routinely for veterinary use.

Therapy

At this time, murine typhus is not recognized as a cause of clinical illness in cats. In pets associated with human cases of disease, treatment with accepted antirickettsial drugs, such as tetracycline, doxycycline, and chloramphenicol, could be considered.

Prevention

Cats should be housed indoors, and flea control should be maintained.

◆ HEMOBARTONELLOSIS

H. felis, previously recognized as a rickettsial agent, has been reclassified in the mycoplasma family. Please refer to Chapters 2, Hemobartonellosis, and 60, Use of the Polymerase Chain Reaction to Detect Hemoparasites, for more information on this infectious disease.

REFERENCES

1. Charpentier F, Groulade P: Probable case of ehrlichiosis in a cat. Bull Acad Vet France 59:287–290, 1986.
2. Bjoersdorff A, Svendenius L, Owens J, et al: Feline granulocytic ehrlichiosis—A report of a new clinical entity and characterisation of the infectious agent. J Small Anim Pract 40:20–24, 1999.
3. Buoro IBJ, Atwell RB, Kipoon JC, et al: Feline anaemia associated with *Ehrlichia*-like bodies in three domestic short-haired cats. Vet Rec 125:434–436, 1989.
4. Neer TM: Canine monocytic and granulocytic ehrlichiosis. In Greene CE (ed): Infectious Diseases of the Dog and Cat, 2nd ed. Philadelphia, WB Saunders, 1998, pp. 139–154.
5. Wen B, Rikihisa Y, Mott J, et al: *Ehrlichia muris* sp. nov., identified on the basis of 16s rRNA base sequences and serological, morphological, and biological characteristics. Int J Syst Bacteriol 45:250–254, 1995.
6. Beaufils JP, Marin-Granel J, Jumelle P: *Ehrlichia* infection in cats: A review of three cases. Prat Med Chir Anim Cie 30:397–402, 1995.
7. Beaufils JP, Marin-Granel J, Jumelle P: Ehrlichiosise feline: A propos de deux cas. Bull Acad Vet France 70:73–80, 1997.
8. Beaufils JP: Ehlichiosis: Clinical aspects in dogs and cats. Compend Contin Educ Pract Vet 19S:57–61, 1997.
9. Buoro IBJ, Nyamwange SB, Kiptoon JC: Presence of *Ehrlichia*-like bodies in monocytes of an adult lioness. Fel Pract 22:36–37, 1994.
10. Jittapalapong S, Jansawan W: Preliminary survey on blood parasites of cats in Bangkhen District Area. Kasetsart J Nat Sci 27:330–335, 1993.
11. Bouloy RP, Lappin MR, Holland CJ, et al: Clinical ehrlichiosis in a cat. J Am Vet Med Assoc 204:1475–1478, 1994.
12. Dawson JE, Abeygunawardena I, Holland CJ, et al: Susceptibility of cats to infection with *Ehrlichia risticii*, causative agent of equine monocytic ehrlichiosis. Am J Vet Res 49:2096–2100, 1988.
13. Lewis GE, Huxsoll DL, Ristic M, et al: Experimentally induced infection of dogs, cats, and nonhuman primates with *Ehrlichia equi*, etiologic agent of equine ehrlichiosis. J Am Vet Med Assoc 36:85–88, 1975.
14. Artursson K, Malmqvist M, Olsson E, et al: Diagnosis of borreliosis and granulocytic ehrlichiosis of horses, dogs, and cats in Sweden. Sven Vet 45:331–336, 1994.
15. Matthewman LA, Kelley PJ, Wray K, et al: Antibodies in cat sera from southern Africa react with antigens of *Ehrlichia canis*. Vet Rec 138:364–365, 1996.
16. Perry BD, Schmidtmann ET, Rice RM, et al: Epidemiology of Potomac horse fever: An investigation into the possible role of non-equine mammals. Vet Rec 125:83–86, 1989.
17. Peavy GM, Holland CJ, Dulta SK, et al: Suspected ehrlichial infection in five cats from a household. J Am Vet Med Assoc 210:231–234, 1997.
18. Chomel BB, Kasten RW, Floyd-Hawkins K, et al: Experimental transmission of *Bartonella henselae* by the cat flea. J Clin Microbiol 34:1952–1956, 1996.
19. Greene CE, Breitschwerdt EB: Rocky Mountain spotted fever, Q fever, and typhus. In Greene CE (ed): Infectious Diseases of the Dog and Cat, 2nd ed. Philadelphia, WB Saunders, 1998, pp. 155–165.
20. Kawahara M, Suto C, Rikihisa Y, et al: Characterization of ehrlichial organisms isolated from a wild mouse. J Clin Microbiol 31:89–96, 1993.
21. Dubey JP, Lappin MR: Toxoplasmosis and neosporosis. In Greene CE (ed): Infectious Diseases of the Dog and Cat, 2nd ed. Philadelphia, WB Saunders, 1998, pp. 493–503.
22. Stubbs CJ, Lappin MR, Holland CJ, et al: Feline ehrlichiosis. J Vet Intern Med 12:230, 1998.
23. Stubbs CJ, Holland CJ, Reif JS, et al: Feline ehrlichiosis: A literature review and serologic survey of 344 cats in the United States. Compend Contin Educ Pract Vet 22:307–318, 2000.
24. Bartsch RC, Greene RT: Post therapy antibody titers in dogs with ehrlichiosis: Follow-up studies on 68 patients treated primarily with tetracycline and/or doxycycline. J Vet Intern Med 10:271–274, 1996.
25. Dawson JE, Biggie KL, Warner CK, et al: Polymerase chain reaction evidence of *Ehrlichia chaffeensis*, an etiologic agent of human ehrlichiosis, in dogs from southeast Virginia. Am J Vet Res 57:1175–1179, 1996.
26. Anderson BE, Dawson JE, Jones DC, et al: *Ehrlichia chaffeensis*, a new species associated with human ehrlichiosis. J Clin Microbiol 29:2838–2842, 1991.
27. Derrick EH: "Q" fever, a new fever entity: Clinical features, diagnosis, and laboratory investigation. Med J Aust 2:281–299, 1937.
28. Pinsky RL, Fishbein DB, Greene CR, et al: An outbreak of cat-associated Q-fever in the United States. J Infect Dis 164:202–204, 1991.
29. Reimer LG: Q-fever. Clin Microbiol Rev 6:193–198, 1993.
30. Randhawa AS, Dieterich WH, Jolley WB, et al: Coxiellosis in pound cats. Fel Pract 4:37–38, 1974.
31. Langley JM, Marrie TJ, Covert DM, et al: Poker players' pneumonia. An urban outbreak of Q fever following exposure to a parturient cat. N Engl J Med 319:354–356, 1988.
32. Marrie TJ, MacDonald A, Durant H, et al: An outbreak of Q fever probably due to contact with a parturient cat. Chest 93:98–103, 1988.
33. Morita C, Katsuyama J, Yanase T, et al: Seroepidemiological survey of *Coxiella burnetii* in domestic cats in Japan. Microbiol Immunol 38:1001–1003, 1994.
34. Azad AF, Radulovic S, Higgins JA, et al: Flea-borne rickettsioses: Ecologic considerations. Emerg Infect Dis 3:319–327, 1997.
35. Higgins JA, Radulovic S, Schriefer MA, et al: *Rickettsia felis*: A new species of pathogenic rickettsia isolated from cat fleas. J Clin Microbiol 34:671–674, 1996.
36. Schriefer ME, Sacci JB, Dumler S, et al: Identification of a novel rickettsial infection in a patient diagnosed with murine typhus. J Clin Microbiol 32:949–954, 1994.
37. Sorvillo FJ, Gondo B, Emmons R, et al: A surburban focus of endemic typhus in Los Angeles county: Association with seropositive domestic cats and opossums. Am J Trop Med Hyg 48:269–273, 1993.
38. Chomel BB: Rickettsial infection in dogs, cats, and humans: An overview. Compend Contin Educ Pract Vet 19:37–41, 1997.

5

◆ Cryptosporidiosis

Christopher A. McReynolds

◆ ETIOLOGY

Cryptosporidium is a coccidian in the phylum Apicomplexa, family Cryptosporidiidae, suborder Eimeria. *Cryptosporidium* species were first described in mice by Tyzzer in 1907.[1] *Cryptosporidium* species were thought to be commensal organisms until *Cryptosporidium parvum* was reported as a cause of bovine neonatal diarrhea in 1971.[2] Subsequently, an abomasum-infecting species presumed to be *Cryptosporidium muris* was reported in adult cows.[2] Natural infections caused by both species are now recognized as a significant cause of gastrointestinal tract disease in a number of mammalian species including rodents, ruminants, and human beings.[3]

In early reports, new *Cryptosporidium* species were named after the host of origin of the oocysts. Subsequent cross-transmission experiments showed lack of host specificity, which invalidated many of the species.[2, 3] Until recently, *C. parvum* and *C. muris* were accepted as the only distinct species in mammals. Based on morphologic characteristics of oocysts, *C. parvum* was thought to be the species transmitted in most instances. Classification of *Cryptosporidium* species is now based on genetic analysis. Species in genotype 1 are those detected only in human beings, whereas species in genotype 2 infect human beings and other mammals and are considered zoonotic.[4] Sequence analysis of polymerase chain reaction (PCR) products from feline *Cryptosporidium* isolates were compared with human and bovine isolates and shown to be different, suggesting that a cat-adapted species exists.[5] Oocysts of the feline isolates are 4.6 μm by 4.0 μm, and so vary morphologically from *C. parvum* as well.[5] One feline *Cryptosporidium* isolate that was not characterized genetically failed to establish infections in mice, rats, guinea pigs, and dogs.[6] Another *Cryptosporidium* species isolated from a cat infected lambs.[7] In a more recent study, the feline genotype was isolated from an infected cow[8] and an infected human being.[9] Cats have been infected experimentally with human and bovine *Cryptosporidium* isolates.[10, 11] Results of these studies suggest that cats harbor a cat-adapted species, *Cryptosporidium felis*, and can be carriers of other *Cryptosporidium* species. Currently, 4 *Cryptosporidium* species are recognized that infect mammals: *C. muris*, *C. parvum*, *C. wrairi*, (guinea pigs only), and *C. felis*.[3]

◆ LIFE CYCLE

Cryptosporidium species are transmitted by the fecal-oral route. The enteric life cycle of *Cryptosporidium* species differs from that of other coccidian parasites in that both thin- and thick-walled oocysts are produced. Thin-walled oocysts rupture in the gastrointestinal tract, resulting in autogenous reinfection. The environmentally resistant, thick-walled oocyst is shed sporulated in the feces, and so is infectious immediately to other hosts.[2] When a mammalian host ingests thick-walled oocysts, 4 sporozoites are released by the action of bile acids and pancreatic enzymes. The liberated sporozoites enter the microvillous border of enterocytes, and become enclosed as trophozoites in parasitiferous vacuoles. The intracellular, extracytoplasmic form matures and undergoes asexual reproduction (schizogony), resulting in production of type I meronts (containing 6 or 8 first-generation merozoites). First-generation merozoites are released into the gastrointestinal lumen and infect other enterocytes, which in turn form more type I or type II meronts (containing 4 second-generation merozoites). Type II meronts undergo gametogony and subsequently sporogony, culminating in the formation of oocysts containing 4 sporozoites.

◆ PATHOGENESIS

In human beings, gastrointestinal, biliary, and respiratory tract infections with *C. parvum* have been documented.[12] In cats, infections have been confined to small intestine and colon.[13-15] Parasitism of enterocytes causes villous atrophy and blunting, crypt hyperplasia, and inflammatory cell infiltration into the lamina propria. Diarrhea results from disruption of the intestinal mucosal architecture, leading to an osmotic diarrhea secondary to malabsorption. Because of the secretory nature of the diarrhea, it is suspected that a cholera-like enterotoxin is produced.[16]

Enteric cryptosporidiosis generally has been believed to be a self-limiting disease in immunocompetent mammals. The severity and duration of clinical disease are dependent both on the immune status of the host and the magnitude of infection. Both humoral and cell-mediated immune responses are necessary to eliminate the protozoan from the mucosal surfaces in immunocompetent mammals.[17] Alteration of secretory immune responses is thought to partially explain the chronic mucosal infections that occur in human beings with AIDS. This hypothesis is supported by studies that show that ruminants develop secretory immunoglobulin A (IgA) responses as the parasite is cleared.[18, 19] Additionally, hyperimmune bovine colostrum has proved partially effective in the treatment of chronic cryptosporidiosis in human beings with AIDS.[20] However, secretory IgA responses alone are ineffective for clearing the parasite in human beings with AIDS.[17, 21] When CD4+ T-lymphocyte counts decrease to less than 140 cells/μl, human immunodeficiency virus (HIV)–positive patients are unable to clear *C. parvum* infection, documenting the importance of cell-mediated immune responses.[22] Cats develop serum and local *C. parvum* IgM, IgG, and IgA after experimental infection.[23] In both experimental and natural infections, chronic carriage of *Cryptosporidium* species has been documented in cats with no apparent underlying cause of immunosuppression.[6, 24]

◆ CLINICAL DISEASE IN CATS

Cryptosporidium species infection was first reported in the domestic cat in 1979.[25] *C. muris* has been documented to infect cats, but the majority of cases of feline cryptosporidiosis are believed due to *C. parvum* or *C. felis*.[3] A number of studies have shown that cats are commonly infected by *Cryptosporidium* species. Epidemiologic studies in Japan and Scotland detected *C. parvum* oocysts in 4 and 8 per cent of random fecal samples, respectively.[26, 27] The majority of cats were asymptomatic.[26–28] In north-central Colorado, *Cryptosporidium* species oocysts or antigens were detected in 5.4 per cent of the cats with diarrhea.[29] Seroprevalence studies from Scotland, Czech Republic, and the United States have shown between 8 and 87 per cent of cats to have antibodies to *Cryptosporidium* species.[28, 30–32] Clinical disease has been attributed to *Cryptosporidium* species infection in a number of cats (Table 5–1). Most clinically affected cats have had chronic small-bowel or mixed-bowel diarrhea. Clinical disease has been detected in both immunosuppressed[14, 15, 33] and immunocompetent cats.[13, 23, 34] In 1 cat, lymphocytic-plasmacytic duodenitis and small intestinal bacterial overgrowth were detected concurrently with *C. parvum* infection.[24] The inflammatory changes resolved when the cat was treated with clindamycin and tylosin, drugs with potential anticryptosporidial activity.

◆ DIAGNOSIS

Diagnosis of *Cryptosporidium* species infection is based primarily on finding oocysts in fecal specimens. The oocysts of *C. parvum* and *C. felis* are approximately 5 μm in diameter, which contributes to the difficulty in diagnosing the infection.[3] Ruminants acutely infected with *C. parvum* will shed between 10^5 and 10^7 oocysts per gram of feces.[19] Results from 2 studies suggest that cats shed be-

Table 5–1. Clinical Reports of Cryptosporidiosis in Cats

Signalment	Clinical Findings	Laboratory Abnormalities	Diagnosis	Treatment and Response	Reference
6-mo-old, kitten	Weight loss, inappetance, chronic diarrhea	Anemia	Fecal smears stained with safranin/methylene blue	No treatment; euthanized	13
6-mo-old, kitten	Thin and chronic diarrhea	Unremarkable	Intestinal biopsy	None/clinical signs resolved 6 wk after initial presentation	13
5-yr-old, MC, DSH	2-wk history of mixed-bowel diarrhea, febrile	FeLV-positive, hypoproteinemia	Necropsy	Amoxicillin and sulfadimethoxine; euthanized 1 wk after initial presentation	14
4-yr-old, FS, DSH	1-yr history of large-bowel diarrhea	FeLV-positive, pleocellular inflammation in the colon	Necropsy	Diarrhea resolved with prednisone; euthanized 16 mo after initial presentation	15
18-mo-old, MC, DSH	2-mo history of mixed-bowel diarrhea	Lymphocytic duodenitis, duodenal bacterial overgrowth	Fecal smear stained with acid-fast stain	Clindamycin gave partial response; clinically resolved with tylosin	24
6-mo-old, DSH	2-mo history of small-bowel diarrhea	Unremarkable	Sucrose flotation	Paromomycin/80% resolution	34
13-yr-old, MC, DSH	4-mo history of small-bowel diarrhea	Intestinal lymphoma diagnosed at necropsy	Fecal smear stained with acid-fast stain	Partial improvement with diet change; euthanized 3 mo after initial presentation	22
16-yr-old, MC, DSH	Weight loss and diarrhea	Intestinal lymphoma	Necropsy	Chemotherapy resolved diarrhea; euthanized 6 wk after initial presentation	33

Abbreviations: DSH, domestic shorthair; FeLV, feline leukemia virus; FS, female, spayed; MC, male, castrated.

tween 10^3 and 10^4 oocysts per gram of feces.[6, 23] This relatively small number of oocysts makes diagnosis of feline cryptosporidiosis difficult with current coprodiagnostic methods. A multitude of fecal flotation or sedimentation techniques and staining procedures have been assessed for diagnostic utility. Acid-fast staining (Acid-fast staining kit, TB Stain Kit K, Becton Dickinson Microbiology Systems, Sparks, MD) of a thin fecal smear (Fig. 5–1) is more sensitive than fecal flotation techniques alone, but 5×10^5 oocysts per gram of formed stool were needed for 100 per cent detection.[35] The use of a fluorescein-labeled monoclonal antibody (IFA) to visualize the oocysts better has emerged as the predominant means for detection of human cryptosporidiosis.[3] Weber and colleagues[35] showed that thresholds of detection of *C. parvum* oocysts in human samples with formalin-ether sedimentation followed by IFA is around 10^4 oocysts per gram of watery stool and 5×10^4 oocysts per gram for formed stool. When staining and concentration techniques were evaluated for use with feline feces, the IFA test was the most sensitive.[36] An IFA kit for detection of *C. parvum* oocysts in feces is available commercially (Merifluor Giardia/*Cryptosporidium*, Meridian Diagnostics, Inc., Cincinnati, OH). Whether these kits detect *C. felis* is currently unknown. Based on sensitivity limits, even the direct IFA test may fail to detect some cases of feline cryptosporidiosis.

Enzyme-linked immunosorbent assay (ELISA) tests are commercially available for detection of *C. parvum*–specific antigen in feces. (ProSpect T, *Cryptosporidium* Microplate Assay, Alexon Trend, Ramsey, MN; Premier *Cryptosporidium*, Meridian, Diagnostics, Inc., Cincinnati, OH; Colour Vue *Cryptosporidium*, Seradyn, Indianapolis, IN). Whether these assays are more sensitive than other techniques when used with cat feces, or whether they detect *C. felis*, is currently unknown. Results of fecal antigen testing do not always correlate to those of oocyst shedding.[29] PCR can be adapted to detect *C. parvum* DNA in human feces, and has a sensitivity limit equivalent to 5×10^2 oocysts per gram of feces.[37] Although ELISA tests for detection of *C. parvum*–specific IgG, IgA, and IgM in feline sera have been developed, positive results document only previous exposure but not necessarily current infection.[23, 30] Cryptosporidiosis in human beings was diagnosed initially by histopathologic documentation of the organism in intestinal biopsy sections. However, this procedure is invasive, and commonly gives false-negative results. The organism was not detected in endoscopically obtained duodenal biopsies in 1 cat.[24]

◆ TREATMENT

A multitude of drugs have been evaluated for the treatment of human and bovine cryptosporidiosis. Unfortunately, very few have shown any consistent clinical efficacy. The broad-spectrum aminoglycoside antibiotic paromomycin has shown the most promising results in AIDS patients with chronic cryptosporidiosis. Paromomycin was reported to clear chronic cryptosporidiosis successfully in 1 cat when administered at 165 mg/kg orally (PO) every (q) 12 hr for 5 days.[34] A recent study implicated paromomycin as a cause of acute renal failure and deafness in cats with hemorrhagic diarrhea, and so it should be used cautiously or only in refractory cases.[38] Tylosin (Tylan, Elanco Products Co., Indianapolis, IN) administered at 11 mg/kg PO q 12 hr for 21 days has resulted in resolution of clinical signs and oocyst shedding in several cats (MR Lappin, unpublished observations).[24] Azithromycin (Zithromax, Pfizer Animal Health, Exton, PA) has been shown to have clinical efficacy in mice infected with *C. parvum*, and may prove to be effective in cats as well.[39] The feline dose is 5 to 10 mg/kg, PO q 12 hr for 7 days. At this time, it is unknown

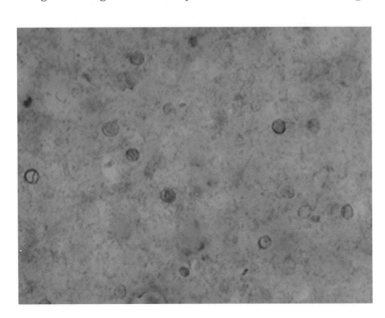

Figure 5–1. *Cryptosporidium parvum* oocysts (4×6 μm) stained by acid-fast stain.

whether treated cats eliminate the infection or are chronically infected.[6, 23]

◆ ZOONOTIC ASPECTS

Clinical cryptosporidiosis is generally self-limiting in immunocompetent individuals, but fatal infection is common in people with AIDS. It is estimated that cryptosporidiosis will develop in 10 to 15 per cent of AIDS patients in the United States.[3] Person-to-person contact with oocysts by fecal-oral contamination or ingesting contaminated water are the most likely routes of exposure.[2, 12] *Cryptosporidium* species infection of people after exposure to infected calves has been recognized for years.[40] Infected human beings and cats have been detected in the same environment,[41, 42] and a research associate developed cryptosporidiosis after exposure to a group of cats experimentally infected with *C. parvum*.[23] In one study, cats were not a risk factor associated with cryptosporidiosis in HIV-infected people, and so the risk of transmission from cats to people likely is very low.[43]

Even though the risk of acquiring cryptosporidiosis from an infected cat is low, care should be taken, particularly in homes with immunosuppressed family members. All cats with diarrhea should be screened for cryptosporidiosis. Because many cats can be subclinical carriers of the organism, new cats entering a home with an immunosuppressed family member should be screened even if healthy. Cryptosporidiosis was most common in cats less than 6 months of age in one study; therefore, an adult cat may be the safest animal to introduce into a home with an immunosuppressed family member.[27] Based on current sensitivity information, direct IFA testing is the most sensitive screening procedure for use with cat feces.

◆ PREVENTION

Cryptosporidium species oocysts are very environmentally resistant and also very infectious. A group of healthy people developed cryptosporidiosis after ingesting only 30 oocysts.[44] Routine disinfectants require extremely long contact with the organism to be effective. Drying, freeze-thawing, boiling, and steam-cleaning can inactivate *Cryptosporidium* species oocysts. Good hygiene should be practiced, scalding water should be used to clean potentially contaminated areas, hands and produce should be washed well when gardening, and water from the environment should be boiled or filtered before ingestion.

REFERENCES

1. Tyzzer E: A sporozoan found in the peptic glands of the common mouse. Proc Soc Exp Biol Med 5:12, 1907.
2. Moore J, Blagburn B, Lindsay D: Cryptosporidiosis in animals including humans. Compend Contin Educ Pract Vet 10:275, 1988.
3. Fayer R, Speer CA, Dubey JP: The general biology of *Cryptosporidium*. *In* Fayer R (ed): *Cryptosporidium* and Cryptosporidiosis. Boca Raton, FL, CRC, 1997, pp. 1–33.
4. Bonnin A, Fourmaux MN, Dubremetz JF, et al: Genotyping human and bovine isolates of *Cryptosporidium parvum* by polymerase chain reaction–restriction fragment length polymorphism analysis of a repetitive DNA sequence. FEMS Microbiol Letters 137:207–211, 1996.
5. Sargent KD, Morgan U, Elliot A, et al: Morphological and genetic characterisation of *Cryptosporidium* oocysts from domestic cats. Vet Parasitol 77:221, 1998.
6. Asahi H, Koyama T, Arai H, et al: Biological nature of *Cryptosporidium* spp. isolated from a cat. Parasitol Res 77:237, 1991.
7. Mtambo MMA, Wright SE, Nash AS, et al: Infectivity of a *Cryptosporidium* species isolated from a domestic cat *(Felis domestica)* in lambs and mice. Res Vet Sci 60:61–63, 1996.
8. Bornay-Llinares FJ, da Silva AJ, Moura INS, et al: Identification of *Cryptosporidium felis* in a cow by morphologic and molecular methods. Appl Environ Microbiol 65:1455–1458, 1999.
9. Pieniazek NJ, Bornay-Llinares FJ, Slemenda SB, et al: New *Cryptosporidium* genotypes in HIV-infected persons. Emerg Infect Dis 5:444–449, 1999.
10. Current WL, Reese J, Ernst JV, et al: Human cryptosporidiosis in immunocompetent and immunodeficient persons: Studies of an outbreak and experimental transmission. N Engl J Med 308:1252, 1983.
11. Pavlasek I: Experimental infection of cat and chicken with *Cryptosporidium* sp. oocysts isolated from a calf. Folia Parasitol (Praha) 30:121, 1983.
12. Ritchie DJ, Becker ES: Update on the management of intestinal cryptosporidiosis in AIDS. Ann Pharmacother 28:767, 1994.
13. Bennett M, Baxby D, Blundell N, et al: Cryptosporidiosis in the domestic cat. Vet Rec 116:73, 1985.
14. Goodwin MA, Barsanti JA: Intractable diarrhea associated with intestinal cryptosporidiosis in a domestic cat also infected with feline leukemia virus. J Am Anim Hosp Assoc 26:365, 1990.
15. Monticello TM, Levy MG, Bunch SE, et al: Cryptosporidiosis in a feline leukemia virus–positive cat. J Am Vet Med Assoc 191:705, 1987.
16. Guarino A, Canani RB, Casola A, et al: Human intestinal cryptosporidiosis: Secretory diarrhea and enterotoxic activity in Caco-2 cell. J Infect Dis 171:976, 1995.
17. Cozon G, Biron F, Jeannin M, et al: Secretory IgA antibodies to *Cryptosporidium parvum* in AIDS patients with chronic cryptosporidiosis. J Infect Dis 169:696, 1994.
18. Hill BD, Blewett AM, Dawson S, et al: Analysis of the kinetics, isotype, and specificity of serum and coproantibody in lambs infected with *Cryptosporidium parvum*. Res Vet Sci 48:76, 1990.
19. Peeters JE, Villacorta I, Vanopdenbosch E, et al: *Cryptosporidium parvum* in calves: Kinetics and immunoblot analysis of specific serum and local antibody responses (immunoglobulin A [IgA], IgG, and IgM) after natural and experimental infection. Infect Immun 60:2309, 1992.
20. Plettenberg D, Stoehr A, Stellbrink HJ, et al: A preparation from bovine colostrum in the treatment of HIV positive patients with chronic diarrhea. Clin Invest 71:42, 1993.
21. Benhamou Y, Kapel N, Hoang C, et al: Inefficacy of intestinal secretory immune response to cryptosporidium in acquired immunodeficiency syndrome. Gastroenterology 108:627, 1995.
22. Flanigan T, Whalen C, Turner J, et al: *Cryptosporidium* infection and CD4 counts. Ann Intern Med 116:840, 1992.
23. McReynolds C, Lappin MR, Spilker MM, et al: *Cryptosporidium parvum* oocyst shedding and serum antibody response in experimentally infected cats. J Vet Intern Med 13:256, 1999.
24. Lappin MR, Dowers K, Edsell D, et al: Cryptosporidiosis and inflammatory bowel disease in a cat. Fel Pract 25:10, 1997.

25. Iseki M: *Cryptosporidium felis* sp. n. (Protozoa: Eimeriorina) from the domestic cat. Jpn J Parasitol 28:285, 1979.

26. Uga S, Matsumura T, Ishibashi K, et al: Cryptosporidiosis in dogs and cats in Hyogo Prefecture, Japan. Jpn J Parasitol 38:139, 1989.

27. Mtambo MMA, Nash AS, Blewett DA, et al: *Cryptosporidium* infection in cats: Prevalence of infection in domestic and feral cats in the Glasgow area. Vet Rec 129:502, 1991.

28. Svobodova V, Konvalinova J, Svobodova M: Coprological and serological findings in dogs and cats with giardiasis and cryptosporidiosis. Acta Vet Brno 63:257, 1994.

29. Hill S, Cheney J, Taton-Allen G, et al: Prevalence of enteric zoonoses in cats. J Am Vet Med Assoc 216:687–692, 2000.

30. Mtambo MMA, Nash AS, Wright SE, et al: Prevalence of specific anti-*Cryptosporidium* IgG, IgM, and IgA in cat sera using an indirect immunofluorescence antibody test. Vet Rec 60:37, 1995.

31. Tzipori S, Campbell I: Prevalence of *Cryptosporidium* antibodies in 10 animal species. J Clin Microbiol 14:455, 1981.

32. McReynolds CA, Lappin M, Ungar B, et al: Regional seroprevalence of *Cryptosporidium parvum*–specific IgG of cats in the United States. Vet Parasitol 80:187, 1998.

33. Lent S, Burkhardt J, Bolka D: Coincident enteric cryptosporidiosis and lymphosarcoma in a cat with diarrhea. J Am Anim Hosp Assoc 29:492, 1993.

34. Barr SC, Jamrosz GF, Hornbuckle WE, et al: Use of paromomycin for treatment of cryptosporidiosis in a cat. J Am Vet Med Assoc 205:1743, 1994.

35. Weber R, Bryan RT, Bishop HS, et al: Threshold of detection of *Cryptosporidium* oocysts in human stool specimens: Evidence for low sensitivity of current diagnostic methods. J Clin Microbiol 29:1323, 1991.

36. Mtambo MM, Nash AS, Blewett DA, et al: Comparison of staining and concentration techniques for detection of *Cryptosporidium* oocysts in cat faecal specimens. Vet Parasitol 45:49–57, 1992.

37. Balatbat AB, Jordan GW, Tang YJ, et al: Detection of *Cryptosporidium parvum* DNA in human feces by nested PCR. J Clin Microbiol 34:1769, 1996.

38. Gookin J, Riviere J, Gilger B, et al: Acute renal failure in four cats treated with paromomycin. J Am Vet Med Assoc 215:1821, 1999.

39. Rehg JE: A comparison of anticryptosporidial activity of paromomycin with that of other aminoglycosides and azithromycin in immunosuppressed mice. J Infect Dis 170:934, 1994.

40. Levine JF, Levy MG, Walker RL, et al: Cryptosporidiosis in veterinary students. J Am Vet Med Assoc 193:1413, 1988.

41. Koch KL, Shankey TV, Weinstein GS, et al: Cryptosporidiosis in a patient with hemophilia, common variable hypogammaglobulinemia, and the acquired immunodeficiency syndrome. Ann Intern Med 99:337, 1983.

42. Egger M, Mai Nguyen X, Schaad UB, et al: Intestinal cryptosporidiosis acquired from a cat. Infection 18:177, 1990.

43. Glaser CA, Safrin S, Reingold A, et al: Association between *Cryptosporidium* infection and animal exposure in HIV infected individuals. J Acquir Immune Defic Syndr Hum Retrovirol 17:79, 1998.

44. Dupont HL, Chappell CL, Sterling CR, et al: The infectivity of *Cryptosporidium parvum* in healthy volunteers. N Engl J Med 332:855, 1995.

6

◆ Cryptococcosis: New Perspectives on Etiology, Pathogenesis, Diagnosis, and Clinical Management

Richard Malik
Gilbert J. Jacobs
Daria N. Love

Cryptococcosis is an important disease of mammals, and generally is considered to be the most common systemic mycosis of cats worldwide.[1] Although the disease is uncommon, it obviously has captured the interest and imagination of small-animal veterinarians, as reflected by the large amount that has been written concerning the condition. Over 70 papers have appeared concerning clinical and pathologic findings in cats with naturally occurring cryptococcosis. The findings have been reviewed comprehensively by a variety of authors.[2–5] Two groups have made a concerted effort to document the diagnosis and treatment of cats with cryptococcosis during the 1990s, the Georgia (United States) group (Linda Medleau, Gilbert Jacobs, Craig Greene, and Jeanne Barsanti) and the Sydney (Australia) group (Richard Malik, Patricia Martin, Denise Wigney, and Daria Love). The study of cryptococcosis in Australia has been facilitated by what we perceive to be a high prevalence compared with other parts of the world, and also by the influence of David Ellis, Tania Pfeiffer, and their collaborators, who have focused attention on the different varieties of *Cryptococcus neoformans* and the association of *C. neoformans* var *gattii* with eucalyptus trees.[6–10]

Rather than recapitulate findings that have been documented thoroughly and reviewed in the literature, we have decided instead to present a review of certain interesting features of this disease, emphasizing recent developments concerning its etiopathogenesis of relevance to feline practitioners. We also would like to highlight the Australian perspective concerning feline cryptococcosis.

◆ ETIOPATHOGENESIS

C. neoformans is a basidiomycetous fungus with 2 varieties, *C. neoformans* var *neoformans* and *C. neoformans* var *gattii*, that differ biochemically, genetically, ecologically, and epidemiologically.[11–13] *C. neoformans* var *neoformans* has a worldwide distribution, whereas var *gattii* has a more restricted distribution, occurring in tropical and subtropical climates. There is strong evidence that several species of Australian eucalyptus trees (including *Eucalyp-*

tus camaldulensis, E. tereticornis, E. rudis, E. blakelyi, and *E. gomphocephala*) provide the natural environmental niche for *C. neoformans* var *gatti*, and are found worldwide wherever var *gattii* has been implicated in disease.[6–10] The environmental niche for var *neoformans* has not been determined, although there may be an association with bird guano[11, 12, 14, 15] or decaying plant matter in the hollows of various fig trees.[16] Most basidiomycetes reproduce sexually in their natural environment, and the teleomorph of *C. neoformans* (*Filobasidiella neoformans*) can be induced to undergo sexual reproduction in the laboratory and produce dikaryotic hyphae, blastoconidia, basidia, and basidiospores.[17] The recent documentation of both α- and a-mating types of *C. neoformans* in *E. tereticornis* trees from pristine Australian environments suggests that this occurs in nature at least for *C. neoformans* var *gattii*.[18] However, other recent work has suggested that *C. neoformans* var *neoformans* may be evolving into an asexual fungus,[19] and that basidiospores may result from haploid (monkaryocytic) fruiting as well as by sexual recombination.[20]

In either case, it seems likely that the basidiospore is the infectious propagule for *C. neoformans*, because this stage of the fungus is adapted to dispersal by air currents and has physicochemical properties that favor adherence to, and penetration into, the respiratory epithelium, thereby facilitating primary infection of the mammalian host.[7, 12] In human beings, the small particle size of the infectious propagule results in the lung being the most likely primary site of infection, as only very small particles are capable of penetrating deep into the lower respiratory tract.[21, 22] However, in cats (and probably also dogs), the nasal cavity usually is the primary site of infection. The reasons for this difference are still a matter of conjecture. It is possible that differences in the anatomy of the nasal passages and paranasal sinuses, or functional differences in the ability of mucociliary clearance mechanisms to deal with different-sized particles in inspired air, may be responsible. Another possibility may be that cats, dogs, and human beings come into contact with different types of infectious propagule. Thus, human individuals may be infected with basidiospores or dehydrated yeast cells small enough to penetrate to the alveoli, whereas cats and dogs may be infected following the deposition of larger infectious propagules or aggregates of organisms from some environmental source, these being preferentially filtered out at the level of the nasal cavity.[23–26]

Human patients with cryptococcosis present typically with neurologic signs referable to meningitis or meningoencephalitis. There is strong circumstantial evidence that after infectious propagules lodge in the lungs, infection disseminates subsequently to the nervous system by way of the blood stream,[11, 12] although the mechanisms by which yeast cells leave the lung to reach the central nervous system hematogenously are the subject of active investigation in several laboratory models. Respiratory involvement usually does not result in symptoms,[11, 21] although lesions may be detected in routine chest radiographs or thoracic computed tomography scans. Cutaneous involvement in human patients is rare, and usually reflects widespread dissemination of infection, typically in the setting of advanced AIDS.[27]

The recent finding[28] in Thailand of nasal colonization of a large percentage of AIDS patients with cryptococcosis, taken together with data from some earlier studies,[29–32] could change our thinking on the pathogenesis of the disease in human beings and bring it closer to the aspects of the disease pathogenesis that seem relevant in cats and dogs. It is our belief that most cases of feline cryptococcosis, at least in Australia, begin as mycotic rhinitis subsequent to possible asymptomatic nasal cavity colonization.[23, 26] When infection ensues (either as a primary event or subsequent to prior colonization), and the rostral portion of the nasal cavity is involved, clinical signs of nasal cavity disease, such as sneezing, epistaxis, and nasal discharge, are conspicuous, and sometimes small granulomatous protuberances

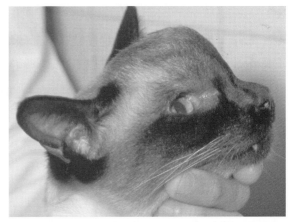

Figure 6–2. A Siamese cat with a long-standing invasive *C. neoformans* var *neoformans* infection of the nasal cavity. The infection has penetrated through the bones overlying the nasal cavity, and the cat's nasal bridge and forehead are swollen markedly. At surgery, this subcutaneous swelling was shown to consist almost exclusively of cryptococcal organisms, rather than host tissue.

can be seen emanating from the nares[33] (Fig. 6–1). If mycotic rhinitis is caused by invasive strains of *C. neoformans*, destruction of adjacent facial bones facilitates spread of infection to contiguous regions, such as the bridge (Fig. 6–2) and side of the nose (Fig. 6–3), the planum nasale, and the hard palate.[33–35] This produces facial distortion, and this type of clinical presentation is strongly suggestive of either fungal rhinosinusitis or nasal neoplasia.

Conversely, when the infection begins in the caudal portion of the nasal cavity, signs of mycotic rhinitis may be subtle or absent, although it is possible to confirm that the nasal cavity is the primary site of infection, using cytology and culture or diagnostic imaging modalities. In some of these cases, infection spreads caudally through the cribriform plate and into the olfactory bulbs and olfactory tracts, thereby giving rise to cryptococcal meningoencephalitis. In these cases, the neuroanatomic proximity to the optic nerves frequently results in the development of cryptococcal optic neuritis.[36]

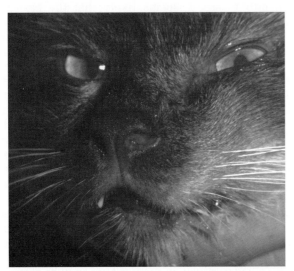

Figure 6–1. A Birman cat with a *Cryptococcus neoformans* var *gattii* infection. The cat has bilateral mycotic rhinitis. Granulomatous inflammation of the nasal mucosa is evident just inside the nostril. This cat was treated successfully using a long course of fluconazole.

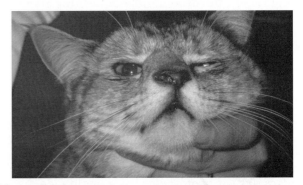

Figure 6–3. This domestic crossbred cat has invasive cryptococcal rhinitis that has extended to involve the subcutaneous tissues on the side of the nose and face. The cat was treated successfully using surgical débridement of the lesion, followed by a long course of fluconazole.

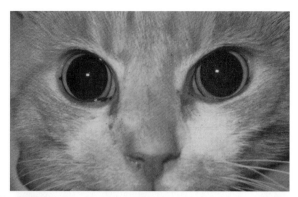

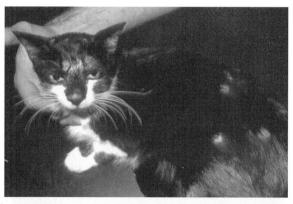

Figure 6–4. Widely dilated pupils in a cat with cryptococcal optic neuritis. Retinitis and a small hemorrhage emanating from the optic disc were evident using indirect ophthalmoscopy. The nasal cavity was shown by culture to be the primary site of infection in this cat. This patient was treated successfully using subcutaneous amphotericin B, flucytosine, and oral fluconazole.

Figure 6–6. Disseminated *C. neoformans* var *neoformans* infection in a feline immunodeficiency virus (FIV)–positive cat. Multiple cutaneous nodules are evident over the head and trunk of the cat. The nasal cavity was demonstrated to be the primary site of infection. This cat was treated successfully using a long course of fluconazole.

Clinically, this is accompanied by widely dilated pupils that respond poorly to light (Fig. 6–4), and ophthalmoscopic findings of swelling of the optic disc, often associated with focal hemorrhage and changes indicative of retinitis. In other cases, caudal nasal cavity involvement gives rise to a mass lesion that occludes one or both choanae (Fig. 6–5), resulting in signs of nasopharyngeal disease such as stertor, snoring, dyspnea, and open-mouth breathing, with or without evidence of neurologic disease.[25] We also have seen cases in which caudal nasal cavity disease has given rise to cryptococcal otitis media, resulting presumably from an ascending infection via the eustachian tube.[37]

As in human beings, multifocal cutaneous involvement in cats (Fig. 6–6) usually reflects hematogenous dissemination from the site of primary infection, most commonly the nasal cavity. An exception is when there is prominent involvement of the nasal planum, in which case, cutaneous involvement merely reflects spread from the nasal cavity

(Fig. 6–7). In a small number of cats, the infection spreads to the mandibular lymph nodes, presumably as a result of lymphatic drainage of organisms from the nasal cavity. Sometimes mandibular lymphadenomegaly may be massive, and requires surgical débridement because of interference with swallowing and breathing (Fig. 6–8). Occasionally, salivary gland infection has been documented, although the route through which organisms reach the glandular tissue has not been determined.

Cryptococcosis can occur in immunocompetent individuals. In Australia, where some of the best epidemiologic work concerning human cryptococcosis has been conducted, about 5 new cases can be expected to occur per million persons per year[38]; the same appears to be true in the United States. In about half of these individuals, no immunologic defect can be detected using sophisticated tests not readily available to veterinary practitioners. In the remaining 50 per cent of cases, there is some discernible defect in cellular immunity, referable to malignancy, cytotoxic chemotherapy, human immunodeficiency virus (HIV) infection, immunosuppressive therapy for immune-mediated diseases, diabe-

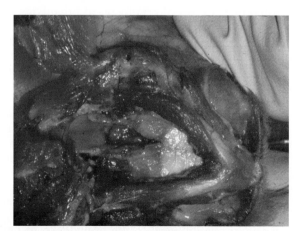

Figure 6–5. Necropsy photograph of a cat that died of cryptococcal meningitis shortly after commencing therapy. The cat has signs of dyspnea and stridor, and the presence of a nasopharyngeal cryptococcal granuloma was confirmed.

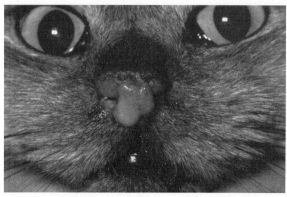

Figure 6–7. Localized involvement of the planum nasale in a cat with cryptococcal rhinitis.

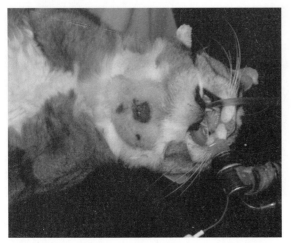

Figure 6–8. Cat with massive cryptococcal mandibular lymphadenomegaly caused by a *C. neoformans* var *neoformans* infection. The lesion was incised and débrided to relieve the cat's discomfort and interference with breathing. The cat was treated successfully using long consecutive courses of fluconazole, and subsequently, ketoconazole.

tes mellitus, sarcoidosis, and other conditions. In inner-city communities with a high prevalence of HIV infection, about 10 per cent of AIDS patients are likely to develop cryptococcosis at some stage in their disease course.[12, 19] Interestingly, whereas patients with HIV/AIDS invariably become infected by *C. neoformans* var *neoformans*, var *gattii* infections tend to occur almost exclusively in immunocompetent individuals.[13, 38, 39] Where we practice in Sydney, about 20 to 30 per cent of infections in human patients are caused by *C. neoformans* var *gattii*, and we see a similar proportion of var *gattii* infections in cats (and dogs). As well as a propensity to cause disease in immunocompetent human hosts, var *gattii* infections tend to be associated with the development of intracranial mass lesion(s), often called cryptococcomas, whereas var *neoformans* infections more typically result in meningitis with little or no involvement of the brain parenchyma.[38, 39] Based on more limited experience, the same would appear to be the case for cats (Figs. 6–9 and 6–10),

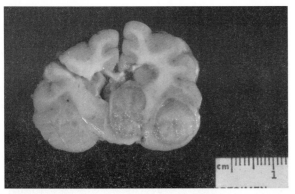

Figure 6–9. Multiple cerebral cryptococcal granulomas in a cat that died as a result of a *C. neoformans* var *gattii* infection. This cat was presented initially with signs of nasal cavity disease.

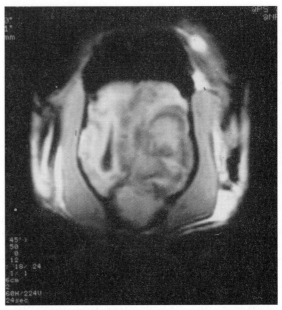

Figure 6–10. T1-weighted magnetic resonance imaging (MRI) scan of a cat with a large intracranial mass lesion. A diagnosis of a cerebral cryptococcal granuloma was possible based on a positive serum cryptococcal antigen titer, and this was later confirmed at necropsy. Similar computed tomography (CT) images have been reported previously in a cat with focal intracranial signs.[72] As a single cryptococcoma can resemble a meningioma in CT or MRI scans, testing for cryptococcal antigen should be performed routinely in such cases, to avoid making the diagnosis at craniotomy.

although there have been exceptions to this generalization.

There may be geographic differences with regard to neurologic pathology in feline cryptococcosis. In the southeastern United States, from cases examined by computed tomographic imaging or necropsy at the University of Georgia, intracranial mass lesions are not typical in the neurologic forms of feline cryptococcosis (Gilbert Jacobs and Craig Greene, unpublished observations).[2] Meningitis or meningoencephalitis are typical. Presumably, this geographic difference in pathologic observations is related to the different varieties of cryptococcal organisms involved, var *neoformans* infection being the most common variety in the southeastern United States.

In cats, factors predisposing to the development of cryptococcosis have not been identified clearly. In Australia, cryptococcosis in cats would appear to be 10 times more common than in dogs from the same geographic region.[23, 24] In North America, there is some evidence that some feline leukemia virus (FeLV)–positive cats develop cryptococcosis as a result of immune dysfunction because these cats are slower to respond or fail to respond to treatment, and are much more likely to suffer relapse compared with FeLV-negative cats.[40] In Australia, we have encountered barely any FeLV-positive cats with cryptococcosis, probably because the prevalence of persistent FeLV infection is so low compared with that in the United States.[41] Although there are several reports of 1 or 2 cats with cryptococcosis allegedly secondary to feline immunodeficiency virus (FIV) infection, larger studies in Australia have failed to produce convincing evidence that cryptococcosis is a feline AIDS-defining infection, and indeed it is considered that coinfection merely reflects the high prevalence of FIV infection in Australian cats. Lymphocyte subset analyses have failed to show lower CD4 cell counts in FIV-positive cats with cryptococcosis than in FIV-negative cats with cryptococcosis.[42] Furthermore, many FIV-positive cats with cryptococcosis can be cured, and do not relapse despite cessation of therapy.[23] Cryptococcosis has been reported very rarely in cats receiving immunosuppressive therapy or cytotoxic chemotherapy as treatment for malignancy. The authors have treated 4 cats with cryptococcosis that subsequently developed malignant lymphoma; a similar association has been the subject of a previous case report.[43] Genetic factors may be involved in the predisposition toward development of feline cryptococcosis, because Siamese cats are significantly overrepresented among reported cases, whereas lifestyle factors may account for the slight preponderance of male cats.[23]

◆ LABORATORY INVESTIGATION

Cryptococcosis should be considered in the differential diagnosis of the following conditions[5]:

- ◆ Nasal discharge
- ◆ Deforming sinonasal disease
- ◆ Nasal planum disease
- ◆ Nasopharyngeal disease
- ◆ Multiple cutaneous nodules (including digital swellings)
- ◆ Peripheral lymphadenomegaly (regional or generalized)
- ◆ Peripheral blindness/optic neuritis/retinitis
- ◆ Intracranial disease, especially vestibular syndromes
- ◆ Spinal cord disease
- ◆ Pulmonary parenchymal disease
- ◆ Pyothorax
- ◆ Middle ear disease

In most of these conditions, definitive diagnosis often is straightforward and based on obtaining representative tissue specimens for cytology, histology, and culture when applicable. Suitable specimens may include nasal swabs, nasal washings, needle aspirates from cutaneous nodules or enlarged lymph nodes, bronchoalveolar lavage specimens, pleural fluid, and cerebrospinal fluid (CSF).

◆ DIAGNOSIS

A definitive diagnosis of cryptococcosis requires the culture and identification of the organism by a reputable laboratory.[44] However, it is possible to obtain a high index of suspicion of cryptococcosis as the etiologic agent in the disease under investigation by demonstrating the characteristic capsulate, narrow-necked budding yeasts in cytologic smears or histology sections. It is worth noting, however, that some var *neoformans* strains have poorly developed capsules in vivo. Serologic assessment also can aid in the diagnosis of cryptococcosis.

Specimen Collection

Because we believe it is important for the management of the case to determine the variety of *C. neoformans* involved and its susceptibility to antifungal agents, our first priority is to obtain a specimen for culture. In our experience, needle aspirates from subcutaneous nodules, enlarged lymph nodes, or skin lesions are the most suitable specimens for culture. If it is not possible to obtain such a specimen, nasal cavity washes may yield an appropriate specimen. These specimens then can be subjected to cytologic examination using DiffQuik and Gram-staining, and submitted for culture. In our laboratory, we have had considerably more success demonstrating organisms in CSF using cytocentrifuged preparations stained with DiffQuik than with India ink preparations. Once the organism has been grown, identification can be made,[45, 46] and the susceptibility to fungal agents can be determined. Cytology and culture are highly sensitive and specific tests if performed as described later.

Culture, Laboratory Identification, and Susceptibility Testing

Most veterinary reports do not emphasize adequately the benefits of obtaining a positive culture in the diagnostic investigation and subsequent management of cryptococcosis cases, nor do they explain techniques likely to achieve this end. Although *C. neoformans* will grow on almost all laboratory media, Sabouraud dextrose agar is preferred when fungi including *C. neoformans* are considered in the differential diagnosis. Standard Sabouraud agar is optimum when culturing a normally sterile site, such as CSF, because antibiotics included in the media may inhibit the growth of some cryptococcal strains. Conversely, when sampling a site normally contaminated by bacteria, such as the nasal cavity, the inclusion of antibiotics in the medium improves the chances for isolating cryptococci. Birdseed agar containing antibiotics also is useful in the diagnosis of cryptococcosis, especially when sampling sites and material expected to be heavily contaminated, such as nasal exudate.[26, 44] Bacteria and other fungi can outgrow *C. neoformans* on the plates; however, the use of birdseed agar containing antibiotics overcomes this problem because the antibiotics suppress growth of contaminating bacteria. At the same time, the medium identifies colonies of *C. neoformans* from other yeasts and filamentous fungi, because they produce a brown-color-effect in the medium adjacent to the yeast colony (Fig. 6–11).

Positive culture helps provide a preliminary indication of the variety of *C. neoformans* involved, because var *gattii* colonies typically are much more mucoid. The biotype can be determined definitively using canavanine glycine bromophenol blue agar.[44, 46] The variety involved has implications with respect to prognosis and clinical management, because var *gattii* infections typically are more severe and more refractory to drug therapy than var *neoformans* infections,[38, 39] and var *gattii* strains tend to be more susceptible to itraconazole than to fluconazole (Richard Malik, unpublished observations).

Fungal susceptibility testing using disc diffusion, Etest strips, or broth microdilution provides useful information concerning therapy. Although not as accurate as bacterial in vitro susceptibility testing, it is our impression that strains that have a low minimum inhibitory concentration for a given drug in vitro tend to be susceptible to the drug in vivo, although the converse is not invariably true.

Indirect Methods of Diagnosis

By definition, this means a diagnosis in which the organism has not been cultured and for which the variety of *C. neoformans* cannot be determined.

These methods include histologic examination of tissues for the presence of yeasts with the typical morphology (capsule elaboration and narrow-necked budding to a smaller daughter cell), and serologic examination for detection of cryptococcal antigen in the blood. In both instances, these methods have the disadvantage of lack of definitive diagnosis and effective treatment indicators. However, serologic investigation is a useful adjunct to the diagnosis, prognosis, and treatment of cryptococcosis.[47, 48] It also is a sensitive and specific means for diagnosis of many cases of cryptococcosis without the necessity of obtaining tissue specimens. This may prove advantageous for establishment of a diagnosis in a patient for which CSF collection may be an unacceptable risk, or when a diagnosis is unlikely but should be excluded. The authors have

seen a number of feline and canine patients whose neurologic status deteriorated markedly after CSF was collected from the cisterna magna, despite the use of contemporary neuroanesthetic regimens. This hardly is surprising, considering that many cases have 1 or more space-occupying intracranial lesions (see Figs. 6–9 and 6–10) with the attendant risk of brain herniation after CSF collection. For this reason, CSF collection should be avoided whenever possible, and the collection of blood for serum cryptococcal antigen testing and nasal swabs for culture are very acceptable alternatives.

Because of the reasons given previously, we routinely take blood for serology from cats. The serologic test for cryptococcosis used in our laboratory detects cryptococcal antigen in the blood. This test utilizes latex particles coated with anticryptococcal antibodies in kit form that is simple, sensitive, specific, and easy to perform by competent laboratory staff. Studies in human and veterinary patients have shown that pretreatment of serum samples with proteinases such as pronase improves the sensitivity and specificity of the cryptococcal antigen testing system. This digestion step is included with some test kits, but should be performed routinely even when the enzyme is not supplied by the manufacturer.[48–50]

Finally, it is worth emphasizing that the nasal cavity of cats occasionally can be colonized asymptomatically by *C. neoformans*.[26] Thus, the diagnosis of cryptococcal rhinitis requires cytologic evidence of inflammation, or abundant organisms, and ideally a positive cryptococcal antigen test result in addition to positive culture.[26]

◆ TREATMENT

One of the reasons for renewed interest in feline cryptococcosis is the availability of a new generation of azole antifungal drugs (e.g., itraconazole, fluconazole, voriconazole) suitable for long-term oral administration.[51–56] Indeed, the main problem in treating cases of cryptococcosis currently is the high cost of drug therapy and the requirement for owners to medicate their cats on a regular basis for a very protracted time.[36] A number of factors affect the therapeutic approach to cats with cryptococcosis, including:

- The duration of the infection
- The extent of local invasion and extent of dissemination
- Tissue involvement, especially the presence or absence of meningoencephalitis
- The variety causing the infection (var *neoformans* versus var *gattii*)
- The in vitro susceptibility of the strain
- FIV and FeLV status
- Age, physical condition, and renal and hepatic function of the patient
- The temperament and appetite of the patient

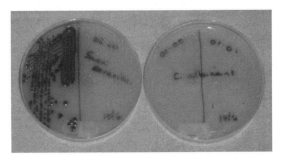

Figure 6–11. *C. neoformans* (left) and *Candida albicans* (right) plated onto Staib bird seed agar. Note the prominent brown-color-effect of *C. neoformans* colonies.

- The financial resources of the owner and the owner's emotional commitment to the cat

Surgical Intervention

We consider that the surgical excision, whenever feasible, of large aggregations of fungus-infected tissues, before or shortly after starting medical therapy, is a prerequisite of successful treatment.[25, 36] For example, cats with extensive involvement of the nasal bridge, large nasopharyngeal masses, or massively enlarged lymph nodes benefit enormously if abnormal tissue is removed surgically early in the course of treatment. This avoids problems with diffusion of antifungal agents into poorly perfused tissues, because these sometimes consist almost exclusively of cryptococcal elements with very little vascularized supportive host tissue.

Therapeutic Agents

Five drugs currently are available for treatment of cryptococcosis in cats, and each has a place in therapy depending on the considerations of each individual case.

Amphotericin B

In our opinion, amphotericin B is the most effective anticryptococcal agent, being the only drug that is unequivocally fungicidal and of proven permanent benefit in central nervous system (CNS) infections.[57-60] However, it must be given parenterally and therefore is inconvenient for outpatient therapy, and is nephrotoxic, although this is at least partially reversible.[61] We consider the combination of amphotericin B and flucytosine to be optimum therapy for cats with severe or widely disseminated disease, especially when there is CNS involvement.[57]

Flucytosine

Flucytosine (Ancotil, Roche) is a useful, effective, and only moderately expensive drug, but because of the rapid development of resistance that occurs when it is used alone, it is employed mainly to improve the efficacy of other antifungal drugs.[62] It is particularly good at penetrating the CSF and blood-brain barriers, and therefore complements amphotericin B effectively in the treatment of cryptococcal meningoencephalitis.[52, 63,-65]

Fluconazole

Fluconazole (Diflucan, Pfizer) is an extremely effective drug for treating cryptococcosis, certainly more effective than ketoconazole for the majority of isolates, with good penetration of the brain, eye, and urinary tract and minimal side-effects. It is, however, so expensive that only very wealthy or dedi-

cated owners can afford it, particularly for long courses of therapy. In such cases, it may be the drug of choice for initial therapy.[23, 54]

Itraconazole

Itraconazole (Sporanox, Janssen-Cilag) probably is the current drug of choice for empirical treatment of most cases of feline cryptococcosis.[40] It is more effective than ketoconazole, with generally fewer side-effects and a higher therapeutic index, and has a pharmacokinetic profile that permits once-daily dosing. Importantly, it has a significant cost advantage over fluconazole, with which it has comparable efficacy for infections outside the CNS, eye, and urinary tract, so that a majority of owners can afford therapy. It reaches high levels in soft tissues and skin, and penetrates the blood-brain barrier to some extent in the presence of meningoencephalitis. As is the case for ketoconazole, itraconazole should be given with food to ensure maximum absorption from the alimentary tract.

Ketoconazole

Ketoconazole is the cheapest of the available drugs, although doses that have efficacy in vivo often result in inappetence and vomiting, especially in cats with capricious appetites.[66]

Management Regimens

Based on these considerations, we suggest the following strategy for managing cases of feline cryptococcosis. First, procure material to culture the organism, determine the variety, and obtain in vitro susceptibility data from a mycology reference laboratory. Second, obtain a serum sample to determine baseline biochemical measurements and FeLV and FIV status, and to permit future measurement of the pretreatment cryptococcal antigen titer (a portion of the sample should be stored frozen, as sequential antigen titers used to monitor therapy ideally should be processed in the same assay run). Third, debulk localized accumulations of fungus-infected tissues surgically, if possible. This may be done at the outset, or after a short period of drug therapy, depending on convenience, the physical status of the patient, and the initial response to treatment.

The subsequent management of each individual case depends on the severity of disease and whether there is involvement of the CNS.

Cats That Are Eating and Have Mild-to-Moderate Disease Without Central Nervous System Involvement

Commence therapy with itraconazole, 50 to 100 mg per cat orally (PO) every (q) 24 hr with food.[40] Medium-sized to large cats should receive 100 mg q 24 hr, whereas cats weighing 3.5 kg or less should receive 50 mg q 24 hr, or 100 mg q 48 hr. Itraconazole capsules may be opened and split into two 50-mg portions using empty gelatin capsules. Alternately, the content of the capsules may be mixed with a small portion of a tasty food treat and given at the start of the meal because the standard formulation of itraconazole has no discernible effect on the texture or palatability of food. Many cats eventually develop reversible liver toxicity during therapy with itraconazole, especially when given high doses. This can take several weeks to months to develop, and is manifest clinically as inappetence to anorexia, sometimes accompanied by vomiting. Invariably, there is a concurrent elevation in serum alanine aminotransferase activity. Itraconazole-induced hepatotoxicity is reversible on discontinuation of the drug, although cats take as long as 7 days to regain their former appetite and demeanor. Once this occurs, it is possible to readminister the drug safely, albeit at a reduced dose, typically 50 per cent of the dose given originally.[40]

Therapy should be continued until the cat appears completely normal, with resolution of all presenting complaints and clinical signs, and eradication of viable organisms from accessible tissues (as assessed by cytology and culture). Typically, this takes 2 to 6 months, although some cases require considerably longer. When this stage has been reached, a second serum sample should be obtained from the patient to determine the extent of the decline in the antigen titer that has occurred as a result of therapy.[48] A 4- to 5-fold reduction suggests successful therapy, and once this has been obtained, we recommend continuing itraconazole (often at a reduced dose) or changing therapy to ketoconazole (50 mg q 24 hr with food) until the antigen titer declines to zero. If the antigen titer has declined but still is substantial, itraconazole therapy should be continued as before because it is very likely that a substantial amount of viable fungus is present in the cat's tissues. If the antigen titer has not declined in spite of therapy, more aggressive therapy should be implemented, as described later. Generally speaking, the cryptococcal antigen titer drops by approximately one 2-fold dilution per month during successful therapy; failure to observe a decline of this order in the antigen titer strongly suggests the need for more aggressive therapy.

At the University of Georgia, if the serum antigen titer decreases from pretreatment values by 2 orders of magnitude by the completion of 3 months of treatment, the likelihood of cure is high.[52] Accordingly, we have used results of sequential serum antigen titers in altering treatment strategies. For example, if serum antigen titers have not changed sufficiently from pretreatment values after 3 months of treatment, we augment treatment with an additional antifungal agent, typically combining amphotericin B with an azole as described in a subsequent section.

Fluconazole may be used in the same way as itraconazole, although currently it is substantially more expensive.[36] It is a very effective agent for treating cryptococcosis, except for some var *gattii* strains that show reduced sensitivity in vitro and in vivo. Even in these cases, however, it usually is possible to cure the patient using high doses of fluconazole. As well as being a very effective agent, it is usually devoid of side-effects. We generally use a dose of 25 to 50 mg per cat PO q 12 hr,[23, 67] for small and large cats, respectively. Some pharmacokinetic studies suggest that lower doses achieve therapeutic blood levels,[68] but it has been our experience that higher doses are required in vivo to successfully treat most cases of cryptococcosis in cats. Fluconazole has an important advantage over itraconazole in reaching effective concentrations in the CNS and CSF, even in the absence of inflammation, and being devoid of hepatic or other toxicities.[54] At present, largely for financial reasons, we tend to reserve the use of fluconazole for cases with CNS involvement, or for cats that show exaggerated hepatotoxicity after itraconazole therapy. The latter subgroup of cats generally does much better on fluconazole.

Cats With Severe Disease, Including All Cats With Meningoencephalitis, and Cases That Have Failed to Respond Adequately to Oral Azole Therapy

Cats with advanced, disseminated, or severe disease, and patients with CNS involvement may improve with oral azole therapy; however, it has been our evolving experience that these cases respond more quickly and do better in the long-term if treated using combination therapy consisting of amphotericin B and flucytosine.[52] If the animals are sufficiently debilitated to require intravenous fluid therapy, we elect to give the amphotericin B intravenously at first. Otherwise, we use a protocol that we have developed over the years in which the amphotericin B is administered 2 or 3 times weekly. Amphotericin B is prepared by adding 10 ml of sterile distilled water to a 50-mg vial of Fungizone (Bristol-Myers Squibb, Princeton, NJ) to produce a 5 mg/ml colloidal suspension. We use Fungizone designed for tissue culture use because it has a cost advantage over the same product formulated for intravenous use in human patients, but is of identical efficacy. Once formulated, the amphotericin B suspension may be stored frozen for up to 4 weeks without detectable loss of efficacy. The vial is thawed when amphotericin B is required, the calculated dose of drug being aspirated aseptically from the vial, which is subsequently refrozen. To prepare a subcutaneous infusion of amphotericin B, a 500-ml bag of 0.45 per cent sodium chloride in 2.5 per cent dextrose is heated in a microwave oven to 40°C, connected to an administration set, and 100 to 150 ml of the fluid is discarded. The calculated dose (0.5 to 0.8 mg/kg; typically 0.4 to 0.8 ml) of the stock amphotericin B suspension is injected into the fluid bag through its injection port. Fluid then

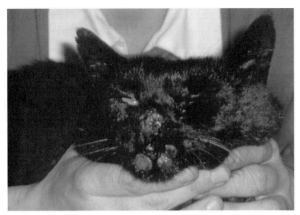

Figure 6–12. A cat with severe, long-standing, disseminated *C. neoformans* var *neoformans* infection before therapy.

is aspirated, and injected back and forth into the syringe repeatedly, to ensure effective transfer of the drug to the bag.

A 19- or 21-gauge needle then is attached to the administration set, inserted into the subcutaneous space between the scapulae roughly on the midline, and the fluid allowed to flow as fast as gravity will permit. Raising the bag of fluid as high as possible facilitates the timely delivery of the subcutaneous infusion, which usually takes 10 to 15 minutes (Figs. 6–12 and 6–13). Usually, the entire volume of fluid (350 to 400 ml) is given in 1 site, although the needle occasionally is repositioned further caudally if the cat displays signs of excessive discomfort after half or more of the fluid has been administered. In general, the subcutaneous infusion is well tolerated by cats that do not resent restraint per se. In fractious cats, sedation using midazolam/ketamine, or light anesthesia using sevoflurane, is necessary.[68a] The infused fluid moves extensively through the subcutaneous space, tending to pool ventrally over several hours before being absorbed.

These infusions are continued 2 to 3 times each week until there has been demonstrable clinical improvement, eradication of organisms from tissue accessible to needle aspiration, and a corresponding

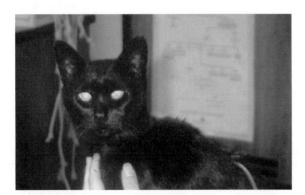

Figure 6–13. The same cat as in Figure 6–12 receiving a subcutaneous infusion of amphotericin B. Note the marked improvement in the appearance of the lesions about the cat's head. The cat also received flucytosine and fluconazole.

decline in the cryptococcal antigen titer. Typically, the cumulative dose of amphotericin B required to effect this clinical improvement is on the order of 10 to 20 mg/kg.[57] Interestingly, it is the cumulative dose of amphotericin B that appears to be important, rather than the period over which the drug is administered. The rationale for using amphotericin B subcutaneously as a dilute suspension is to delay its absorption into the systemic circulation, thereby avoiding the high peak blood levels that result in nephrotoxicity. Delivering amphotericin B together with a large volume of fluid (and sodium) reduces further the tendency toward renal damage, because of the protective effect of the ensuing mild diuresis.[69, 70] It is possible therefore to administer larger and thus more effective quantities of amphotericin B using this protocol than have been administered traditionally, and to do so without producing substantial azotemia. It is prudent, however, to monitor serum urea and creatinine concentrations repeatedly during therapy on a regular basis, and to discontinue amphotericin B infusions temporarily if azotemia develops. Owners also are advised to add a small amount of salt to the cat's diet because this is thought to minimize further the propensity for nephrotoxicity.[69]

Flucytosine is administered simultaneously with amphotericin B because this combination has been shown convincingly to have a synergistic action against *C. neoformans* in human patients.[63–65] Flucytosine is administered at a dose of 250 mg (1/2 tablet) PO q 8 hr, for small to normal-sized cats. In contrast to dogs in which it consistently produces systemic malaise associated with severe cutaneous drug eruptions,[71] in our experience this drug is uniformly well tolerated in cats. In some patients with neurologic signs, fluconazole is administered also, although generally we reserve the use of the azoles for a later stage in therapy.

Amphotericin B is continued on a 2 or 3 times a week basis. If animals are hospitalized, treatment is often given on a Monday, Wednesday, and Friday schedule, whereas cases treated on an outpatient basis generally receive 2 infusions per week for the convenience of the owners. The weekly dose of amphotericin B should not exceed 1.6 mg/kg. Once this therapy is initiated, it usually is continued for at least 6 to 12 weeks, at which time the patient is usually well enough to be discharged on follow-up oral azole therapy. In some cases, a further course of amphotericin B infusions is required at a later time; for example, if the decline in the antigen titer is not sustained during azole therapy.

Based on our experience of managing numerous cases of cryptococcosis in cats, dogs, ferrets, and koalas, there is no doubt that combination therapy using amphotericin B and flucytosine represents more effective therapy for cryptococcosis than oral therapy using either itraconazole or fluconazole. We recommend this regimen, therefore, for severe or intractable cases, and cases with neurologic involvement. However, treatment using this combination requires much more effort and dedication from both the owner and the veterinary team, and involves more morbidity and hospitalization time for the patient. It has been our observation that many patients with cryptococcal meningoencephalitis deteriorate during initial treatment using amphotericin B and flucytosine. In these patients, very short courses of short-acting glucocorticoids such as prednisolone are sometimes necessary to get them through this transient crisis period in which increased intracranial pressure occurs subsequent to death of organisms and the associated inflammatory response in the brain of the host.

One of the greatest challenges in treatment of feline cryptococcosis cases is to ensure that the infection is eliminated from the patient. Serial antigen titer determinations are most useful in this regard[5, 47, 48, 52] because the patient typically improves clinically long before viable fungus is completely eliminated from the body. This is especially true during monotherapy with azoles, which generally are considered fungistatic and therefore rely on phagocytosis and a directed cell-mediated immune response to eliminate cryptococci from the host tissues. Having experienced several disease recurrences as long as 6 years after apparently successful therapy, we now recommend continuing antifungal therapy until the cryptococcal antigen titer is zero. In severe cases, this may take a very considerable period of time (up to 2 years from the initiation of therapy). In these circumstances, often only 1 drug is prescribed, and in some cases, ketoconazole is chosen over itraconazole in the interests of economy. Patients that have received a large cumulative dose of amphotericin B along with flucytosine generally require a shorter duration of therapy, presumably because the combination is fungicidal, and residual antigen titers reflect dead fungus undergoing phagocytosis. We have had the opportunity of demonstrating this effect in a cat with severe neurologic signs that improved with therapy, but had persisting severe neurologic deficits that necessitated euthanasia. At necropsy, gelatinous cryptococcal material was observed replacing the olfactory tracts and olfactory bulbs, although culture of the material collected was negative.

◆ PROGNOSIS

The prognosis for most cats with cryptococcosis is excellent, given diligent, cooperative owners prepared to dose their cats for several months and pay for the costs of medication and monitoring.

Cats with long-standing extensive disease have a less favorable prognosis than cats diagnosed early with mild signs of disease, although even long-standing cases with severe disseminated disease may be cured with appropriate therapy. Cats with neurologic signs always have a guarded prognosis, although many (perhaps 70 per cent) can be treated successfully using aggressive treatment regimens, typically with combination therapy consisting of amphotericin B and flucytosine, and possibly also an azole.[1, 5, 51, 52] Two additional considerations apply to cats with cryptococcal meningoencephalitis. First, the neurologic status of these cats often deteriorates soon after starting therapy, presumably because death of cryptococci and the resulting inflammation give rise to a dangerous increase in intracranial pressure. Second, there can be permanent neurologic deficits (such as blindness and gait abnormalities) after successful therapy.

Cats in which a positive FeLV status is confirmed on 2 consecutive occasions have a poor long-term prognosis,[52] and drug therapy for cryptococcosis in these cases usually does not have curative intent, but rather should be considered as palliative. On the other hand, at least in Australia, FIV-positive cats generally can be cured despite their FIV status, although some need more prolonged courses of treatment than FIV-negative patients to effect a cure.

◆ PUBLIC HEALTH CONCERNS

Cryptococcosis is not considered to be a zoonotic disease; therefore, infected cats pose no public health threat to their owners or veterinarians.[11] The organism does not aerosolize from sites of tissue infection, so the disease cannot be spread between people or animals.[11] The major public health significance of infected cats is that they may act as a sentinel species for human beings, in that their source of exposure to infectious propagules also is a potential source of exposure for people and other mammals.

◆ CONCLUDING COMMENTS AND FUTURE DIRECTIONS

The diagnosis and treatment of cats with cryptococcosis remain a challenge for feline practitioners, although the availability of drugs such as fluconazole and itraconazole, and new strategies for delivering older drugs like amphotericin B, have resulted in a much improved prognosis for our patients. A high index of suspicion for this infection is required, especially in cats with nasal cavity and neurologic disease, because early diagnosis markedly improves the chances for a successful outcome. The cost of therapy is likely to decline over time as the new azoles come out of patent, whereas new formulations of amphotericin B using delivery systems such as liposomes or lipid emulsions will further improve the prognosis for feline cryptococcosis.[5] Although well-documented trials have yet to be conducted, many human infectious disease physicians consider liposomal amphotericin B to be a significant advance over the deoxycholate formulation, due to increased efficacy, reduced toxicity, and thus a greater therapeutic index. Unfortunately, the very high cost of this formulation makes it difficult to use in a veterinary setting, even in cats, because strategies to use the contents of a reconstituted vial economically have not been described.

REFERENCES

1. Malik R, Wigney DI, Martin P, et al. Veterinary aspects of cryptococcosis. *In* Proceedings of the Second International Conference on Cryptococcus and Cryptococcosis. L29. Milan, Italy, 1993, p. 74.
2. Medleau L, Barsanti J: Cryptococcosis. *In* Greene CE (ed): Infectious Diseases of the Dog and Cat, 1st ed. Philadelphia, WB Saunders, 1990, pp. 687–695.
3. Ackerman L: Feline cryptococcosis. Compend Contin Educ Pract Vet 10:1049–1055, 1988.
4. Pederson NC (ed): Cryptococcosis. *In* Infectious Diseases of the Cat. Goleta, CA, American Veterinary Publications, 1988, pp. 255–261.
5. Jacobs GJ, Greene CE, Medleau L: Feline and canine cryptococcosis. Waltham Focus 8:21–27, 1998.
6. Ellis DH, Pfeiffer TJ: Natural habitat of *Cryptococcus neoformans* var. *gattii*. J Clin Microbiol 228:1642–1644, 1990.
7. Ellis DH, Pfeiffer TJ: Ecology, life cycle and infectious propagule of *Cryptococcus neoformans*. Lancet 336:923–925, 1990.
8. Ellis DH, Pfeiffer TJ: The ecology of *Cryptococcus neoformans*. Eur J Epidemiol 8:321–325, 1992.
9. Pfeiffer TJ, Ellis DH: Environmental isolation of *Cryptococcus neoformans* var. *gattii* from *Eucalyptus tereticornis*. J Med Vet Mycol 30:407–408, 1992.
10. Pfeiffer TJ, Ellis DH: Additional eucalyptus hosts of *Cryptococcus neoformans* var. *gattii* (Abstract p5.6). *In* International Meeting and Exhibition of Australian and New Zealand Societies for Microbiology, Christchurch, New Zealand, 1996, p. A53.
11. Diamond RD: *Cryptococcus neoformans*. *In* Mandell GL, Douglas RG, Bennett JE (eds): Principles and Practice of Infectious Diseases, 3rd ed. New York, Churchill Livingstone, 1990, pp. 1980–1989.
12. Levitz SM: The ecology of *Cryptococcus neoformans* and the epidemiology of cryptococcosis. Rev Infect Dis 13:1163–1169, 1991.
13. Kwon-Chung KJ, Bennett JE: Epidemiologic differences between the two varieties of *Cryptococcus neoformans*. Am J Epidemiol 120:123–130, 1984.
14. Denton JF, DiSalvo AF: The prevalence of *C. neoformans* in various natural habitats. Sabouraudia 6:213–217, 1968.
15. Emmons CW: Saprophytic sources of *Cryptococcus neoformans* associated with the pigeon (*Columba livia*). Am J Hyg 62:227–232, 1955.
16. Lazera MS, Pires FDA, Camillo-Coura L, et al: Natural habitat of *Cryptococcus neoformans* var. *neoformans* in decaying wood forming hollows in living trees. J Med Vet Mycol 34:127–131, 1996.
17. Kwon-Chung KJ: Morphogenesis of *Filobasidiella neoformans*, the sexual state of *Cryptococcus neoformans*. Mycology 68:821–833, 1976.
18. Halliday CL, Bui T, Krockenberger M, et al: Presence of α and **a** mating types in environmental and clinical collections of *Cryptococcus neoformans* var. *gattii* from Australia. J Clin Microbiol 37:2920–2926, 1999.
19. Franzot SP, Hamdan JS, Currie BP, Casadevall A: Molecular epidemiology of *Cryptococcus neoformans* in Brazil and the United States: Evidence for both local genetic differences and a global clonal population structure. J Clin Microbiol 35:2243–2251, 1997.
20. Wilkes BL, Mayorga ME, Edman U, Edman JC: Dimorphism and haploid fruiting in *Cryptococcus neoformans*: Association with the alpha-mating type. Proc Nat Acad Sci U S A 93:7327–7331, 1996.
21. Warr W, Bates JH, Stone A: The spectrum of pulmonary cryptococcosis. Ann Intern Med 69:1109–1116, 1968.
22. Sukroongreung S, Kitiniyom K, Nilakul C, Tantimavanich S: Pathogenicity of basidiospores of *Filobasidiella neoformans* var. *neoformans*. Med Mycol 36:419–424, 1998.
23. Malik R, Wigney DI, Muir DB, et al: Cryptococcosis in cats: Clinical and mycological assessment of 29 cases and evaluation of treatment using orally administered fluconazole. J Med Vet Mycol 30:133–144, 1992.
24. Malik R, Dill-Macky E, Martin P, et al: Cryptococcosis in dogs: A retrospective study of 20 consecutive cases. J Med Vet Mycol 33:291–297, 1995.
25. Malik R, Martin P, Wigney DI, et al: Nasopharyngeal cryptococcosis. Aust Vet J 75:483–488, 1997.
26. Malik R, Wigney DI, Muir D, et al: Asymptomatic carriage of *Cryptococcus neoformans* in the nasal cavity of dogs and cats. J Med Vet Mycol 35:27–31, 1997.
27. Eng RHK, Bishburg E, Smith SM, Kapila R: Cryptococcal infections in patients with acquired immune deficiency syndrome. Am J Med 81:19–23, 1986.
28. Skroongreung S, Eampokalap B, Tansuphaswadikul S, et al: Recovery of *Cryptococcus neoformans* from the nasopharynx of AIDS patients. Mycopathologia 143:131–134, 1999.
29. Briggs DR, Barney PL, Bahu RM: Nasal cryptococcosis. Arch Otolaryngol 100:390–392, 1974.
30. Norris JC, Armstrong WB: Membranous cryptococcic nasopharyngitis (*Cryptococcus neoformans*). Arch Otolaryngol 60:720–722, 1954.
31. Dixon DM, Polak A: *In vivo* and *in vitro* studies with an atypical rhinotropic isolate of *Cryptococcus neoformans*. Mycopathologia 96:33–40, 1986.
32. Kuttin ES, Feldman M, Nyska A, et al: Cryptococcosis of the nasopharynx in mice and rats. Mycopathologia 101:99–104, 1988.
33. Wilkinson GT: Feline cryptococcosis: A review and seven case reports. J Small Anim Pract 20:749–768, 1979.
34. Legendre AM, Gompf R, Bone D: Treatment of feline cryptococcosis with ketoconazole. J Am Vet Med Assoc 181:1541–1542, 1982.
35. Medleau L, Hall EJ, Goldschmidt MH, Irby N. Cutaneous cryptococcosis in three cats. J Am Vet Med Assoc 187:169–170, 1985.
36. Malik R, Martin P, Wigney DI, Love DN: Diagnosis and treatment of cryptococcosis in cats. *In* Proceedings 243 of the Postgraduate Committee in Veterinary Science, The University of Sydney, 1995, pp. 49–54.
37. Beatty J, Barrs VR, Swinney GR, et al: Peripheral vestibular disease associated with cryptococcosis in three cats. J Fel Med Surg 2:29–34, 2000.
38. Speed B, Dunt D: Clinical and host differences between infections with the two varieties of *Cryptococcus neoformans*. Clin Infect Dis 21:28–34, 1995.
39. Mitchell DH, Sorrell TC, Allworth AM, et al: Cryptococcal disease of the CNS in immunocompetent hosts: Influence of cryptococcal variety on clinical manifestations and outcome. Clin Infect Dis 20:611–616, 1995.
40. Medleau L, Jacobs GJ, Marks MA: Itraconazole for the treatment of cryptococcosis in cats. J Vet Intern Med 9:39–42, 1995.
41. Malik R, Kendall K, Cridland J, et al: Prevalences of feline leukaemia virus and feline immunodeficiency virus infections in cats in Sydney. Aust Vet J 75:323–327, 1997.
42. Walker C, Malik R, Canfield PJ: Analysis of leucocytes and lymphocyte subsets in cats with naturally occurring cryptococcosis but differing feline immunodeficiency virus status. Aust Vet J 72:93–96, 1995.
43. Madewell BR, Holmberg CA, Ackerman N: Lymphosarcoma and cryptococcosis in a cat. J Am Vet Med Assoc 175:65–68, 1979.
44. Dimech WJ: Diagnosis, identification and epidemiology of *Cryptococcosis neoformans* infection. Aust J Med Lab Sci 12:13–21, 1990.
45. Healy ME, Dillavou CL, Taylor GE: Diagnostic medium containing inositol, urea and caffeic acid for selective growth of *Cryptococcus neoformans*. J Clin Microbiol 6:387–391, 1977.
46. Kwon-Chung KJ, Polacheck I, Bennett JE: Improved diagnostic medium for separation of *Cryptococcus neoformans* var *neoformans* (serotypes A & D) and *Cryptococcus neoformans*

var *gattii* (serotypes B & C). J Clin Microbiol 15:535–537, 1982.

47. Medleau L, Marks MA, Brown J, Borges WL: Clinical evaluation of a cryptococcal antigen latex agglutination test for diagnosis of cryptococcosis in cats. J Am Vet Med Assoc 196:1470–1473, 1990.

48. Malik R, McPetrie R, Wigney DI, Love DN: Use of the cryptococcal latex agglutination antigen test for diagnosis and monitoring of therapy in veterinary patients with cryptococcosis. Aust Vet J 74:358–364, 1996.

49. Gray LD, Roberts GD: Experience with the use of pronase to eliminate interference factors in the latex agglutination test for cryptococcal antigen. J Clin Microbiol 26:2450–2451, 1988.

50. Hamilton JR, Noble A, Denning DW, Stevens DA: Performance of cryptococcus antigen latex agglutination kits on serum and cerebrospinal fluid specimens of AIDS patients before and after pronase treatment. J Clin Microbiol 29:333–339, 1991.

51. Berthelin CF, Legendre AM, Bailey CS, et al: Cryptococcosis of the nervous system in dogs. Part 2: Diagnosis, treatment, monitoring and prognosis. Prog Vet Neurol 5:136–146, 1994.

52. Jacobs GJ, Medleau L, Calvert CC, et al: Cryptococcal infection in cats: Factors influencing treatment outcome, and results of sequential serum antigen titers in 35 cats. J Vet Intern Med 11:1–4, 1997.

53. Denning DW, Stevens DA: New drugs for systemic fungal infections. BMJ 299:407–408, 1989.

54. Grant SM, Clissold SP: Fluconazole. A review of its pharmacodynamic and pharmacokinetic properties and therapeutic potential in superficial and systemic mycoses. Drugs 39:877–916, 1990.

55. Sugar AM, Stern JJ, Dupont B. Overview: Treatment of cryptococcal meningitis. Rev Infect Dis 12(Suppl 3):S338–S348, 1990.

56. Bodey GP: Azole antifungal agents. Clin Infect Dis 14(Suppl 1):S161–S169, 1992.

57. Malik R, Craig AJ, Martin P, et al: Combination chemotherapy of cryptococcosis using subcutaneously administered amphotericin B. Aust Vet J 73:124–128, 1996.

58. Gallis HA, Drew RH, Pickard WW: Amphotericin B: 30 years of clinical experience. Rev Infect Dis 12:308–329, 1990.

59. Larsen RA, Leal ME, Chan LS: Fluconazole compared with amphotericin B plus flucytosine for cryptococcal meningitis in AIDS. A randomised trial. Ann Intern Med 113:183–187, 1990.

60. Just-Nubling G, Heise W, Ganger G, et al: Initial triple combination of amphotericin B, flucytosine and fluconazole in AIDS patients with acute cryptococcal meningitis. *In* Proceedings of the Second International Conference on Cryptococcus and Cryptococcosis, 1993, P 7–6, p. 130.

61. Miller RP, Bates JH: Amphotericin B toxicity: A follow-up report of 53 patients. Ann Intern Med 71:1089–1095, 1969.

62. Bennett JE: Flucytosine. Ann Intern Med 86:319–322, 1977.

63. Bennett JE, Dismukes WE, Duma RJ, et al: A comparison of amphotericin B alone and combined with flucytosine in the treatment of cryptococcal meningitis. N Engl J Med 301:126–131, 1979.

64. Dismukes WE, Cloud G, Gallis HA, et al: Treatment of cryptococcal meningitis with combination amphotericin B and flucytosine for four as compared to six weeks. N Engl J Med 317:334–341, 1987.

65. Utz JP, Garriques IL, Sande MA, et al: Therapy of cryptococcosis with a combination of flucytosine and amphotericin B. J Infect Dis 132:368–373, 1975.

66. Greene CE: Antifungal chemotherapy. *In* Greene CE (ed): Infectious Diseases of the Dog and Cat, 1st ed. Philadelphia, WB Saunders, 1990, pp. 649–658.

67. Craig AC, Ramzan I, Malik R: Pharmacokinetics of intravenous and oral fluconazole in cats. Res Vet Sci 57:372–376, 1994.

68. Vaden SL, Heit MC, Manaugh C, Riviere J: Fluconazole in cats: Pharmacokinetics following intravenous and oral administration and penetration into cerebrospinal fluid, aqueous humour and pulmonary epithelial lining fluid. J Vet Pharmacol Ther 20:181–186, 1997.

68a. Tzannes S, Govendir M, Zaki S, et al: The use of sevoflurane in a 2:1 mixture of nitrous oxide and oxygen for rapid mask induction of anaesthesia in the cat. J Fel Med Surg 2:83–90, 2000.

69. Branch RA: Prevention of amphotericin B–induced renal impairment: A review on the use of sodium supplementation. Arch Intern Med 148:2389–2394, 1988.

70. Rubin SI: Nephrotoxicity of amphotericin B. *In* Kirk, RW (ed): Current Veterinary Therapy IX. Philadelphia, WB Saunders, 1986, pp. 1142–1146.

71. Malik R, Medeiros C, Wigney DI, Love DN: Suspected drug eruption in seven dogs during administration of flucytosine. Aust Vet J 74:285–288, 1996.

72. Glass E, deLahunta A, Kent M, et al: A cryptococcal granuloma in the brain of a cat causing focal signs. Prog Vet Neurol 7:141–144, 1996.

7

◆ Update on the Diagnosis and Management of Feline Herpesvirus-1 Infection

David J. Maggs

Vaccines for feline herpesvirus type 1 (FHV-1) have been used widely for a number of years, and more recently an increasing array of antiviral agents has become available for treating cats infected with this virus. Despite these advances, the broad spectrum of acute and chronic clinical syndromes associated with FHV-1 remains a significant and sometimes frustrating problem in modern veterinary practice. The reasons for this dilemma are many and diverse; however, principal among them is difficulty detecting and interpreting the significance of viral presence in diseased cats. Even if we assumed that current diagnostic techniques afforded perfect sensitivity and specificity, the ability of this virus to remain sequestered from antiviral agents and the immune-mediated pathology associated with FHV-1 infection create unique therapeutic challenges. Despite this, some significant advances in the diagnosis and management of FHV-1 have been made in recent years. This chapter is intended to highlight such information while briefly reviewing some clinically relevant virologic and pathogenetic features.

◆ ETIOLOGY

FHV-1 is a large DNA virus that is a major cause of respiratory and ocular disease in felidae only. Recent seroprevalence studies reveal that over 90 per cent of cats have been exposed to this virus.[1] Although the virus has worldwide distribution, it appears to demonstrate little genomic diversity, suggesting that diagnostic and treatment modalities should be universally applicable. FHV-1 is a representative member of the alphaherpesvirus subfamily whose members demonstrate remarkable predictability in their biologic behavior. The alphaherpesviruses tend to be highly species-specific, environmentally labile viruses with marked epithelial tropism. Following rapid replication in peripheral epithelial cells, life-long latency within neural tissues develops in most infected individuals; recrudescent disease occurs in a small percentage. The best studied of the subfamily is the analogous human virus—herpes simplex virus type 1 (HSV-1). The basic and clinical research data generated for HSV-1 have provided useful diagnostic and therapeutic insights into FHV-1. However, occasional areas of biologic diversity have been demonstrated between the 2 viruses, and these must be considered

before applying data generated for one viral or host species to another.

◆ EPIDEMIOLOGY

FHV-1 is extremely labile within the environment, surviving between 12 and 18 hours depending on the degree of desiccation. Thus, the major mechanism of infection is direct mucosal transfer of virus between cats via sneezed macrodroplets. Cats have been demonstrated to sneeze these particles over a distance of 1.3 m; however, aerosolization of virus during normal respiratory movements is considered unlikely.[2] Because FHV-1 is sensitive to all commonly used disinfectants, transfer of virus via fomites is easy to avoid with adequate hygiene.

It has been estimated that at least 80 per cent of FHV-1–infected cats become life-long carriers of the virus within the trigeminal ganglia, and that at least half of these are of epidemiologic importance owing to reactivation and shedding of virus.[3] Such episodes of reactivation may be stimulated by stress such as rehousing, intercurrent illness, or changes in the human or pet population within a household. Administration of glucocorticoids is a very reliable method of reactivating latent virus under experimental conditions; this also may occur in clinical veterinary practice. Viral shedding initiated by stress associated with pregnancy, parturition, and lactation is an epidemiologically ingenious method by which this virus is perpetuated between generations. Of particular importance in the spread of FHV-1 are episodes of apparently spontaneous and often subclinical reactivation, which are estimated to occur in 1 per cent of carrier cats on any given day.[3] Detection and isolation of such cats are very difficult, and yet these animals are probably of greater epidemiologic significance than other individuals within a multicat household that may attract more attention owing to more overt clinical signs. As is discussed later in this chapter, current treatments and vaccines may do little to decrease shedding of virus in carrier cats.

◆ PATHOGENESIS

After primary inoculation of oral, nasal, or conjunctival mucosa, there is an initial period of rapid replication within epithelial cells, causing cytolysis.

This sometimes can be observed directly in the cornea as the pathognomonic dendritic ulcers. This phase of cell destruction also causes rhinitis and conjunctivitis. If cytolysis is severe enough to cause ulceration of mucosal surfaces, serosanguineous ocular or nasal discharge may be seen. Exposure of conjunctival substantia propria and corneal stroma permits formation of adhesions between these tissues (symblepharon) (Fig. 7–1). If viral infection occurs before the eyelids open, large amounts of inflammatory debris may accumulate in the conjunctival sac (conjunctivitis neonatorum). Transient keratoconjunctivitis sicca also has been associated with primary FHV-1 infection.[4] Given the epitheliotropism of FHV-1, this may represent a primary lacrimal adenitis. Alternatively, ductal occlusion secondary to inflammation of surrounding tissues or accumulation of debris may be responsible. Erosion of the nasal mucosa exposes underlying bone and cartilage. Subsequent distortion and remodeling of these tissues may be associated with chronic rhinosinusitis.

Primary disease usually is self-limiting within 10 to 20 days; however, during this period, viral latency is established in the majority of cats (Fig. 7–2). Latent virus may be detected in trigeminal ganglia within 4 days of primary infection.[5] As with other alphaherpesviruses, viremia does not occur, and FHV-1 is believed to reach the sensory ganglia following ascent of the sensory axons of the trigeminal nerve. Latency describes a period of viral quiescence, and may be defined clinically, histologically, virologically, or molecularly. Combining these definitions, *latency* may be characterized as a period during which there is no clinical evidence of disease, no histologically detectable inflammation peripherally or within ganglia, no detectable virus using standard culture techniques, and limited viral transcriptional activity.[6]

Intermittent, and usually recurrent, episodes of viral reactivation from the latent state may be followed by centrifugal spread of virus back along the sensory axons to peripheral epithelia in some animals (see Fig. 7–2). When these episodes of reactivation are associated with clinically evident disease at peripheral sites, this is termed *recrudescence.* Whereas many pharmacologic and environmental triggers for reactivation are recognized, the molecular basis by which this occurs remains an area of intense research. Once reactivated virus reaches respiratory or ocular epithelial tissue, it may cause recrudescent disease, or viral shedding may occur without clinical signs. Currently, predicting which cats within a population are going to suffer recrudescent disease is not possible. The important concept is that whereas the majority of hosts appear to become latently infected, a minor percentage of them are affected by chronic or recurrent herpetic disease.

Primary infection, neural latency, and recrudescent infection are the classically described phases of in vivo alphaherpesvirus activity. Recently, more sensitive viral detection methods such as the polymerase chain reaction (PCR) have demonstrated virus in peripheral sites for protracted periods after initial infection.[7–9] These findings have led to the suggestion that an additional viral state may exist (see Fig. 7–2). This state has been termed *extraneural latency* or *persistence,* depending on whether associated local inflammation can be demonstrated. The involvement of this putative viral state in chronic herpes-associated diseases such as stromal keratitis, chronic conjunctivitis, feline eosinophilic keratitis, and corneal sequestration is an area currently under investigation.

FHV-1 induces tissue damage via 2 classical mechanisms—as a direct result of viral replication (cytolysis) or indirectly through immunopathologic processes mediated by inflammatory cells. The most striking example of immunopathologic herpetic disease in cats is stromal keratitis. This is an uncommon response of some cats to infection with FHV-1 and involves infiltration of the corneal stroma with inflammatory cells (primarily lymphocytes). Chronic inflammatory changes, especially fibrosis and vascularization, ultimately can cause blindness.[10] Of central importance to the pathogenesis and understanding of this disease is identification of the antigenic stimuli for this immune response. Strong experimental evidence suggests that persistent viral antigen gains access to the stroma during periods of protracted ulceration and is cleared ineffectually, leading to immune-mediated tissue damage.[10] A similar mechanism may well be important in the pathogenesis of chronic rhinosinusitis in cats, but this has not been examined.

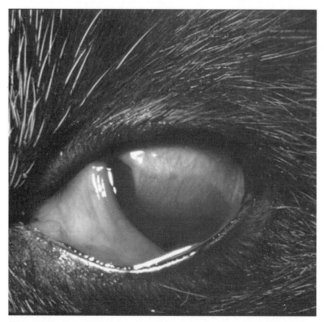

Figure 7–1. Symblepharon (conjunctival and corneal adhesion) is a relatively common complication of severe primary feline herpesvirus type 1 (FHV-1) infection. Here, fornical conjunctiva has adhered to the superior cornea.

◆ CLINICAL SIGNS

A diverse range of clinical signs and diseases has been attributed to FHV-1 infection. These may be

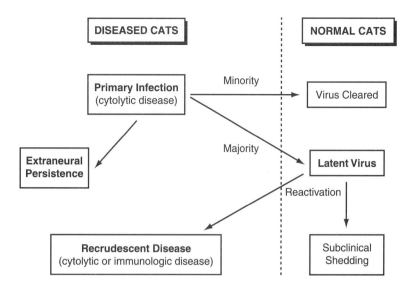

Figure 7–2. Pathogenesis of FHV-1. Traditionally, 3 phases of viral activity have been described for FHV-1: primary infection, neural latency, and recrudescent infection. Recent evidence suggests that extraneural latency and/or persistence of virus also may occur.

considered as 3 broad groups: those associated with primary infection, those associated with recrudescent or persistent infection, and a collection of disorders purportedly due to FHV-1 infection. With further insights into the pathogenetic mechanisms of this virus, more sensitive diagnostic assays, and better clinical studies, there has been a gradual shift of diseases from the last category to one of the first 2; therefore, these should not be seen as strictly delineated categories.

Primary Disease

Primary FHV-1 infection generally is limited to the upper respiratory tract and eyes, with rhinitis and conjunctivitis predominating. Nasal and ocular discharges are serous at first, but may become blood-stained if conjunctival ulceration is severe (Fig. 7–3). With disease progression and recruitment of immunologic cells, particularly neutrophils, discharges usually become mucopurulent. Sneezing is a consistent sign at this stage of the disease. Systemic signs such as fever, malaise, and anorexia also are common, particularly in young animals. Rare cases of mortality have been associated with lower respiratory tract compromise in young kittens; however, the majority of cases are self-limiting. Ocular signs in the acute form of the disease usually are bilateral, although not necessarily symmetric in degree or timing of involvement.

Conjunctivitis is characterized by marked hyperemia with minimal to moderate chemosis. Corneal infection is seen with primary FHV-1 infection but is less common than conjunctivitis, which reflects the marked tissue tropism of the virus.[10] Dendritic corneal ulcers may begin as multiple, superficial pinpoint ulcers that later tend to become arranged in lines with or without branching and are considered pathognomonic for FHV-1 infection. Dendritic ulcers, however, occur relatively early in the disease course and may be subtle, and so are recognized

relatively infrequently. Corneal ulcers are associated with marked corneal pain evident as blepharospasm, epiphora, and occasionally spastic entropion. FHV-1–associated ulcers may coalesce to form larger, geographic ulcers that are more obvious.

Recrudescent or Persistent Disease

In contrast to the relatively typical, dramatic, and self-limiting clinical signs observed during primary FHV-1 infection, a diverse array of clinical signs of varying severity and chronicity may be seen during recrudescent or persistent disease syndromes. Clinically detectable keratoconjunctivitis may be mini-

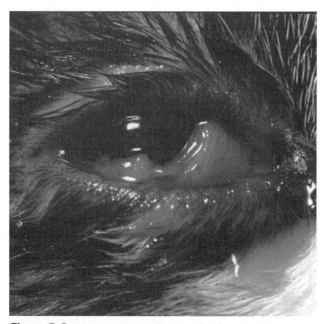

Figure 7–3. Primary FHV-1 infection. This kitten is demonstrating signs of severe primary FHV-1 infection. The serosanguineous discharge arises from ulceration of the conjunctival epithelium secondary to viral cytolysis. Purulent discharge also is evident and reflects neutrophilic infiltration. Signs are bilateral.

mal at this stage, and frequently seems disproportionate relative to the severity of ocular discomfort described by the owner or evident on examination. Conjunctivitis, rhinosinusitis, and keratitis are the dominant diseases associated with FHV-1 persistence or recrudescence. Often, it seems that disease of one of these tissues will dominate the clinical picture, occasionally in the complete absence of any signs of disease at other sites. In contrast to primary infection, disease is commonly unilateral. Conjunctivitis is usually mild and may exhibit a waxing-waning course. As with primary infection, hyperemia tends to be more obvious than chemosis. Sometimes the major clinical and historical finding will be persistent ocular discharge. Some authors believe that a dried brown discharge is particularly characteristic of herpetic conjunctivitis. Chronic herpetic keratitis may be ulcerative; however, non-ulcerative keratitis with stromal infiltration by inflammatory cells and blood vessels, and culminating in fibrosis and scarring, is more common. This lends a yellowish white hue to the cornea and may become severe enough to obstruct visualization of intraocular structures. Deep and superficial vascularization occurs frequently. Corneal and conjunctival irritation may cause significant blepharospasm, and FHV-1 infection should be suspected in cats presented with spastic entropion. The role of FHV-1 in chronic rhinosinusitis remains unresolved. Affected cats are presented for sneezing, stertorous respiration, and mucopurulent or blood-tinged nasal discharge. Chronic mucosal inflammation may be associated with distortion and remodeling of the turbinates. Tissue damage may predispose cats to excessive mucus production or ineffective clearing of secretions and development of secondary infections, particularly bacterial overgrowth. Whether active viral replication or immunopathology is involved at this point deserves further investigation.

FHV-1–Associated Syndromes

A number of ocular syndromes may be associated with FHV-1 infection. Proving a causal association between FHV-1 and these syndromes is made difficult by a number of aspects of viral behavior. First, FHV-1 can persist in epithelial tissues after primary infection without causing overt clinical signs.[9] Second, FHV-1 recrudescence can occur in the absence of clinical signs.[3] Finally, recrudescence can be elicited by sensory nerve stimulation, and thus viral presence in an inflamed eye may result from, rather than be the cause of, the primary inflammatory process.[11] With those qualifications, the following syndromes are suspected to be associated with FHV-1, because FHV-1 is detected significantly more frequently in tissues from cats with these diseases than from normal cats.

Corneal Sequestration

Corneal sequestration is an enigmatic disease of cats with a characteristic clinical appearance (Fig. 7–4).

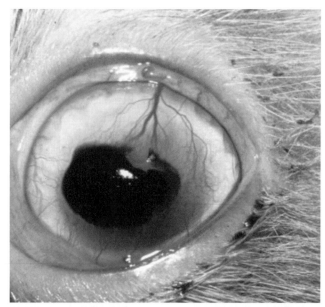

Figure 7–4. Feline corneal sequestration in a 1-year-old Himalayan cat. The black, central plaque is sequestered, necrotic corneal collagen. Note the associated corneal vascularization and edema. FHV-1 DNA has been detected in approximately 50 per cent of these lesions.

It is reported frequently in Himalayan and Persian cats, but may occur in any breed. An amber-to-black plaque develops in the central-to-paracentral cornea, and frequently is associated with blepharospasm, epiphora, and keratoconjunctivitis. Histologically, the lesion consists of an area of stroma that has undergone coagulation necrosis and has become sequestered from surrounding viable stroma. The characteristic color is due to a soluble pigment presumably present in the tear film. The onset is usually gradual, and in most cases a period of chronic corneal ulceration is noted before sequestrum formation. FHV-1 frequently is suspected as the cause of preceding chronic ulceration, and experimentally, sequestra can be induced in cats infected with FHV-1, especially when glucocorticoids have been administered.[4] More recently, FHV-1 DNA was demonstrated in 55 per cent of 156 corneal sequestrum biopsies.[12] By comparison, only 6 per cent of normal corneas contained viral DNA. When compared with domestic breed cats, FHV-1 DNA was isolated from significantly fewer corneal sequestra from brachycephalic cats. This suggests that corneal sequestration may be induced by ulcerative stimuli other than FHV-1, and that the conformation of cats with more exposed eyes predisposes them to a variety of other causes in addition to FHV-1.

Feline Eosinophilic Keratitis

In the same study, FHV-1 DNA was detected in corneal scrapings from 76 per cent of 59 cats with feline eosinophilic keratitis.[12] This is a proliferative keratitis characterized clinically by chronic, progressive development of a pink, raised lesion begin-

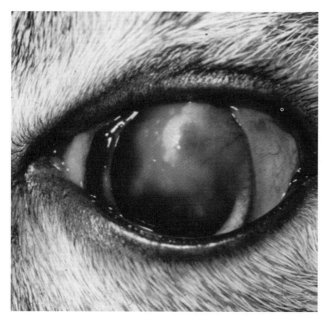

Figure 7–5. Feline eosinophilic keratitis is a raised, somewhat chalky plaque with surrounding areas of corneal ulceration and neovascularization. FHV-1 DNA has been detected in approximately 75 per cent of these lesions.

ning at the limbus and spreading over 1 or both corneas (Fig. 7–5). Histologically, focal stromal accumulations of eosinophils and mast cells, along with a diffuse infiltration of lymphocytes, plasma cells, macrophages, and neutrophils, are seen in association with corneal neovascularization. Although this study did not provide definitive proof of a causal association between FHV-1 and eosinophilic keratitis or corneal sequestration, the implantation of viral antigen within the corneal stroma would be a potent drive for such immune-mediated pathology. Future studies using in situ PCR may assist in localizing viral DNA in biopsy specimens from cats with these diseases.

Idiopathic Uveitis

Recently, PCR was used to demonstrate FHV-1 DNA in aqueous humor samples from cats with idiopathic uveitis.[13] This study also examined intraocular production of FHV-1–specific antibody, and determined that only cats with uveitis produced intraocular FHV-1–specific antibody. Further, cats with idiopathic uveitis produced significantly greater concentrations of intraocular FHV-1–specific antibodies than cats with toxoplasmic uveitis. Jointly, these data indicate that intraocular infection with FHV-1 does occur, and that this virus may be associated with uveitis in some cats. Further studies will be required to establish whether the association is causal, and if so, whether viral replication within intraocular epithelia or immune-mediated pathology is responsible for uveal inflammation. This information will be important in guiding therapeutic decisions.

◆ DIFFERENTIAL DIAGNOSES

Major Pathogens

There are 3 major pathogens that are the most likely differential diagnoses for a cat with acute upper respiratory tract and ocular disease: FHV-1, feline calicivirus (FCV), and *Chlamydia psittaci.* The 2 viruses have approximately equal prevalence and are estimated to account for about 90 per cent of all feline upper respiratory infections, whereas *Chlamydia* is thought to be less common.[14] Table 7–1 summarizes the major signs that assist in the clinical differentiation of these 3 agents. Primary FHV-1 infection is suggested by a more severely affected animal with marked sneezing and keratoconjunctivitis; presence of ulcerative keratitis is particularly pathognomonic. FCV typically produces a less severe upper respiratory syndrome, but commonly induces ulceration of the nasal planum or oral cavity, especially the tongue. FCV is not a significant conjunctival pathogen and does not cause keratitis. *C. psittaci* can cause conjunctivitis in cats. However, its incidence appears to show some seasonal variation, and the organism can be isolated from the conjunctival fornix of apparently normal cats.[15] Chlamydiosis originally was associated with severe lower respiratory tract signs; however, experimental studies and the identification of the respiratory viruses have confirmed that the predominant clinical syndrome is one of persistent, recurrent conjunctivitis with or without rhinitis.[16] Conjunctivitis may be unilateral at first but frequently becomes bilateral. Chemosis is predominant, and follicular hyperplasia can be a feature of more chronic disease. Keratitis is not a feature of chlamydial disease. Coinfection with FHV-1 and *C. psittaci* is demonstrated rarely.[15, 17]

Minor Pathogens

The importance of *Mycoplasma* as a primary ocular pathogen remains controversial. Although *Myco-*

Table 7–1. Clinical Signs That May Assist With the Differential Diagnosis of Acute Rhinitis and Keratoconjunctivitis in Cats

Clinical Signs	FHV-1	FCV	*Chlamydia*
Malaise/anorexia	+ + +	+ +	±
Sneezing	+ + +	+	+ +
Nasal discharge	+ + +	+ +	+ +
Oral ulceration	–	+ + +	–
Ptyalism	+	+ + +	±
Ocular discharge	+ + +	+	+ +
Conjunctivitis	+ + + (Hyperemic)	–	+ + + (Chemotic)
Keratitis	+ + +	–	–

Abbreviations: FCV, feline calicivirus; FHV-1, feline herpesvirus-1.
Modified from Gaskell RM, Dawson S: Viral-induced upper respiratory tract disease. *In* Chandler EA, Gaskell CJ, Gaskell RM (eds): Feline Medicine and Therapeutics, 2nd ed. Boston, Blackwell Scientific, 1994, p. 458.

plasma species can be found in conjunctival fornices of normal cats, they are found more frequently in cats with conjunctivitis. Infection can be induced after experimental inoculation, especially in younger kittens, but disease usually is mild and self-limiting. Signs of lower respiratory tract involvement and keratitis usually are absent. Although natural transfer of infection from inoculated cats to cohabiting cats can occur, clinical disease is not apparent in the naturally infected cats.[18] Mycoplasmal conjunctivitis has been described as unilateral or bilateral with initially hyperemic but later paler, chemotic conjunctival surfaces. Lymphoid follicles and papillary hypertrophy are reported. Ocular discharge initially is serous, but can become mucopurulent and occasionally form pseudomembranes.

Bacteria are common secondary invaders of both the feline conjunctival sac and the feline upper respiratory system. Their primary significance is questionable, however, in an otherwise healthy eye. *Bordetella bronchiseptica* may be an exception. This organism has been associated with respiratory disease, especially in cats in more crowded environments.[19] Some affected cats have had ocular signs such as conjunctivitis; however, the exclusion of other known causes of conjunctivitis is essential before more definitive comments can be made regarding this organism's primary role in feline ocular surface disease. Coinfection with feline leukemia virus or feline immunodeficiency virus could potentiate other infectious diseases; however, clinically and experimentally, the relationship seems to be of relatively minor importance.[17, 20]

◆ DIAGNOSIS

A major paradox exists with respect to the diagnosis of FHV-1. Cats experiencing primary FHV-1 infection shed virus in sufficient quantities that viral detection is relatively easy. However, clinical signs during this phase of infection tend to be characteristic and self-limiting, making definitive diagnosis less necessary. By contrast, the diversity and ambiguity of clinical signs of the more chronic FHV-1–associated syndromes make viral identification important if specific antiviral therapy is to be attempted; however, the virus is difficult to detect. The diagnosis of FHV-1 in individual cats represents one of the greatest challenges in the management of chronic FHV-1–related diseases. Although the extreme sensitivity of PCR has improved detection of virus, it also has confirmed that virus can be demonstrated in a number of apparently normal cats.[8, 9, 12, 13] This must be considered when interpreting results of this assay in diseased cats. However, from a clinical standpoint, the relevant issue relates to those cases in which FHV-1 is present in a cat with evidence of disease. The clinician then must consider whether specific antiviral treatment is warranted regardless of whether the virus is there as a cause or an effect of the primary disease process. The assays in common use for the diagnosis of FHV-1 rely on demonstration of an immunologic response (usually in serum) to the organism, or detection of the virus by culture (virus isolation), the immunofluorescent antibody (IFA) test, or PCR.

FHV-1 seroprevalence generally is high in the feline population because of the ubiquitous nature of the virus and the frequency with which vaccination is practiced. Therefore, presence or absence of a titer is not useful in the diagnosis of FHV-1 in individual cats. Serum neutralization (SN) and enzyme-linked immunosorbent assay (ELISA) titer magnitudes have been shown to vary greatly but independent of the presence or absence of clinical evidence of FHV-1–related disease.[1]

Virus isolation (VI) may be attempted from oropharyngeal or conjunctival swab samples placed in viral transport media, and transported promptly on ice to a laboratory where they are grown in cell culture and examined daily for the characteristic cytopathic effect. Primary limitations include the delay in receiving a diagnosis, and false-negative results in cats with chronic disease that presumably are shedding relatively little virus. Samples should be collected using Dacron or cotton swabs, because calcium alginate swabs can inhibit viral growth. Samples must be collected before application of fluorescein or rose bengal stains, which can inhibit viral replication. For IFA testing, conjunctival or corneal cells collected by scraping are spread as thinly as possible on a microscope slide. After air-drying, slides are sent to a laboratory for direct or indirect IFA testing. An experienced technician assesses cells for the presence of specific perinuclear or cell membrane fluorescence. It is important to collect samples before the instillation of fluorescein dye, because this will interfere with the interpretation of the IFA test.

The results of VI and IFA were assessed prospectively in a large group of healthy cats and cats with signs of primary or recrudescent FHV-1 infection.[1] Owing to the relatively high frequency with which FHV-1 could be detected by VI and by IFA in samples collected from clinically normal cats, there was no significant difference in viral detection rates between diseased cats and healthy cats. Consequently, sensitivity, specificity, negative predictive value, and positive predictive value never simultaneously exceeded 50 per cent for either assay. However, FHV-1 was never detected by both methods in healthy cats, and so negative results in both tests may allow exclusion of the diagnosis.

PCR involves the isolation and amplification of specific target areas of DNA from a background of host and irrelevant DNA. Owing to repeated doubling of DNA during each cycle, the amount of target DNA can be amplified exponentially. This creates exquisite sensitivity but also requires exemplary laboratory conditions and strict adherence to protocols, especially the inclusion of positive and negative controls. A number of different protocols for

FHV-1 PCR have been described in the literature, and some of these are available on a commercial basis.[8, 9, 15, 20–22] Because FHV-1 is an obligate intracellular organism, the more host cells that are submitted, the more chance that viral DNA will be detected. With respect to ocular samples, this means that biopsies (conjunctival "snip" biopsies or keratectomy specimens) would be expected to contain more DNA than cytologic scrapings, which in turn would contain more DNA than swab specimens. This information, along with the fact that up to 31 per cent of normal conjunctival samples[21, 22] and 6 per cent of normal corneal samples[12] may contain FHV-1 DNA, dictates that positive test results be interpreted in light of laboratory normals for the same tissue type that is submitted.

Cytology may be useful in the diagnosis of cats with chronic conjunctivitis; however, it has little specific merit for the diagnosis of FHV-1. The majority of cats with FHV-1 conjunctivitis demonstrate nonspecific, neutrophilic inflammation. The major indication for cytologic assessment of conjunctival scrapings is detection of chlamydial or mycoplasmal inclusion bodies.

◆ TREATMENT

Supportive Therapy

Supportive therapy is the mainstay of treatment for primary FHV-1 infections, because these usually are self-limiting. Major goals of supportive therapy should be prevention of secondary bacterial infection, especially of the lower respiratory tract, and maintenance of adequate nutrition, hydration, and patient comfort. A warm, humid, and well-ventilated environment is essential. The eyes and nares should be kept clear of discharge both for patient comfort and to allow better penetration and efficacy of topical medications. Nebulization, steam inhalation, and adequate hydration will aid in the loosening and expectoration of secretions. Supplementation of the tear film with lubricant drops or ointments should be considered, particularly in cats with keratoconjunctivitis sicca. Appetite may be stimulated by offering warmed, strongly flavored, and aromatic foods. Systemic and ophthalmic antibiotics should be considered to control secondary bacterial infection and to limit chronic sequelae. Tetracyclines or chloramphenicol are effective against *C. psittaci, Mycoplasma* species, and many other common ocular and respiratory pathogens; however, the potential for tetracyclines to discolor the teeth of young cats should not be overlooked. Azithromycin is a relatively new antichlamydial drug that accumulates preferentially within human ocular tissues. Therapeutic concentrations have been demonstrated for 4 days in tears and for 14 days in conjunctiva after a single oral dose.[23] Azithromycin also is absorbed rapidly and effectively after oral dosing in cats, and protracted tissue

half-lives have been demonstrated; however, conjunctiva was not assayed specifically.[24] Initial anecdotal evidence suggests that this drug may be useful for the treatment of cats with chlamydial conjunctivitis. The antibiotics in commonly used "triple antibiotic" ophthalmic preparations (neomycin, polymyxin, bacitracin/gramicidin) are not reliable for treatment of *C. psittaci* or *Mycoplasma* species.

Glucocorticoid administration can induce several deleterious effects in cats acutely infected with FHV-1, including deeper and more persistent corneal ulcers, corneal edema, corneal vascularization, sequestrum formation, and extension of the viral-shedding period.[4] For these reasons, topical or systemic glucocorticoids should never be used in cats with acute FHV-1 infections. The effect of nonsteroidal anti-inflammatory agents and cyclosporine on acute FHV-1 infections has not been examined; however, whenever ulceration or other evidence of active lytic infection is observed, anti-inflammatory medications of any type would appear to be ill-advised because they may potentiate antigen persistence and encourage penetration into the corneal stroma.

Antiviral Agents

Currently, there are no antiherpetic drugs approved for veterinary use in the United States. However, antiviral agents should be considered when signs are severe, persistent, or recurrent, or when there is corneal involvement, particularly ulceration. Because epithelial replication, latency and reactivation, and persistence are such interdependent and sequential phases of herpetic disease, interruption of any stage might be expected to limit viral association with subsequent disease. Therefore, aggressive treatment of FHV-1 may limit disease progression and minimize frequency and severity of recurrences. Some important general concepts about antiviral agents assist with selection and expectations of this class of drugs. Because viruses reside intracellularly and utilize host cellular machinery, antiviral agents tend to induce greater host toxicity than do antibacterial drugs. This rarely limits topical application of these drugs, but may severely limit systemic use. Most antiviral agents in common use are virostatic, and therefore require relatively frequent dosing or topical application. In some cases, hourly application of ophthalmic preparations is recommended for at least the first 24 hours of therapy.

The effect of 4 antiviral drugs on FHV-1 replication in vitro has been studied and the relative potency reported as trifluridine >> idoxuridine > vidarabine >> acyclovir.[25] These drugs have received relatively widespread clinical use over a number of years—the first 3 as topical agents and acyclovir as a systemic drug. In some countries, acyclovir also is available as an ophthalmic medication; however, reports of its veterinary use appear to be lacking at this time. Idoxuridine (Herplex or

Stoxil) no longer is commercially available, but compounding pharmacists can formulate a 0.1 per cent ophthalmic solution.

The superior potency and corneal penetration of trifluridine suggest that it should be the first choice for topical therapy. However, cats often show marked aversion to application of this drug, suggesting that it is irritating. It is available as a 1 per cent solution (Viroptic), and recently was released in less expensive generic preparations. Trifluridine should be applied every hour for the first day and every 4 hours thereafter. Idoxuridine may be a more practical choice in veterinary patients owing to high clinical efficacy, lower cost, and reduced irritancy. Treatment with idoxuridine initially is recommended every 2 to 4 hours. Vidarabine is available as a 3 per cent ointment (Vira-A), and use of an ointment may be particularly helpful when kerato-conjunctivitis sicca is apparent. Treatment is recommended at least 4 times daily. Therapy with any of these drugs should be continued for at least 1 week beyond resolution of ocular lesions. Typically, this is for 2 to 3 weeks. An apparent "rebound" of clinical signs has been reported when treatment of HSV-1 infections is terminated in human beings. This does not appear to be a frequent or severe problem in cats, but should be considered in cats with rapidly worsening disease immediately after treatment is terminated.

Acyclovir (Zovirax) is the only systemic antiherpetic drug that has received adequate clinical and research attention in veterinary medicine. Acyclovir must be phosphorylated before activation, with the initial phosphorylation step catalyzed by viral thymidine kinase. It appears that the capacity of FHV-1 thymidine kinase is limited in this regard when compared with HSV-1, leading to unexpectedly poor efficacy against FHV-1 relative to HSV-1. Poor bioavailability further limits use of this drug in cats.[26] Cats receiving doses as high as 100 mg/kg failed to attain plasma acyclovir concentrations that approximate the median effective dose for FHV-1, and some cats showed toxic effects at this dose. The principal toxic effects seen in cats are leukopenia and anemia. Although normalization of the complete blood count usually accompanies withdrawal of acyclovir therapy and appropriate supportive care, toxicity significantly influences the choice of this drug for treatment of FHV-1 in cats. Current recommendations are that treatment should not be initiated in cats with leukopenia, and a complete blood count should be examined regularly throughout the treatment period. Valacyclovir is an acyclovir pro-drug that has superior bioavailability in cats, but does not reduce viral replication. In addition, valacyclovir can induce fatal myeloid dysplasia and subsequent leukopenia and should not be used in cats.[27]

Novel antiviral agents currently are being investigated owing to emergence of acyclovir-resistant strains of HSV-1, and to increasing morbidity and frequency of herpetic infections in immuno-compromised human beings. Because these drugs are likely to be unrelated pharmacologically to acyclovir, it is possible that veterinarians will gain some useful drugs for the treatment of FHV-1 in this process. However, awareness that some drugs developed for treatment of HSV-1 have proved to be ineffectual or even fatal in cats infected with FHV-1 will necessitate careful investigation of these new therapies before their widespread clinical use.

Adjunctive Therapies

Cats that experience frequent herpetic recurrences can be extremely frustrating to treat. The unpredictable nature of recrudescent disease episodes has led some practitioners to use chronic antiviral therapy to minimize clinical signs in these patients. However, efficacy, toxicity, availability, and cost of many antiviral agents can make this an unrealistic option. This has led to increasing interest in adjunctive therapies for the treatment of FHV-1. Lysine has been used to limit herpetic episodes in human beings by antagonizing the availability of arginine, which is an essential amino acid for viral protein synthesis. Human patients, therefore, have been advised to minimize arginine intake while taking lysine.[28] Early data suggest that lysine may exert a similar effect on FHV-1 replication in vitro, but also only in the presence of low concentrations of arginine.[29] This interaction was a concern in cats, given their exquisite sensitivity to arginine deficiency. However, a preliminary study suggested that oral administration of lysine provided a safe and effective means for reducing spontaneous ocular viral-shedding rate in cats latently infected with FHV-1 without inducing significant changes in plasma arginine levels.[30] The current recommendation is to administer 250 mg of lysine orally every (q) 12 hr.

Interferons are a group of related cytokines that have diverse immunologic and antiviral functions. Interferon alpha (INF-α) is released by white blood cells during viral infection and appears to decrease cell-to-cell spread of virus. Numerous studies suggest that INF-α may have a role in the control of alphaherpesvirus infections, particularly during the acute phase. Specifically, oral administration of low doses of INF (5 or 25 units daily) has been associated with reduced clinical disease but not decreased FHV-1 shedding rates.[31] INF-α is unstable once thawed, which should be addressed with respect to dispensing practices for this drug. In vitro data suggest that human recombinant INF-α reduces by a factor of 8 the concentration of acyclovir required to inhibit FHV-1 in tissue culture.[32] At this time, INF-α and lysine should be considered adjunctive therapies either to potentiate other treatments or to lessen the likelihood of FHV-1 recrudescence. Further controlled studies are required to verify whether these drugs exert any clinically useful effects in cats affected by chronic or recrudescent herpesvirus infection.

Controlled studies in HSV-1 support the use of corticosteroids and other anti-inflammatory agents in treatment of chronic immunologic herpetic disease, usually in conjunction with a potent antiviral agent. Owing to its relatively specific T-cell suppression, cyclosporine has been a useful adjunct to antiviral therapy in more chronic, immune-mediated herpetic disease.[33] However, use of these drugs in chronic feline herpetic disease has been studied inadequately.

Treatment of Chronic Rhinitis

The role of FHV-1 in chronic rhinosinusitis is largely speculative, therefore treatment currently is symptomatic. To maintain hydration of the nasal cavity and enhance removal of nasal mucus, saline nasal drops may be used daily in the nostrils. Systemic antibiotics are recommended to treat secondary infection. Whereas antibiotics frequently reduce the severity of nasal discharge, signs usually return after cessation of treatment. If turbinate involvement is suspected, prolonged courses of appropriate antibiotics (16 weeks) may be necessary. The efficacy of antiviral medications in treating nasal disease is unknown. One study showed no significant difference between clinical improvement in cats treated subcutaneously with 10 mg/kg acyclovir q 8 hr for 7 days when compared with controls.[34]

◆ CONTROL AND VACCINATION

The diagnosis of herpes-related disease in 1 cat from a multicat household frequently elicits questions from owners regarding the need to "quarantine" such animals. Cats suffering primary infection and presumably shedding large quantities of virus probably should be isolated while showing clinical signs. By contrast, chronically affected cats, especially those demonstrating immunopathologic syndromes, probably do not need to be isolated because they are unlikely to be shedding virus in significant quantities and because other felids within the household are likely already infected. The disadvantages of the stress of any major management changes, especially in large groups or catteries, must also be weighed against any advantage gained from isolation of affected animals.

The principal method of control of FHV-1 in the general feline population has been vaccination. Undoubtedly, one of the reasons this has been relatively successful is the genetic homogeneity of the virus even when isolates from different continents are compared. Recent recommendations for reduced vaccination frequency have promoted renewed consideration of the cost-benefit ratio of vaccination, along with safety and efficacy of the products used. In the case of FHV-1, a number of points are of particular relevance. First, FHV-1 generally causes self-limiting disease with high morbidity but rare mortality. Second, the majority of cats become lifelong but "silent" carriers of the virus, and the ability of vaccines to reduce establishment of latency or frequency of reactivation has not been shown. Lastly, many chronic FHV-1–related diseases may represent an exuberant or aberrant immune response to viral antigen rather than an inadequate protective response. As such, frequent stimulation of humoral and cell-mediated immunity may be contraindicated. Any effect that reduced FHV-1 vaccination frequency may exert on the epidemiology of FHV-1–related disease remains to be seen.

Current vaccination strategies for FHV-1 include the use of modified-live, inactivated, or genetically modified virus administered by injection (subcutaneously or intramuscularly) or topically (conjunctivally or intranasally). Mucosally administered vaccines appear to have certain merit in the prevention of FHV-1 because the virus gains entry, replicates, and recurs at mucosal sites and because mucosal associated lymphoid tissue of the conjunctiva and respiratory tract fulfills distinct and frequently advantageous immunologic functions (Table 7–2). Mucosal vaccination induces systemic immunity and mucosal immunity both at the site of inoculation and at distant mucosal sites. The onset of mucosal immunity is relatively rapid, with development of partial immunity within 2 days and complete immunity in approximately 4 days.[35] It is suggested that maternal immunity is less likely to interfere with mucosal vaccination than systemic vaccination, allowing relatively early vaccination of kittens believed to be at risk. When compared with injectable vaccines, mucosal vaccination is believed to be associated with a higher but infrequent (1.6 to 4.3 per cent) rate of very mild side-effects. Of major current interest is the role of the various vaccine viruses and adjuvants in the formation of postvaccinal sarcomas (see Chapters 1, Update on Vaccine-Associated Sarcomas and Current Vaccine Recommendations, and 69, Update on Vaccine-Associated Sarcomas). Whereas the involvement of other vaccines appears more likely, the development of postvaccinal sarcomas that are spatially and temporally

Table 7–2. Comparison of the Mucosal and Systemic Routes of Feline Herpesvirus-1 Vaccination

Feature	Vaccine Route	
	Mucosal	*Systemic*
Onset of immunity	Rapid	Slower
Postvaccinal sarcoma	Not recognized	Possible
Postvaccinal disease	2–4%	Rare
Potential for spread of vaccine virus	Possible	Unlikely
Generation of mucosal immunity	+	?
Generation of systemic immunity	+	+
Anamnestic response demonstrated	?	+

related to trivalent (panleukopenia/calicivirus/herpesvirus) vaccine administration has been reported.[36] Mucosal administration of vaccines would be expected to militate against postvaccinal sarcoma formation.

Until recently, vaccine studies have tended to emphasize the dramatic reduction in severity of clinical disease when animals are challenged at varying periods after vaccination. Most FHV-1 vaccines show good efficacy if this is the only criterion assessed. However, little attention has been given to vaccine effect on establishment of latency or limitation of future shedding. Latency and shedding of either the vaccine or challenge strains may be of particular epidemiologic importance with FHV-1. These issues were examined in a study in which cats were vaccinated topically with a temperature-sensitive mutant virus and monitored for FHV-1 shedding using VI and PCR for 13 weeks.[37] During this period, half of the cats were challenged with a field strain at 28 days after vaccination, and viral reactivation was induced in all cats at 56 days after vaccination. All cats shed the vaccine virus from oropharyngeal or conjunctival tissues at multiple times after vaccination, most for the duration of the experiment (13 weeks). Vaccination did not significantly reduce the amount of virus shed after challenge, and vaccine virus accounted for 32 per cent of all virus shed. Vaccination also did not significantly reduce the amount of virus shed after reactivation. At necropsy, vaccine virus was identified in the same tissues and at the same frequency as wild-type virus. Persistent or latent virus was detected in neuronal (trigeminal ganglia, optic nerve, olfactory bulb) and extraneuronal (cornea, nasal turbinates, and tonsil) sites. Taken together, these data suggest that this intranasal vaccination did reduce clinical evidence of disease, but did not limit establishment of latency, reactivation from latency, or viral shedding after challenge. The finding that vaccine virus itself establishes latency and is shed from conjunctival fornices and the oropharynx suggests that it could be a source of antigen and cause or exacerbate chronic herpetic disease, or be detected by diagnostic assays and alter their interpretation.

A recent study of duration of immunity for FHV-1 vaccination administered subcutaneously to young kittens provides further interesting information.[38] Whereas antibody titers appeared to wane rapidly between 6 and 7.5 years, cats showed a rapid and exaggerated anamnestic humoral response on challenge even in the absence of a detectable prechallenge titer. Even 7.5 years after vaccination, clinical evidence of disease after challenge was reduced by approximately half and fatalities were prevented. Importantly, though, from an epidemiologic standpoint, vaccination did not reduce the amount or duration of virus shed after challenge.

The perfect vaccine for FHV-1 would prevent clinical evidence of disease and block establishment of latency in cats challenged with wild-type virus for a long period after vaccination. Additionally, it would do this without causing adverse side-effects and without establishing latency and being shed itself. Currently, such a vaccine does not exist. Given the constraints and advantages of the currently available vaccines, results of these 2 studies appear to support current recommendations for reduction in FHV-1 vaccination frequency.

REFERENCES

1. Maggs DJ, Lappin MR, Reif JS, et al: Evaluation of serologic and viral detection methods for diagnosing feline herpesvirus-1 infection in cats with acute respiratory or chronic ocular disease. J Am Vet Med Assoc 214:502–507, 1999.
2. Wardley RC, Povey RC: The pathology and sites of persistence associated with three different strains of feline calicivirus. Res Vet Sci 23:15–19, 1977.
3. Gaskell RM, Povey RC: Experimental induction of feline viral rhinotracheitis virus re-excretion in FVR recovered cats. Vet Rec 100:128–133, 1977.
4. Nasisse MP, Guy JS, Davidson MG, et al: Experimental ocular herpesvirus infection in the cat. Sites of virus replication, clinical features and effects of corticosteroid administration. Invest Ophthalmol Vis Sci 30:1758–1768, 1989.
5. Nasisse MP, Davis BJ, Guy JS, et al: Isolation of feline herpesvirus 1 from the trigeminal ganglia of acutely and chronically infected cats. J Vet Intern Med 6:102–103, 1992.
6. Hill TJ: Herpes simplex virus latency. In Roizman B (ed): The Herpesviruses, vol. 3. New York, Plenum, 1985, pp. 175–240.
7. Maggs DJ, Chang E, Nasisse MP, et al: Persistence of herpes simplex virus type 1 DNA in chronic conjunctival and eyelid lesions of mice. J Virol 72:9166–9172, 1998.
8. Weigler BJ, Babineau CA, Sherry B, et al: High sensitivity polymerase chain reaction assay for active and latent feline herpesvirus-1 infections in domestic cats. Vet Rec 140:335–338, 1997.
9. Reubel GH, Ramos RA, Hickman MA, et al: Detection of active and latent feline herpesvirus 1 infections using the polymerase chain reaction. Arch Virol 132:409–420, 1993.
10. Nasisse MP, English RV, Tompkins MB, et al: Immunologic, histologic, and virologic features of herpesvirus-induced stromal keratitis in cats. Am J Vet Res 56:51–55, 1995.
11. Anderson WA, Margruder B, Kilbourne ED: Induced reactivation of herpes simplex virus in healed rabbit corneal lesions. Proc Soc Exp Biol Med 107:628–632, 1961.
12. Nasisse MP, Glover TL, Moore CP, et al: Detection of feline herpesvirus 1 DNA in corneas of cats with eosinophilic keratitis or corneal sequestration. Am J Vet Res 59:856–858, 1998.
13. Maggs DJ, Lappin MR, Nasisse MP: Detection of feline herpesvirus–specific antibodies and DNA in aqueous humor from cats with or without uveitis. Am J Vet Res 60:932–936, 1999.
14. Ott RL: Viral diseases. In Catcott EJ (ed): Feline Medicine and Surgery, 2nd ed. Santa Barbara, CA, American Veterinary Publications, 1975, p. 19.
15. Sykes JE, Anderson GA, Studdert VP, et al: Prevalence of feline Chlamydia psittaci and feline herpesvirus 1 in cats with upper respiratory tract disease. J Vet Intern Med 13:153–162, 1999.
16. Sykes JE, Studdert VP, Browning GF: Comparison of the polymerase chain reaction and culture for the detection of feline Chlamydia psittaci in untreated and doxycycline-treated experimentally infected cats. J Vet Intern Med 13:146–152, 1999.
17. Nasisse MP, Guy JS, Stevens JB, et al: Clinical and laboratory findings in chronic conjunctivitis in cats: 91 cases (1983–1991). J Am Vet Med Assoc 203:834–837, 1993.
18. Haesebrouck F, Devriese LA, van Rijssen B, et al: Incidence and significance of isolation of Mycoplasma felis from conjunctival swabs of cats. Vet Microbiol 26:95–101, 1991.
19. Welsh RD: Bordetella bronchiseptica infections in cats. J Am Anim Hosp Assoc 32:153–158, 1996.

20. Reubel GH, George JW, Barlough JE, et al: Interaction of acute feline herpesvirus-1 and chronic feline immunodeficiency virus infections in experimentally infected specific pathogen free cats. Vet Immunol Immunopathol 35:95–119, 1992.
21. Stiles J, McDermott M, Willis M, et al: Use of nested polymerase chain reaction to identify feline herpesvirus in ocular tissues from clinically normal cats and cats with corneal sequestra or conjunctivitis. Am J Vet Res 58:338–342, 1997.
22. Burgesser KM, Hotaling S, Schiebel A, et al: Comparison of PCR, virus isolation, and indirect fluorescent antibody staining in the detection of naturally occurring feline herpesvirus infections. J Vet Diagn Invest 11:122–126, 1999.
23. Tabbara KF, Al-Kharashi SA, Al-Mansouri SM, et al: Ocular levels of azithromycin. Arch Ophthalmol 116:1625–1628, 1998.
24. Hunter RP, Lynch MJ, Ericson JF, et al: Pharmacokinetics, oral bioavailability and tissue distribution of azithromycin in cats. J Vet Pharmacol Ther 18:38–46, 1995.
25. Nasisse MP, Guy JS, Davidson MG, et al: In vitro susceptibility of feline herpesvirus-1 to vidarabine, idoxuridine, trifluridine, acyclovir, or bromovinyldeoxyuridine. Am J Vet Res 50:158–160, 1989.
26. Owens JG, Nasisse MP, Tadepalli SM, et al: Pharmacokinetics of acyclovir in the cat. J Vet Pharmacol Ther 19:488–490, 1996.
27. Nasisse MP, Dorman D, Weigler BJ, et al: Effects of valacyclovir in cats infected with feline herpesvirus 1. Am J Vet Res 58:1141–1144, 1997.
28. Griffith RS, Walsh DE, Myrmel KH, et al: Success of L-lysine therapy in frequently recurrent herpes simplex infection. Dermatologica 175:183–190, 1987.
29. Maggs DJ, Collins BK, Thorne JG, et al: Effects of L-lysine and L-arginine on in vitro replication of feline herpesvirus type-1. Am J Vet Res (in press).
30. Maggs DJ, Nasisse MP: Effects of oral L-lysine supplementation on the ocular shedding rate of feline herpesvirus (FHV-1) in cats. Proceedings American College of Veterinary Ophthalmologists, 28th Annual Meeting, Santa Fe, NM, November 1997.
31. Nasisse MP, Halenda RM, Luo H: Efficacy of low dose oral, natural human interferon alpha (nHuIFNα) in acute feline herpesvirus 1 (FHV-1) infection, a preliminary dose determination trial. Proceedings American College of Veterinary Ophthalmologists, 27th Annual Meeting, Newport, RI, November 1996.
32. Weiss RC: Synergistic antiviral activities of acyclovir and recombinant human leukocyte (alpha) interferon on feline herpesvirus replication. Am J Vet Res 50:1672–1677, 1989.
33. Gunduz K, Ozdemir O: Topical cyclosporine as an adjunct to topical acyclovir treatment in herpetic stromal keratitis. Ophthalmic Res 29:405–408, 1997.
34. Harder TC, Findik A, Nolte I, et al: Investigation of the spectrum of viral causative agents within the scope of the upper respiratory disease complex in cats. Treatment experiments with the antiherpesvirus agent acyclovir (Zovirax). Kleintier-Prax 39:93–106, 1994.
35. Cocker FM, Gaskell RM, Newby TJ, et al: Efficacy of early (48 and 96 hour) protection against feline viral rhinotracheitis virus following intranasal vaccination with a live temperature sensitive mutant. Vet Rec 114:353–354, 1984.
36. Burton G, Mason KV: Do postvaccinal sarcomas occur in Australian cats? Aust Vet J 75:102–106, 1997.
37. Weigler BJ, Guy JS, Nasisse MP, et al: Effect of a live attenuated intranasal vaccine on latency and shedding of feline herpesvirus 1 in domestic cats. Arch Virol 142:2389–2400, 1997.
38. Scott FW, Geissinger CM: Long-term immunity in cats vaccinated with an inactivated trivalent vaccine. Am J Vet Res 60:652–658, 1999.

8

◆ Feline Spongiform Encephalopathy and Borna Disease

Danièlle Gunn-Moore

David A. Harbour

Since about 1990, there has been a dramatic increase in our recognition and understanding of infectious diseases that can affect the central nervous system (CNS). This results largely from advances in molecular technology, which have improved our ability to detect pathogens within the CNS. New infectious diseases have been recognized in most animal species, and our understanding of the etiopathogenesis of previously discovered infections is expanding. By studying the genetic relationship among these pathogens, and performing infectivity studies, a number of infectious agents have been identified that can cross species barriers and raise the possibility of zoonotic infection. Two such diseases are discussed in this chapter; feline spongiform encephalopathy (FSE) and Borna disease (BD). In both cases, the agents can infect a number of mammalian species, including human beings. Both infections have a poorly understood etiopathogenesis, and both may result in terminal neurologic disease. See Table 8–1 for a summary of FSE and feline BD.

◆ FELINE SPONGIFORM ENCEPHALOPATHY

FSE was first recognized in 1990 during the bovine spongiform encephalopathy (BSE) epidemic in the United Kingdom.[1–3] FSE is one of a group of naturally occurring transmissible spongiform encephalopathies (TSEs). TSEs occur in many mammalian species, including human beings.[4] Most TSEs are seen in ruminants, with scrapie in sheep and goats, BSE in cattle, and similar diseases being seen in a number of captive exotic ungulates.[5, 6] TSEs also have been seen in mink (transmissible mink encephalopathy)[7]; captive exotic cat species, including cheetah,[6, 8, 9] puma,[6, 10] lion (AL Meredith, University of Edinburgh, personal communication, 1999), ocelot, and tiger [10a]; and possibly, ostrich.[8] TSEs in human beings include Creutzfeldt-Jakob disease (CJD), Gerstmann-Sträussler-Scheinker disease (GSS), and kuru.[11] Experimentally, TSEs can be transmitted to an even wider range of species, including rodents and nonhuman primates.[12–14] Whereas the widespread interest in TSEs developed only recently, mainly associated with the BSE epidemic and the recognition of a variant CJD (vCJD), this type of disease is far from new. Historical records show that scrapie was first recognized almost 300 years ago.[15]

Epizootiology

TSEs have been seen in many countries throughout the world. However, whereas scrapie and human TSEs have a widespread distribution, BSE has been seen mainly in Europe, particularly in the United Kingdom. The situation with FSE is similar to that with BSE, with all but 3 cases in domestic cats being seen in Great Britain. All 3 of these cases occurred on continental Europe, and 2 of the cats were believed to have been fed British cat food or had access to bovine offal.[10a, 16] The other was a cat in Italy. This cat was unusual, because it and its owner appear to have been affected by a strain of TSE that is associated more typically with spontaneous CJD.[17] However, the accuracy of the diagnosis for both the cat and its owner has since been questioned.[10a] All of the captive exotic felids that have developed FSE have been fed on tissue from British cattle (AL Meredith, University of Edinburgh, personal communication, 1999).[6, 8–10]

In order to understand the epizootiology of FSE, it is necessary to understand how BSE is believed to have originated. BSE was first reported in 1987, in the United Kingdom.[18] It is believed to have resulted from the inclusion of scrapie-infected sheep carcasses, in the form of meat and bonemeal, into feedstuffs for cattle.[19] A change in the rendering process of meat and bonemeal had enabled the TSE agent, which is highly heat-resistant, to survive the processing procedures.[19] Transmitting the scrapie agent through cattle is believed to have altered its pathogenicity, making it more infectious to cattle (and cats). Cattle succumbing to BSE were then included into the meat and bonemeal, thereby amplifying the transmission and spreading the infection.[19, 20] Once this epidemiologic pattern was determined, the feeding of meat and bonemeal to ruminants was banned in 1988. After a delay of 5 to 7 years, which is believed to be the incubation period for this infection, the incidence of BSE began to plateau and then fall.[21, 22]

The agent responsible for FSE is believed to be the same as for BSE. In mouse inoculation studies, the FSE and BSE agents have the same incubation period, whereas the scrapie agent is different.[14, 22a] The BSE agent is believed to have entered the U.K. cat population in pet food containing contaminated meat and bonemeal. To prevent further exposure, the Pet Food Manufacturers Association recommended to its members in 1988 that "specified bo-

Table 8–1. Comparison of Feline Spongiform Encephalopathy and Feline Borna Disease

	FSE	**Feline Borna Disease**
Etiology	PrP-res	BDV
Signalment	Adult cats, no breed predisposition; youngest 2 yr; perhaps seen more in males	Adult cats, no breed predisposition; youngest 5 mo; seen more in males
Transmission	Unknown—probably BSE agent in food	Unknown—probably BDV from asymptomatic carriers; rodents?
Incubation period	Unknown	Unknown
Geographic distribution	Great Britain	Northern and central Europe; Great Britain; worldwide?
Clinical signs (in descending order of incidence)	Ataxia: (~100%), often with hypermetria, and crouching gait	Ataxia: (~100%), often with hypermetria, and crouching gait
	Behavioral changes: (100%); increased aggression or timidity	Behavioral changes: (100%); increased aggression or timidity
	Hyperesthesia: to touch, and/or light and sound	Fever
	Polyphagia	Hyperesthesia: to touch, and/or light and sound
	Altered grooming: either increased or decreased	Intermittent pupil dilatation and staring expression
	Hypersalivation	Altered grooming: either increased or decreased
	Muscle fasciculations	Hypersalivation
	Polydipsia	Muscle fasciculations
	Intermittent pupil dilatation and staring expression	Inability to judge distances
	Inability to judge distances	Polyphagia/polydipsia
	Inability to retract claws	Inability to retract claws
	Unusual head position or carriage	Seizures
	Jaw chattering/head pressing	Constipation
Duration of disease	Progressive deterioration warranting euthanasia in weeks to months of onset of clinical signs	Usually progressive deterioration warranting euthanasia in weeks to months of onset of clinical signs; occasional cases are more chronic, or episodic
Diagnosis	Histopathology of CNS	Histopathology of CNS
Pathology	Vacuolar changes in gray matter of CNS	Nonsuppurative meningoencephalomyelitis
Zoonotic risk	Negligible?	Unknown

Abbreviations: BDV, Borna disease virus; BSE, bovine spongiform encephalopathy; CNS, central nervous system; FSE, feline spongiform encephalopathy; PrP-res, prion-protein isolated from transmissible spongiform encephalopathy–infected individuals.

vine offal" be banned from inclusion in pet food; this later became law. Subsequent changes to the handling of offal material should have removed any further risk of cats being exposed to the BSE agent in commercial pet food.

Since its recognition in 1990, 87 cases of FSE have been confirmed. The majority of these were seen between 1990 and 1994. Since that time, there has been a general decline in the number of cases, and there have been no new cases reported since early 1999 (Fig. 8–1) (JW Wilesmith, Central Veteri-

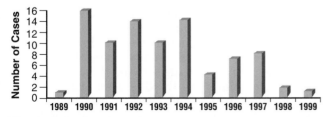

Figure 8–1. Incidence of feline spongiform encephalopathy (FSE) cases in cats in Great Britain by year of onset of clinical signs. (From Wilesmith JW, personal communication, cases confirmed by June 2000.)

nary Laboratory, Weybridge, England, personal communication, 2000). This pattern of disease supports the hypothesis that FSE is caused by the BSE agent. It shows that after a time interval representing the incubation period of the disease, the removal of specified bovine offal from the diet of cats in the United Kingdom resulted in a marked reduction in the incidence of FSE. Consistent with this hypothesis, a retrospective study of brain sections from cats with neurologic disease, which had been euthanized between 1975 and 1990, revealed no cases of FSE before 1990.[23] Because very few domestic cats are subject to routine post-mortem examination, it is likely that the total number of FSE cases has been underestimated.

Although the natural routes of TSE transmission are unclear, in animals ingestion appears to be most common. Whereas maternal transmission may occur in some species,[24] there is no evidence of it occurring in cats.[23] TSE diseases are not only infectious but also can be transmitted genetically in some cases. However, whereas this is true of certain human TSEs (e.g., GSS)[11] and for scrapie in sheep,[4] it does not appear to be the case for BSE or FSE, which appear to be transmitted only by infection.[19, 23]

Consistent with a food-related disease, FSE shows no breed predisposition, and cats from all types of households have been affected. Although FSE has been seen in both genders, it has been seen more frequently in males.[10a, 23] The mean age at onset is approximately 5 to 7 years. However, a wide age range of cats has been affected, from 2 to 14 years of age.[1–3, 10a, 16]

Etiopathogenesis

The etiology of TSEs is poorly understood. The TSE agent has biologic and physiochemical characteristics unlike those of any other microorganism. All TSE diseases are characterized by the accumulation of an abnormal isoform of a host-coded protein, the prion-protein (PrP). PrP is found in all animals; it is a cell-surface glycoprotein of unknown significance. However, whereas the PrP isolated from normal individuals (PrPc) and the PrP isolated from TSE infected individuals (PrP-res) have the same amino acid sequence and secondary structure, PrPc is totally degraded by proteinase K, and PrP-res resists digestion. Once present, PrP-res is believed to induce additional copies of itself by interacting with normal PrPc. In doing this, PrP-res acts as an infectious agent.[25] Once the host-coded PrPc has been transformed to PrP-res, it accumulates in fibrils (scrapie-associated fibrils [SAF]), and this leads to disease.[4]

Although the pathogenesis of FSE is largely unknown, it is thought to be similar to that seen in other TSE diseases. In natural scrapie infection, in which the agent is believed to be transmitted largely orally, the agent can be detected within the lymphoreticular system, including the tonsils, spleen, and lymph nodes, for a variable period of time before the development of clinical signs.[26] It has been hypothesized that the infection spreads from these areas, along the sympathetic and enteric nerves, to the midthoracic spinal cord and then to the brain.[27] The migration of the agent and the transformation of PrPc to PrP-res take time; hence, all TSE diseases have prolonged incubation periods. Once the TSE agent has induced the change in PrP, the accumulation of SAF results in vacuolar degeneration of the CNS. Because PrP is host-coded, the accumulation of SAF induces no immune response.[28, 29]

Clinical and Pathologic Findings

FSE is characterized by a long asymptomatic incubation period followed by an insidious onset of clinical signs. It is characterized by progressive behavioral and motor disturbances. Cases may present with progressive hindlimb ataxia; increased aggression or affection; hyperesthesia to touch, sound, or light; altered grooming patterns; increased saliva-

tion; dilated pupils with an unusual staring expression; polyphagia and/or polydipsia; abnormal head posture; muscle fasciculations; and/or an inability to retract claws.[1–3, 16, 23] Behavioral changes usually have been noted first, followed by progressive locomotor dysfunction. The cats tend to show ataxia, with dysmetria or hypermetria, which often leads to an erratic crouching gait and an inability to judge distances.[3, 16] The disease generally is progressive, warranting euthanasia within 8 to 12 weeks of the onset of clinical signs.[3] There is no effective treatment.

Pre-mortem diagnosis rarely is possible. Although clinical signs may be suggestive of FSE, and nonspecific tests, like electroencephalography or magnetic resonance imaging, may indicate the presence of diffuse CNS disease, specific tests generally are lacking. A number of possible ante-mortem tests have been developed for the diagnosis of scrapie, for example, the detection of PrP-res in tonsillar biopsies.[26] However, these assays have not, to the authors' knowledge, been assessed in the diagnosis of FSE. Significant abnormalities have not been detected in cerebrospinal fluid.[23] Diagnosis of FSE usually is made by histopathologic examination of the brain (formalin-fixed tissue), and the ultrastructural detection of SAF in brain extracts (fresh frozen brain or spinal cord).[30] After euthanasia, any case suspected of having FSE should have a full post-mortem examination performed by a trained veterinary pathologist. On confirmation of cases in the United Kingdom, the Ministry of Agriculture, Farming, and Fisheries (MAFF) should be contacted.

Pathologic changes are confined to the CNS and consist of variable degrees of neurophil vacuolation, vacuolation of the neuronal parenchyma, and an astrocytic response. Changes generally are bilaterally symmetric, and are particularly evident in the gray matter of the thalamus, basal ganglia, and the cerebral and cerebellar cortices. More advanced cases may show neuronal loss and more striking gliosis. There are no inflammatory changes (Fig. 8–2). Fibrils analogous to SAF may be seen on electron microscopy.[3, 31, 32]

Zoonotic Risk

Although it is generally difficult to transmit a TSE agent from 1 species to another by mouth, BSE appears to have been transmitted naturally, not only to cats, captive exotic felids, and captive exotic ungulates, but also to human beings, as vCJD.[6, 33] With the introduction of strict laws regulating the slaughter and rendering of ruminants in the United Kingdom, and the overall decline in the incidence of BSE, the possibility of the BSE agent continuing to be included in the food chain is extremely small. However, because the incubation period is long and variable, we are likely to continue to see new cases of vCJD for a few years to come.

It is very unlikely that cats present a zoonotic

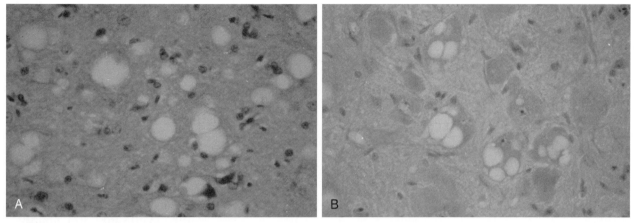

Figure 8–2. Histopathology of FSE. *A,* Vacuolation of gray matter. Head of the caudate nucleus, rostral to optic chiasma. Hematoxylin and eosin (H&E), ×30. *B,* Multiple vacuolated neurons. Raphe nucleus, medulla oblongata. H&E, ×30. (*A* and *B,* Courtesy of Dr. G. Pearson, University of Bristol, England.)

risk. Not only is the disease now extremely rare, it was never very common, and the likelihood of FSE-infected brain or spinal cord entering the human food chain is almost nonexistent.

◆ FELINE BORNA DISEASE

BD was first described over 200 years ago as a fatal neurologic disease affecting horses in southern Germany.[34] BD still is seen predominantly in horses and sheep in endemic areas of Germany and Switzerland. However, in addition to horses and sheep, natural infections also have been seen in cats, ostriches, and occasionally, rabbits, cattle, goats, deer, and dogs.[35–43] Experimentally, Borna disease virus (BDV) can be transmitted to a wide variety of species, including birds, rodents, and monkeys.[36, 42, 44] BD in cats, which is also known as "staggering disease," was first described in Sweden.[45] It was later shown to be caused by BDV infection.[46]

Epizootiology

The exact geographic distribution of BDV is uncertain, but serologic evidence of infection has been documented in central and northern Europe, North America, the United Kingdom, Japan, Iran, and Israel.[47–51] With increasing knowledge, particularly from serologic surveys or surveys looking for BDV RNA within peripheral blood samples, we now know that BDV infection is often asymptomatic.[46, 52] For example, in the United Kingdom 6 per cent of cats with no evidence of CNS disease had antibodies against BDV,[50] and in a recent study of sera from 654 ill cats submitted for feline immunodeficiency virus, feline leukemia virus, and feline infectious peritonitis virus testing, 8.9 per cent were seroposi-

tive for BDV (Harbour DA, Ingham TJ, and Sibson JM, unpublished results, 1999). The prevalence of seropositivity increased steadily with age of cat. In Japan, 13 per cent of healthy, randomly selected cats were positive for BDV RNA by reverse transcription-polymerase chain reaction (RT-PCR).[47] However, whereas BDV may be detected in many normal cats, BDV RNA or antibodies against BDV are seen most frequently in cats with neurologic disease. Of cats with undefined neurologic disorders, 13 per cent and 35 per cent were BDV antibody–positive in Germany[53] and the United Kingdom,[50] respectively. Fatal BD is seen most commonly as a rare isolated event. However, occasionally it can be seen in large outbreaks, even in cats, in which as many as 30 to 40 cases may be seen in a week.[54]

Natural BD ("staggering disease") has been reported in over 100 cats.[38, 54–56] It is recognized most frequently in male cats, with no particular breed predisposition. Whereas a wide age range of cats may be affected (from 5 months to 11 years of age), young adults appear to be most at risk.[38, 54, 55] Affected cats usually have been allowed to roam outdoors, particularly in rural or woodland areas.[54–56] Whereas most documented cases of feline BD have originated from northern and central Europe, probable cases of BD also have been seen in other countries.[50] Given the difficulty in making a pre-mortem diagnosis, and the low index of suspicion, it is likely that BD is underdiagnosed.

The natural reservoir host of BDV is not known. However, because the virus can infect so many different species, a single reservoir may not be required. Hunting mice appears to be a risk factor in feline BD. It has been suggested, therefore, that rodents may be subclinically infected with BDV and may act as viral carriers.[56] Although, to the authors' knowledge, BDV has not yet been confirmed within wild rodent populations, it is known to cause persistent infections in experimentally inoculated rats and mice.[57, 58] In support of this theory, outbreaks of BD tend to show a seasonal pattern, with most cases occurring during spring, summer, and early autumn, times when the purported wildlife reservoir is most active. Also, the number of cases of BD has been seen to fall after a very cold winter, when the wildlife reservoir may be expected to have been depleted.[56]

Most natural infections are believed to be transmitted via saliva or nasal secretions from clinically affected animals or apparently normal virus carriers.[59] Subclinical carriers with life-long infection have been found in almost all susceptible species.[36, 52] Most animals probably become infected by direct contact with secretions or via contaminated food or water. However, in horses, colostrum and milk also may play a role,[42] and experimentally, in rats, oral infection was shown to be possible.[36]

Etiopathogenesis

BDV is a novel, single-stranded RNA virus that replicates within the nucleus of infected cells and represents the sole member of the Bornaviridae family of the order Mononegavirales.[60–62] After intranasal inoculation, the neurotropic BDV is disseminated by intra-axonal transport. The virus usually appears within the brain in 3 to 5 days, and has a predilection for the limbic system.[63, 64] In later stages of infection, BDV diffuses centrifugally, via peripheral nerves, to other body systems. It then may be found in the salivary glands, mammary glands, nasal mucosa, and kidneys.[42, 64, 65] BDV infection usually is limited by the development of neutralizing antibody.[46]

It is not clear at this time whether there is a single biotype of BDV that can infect and cause disease in a wide range of species, or whether there are species-specific biotypes.[66] However, sequence analysis of a number of BDV isolates has shown the virus to be very stable genetically, supporting the hypothesis that there is a single biotype.[65, 67] Whereas there appears to be a degree of host-species adaptation, BDV from 1 species can be used successfully to experimentally infect different mammalian species.[46]

The degree of genetic conservation suggests that BDV does not need to mutate to exist within its hosts. This degree of virus-host adaptation usually is seen in viruses that are evolutionarily very old.[52] This, coupled with serologic evidence of an almost worldwide distribution, supports the hypothesis that BDV is a ubiquitous virus that is very well adapted to its various host species. In most cases, infection with BDV causes little or no sign of disease. It is only when a host is particularly susceptible, or mounts an abnormal response to the virus, that clinical signs develop.[42, 52]

Whether or not an infected individual develops clinical disease, along with the exact nature, severity, and duration of the disease, is determined by a number of interacting factors. These include the age and genetic background of the host, the dose and strain of the virus, and the route of infection.[42, 46, 52, 64, 68] The effect of age can be seen from studies in Lewis rats. When infected with BDV as neonates, these rats fail to produce a nonsuppurative encephalitis despite high levels of virus within their brain, but later develop behavioral disorders associated with altered memory and learning[69] and are hyperreactive to aversive stimuli, possibly as a result of chronic emotional abnormalities.[70] In contrast, adult rats show far more severe disease with marked behavioral and stereotypic changes. Some then develop a severe obesity syndrome, and almost all develop premature senescence.[71] More generally, animals exposed to a high dose of virus tend to develop an efficient immune response and eliminate the virus, whereas those exposed to a lower dose have a delayed immune response, which allows viral replication to proceed and encephalitis to develop.[68] If an animal is infected with a BDV strain that is adapted to that species, it tends to produce a more effective immune response than when infected with a BDV strain that has been isolated from a different host species.[46] The effect of route of infection can be seen in cats infected intracerebrally with BDV; these cats develop a different distribution of inflammatory changes within their CNS than is seen classically in natural infections.[46] The exact role of these various factors in the development of natural feline BD has not been determined.

The pathogenesis of feline BD still is poorly understood. From experimental infection studies, it is known that whereas BDV infection may induce acute disease, most clinically affected cats recover from this phase of infection, and seroconvert to BDV-positive. Fatal disease is rare.[46]

Clinical and Pathologic Findings

"Staggering disease" is characterized by behavioral and motor disturbances resulting from meningoencephalomyelitis. In experimental infections, clinical signs included protrusion of the third eyelid, behavioral changes, circling, ataxia, and tremors.[46] Naturally infected cats may present with progressive hindlimb ataxia (Fig. 8–3), loss of appetite, fever, increased affection toward the owner, unusual staring expression, apparent pain over the sacrum, seizures, increased salivation, increased aggression, an inability to retract claws, and hypersensitivity to light and sound.[53–55] Disease usually is progressive, warranting euthanasia within 1 week to 6 months from the onset of clinical signs.[54, 55] Animals that survive the initial episode may remain chronically infected, and may experience recurrent episodes of disease.[46] This is similar to BD in horses.[65]

Pre-mortem diagnosis can be difficult. In most cases, detection of typical clinical signs in a cat from an endemic area will result in a presumptive

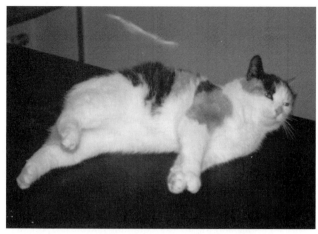

Figure 8–3. Cat with "staggering disease"/feline Borna disease shows paralysis of the hindlimbs. (Courtesy of Dr. A.-L. Burg, Swedish University of Agricultural Sciences, Uppsala, Sweden.)

diagnosis of BD. Detection of serum antibodies is not reliable. Although raised serum antibodies may be present in some cats with BD (approximately 40 per cent),[53] other affected cats may be antibody negative.[38, 46, 47, 50, 55] Although clinical signs of BD

tend to develop at the same time that BDV RNA can be detected within the peripheral white blood cells,[66] the detection of BDV RNA within peripheral blood does not necessarily reflect the extent of the viral load in the CNS.[47] Routine serum biochemistry and hematology generally are unremarkable, although some cats may show a leukopenia, and mild elevations in glucose and alanine aminotransferase activity.[46, 54] Cerebrospinal fluid analysis may show increased protein concentrations and a leukocytosis, with mononuclear cells predominating.[46]

The primary histopathologic lesions include a nonsuppurative meningoencephalomyelitis, with neuronophagia, microgliosis, and heavy perivascular cuffing by mononuclear cells (Fig. 8–4). Neurons in affected areas usually appear to be unaffected, but may contain inclusion bodies within their nuclei.[46, 72] Disease may result from a T-cell–dependent immune mechanism.[44] Lesions are particularly evident in the gray matter of the cerebral hemispheres, the limbic system, and the brain stem.[38, 54, 72] BDV antigen and RNA usually can be detected within the inflamed areas.[46] However, because cats harbor less BDV RNA than horses, in situ hybridization or immunohistochemistry may fail to detect the virus, and more sensitive assays, such as

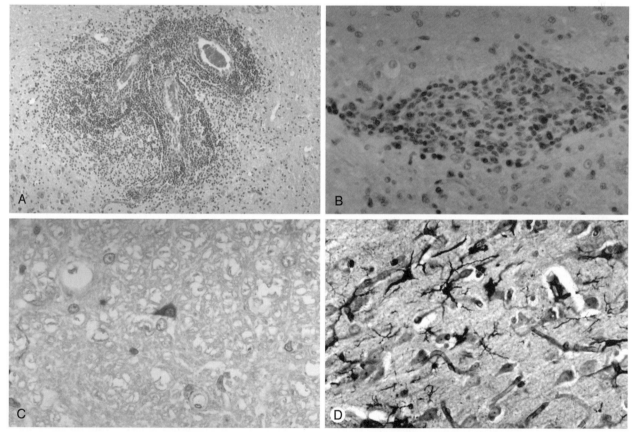

Figure 8–4. Histopathology of "staggering disease"/feline Borna disease. *A,* Mononuclear adventitial and perivascular cuffs in the thalamus of a cat with Borna disease. H&E, ×168. *B,* Immunoglobulin G–containing plasma cells within an adventitial cuff, mesencephalon of a cat with Borna disease. Peroxidase-antiperoxidase technique, ×420. *C,* Borna disease virus antigen in a neuron in the pons of a cat with Borna disease. Polyclonal antibody, avidin-biotin-complex technique, ×672. *D,* Infiltration of microglial cells in the cerebral cortex of a cat with Borna disease. Gallyas impregnation technique, ×420. (*A–D,* Courtesy of Dr. A.-L. Burg, Swedish University of Agricultural Sciences, Uppsala, Sweden.)

nested RT-PCR, may be necessary to confirm the diagnosis.[38, 73, 74]

A number of other nonsuppurative encephalitides also have been described in cats. Some of these appear to have a viral origin, and to some extent, resemble BD in their clinical appearance and/or pathologic changes.[54, 75–77] Although it has been suggested that BDV may be responsible for at least some of these disorders, more cases need to be studied before a causal relationship can be proved. Because BDV can be found in the CNS of some clinically normal individuals,[50] its presence, per se, within the CNS of a cat showing neurologic disease does not prove that it is the cause of the disorder.

Zoonotic Risk

It is unclear at this time what role BDV may play in the induction of human disease. Antibodies against BDV, viral proteins, and RNA have been found in human beings in Europe, North America, and Asia. A higher prevalence of infection is seen in patients with neurologic or psychiatric disorders, particularly schizophrenia and uni- or bipolar disorders.[78–83] However, because the virus also has been detected in clinically normal patients,[84] a role for BDV in the development of these complex psychiatric disorders still has to be proved.

The apparent presence of a single virus genotype, the presence of BDV infection in many domestic species, and evidence of cross-species transfer, all raise the possibility of zoonotic spread. However, whereas animal species may pose a potential risk to human beings, finding BDV RNA in blood from normal human blood donors suggests that human beings perhaps may be as much at risk from horizontal spread between human beings.[49] Considerably more investigation needs to be performed before the zoonotic potential of BDV can be determined.

REFERENCES

1. Leggett MM, Dukes J, Pirie HM: A spongiform encephalopathy in a cat. Vet Rec 127:586–588, 1990.
2. Wyatt JM, Pearson GR, Smerdon TN, et al: Spongiform encephalopathy in a cat. Vet Rec 126:513, 1990.
3. Wyatt JM, Pearson GR, Smerdon TN, et al: Naturally occurring scrapie-like spongiform encephalopathy in five domestic cats. Vet Rec 129:233–236, 1991.
4. Kimberlin RH: Transmissible spongiform encephalopathies in animals. Can J Vet Res 54:30–37, 1990.
5. Wells GAH, McGill IS: Recently described scrapie-like encephalopathies in animals: Case descriptions. In Bradley R, Savey M, Marchant B (eds): Sub-Acute Spongiform Encephalopathies. Current Topics in Veterinary Medicine and Animal Science, vol. 55. Dordrecht, The Netherlands, Kluwer Academic, 1991, pp. 11–24.
6. Kirkwood JK, Cunningham AA: Epidemiological observations on spongiform encephalopathies in captive wild animals in the British Isles. Vet Rec 135:296–303, 1994.
7. Hartsough GR, Burger D: Encephalopathy of mink. I. Epizootiology and clinical observations. J Infect Dis 115:387–392, 1965.
8. Kirkwood JK, Cunningham AA, Flach EJ, et al: Spongiform encephalopathy in another captive cheetah (Acinonyx jubatus): Evidence for variation in susceptibility or incubation periods between species? J Zoo Wildl Med 24:577–582, 1995.
9. Baron T, Belli P, Madec JY, et al: Spongiform encephalopathy in an imported cheetah in France. Vet Rec 141:270–271, 1997.
10. Willoughby K, Kelly DF, Lyon DG, Wells GAH: Spongiform encephalopathy in a captive puma (Felis concolor). Vet Rec 131:431–434, 1992.
10a. Wilesmith JW: Central Veterinary Laboratory, Weybridge, England, personal communication, 2000.
11. Brown P: Transmissible spongiform encephalopathies in humans: Kuru, Creutzfeldt-Jakob disease, Gerstmann-Sträussler-Scheinker disease. Can J Vet Res 54:38–41, 1990.
12. Gibbs CJ, Gajdusek DC: Experimental subacute spongiform virus encephalopathies in primates and other laboratory animals. Science 182:67–69, 1973.
13. Baker HF, Ridley RM, Wells GAH: Experimental transmission of BSE and scrapie to the common marmoset. Vet Rec 132:403–406, 1993.
14. Fraser H, Pearson GR, McConnell I, et al: Transmission of feline spongiform encephalopathy to mice. Vet Rec 134:449, 1994.
15. Parry HB: Scrapie Disease in Sheep, edited by Oppenheimer DR. London, Academic, 1983, p. 31.
16. Bratberg B, Ueland K, Wells GAH: Feline spongiform encephalopathy in a cat in Norway. Vet Rec 136:444, 1995.
17. Zanusso G, Nardelli E, Zosati A, et al: Simultaneous occurrence of spongiform encephalopathy in a man and his cat in Italy. Lancet 352:1116–1117, 1998.
18. Wells GAH, Scott AC, Johnson CT, et al: A novel progressive spongiform encephalopathy in cattle. Vet Rec 121:419–420, 1987.
19. Wilesmith JW, Wells GAH, Cranwell MP, Ryan JBM: Bovine spongiform encephalopathy: Epidemiological studies. Vet Rec 123:638–644, 1988.
20. Wilesmith JW, Ryan JB, Atkinson MJ: Bovine spongiform encephalopathy: Epidemiological studies on the origin. Vet Rec 128:199–203, 1991.
21. Hoinville LJ: Decline in the incidence of BSE in cattle born after the introduction of the "feed ban." Vet Rec 134:274–275, 1994.
22. Wilesmith JW, Ryan JB: Bovine spongiform encephalopathy: Observations on incidence during 1992. Vet Rec 132:300–301, 1993.
22a. Bruce ME, Chree A, McConnell I, et al: Transmission of bovine spongiform encephalopathy and scrapie to mice: Strain variation and the species barrier. Philos Trans R Soc Lond B Biol Sci 343:405–411, 1994.
23. Gruffydd-Jones TJ, Galloway PE, Pearson GR: Feline spongiform encephalopathy. J Small Anim Pract 33:471–476, 1991.
24. Donnelly CA: Maternal transmission of BSE: Interpretation of the data on the offspring of BSE-affected pedigree suckler cows. Vet Rec 142:579–580, 1998.
25. Prusiner SB: Genetic and infectious prion diseases. Arch Virol 50:1129–1153, 1993.
26. Schreuder BEC, van Keulen LJM, Vromans MEW, et al: Tonsillar biopsy and PrPSc detection in the preclinical diagnosis of scrapie. Vet Rec 142:564–568, 1998.
27. Hadlow WJ, Kennedy RC, Race RE: Natural infection of Suffolk sheep with scrapie virus. J Infect Dis 146:657–664, 1982.
28. Bolton DC, McKinley MP, Prusiner SB: Identification of a protein that purifies with scrapie prion. Science 218:1309–1311, 1982.
29. Chesebro B, Race R, Wehrly K, et al: Identification of scrapie prion protein–specific mRNA in scrapie-infected and uninfected brain. Nature 315:331–333, 1985.
30. Gibson PH, Somerville RA, Fraser H, et al: Scrapie associated fibrils in the diagnosis of scrapie in sheep. Vet Rec 120:125–127, 1987.
31. Pearson GR, Gruffydd-Jones TJ, Wyatt JM, et al: Feline spongiform encephalopathy. Vet Rec 128:532, 1991.
32. Pearson GR, Wyatt JM, Gruffydd-Jones TJ, et al: Feline spongiform encephalopathy: Fibril and PrP studies. Vet Rec 131:307–310, 1992.

33. Collinge J, Sidle KCL, Meads J, et al: Molecular analysis of prion strain variation and the etiology of new variant CJD. Nature 383:685–690, 1996.

34. Abildgaard PC: Handbuch von den gewöhnlichsten Krankheiten der Pferde, des Hornivichee, der Schafe und Schweine, sammt der bequemsten und wohlfellesten Art sie zu heilen. Zum Gebrauch des Landmanns. Vienna, JT Edlen von Tratthern, 1785.

35. Nicolau S, Galloway IA: Borna disease and enzootic encephalomyelitis of sheep and cattle. Special Reports Series. Medical Research Council 121:7–90, 1928.

36. Ludwig H, Bode L, Gosztonyi G: Borna disease: A persistent virus infection of the central nervous system. Progr Med Virol 35:107–151, 1988.

37. Lundgren AL, Czech G, Bode L, Ludwig H: Natural Borna disease in domestic animals other than horses and sheep. J Vet Med B40:298–303, 1993.

38. Lundgren AL, Zimmermann W, Bode L, et al: Staggering disease in cats: Isolation and characterization of the feline Borna virus. J Gen Virol 76:2215–2222, 1995.

39. Malkinson M, Weisman Y, Ashash E, et al: Borna disease in ostriches. Vet Rec 133:304, 1993.

40. Malkinson M, Weisman Y, Perl S, Ashash E: A Borna-like disease of ostriches in Israel. In Koprowski H, Lipkin WI (eds): Borna Disease. Current Topics in Microbiology and Immunology, vol. 190. Berlin, Springer-Verlag, pp. 31–38, 1995.

41. Bode L, Durrwald R, Ludwig H: Borna virus infections in cattle associated with fatal neurological disease. Vet Rec 135:283–284, 1994.

42. Rott R, Becht H: Natural and experimental Borna disease in animals. In Koprowski H, Lipkin WI (eds): Borna Disease. Current Topics in Microbiology and Immunology, vol. 190. Berlin, Springer-Verlag, pp. 15–30, 1995.

43. Weissenbock H, Nowotny N, Caplazi P, et al: Borna disease in a dog with lethal meningoencephalitis. J Clin Microbiol 36:2127–2130, 1998.

44. Narayan O, Herzog S, Frese K, et al: Pathogenesis of Borna disease in rats: Immune-mediated viral ophthalmoencephalopathy causing blindness and behavioural abnormalities. J Infect Dis 148:305–315, 1983.

45. Kronevi T, Nordstrom M, Moreno W, Nilsson PO: Feline ataxia due to nonsuppurative meningoencephalomyelitis of unknown aetiology. Nord Vet Med 26:720–725, 1974.

46. Lundgren AL, Johannisson A, Zimmermann W, et al: Neurological disease and encephalitis in cats experimentally infected with Borna virus. Acta Neuropathol 93:391–401, 1997.

47. Nakamura Y, Asahi S, Nakaya T, et al: Demonstration of Borna disease virus RNA in peripheral blood mononuclear cells derived from domestic cats in Japan. J Clin Microbiol 34:188–198, 1996.

48. Richt JA, Pfeuffer I, Christ M, et al: Borna disease virus infection in animals and humans. Emerg Infect Dis 3:343–352, 1997.

49. Takahashi H, Nakaya T, Nakamura Y, et al: Higher prevalence of Borna disease virus infection in blood donors living near thoroughbred horse farms. J Med Virol 52:330–335, 1997.

50. Reeves NA, Helps CR, Gunn-Moore DA, et al: Natural Borna disease virus infection in cats in the United Kingdom. Vet Rec 143:523–526, 1998.

51. Weissenbock H, Suchy A, Caplazi P, et al: Borna disease in Austrian horses. Vet Rec 143:21–22, 1998.

52. Ludwig H, Bode L: The neuropathogenesis of Borna disease virus infections. Intervirology 40:185–197, 1997.

53. Lundgren AL, Ludwig H: Clinically diseased cats with nonsuppurative meningoencephalomyelitis have Borna disease virus–specific antibodies. Acta Vet Scand 34:101–103, 1993.

54. Strom B, Andren B, Lundgren AL: Idiopathic non-suppurative meningoencephalo-myelitis (staggering disease) in the Swedish cat: A study of 33 cases. Svensk Veterinar Tindning 44:19–24, 1992 (translation published in Eur J Companion Anim Pract 3:9–13, 1992).

55. Nowotny N, Weissenbock H: Description of feline nonsuppurative meningoencephalomyelitis ("staggering disease") and studies of its etiology. J Clin Microbiol 33:1668–1669, 1995.

56. Berg AL, Reid-Smith R, Larsson M, Bonnett B: Case control study of feline Borna disease in Sweden. Vet Rec 142:715–717, 1998.

57. Kao M, Ludwig H, Gosztonyi G: Adaptation of Borna disease virus to the mouse. J Gen Virol 65:1845–1849, 1984.

58. Herzog S, Frese K, Rott R: Studies on the genetic control of resistance of black hooded rats to Borna disease. J Gen Virol 72:535–540, 1991.

59. Richt JA, Herzog S, Haberzettl K, Rott R: Demonstration of Borna disease virus–specific RNA in secretions of naturally infected horses by the polymerase chain reaction. Med Microbiol Immunol (Berl) 182:293–304, 1993.

60. Briese T, de la Torre JC, Lewis A, et al: Borna disease virus, a negative-strand RNA virus, transcribes in the nucleus of infected cells. Proc Natl Acad Sci U S A 89:11486–11489, 1992.

61. Briese T, Lipkin WI, de la Torre JC: Molecular biology of Borna disease virus. In Koprowski H, Lipkin WI (eds): Borna Disease. Current Topics in Microbiology and Immunology vol. 190. Berlin, Springer-Verlag, 1995, pp. 1–16.

62. Cubitt B, de la Torre JC: Borna disease virus (BDV), a nonsegmented RNA virus, replicates in the nucleus of infected cells where infectious BDV ribonucleoproteins are present. J Virol 68:1371–1381, 1994.

63. Carbone KM, Duchala CS, Griffin JW, et al: Pathogenesis of Borna disease in rats: Evidence that intra-axonal spread is the major route for virus dissemination and the determination of disease incubation. J Virol 61:3431–3440, 1987.

64. Gosztonyi G, Ludwig H: Borna disease—Neuropathology and pathogenesis. In Koprowski H, Lipkin WI (eds): Borna Disease. Current Topics in Microbiology and Immunology, vol. 190. Berlin, Springer-Verlag, 1995, pp. 39–73.

65. Gonzalez-Dunia D, Sauder C, de la Torre JC: Borna disease virus and the brain. Brain Res Bull 44:647–664, 1997.

66. Bode L, Ludwig H: Clinical similarities and close genetic relationship of human and animal Borna disease virus. Arch Virol Suppl 13:167–182, 1997.

67. Cubitt B, Oldstone C, de la Torre JC: Sequence and genome organisation of Borna disease virus. J Virol 68:1382–1396, 1994.

68. Oldach D, Zink MC, Pyper JM, et al: Induction of protection against Borna disease by inoculation with high-dose-attenuated Borna disease virus. Virology 206:426–434, 1995.

69. Dittrich W, Bode L, Ludwig H, et al: Learning deficiencies in Borna disease virus–infected but clinically healthy rats. Biol Psychiatr 26:818–828, 1989.

70. Pletnikov MV, Rubin SA, Schwartz GJ, et al: Persistent neonatal Borna disease virus (BDV) infection of the brain causes chronic emotional abnormalities in adult rats. Physiol Behav 66:823–831, 1999.

71. Narayan O, Herzog S, Frese K, et al: Behavioural disease in rats caused by immunopathological responses to persistent Borna virus in the brain. Science 220:1401–1403, 1983.

72. Lundgren AL: Feline non-suppurative meningoencephalomyelitis. A clinical and pathological study. J Comp Pathol 107:411–425, 1992.

73. Lundgren AL, Lindberg R, Ludwig H, Gosztonyi G: Immunoreactivity of the central nervous system in cats with a Borna disease–like meningoencephalomyelitis (staggering disease). Acta Neuropathol 90:184–193, 1995.

74. Lundgren AL: Borna disease in cats. Vet Rec 145:87, 1999.

75. Hoff EJ, Vandevelde M: Non-suppurative encephalomyelitis in cats suggestive of a viral origin. Vet Pathol 18:170–180, 1981.

76. Berg AL, Berg M: A variant form of feline Borna disease. J Comp Pathol 119:323–331, 1998.

77. Vandevelde M: Neurologic diseases of suspected infectious origin. In Greene CE (ed): Infectious Diseases of the Dog and Cat. Philadelphia, WB Saunders, 1998, pp. 530–539.

78. Rott R, Herzog S, Fleischer B, et al: Detection of serum antibodies to Borna disease virus in patients with psychiatric disorders. Science 228:755–756, 1985.

79. Bode L, Riegel S, Lange W, Ludwig H: Human infection with Borna disease virus: Seroprevalence in patients with chronic diseases and healthy individuals. J Med Virol 36:309–315, 1992.

80. Bode L, Durrwald R, Rantam FA, et al: First isolates of infectious human Borna disease virus from patients with mood disorders. Mol Psychiatry 1:200–212, 1996.
81. Salvatore M, Morzunov S, Schwemmle M, Lipkin WI: Borna disease virus in brains of North American and European people with schizophrenia and bipolar disorder. Lancet 349:1813–1814, 1997.
82. Iwahashi K, Watanabe M, Nakamura K, et al: Clinical investi-gation of the relationship between Borna disease virus (BDV) infection and schizophrenia in 67 patients in Japan. Acta Psychiatr Scand 96:412–415, 1997.
83. Hatalski CG, Lewis AJ, Lipkin WI: Borna disease. Emerg Infect Dis 3:129–135, 1997.
84. Haga S, Yoshimura M, Motoi Y, et al: Detection of Borna disease virus genome in normal human brain tissue. Brain Res 770:307–309, 1997.

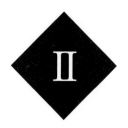

Gastrointestinal System

Albert E. Jergens, Editor

◆ Contrast Radiography for Evaluation of the
  Gastrointestinal Tract 73
◆ Approach to the Icteric Cat 87
◆ Gastric *Helicobacter* Infection 91
◆ Diseases of the Esophagus 99
◆ Update on Antiemetic Therapy 107
◆ The Gastrointestinal Tract and Adverse
  Reactions to Food 113
◆ Cytologic Evaluation of Fine-Needle Liver Biopsies . . 118
◆ Clinical Approach to Chronic Diarrhea 127

Still-Current Information Found in *Consultations in Feline Internal Medicine 2*:
Regurgitation: Diagnosis and Management (Chapter 10), p. 65
Inflammatory Bowel Disease (Chapter 11), p. 75
Hepatic Lipidosis (Chapter 13), p. 87
Gastrointestinal Endoscopy (Chapter 16), p. 119
Thyroid Function Testing (Chapter 19), p. 143
Nutritional Management of the Allergic Patient (Chapter 26), p. 201

Still-Current Information Found in *Consultations in Feline Internal Medicine 3*:
Clinical Approach to Chronic Vomiting (Chapter 10), p. 61
Inflammatory Liver Disease (Chapter 11), p. 68
Acute Pancreatitis (Chapter 13), p. 91
Gastrointestinal Endoscopic Biopsy Techniques (Chapter 16), p. 113
Food Hypersensitivity: New Recommendations for Diagnosis and Management (Chapter 28), p. 209

Elsewhere in *Consultations in Feline Internal Medicine 4*:
Hemobartonellosis (Chapter 2), p. 12
Cat Ownership by Immunosuppressed People (Chapter 3), p. 18
Cryptosporidiosis (Chapter 5), p. 34
Complications of Therapy for Hyperthyroidism (Chapter 19), p. 151
APUDomas: Pheochromocytoma, Insulinoma, and Gastrinoma (Chapter 23), p. 181
Medical Management of Chronic Renal Failure (Chapter 44), p. 328

Acquired Myasthenia Gravis and Other Disorders of the Neuromuscular Junction (Chapter 48), p. 374

Update on Cytauxzoonosis (Chapter 55), p. 436

Transfusion Medicine (Chapter 58), p. 461

Use of the Polymerase Chain Reaction to Detect Hemoparasites (Chapter 60) p. 479

Gastrointestinal Lymphoma and Inflammatory Bowel Disease (Chapter 63), p. 499

Chemotherapeutic Challenges: Special Considerations and New Agents (Chapter 65), p. 521

Approach to Oral Tumors (Chapter 66), p. 526

Evaluation and Treatment of Cranial Mediastinal Masses (Chapter 68), p. 533

Diagnostic Imaging of Neoplasia (Chapter 70), p. 548

9

◆ Contrast Radiography for Evaluation of the Gastrointestinal Tract

Kristina G. Miles

Radiographic evaluation of the feline gastrointestinal tract and surrounding structures should begin by obtaining right lateral recumbent and ventrodorsal survey films. Radiographic contrast studies may be performed when significant changes cannot be identified or differentiated after careful assessment of the initial films. Indications for the use of gastrointestinal contrast studies in cats include (1) confirmation or differentiation of suspected disease, (2) determination of the extent of involvement of a known abnormality, (3) attempts to identify the organ of origin of a soft-tissue mass, and (4) aids in the selection of medical or surgical therapy for a specific disease process.

◆ ESOPHAGUS

Normal Anatomy

The cervical esophagus is located dorsal to the trachea on lateral radiographic views. The position of the esophagus becomes slightly more ventral at the thoracic inlet. This anatomic relationship can create a soft-tissue opacity along the dorsal margin of the trachea that should not be mistaken for an abnormality. The caudal portion of the esophagus is positioned midway between the aorta and the caudal vena cava. The esophagus lies to the left of the trachea on dorsoventral or ventrodorsal views, and is superimposed partially with the thoracic vertebrae. The position of the esophagus becomes more midline at the level of the tracheal bifurcation. The descending aorta courses to the left of the esophagus, and may indent its margin.

The soft-tissue margins of the normal collapsed esophagus are not seen on survey radiographs owing to border effacement with the surrounding mediastinum or cervical muscles. However, a dilated esophagus containing a gas and/or fluid opacity may be observed (Fig. 9–1). Aspiration pneumonia is a common sequela to megaesophagus owing to either congenital or acquired causes.

Esophagram

Suspected luminal and mucosal esophageal lesions often are evaluated more accurately with a barium contrast agent. A single-step barium esophagram requires per os administration of a thick barium paste to coat the esophageal mucosa. Barium paste typically will persist along the mucosal folds while the patient is positioned and 1 or more radiographs are obtained. Right lateral recumbent and right ventrodorsal oblique projections are obtained most commonly. If contrast is not seen in the gastric lumen on initial radiographs, the patient may be held with forelimbs elevated for 5 to 10 minutes and the films repeated. Passage of the contrast material through the lower esophageal sphincter with the aid of gravity helps evaluate sphincter patency.

Visualization of a very small amount of contrast material immediately caudal to the upper esophageal sphincter, at the thoracic inlet, and/or over the heart base is considered normal on esophagram films. Parallel longitudinal mucosal folds are seen in the cranial two-thirds of the feline esophagus after contrast agent administration. The caudal one-third of the esophagus exhibits a "herringbone" pattern owing to the redundant mucosa associated with the change from skeletal to smooth muscle (Fig. 9–2).

A 3-step barium esophagram also may be performed. A liquid barium preparation is administered initially to determine whether a complete obstruction or other marked abnormality is present. Unfortunately, liquid barium does not adhere well to the esophageal mucosa, and may result in a false-negative study. Barium paste is administered during the second phase of evaluation to assess more fully the esophageal mucosa. Lastly, a barium meal may be given to demonstrate a partial esophageal obstruction or a difference in ability to swallow solids versus liquids. Patient refusal is a significant disadvantage of the barium meal.

Use of chemical restraint will alter esophageal motility, and should be avoided. Esophagrams should not be performed with the patient under general anesthesia, because false-positive results are common and the risk of contrast agent aspiration is increased. Either ionic or nonionic water-soluble contrast agents may be used in lieu of barium when esophageal perforation is suspected. However, small tears are more likely to be identified with conventional liquid barium.

Motility disorders are best evaluated with fluoroscopy. The dynamics of the entire swallowing mechanism may be assessed, and the severity of any segmental or generalized abnormalities may be staged. Gastroesophageal reflux generally involves only the caudal portion of the esophagus, and is

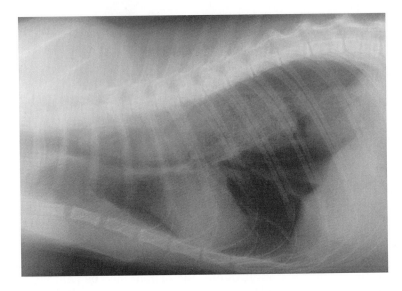

Figure 9–1. Survey thorax, lateral view. A large, tubular structure with a mottled opacity of soft tissue/fluid mixed with air lies dorsal to the heart base. The trachea is displaced ventrally. A cloth diaper was removed via gastrotomy. (Courtesy of the Veterinary Teaching Hospital, University of Missouri–Columbia.)

reported to occur in healthy animals.[1] One or 2 gastroesophageal reflux events observed during an esophagram may be within normal limits if the contrast material is cleared from the esophagus with the next swallow. Chronic gastroesophageal reflux may result in distal esophagitis.

A regional esophageal dilatation is most likely to be seen cranial to an intraluminal or an extrinsic obstruction (Fig. 9–3). The portion of the esophagus caudal to an obstruction may, or may not, be normal, and also should be evaluated. Esophageal foreign bodies lodge most commonly at the thoracic inlet, at the base of the heart, or at the esophageal hiatus near the diaphragm.

◆ STOMACH

Normal Anatomy

The gastric axis may be assessed subjectively on a lateral view by drawing a line from the fundus through the gastric body to the pylorus. A normal gastric axis will be positioned somewhere between a line parallel to the ribs and a line perpendicular to the thoracic vertebrae dorsal to the stomach (Fig. 9–4). Gastric axis position cannot be evaluated when localization of the fundus and pylorus is lost owing to a lack of luminal contrast.

Unlike dogs, the feline pylorus is located near midline on a ventrodorsal view. This position creates a J-shaped gastric silhouette that should not be mistaken for stomach displacement. Gastric wall thickness cannot be assessed reliably on survey films owing to variability in gastric distention with fluid and digesta, as well as border effacement of the serosal margin with adjacent soft-tissue structures, such as the liver.

Modified Pneumogastrogram

Additional evaluation of the stomach often may be obtained simply by adding a left lateral recumbent view to the baseline survey films. Any air present in the lumen will be located in the pylorus on a left lateral recumbent view (Fig. 9–5). Additional air may be introduced into the stomach with an orogastric tube if the volume of this negative contrast

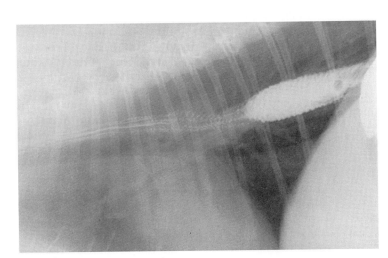

Figure 9–2. Barium paste esophagram, lateral view, close-up. The normal "herringbone" pattern of the feline caudal esophagus can be compared with the longitudinal mucosal folds of the more proximal esophagus. The slight increase in caudal esophageal diameter was transient, caused by passage of the contrast bolus.

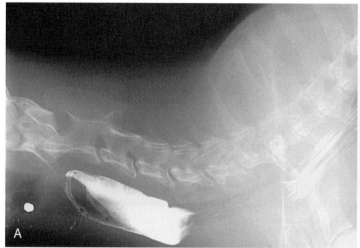

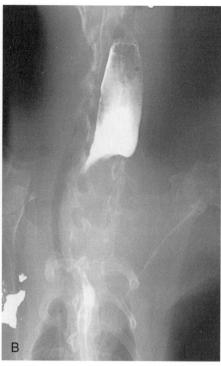

Figure 9–3. Barium paste esophagram, lateral *(A)* and ventrodorsal *(B)* views. The cranial cervical esophagus is distended abnormally owing to partial obstruction by a left-side, caudal cervical soft-tissue mass. In addition, the trachea is displaced to the right on *B*. After fine-needle aspiration and cytology, the mass was determined to be an enlarged lymph node. *Diagnosis: lymphosarcoma.* Metal opacities seen on the radiographs are bullet fragments, in this case an incidental finding.

material is considered inadequate. Total volume of air to be introduced is somewhat subjective, but should not exceed 10 ml/kg.

Upper Gastrointestinal Series

A positive contrast study often is required for complete evaluation of the stomach and small intestines. Lateral and ventrodorsal survey radiographs should be obtained before the initiation of any radiographic contrast procedure. The upper gastrointestinal (UGI) contrast agent of choice is a 30 to 50 per cent weight-per-volume barium sulfate suspension. A nonionic, water-soluble positive contrast medium, such as iohexol, may be used instead of barium,[2, 3] particularly if a gastrointestinal perforation is suspected. Iohexol is preferred over osmotically active ionic agents, but is more expensive. Ionic contrast medium is contraindicated in patients with chronic fluid loss from vomiting, diarrhea, or dehydration.[4] The use of anticholinergic drugs[5] or sedatives before a UGI contrast study should be avoided, because many tranquilizers can alter gastrointestinal motility. Shortened gastrointestinal transit times have been reported with administration of ketamine alone or in combination with acepromazine.[6]

The stomach, intestines, and colon should be free of ingesta and fecal material before beginning a UGI study. Digesta will create unusual filling defects within the barium contrast that can be mistaken for abnormalities, and also may obscure true mucosal

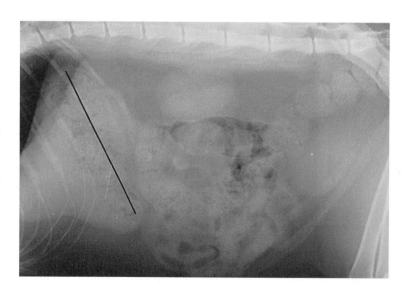

Figure 9–4. Survey abdomen, lateral view. A normal feline gastric axis line extends from the fundus through the body to the pylorus *(black line).* This axis line may be parallel to the ribs, perpendicular to the vertebral bodies immediately dorsal to the stomach, or at any angle between these 2 parameters.

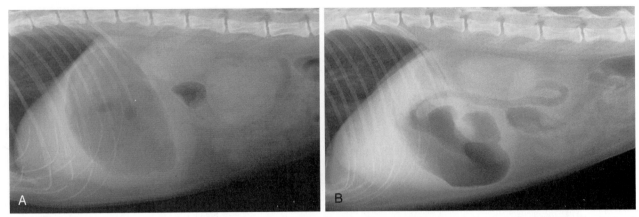

Figure 9–5. Survey abdomen. *A*, Air is present in the fundus, but the pyloric region of the stomach is poorly defined owing to border effacement with fluid in the gastric lumen on the right lateral recumbent view. *B*, Air fills the pylorus on the left lateral view, and provides radiographic contrast to the asymmetrically thickened wall. *Diagnosis: anaplastic tumor of the gastric wall.*

changes. To minimize these entrapments, food typically is withheld from the patient for 12 to 24 hours before the UGI study.

Recent patient anorexia does not guarantee a lack of fecal material in the colon. Survey radiographs will readily demonstrate the presence of fecal material in the colon that may obscure visualization of small-bowel loops and other structures. Tepid saline solution enemas (20 ml/kg body weight) used to cleanse the colon should be administered at least 2 hours before the contrast study to minimize the radiographic appearance of air and fluid that is introduced.

One common technical error that occurs when performing a UGI series is use of an inadequate volume of contrast material. Ten to 12 ml/kg of a 30 to 50 per cent liquid barium sulfate suspension should be administered via orogastric tube. Alternative routes of administration include use of a nasogastric tube, or contrast material may be placed in the buccal pouch via a syringe. Per os administration of contrast material requires more time to complete, and a significant volume of contrast agent may not be swallowed. Contrast material smeared inadvertently on the hair coat may create film artifacts that must be differentiated from true abnormalities.

Radiographs should be obtained immediately after introduction of contrast material (time zero), and at 15 and 30 minutes and 1 hour after contrast agent administration. Additional radiographs may be required if contrast material is not present in the colon by the time the 1-hour films are obtained. Right lateral and ventrodorsal projections are standard; however, all 4 radiographic views (dorsoventral, ventrodorsal, left lateral, and right lateral) should be obtained at time zero if gastric disease is suspected. Evaluation of gastric peristalsis requires videofluoroscopy.

Normal gastric transit usually begins immediately. However, movement of contrast material into the duodenum may be delayed for 15 to 30 minutes owing to patient stress.[7] Longer delays are considered abnormal. The stomach typically contains little contrast agent 1 hour after administration of contrast material (Fig. 9–6). Small-intestine transit time of liquid barium varies between 30 and 60 minutes after contrast agent administration in most normal cats.[8]

A double-contrast gastrogram is most useful for evaluation of radiolucent gastric foreign bodies and gastric mucosal lesions (gastritis, ulceration, neoplasia). A smaller dose of barium sulfate and large volume of negative contrast material (air) is introduced into the gastric lumen. Gastric emptying may be delayed by administration of an anticholinergic drug, such as glucagon, before the double-contrast study to maintain adequate gastric distention.[4, 5, 9] As a result, normal gastric emptying cannot be assessed.

Other diagnostic methods used to evaluate the gastrointestinal tract include ultrasonography, endoscopy, and oral administration of nondigestable barium-impregnated spheres[10] to determine the transit time of solids. The latter technique may be useful in specific patients with gastric motility disorders, but is performed much less commonly than the barium UGI series. Transit time of these radiopaque markers in dogs may be affected by sphere diameter, particularly at the pylorus and ileocolic junction, as well as the digestibility of the meal with which these are introduced.[11] Similar findings may be observed in cats,[12] and could result in misinterpretation. Scintigraphic imaging after ingestion of a radionuclide-labeled meal remains the most accurate method for detecting motility abnormalities.[13]

Table 9–1. Normal Feline Small-Intestine Diameter Estimation Techniques

SID = 1–1.5 central height of second lumbar vertebral body
SID = 2–3× width of proximal T11 rib
SID = 10–12 mm maximum

Abbreviation: SID, small-intestine diameter.

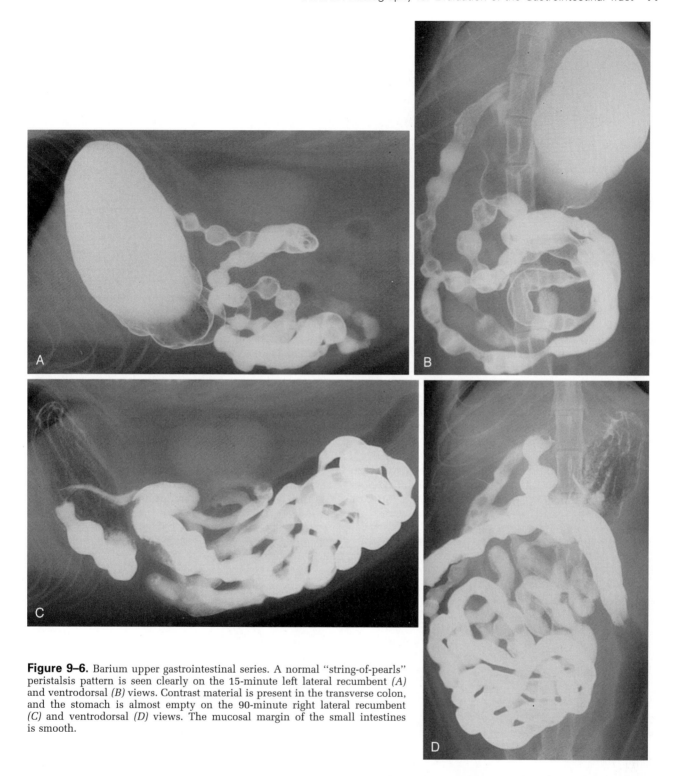

Figure 9–6. Barium upper gastrointestinal series. A normal "string-of-pearls" peristalsis pattern is seen clearly on the 15-minute left lateral recumbent *(A)* and ventrodorsal *(B)* views. Contrast material is present in the transverse colon, and the stomach is almost empty on the 90-minute right lateral recumbent *(C)* and ventrodorsal *(D)* views. The mucosal margin of the small intestines is smooth.

However, availability of this option is limited to facilities that offer digital nuclear medicine studies.

◆ SMALL INTESTINE
Normal Anatomy

The diameter of feline small-intestine loops may be assessed with various techniques. One method described for cats and dogs compares small-intes-tine diameter with the central height of the second lumbar vertebra on the lateral view.[14] Another rule-of-thumb method is described for dogs.[15] The more uniform body size of feline patients has allowed a maximum small-bowel diameter standard to be determined.[8] Personal observations suggest that the diameter of the normal feline small intestine falls between 1 and 1.5 times the central height of the second lumbar vertebral body (Table 9–1).

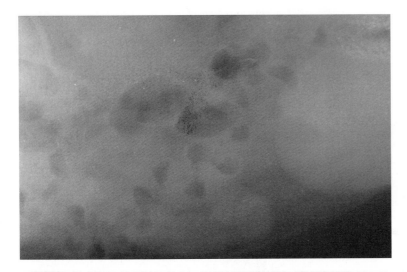

Figure 9–7. Survey abdomen, lateral view, close-up. A dot-dash pattern of bizarre gas bubbles is present in the small intestine. *Diagnosis: linear foreign body.* The string was removed surgically. (Courtesy of Angell Memorial Animal Hospital, Boston.)

The volume of radiolucent gas seen within the feline small intestine typically is much less than that found in dogs.[8] However, dyspnea or vomiting, with resultant aerophagia, may increase the amount of air present in the gastrointestinal tract. Gas within normal small intestines tends to present an ovoid or curvilinear pattern. The presence of gas bubbles with bizarre shapes is a nonspecific finding that may be seen occasionally with abnormalities such as linear foreign bodies (Fig. 9–7).

Serial survey radiographs may be useful for evaluation of nonspecific changes in small-bowel size or gas patterns in clinically stable patients. Abnormalities that repeat on multiple views over time, or

that become more pronounced, are identified more readily. When survey radiographs are inconclusive and clinical signs persist, a UGI series may be performed to determine the underlying cause of small-intestine distention (Fig. 9–8). However, a contrast agent study may not be required before exploratory celiotomy if survey films are highly suggestive of a mechanical obstruction (Fig. 9–9).

Upper Gastrointestinal Series

As with the stomach, small-intestine wall thickness cannot be determined accurately on survey radio-

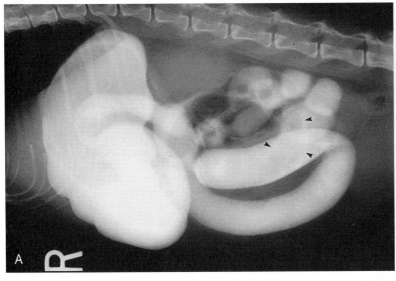

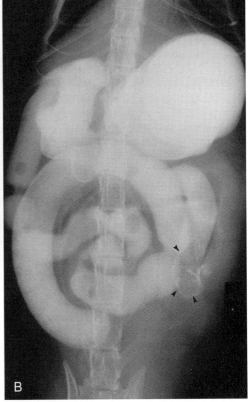

Figure 9–8. Barium upper gastrointestinal series, lateral *(A)* and ventrodorsal *(B)* views. Two hours after contrast medium administration, a large volume of barium is still observed in the gastric lumen, without contrast medium present in the colon. Several small-intestine loops are abnormally distended, but evidence of peristalsis also is observed. An irregular radiolucent filling defect *(arrowheads)* is noted within one small-intestine segment. *Diagnosis: mechanical obstruction caused by an intraluminal foreign body.*

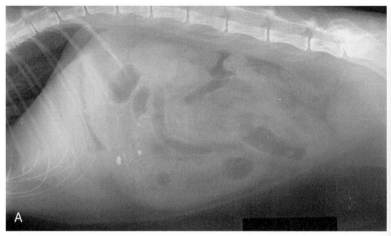

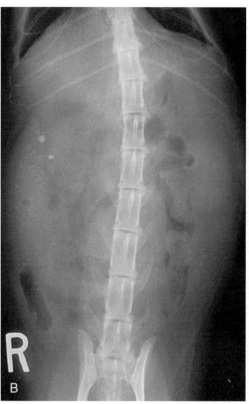

Figure 9–9. Survey abdomen, lateral *(A)* and ventrodorsal *(B)* views. An abnormally distended small-intestine loop filled with digesta and gas suggests a mechanical obstruction. Other small-intestine loops vary in size, from enlarged, but less distended, to within normal limits. Exploratory laparotomy revealed a small intramural mass of the jejunum immediately aboral to the most distended intestinal segment. *Diagnosis: small-intestine adenocarcinoma.*

graphs alone. Barium UGI contrast agent studies provide additional diagnostic information concerning the small-intestine mucosal surface, wall thickness, and luminal filling defects (Fig. 9–10). Barium may be seen in the colon as early as 30 to 60 minutes after contrast agent administration in the majority of normal cats.[8]

In cats, normal increased segmentation of the duodenum may create a "string-of-pearls" or beaded appearance on the UGI series that will not be seen on survey films. Pronounced muscular contractions produce a series of foci where the lumen is collapsed. Longitudinal folds of mucosa seen at these foci may produce a "pseudostring" appearance,[16] alternating with the distended beaded segments of duodenum on the feline UGI images. These normal findings should not be mistaken for the more asymmetric "accordion" plication produced by linear foreign bodies (Fig. 9–11). Abnormal distention of small-intestine loops may be categorized by the severity of distention and by the number of loops affected (Table 9–2).

Use of iohexol, a nonionic contrast agent, for radiographic evaluation of the stomach and small bowel in cats also has been described.[2, 3] A dose of 10 ml/kg of a 240 mg iodine/ml contrast solution, given per os as a 1:3 or 1:2 dilution with saline, should provide good visualization of the gastrointestinal tract with no adverse side-effects.[3] Undiluted, oral administration of iohexol in cats can cause vomiting.[3] Gastric emptying time and small-intestine transit time typically are rapid (30 to 60 minutes).[2, 3]

◆ COLON

Normal Anatomy

A commonly accepted rule of thumb used to determine normal colonic size compares colon diameter with the length of L7 on the lateral view. A colon diameter less than or equal to the length of the L7 body is within normal limits. Colon diameters greater than 1.5 times the length of L7 are considered abnormal (Fig. 9–12). A colonic diameter greater than the length of L7 but less than 1.5 times the L7 length falls into a gray zone that is considered acceptable only if transient.

The normal descending colon is a fairly mobile

Table 9–2. Abnormal Distention of Small-Intestine Loops Classified by Degree of Distention and Number of Loops Affected*

Classification	Primary Differential Diagnoses	Treatment
Mild focal	Partial mechanical obstruction Linear foreign body	Surgery
Severe focal	Complete mechanical obstruction	Surgery
Mild generalized	Functional dilatation due to mucosal or serosal inflammation	Medical
Severe generalized	Complete functional dilatation—rare	Emergency surgery

*Focal = 1–3 loops; generalized ≥ 4 loops.

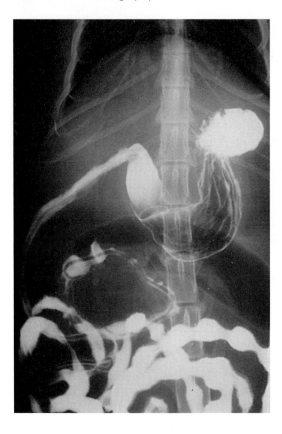

Figure 9–10. Barium upper gastrointestinal contrast study, ventrodorsal view. Thin, tubular radiolucent filling defects with smooth walls and tapered tips are present within the duodenum and other portions of the small intestine. Fecal flotation was positive for nematode *(Ascaris)* eggs.

structure, and can be displaced easily to the right of midline by a distended urinary bladder. This variation of colon position should not be mistaken for an abnormality. Also, the ileocolic junction is the narrowest part of the gastrointestinal tract caudal to the pylorus. Intestinal foreign bodies that pass beyond this level usually are capable of traversing the colon and being eliminated from the body.

Pneumocolon

The use of endoscopic techniques essentially has replaced the barium enema for diagnosis of colonic mucosal disease. However, a modified contrast agent study of the large bowel may be performed by introducing air into the rectum via a pliable feeding tube and large syringe. A pneumocolon provides a low

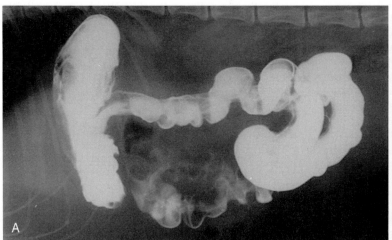

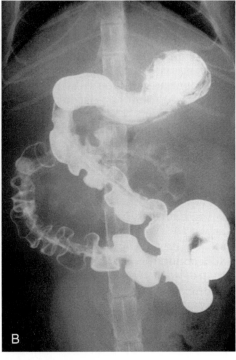

Figure 9–11. Barium upper gastrointestinal contrast study, right lateral *(A)* and ventrodorsal *(B)* views. Radiographs obtained 15 minutes after contrast medium administration demonstrate the asymmetric pleating of the proximal small intestine as it "climbs" along a linear foreign body. The string was removed surgically. (*A* and *B*, Courtesy of Angell Memorial Animal Hospital, Boston.)

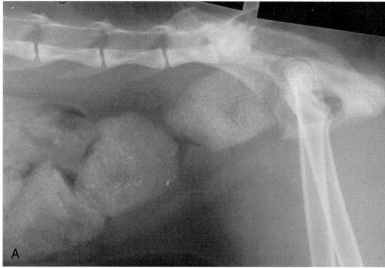

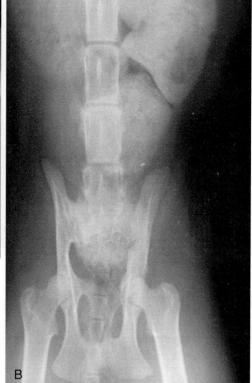

Figure 9–12. Survey caudal abdomen, lateral *(A)* and ventrodorsal *(B)* views. The descending colon is distended excessively with well-formed fecal material and gas. The pelvic canal is narrowed abnormally owing to malalignment of healed pelvic fractures.

patient stress technique for rapid evaluation of colonic position in cats with suspected caudal abdominal masses, or in cases in which differentiation of small- and large-bowel segments is difficult (Fig. 9–13). However, a pneumocolon does not provide reliable evaluation of the colonic mucosa.

Peritoneography

A small volume of water-soluble positive contrast material may be introduced into the peritoneal space to delineate serosal and peritoneal margins. Peritoneography, or celiography, is performed most commonly to aid in assessment of diaphragmatic integrity.[17–19] Nonionic contrast agents (iohexol, iopamidol) are less likely to be associated with adverse side-effects, such as hypovolemia and hypersensitivity reaction, that may be seen with ionic contrast agents.

The skin of the left caudoventral abdomen should be prepared in a standard fashion before contrast agent administration. Sedation typically is not required. A small, blunt-tipped cephalic vein catheter may be used to introduce 1 to 2 ml/kg of the water-soluble positive contrast agent into the peritoneal space.[17–19] The catheter may be placed in the left caudal abdominal quadrant at the midpoint between the midline and the lateral body wall, thereby avoiding the falciform fat pad. The catheter should be aspirated before contrast agent administration to ensure that the tip has not been placed into a hollow viscus or blood vessel. The patient may be rolled gently or elevated partially to help disperse the contrast material throughout the peritoneal space. Horizontal-beam views may be useful in combination with this contrast technique.

The positive contrast material will remain in the peritoneal space if integrity of the diaphragm is intact (Fig. 9–14). Contrast material will extravasate through the diaphragm if a traumatically induced tear or congenital hernia is present. A false-negative study could be obtained if a chronic diaphragmatic lesion is occluded by adhesions or other material.

◆ ANCILLARY STRUCTURES

Liver

There is no reliable, direct radiographic method for determining liver size. The size of the feline hepatic silhouette may be evaluated very subjectively based on the distance the margins extend caudal to the rib cage. The caudoventral margin of the liver may, or may not, extend slightly beyond the costal arch on the lateral view, and still be within normal limits. Unfortunately, this method of hepatic size evaluation has no specific range of normal. A mild increase in liver size also may be suspected by rounding of the normally crisp hepatic margins, and by displaced adjacent structures.

Evaluation of indirect signs of hepatomegaly is very important in patients that have poor abdominal detail. When present, the gastric axis on the lateral view may provide an indirect assessment of hepatic

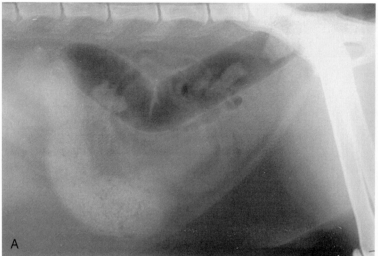

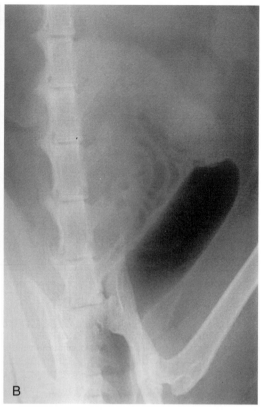

Figure 9–13. Pneumocolon, right lateral *(A)* and ventrodorsal oblique *(B)* views. The column of radiolucent air filling the descending colon ends abruptly at the level of L5 on *B*. The descending colon proximal to this site is abnormally distended with fecal material and gas and can now be differentiated from small intestine. *Diagnosis: annular adenocarcinoma of the colonic wall.* (*A* and *B*, Courtesy of Angell Memorial Animal Hospital, Boston.)

size. A gastric axis that is displaced caudodorsally provides evidence of hepatomegaly. A gastric axis displaced cranially suggests microhepatica or a decrease in abdominal liver tissue due to a diaphragmatic hernia. A large falciform fat pad is seen commonly ventral to the liver on the lateral view in cats, and should not be mistaken for an abnormal mass. Unlike dogs, retroperitoneal fat commonly produces a wide separation between the right kidney and the caudate lobe of the liver in cats. Also, a greater proportion of the liver in cats than in dogs lies to the right of midline.

Portography

Operative mesenteric venography is performed most commonly to aid in identification of portosystemic shunts (Fig. 9–15). The procedure is invasive, requiring sterile preparation and incision of the ventral abdomen to exteriorize a jejunal loop. Catheterization of a jejunal vein allows a rapidly injected bolus of a water-soluble positive contrast agent to be introduced for visualization of the portal vein system. A series of lateral radiographic views is obtained as the final milliliter of contrast agent is injected (total dose of 1 to 2 ml/kg).[20–22] The use of a rapid film changer and fluoroscopy allows more precise timing of film exposure, but a short series of 3 to 6 films can be obtained with brisk manual changing of cassettes. A second contrast agent injection is required if ventrodorsal images are desired.

Gallbladder

The gallbladder lies in a fossa of the right medial liver lobe in cats, and usually is not distinguishable as a separate radiographic shadow. Increased opacity in the region of the gallbladder may be caused by mineralized choleliths, or by mineralization of the gallbladder wall owing to chronic disease or neoplasia. Only a small percentage of choleliths that contain calcium will be seen on survey radiographs. A radiopaque structure in the area of the gallbladder also may be due to a superimposed intestinal loop or mineralization of the hepatic parenchyma. Suspected choleliths should be confirmed with ultrasonography, a UGI series, and/or cholecystography.

The gallbladder may be seen as an ovoid mass protruding caudal to the liver if severely distended (Fig. 9–16). Such a soft-tissue opacity must be differentiated from a normal fluid-filled pylorus or hepatic mass. A left lateral view will allow the pylorus to fill with radiolucent gas and help rule out this structure. Gallbladder distention occurs most commonly when the common bile duct is obstructed owing to cholelithiasis, chronic pancreatitis, or primary or secondary neoplasia.

Recognition of gallbladder and biliary tree diseases other than advanced neoplasia or obstruction requires a special contrast agent study, ultrasonography, and/or nuclear scintigraphy. Positive-contrast cholecystography requires the use of specific oral or intravenous contrast medium and delayed timing

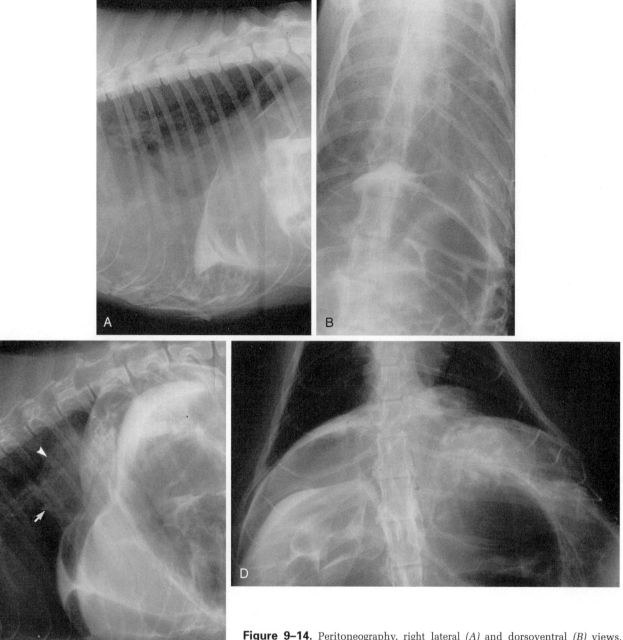

Figure 9–14. Peritoneography, right lateral *(A)* and dorsoventral *(B)* views. Positive contrast material can be seen in the left ventral pleural space owing to a traumatic diaphragmatic tear. Pleural effusion also is present, obscuring the margins of the cardiac silhouette. *C* and *D*, By comparison, the positive contrast material remains trapped in the peritoneal space in this second cat with a caudal pulmonary mass *(arrows in C)*.

for post-contrast administration films.[23] Although no anesthesia or special equipment is required, it may be difficult to obtain consistently good opacification of the gallbladder. Noninvasive ultrasonography is considered more sensitive for detection of liver and biliary disease than radiographic examinations, and is the imaging modality of choice, if available.

Pancreas

The left lobe of the pancreas lies caudal to the gastric body's greater curvature and cranial to the transverse colon. The right lobe is adjacent to the mesenteric border of the proximal duodenum. On a ventrodorsal projection, the pancreas is located

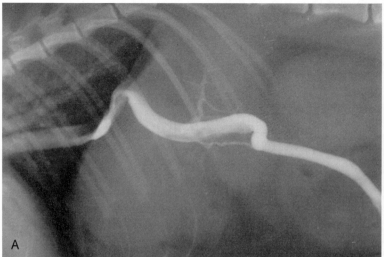

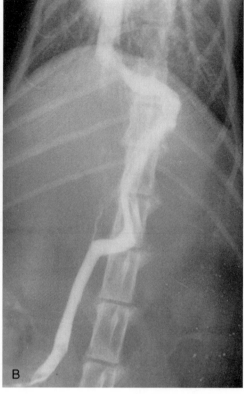

Figure 9–15. Operative mesenteric portogram, right lateral *(A)* and ventrodorsal *(B)* views. A single large extrahepatic shunt vessel communicates between the portal vein and the caudal vena cava, slightly to the left of midline. A small amount of contrast material is present within scattered parenchymal portal vein branches.

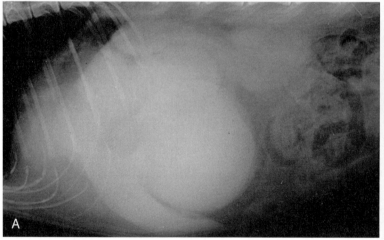

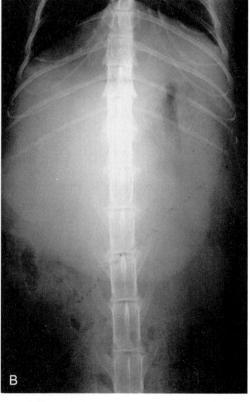

Figure 9–16. Survey abdomen. *A*, A smooth, circular soft-tissue mass is seen caudal to the hepatic lobar margins and ventral to the stomach on the right lateral view. *B*, The edges of the centrally located mass are less distinct on the ventrodorsal view. Surgical exploration revealed a markedly distended gallbladder with obstruction of the common bile duct by multiple small radiolucent choleliths. (*A* and *B*, Courtesy of Rowley Memorial Animal Hospital, Springfield, MA.)

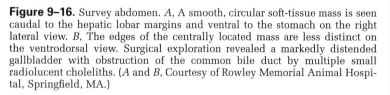

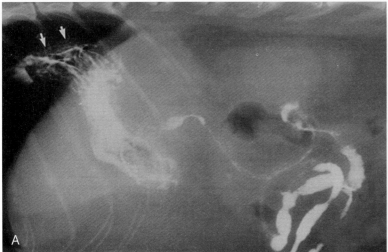
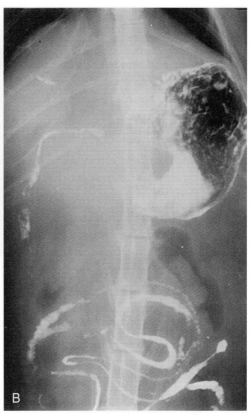

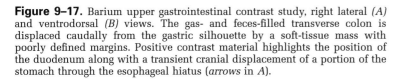

Figure 9–17. Barium upper gastrointestinal contrast study, right lateral *(A)* and ventrodorsal *(B)* views. The gas- and feces-filled transverse colon is displaced caudally from the gastric silhouette by a soft-tissue mass with poorly defined margins. Positive contrast material highlights the position of the duodenum along with a transient cranial displacement of a portion of the stomach through the esophageal hiatus (*arrows* in *A*).

primarily in the right cranial quadrant of the abdomen. The normal pancreas is not identified on survey films, and can be evaluated only indirectly on radiographs by changes in the opacity and serosal detail of the right cranial quadrant of the abdomen, and by positioning of adjacent structures.

An increase in radiographic opacity in the area of the pancreas often is difficult to identify because this quadrant is the most radiopaque area of the abdomen on the ventrodorsal view. Two anatomic changes most often associated with enlargement of the pancreas are widening of the duodenal flexure, and separation of the stomach and transverse colon. A concave caudal gastric border caused by the presence of a pancreatic mass also may be observed. A "fixed" bowel loop may be caused by adhesions after pancreatitis, or by neoplasia. However, these radiographic changes are merely suggestive, and not pathognomonic. A UGI series may be useful in delineating displaced portions of the stomach or duodenum (Fig. 9–17). Ultrasonographic evaluation is useful in visualizing larger pancreatic parenchymal masses.

REFERENCES

1. Gorbach SL: Bismuth therapy in gastrointestinal disease. Gastroenterology 99:863–875, 1990.
2. Williams J, Biller DS, Miyabayashi T, et al: Evaluation of iohexol as a gastrointestinal contrast medium in normal cats. Vet Radiol Ultrasound 34:310–314, 1993.
3. Agut A, Sanchezvalverde MA, Torrecillas FE, et al: Iohexol as a gastrointestinal contrast medium in the cat. Vet Radiol Ultrasound 35:164–168, 1994.
4. Owens JM, Biery DN: Radiographic contrast procedures. *In* Owens JM, Biery DN (eds): Radiographic Interpretation for the Small Animal Clinician. Baltimore, Williams & Wilkins, 1999, pp. 15–26.
5. Hall JA, Twedt DC, Burrows CF: Gastric motility in dogs. Part II. Disorders of gastric motility. Compend Contin Educ Pract Vet 12:1373–1390, 1990.
6. Hogan PM, Aronson E: Effect of sedation on transit time of feline gastrointestinal contrast studies. Vet Radiol 29:85–88, 1988.
7. O'Brien T: Small intestine. *In* O'Brien T (ed): Radiographic Diagnosis of Abdominal Disorders in the Dog and Cat. Philadelphia, WB Saunders, 1978, pp. 279–351.
8. Morgan JP: The upper gastrointestinal examination in the cat: Normal radiographic appearance using positive-contrast medium. Vet Radiol 22:159, 1981.
9. Willard MD: Diagnostic tests for the alimentary tract. *In* Nelson RW, Couto CJ (eds): Small Animal Internal Medicine. St. Louis, Mosby, 1998, pp. 368–389.
10. Chandler ML, Guilford WG, Lawoko CRO, et al: Gastric emptying and intestinal transit times of radiopaque markers in cats fed a high-fiber diet with and without low-dose intravenous diazepam. Vet Radiol Ultrasound 40:3–8, 1999.
11. Nelson OL, Jergens AE, Miles KG, et al: Gastric emptying in healthy dogs consuming a commercial kibble ration as assessed by barium-impregnated polyethylene spheres. (submitted for publication).
12. Myers NC, Kirk CA, Jewell DE, et al: Assessment of gastric emptying time in cats using nuclear imaging and radiopaque markers (Abstract). J Vet Intern Med 10:158, 1996.
13. Goggin JM, Hoskinson JJ, Butine MD, et al: Scintigraphic assessment of gastric emptying of canned and dry diets in healthy cats. Am J Vet Res 59:388–392, 1998.
14. Jergens AE, Moore FM, Haynes JS, et al: Idiopathic inflammatory bowel disease in dogs and cats: 84 cases (1987–1990). J Am Vet Med Assoc 201:1603–1608, 1992.
15. Owens JM, Biery DN: Gastrointestinal system. *In* Owens JM,

Biery DN (eds): Radiographic Interpretation for the Small Animal Clinician. Baltimore, Williams & Wilkins, 1999, pp. 223–260.

16. McNeel SV, Riedesel EA: The small bowel. *In* Thrall DE (ed): Textbook of Veterinary Diagnostic Radiology. Philadelphia, WB Saunders, 1998, pp. 540–557.

17. Norsworthy GD: Contrast radiography in cats: Practical procedures for private practice. Vet Med 90:862–868, 1995.

18. Stickle RL: Positive-contrast celiography (peritoneography) for the diagnosis of diaphragmatic hernia in dogs and cats. J Am Vet Med Assoc 185:295–298, 1984.

19. Rendano VT: Positive contrast peritoneography: An aid in the radiographic diagnosis of diaphragmatic hernia. J Am Vet Radiol Soc 20:67–73, 1979.

20. Birchard SJ: Surgical management of portosystemic shunts in dogs and cats. Compend Contin Educ Pract Vet 6:795–802, 1984.

21. Ewing GO, Suter PF, Bailey CS: Hepatic insufficiency associated with congenital anomalies of the portal vein in dogs. J Am Anim Hosp Assoc 10:463–476, 1974.

22. Barrett RE, Delahunta A, Roenigk WJ, et al: Four cases of congenital portacaval shunt in the dog. J Small Anim Pract 17:71–85, 1976.

23. Carlisle CH: A comparison of technics for cholecystography in the cat. J Am Vet Radiol Soc 18:173–176, 1977.

10
◆ Approach to the Icteric Cat

Joseph Taboada

Bilirubin is the major pigment in bile. It is produced as the catabolic byproduct of hemoproteins and excreted via a hepatobiliary route. Accumulation of bilirubin, due to either accelerated hemoprotein catabolism or reduced bilirubin clearance, will result in hyperbilirubinemia and, subsequently, icterus. Icterus first can be detected as a yellowish discoloration of plasma or serum that usually is apparent as bilirubin concentrations reach 1.0 to 2.0 mg/dl. As bilirubin concentrations reach 2.0 to 3.0 mg/dl, icterus becomes apparent in soft tissues such as mucous membranes, sclerae, and skin. In cats, the oropharyngeal mucosa and the inner pinnae of the ears are valuable sites to evaluate for icterus. The term *jaundice* often is used to refer to the yellow appearance when it is clinically apparent in the soft tissues.

Icterus is a common problem encountered in feline practice. The challenge to the veterinarian when faced with the icteric cat is to establish a differential diagnosis and diagnostic plan that are reflective of where the derangement in bilirubin metabolism is occurring. This is best accomplished when bilirubin metabolism and the pathophysiology of hyperbilirubinemia are well-understood.

◆ PATHOPHYSIOLOGY OF HYPERBILIRUBINEMIA

Hemoprotein catabolism and bilirubin metabolism occur at a constant steady rate in healthy cats. Minor, short-lived disruptions in these pathways may occur without the development of icterus, but more extensive disruptions overwhelm the ability of the catabolic and excretory pathways to handle bilirubin. Once this happens, increases in urine, serum, or plasma, and subsequently, tissue-associated bilirubin rapidly become apparent.

Bilirubin is formed as a byproduct of hemoprotein catabolism. The primary source of hemoprotein is hemoglobin from senescent erythrocytes. To a lesser extent, hemoglobin from ineffective erythropoiesis, myoglobin from turnover of myocytes in muscle, and catabolism of a number of short-half-life hemoprotein enzymes and cytochromes collectively contribute hemoprotein that eventually is metabolized to bilirubin. Hemoglobin from senescent erythrocytes makes up approximately two-thirds of the hemoprotein being catabolized; most of the remainder is accounted for by the many short-lived hemoproteins, with myoglobin typically making up only a small fraction of the total.

When erythrocytes become senescent, they are phagocytized and degraded by the mononuclear phagocytic cells of the spleen, liver, and bone marrow. When intravascular hemolysis occurs, the hemoprotein is bound initially to haptoglobin, an acute-phase reactant transport protein synthesized in the liver, for transport to the phagocytic cells. Once in cells of the mononuclear phagocytic system, the hemoprotein is cleaved enzymatically by heme oxygenase to form biliverdin, and then is reduced via biliverdin reductase to bilirubin. The bilirubin at this time is referred to as *unconjugated* or *indirect bilirubin*. The phagocytic cells release this unconjugated bilirubin into the circulation, where it is bound rapidly to albumin in a reversible manner for transport to the liver. Albumin has a high binding affinity for unconjugated bilirubin, which limits glomerular filtration. Unbound unconjugated bilirubin is readily miscible with phospholipids and will distribute readily into the intracellular space where it can produce toxic consequences. Although very rarely a problem in cats, this unconjugated bilirubinemia may induce central nervous system toxicity and cause seizures and hyperthermia in neonatal kittens.

In normal cats, the liver appears to be the only organ removing bilirubin from the plasma. Albumin-bound unconjugated bilirubin is extracted from plasma by hepatocytes via a carrier-mediated process or via high affinity domains in the hepatocellular membrane. Organic anions such as indocyanine green and sulfobromophthalein interact competitively with bilirubin for transmembrane transport, but bile acids do not. This process does not appear to be significantly dependent on hepatic perfusion. Even severe impairment of hepatic perfusion, as might occur in cats with congenital portosystemic shunts, rarely results in the development of increased plasma concentrations of bilirubin.

Once in the hepatocyte, bilirubin binds to a number of different storage proteins until it can be conjugated in the smooth endoplasmic reticulum. Conjugation, primarily with glucuronic acid and to lesser extent with simple sugars, is a very efficient process. At this point, the bilirubin is referred to as *conjugated* or *direct bilirubin*. Both unconjugated and conjugated bilirubin are able to flux bidirectionally across the hepatocyte membrane, which contributes to the measured plasma concentration. Conjugated bilirubin in plasma also is rapidly bound to albumin, but with an affinity that is less than that for unconjugated bilirubin. A small amount of free conjugated bilirubin thus is available for glomerular filtration and tubular reabsorption. The renal tubular threshold for bilirubin in cats is approximately 9 times higher than in dogs; therefore, cats, unlike dogs, do not demonstrate bilirubinuria without an associated hyperbilirubinemia. Bilirubinuria is both a sensitive and a specific indicator of abnormal bilirubin metabolism in cats, and thus, always warrants evaluation for hepatobiliary or hemolytic disease.

Conjugated bilirubin is excreted via an energy-dependent, carrier-mediated process across the canalicular membrane of the hepatocyte into the canaliculus. Transport of conjugated bilirubin from the liver cell to the canalicular bile is a saturable process that is susceptible to a variety of physiologic insults, and is the rate-limiting step in bilirubin metabolism. A number of disease processes seemingly unrelated to hemolytic or hepatobiliary disease exert an influence on bilirubin metabolism by interfering with canalicular membrane transport. Conditions such as septicemia and pancreatitis and the influence of a number of drugs can reduce conjugated bilirubin excretion via such mechanisms.

The liver has a large reserve capacity for bilirubin excretion, and the capacity of the liver to metabolize and maintain normal plasma bilirubin concentration is greater than for many other hepatic functions. Most hepatobiliary causes of hyperbilirubinemia therefore are due to cholestasis or canalicular biliary transport aberrations as opposed to hepatocellular dysfunction per se.

Once bile with the accompanying conjugated bilirubin is excreted into the intestine, bilirubin is deconjugated and hydrogenated by colonic bacteria eventually to form a group of colorless tetrapyrroles collectively referred to as *urobilinogen*. Small amounts of urobilinogen are absorbed into the portal circulation, where they are extracted and re-excreted by the liver. Approximately 5 per cent of this urobilinogen escapes hepatic re-uptake and is excreted in the urine. Despite this step in bilirubin metabolism, the measurement of urinary urobilinogen via urine dipsticks is neither a sensitive nor a specific indicator of bile-duct patency, and is not useful clinically. Fecal urobilinogen is oxidized further to the pigmented compounds urobilin and stercobilin, which impart the normal brown color on stool. Either a complete bile duct obstruction or a lack of normal intestinal bacterial activity may result in a lack of pigment production and a gray-appearing, "acholic" stool.

◆ PHYSICAL EXAMINATION AND LABORATORY TESTING

Icterus generally is noted on physical examination. Typically, serum bilirubin concentrations of greater than 2.5 mg/dl are necessary before the icterus is apparent clinically. The yellow discoloration generally is seen most easily on the mucous membranes of the pharyngeal and oral soft tissues, although as the bilirubin concentrations increase, the icterus becomes apparent on all visible soft-tissue surfaces. When bilirubin concentrations are only mildly increased, icterus may not be apparent until the blood is evaluated and plasma is noted to be icteric. Some laboratories report icterus in a semiquantitative manner by referring to an *icterus index*. The icterus index is determined by comparing the color of the plasma from a hematocrit tube to a set of standards that progress from clear to bright yellow. In this index, less than 5 is considered normal (clear) with increasing increments of 5 being used to describe progressively more yellow plasma appearance. For example, a cat with normal-appearing plasma may be said to have an icterus index of less than 5, whereas a cat with severe icterus may be described as having an icterus index of 20. Icterus indices of 5 or 10 would indicate less severe icterus. Measurement of bilirubin concentration will be reflected most accurately on a chemistry panel. Normal concentrations in cats typically are between 0.1 and 0.3 mg/dl, and are fairly consistent from one laboratory to the next. Serum concentrations generally are reported as total bilirubin, meaning that both conjugated and unconjugated bilirubin are being measured. Conjugated and unconjugated bilirubin, reported as separate indices, are of little clinical utility in cats.

Most icteric cats will present to the veterinarian for anorexia, weakness, or other nonspecific or gastrointestinal clinical signs. Recognition of icterus causes the clinician to consider disease processes that increase bilirubin production (hemolytic diseases referred to as a *prehepatic process*), or decrease bilirubin clearance and excretion (hepatobiliary disease referred to as *hepatic* or *posthepatic processes*).

◆ DIAGNOSTIC TESTS

The most important initial evaluation to perform on the icteric cat is to assess for the presence or absence of anemia. A hematocrit, together with a total plasma protein concentration, generally will allow the clinician to define the cause of the icterus as either a prehepatic or a hepatic/posthepatic problem. Generally, a hematocrit of less than 20 per cent will signify that the cause for the icterus is likely hemolysis. If the anemia is less severe, then it is more difficult to make that assumption, because many hepatic diseases are accompanied by a mild-to-moderate nonregenerative anemia. A complete blood count will give added information relative to the cause of an anemia. Hemolytic processes generally are characterized by a decreased hematocrit with a normal total plasma protein concentration. If both the hematocrit and the plasma protein are decreased in an icteric cat, gastrointestinal blood loss associated with liver disease should be considered as a possibility. Hemolytic anemias usually are regenerative, with reticulocytosis, nucleated red blood cells, poikilocytosis, and anisocytosis present.

It is important to remember when assessing for regeneration that acute hemolytic anemias initially will be nonregenerative, because it takes from 2 to 4 days for a significant regenerative response to be generated. That said, most hemolytic processes occur over a number of days before presentation to the veterinarian, so that an obvious regenerative response is apparent at the time of the initial evaluation. A neutrophilic leukocytosis with a moderate-to-marked left shift may be seen, especially in immune-mediated hemolytic anemia. The severity of the left shift and of the reticulocytosis generally is less than that seen in dogs. Assessment of a serum biochemistry panel may be helpful in evaluating the cat for potential hepatic or posthepatic disease, but it should be remembered that severe anemia will often cause centrolobular hepatocellular degeneration and/or necrosis that will result in increased transaminase and cholestatic enzyme activity. A urinalysis is helpful in confirming icterus in cats when only mild increases in bilirubin concentration are present. Because the renal threshold for bilirubin in cats is high, and unlike dogs, the feline kidney is unable to conjugate and excrete bilirubin, any evidence of bilirubinuria is a significant indicator of hyperbilirubinemia.

When icterus is present without an accompanying anemia, the cat should be evaluated for hepatic or posthepatic biliary disease. Abdominal ultrasonography is the most useful noninvasive test to differentiate between hepatic and posthepatic causes of icterus. Dilated and tortuous common and/or hepatic bile ducts would be suggestive of biliary tract obstruction.[1] Choleliths, biliary or peribiliary masses, and pancreatitis are other potential posthepatic causes that may be evident. If no evidence of biliary obstruction is noted, hepatic disease should be suspected.

◆ DIFFERENTIAL DIAGNOSIS

Prehepatic Causes (Hemolysis)

Hemolytic causes of icterus are less common in cats than in dogs. The most common cause for hemolysis in cats is *Haemobartonella felis* infection (see Chapters 2, Hemobartonellosis, and 60, Use of the Polymerase Chain Reaction to Detect Hemoparasites). *Haemobartonella* organisms may be observed as epicellular parasites on the red blood cells. They are present intermittently on blood smears from infected cats, so multiple smears from blood drawn at different times should be examined. Less common hemoparasites causing hemolysis and icterus in cats include *Cytauxzoon felis* (see Chapter 55, Update on Cytauxzoonosis), *Babesia felis*, *Babesia herpailuri*, and *Babesia pantherae*. Feline leukemia virus also has been associated with hemolytic anemia.

Toxic causes of hemolysis often are associated with oxidative injury and Heinz body formation. Feline erythrocytes are very sensitive to oxidative injury. Toxins causing hemolysis in cats include zinc, copper, onion, methylene blue, acetaminophen, D-L-methionine, benzocaine, and propylene glycol.

Immune-mediated causes of hemolysis are uncommon in cats.[2] Idiopathic immune-mediated hemolytic anemia or anemia associated with systemic lupus–like disease is seen occasionally. Neoplasia, feline leukemia virus infection, or drug/hapten-related hemolytic anemias should be considered. Incompatible blood transfusion and the presence of alloantibodies in the neonate causing neonatal isoerythrocytolysis are additional immunologically related causes of hemolysis (see Chapter 58, Transfusion Medicine).

Microangiopathic causes of hemolysis also are uncommon in cats. The 2 primary causes in dogs are splenic hemangiosarcoma and caval syndrome associated with heartworm disease. In cats, disseminated intravascular coagulation may induce a microangiopathic anemia. A coagulation panel consisting of a prothrombin time, partial thromboplastin time, or D-dimer assay and fibrinogen would be of value in ruling out disseminated intravascular coagulation. Hypophosphatemia may result in hemolysis.[3, 4] In cats, hypophosphatemia may be seen as a complication of insulin therapy or as a result of enteral refeeding. Refeeding-induced hypophosphatemia is seen most often in cats with hepatic lipidosis.

Inherited in-born errors of metabolism resulting in hemolysis are not as well described in cats as in dogs. Pyruvate kinase deficiency has been reported in the Abyssinian and Somali breeds (see Chapter 61, Hereditary Erythrocyte Disorders).

Hepatic Causes

Hepatic causes of icterus are more common in cats than either pre- or posthepatic causes. Hepatic lipidosis is the most common liver disease of cats in the United States, and most cats with this disease are icteric. Hepatic lipidosis may occur secondary to a variety of metabolic derangements or may be of a primary idiopathic origin. Whereas biopsy is necessary for definitive diagnosis of hepatic lipidosis, fine-needle aspiration cytology is useful in most cases (see Chapter 15, Cytologic Evaluation of Fine-Needle Liver Biopsies). The prognosis for cats with hepatic lipidosis generally is good when aggressive enteral nutritional support is supplied.[5]

Cholangiohepatitis and lymphocytic portal hepatitis are common inflammatory liver diseases of cats that often cause icterus.[6] Together, these inflammatory liver diseases are almost as common as hepatic lipidosis.[7] Biopsy for histopathology and bacterial culture is important in the diagnosis of these conditions. Cholangiohepatitis also may be associated with pancreatitis and inflammatory bowel disease.[8] Pancreatitis can contribute to icterus via both hepatic and posthepatic mechanisms.[9] A subset of cats with cholangiohepatitis will have bacterial infection (especially gram-negative and anaerobic bacteria) as part of the pathogenesis. Both gram-negative and gram-positive septicemia can result in icterus associated with a reversible functional abnormality of the canalicular membrane, even if the liver is not the primary site of infection. Histoplasmosis is the most common fungal cause of infectious hepatitis. Other infectious diseases such as blastomycosis, sporotrichosis, systemic aspergillosis, toxoplasmosis, neosporosis, and *Hepatozoon canis*–like infections also affect the liver on rare occasions. Feline infectious peritonitis is an important viral cause of hepatic icterus. A feline infectious peritonitis–induced pyogranulomatous vasculitis affecting the hepatic vasculature may or may not be associated with abdominal effusion. Fever and multisystemic signs often accompany icterus in cats with feline infectious peritonitis.

Lymphosarcoma is an important neoplastic cause of hepatic icterus. Lymphosarcoma may occur in the livers of cats with diffuse disease, gastrointestinal disease, or disease limited primarily to the liver. Neoplastic lymphocytes tend to infiltrate the liver diffusely and generally are demonstrated easily by biopsy or fine-needle aspiration cytology (see Chapter 15, Cytologic Evaluation of Fine-Needle Liver Biopsies). Hepatocellular carcinoma can occur as a solitary lesion, as multifocal lesions, or as diffuse infiltration of large portions of the liver. Multiple liver lobe involvement is seen in cats more often than in dogs. Icterus is noted in about one-third of cats with primary liver tumors.

Cirrhosis as an end-stage of chronic inflammatory disease is rare in cats compared with other species. Hepatic fibrosis may be seen in cats with sclerosing cholangitis, an unusual disease that is thought to be a severe form of chronic cholangiohepatitis. The lesions seen are very similar to those observed in primary sclerosing cholangitis in human beings, a disease with an immune-mediated pathogenesis. Cats with sclerosing cholangitis usually have ascites as a significant clinical finding. Icterus is variably present.

Hepatic amyloidosis is a progressive systemic disease associated with extracellular deposition of insoluble fibrillar proteins that eventually results in organ dysfunction. It is a familial disorder in Abyssinian, Oriental, and Siamese cats. The liver, spleen, kidneys, and adrenal glands typically are affected. Whereas Abyssinian cats typically show signs of renal dysfunction, Oriental and Siamese cats are more likely to show signs of hepatic disease.

Toxic causes of hepatic icterus in cats usually are associated with administration of therapeutic agents. Commonly used drugs in cats that have been shown to cause hepatic injury include diazepam, methimazole, glipizide, itraconazole, and ketoconazole. Acetaminophen is an antipyretic/analgesic readily available in most households. Cats are highly sensitive to the toxic effects of this drug, which causes methemoglobinemia, Heinz body formation, and hepatocellular necrosis.

Posthepatic Causes

Posthepatic icterus is less common in cats than in dogs. Nonneoplastic obstructive processes include cholelithiasis, biliary and pancreatic pseudocysts, mucoceles, diaphragmatic hernia, and liver flukes. Cholelithiasis is seen most often in cats with cholangiohepatitis. The choleliths may be apparent radiographically. In areas such as Florida, Hawaii, Puerto Rico, and the Caribbean, the liver fluke, *Platynosomum fastosum*, is an important cause of posthepatic icterus. *Amphimerus pseudofelineus* also has been associated with obstructive cholangitis and cholangiohepatitis, and is endemic to a wider range. Neoplasia of the bile duct and peribiliary tissues are unusual causes of posthepatic icterus. Lymphosarcoma, bile duct carcinoma, and pancreatic carcinoma should be considered. Bile peritonitis after biliary trauma or necrotizing cholecystitis also may result in icterus.

REFERENCES

1. Leveille R, Biller D, Shiroma J: Sonographic evaluation of the common bile duct in cats. J Vet Intern Med 10: 296–299, 1996.
2. Day M: Immune-mediated hemolytic anemia. Vet Q 20:39–40, 1998.
3. Adams L, Hardy R, Weiss D, et al: Hypophosphatemia and hemolytic anemia associated with diabetes mellitus and hepatic lipidosis in cats. J Vet Intern Med 7:266–271, 1993.
4. Justin R, Hohenhaus A: Hypophosphatemia associated with enteral alimentation in cats. J Vet Intern Med 9:228–233, 1995.
5. Center S, Crawford M, Guida L, et al: A retrospective study of 77 cats with severe hepatic lipidosis: 1975–1990. J Vet Intern Med 7:349–359, 1993.
6. Gagne J, Weiss D, Armstrong P: Histopathologic evaluation of feline inflammatory liver disease. Vet Pathol 33:521–526, 1996.
7. Day D: Feline cholangiohepatitis complex. Vet Clin North Am Small Anim Pract 25:275–285, 1995.
8. Weiss D, Gagne J, Armstrong P: Relationship between inflammatory hepatic disease and inflammatory bowel disease, pancreatitis, and nephritis in cats. J Am Vet Med Assoc 209:1114–1116, 1996.
9. Steiner J, Williams D: Feline exocrine pancreatic disorders. Vet Clin North Am Small Anim Pract 29:551–575, 1999.

11

◆ Gastric *Helicobacter* Infection

Kenneth W. Simpson
Dalit Strauss-Ayali
Reto Neiger

The discovery of the association of *Helicobacter pylori* with gastritis, peptic ulcers, and gastric neoplasia has led to fundamental changes in the understanding of gastric disease in human beings.[1–3] The presence of spiral bacteria in the stomachs of animals has been known for over a century,[4–6] and gastric spiral organisms have been documented in dogs, cats,[7–13] ferrets, monkeys, cheetahs, pigs, cows, predatory cats, and foxes, among other species.[14] Relatively little attention has been paid to the pathogenicity of *Helicobacter* species other than *H. pylori*; *H. mustelae* has been associated with gastritis and peptic ulcers in ferrets, *H. acinonychis* with severe gastritis in cheetahs, and *H. heilmannii* with gastric ulcers in pigs.[14] This review summarizes our current knowledge of gastric *Helicobacter* species infection in cats.

◆ *HELICOBACTER* SPECIES INFECTING THE STOMACHS OF CATS

Helicobacter species are gram-negative, microaerophilic, curved to spiral-shaped, motile bacteria that, along with *Campylobacter* and *Arcobacter*, belong to a distinct phylum within the class Proteobacteria of the eubacteria.[15] Gastric *Helicobacter*-like organisms (HLO) found in pet cats are much larger (0.5 × 5 to 12 μm) than *H. pylori* (0.5 × 1.5 to 3 μm) (Fig. 11–1). Electron microscopy has revealed that HLO, which appear uniform by light microscopy, can have very different morphology.[11] However, because bacterial morphology is not a definitive means of distinguishing different HLO, precise identification of *Helicobacter* species relies mainly on genetic analyses and culture with conventional phenotype testing or protein profiling.[16–19]

To date, *Helicobacter felis*, *Helicobacter pametensis*, and an *H. heilmannii*–like bacterium have been identified in the stomachs of pet cats.[12, 17, 20] The first large HLO cultured was named *H. felis* owing to its isolation from a cat stomach,[20] but it also can be found in dogs[17] and human patients.[21] It has sparsely distributed periplasmic fibers appearing singly or in groups of 2, 3, or 4 on the crest of the helical body (Fig. 11–2). *H. pametensis* has been isolated from the stomach of 1 cat.[12]

H. pylori has been cultured from a group of laboratory cats,[22] and is much smaller (0.5 × 1.5 to 3 μm), curved or S-shaped, and easily distinguished by light microscopy (see Fig. 11–1). Uncultivable large gastric spiral organisms, which lack periplasmic fibrils or have a small fiber in the valley of the helical body (see Fig. 11–2), are perhaps the most common HLO found in cats.[12, 13] By comparison of their 16S rRNA sequence, these organisms are considered members of the genus *Helicobacter*, and some were subsequently named "*H. heilmannii*" in honor of the German pathologist Konrad Heilmann.[24] It is likely that "*H. heilmannii*" encompasses several different *Helicobacter* species. Only recently, one "*H. heilmannii*" strain was isolated in Denmark and typed based on its 16S rRNA sequence.[25]

◆ PREVALENCE AND TRANSMISSION

Recent studies suggest a high prevalence of gastric *Helicobacter* infection in cats. HLO have been observed in gastric biopsies from 41 to 100 per cent of clinically healthy cats and from 57 to 100 per cent of vomiting cats (Table 11–1).

Interestingly, Yamasaki and coworkers[26] found a lower prevalence in sick cats than in healthy cats.

Table 11–1. Prevalence of Gastric *Helicobacter*-Like Organisms in Cats

Infected (%)	Cats (n)	Reference
Healthy		
100	12	Weber, 1958[11]
41	29	Geyer, 1993[8]
97	32 stray	Otto, 1994[10]
100	25 stray	El-Zaatari, 1997[27]
100	15*	Papasouliotis, 1997[13]
90	10	Yamasaki, 1998[26]
94	32*	De Majo, 1998[28]
91	58	Neiger, 1998[12]
100	15	Norris, 1999[23]
Sick		
57	60	Geyer, 1993[8]
76	127	Hermanns, 1995[9]
64	33	Yamasaki, 1998[26]
100	24	Papasouliotis, 1997[13]

*Colony cats.

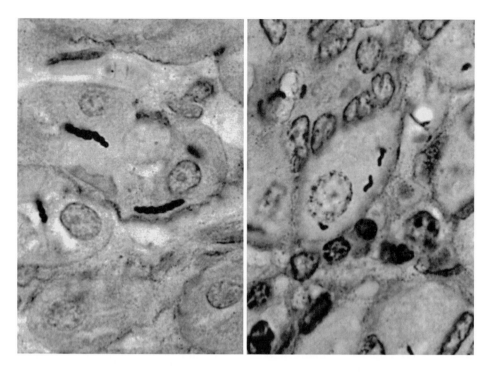

Figure 11–1. Light microscopy of *Helicobacter felis* (*left*) and *Helicobacter pylori* (*right*) in gastric biopsies from infected cats. Although typically observed on the mucus and within gastric pits, spiral organisms also can be detected within the cytoplasm of gastric cells.

Possible explanations for this finding could be the recent use of antibiotics in sick animals or perhaps a protective immune response.

Few reports mention the prevalence of specific *Helicobacter* species in the stomach of cats, because identification of the organism requires specialized techniques. *H. felis* has been cultured from 3 of 21 *Helicobacter*-infected cats in Finland,[17] whereas "*H. heilmannii*" was identified by polymerase chain reaction (PCR) in 38 of 49 Swiss cats.[12] Results of PCR studies in *Helicobacter*-infected cats in the United States have identified 9 of 17 cats with "*H. heilmannii*," 1 of 17 with *H. felis*, 3 of 17 coinfected with *H. felis* and "*H. heilmannii*," and 4 cats with unclassified *Helicobacter* species (K. Simpson and D. Strauss-Ayali, unpublished results, 1999).

The mode of transmission and time of acquisition of *Helicobacter* is unclear. A fecal-oral spread is hypothesized by some investigators because *H. pylori* can be cultured from cat feces, and suboptimum sanitary conditions in underdeveloped countries might favor such a transmission in people.[29, 30] Oral-oral spread is hypothesized by others, because *H. pylori* can be found in the saliva of infected cats, and because infected human beings and their spouses have a higher prevalence.[30] However, the recent isolation of *H. pylori* from surface water in the United States and Sweden[31, 32] suggests that water-borne infection is likely to be an important route, particularly when considering that *H. pylori* is more resistant to chlorination than *Escherichia coli*.

It appears that *Helicobacter* infections in cats are acquired early in life. In a breeding colony of queens infected with *H. pylori*, 9 of 17 kittens were infected at 6 to 8 weeks of age (K. Simpson and A. Gerold, unpublished observations, 1999). Cats as young as 6 weeks of age were already positive utilizing the ^{13}C-urea breath test (R. Neiger, unpublished observations, 1999). Thus, *Helicobacter* infection can be acquired at a very young age.

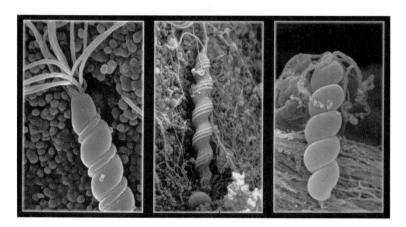

Figure 11–2. Electron microscopic appearance of the large gastric spirals *Helicobacter heilmannii*, *Helicobacter felis*, and *Helicobacter bizzozeronii* (*left to right*).

◆ PUBLIC HEALTH

Owing to the discovery of cats harboring *H. pylori* in a research colony[22] as well as in China[33] and based on 1 report in France,[34] cats may be a potential natural reservoir of *H. pylori* and might pose a zoonotic risk. Preliminary findings of 1 epidemiologic study of *H. pylori*–positive farm workers showed significantly more contact with cats than with other animals.[35] However, 2 studies evaluating *H. pylori* antibodies in cat owners, and comparing them with people without contact with cats, showed no increased risk in the first population.[36, 37] A study in veterinarians was equally negative for an increased risk of acquiring an *H. pylori* infection from pets.[38] Finally, it has not been possible to isolate *H. pylori* from stray and pet cats in various studies,[12, 17, 23, 27] suggesting that *H. pylori* infection in cats may be an anthroponosis—an animal infection with a human pathogen.

Several reports in human patients have assumed a possible zoonotic transmission of large HLO from dogs or cats.[39] Only recently, an identical "*H. heilmannii*" organism, defined by PCR and urease-B gene sequencing, has been found in a patient and 1 of his cats.[40] The possible risk of transmission of large gastric HLO to human patients is rather small, considering the more than 90 per cent prevalence in dogs and cats and the rare (<0.5 per cent) occurrence in human beings. Notwithstanding, proper hygienic control is necessary to keep the risk to a minimum.

◆ PATHOGENICITY

The role of *Helicobacter* species in the pathogenesis of gastric disease in cats still is under debate. Obvious clinical signs of infection are absent in the majority of infected cats, and few studies have investigated the cellular and immunologic consequences of infection. A clear definition of disease also is required—is it tissue injury and/or clinical manifestation?

This situation contrasts with that in human patients, in whom there is extensive evidence implicating *H. pylori* in the pathogenesis of chronic superficial gastritis. Eradication of *H. pylori* by antimicrobial therapy cures gastritis, and the titer of anti–*H. pylori* antibodies decreases with time. A plethora of reports have shown many putative mechanisms by which *H. pylori* alters gastric physiology[29, 41, 42]—for example, by inducing gastric inflammation, disrupting the gastric mucosal barrier (e.g., disrupting phospholipases, secreting vacuolating cytotoxins, inducing apoptosis), or altering the gastric-secretory axis (e.g., by decreasing somatostatin release, inducing hypergastrinemia, diminishing the responsiveness of parietal cells). *H. pylori* infection in human beings has been associated with the production of the proinflammatory cytokines interleukin (IL)-1β, IL-6, IL-8, and tumor necrosis factor-alpha (TNF-α).[43, 44] The production of these proinflammatory cytokines has been linked to alterations in gastrin, somatostatin, and acid secretion, and to the genesis of gastritis and ulceration.[43, 45, 46]

Infection with *Helicobacter* species also predisposes human beings to the development of gastric cancer.[2, 3] The precise mechanism of carcinogenesis is unclear, but it may involve the induction of nitric oxide synthetase by proinflammatory cytokines with subsequent nitric oxide production and nitrosamine formation.[47] It also may involve a decrease in apoptosis relative to cell proliferation.[48]

◆ INFLAMMATION AND GASTRIC FUNCTION

Naturally Acquired Infections

Histologic findings in infected as well as uninfected cats vary from a "normal" gastric mucosa to mild or moderate chronic gastritis.[7–10, 12, 13, 23, 26, 28] A correlation between the presence of HLO and the extent of histopathologic changes was demonstrated in one study,[9] and Happonen and colleagues[7] found lymphocyte aggregates only in HLO-positive cats, which also had more lymphocytes in the fundus and corpus than HLO-negative cats. Interestingly, in a recent study, glandular degeneration was more frequent in the fundi of cats with HLO than those without HLO, but gastric fibrosis and lymphocytic-plasmacytic enteritis were similar.[26] A more severe gastritis, characterized by marked lymphoid follicular hyperplasia and infiltration of neutrophils and eosinophils, has been observed in cats with *H. pylori* infection.[22] To date, gastric function has not been evaluated in cats colonized with large HLO. Changes in gastric acid secretion and serum gastrin, which are known to occur in human beings with *H. pylori* infection, have not been demonstrated in cats with *H. pylori* infection.

Although multiple studies have evaluated gastric histopathology, the lack of standardized criteria to define histologic changes makes comparison between different studies difficult. The high prevalence of infection in cats also makes it difficult to find a suitable negative control group and to define *normal mucosa*. Furthermore, because most studies have used only limited diagnostic tests with limited sensitivity, comparisons of colonized with noncolonized animals may have been inaccurate. Finally, the presence of multiple species of HLO complicates the investigation of pathogenicity.

Experimental Studies

There are relatively few experimental studies of *Helicobacter* infection in cats. Specific-pathogen–free (SPF) cats have been infected with *H. felis* and *H. pylori*.[49–51] Five SPF *Helicobacter*-free cats were studied before and for 1 year after inoculation with

H. felis.[49] Four SPF-uninfected cats served as controls. Lymphoid follicular hyperplasia, atrophy, and fibrosis were observed primarily in the pylorus of infected cats. Mild mononuclear inflammation was detected in both infected and uninfected cats, but was more extensive in infected cats, with inflammation throughout the stomach. Eosinophilic infiltrates were observed only in infected cats. No upregulation of antral mucosal IL-1α, IL-1β, or TNF-α was detected by reverse transcriptase polymerase chain reaction (RT-PCR) in any cats. The gastric secretory axis, assessed by fasting plasma gastrin and pentagastrin-stimulated gastric acid secretion, was similar in both infected and uninfected cats.

In SPF cats infected with 2 different *H. pylori* strains (cytotoxin-associated protein *cagA* present or absent), chronic gastritis was observed 4 to 7 months after infection.[50, 51] Multifocal lymphoplasmacytic follicles were prominent in the antrum and body of infected cats. Serologic responses observed in SPF cats infected with *H. pylori* and *H. felis* demonstrated that some cats did not seroconvert (immunoglobulin [Ig] G) until 6 months after infection, and had titers 2- to 15-fold greater than baseline.[49, 51]

◆ DIAGNOSIS

Diagnostic tests consist of invasive tests (culture, histopathology, touch cytology, rapid-urease test, electron microscopy, PCR), which require a gastric tissue sample, and noninvasive tests (urea breath and blood tests, serology).[12, 52]

Invasive Tests

Culture

Culture of *Helicobacter* species is a difficult and insensitive means of confirming infection. Only *H. felis* was cultured from 3 of 21 *Helicobacter*-infected cats in Finland.[17] The designation "*H. heilmannii*"–like organism has been suggested for uncultured *Helicobacter* species without periplasmic fibers.[23] Positive culture is the only means of evaluating antimicrobial sensitivity.

Histopathology

Histopathology depends on the visual identification of *Helicobacter* organisms in gastric tissue. Silver stains,[12] Giemsa,[8, 9] or toluidine blue[7] will enhance the visibility of HLO when colonization density is low. Owing to the patchy distribution, several biopsies from antrum, corpus, and cardia should be evaluated. The development of a visual analogue scale for gastric biopsy specimens may make future comparison between various studies possible.[53]

Impression Smears/Touch Cytology

Impression smears or touch cytology with gram or DiffQuik staining is a simple, rapid, and sensitive diagnostic test for diagnosing infection with HLO.[12, 13, 53] However, the extent of a concurrent gastritis or lymphoid follicular hyperplasia cannot be determined reliably.

Biopsy Urease Test

The biopsy urease test is based on the production of urease by gastric *Helicobacter* species.[14] A gastric biopsy is incubated in urea broth containing phenol red as a pH indicator. As urease breaks down urea into ammonia, the pH rises and a color change occurs. Other urease-producing bacteria in the stomach (e.g., *Proteus* species) can cause a false-positive reading. Diagnosis in pets is obtained normally within 1 to 3 hours.

Electron Microscopy

Electron microscopy has been advocated to differentiate *Helicobacter* species on the basis of typical morphologic criteria. However, cultured *Helicobacter* species may lose their typical in vivo morphologic characteristics.[17, 54]

Polymerase Chain Reaction

DNA extracted from gastric tissue or juice can be subjected to PCR with *Helicobacter* genus–specific primers and *Helicobacter* species–specific primers, enabling diagnosis as well as identification of the *Helicobacter* species.[12, 55] Primers are derived mostly either from the urease gene or from the 16S rRNA gene. PCR products subsequently can be cloned and sequenced, or analyzed by restriction fragment length polymorphism, to identify the species and strain.[40]

For the diagnosis of naturally acquired *Helicobacter* infection in dogs and cats, touch cytology, rapid-urease test, and histopathology appear to be highly accurate.[12, 53] When colonization density is low, impression smears and PCR seem more accurate than a modified Steiner stain and rapid-urease test. Multiple biopsies always should be acquired, not only from the fundus but also from the cardia and antrum/pylorus area, owing to the patchy distribution of gastric *Helicobacter* species. Owing to this pattern and the requirement of a gastric biopsy, there is a clear need for less invasive methods of diagnosing infection. In people, noninvasive diagnosis of *H. pylori* has been achieved using serology or the urea breath test. The former is used largely as a screening test, whereas the latter test also is used to confirm eradication after treatment.

Noninvasive Tests

Serology

Enzyme-linked immunosorbent assay (ELISA) and immunoblotting are used frequently as diagnostic tools in human clinics and for epidemiologic studies. The most accurate ELISA test kits are based on a variety of semipurified antigens derived from *H. pylori*, and measure circulating IgG in serum. Immunoblotting has been used to define the immunogenic moieties of *H. pylori* or to investigate equivocal ELISA test results. Serodiagnosis in cats represents a challenge, because they can harbor several *Helicobacter* species.[17] A recent study evaluated immunoblotting and ELISA in serum samples from naturally infected dogs and from uninfected SPF dogs.[56] Kinetic ELISA results and number of bands per lane on an immunoblotting test were significantly higher for samples from infected dogs than those from uninfected dogs. A report of serology in cats has been published, although the results are difficult to interpret as the presence or absence of HLO in the stomach was not ascertained.[57] Serology has limited utility as an aid in demonstrating therapeutic success in human patients, because titers may not decrease for 6 months or more after the infection has been cleared, although recent studies in human beings show that a drop in antibody titers is consistent with eradication.

Urea Breath and Blood Tests

Urea breath and blood tests use urea labeled with isotopically stable ^{13}C or radioactive ^{14}C. Ingested labeled urea is cleaved to ammonia by urease produced by *Helicobacter* species. The released labeled C-atoms are absorbed into the circulation and exhaled. Exhaled air is collected, and with ^{13}C-urea, the ratio of $^{13}CO_2$ to $^{12}CO_2$ is measured by mass spectrometry, while the amount of radioactive CO_2 is analyzed with ^{14}C-urea.[58, 59] The ratio of $^{13}CO_2$ to $^{12}CO_2$ also can be measured in a blood sample.[58] The ^{13}C-urea breath and blood test has been evaluated in cats.[12, 59] Because the urea breath test demonstrates actual *Helicobacter* colonization, it is the preferred noninvasive method to document a successful eradication in human beings and animals. However, proton pump inhibitors and H_2-receptor antagonists decrease the urease activity of *Helicobacter* species; therefore, the time of testing after antibiotic and antisecretory usage is important. A gap of at least 2 to 5 days after cessation of antisecretory therapy should be maintained. Furthermore, low levels of colonization might be missed by testing earlier than 4 to 8 weeks after therapy.[58, 59]

◆ TREATMENT

The National Institutes of Health and the European *H. pylori* study group recommend that all people with peptic ulcers and *H. pylori* infection be treated for their infection. Eradication is not recommended for *H. pylori*–infected asymptomatic persons.[60] An acid-secretory inhibitor, drug-potentiated triple therapy for 2 weeks (e.g., clarithromycin, amoxicillin, bismuth plus ranitidine) or double therapy for 1 week (e.g., metronidazole or amoxicillin, clarithro-

mycin plus omeprazole or lansoprazole) show eradication rates of greater than 90 per cent in human patients.

Whether antimicrobial therapy should be instituted in cats with gastritis or ulcer disease is unknown at present. The authors consider the therapy indicated in cats with gastritis and *Helicobacter* infection before immunosuppressive therapy. Current treatment protocols are based on those found to be effective in human beings infected with *H. pylori*. An uncontrolled treatment trial of dogs and cats with gastritis and *Helicobacter* infection showed that clinical signs in 90 per cent of 63 dogs and cats responded to treatment with a combination of metronidazole, amoxicillin, and famotidine, and that 74 per cent of 19 animals re-endoscoped had no evidence of *Helicobacter* in gastric biopsies.[61] Unfortunately, those promising results regarding the eradication of *Helicobacter* species have not been borne out by more controlled studies in asymptomatic *Helicobacter*-infected cats. Treatment combinations that have been evaluated critically are (1) clarithromycin (30 mg orally [PO] every [q] 12 hr for 4 days), metronidazole (30 mg PO q 12 hr for 4 days), ranitidine (10 mg PO q 12 hr for 4 days), and bismuth (20 mg PO q 12 hr for 4 days) (CMRB) in *H. heilmanni*–infected cats and (2) azithromycin (30 mg PO q 24 hr for 4 days), tinidazole (100 mg PO q 24 hr for 4 days), ranitidine (20 mg PO q 24 hr for 4 days), and bismuth (40 mg PO q 24 hr for 4 days) (ATRB) in *H. heilmanni*–infected cats. Re-evaluation of infection status at 10 days after treatment revealed 11 of 11 CMRB- and 4 of 6 ATRB-treated cats to be *Helicobacter*-free on the basis of histology and ^{13}C-urea breath testing.[59] However, at 42 days after completing antimicrobial therapy, 4 of 11 CMRB and 5 of 6 ATRB cats were found to be reinfected. A transient effect of combination therapy (amoxicillin 20 mg/kg PO q 8 hr for 21 days, metronidazole 20 mg/kg PO q 8 hr for 21 days, and omeprazole 0.7 mg PO q 24 hr for 21 days) on bacterial colonization also has been observed in 6 cats with *H. pylori* infection. Further analysis of gastric biopsies from *H. pylori*–infected cats using PCR and *Helicobacter*-specific primers revealed persistence of *Helicobacter* DNA in gastric biopsies that appeared negative on histology and urease testing.[55] These studies suggest that antibiotic regimens that are effective against *H. pylori* in people may cause only transient suppression, rather than eradication, of gastric *Helicobacter* species in cats. Further controlled trials of antibiotic therapy in infected cats, particularly symptomatic patients with gastritis and *Helicobacter* infection, clearly are required before statements regarding the merit of treating gastric *Helicobacter* species can be made.

The morbidity and mortality associated with *H. pylori* infection in people has made it desirable to prevent rather than treat infection. Oral vaccination has been successful in preventing and treating *Helicobacter* infections in mice, and much research is now being undertaken to develop a vaccine for human beings. Once more is known about the relationship of *Helicobacter* species to disease in cats, a similar strategy may be equally desirable, particularly because eradicating infection transiently with antibiotics, without evoking a protective immune response, may be futile.

REFERENCES

1. Warren JR, Marshall BJ: Unidentified curved bacilli of gastric epithelium in active chronic gastritis. Lancet 1:1273–1275, 1983.
2. Parsonnet J, Friedman GD, Vandersteen DP, et al: *Helicobacter pylori* infection and the risk of gastric carcinoma. N Engl J Med 325:1127–1131, 1991.
3. Wotherspoon AC, Ortiz-Hidalgo C, Falzon MR, Isaacson PG: *Helicobacter pylori*–associated gastritis and primary B-cell gastric lymphoma. Lancet 338:1175–1176, 1991.
4. Rappin J: Contribution à l'étude des bactéries de la bouche à l'état normal (1881). *In* Breed RS, Murray EGD, Hitchens AP (eds): Bergey's Manual of Determinative Bacteriology, 6th ed. Baltimore, Williams & Wilkins, 1948, p. 217.
5. Bizzozero G: Sulla presenza di batteri nelle ghiandole rettali, e nelle ghiandole gastriche del cane. Atti R Accad Sci Torino 28:249–251, 1893.
6. Salomon H: Über das Spirillium des Säugetiermagens und sein Verhalten zu den Belegzellen. Zentralbl Bakteriol [Naturwiss] 19:433–441, 1896.
7. Happonen I, Saari S, Castren L, et al: Occurrence and topographical mapping of gastric *Helicobacter*-like organisms and their association with histological changes in apparently healthy dogs and cats. Zentrabl Veterinarmed 43:305–315, 1996.
8. Geyer C, Colbatzky F, Lechner J, Hermanns W: Occurrence of spiral-shaped bacteria in gastric biopsies of dogs and cats. Vet Rec 133:18–19, 1993.
9. Hermanns W, Kregel K, Breuer W, Lochner J: *Helicobacter*-like organisms: Histopathological examination of gastric biopsies from dogs and cats. J Comp Pathol 112:307–318, 1995.
10. Otto G, Hazell SL, Fox JG, et al: Animal and public health implications of gastric colonization of cats by *Helicobacter*-like organisms. J Clin Microbiol 32:1043–1049, 1994.
11. Weber AF, Hasa O, Sautter JH: Some observations concerning the presence of spirilla in the fundic glands of dogs and cats. Am J Vet Res 19:677–680, 1958.
12. Neiger R, Dieterich C, Burnens AP, et al: Detection and prevalence of *Helicobacter* infection in pet cats. J Clin Microbiol 36:634–637, 1998.
13. Papasouliotis K, Gruffydd-Jones TJ, Werrett G, et al: Occurrence of "gastric *Helicobacter*-like organisms" in cats. Vet Rec 140:369–370, 1997.
14. Fox JG, Lee A: The role of *Helicobacter* species in newly recognized gastrointestinal tract diseases of animals. Lab Anim Sci 47:222–255, 1997.
15. Vandamme P, Goossens H: Taxonomy of *Campylobacter, Arcobacter*, and *Helicobacter*: A review. Zentralbl Bakteriol [Naturwiss] 276:447–472, 1992.
16. Jalava K: Taxonomic studies on canine and feline gastric *Helicobacter* species. PhD Thesis, University of Helsinki, Helsinki, Finland, 1999.
17. Jalava K, On SLW, Vandamme P, et al: Isolation and identification of *Helicobacter* spp. from canine and feline gastric mucosa. Appl Environ Microbiol 64:3998–4006, 1998.
18. Jalava K, Hielm S, Hirvi U, Hänninen M: Evaluation of a molecular identification scheme based on 23S rRNA gene polymorphisms for differentiation of canine and feline gastric *Helicobacter* spp. Lett Appl Microbiol 28:269–274, 1999.
19. Handt LK, Fox JG, Stalis IH, et al: Characterization of feline *Helicobacter pylori* strains and associated gastritis in a colony of domestic cats. J Clin Microbiol 33:2280–2289, 1995.
20. Lee A, Hazell SL, O'Rourke JL, Kouprach S: Isolation of a spiral-shaped bacterium from the cat stomach. Infect Immun 56:2843–2850, 1988.
21. Germani Y, Dauga C, Duval P, et al: Strategy for the detection of *Helicobacter* species by amplification of 16S rRNA genes and identification of *H. felis* in a human gastric biopsy. Res Microbiol 148:315–326, 1997.
22. Handt LK, Fox JG, Dewhirst FE, et al: *Helicobacter pylori* isolated from the domestic cat: Public health implications. Infect Immun 62:2367–2374, 1994.
23. Norris CR, Marks SL, Eaton KA, et al: Healthy cats are commonly colonized with "*Helicobacter heilmannii*" that is associated with minimal gastritis. J Clin Microbiol 37:189–194, 1999.
24. Heilmann KL, Borchard F: Gastritis due to spiral shaped bacteria other than *Helicobacter pylori*: Clinical, histological and ultrastructural findings. Gut 32:137–140, 1991.
25. Andersen LP, Boye K, Blom J, et al: Characterization of a culturable "*Gastrospirillum hominis*" (*Helicobacter heilmannii*) strain isolated from the human gastric mucosa. J Clin Microbiol 37:1069–1076, 1999.
26. Yamasaki K, Suematsu H, Takahashi T: Comparison of gastric lesions in dogs and cats with and without gastric spiral organisms. J Am Vet Med Assoc 212:529–533, 1998.
27. El-Zaatari FAK, Woo JS, Badr A, et al: Failure to isolate *Helicobacter pylori* from stray cats indicates that *H. pylori* in cats may be an anthroponosis—An animal infection with a human pathogen. J Med Microbiol 46:372–376, 1997.
28. De Majo M, Pennisi MG, Carbone M, et al: Occurrence of *Helicobacter* spp. in gastric biopsies of cats living in different kinds of colonies. Eur J Comp Gastroenterol 3:13–18, 1998.
29. Dunn BE, Cohen H, Blaser MJ: *Helicobacter pylori*. Clin Microbiol Rev 10:720–741, 1997.
30. Fox JG, Perkins SE, Yan L, et al: Local immune response in *Helicobacter pylori*–infected cats and identification of *H. pylori* in saliva, gastric fluid and feces. Immunology 88:400–406, 1996.
31. Hulten K, Enroth H, Nyström L, Engstrand L: Presence of *Helicobacter* species DNA in Swedish water. J Appl Microbiol 85:282–286, 1998.
32. Hegarty JP, Dowd MT, Baker KH: Occurrence of *Helicobacter pylori* in surface water in the United States. Appl Environ Microbiol (submitted).
33. Dianyuan Z, Haitao Y: Epidemiology of *Helicobacter pylori* infection in the People's Republic of China. Chin Med J 108:304–313, 1995.
34. Lecoindre P: About a case of *Helicobacter pylori* gastritis in a pet cat: Public health implications (Abstract). Proceeding European Society of Veterinary Internal Medicine Forum, Veldhoven, Belgium, 1996, p. 45.
35. Thomas DR, Salmon RL, Meadows D, et al: Incidence of *Helicobacter pylori* in farmworkers and the role of zoonotic spread (Abstract). Gut 37(Suppl 1):A24, 1995.
36. Ansorg R, Heintschel von Heinegg E, von Recklinghausen G: Cat owners' risk of acquiring a *Helicobacter pylori* infection. Zentralbl Bakteriol 283:122–126, 1995.
37. Webb PM, Knight T, Elder J, et al: Is *Helicobacter pylori* transmitted from cats to humans? Helicobacter 1:79–81, 1996.
38. Neiger R, Schmassmann A, Seidel KE: Antibodies against *Helicobacter pylori* and *Helicobacter felis* in veterinarians (Abstract). Gastroenterol Int 11:127, 1998.
39. Meining A, Kroher G, Stolte M: Animal reservoirs in the transmission of *Helicobacter heilmannii*. Scand J Gastroenterol 33:795–798, 1998.
40. Dieterich C, Wiesel P, Neiger R, et al: Presence of multiple "*Helicobacter heilmannii*" strains in an individual suffering from ulcers and his two cats. J Clin Microbiol 36:1366–1370, 1998.
41. Lee A, Mitchell H: Basic bacteriology of *H. pylori*: *H. pylori* colonization factors. *In* Hunt RH, Tytgat GNJ (eds): *Helicobacter pylori*: Basic Mechanisms to Clinical Cure. Dordrecht, The Netherlands, Kluwer Academic, 1993, pp. 59–72.
42. Michetti P, Wadström T, Kraehenbuhl J-P, et al: Frontiers in *Helicobacter pylori* research: Pathogenesis, host response, vaccine development and new therapeutic approaches. Eur J Gastroenterol Hepatol 8:717–722, 1996.
43. Yamaoka Y, Kita M, Kodama T, et al: Expression of cytokine

mRNA in gastric mucosa with *Helicobacter pylori* infection. Scand J Gastroenterol 30:1153–1159, 1995.

44. Noach LA, Bosma NB, Jansen J, et al: Mucosal tumor necrosis factor-α, interleukin-1b, and interleukin-8 production in patients with *Helicobacter pylori* infection. Scand J Gastroenterol 29:425–429, 1994.

45. Beales ILP, Post L, Calam J, et al: Tumour necrosis factor alpha stimulates gastrin release from canine and human antral G cells: Possible mechanism of the *Helicobacter pylori*–gastrin link. Eur J Clin Invest 26:609–611, 1996.

46. Beales I, Blaser MJ, Srinivasan S, et al: Effect of *Helicobacter pylori* products and recombinant cytokines on gastrin release from cultured canine G cells. Gastroenterology 113:465–471, 1997.

47. Mannick EE, Bravo LE, Zarama G, et al: Inducible nitric oxide synthase, nitrotyrosine, and apoptosis in *Helicobacter pylori* gastritis: Effects of antibiotics and antioxidants. Cancer Res 56:3238–3243, 1996.

48. Peek RM, Jr., Moss SF, Tham KT, et al: *Helicobacter pylori* cagA + strains and dissociation of gastric epithelial cell proliferation from apoptosis. J Natl Cancer Inst 89:863–868, 1997.

49. Simpson KW, Strauss-Ayali D, Scanziani E, et al: *Helicobacter felis* infection is associated with lymphoid follicular hyperplasia and mild gastritis but normal gastric secretory function in cats. Infect Immun 68:779–790, 2000.

50. Perkins SE, Fox JG, Marini RP, et al: Experimental infection in cats with a cagA + human isolate of *Helicobacter pylori*. Helicobacter 3:225–235, 1998.

51. Fox JG, Batchelder M, Marini RP, et al: *Helicobacter pylori*–induced gastritis in the domestic cat. Infect Immun 63:2674–2681, 1995.

52. Happonen I, Saari S, Castren L, et al: Comparison of diagnostic methods for detecting gastric *Helicobacter*-like organisms in dogs and cats. J Comp Pathol 115:117–127, 1996.

53. Happonen I, Linden J, Saari S, et al: Detection and effects of helicobacters in healthy dogs and dogs with signs of gastritis. J Am Vet Med Assoc 213:1767–1774, 1998.

54. Fawcett PT, Gibney KM, Vinette KMB: *Helicobacter pylori* can be induced to assume the morphology of *Helicobacter heilmannii*. J Clin Microbiol 37:1045–1048, 1999.

55. Perkins SE, Yan LL, Shen Z, et al: Use of PCR and culture to detect *Helicobacter pylori* in naturally infected cats following triple antimicrobial therapy. Antimicrob Agents Chemother 40:1486–1490, 1996.

56. Strauss-Ayali D, Simpson KW, Schein AH, et al: Serologic discrimination of dogs infected with gastric *Helicobacter* spp. and uninfected dogs. J Clin Microbiol 37:1280–1287, 1999.

57. Seidel KE, Stolte M, Lehn N, et al: Antibodies against *Helicobacter felis* in sera of cats and dogs. Zentralbl Veterinarmed [B] 46:181–188, 1999.

58. Cornetta A, Simpson KW, Strauss-Ayali D, et al: Evaluation of a ^{13}C-urea breath test for detection of gastric infection with *Helicobacter* spp. in dogs. Am J Vet Res 59:1364–1369, 1998.

59. Neiger R, Seiler G, Schmassmann A: Use of a urea breath test to evaluate short-term treatments for cats naturally infected with *Helicobacter heilmannii*. Am J Vet Res 60:880–883, 1999.

60. Tytgat GNJ: Current indications for *Helicobacter pylori* eradication therapy. Scand J Gastroenterol 31(Suppl 215):70–73, 1996.

61. DeNovo RC, Magne ML: Current concepts in the management of *Helicobacter* associated gastritis. Proceedings 13th American College of Veterinary Internal Medicine Forum, Lake Buena Vista, FL, 1995, pp. 57–61.

12

◆ Diseases of the Esophagus

Albert E. Jergens

Diseases of the feline esophagus encompass a spectrum of obstructive lesions, inflammatory/degenerative disorders, and motility disturbances[1] (Fig. 12–1). Although less prevalent than disorders affecting the canine esophagus, feline esophageal diseases are equally problematic to the clinician with regard to diagnostic and therapeutic strategies. Data describing the most common disorders seen in clinical practice, including esophageal foreign bodies, esophagitis, and esophageal stricture, are notably sparse. This chapter highlights a practical approach to the diagnosis and therapy of feline esophageal diseases. Additionally, a technique for balloon catheter dilatation of esophageal strictures used successfully by the author is described.

◆ CLINICAL FINDINGS

History and Clinical Signs

Cats with esophageal diseases have variable signs depending on the chronicity and extent of esophageal dysfunction. In general, regurgitation, dysphagia, excessive salivation, and weight loss are reported most frequently by owners. Alterations in appetite, odynophagia (painful swallowing), and respiratory signs are observed less commonly. Differentiating vomiting from regurgitation is a salient consideration, because the diagnostic strategies for each sign are widely divergent. *Regurgitation* is defined as a passive retrograde expulsion of ingesta from the oral cavity with few (if any) prodromal signs. Regurgitated material is undigested, devoid of bile-staining, and often coated with mucus. The immediate ejection of food may have localizing value for proximal esophageal disorders, whereas regurgitation several hours after eating suggests distal esophageal disease or generalized dilatation. In contrast, *vomiting* is a centrally mediated, active reflex event characterized by premonitory signs of nausea, retching, and forceful abdominal contractions. Furthermore, vomited material often is bile-stained, is noncylindrical, and may contain partially digested food. Generally, it is easier to distinguish vomiting from regurgitation in cats than in dogs.

Pertinent questions for consideration in cats suspicious for esophageal disease include:

1. At what age did signs begin?
2. Are the signs associated with eating and/or drinking?
3. Are signs progressive—if so, acutely or more insidiously?
4. Has there been a significant exposure risk to caustic agents or foreign objects?
5. Is there history of a recent anesthetic event?

Several "generalizations" concerning historical clues and their correlation to specific feline esophageal disorders may be made. Congenital problems are exceedingly uncommon; the exception being Siamese-related breeds that may be at risk for idiopathic esophageal dilatation. Younger animals are more likely to ingest foreign objects, whereas acquired disorders such as esophagitis, neoplasia, and periesophageal lesions are most prevalent in middle-aged and older cats. Acute onset of signs is consistent with the presence of a foreign object or acute esophagitis. Mass lesions and esophageal stricture generally cause chronic signs characterized by progressive intolerance to solid foods. Evidence of pain during swallowing is seen with esophagitis and luminal foreign bodies, but is observed uncommonly with motility disturbances.

Physical Examination

The physical examination findings in many cats with esophageal diseases are unremarkable. A careful oral cavity evaluation should be performed in cats with profuse salivation or in those with histories suspicious for foreign-body ingestion. Look for evidence of linear foreign bodies under the base of the tongue. Pain elicited on neck palpation may occur with luminal foreign bodies and esophagitis. Reduced lean muscle mass is evident in cats with chronic disorders such as stricture or neoplasia. Chest auscultation usually is normal, but should be performed to assess for evidence of aspiration pneumonia.

◆ DIAGNOSING THE PROBLEM

Radiography

Radiographic imaging is an essential component for diagnosing and differentiating feline esophageal diseases. Survey radiographs are useful in the identification of radiopaque foreign bodies and masses, whereas static contrast procedures may further characterize mucosal detail and luminal patency. If fluoroscopy is available, evaluation of dynamic esoph-

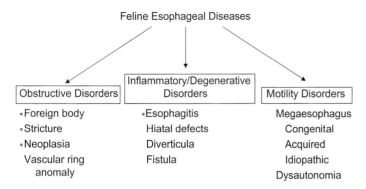

Feline Esophageal Diseases

Obstructive Disorders	Inflammatory/Degenerative Disorders	Motility Disorders
*Foreign body	*Esophagitis	Megaesophagus
*Stricture	Hiatal defects	Congenital
*Neoplasia	Diverticula	Acquired
Vascular ring anomaly	Fistula	Idiopathic
		Dysautonomia

* Clinically prevalent disorder

Figure 12–1. Classification of feline esophageal diseases. (Modified from Twedt DC: Diseases of the esophagus. *In* Ettinger SJ, Feldman EC [eds]: Textbook of Veterinary Internal Medicine. Philadelphia, WB Saunders, 1995, p. 1124.)

ageal motility with barium contrast agents also may be performed. Keys to proper radiographic evaluation include: (1) imaging of the complete esophagus; (2) performance of both lateral and ventrodorsal projections on survey films; and (3) adherence to good technique when performing an esophagram.

Survey radiography may suggest clues to esophageal disease such as radiopaque intraluminal objects, displacement of adjacent structures caused by esophageal disease, and the presence of intraluminal air (Fig. 12–2). Segmental or generalized retention of air may be seen with luminal obstruction, esophagitis, and megaesophagus.[2] Air accumulation also may result from nonpathologic processes including aerophagia (seen with excitement/restraint) and as a consequence of general anesthesia.[3] Static contrast procedures serve to highlight mucosal de-

tail, intraluminal patency, and periesophageal compression as caused by mass lesions. Details on the utility of contrast radiography in diagnosing feline gastrointestinal disorders may be found in Chapter 9, The Role of Contrast Radiography in the Diagnosis of Gastrointestinal Tract Disease.

Ultrasonographic evaluation of the cervical esophagus and thorax may assist in the detection of periesophageal masses such as lymphosarcoma.

Esophagoscopy

Endoscopic examination of the esophagus is an extremely useful diagnostic technique. Whereas radiography is the best method for documenting motility disturbances, esophagoscopy provides a de-

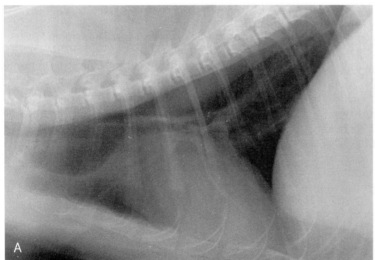

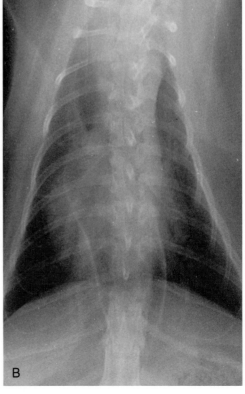

Figure 12–2. Lateral *(A)* and ventrodorsal *(B)* thoracic radiographs in a 1-year-old cat with congenital megaesophagus. Note the generalized dilatation of the esophagus with air.

finitive means for diagnosis of conditions involving the esophageal mucosa or abnormalities within the lumen, such as foreign body, esophagitis, stricture, and neoplasia. Distinct advantages of esophagoscopy include direct assessment of mucosal surfaces, targeted procurement of tissue and cytologic specimens for pathologic interpretation, performance of interventional procedures (e.g., extraction of intraluminal foreign bodies, balloon catheter dilatation of strictures), and examination of the remainder (stomach and small intestine) of the upper gastrointestinal tract.

A standard 7.8- to 9.8-mm flexible endoscope with 4-way tip deflection and a large (preferably 2.8 mm in diameter) accessory channel is the instrument of choice for esophagoscopy. The accessory instruments needed for successful endoscopic examination include foreign-body retrieval graspers, a balloon dilatation catheter, serrated-jaw biopsy forceps (rarely required), and guarded cytology brushes. Excellent summaries on the endoscopic appearances of the normal feline esophagus have been published.[4, 5] Abnormal findings may include intraluminal foreign objects, mass lesions (neoplastic most commonly), esophagitis, stricture, focal or generalized dilatation, and perforation. The endoscopic appearances of select mucosal disorders are discussed more fully later. Esophageal biopsy usually is *not* required for diagnosis of esophageal disease, with the exception of intraluminal mass lesions.

Miscellaneous Diagnostic Tests

Routine laboratory tests (complete blood count, serum chemistry profile, urinalysis, fecal examination) rarely are useful in determining the causes of regurgitation. Rather, they may assess the presence of systemic or metabolic disease and provide clues to complications (e.g., nonregenerative anemia of chronic disease, leukocytosis associated with aspiration pneumonia) directly attributable to esophageal dysfunction.

◆ ESOPHAGEAL OBSTRUCTION

Esophageal Foreign Bodies

Cats may ingest a variety of digestible and nondigestible objects that may cause esophageal obstruction. Linear foreign objects, sewing needles, and small play toys are encountered most frequently. Foreign bodies typically lodge in anatomically narrow locations, such as the thoracic inlet, base of the heart, or esophageal hiatal region, with the latter 2 sites being most common. Complications of foreign-body ingestion include intraluminal obstruction, mucosal ischemia due to pressure from the impinged object, and a spectrum of potential postextraction complications (Table 12–1). Esophageal foreign bodies should be removed promptly.

Table 12–1. Potential Complications Associated With Esophageal Foreign Bodies

Intraluminal obstruction	Diverticula
Mucosal ischemia	Fistula
Stricture	Motility disturbances
Mucosal laceration	Esophageal perforation

Clinical Signs

Excessive salivation (sometimes blood-tinged), odynophagia, and anorexia are prominent signs in many cats. Cervical pain may be evident with objects lodged in the cervical esophagus. Fever is seen in association with mediastinal or pulmonary infections. Clinical signs occur acutely in most instances.

Diagnostic Tests

Diagnosis of a retained foreign body may be apparent from the history. Has the cat gotten into the garbage or is there a favorite toy missing? Survey radiographs of the cervical esophagus and thorax are useful in detecting radiopaque objects and intraluminal accumulations of air. Films should be evaluated critically for evidence of esophageal perforation such as pneumomediastinum or pleural effusion. Radiolucent intraluminal foreign bodies (e.g., cloth, wood, plastic) may be identified only after administration of positive contrast agents or by performing esophagoscopy.

Treatment

Endoscopic removal of the foreign body is the treatment of choice. Factors affecting the feasibility of successful endoscopic removal include the size of the foreign object, the grasping strength of the retrieval instrument, the angularity of the object, and the extent of mucosal trauma present.[6] Use of a flexible endoscope is preferred because it provides greater intraluminal maneuverability around objects, and it may accommodate a variety of different grasping instruments (Fig. 12–3). The choice of which type of grasping instrument to use is dictated largely by personal preference. I most frequently use a rat-tooth instrument for sewing needles or cloth linear foreign bodies, and a basket-type forceps for angular objects such as bones. Foreign bodies that may not be retracted out of the mouth sometimes may be advanced into the stomach and subsequently removed. After the foreign object is extracted, the esophageal mucosa should be examined carefully for trauma, including perforation. Surgery is required if endoscopic retrieval fails or if perforation occurs.

Medical management of esophagitis is indicated in most cats after foreign-body removal (see section on esophagitis later in this chapter). The prognosis for cats with esophageal foreign bodies is good to excellent, especially with prompt endoscopic removal.

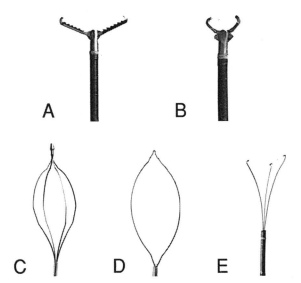

Figure 12–3. Various endoscopic foreign-body grasping instruments. *A,* Alligator jaw forceps. *B,* Rat-tooth (sharp) forceps. *C,* Basket forceps. *D,* Oval snare forceps. *E,* Three-prong forceps.

Esophageal Stricture

Esophageal stricture is a circumferential narrowing of the esophageal lumen caused by muscular inflammation and resultant scar tissue formation. Strictures may occur anywhere along the length of the esophagus, but are observed most commonly in the midthoracic esophagus near the heart. Primary causes for stricture include anesthesia-induced gastroesophageal (GE) reflux, foreign bodies, esophageal surgery, and malignant neoplasia.[7] Most of the cases that I have seen presumably occurred in association with caustic GE reflux during a general anesthetic event. The time period from severe mucosal inflammation to esophageal stenosis is surprisingly short (e.g., 1 to 3 weeks).[8]

Clinical Signs

Classic signs of esophageal dysfunction are observed including regurgitation, dysphagia, and a gradual intolerance to solid foods compared with liquids and gruel-consistency diets. Regurgitation episodes generally occur shortly after eating. It is noteworthy that signs are progressive and may include weight loss in spite of a good or even ravenous appetite. Physical examination often is unremarkable.

Diagnostic Tests

A diagnosis often is suggested by a clinical history of recent surgery or foreign-body ingestion. Survey thoracic radiographs usually are unremarkable unless concurrent aspiration pneumonia is present. Positive contrast studies (e.g., an esophagram using liquid barium alone or barium mixed with food) are required to demonstrate esophageal luminal stenosis. A variable degree of esophageal dilatation proximal to the stricture may be observed (Fig. 12–4). Contrast radiography also delineates the number and location of strictures. Endoscopically, benign strictures appear as smooth circumferential narrowings caused by fibrous connective tissue. The esophageal lumen at the stricture site is smooth, typically less than 5 mm in diameter, and indistensible, which impedes passage of the endoscope. A distinct fibrous ring around the proximal opening of the stricture is sometimes visualized (Fig. 12–5). In contrast, the mucosa surrounding malignant strictures is hemorrhagic, friable, or ulcerated. Besides confirming the site and severity of stricture, esophagoscopy allows for procurement of tissue/cytologic specimens and performance of balloon catheter dilatation.

Treatment

Benign strictures are best treated by mechanical dilatation using a balloon catheter under endoscopic guidance.[9–11] These catheters exert radial stretching forces rather than longitudinal shearing forces because they are positioned stationary within the stricture during dilatation. Commercially available polyethylene balloon catheters (Rigiflex Balloon Dilator, Microvasive, Watertown, MA) come in a variety of lengths and diameters, and are relatively inexpensive and reusable. A balloon catheter with a maxi-

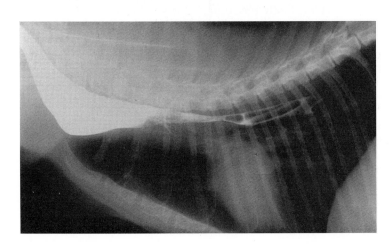

Figure 12–4. Esophagram—lateral thoracic radiograph. An esophageal stricture is causing abrupt attenuation of flow of liquid contrast medium (over the heart) and esophageal dilatation proximal to the strictured site.

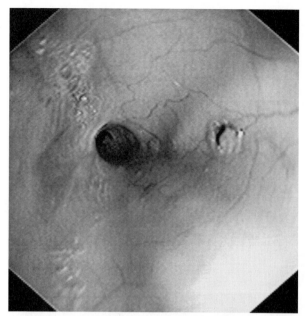

Figure 12–5. Endoscopic appearance of a benign esophageal stricture. The lumen is narrowed circumferentially with a fibrous ring evident around the proximal opening.

mum diameter of 18 mm and 8 cm in length is ideal for most feline strictures. Principles of successful balloon dilatation therapy are outlined in Table 12–2. Note that separate but progressive dilatations are performed during anesthesia. The majority of cats will require multiple (e.g., 2 to 3) procedures to maintain luminal patency and prevent restricturing (Fig. 12–6). Patients with active esophagitis may need additional dilatation procedures.[11] Therapy for postdilatory esophagitis is mandatory (see section on esophagitis later in this chapter). Esophageal perforation is an uncommon complication that generally responds to conservative medical therapy.[12]

Neoplasia

Esophageal cancer occurs uncommonly in cats.[13] Tumors of the esophagus may present as primary

Table 12–2. Principles of Esophageal Balloon Dilatation Therapy

1. Procure an appropriate-sized (18 mm outside diameter, 8-cm-long) balloon dilatation catheter. Use of a pressure monitor* is advised.
2. Pass the dilatation catheter *alongside* the endoscope, and position the middle of the catheter over the stricture. Passing the catheter through the accessory channel damages the catheter and shortens its lifespan.
3. Slowly inflate the catheter using 3 *separate but progressive* dilatations during anesthesia. Hold each dilatation for 3 minutes before deflating. Closely monitor for excessive mucosal hemorrhage or tearing.
4. Multiple (2–4) dilatation procedures generally are required to maintain luminal patency. Repeat as needed at 48-hour intervals.
5. Medical management of postdilatation esophagitis is required.

*LaVeen Inflator, Microvasive, Watertown, MA.

esophageal, periesophageal, or metastatic lesions. Squamous cell carcinoma is the most common primary neoplasm observed; lymphosarcoma is encountered predominantly as a periesophageal mass that may invade the mucosal surface. Organ dysfunction is attributable to direct mechanical obstruction and disturbances in motility caused by neoplastic infiltration.

Clinical Signs

Dysphagia (with marked intolerance to solids), regurgitation, hypersalivation, and anorexia with weight loss are observed most frequently in aged cats. Clinical signs typically are chronic and progressive over several weeks to months. Cats with periesophageal tumors may have histories or examination findings suggestive of aspiration pneumonia. Physical examination usually reveals generalized debilitation and weight loss.

Diagnostic Tests

Radiography and esophagoscopy often are combined for diagnosis of esophageal neoplasia. Periesophageal neoplasia may be diagnosed by survey radiography and ultrasonography of the neck and thorax. Contrast radiography is useful in detecting gross mucosal irregularities and intraluminal stenosis associated with malignant stricture. Endoscopy with biopsy/cytology usually is required for a definitive diagnosis. Squamous cell carcinoma often appears as a proliferative mass along the mucosa, whereas lymphosarcoma (Fig. 12–7) has a smooth and eroded appearance endoscopically. Note that endoscopic biopsy of the esophagus is difficult, and that only superficial epithelia may be obtained. Endoscopic exfoliative cytology is a useful adjunct to mucosal biopsy in the diagnosis of esophageal squamous cell carcinoma and lymphosarcoma.

Treatment

The prognosis for esophageal neoplasia generally is poor. Treatment options are limited for squamous cell carcinoma because the mucosal lesions are quite advanced at the time of diagnosis and often locally aggressive. Periesophageal lymphosarcoma is quite responsive to LCOP (L-asparaginase, cyclophosphamide, Oncovin [vincristine], prednisone) or COP (cyclophosphamide, Oncovin, prednisone) chemotherapy.

◆ MEGAESOPHAGUS

Megaesophagus denotes generalized esophageal dilatation with hypomotility. Both congenital and adult-onset forms of megaesophagus are rare in cats. Most cases of adult-onset megaesophagus are idiopathic; for example, feline dysautonomia represents a generalized autonomic neuropathy that may cause

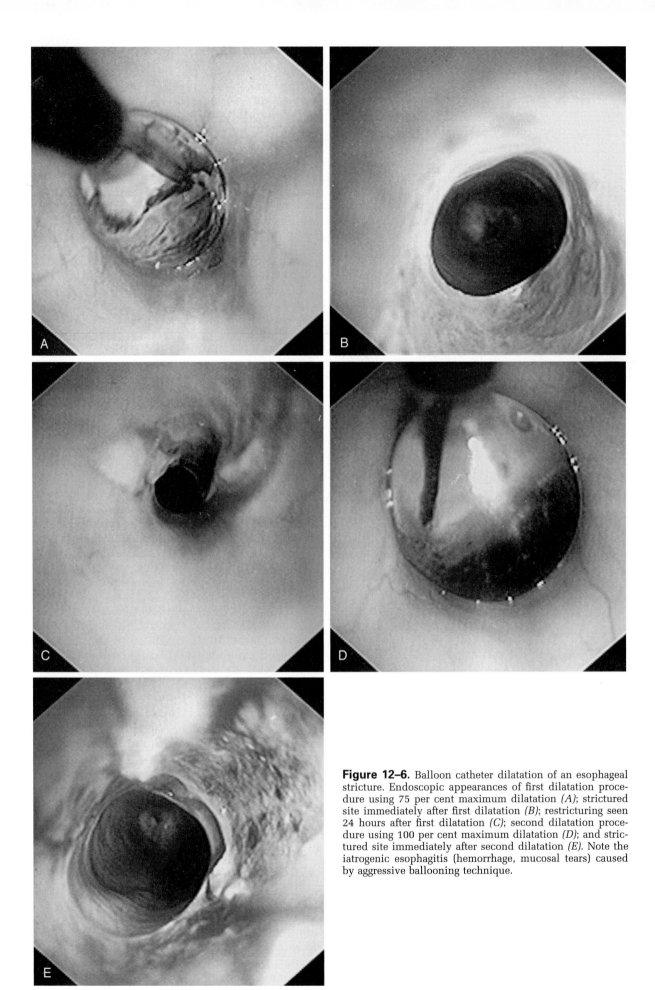

Figure 12–6. Balloon catheter dilatation of an esophageal stricture. Endoscopic appearances of first dilatation procedure using 75 per cent maximum dilatation *(A)*; strictured site immediately after first dilatation *(B)*; restricturing seen 24 hours after first dilatation *(C)*; second dilatation procedure using 100 per cent maximum dilatation *(D)*; and strictured site immediately after second dilatation *(E)*. Note the iatrogenic esophagitis (hemorrhage, mucosal tears) caused by aggressive ballooning technique.

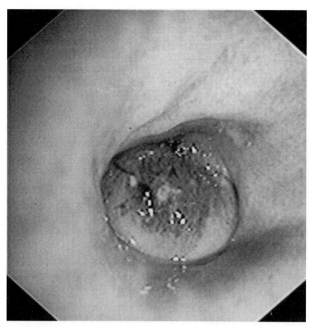

Figure 12–7. Endoscopic appearance of lymphosarcoma in a 5-year-old cat. The tumor is projecting into the lumen as a peri-esophageal mass and was diagnosed readily by brush cytology.

progressive regurgitation, esophageal hypomotility, and megaesophagus[14, 15] (see Chapter 49, Dysautonomia Revisited).

Clinical Signs

Regurgitation is the predominant sign. The timing of regurgitation episodes after eating is extremely variable. Affected cats may show systemic signs (anorexia, depression, and constipation with dysautonomia), or may exhibit no other abnormalities. Moist crackles may be auscultated in cats with aspiration pneumonia.

Diagnostic Tests

Thoracic radiography easily confirms generalized esophageal dilatation with air, fluid, and/or ingesta. If survey films are inconclusive, an esophagram that also evaluates motility should be performed. Routine hematology, serum biochemical analysis, and urinalysis may identify potential causes for esophageal hypomotility (e.g., lead intoxication or hypoadrenocorticism), but often are unremarkable. A clinical diagnosis of feline dysautonomia usually is made on characteristic historical and physical examination findings and confirmed by specialized autonomic function tests[15] (see Chapter 49, Dysautonomia Revisited).

Treatment

Medical therapy largely is symptomatic, and includes elevating feedings, feeding multiple small meals to minimize dilatation/aspiration, varying the consistency of the food, and providing adequate nutrition. Aspiration pneumonia is treated with broad-spectrum antibiotics. Although controversial, administering cisapride may be of value in augmenting distal esophageal peristalsis in cats.[16] Supportive care is first-line therapy for feline dysautonomia. In general, the prognosis for idiopathic megaesophagus is guarded, whereas dysautonomia carries a poor long-term prognosis.

◆ ESOPHAGITIS

Inflammation of the esophageal mucosa may occur from acute or chronic insults. Potential causes include injury from esophageal foreign bodies, GE reflux, persistent vomiting, hiatal defects, malpositioned nasogastric/pharyngostomy tubes, and thermal or chemical insults.[1, 17] Anesthetic-associated GE reflux is the most common cause for esophagitis in my feline practice. Mild esophagitis (most common) is limited to the mucosa, and heals quickly without fibrosis. Severe esophagitis extends into the muscular layer, and may cause erosion/ulceration and stricture formation.

Clinical Signs

Signs vary with the severity of esophageal inflammation. Cats with mild esophagitis may be asymptomatic. Moderate-to-severe esophagitis causes anorexia, dysphagia, odynophagia, and hypersalivation. Regurgitation usually is intermittent. Thick, ropy saliva that is blood-tinged is observed with active lesions. Gradual weight loss occurs with chronicity.

Diagnostic Tests

A diagnosis of esophagitis is suspected in cats with suggestive histories. Survey radiographs often are unremarkable. Liquid barium contrast procedures may show deranged esophageal motility and gross mucosal irregularities. Endoscopic examination is the most reliable means to diagnose esophagitis.[5] Lesions are most prominent in the distal esophagus adjacent to the lower esophageal sphincter. Mild cases often appear normal endoscopically, but subtle lesions such as mild erythema and focal erosions also may be seen. Severe esophagitis manifests as marked erythema, multifocal erosions, and mucosal irregularity (e.g., increased granularity). Concurrent GE reflux also may be seen with active lesions (Fig. 12–8). Esophagitis is an endoscopic diagnosis and rarely requires histologic confirmation, in the author's opinion.

Treatment

Cats with mild esophagitis may be treated by dietary modification alone. Oral food intake may be withheld for 24 to 48 hours, and once feeding resumes, diets that are fat-restricted but high in protein

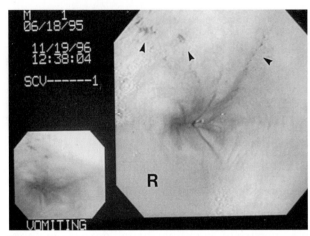

Figure 12–8. Endoscopic appearance of esophagitis in a 1-year-old cat with a history of chronic vomiting. Subtle yet obvious mucosal erosions *(arrowheads)* are evident along with lesion due to gastroesophageal reflux (R) in the distal esophagus.

should be fed. Cats having severe esophagitis will require gastrostomy tube placement for nutritional support and to bypass the inflamed esophagus.

Empirical medical therapy is indicated in cats with moderate-to-severe disease. Sucralfate suspensions (0.5 g crushed in 5 to 10 ml H_2O by mouth every [q] 8 hr) may be used alone because they provide excellent cytoprotection and promote mucosal healing. Gastric acid secretory inhibitors (e.g., cimetidine, 5 to 10 mg/kg PO or intravenously [IV] q 8 hr; ranitidine, 3.5 mg/kg PO or 2.5 mg/kg IV q 12 hr; or omeprazole, 0.7 mg/kg PO q 24 hr) also are used to prevent further reflux injury to the esophagus. Promotility drugs (e.g., metoclopramide, 0.2 to 0.4 mg/kg PO q 8 hr, or cisapride, 0.1 to 1.0 mg/kg PO q 8 to 12 hr) enhance gastric emptying and increase lower esophageal sphincter tone, which reduces the likelihood of GE reflux. Mild lesions are treated for 5 to 7 days. Moderate-to-severe esophagitis is treated for 3 to 4 weeks. The prognosis in most cases of esophagitis is good with appropriate medical management. However, complications, including segmental or generalized hypomotility and stricture, may arise with severe disease.

REFERENCES

1. Twedt DC: Diseases of the esophagus. *In* Ettinger SJ, Feldman EC (eds): Textbook of Veterinary Internal Medicine. Philadelphia, WB Saunders, 1995, pp. 1124–1142.
2. Watrous BJ: The esophagus. *In* Thrall DE (ed): Textbook of Veterinary Diagnostic Radiology. Philadelphia, WB Saunders, 1994, pp. 234–252.
3. Guilford WG, Strombeck DR: Diseases of swallowing. *In* Guilford WG, Center SA, Strombeck DR, et al (eds): Strombeck's Small Animal Gastroenterology. Philadelphia, WB Saunders, 1996, pp. 211–238.
4. Leib MS: Gastrointestinal endoscopy. *In* August JR (ed): Consultations in Feline Internal Medicine, vol. 2. Philadelphia, WB Saunders, 1994, pp. 119–126.
5. Tams TR: Esophagoscopy. *In* Tams TR (ed): Small Animal Endoscopy. St. Louis, CV Mosby, 1990, pp. 47–88.
6. Tams TR: Endoscopic removal of gastrointestinal foreign bodies. *In* Tams TR (ed): Small Animal Endoscopy, 2nd ed. St. Louis, Mosby, 1999, pp. 247–295.
7. Jergens AE: Diseases of the esophagus. *In* Morgan RV (ed): Handbook of Small Animal Practice. Philadelphia, WB Saunders, 1997, pp. 323–333.
8. Zawie DA: Esophageal strictures. *In* Kirk RW (ed): Current Veterinary Therapy X: Small Animal Practice. Philadelphia, WB Saunders, 1989, pp. 904–906.
9. Burk RL, Zawie DA, Garvey MS: Balloon catheter dilation of intraluminal strictures in the dog and cat: A description of the procedure and a report of six cases. Semin Vet Med Surg 2:241–247, 1987.
10. Harai BH, Johnson SE, Sherding RG: Endoscopically guided balloon dilatation of benign esophageal strictures in 6 cats and 7 dogs. J Vet Intern Med 9:332–335, 1995.
11. Melendez LD, Twedt DC, Weyrauch EA, et al: Conservative therapy of esophageal strictures using balloon catheter dilatation (Abstract). J Vet Intern Med 12:205, 1998.
12. Willard MD, Delles EK, Fossum TW: Iatrogenic tears associated with ballooning of esophageal strictures. J Am Anim Hosp Assoc 30:431–435, 1994.
13. Withrow SJ: Esophageal cancer. *In* Withrow SJ, MacEwen EG (eds): Small Animal Clinical Oncology. Philadelphia, WB Saunders, 1996, pp. 241–243.
14. Sharp NJH, Nash AS, Griffiths IR: Feline dysautonomia (the Key-Gaskell syndrome): A clinical and pathological study of forty cases. J Small Anim Pract 25:599–615, 1984.
15. Guilford WG, O'Brien DP, Allert A, et al: Diagnosis of dysautonomia by autonomic nervous system function testing. J Am Vet Med Assoc 193:823–828, 1988.
16. Washabau RJ, Hall JA: Cisapride. J Am Vet Med Assoc 207:1285–1288, 1995.
17. Sherding RG, Johnson SE, Tams TR: Esophagoscopy. *In* Tams TR (ed): Small Animal Endoscopy. St. Louis, Mosby, 1999, pp. 39–96.

13

◆ Update on Antiemetic Therapy

Robert J. Washabau

Emesis, or vomiting, is a complex reflex pathway that has evolved to protect animals from ingested toxins. Whereas it is undoubtedly protective, emesis is important medically because of the large number of conditions that may cause or be associated with it. Emesis may occur with such diverse conditions as inflammatory bowel disease, gastrointestinal obstruction, pancreatitis, hepatobiliary disease, diabetic ketoacidosis, thyrotoxicosis, uremia, and motion sickness. (The medical work-up of the vomiting cat has been outlined in a previous volume of this text.[1]) Aspiration pneumonia, fluid and electrolyte depletion, and acid-base disturbances all are potentially serious consequences of vomiting, hence the great need to understand the pathophysiologic mechanisms, pharmacology, and therapy of vomiting in each of these disorders.

◆ MECHANISMS OF VOMITING: HUMORAL AND NEURAL PATHWAYS

Our current understanding of the physiology of emesis is dominated by concepts elaborated in the early 1950s by Borison and Wang.[2, 3] In their 2-component model, vomiting is believed to occur through activation of a humoral or neural pathway (reviewed in ref. 4; Fig. 13–1). In this model, vomiting occurs through activation of the chemoreceptor trigger zone (CRTZ) by blood-borne substances *(humoral pathway)*, or through activation of the emetic center by vagosympathetic, CRTZ, vestibular, or cerebrocortical neurons *(neural pathway)*. Thus, activation of the CRTZ by circulating emetogenic substances (e.g., uremic toxins, cardiac glycosides, ammonia and other hepatoencephalopathic toxins, endotoxins, and apomorphine) is abolished by CRTZ antagonism, but not by vagotomy, sympathectomy, or emetic center antagonism. In contrast, neural activation of the emetic center by gastrointestinal disease (e.g., inflammation and infection) is abolished by vagotomy, sympathectomy, and emetic center antagonism, but not by CRTZ antagonism. Many experimental data have been readily explained by this 2-component model.[2, 3] The Borison-Wang model is not without challenge, however; it has been suggested that there are parallel mechanisms for the initiation of emesis in response to any stimulus, and it is the sum of these inputs that drives the emetic response.[5] In other words, emesis need not be simply an either/or response. The concept of a discrete emetic center also has been seriously challenged. Based on more recent electrophysiologic studies, a model of sequential activation of a series of effector nuclei has been proposed that does not require a discrete emetic center.[5] Despite contemporary re-examination, there still is good agreement on 2 general patterns of emesis, 1 humoral and the other neural.

Many of the spontaneous vomiting disorders of domestic cats, particularly those of the primary gastrointestinal tract, are believed to result from activation of the neural pathway. Vomiting associated with primary gastrointestinal tract disease (e.g., inflammation, infection, malignancy, toxicity) results from activation of visceral receptors, afferent neurons, and the emetic center. Efferent information transmitted back to the gastrointestinal tract stimulates the motor correlates of vomiting (retrograde duodenal and gastric contractions, relaxation of the caudal esophageal sphincter, gastroesophageal reflux, opening of the proximal esophageal sphincter, and evacuation of gastrointestinal contents).[6] A neural pathway also may be involved in vomiting associated with motion sickness. Motion within the semicircular canals is transduced to vestibulocochlear neurons that synapse ultimately in the CRTZ or emetic center. Cats experience motion sickness just like dogs, although the neuroanatomy and pharmacology appear to be somewhat different between the 2 species.[7-9] Histaminergic neurons and the CRTZ are involved in motion sickness in dogs, whereas neither is involved in motion sickness in cats.[7-9] A neural pathway involving cerebrocortical neurons may be involved in vomiting disorders associated with anxiety or anticipation, but these probably are more important in human beings.

The essential component of the humoral pathway is the CRTZ located within the area postrema that is sensitive to blood-borne substances. Receptors within the CRTZ may be activated by many endogenous (e.g., uremic toxins, hepatoencephalopathic toxins, or endotoxins) and exogenous (e.g., digitalis glycosides, apomorphine) blood-borne substances. Most pharmacologic approaches to antiemetic therapy have been based on neurotransmitter-receptor interactions at the CRTZ, emphasizing the humoral pathway of emesis.[4] The neural pathway has received much less emphasis, even though it is a

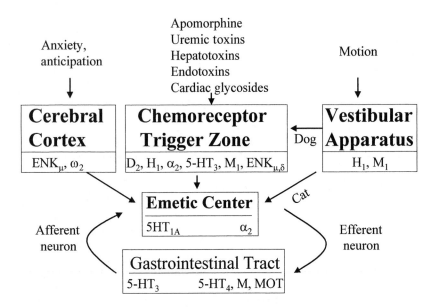

Figure 13–1. Humoral and neural pathways for emesis. α, alpha-adrenergic; D, dopamine; ENK, enkephalin; H, histamine; 5-HT, 5-hydroxytryptamine; M, muscarinic cholinergic; MOT, motilin; ω, benzodiazepine.

much more important pathway in many spontaneous vomiting disorders.

◆ PHARMACOLOGY OF VOMITING: NEUROTRANSMITTERS AND RECEPTORS

Chemoreceptor Trigger Zone

Neurochemical studies in cats (and dogs) have demonstrated the presence of several neurotransmitters: dopamine, norepinephrine, 5-hydroxytryptamine (5-HT, serotonin), acetylcholine, histamine, and enkephalins (ENKs); their respective receptors or binding sites: D_2-dopaminergic, α_2-adrenergic, 5-HT_3-serotonergic, M_1-cholinergic, H_1- and H_2-histaminergic, and ENK_μ and ENK_δ enkephalinergic; and their respective synthetic or degradable enyzmes: dihydroxyphenylalanine (DOPA) decarboxylase, dopamine β hydroxylase, 5-HT decarboxylase, choline acetyltransferase, histidine decarboxylase, and enkephalinase.[10] Some neurotransmitter-receptor systems probably are more important than others. For example, apomorphine, a D_2-dopamine receptor agonist, is a potent emetic agent in dogs, but it does not readily induce emesis in cats.[11] This finding has 2 important implications: (1) CRTZ D_2-dopamine receptors are not as important in mediating humoral emesis in cats, and (2) D_2-dopamine receptor antagonists (e.g., metoclopramide) are not as useful as antiemetic agents in cats. Xylazine, an α_2-adrenergic agonist, is a more potent emetic agent in cats than in dogs.[11, 12] Xylazine's effect suggests that α_2-adrenergic antagonists may be more useful antiemetic agents than D_2-dopamine antagonists in cats.[8] Cancer chemotherapy (e.g., cisplatinum, doxorubicin, cyclophosphamide)–induced emesis is mediated by activation of 5-HT_3 receptors in the CRTZ of cats,[10, 13–15] whereas visceral and vagal afferent 5-HT_3 recep-

tors may be involved more importantly in dogs.[16] Antagonists of the 5-HT_3 receptor are efficacious in the prevention of emesis associated with cisplatinum and other chemotherapy in cats[13–15] and dogs.[17] Finally, whereas histamine and H_1- and H_2-histaminergic receptors have been demonstrated in the CRTZ of dogs, they have not to date been demonstrated in cats. Histamine is a potent emetic agent in dogs, but cats seem resistant to its emetic effects.[10, 11] H_1-Histaminergic antagonists (e.g., diphenhydramine) are ineffective antiemetic agents for motion sickness in cats.[9]

Emetic Center

At the present time, the 5-HT_{1A}- and α_2-adrenergic receptors are the only documented receptors involved in the regulation of emesis at the level of the emetic center. It has been shown that agonists of the 5-HT_{1A} receptor (e.g., flesinoxan, 8-OH-DPAT, buspirone) suppress emesis associated with motion sickness in cats.[18] These drugs have not been approved for use in cats, however. The α_2-adrenergic receptor, conversely, may be antagonized with currently available antiemetic drugs. The emetic center α_2 receptor, as well as the CRTZ α_2 receptor, may be antagonized by a pure α_2 antagonist (e.g., yohimbine), or by mixed α_1-α_2-antagonists (e.g., prochlorperazine and chlorpromazine).[12] It is likely, however, that most of the antiemetic effect of the α receptor antagonists results from antagonism of the CRTZ α_2-adrenergic receptor.[12, 19]

Vestibular Apparatus

Muscarinic M_1 receptors and acetylcholine have been demonstrated in the vestibular apparatus of cats. Mixed M_1-M_2-antagonists (e.g., atropine) and pure M_1 antagonists (e.g., pirenzepine) inhibit motion sickness in cats. It is not clear, however, whether the antiemetic effect of these drugs is due solely to M_1-receptor antagonism at the vestibular apparatus. Other sites (e.g., cerebral cortex, reticular formation, area postrema) of antagonism are possible.[10]

Cerebral Cortex

Opioids (e.g., cannabinoids and nabilone) and benzodiazepines (e.g., diazepam and lorazepam) have been used to reduce anticipatory nausea and vomiting in human beings undergoing cytotoxic drug therapy. Cerebrocortical opioid and benzodiazepine receptors have been implicated, but have not been characterized very well pharmacologically. These receptors will likely be of minor significance in the pathogenesis of most vomiting disorders in cats.[4, 10, 11]

Gut Afferents

There are a number of different mechanisms by which stimuli arising from the gastrointestinal tract cause emesis. For example, ingested toxins, cell degeneration or necrosis, inflammation, luminal distention, chemotherapy, and radiation therapy all induce emesis. Of the many receptors found in the gastrointestinal tract, $5\text{-}HT_3$ receptors likely play an important role in the initiation of emesis.[10] It is now well-established that cytotoxic drugs cause 5-HT release from enterochromaffin cells in the gastrointestinal tract, which then activates $5\text{-}HT_3$ receptors in afferent vagal fibers (dog)[16] or the CRTZ (cat).[13–15] Vomiting induced by 5-HT release and $5\text{-}HT_3$ receptor activation is abolished by pretreatment with 5-HT_3 antagonists (e.g., ondansetron, granisetron, and tropisetron).[13, 17] Metoclopramide is a weak antagonist of $5\text{-}HT_3$ receptors, but does not seem to be very effective in preventing chemotherapy-induced emesis.[20] It remains to be determined whether other gastrointestinal tract pathologies (e.g., inflammation, infection, malignancy, toxicity) are associated with 5-HT release and $5\text{-}HT_3$-receptor activation.

Gut Efferents

Vagal efferent and myenteric neurons initiate the complex excitation and inhibition of visceral smooth muscle (e.g., retrograde duodenal and gastric contractions, relaxation of the caudal esophageal sphincter, gastroesophageal reflux, opening of the proximal esophageal sphincter, and evacuation of gastrointestinal contents) that culminate in emesis. A number of receptors have been identified on myenteric neurons and gastrointestinal smooth-muscle cells that regulate gastric emptying and/or intestinal transit. These include $5\text{-}HT_4$ serotonergic (neuronal),[21–23] D_2-dopaminergic (neuronal),[23, 24] M_2-cholinergic (smooth muscle),[23] and motilin (smooth

muscle—dog only)[23, 25] receptors. Cisapride, a substituted benzamide, facilitates gastric emptying by activating presynaptic neuronal $5\text{-}HT_4$ receptors.[22, 26] Cisapride probably is the best example of a $5\text{-}HT_4$ gastrointestinal prokinetic agent, but it was withdrawn from the American market in July 2000. Metoclopramide is a weak gastric prokinetic agent in cats, and is believed to facilitate gastric emptying via agonism of $5\text{-}HT_4$-serotonergic receptors,[22] or via antagonism at D_2-dopamine receptors.[24] Canine gastric emptying also is regulated by motilin, a hormone that is released episodically from gastrointestinal endocrine cells. Motilin initiates phase III of the migrating myoelectric complex and facilitates gastric emptying during the fasting state. Low doses of erythromycin (0.5 to 1.0 mg/kg every [q] 8 hr orally [PO] or intravenously [IV]) have been shown to stimulate motilin release and facilitate gastric emptying in dogs.[23, 25, 27] The role of motilin in the regulation of feline gastric emptying is understood incompletely. Motilin-like macrolide antibiotics increase tone in the feline caudal esophageal sphincter,[28] but their role in the regulation of gastrointestinal motility is understood incompletely.

◆ ANTIEMETIC CLASSIFICATION
(Table 13–1)

A number of antiemetic drugs have been formulated based on the aforementioned neurotransmitter-receptor systems. These drugs may be classified as α_2-adrenergic antagonists, D_2-dopaminergic antagonists, H_1- and H_2-histaminergic antagonists, M_1-muscarinic cholinergic antagonists, and $5\text{-}HT_3$-serotonergic antagonists. The $5\text{-}HT_4$-serotonergic agonists are not direct antiemetic drugs per se, but may have an indirect antiemetic effect by promoting gastrointestinal motility. Several important points should be made about these classifications.

1. *Some drugs have several mechanisms of antiemesis.* Metoclopramide antagonizes D_2-dopaminergic and $5\text{-}HT_3$-serotonergic receptors, and acts as a weak agonist at $5\text{-}HT_4$ receptors. The antiemetic properties of metoclopramide relate to D_2-dopaminergic receptor antagonism at the CRTZ, whereas the weak prokinetic effect relates to $5\text{-}HT_4$-serotonergic receptor agonism.[11, 26] Combined antiemetic and prokinetic therapy may prove useful in treating refractory cases of vomiting. The phenothiazines (e.g., chlorpromazine and prochlorperazine) are antagonists of α_1- and α_2-adrenergic receptors, but they also antagonize D_2-dopaminergic, H_1- and H_2-histaminergic, and muscarinic cholinergic receptors.[10] Thus, it may be difficult to discern the exact locus of a drug's antiemetic effect.
2. *Some drugs are nonselective with regard to receptor subtype.* Atropine, for example, may be useful in the therapy of motion sickness because it crosses the blood-brain barrier and antagonizes

Table 13–1. Antiemetic Classifications

Classification	Examples	Anatomic Site(s) of Action	Dosage	Side-Effects
α_2-Adrenergic antagonists	Prochlorperazine* (Compazine, SmithKline)	CRTZ, emetic center	0.5 mg/kg q 8 hr SQ, IM	Hypotension, sedation
	Chlorpromazine* (Thorazine—SmithKline)	CRTZ, emetic center	0.2–0.4 mg/kg q 8 hr SQ	Hypotension, sedation
	Yohimbine (Yobine—Lloyd Laboratories)	CRTZ, emetic center	0.25–0.5 mg/kg q 12 hr SQ, IM	Hypotension, sedation
D_2-Dopaminergic antagonists	Metoclopramide* (Reglan—Robins)	CRTZ, GI smooth muscle	0.2–0.4 mg/kg q 6 hr PO, SQ, IM; or 1–2 mg/kg/24 hr continuous IV infusion	Extrapyramidal signs
	Domperidone*† (Motilium—Janssen Pharmaceutica)	GI smooth muscle	0.1–0.3 mg/kg q 12 hr IM, IV	None reported
H_1-Histaminergic antagonists	Diphenhydramine*‡ (Benadryl—Parke-Davis)	CRTZ	2–4 mg/kg q 8 hr PO, IM	Sedation
	Dimenhydrinate*‡ (Dramamine—Searle)	CRTZ	4–8 mg/kg q 8 hr PO	Sedation
	Chlorpromazine* Prochlorperazine*			
M_1-Cholinergic antagonists	Pirenzepine*† Chlorpromazine* Prochlorperazine*	Vestibular apparatus, CRTZ, other sites?		
5-HT$_3$-Serotonergic antagonists	Ondansetron* (Zofran—Glaxo Wellcome)	CRTZ, vagal afferent neurons	0.5–1.0 mg/kg q 12–24 hr PO, or 0.5–1.0 mg/kg PO 30 min before chemotherapy	Sedation, lip-licking, head-shaking
5-HT$_4$-Serotonergic agonists	Cisapride*§ (Propulsid, Janssen Pharmaceutica)	Myenteric neurons	0.1–0.5 mg/kg q 8 hr PO	None reported

Abbreviations: CRTZ, chemoreceptor trigger zone; GI, gastrointestinal; 5-HT$_3$, 5-hydroxytryptamine$_3$; 5-HT$_4$, 5-hydroxytryptamine$_4$; IM, intramuscular; IV, intravenous; PO, by mouth; q, every; SQ, subcutaneous.
*Not approved for use in cats or dogs.
†Not available in the United States.
‡More useful in dogs.
§No longer marketed in the United States.

M_1-cholinergic receptors involved in the pathogenesis of motion sickness. However, atropine is a mixed cholinergic receptor antagonist that also binds M_2- and M_3-cholinergic receptors. Antagonism of gastrointestinal smooth-muscle M_2-cholinergic receptors may result in delayed gastric emptying and ileus. This especially is true of atropine, aminopentamide, and isopropamide, which is the reason that these drugs usually are contraindicated in the therapy of vomiting disorders. Pirenzepine is a more highly selective M_1-cholinergic antagonist, although it is currently available only in Canada and Europe.[29]

3. *Most of these drugs have not been approved for use in cats.* Of the 14 antiemetic drugs discussed in this chapter, only yohimbine (an α_2-adrenergic antagonist) has been approved for use in dogs and cats.

◆ RATIONAL USE OF ANTIEMETIC AGENTS IN THE DIAGNOSED PATIENT
Motion Sickness

The neuronal pathways for motion sickness are still characterized incompletely, but motion sickness is believed to arise from stimulation of labyrinthine structures in the inner ear. The CRTZ and H_1-histaminergic receptors are involved in this pathway in dogs, but apparently they are involved less importantly in cats.[7, 8] Histamine receptors are not expressed in the feline CRTZ,[9] cats are insensitive to the emetic effects of histamine,[10, 11] and H_1-histaminergic receptor antagonists like diphenhydramine are ineffective in treating motion sickness in cats.[9] Motion sickness in cats probably is best treated with an α-adrenergic antagonist (e.g., chlorpromazine) instead of a pure H_1-histaminergic antagonist.[4, 7–9]

Uremia

Vomiting associated with uremia has both central and peripheral components. The central component of uremic vomiting is associated with activation of CRTZ D_2-dopaminergic receptors by circulating uremic toxins. The central component is best treated with a D_2-dopaminergic antagonist, for example, metoclopramide. The peripheral component of uremic vomiting is associated with uremic gastritis, and is best treated with acid-secretory inhibitors (e.g., cimetidine 5 to 10 mg/kg q 8 hr IV; ranitidine 1 to 2 mg/kg q 12 hr IV; omeprazole 0.7 mg/kg q

12 hr PO) to diminish gastric parietal cell H^+ ion secretion, and with chemical diffusion barriers (e.g., sucralfate 0.25 to 0.5 g q 8 to 12 hr PO) to provide a barrier to H^+ ion backdiffusion.[30, 31]

Cancer Chemotherapy

Certain cancer chemotherapies (e.g., cisplatinum, cyclophosphamide) are associated with a high incidence of vomiting. Chemotherapy-induced emesis is mediated by 5-HT_3-serotonergic receptors, either in the CRTZ or in vagal afferent neurons. Antagonists of the 5-HT_3-serotonergic receptor (e.g., ondansetron, granisetron, tropisetron) abolish the vomiting associated with cisplatinum administration in cats.[10, 13–15] Although metoclopramide has some 5-HT_3-antagonistic properties, it has not proved very useful in chemotherapy-induced emesis.[20]

Delayed Gastric-Emptying Disorders

Disorders of delayed gastric emptying (e.g., gastritis, metabolic derangements, postoperative gastric dilatation and volvulus) may cause an animal to experience nausea and vomiting.[23, 32] Treatment of these disorders with cholinomimetic agents has been associated with untoward side-effects. Contemporary therapy consists of 5-HT_4-serotonergic agonists (e.g., cisapride, metoclopramide), cholinesterase inhibitors (e.g., ranitidine or nizatidine), and motilin agonists (e.g., low-dose erythromycin—dog only).[32, 33] Cisapride is superior to metoclopramide in the treatment of gastric-emptying disorders of cats and dogs; however, the drug was withdrawn from the American market in July 2000. Ranitidine and nizatidine inhibit acetylcholinesterase activity in addition to their effects on histamine H_2 receptors in the gastric mucosa.[34] Both drugs (ranitidine and nizatidine) stimulate gastric emptying in cats and dogs.[32, 34] Cimetidine and famotidine are without this prokinetic effect. Erythromycin stimulates phase III migrating myoelectric complex activity in dogs,[27] but the migrating spike complex activity of cats is under different physiologic regulation.[35]

◆ RATIONAL USE OF ANTIEMETIC AGENTS IN THE UNDIAGNOSED PATIENT

Antiemetic therapy in an undiagnosed patient may be appropriate when 1 or more of the following criteria have been satisfied: (1) the vomiting is frequent or severe enough to make the animal feel uncomfortable; (2) persistent vomiting places the animal at risk for aspiration pneumonia or acid-base and electrolyte disturbances; (3) the animal is not suffering from gastrointestinal obstruction or toxicity; or (4) the client does not desire a definitive

Rational Use of Anti-Emetic Agents in the Undiagnosed Patient

α₂ **Adrenergic Antagonists**
↓
D₂ **Dopaminergic Antagonists**
↓
5–HT_3 **Serotonergic Antagonists**

Figure 13–2. Rational use of antiemetic agents in the undiagnosed patient. α, alpha-adrenergic; D, dopamine; 5-HT, 5-hydroxytryptamine.

diagnosis. When these criteria have been met, a systematic approach to antiemesis should be followed (Fig. 13–2; see also Table 13–1).

◆ IRRATIONAL USE OF ANTIEMETIC AGENTS

Antiemetics may be inappropriate in any or all of the following situations: (1) *gastrointestinal infection*: antiemetics may prolong gastrointestinal infections, particularly bacterial infections; (2) *gastrointestinal obstruction*: some antiemetic agents have peripheral gastrointestinal prokinetic effects that, if used, could accelerate gastrointestinal motility against a fixed obstruction; (3) *gastrointestinal toxicity*: antiemetic agents used in this circumstance could prevent the animal from eliminating the ingested toxin; (4) *systemic hypotension*: the classic phenothiazines (mixed α₁-α₂-antagonists) could exacerbate preexisting hypotension by antagonizing α₁ receptors on vascular smooth muscle; and (5) *epilepsy*: the classic phenothiazines tend to lower the threshold for seizure activity.

REFERENCES

1. Hall JA: Clinical approach to chronic vomiting. *In* August JR (ed): Consultations in Feline Internal Medicine, vol. 3. Philadelphia, WB Saunders, 1997, pp. 61–67.
2. Borison HL, Wang SC: Physiology and pharmacology of vomiting. Pharmacol Rev 5:193–230, 1953.
3. Wang SC, Borison HL: A new concept of organization of the central emetic mechanism: Recent studies on the sites of action of apomorphine, copper sulfate, and cardiac glycosides. Gastroenterology 22:1–12, 1952.
4. Washabau RJ, Elie ME: Antiemetic therapy. *In* Bonagura JD (ed): Current Veterinary Therapy XII. Philadelphia, WB Saunders, 1995, pp. 679–684.
5. Harding RK: Concepts and conflicts in the mechanism of emesis. Can J Physiol Pharmacol 68:218–220, 1990.
6. Lang IM, Sarna SK, Condon RE: Gastrointestinal motor correlates of vomiting in the dog: Quantification and identification as an independent phenomenon. Gastroenterology 90:40–47, 1986.
7. Borison HL, Borison R: Motion sickness reflex arc bypasses the area postrema in cats. Exp Neurol 92:723–737, 1986.

8. Lucot JB, Crampton GH: Xylazine emesis, yohimbine and motion sickness susceptibility in the cat. J Pharmacol Exp Ther 237:450–455, 1986.

9. Lucot JB, Takeda T: α-Fluoromethylhistidine but not diphenhydramine prevents motion-induced emesis in the cat. Am J Otorhinolaryngol 13:176–180, 1992.

10. Beleslin DB: Neurotransmitter receptor subtypes related to vomiting. *In* Bianchi AL (ed): Mechanisms and Control of Emesis. Paris, Inserm, 1992, p. 11.

11. King GL: Animal models in the study of vomiting. Can J Physiol Pharmacol 68:260–268, 1990.

12. Lang IM, Sarna SK: The role of adrenergic receptors in the initiation of vomiting and its gastrointestinal motor correlates in the dog. J Pharmacol Exp Ther 263:395–403, 1992.

13. Smith WL, Callaham EM, Alphin RS: The emetic activity of centrally administered cisplatin in cats and its antagonism by zacopride. J Pharm Pharmacol 40:142–146, 1988.

14. Lucot JB: Blockade of 5-hydroxytryptamine₃ receptors prevents cisplatin-induced but not motion or xylazine-induced emesis in the cat. Pharmacol Biochem Behav 32:207–212, 1989.

15. Costall B, Naylor RJ: Neuropharmacology of emesis in relation to clinical response. Br J Cancer 66(Suppl XIX):S2–S8, 1992.

16. Fukui H, Yamamoto M, Sato S: Vagal afferent fibers and peripheral 5-HT₃ receptors mediate cisplatin-induced emesis in dogs. Jap J Pharmacol 59:221–226, 1992.

17. Tucker ML, Jackson MR, Scales MDC, et al: Ondansetron: Pre-clinical safety evaluation. Eur J Cancer Clin Oncol 25:S79–S93, 1989.

18. Lucot JB: Prevention of motion sickness by 5-HT₁A agonists in cats. *In* Bianchi AL (ed): Mechanisms and Control of Emesis. Paris, Inserm, 1992, p. 195.

19. Hikasa Y, Takase K, Ogasawara S: Evidence for the involvement of α₂-adrenoceptors in the emetic action of xylazine in cats. Am J Vet Res 50:1348–1351, 1989.

20. Gyllys JA, Doran KM, Buyniski JP: Antagonism of cisplatin induced emesis in the dog. Res Commun Chem Pathol Pharmacol 23:61–68, 1979.

21. Washabau RJ, Hall JA: Clinical pharmacology of cisapride. J Am Vet Med Assoc 207:1285–1288, 1995.

22. Washabau RJ, Hall JA: Gastrointestinal prokinetic therapy: Serotonergic drugs. Compend Contin Educ Pract Vet 19:473–480, 1997.

23. Washabau RJ, Hall JA: Diagnosis and management of gastrointestinal motility disorders in dogs and cats. Compend Contin Educ Pract Vet 19:721–734, 1997.

24. Hall JA, Washabau RJ: Gastrointestinal prokinetic therapy: Dopaminergic antagonistic drugs. Compend Contin Educ Pract Vet 19:214–221, 1997.

25. Hall JA, Washabau RJ: Gastrointestinal prokinetic therapy: Motilin-like drugs. Compend Contin Educ Pract Vet 19:281–288, 1997.

26. Gullikson GW, Loeffler RF, Virina AM: Relationship of serotonin-3 receptor antagonist activity to gastric emptying and motor-stimulating actions of prokinetic drugs in dogs. J Pharmacol Exp Ther 258:103–109, 1991.

27. Itoh Z: Erythromycin mimics exogenous motilin in gastrointestinal contractile activity in the dog. Am J Physiol 247:G688–G694, 1984.

28. Greenwood B, Dieckman D, Kirst HA, et al: Effects of LY267108, an erythromycin analogue derivative, on lower esophageal sphincter function in the cat. Gastroenterology 106:624–628, 1994.

29. Coruzzi G, Adami M, Bertaccini G: Gastric antisecretory activity of telenzepine, a new M₁ selective muscarinic antagonist: Comparison with pirenzepine in the cat. Arch Intern Pharmacodyn Ther 302:232–241, 1989.

30. Washabau RJ: Gastrointestinal hemorrhage: Approach to patients (Part I). Compend Contin Educ Pract Vet 18:1317–1325, 1996.

31. Washabau RJ: Gastrointestinal hemorrhage: Causes and therapy (Part II). Compend Contin Educ Pract Vet 18:1327–1337, 1996.

32. Hall JA, Washabau RJ: Diagnosis and therapy of gastrointestinal motility disorders. Vet Clin North Am Small Anim Pract 29:377–395, 1999.

33. Hall JA, Washabau RJ: Gastric prokinetic agents. *In* Bonagura JD (ed): Current Veterinary Therapy XIII. Philadelphia, WB Saunders, 2000, pp. 614–616.

34. Hall JA, Washabau RJ: Gastrointestinal prokinetic therapy: Acetylcholinesterase inhibitors. Compend Contin Educ Pract Vet 19:615–621, 1997.

35. De Vos W: Migrating spike complex in the small intestine of the fasting cat. Am J Physiol 265:G619–G627, 1993.

14

◆ The Gastrointestinal Tract and Adverse Reactions to Food

W. Grant Guilford

◆ ADVERSE REACTIONS TO FOOD (FOOD SENSITIVITY)

Terminology

Adverse reactions to food comprise a variety of subclassifications: dietary indiscretion, food allergies, food anaphylaxis, food idiosyncrasy, food intolerances, food poisoning, metabolic adverse reactions to food, and pharmacologic reactions to food. The terminology applied previously to the various subclassifications of adverse reactions to food has been misleading. To rectify this situation, the terms and definitions listed in Table 14–1 were recommended by the American Academy of Allergy and Immunology.[1] These terms also are preferred for description of adverse reactions to food in animals.[2]

Pathogenesis

In general, the pathogenic mechanisms that lead to an adverse reaction (allergy or intolerance) include interaction of the food with a biologic amplification system that leads to inflammation and the generation of clinical signs. The amplification system varies considerably with the inciting agent, but may include the immune system, the arachidonic acid cascade, the complement cascade, chemotaxis of phagocytes, and generation of kinins. At times, sufficient toxic material may be present in the food to produce clinical signs without need for amplification.

Clinical Signs

The signs usually are dermatologic or gastrointestinal,[3–7] but other body systems occasionally are affected. In cats, the most frequent gastrointestinal manifestations are vomiting and diarrhea. The vomiting usually is infrequent, occurring less than once daily in most cats.[7] Some food-sensitive cats vomit food within minutes of eating, whereas others vomit food many hours later. Many food-sensitive cats with diarrhea have evidence of large-bowel dysfunction (mucus and fresh blood in the feces and/or excessive straining to defecate). Dermatologic signs need not be present to attribute a gastrointestinal abnormality to food sensitivity, but the concurrent appearance of clinical signs in these body systems should raise the index of suspicion for food sensitivity.

Differential Diagnosis

Adverse reactions to food usually are suspected when a pet owner or veterinarian establishes a historical association between the ingestion of a certain foodstuff and the appearance of clinical signs. Several abdominal disorders other than food sensitivity may be associated with acute signs after food ingestion. Examples include chronic gastritis, pancreatitis, biliary neoplasia, and esophagitis. These disorders usually can be differentiated from food sensitivity because the initiating food is often nonspecific, and the response to the elimination diet usually is not rapid or complete.

Diagnosis

The diagnosis of an adverse reaction to a food is confirmed by elimination-challenge trials. In food-sensitive patients, resolution of clinical signs occurs after elimination of the responsible food from the diet, followed by recrudescence of the signs when the patient is rechallenged with the food. Subsequent resumption of the elimination diet should alleviate the signs again.

Correct design of elimination-challenge trials is imperative for reliable diagnosis. The initial elimination period chosen usually is 2 to 4 weeks in duration. This period is sufficient for resolution of the clinical signs in the majority of food-sensitive cats. In a recent Massey University study of cats with gastrointestinal adverse reactions to foods, the clinical signs of all affected cats had resolved within 2 to 3 days of beginning the elimination diet.[7] In chronic relapsing conditions (e.g., inflammatory bowel disease), the elimination period chosen must be longer than the usual symptom-free period of the patient to allow reliable assessment of the contribution of food sensitivity to the patient's signs.[8]

Once the clinical signs have resolved (or partially resolved), the patient is rechallenged with its old diet. Failure to rechallenge a suspected food-sensitive cat will lead to marked overdiagnosis of food sensitivity.[7] If signs recur after rechallenge and then resolve for a second time once the patient is fed the elimination diet again, a diagnosis of food sensitiv-

Table 14–1. Adverse Reactions to Food: Preferred Terminology

Adverse reaction to food (food sensitivity): general term for a clinically abnormal response attributed to an ingested food or food additive

Dietary indiscretion: adverse reactions as a result of such behaviors as gluttony, pica, or ingestion of indigestible materials

Food allergy (hypersensitivity): adverse reaction to a food or food additive with a proven immunologic basis

Food anaphylaxis: acute food allergy with systemic consequences resulting from an immunoglobulin E–mediated release of chemical mediators

Food idiosyncrasy: quantitatively abnormal response to a food substance or additive that resembles a hypersensitivity response but does not involve immune mechanisms

Food intolerance: abnormal response to an ingested food or food additive that does not have an immunologic basis. It includes idiosyncratic, metabolic, pharmacologic, and toxic responses to foods

Food poisoning: direct nonimmunologic action on the host of a toxin contained within the food or released by organisms contaminating the food

Metabolic adverse reactions to food: adverse reactions as a result of an effect of the substance on the metabolism of the host, or as a result of defective metabolism of the host, or as a result of defective metabolism of the nutrient by the host

Pharmacologic reactions to food: adverse reactions as a result of a druglike or pharmacologic effect in the host

ity is made. Further cycles of elimination-challenge trials may be undertaken then in an attempt to identify the food ingredients responsible. Reintroduction of the offending food usually causes recurrence of clinical signs within a few hours to 4 days.

The constituents of a suitable elimination diet are determined primarily by diet history. As a general rule, the protein and carbohydrate source chosen should not have formed a significant part of the cat's diet in the previous 6 months. In the author's opinion, commercial, selected-protein diets are effective elimination diets, provided they are purchased from a reputable manufacturer and that a careful dietary history is taken to ensure that the proteins in the elimination diet are indeed novel to the cat. The constituents of the challenge diet(s) also should be chosen primarily from dietary history. The most likely foods responsible are those commonly found in the cat's diet.

To reiterate, such dietary trials confirm or rule out adverse reactions to food but do not indicate the underlying mechanism. To make a diagnosis of food allergy, the clinician must go on to establish that the adverse reaction has an immunologic basis.[2, 8] The latter step often is omitted from the diagnostic evaluation because the management of most patients will not be greatly altered whether the clinical signs result from food allergy or from food intolerance.

◆ FOOD ALLERGY (FOOD HYPERSENSITIVITY)

Food allergy is an adverse reaction to a food with a proven immunologic basis.

Chemistry of Food Allergens

Food allergens are almost exclusively proteins, and in particular glycoproteins with a molecular weight in the range of 10,000 to 40,000 daltons.[1] Although all food proteins are antigenic, often only a small component of the total protein content of a food is allergenic. The reasons for the propensity of some allergens to produce a hypersensitivity response (particularly type I) are incompletely understood. Most food allergens are partially resistant to heat and digestion, 2 properties that help ensure the maintenance of antigenicity. Furthermore, there are apparently other as yet undefined physicochemical properties that result in the higher allergic potential of some proteins, such as shellfish and nuts, in some species.[9]

Common Food Allergens

Foods responsible for allergy in cats often reflect the most prevalent foods in their diet. Fish and dairy products have been incriminated previously,[3, 4] whereas at Massey University the most prevalent allergens causing gastrointestinal adverse reactions to foods in cats were beef, wheat, and corn gluten.[7] Most food sensitivities affecting the skin are due to single foods. In contrast, multiple allergies to foods are quite common in animals suffering from gastrointestinal diseases.[7]

Etiopathogenesis

A food protein has the potential to incite an allergic response if it is digested incompletely in the bowel, absorbed across the mucosa intact in excessive quantities, and then escapes to the systemic lymphoid tissue. Alternatively, the allergic response may result if a small amount of antigen encounters a defective suppressor arm of the gut-associated lymphoid tissue. In either case, the result is the stimulation of the synthesis of immunoglobulins (Ig), such as IgE and IgG, and the sensitization of peripheral lymphocytes, both of which can generate immunosensitivity to the food antigen rather than the usual situation of tolerance.

Immediate hypersensitivities to food occur within a few minutes to several hours of ingestion of the offending antigen.[10] In most species, immediate hypersensitivity responses are mediated by IgE-induced degranulation of mast cells, and this also probably is true of cats. The mediators released by mast cell degranulation cause loss of fluid, plasma proteins, and even blood from the capillaries into the lumen of the gut. The mediators stimulate intestinal mucus and chloride secretion, and cause mucosal disaccharidase and motility derangements.[10–12]

Intermediate hypersensitivities to food occur several hours after antigen ingestion. They appear to be frequent in cats, judging by the usual time of occurrence of adverse reactions after food challenges. Intermediate reactions are a poorly defined intergrade between immediate and delayed reactions. Intermediate hypersensitivity responses probably are the result of a late-phase response to IgE-mediated mast cell degranulation and/or a type III hypersensitivity response to immune complexes.

Delayed hypersensitivity responses to food are considered by some investigators to be the most prevalent classification of food allergy in human beings. In spite of their probable importance, delayed hypersensitivities remain poorly documented in clinical situations. The prevalence of delayed hypersensitivity responses to food in cats is unknown.

Epidemiology and Clinical Signs

Food allergy usually is nonseasonal (in contrast to many inhalation allergies), and often occurs suddenly after months or years of consuming the diet containing the inciting foodstuff.[3, 4] A wide age range of patients may be affected, including cats as young as 2 to 6 months.[3, 4] No breed or gender predilections have been established.[3, 4, 7]

The clinical signs of food allergy are the same as those described for adverse reactions to foods (see earlier). The specific clinical signs manifested in an individual cat depend on the level of the gastrointestinal tract affected. Every level of the gastrointestinal tract (including the oral cavity, stomach, small intestine, and large intestine) may be affected by food allergies. The signs seen in an affected cat usually are uniform in manifestation, and occur consistently on subsequent rechallenges.

Diagnosis

The diagnosis of food allergy requires that an adverse reaction to a food be proved to have an immune-mediated basis. This is not a simple matter. The enormous number of possible dietary allergens is one stumbling block. Furthermore, whether or not an animal manifests clinical signs after ingesting an allergen to which it is sensitive may depend on a number of different factors, including synergism with sensitivities to other allergens, and emotional and various environmental factors that may influence the "allergy threshold." Another problem is the high incidence of asymptomatic sensitization, whereby patients demonstrate positive immunologic tests to food antigens but do not show signs on subsequent challenge with the incriminated food. It is important to realize that a positive reaction to an allergy test is an immunologic phenomenon that must not be the only basis for diagnosis. Both positive and negative results provide only a part of the accumulated evidence in the clinician's final judgment.

There are no routine laboratory tests that differen-

tiate food-allergic from non–food-allergic cats.[7] A persistent eosinophilia is present in approximately one-third of cats with food allergies, but also occurs in cats with gastrointestinal signs not due to food allergy.[7]

Skin testing has poor accuracy for the prediction of adverse reactions to foods in most veterinary studies,[13] and is not recommended in cats.

The concentration of food-specific IgE in the serum can be measured by a radioallergosorbent test (RAST) or enzyme-linked immunosorbent assay (ELISA). As with skin tests, RAST and ELISA can diagnose only 1 form of food sensitivity (immediate hypersensitivity mediated by IgE), and therefore, axiomatically, cannot be used to screen for all adverse reactions to foods. The diagnostic value of in vitro tests for food-specific IgE antibodies varies widely in reported human studies.[14] However, a positive challenge test along with an elevated IgE level to a food protein strongly implies food allergy (rather than intolerance) to that protein.[14] Because of the high incidence of asymptomatic sensitization, a positive RAST or ELISA test alone does not permit a diagnosis of food allergy to a particular protein.[14] Unfortunately, in a recent study of food-sensitive cats with chronic gastrointestinal problems, there was little evidence to support the diagnostic utility of a commercial feline food-specific IgE assay (Bio-Medical Services, Austin, TX).[7]

Gastroscopic food-sensitivity testing has been used to diagnose food allergies in human beings and dogs, but has not proved useful in cats.[7, 15]

Gastrointestinal biopsy specimens cannot be used to confirm food allergy because many of the acute changes, such as edema, are transient or not detectable by light microscopy.[10] Furthermore, in chronic food-allergic conditions, there are no pathognomonic histologic features that differentiate food hypersensitivity from the other causes of chronic intestinal inflammation.[12] Eosinophils have been found in rectal scrapes from food-sensitive cats.[6] Eosinophilic infiltration is suggestive of food allergy but not pathognomonic. The majority of cats with food sensitivity do not have eosinophilic gastrointestinal infiltrates.[7] Repeated gastrointestinal biopsy specimens acquired during elimination-challenge trials are of considerably more diagnostic value than single biopsy specimens.[16]

Pathologic Findings

The histologic changes in food-sensitive cats are diverse, nonspecific, and of variable severity. They include lymphocytic-plasmacytic and/or eosinophilic gastritis, enteritis, or colitis.[7, 17] The small intestine of a cat allergic to milk showed congestion, edema, villus degeneration, hemorrhage, and an increase in the number of plasma cells after 4 days of milk challenge.[18] The histologic features of food protein–induced enteropathies usually are patchy, and the villus atrophy partial rather than complete.[10] At times, the histologic changes of food sensitivity are reminiscent of gastrointestinal lymphoma[19] (see Chapter 63, Gastrointestinal Lymphoma and Inflammatory Bowel Disease).

Treatment

Treatment is dependent on identification of the responsible food proteins by elimination-challenge diets. These antigens then should be omitted from the diet for a minimum of 6 months. Care should be taken to ensure that the therapeutic diet remains balanced, palatable, and practical. Ninety per cent of homemade elimination diets are not nutritionally adequate.[20] Acquisition of food allergy to the protein source in the therapeutic diet can occur, and may be responsible for a recurrence of signs.

Antihistamines (H_1 blockers) administered before meals may decrease some of the systemic manifestations of food hypersensitivity, but usually do not prevent gastrointestinal signs.[2] Corticosteroids are reserved for the induction of a more rapid remission in severe conditions, such as allergic chronic gastroenteropathies, and for those patients in which avoidance of the offending antigen is impossible. Animals with food allergy do not respond as consistently to anti-inflammatory doses of corticosteroids as do those with atopy, but usually will show partial improvement. Hyposensitization therapy, through either oral or parenteral routes, has no proven benefit in food hypersensitivity.

◆ FOOD INTOLERANCES

Food Idiosyncrasy

A wide variety of food additives has been noted to produce adverse reactions to food in susceptible people. These reactions can mimic food allergies closely. One distinguishing feature is that they usually do not require prior sensitization, and thus may occur on the first exposure to the inciting agent. By far, the majority of reactions to food additives are due to idiosyncratic food intolerances and not immunologic mechanisms. The reactions may be dermatologic, respiratory, gastrointestinal, or behavioral.[21]

The prevalence of adverse reactions to food additives has been estimated to range from 0.15 to 0.3 per cent of the total human population.[21] The same reactions are likely to occur in cats, but are poorly documented. Diagnosis of food idiosyncrasy most often requires the use of elimination-challenge diets. No in vitro tests are available. It is difficult to rule out an immunologic basis to a food idiosyncrasy. RASTs for food additives are not available, and skin testing using chemicals, many of which are known contact irritants, has received little evaluation.

The mechanisms by which these chemical additives produce such clinical signs without involve-

ment of the immune system are a matter of continuing investigation. Suggested possibilities include triggering of eicosanoid pathways, alteration of cell-membrane permeability, inhibition of enzymes, direct release of histamine, changes in neurotransmitter levels, and independent activation of the complement and kinin cascades.

Anaphylactoid Reactions to Food

Anaphylactoid reactions mimic anaphylactic reactions, yet laboratory tests fail to establish an immune basis. Anaphylactoid reactions may occur in cats after ingestion of spoiled scombroid fish (such as tuna, mackerel, or mahi-mahi) that contain large amounts of histamine. The contamination of the fish with bacteria results in microbial decarboxylation of histidine to yield histamine.

Pharmacologic Reactions to Food

A number of foods contain vasoactive amines and other pharmacologically active substances capable of inducing a wide variety of signs that particularly affect the gastrointestinal tract and nervous system.[22] The vasoactive amines include tyramine, tryptamine, phenylethylamine, dopamine, norepinephrine, serotonin, and histamine.[22] They usually are produced by bacterial decarboxylation of amino acids. Tyramine is common in cheese, histamine in spoiled tuna, and phenylethylamine in chocolate.[1, 22]

Psychoactive agents and stimulants are contained in some foods. The most important example is chocolate toxicosis resulting from methylxanthines. Another example is myristin in nutmeg.

Metabolic Adverse Reactions to Food

Metabolic adverse reactions to food usually occur only in a susceptible subpopulation. Reasons for susceptibility to a particular food include disease states, malnutrition, and inborn errors of metabolism.[22] The diarrhea, bloating, and abdominal discomfort that occur after ingestion of milk by cats with lactose intolerance constitute a metabolic adverse reaction that is relatively common. Inborn errors of metabolism collectively are an important cause of metabolic adverse reactions to food in human beings, and also occur in animals (for example, urea cycle enzyme deficiencies).

Food Poisoning

Food poisoning is an occasional cause of gastrointestinal signs in cats. The diagnosis of food poisoning usually is made when a pet is suspected to have eaten inadequately prepared, spoiled, or contaminated food. Clinical signs will occur within a few hours of ingestion when the poisoning is due to a toxin inherent to the food or to a secreted toxin derived from a microorganism. More delayed signs result if the food poisoning is due to a microorganism that must colonize the bowel for pathogenicity.[1] Ingestion of a variety of toxic plants mistaken as food can cause poisoning.

REFERENCES

1. Anderson JA, Sogu DD (eds): Adverse reactions to foods. National Institutes of Health Publication No. 84-2442. Bethesda, MD, National Institutes of Health, July 1984.
2. Halliwell REW: Management of dietary hypersensitivity in the dog. J Small Anim Pract 33:156–160, 1992.
3. Walton GS: Skin responses in the dog and cat to ingested allergens: Observations on one hundred confirmed cases. Vet Rec 81:709–713, 1967.
4. White SD, Sequoia D: Food hypersensitivity in cats: 14 cases (1982–1987). J Am Vet Med Assoc 194:692–695, 1989.
5. Denis S, Paradis M: Food allergies in dogs and cats. Part 2: Retrospective study. Med Vet Que 24:15–20, 1994.
6. Guaguere E: Food intolerance in cats with cutaneous manifestations: A review of 17 cases. Eur J Comp Anim Pract 5:27–35, 1995.
7. Guilford WG, Jones BR, Markwell PJ, et al: Food sensitivity in cats with chronic idiopathic gastrointestinal problems. J Vet Intern Med (in press).
8. Bahna SL: Practical considerations in food challenge testing. Immunol Allergy Clin North Am 11:843–850, 1991.
9. Sampson HA: Immunologic mechanisms in adverse reactions to foods. Immunol Allergy Clin North Am 11:701–716, 1991.
10. Patrick MK, Gall DG: Protein intolerance and immunocyte and enterocyte interaction. Pediatr Clin North Am 35:17–34, 1988.
11. Curtis GH, Patrick MK, Catto-Smith AG, Gall DG: Intestinal anaphylaxis in the rat. Effect of chronic antigen exposure. Gastroenterology 98:1558–1566, 1990.
12. Gryboski JD: Gastrointestinal aspects of cow's milk protein intolerance and allergy. Immunol Allergy Clin North Am 11:733–797, 1991.
13. Foster AP, O'Dair H: Allergy testing for skin disease in the cat: In vivo versus in vitro tests. Vet Dermatol 4:111–115, 1993.
14. Ownby DR: In vitro assays for the evaluation of immunologic reactions to foods. Immunol Allergy Clin North Am 11:851–862, 1991.
15. Guilford WG, Strombeck DR, Frick O, Lawoko C: Development of gastroscopic food sensitivity testing in dogs. J Vet Intern Med 8:414–422, 1994.
16. Proujansky R, Winter HS, Walker WA: Gastrointestinal syndromes associated with food sensitivity. Adv Pediatr 35:219–238, 1988.
17. Nelson RW, Dimperio ME, Long GG: Lymphocytic-plasmacytic colitis in the cat. J Am Vet Med Assoc 184:1133–1135, 1984.
18. Walton GS, Parish WE, Coombs RAA: Spontaneous allergic dermatitis and enteritis in a cat. Vet Rec 83:35–41, 1968.
19. Wasmer ML, Willard MD, Helman RG, Edwards JF: Food intolerance mimicking alimentary lymphosarcoma. J Am Anim Hosp Assoc 31:463–466, 1995.
20. Roudebush P, Cowell CS: Results of a hypoallergenic diet survey of veterinarians in North America with a nutritional evaluation of homemade diet prescriptions. Vet Dermatol 3:23–28, 1992.
21. Hannuksela M, Haahtela T: Hypersensitivity reactions to food additives. Allergy 42:561–575, 1987.
22. Furukawa CT: Nonimmunologic food reactions that can be confused with allergy. Immunol Allergy Clin North Am 11:815–829, 1991.

15

◆ Cytologic Evaluation of Fine-Needle Liver Biopsies

Michele Menard
Marc Papageorges

Cats with different liver disorders often present with similar clinical signs and laboratory abnormalities, and a definitive diagnosis requires a liver biopsy.[1, 2] Ultrasonography, currently the best imaging technique to evaluate the liver, provides useful anatomic information, but frequently lacks the sensitivity and specificity necessary to obtain final diagnoses.[3, 4] This modality is ideal to guide fine-needle biopsies (FNBs), however, and the combination of ultrasonography and cytopathology is a powerful diagnostic tool when skillful sonographers and cytopathologists work as a team. The ultrasound examination provides macroscopic information, and cytology provides microscopic information.[5] The advantages of FNBs are numerous; they are fast, minimally invasive, and affordable, can be performed on inpatients and outpatients, and are well accepted by clients (and patients). The risk of serious complications is less than 1 per cent.[6–8]

To obtain a high diagnostic yield with liver cytology, a sample of good quality, a complete history including pertinent blood work and ultrasound findings, and an experienced cytopathologist are necessary.[6, 7, 9, 10] When sonographers and cytopathologists master their art, large-scale studies have shown that diagnostic yields can exceed 90 to 95 per cent.[6–8, 10] Poor correlation between cytology and histopathology was reported in a small study of 25 dogs and 7 cats.[11] In that study, none of the 3 cases of hepatic lipidosis was confirmed by cytology. A similar comparative study of 27 dogs and 32 cats showed a good correlation between cytology and histopathology for hepatic lipidosis and neoplasia, but inflammation was often missed with cytology.[11a] Such results, compared with our experience and the high diagnostic yield reported in the human literature, emphasize the importance of experience and sample quality.

Cytopathology of internal organs including the liver is a rapidly growing field in human medicine.[5, 7, 8, 10, 12] The literature in veterinary medicine concerning cytopathology of the liver is scarce.[13–15] Whether to use fine-needle, core, or surgical wedge hepatic biopsies is a controversial issue in veterinary medicine. Some authors recommend surgical wedge biopsy as a routine procedure for liver biopsies.[16] Others prefer using FNBs first, because this procedure is less invasive, and if a diagnosis is not obtained, more invasive methods of hepatic biopsy are used later.[2, 5–9, 12, 17, 18] This debate is likely to continue until clinicians improve the quality of their FNBs, and more cytopathologists become experienced with liver cytology. In our cytopathology practice, we read 10 to 15 ultrasound-guided, fine-needle liver biopsies daily sent to us by various sonographers, and in our experience, the diagnostic yield clearly correlates with the ability to obtain good biopsies. Once the FNB technique is mastered, the diagnostic yield exceeds 90 per cent.

◆ FINE-NEEDLE BIOPSY TECHNIQUE

A good biopsy technique is essential to obtain a high diagnostic yield.[6, 9] If the sample is poorly cellular or diluted excessively by blood, evaluation for inflammation is not possible, and neoplasia can be missed. We prefer a nonaspiration technique for the following reasons: reduced hemodilution, increased numbers of diagnostic cells, and better evaluation of inflammation. Those are critical factors because approximately 50 per cent of liver diseases in cats are inflammatory.[19, 20] We also use an extension set for intravenous lines between the syringe and the needle. The extension set makes it easier to hold the needle, allows more precise sampling, reduces risk of laceration, and expedites the transfer of the sample onto glass slides. The syringe and extension set can be used multiple times until they become contaminated with tissue and/or blood.

The decision to use sedation or general anesthesia is dictated by potential coagulation defects and the temperament and/or mental status of the animal. Short-term anesthesia enables a more thorough examination of the liver and abdominal cavity, and decreases the risk of laceration during biopsies. We perform most of our ultrasound-guided fine-needle hepatic biopsies under short-term anesthesia. Although abnormalities in coagulation profiles may be associated with hepatic disease, complications are rare with this technique, and a prebiopsy coagulation profile is not performed routinely.[21]

We use 22-gauge needles. Regular 1.5-inch needles work well for most cats, but if the patient is obese or the liver is small, 2.5- or 3.5-inch spinal needles make it easier to reach the liver and obtain a cellular sample. The needle is connected to a 12-

ml syringe via an 84-cm flexible extension set for intravenous lines, and the syringe is prefilled with 5 to 10 ml of air. The syringe, connected to the extension set, is hung around the neck of the operator, and the needle hub is held like a pen to allow precise manipulations. We use alcohol rather than ultrasound gel as a coupling agent for most of our biopsies, because ultrasound gel stains dark purple and can interfere with smear evaluation. If ultrasound gel is used, it is important to keep the biopsy site and fingers free of gel.

After determining the optimum needle path, the needle tip is positioned within the liver. The needle tip then is moved rapidly back and forth 8 to 10 times within the same path. A common mistake is to move the needle slowly or to use short needle passes, which does not detach a sufficient number of cells. Long needle passes are better, but the needle tip must remain within the liver at all times during this part of the procedure. The needle is then withdrawn, and the biopsy material contained within the needle is expelled immediately on glass slides using the syringe that had been prefilled with air.

A gentle squash preparation technique should be used to make the smears. This technique keeps the liver cells at the center and displaces blood to the periphery, which greatly facilitates evaluation for inflammation. The smears are air-dried immediately, preferably using a blow dryer. Unstained hepatic smears of good quality have a central area of whitish granular material that represents liver cells, surrounded by a rim of peripheral blood. In many cases, there is a very small amount of peripheral blood. For the occasional cases in which the sample is excessively hemodiluted, only 1 or 2 smears are made, and the remainder of the sample is discarded. If the smears are composed of clear fatty material only, the needle most likely has remained in perihepatic fat, and did not penetrate the liver.

Three to 5 cellular biopsies of different areas of the liver are obtained. If focal lesions are observed, they should be sampled in addition to the hepatic parenchyma, and the smears should be labeled accordingly.

◆ RETROSPECTIVE STUDY OF 610 CASES PERFORMED AT VETERINARY DIAGNOSTIC IMAGING & CYTOPATHOLOGY, P.C., BETWEEN 1992 AND 1998

Six hundred and ten feline liver ultrasonographic examinations combined with ultrasound-guided FNBs were performed and evaluated between 1992 and 1998 at Veterinary Diagnostic Imaging & Cytopathology, P.C. The results were distributed as follows: 281 (46 per cent) inflammatory, 273 (44 per cent) lipidosis, 112 (18 per cent) neoplasia, 20 (3 per cent) others, and 13 (2.1 per cent) inconclusive. More than 1 type of liver disease was present in 14 per

cent of the cats. In the 273 cases of hepatic lipidosis, lipidosis was the only hepatic abnormality in 184 (67 per cent) cats. Fifty-one (19 per cent) cats had lipidosis and lymphocytic/plasmacytic hepatitis, 15 (5 per cent) had lipidosis and suppurative hepatitis, and 23 (8 per cent) had lipidosis and neoplasia. Neoplasia included hepatocellular carcinoma (9 [8 per cent]), hepatocellular adenoma or well-differentiated hepatocellular carcinoma of low-grade malignancy (7 [6 per cent]), cholangiocarcinoma (19 [17 per cent]), biliary cystadenoma (3 [3 per cent]), carcinoma of undetermined origin (10 [9 per cent]), lymphoma (37 [33 per cent]), large granular lymphocyte lymphoma (10 [9 per cent]), myeloproliferative disease (2 [2 per cent]), systemic mastocytosis (4 [4 per cent]), and metastatic neoplasia (11 [10 per cent]). The 281 cases of inflammatory liver disease were classified as lymphocytic/plasmacytic (144 [51 per cent]), mixed suppurative and lymphocytic/plasmacytic (53 [19 per cent]), suppurative (73 [26 per cent]), suppurative with sepsis (6 [2 per cent]), and pyogranulomatous (5 [2 per cent]). The miscellaneous category included cholestatic liver disease (4), vacuolar hepatopathy (8), normal (3), necrosis (1), benign nodule (3), and benign cyst (1).

The reasons for inconclusive biopsies included insufficient cellularity (5) and inability to differentiate between a chronic lymphocytic lymphoma and severe lymphocytic hepatitis without plasma cell infiltration (2) or between an early, well-differentiated cholangiocarcinoma, a bile duct adenoma, and severe biliary hyperplasia (6).

Two cats (0.3 per cent) died after the procedure. Both cats had severe hepatic lipidosis, and were severely debilitated. Serosanguineous fluid was present in the abdominal cavity of 1 cat at necropsy. A necropsy was not performed on the second cat.

In a retrospective study of 175 feline hepatic surgical biopsies between 1983 and 1993 at the University of Minnesota Veterinary Teaching Hospital, 26 per cent were classified as cholangitis/cholangiohepatitis, 49 per cent as lipidosis, 10 per cent as neoplasia, and 15 per cent as others.[22] The differences between these 2 studies may be explained by the different populations evaluated (referral cases versus general practices for our study), by geographic differences, and by the different number of cases.

◆ CYTOLOGY

Normal Liver

FNBs from normal livers contain several large clusters of hepatocytes with occasional clusters of benign biliary epithelial cells. Normal hepatocytes are large round-to-polygonal cells characterized by a moderate-to-large amount of basophilic cytoplasm, with a faint eosinophilic granulation and occasional greenish bile pigments; medium-sized round, often centrally located nuclei with granular chromatin; a

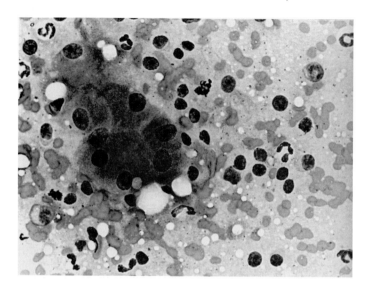

Figure 15–1. Lymphocytic/plasmacytic inflammatory liver disease. Hepatocytes are of normal morphology, and do not show significant vacuolar degeneration or intracellular cholestasis. There are several small lymphocytes surrounding the cluster of hepatocytes, with occasional plasma cells and neutrophils. Dip Quick stain, 500×.

single small to medium-sized nucleolus; and mild-to-moderate anisocytosis and anisokaryosis. Few sheets of biliary epithelial cells are usually present. They are small cells with a small amount of basophilic, often vacuolated cytoplasm; high nuclear-cytoplasmic ratio; small, round, dark nuclei, no nucleoli; and mild anisocytosis and anisokaryosis. Although occasional neutrophils, small lymphocytes, and plasma cells may be observed, significant infiltration by inflammatory cells surrounding the clusters of hepatocytes is absent with normal hepatic FNBs.

Inflammatory Liver Disease

High-quality smears with several large clusters of hepatocytes and minimum peripheral blood contamination are necessary to detect and determine the severity of inflammation. Whether inflammation involves the bile ducts and/or hepatic parenchyma cannot be established with cytology because of lack of architecture. Feline inflammatory liver diseases were classified as lymphocytic/plasmacytic (Fig. 15–1), mixed suppurative and lymphocytic/plasmacytic (Fig. 15–2), suppurative (Fig. 15–3), and pyogranulomatous, depending of the predominant type of inflammatory cells infiltrating the liver. Inflammatory cells usually are present between, rather than within, the large clusters of hepatocytes. With lymphocytic/plasmacytic inflammation, the inflammatory infiltrate is composed of a predominance of small lymphocytes with a smaller number of plasma cells and occasional neutrophils. The infiltrate with mixed lymphocytic/plasmacytic and suppurative inflammation is composed of a mixture of neutrophils, small lymphocytes, and a variable number of plasma cells. With suppurative inflammation, the infiltrate is composed of a predominance of neutrophils with occasional small lymphocytes and plasma cells. Few cases of suppurative hepatitis show evidence of a bacterial infection. Most cases of pyogranulomatous hepatitis in our area are secondary to feline infectious peritonitis, and show infiltration of the liver by multiple large clusters of macrophages and neutrophils (pyogranu-

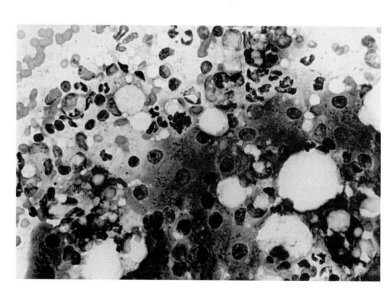

Figure 15–2. Mixed suppurative and lymphocytic/plasmacytic inflammatory liver disease. Hepatocytes show mild-to-moderate intracellular accumulation of bile pigments. A large number of small lymphocytes and neutrophils surround the clusters of hepatocytes, with occasional plasma cells and macrophages. Dip Quick stain, 500×.

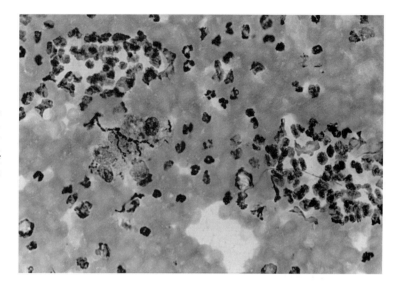

Figure 15–3. Suppurative inflammatory liver disease with sepsis. The sample is fairly diluted with blood. Inflammation was confirmed based on the severe infiltration by neutrophils with occasional rod-shaped bacteria in chains. There is a single small cluster of hepatocytes with extracellular bile casts. Dip Quick stain, 500×.

lomas). Fungal diseases, particularly if endemic to the area, also should be a primary consideration with pyogranulomatous hepatitis. The hepatocytes may show mild-to-moderate fine vacuolar degeneration with mild-to-moderate intracellular accumulation of bile pigments. Bile casts may be present if the inflammation is suppurative or pyogranulomatous. The casts usually are absent with lymphocytic/plasmacytic inflammation. Cats with liver fluke infestation (seen in Florida and Hawaii) show an inflammatory infiltrate composed of a mixture of eosinophils, macrophages, neutrophils, and lymphocytes, with a variable number of fluke eggs. This infiltrate often is associated with lakes of mucoid material suggestive of dilated bile duct contents.

Hepatic Lipidosis

The hepatocytes show moderate-to-severe intracytoplasmic distention by sharply demarcated clear lipid vacuoles of variable sizes with mild-to-moder-ate intracellular accumulation of bile pigments (Fig. 15–4). Several clear lipid droplets are present between the hepatocytes. Extracellular bile casts are common with severe hepatic lipidosis. Concurrent inflammation or hepatic neoplasia is present in approximately 35 per cent of cats with hepatic lipidosis (Figs. 15–5 to 15–7).

Hepatic Neoplasia

Cholangiocarcinomas are the most common malignant hepatobiliary tumors in cats.[23, 24] Multiple liver lobe involvement is common. The smears show severe infiltration by tight clusters of small to medium-sized epithelial cells showing a small amount of basophilic cytoplasm with occasional small, clear vacuoles, high nucleocytoplasmic ratio, medium-sized round-to-oval nuclei with dark chromatin, 1 to 3 small to medium-sized nucleoli, and moderate anisocytosis and anisokaryosis (Fig. 15–8). Cholangiocarcinomas of low-grade malignancy, bile duct

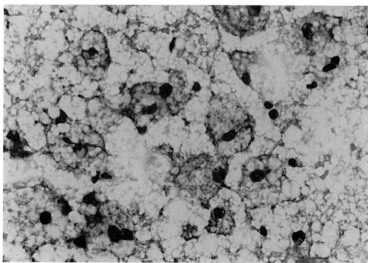

Figure 15–4. Hepatic lipidosis. Hepatocytes show severe intracytoplasmic infiltration by clear lipid vacuoles of variable sizes. Dip Quick stain, 500×.

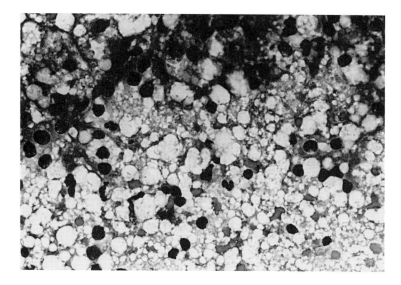

Figure 15–5. Hepatic lipidosis and lymphocytic/plasmacytic inflammatory liver disease. Hepatocytes show severe intracytoplasmic infiltration by clear lipid vacuoles of variable sizes. Several small lymphocytes and occasional neutrophils and plasma cells surround the clusters of hepatocytes. Dip Quick stain, 500×.

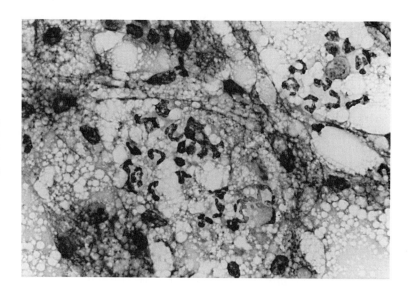

Figure 15–6. Hepatic lipidosis and suppurative inflammatory liver disease. Hepatocytes show severe intracytoplasmic infiltration by clear lipid vacuoles of variable sizes. Several neutrophils and occasional small lymphocytes are associated with the clusters of hepatocytes. Dip Quick stain, 500×.

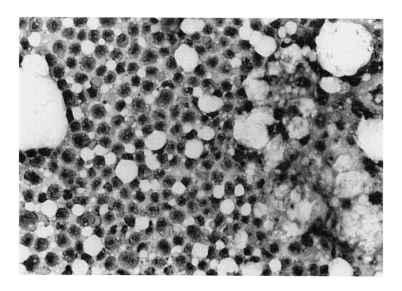

Figure 15–7. Hepatic lipidosis and lymphoma. Hepatocytes (to the right) show severe intracytoplasmic infiltration by clear lipid vacuoles of variable sizes. There is severe infiltration by large lymphoblasts, with a rim of basophilic, often vacuolated cytoplasm; large, round nuclei with slightly clumped chromatin; and 1 to 3 prominent nucleoli. Dip Quick stain, 500×.

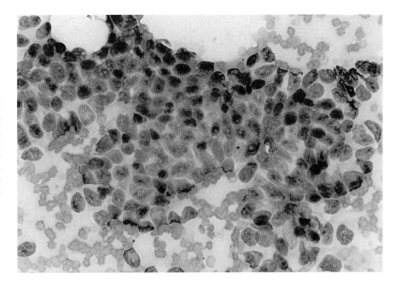

Figure 15–8. Cholangiocarcinoma. The liver from this cat appeared fairly normal on ultrasonography. On multiple fine-needle biopsies, there was severe infiltration by large sheets of small to medium-sized neoplastic cells showing a small amount of basophilic cytoplasm, high nucleocytoplasmic ratio, small to medium-sized nuclei with fine granular chromatin, and 1 to 3 small to medium-sized nucleoli. Very few hepatocytes were present on the smears (there are none on this figure). Dip Quick stain, 500×.

adenoma, and severe biliary hyperplasia may be difficult to differentiate cytologically, and may require a surgical biopsy or follow-up ultrasonographic examination.

Biliary cystadenomas are uncommon benign liver tumors of older cats that may occur as unifocal or multifocal cystic lesions on ultrasonographic examination.[25, 26] The ultrasound-guided needle biopsies are composed mainly of cystic fluid, which gives a pale blue background, with scattered sheets of benign round-to-polygonal epithelial cells showing a moderate amount of pale gray cytoplasm, small to medium-sized round-to-oval nuclei with fine granular chromatin, occasional small nucleoli, and mild anisocytosis and anisokaryosis (Fig. 15–9).

Hepatocellular carcinomas of high-grade malignancy can be confirmed cytologically. They are composed of large hepatocytes showing prominent criteria for malignancy, including high nuclear-cytoplasmic ratio, large nuclei with coarse granular chromatin, prominent multiple nucleoli with frequent pleomorphic macronucleoli, and severe ani-

socytosis and anisokaryosis (Fig. 15–10). Well-differentiated hepatocellular carcinomas of low-grade malignancy may be difficult to differentiate from benign nodules of hepatocellular regeneration and hepatocellular adenomas. The diagnosis in these cases is based on the combination of cytology, which is suggestive of a well-differentiated hepatocellular carcinoma of low-grade malignancy or hepatocellular adenoma, and ultrasonographic examination findings. A well-defined and noninvasive mass on ultrasonographic examination suggests a hepatocellular adenoma or a benign regeneration nodule. A poorly defined mass that appears invasive suggests a hepatocellular carcinoma. This distinction, however, can be subjective.

Lymphoma is the most common hepatic neoplasia in cats. Most lymphomas are of the acute lymphoblastic form, with severe infiltration of the liver by large lymphoblasts showing a rim of deeply basophilic, often vacuolated cytoplasm; large, dark, round nuclei; and 1 to 3 prominent nucleoli (Fig. 15–11). Occasional cases of chronic lymphocytic

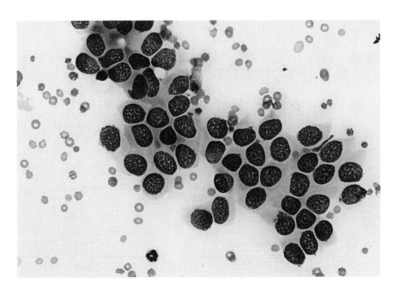

Figure 15–9. Biliary cystadenoma. A single large, well-defined, cystic mass was detected on ultrasonography. The smears consisted of a moderate number of erythrocytes, with a few sheets of small round-to-polygonal epithelial cells showing a moderate amount of pale gray cytoplasm; small, round nuclei with clumped chromatin; no nucleoli; and mild anisocytosis and anisokaryosis. Dip Quick stain, 500×.

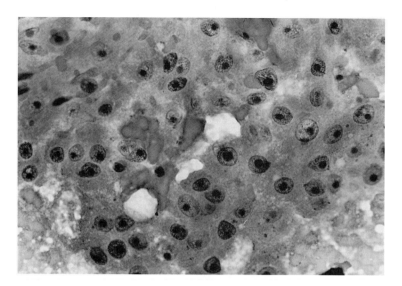

Figure 15–10. Hepatocellular carcinoma. A large liver mass was present on ultrasonography. The smears from this mass consisted of young hepatocytes showing increased cytoplasmic basophilia, increased nucleocytoplasmic ratio, large round-to-oval nuclei with fine-to-coarse chromatin, a single large nucleolus, and moderate anisocytosis and anisokaryosis. Dip Quick stain, 500×.

lymphomas (rare form of hepatic lymphomas in cats) may be difficult to differentiate from severe lymphocytic hepatitis with minimum plasma cell infiltration. Lymphomas of large granular lymphocytes are characterized by infiltration of the liver by medium-sized lymphocytes showing a moderate amount of pale gray cytoplasm containing a variable number of eosinophilic granules, often surrounded by a clear halo, medium-sized round-to-oval nuclei with fine granular chromatin, and no nucleoli. In addition to hepatic infiltration, intestinal and/or mesenteric lymph node involvement is common with lymphomas of large granular lymphocytes. Splenic mast-cell tumors often metastasize to the liver, with severe hepatic mast-cell infiltration. The mast-cell granules may stain purple, or appear as small, clear vacuoles with Wright staining (Fig. 15–12).

Ultrasonographic examination of the liver is very useful to detect focal lesions. As opposed to dogs, benign regenerative nodules are rare in cats, and most focal lesions should be biopsied. Metastatic sarcomas and carcinomas usually exfoliate well, and ultrasonographic examination often will identify the primary tumor within the abdominal cavity as well as metastatic lesions to the liver (Fig. 15–13). A number of carcinomas involving the liver are not sufficiently differentiated to distinguish between a primary hepatic tumor and metastatic disease.

Because diffuse hepatic neoplasia may appear normal on ultrasonography, and because liver enzymes are not sensitive in cats, liver FNBs should be considered when evaluating occult neoplasia. If neoplastic cells are not seen on several good FNB smears, diffuse hepatic neoplasia may be ruled out with a high degree of confidence.

Others

Occasional liver FNBs show severe cholestasis characterized by intracellular accumulation of bile pigments and/or extracellular bile casts as a single abnormality (Fig. 15–14). These can be secondary to a

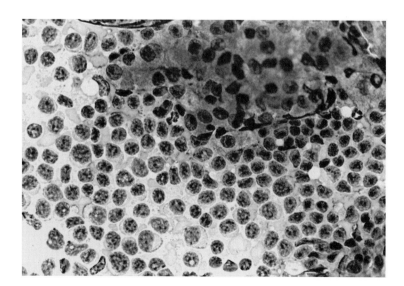

Figure 15–11. Hepatic lymphoma. Hepatocytes show mild cytoplasmic fine vacuolar degeneration. There is severe infiltration by a single population of large lymphoblasts, with a rim of basophilic cytoplasm; large, round nuclei with slightly clumped chromatin; and 1 to 3 prominent nucleoli. Dip Quick stain, 500×.

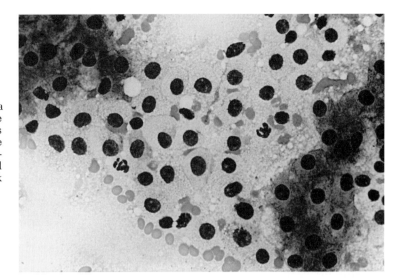

Figure 15–12. Disseminated mast cell neoplasia with severe hepatic infiltration by mast cells. The granules did not stain in this case, and appear as numerous intracytoplasmic small, clear vacuoles. The cytoplasm is abundant, and nuclei are small to medium-sized without nucleoli. Hepatocytes show mild cytoplasmic fine vacuolar degeneration. Dip Quick stain, 500×.

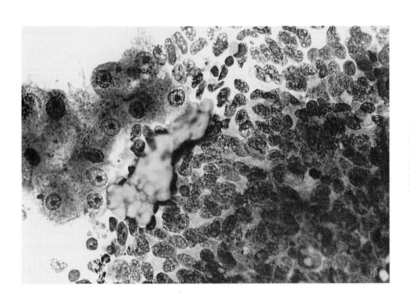

Figure 15–13. Metastatic sarcoma. An intestinal mass and hepatic nodules were found on ultrasonography. Fine-needle biopsies of the intestinal mass showed a sarcoma. Clusters of oval-to-spindle-shaped neoplastic cells of morphology similar to the intestinal mass were present on fine-needle biopsies of the hepatic nodules, confirming the presence of metastasis. Dip Quick stain, 500×.

Figure 15–14. Severe hepatic cholestasis. Hepatocytes show mild-to-moderate intracellular accumulation of bile pigments with numerous extracellular bile casts. Dip Quick stain, 500×.

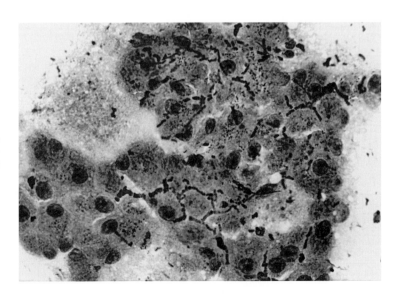

posthepatic obstruction of bile flow, hepatotoxicity, or hemolytic anemia.

In contrast to dogs, vacuolar hepatopathies (fine vacuolar degeneration of the cytoplasm without other hepatic abnormalities) are rare in cats. The vacuolar degeneration is a nonspecific degenerative change that can be secondary to hypoxia (cardiac disease or hypovolemia), hepatotoxicity (endogenous or exogenous), or hyperthyroidism. Steroid-induced hepatopathies are very rare in cats.

◆ CONCLUSION

Liver cytology can be a powerful diagnostic tool, but its efficiency depends on 3 factors: the quality of the sample, the cytopathologist, and the communication between clinician and cytopathologist.

With adequate training and attention to detail, ultrasound-guided FNB of the liver can provide fast and accurate diagnoses, and circumvent procedures that have much higher morbidity and cost.

REFERENCES

1. Dial SM: Clinicopathologic evaluation of the liver. Vet Clin North Am Small Anim Pract 25:257–273, 1998.
2. Kerwin SC: Hepatic aspiration and biopsy techniques. Vet Clin North Am Small Anim Pract 25:275–291, 1995.
3. Partington BP, Biller DS: Hepatic imaging with radiology and ultrasound. Vet Clin North Am Small Anim Pract 25:305–335, 1995.
4. Newell SM, Selcer BA, Girard E, et al: Correlations between ultrasonographic findings and specific hepatic diseases in cats: 72 cases (1985–1997). J Am Vet Med Assoc 213:94–98, 1998.
5. Ducatman BS: Fine needle aspiration of the liver and pancreas. *In* Atkinson BF (ed): Atlas of Diagnostic Cytopathology. Philadelphia, WB Saunders, 1992, pp. 317–350.
6. Menard M, Papageorges M: Ultrasound-guided liver fine needle biopsies: Results of 1,408 cases. Proceedings 16th American College of Veterinary Internal Medicine Forum, May 22–25, 1998, pp. 598–600.
7. Kocjan GIL: Pancreas, liver and extrahepatic bile ducts. *In* Atlas of Diagnostic Cytopathology, 2nd ed. New York, Churchill Livingstone, 1997, pp. 184–206.
8. Cibas ES, Ducatman BS: Abdomen and retroperitoneum. *In* Cytology: Diagnostic Principles and Clinical Correlates. Philadelphia, WB Saunders, 1996, pp. 297–335.
9. Ljung BM, Geller DA: Fine-needle aspiration techniques for biopsies of deep-seated impalpable targets: A primer for radiologists. AJR 171:325–328, 1998.
10. Tao LC: Liver and pancreas. *In* Bibbo M. (ed): Comprehensive Cytopathology, 2nd ed. Philadelphia, WB Saunders, 1997, pp. 827–863.
11. Fondacaro JV, Gulfpin VO, Powers BE, et al: Diagnostic correlation of liver aspiration cytology with histopathology in dogs and cats with liver disease. Proceedings of the 17th American College of Veterinary Internal Medicine, Forum, Chicago, 1999, p. 254.
11a. Roth L: Comparison of liver cytology interpretation and biopsy diagnosis. Vet Pathol 36:5, 1999.
12. Teot LA, Geisinger KR: Fine needle aspiration of the liver and pancreas. *In* Atkinson BF, Silverman JF (eds): Atlas of Difficult Diagnoses in Cytopathology. Philadelphia, WB Saunders, 1998, pp. 327–349.
13. Blue JT, French TW, Meyer DJ: The liver. *In* Cowell RL, Tyler RD, Meinkoth JH (eds): Diagnostic Cytology and Hematology of the Dog and Cat, 2nd ed. St. Louis, Mosby, 1999, pp. 183–194.
14. Alleman AR: Cytologic evaluation of the liver. Proceedings of the 15th American College of Veterinary Internal Medicine, Forum, Lake Buena Vista, FL, 1997, pp. 4–6.
15. Kristensen A, Weiss DJ, Klausner JS, et al: Liver cytology in cases of canine and feline hepatic disease. Compend Contin Educ Pract Vet 12:797–808, 1990.
16. Roth L, Meyer DJ: Interpretation of liver biopsies. Vet Clin North Am Small Anim Pract 25:293–303, 1995.
17. Hubbard BS, Vulgamot JC: Feline hepatic lipidosis. Compend Contin Educ Pract Vet 14:459–464, 1992.
18. Hughes D, King LG: The diagnosis and management of acute liver failure in dogs and cats. Vet Clin North Am Small Anim Pract 25:437–460, 1995.
19. Menard M, Papageorges M: Fine-needle biopsies: How to increase diagnostic yield. Compend Contin Educ Pract Vet 19:738–740, 1997.
20. Menard M, Papageorges M: Technique for ultrasound-guided fine needle biopsies. Vet Radiol 36:137–138, 1995.
21. Thomas JS, Green RA: Clotting times and antithrombin III activity in cats with naturally developing diseases: 85 cases (1984–1994). J Am Vet Med Assoc 213:1290–1295, 1998.
22. Gagne JM, Weiss DJ, Armstrong PJ: Histopathologic evaluation of feline inflammatory liver disease. Vet Pathol 33:521–526, 1996.
23. Patnaik AK: A morphologic and immunocytochemical study of hepatic neoplasms in cats. Vet Pathol 29:405–415, 1992.
24. Hammer AS, Sikkeman DA: Hepatic neoplasia in the dog and cat. Vet Clin North Am Small Anim Pract 25:419–435, 1995.
25. Nyland TG, Koblik PD, Tellyer SE: Ultrasonographic evaluation of biliary cystadenomas in cats. Vet Radiol 40:300, 1999.
26. Adler R, Wilson DW: Biliary cystadenoma of cats. Vet Pathol 32:415–418, 1995.

16

◆ Clinical Approach to Chronic Diarrhea

Jean A. Hall

Diarrhea is a common clinical problem in cats. Although a variety of clinical signs may be caused by intestinal disorders (e.g., anorexia, weight loss, vomiting, or abdominal pain), diarrhea is the most consistent clinical sign of intestinal disease in cats.[1, 2] By definition, *diarrhea* is an abnormal increase in the fluidity, frequency, or volume of feces resulting from excessive fecal water content.

When assessing a cat with diarrhea, it is necessary to first differentiate acute from chronic problems. *Acute diarrhea* develops in a previously healthy cat, lasts for a few days to weeks, and resolves without further complications. Acute diarrhea usually is caused by simple dietary indiscretion, parasites, or infectious diseases.[3] *Chronic diarrhea* persists for more than 3 weeks, or has a pattern of episodic recurrence. Most intoxications, medication side-effects, and some infectious agents (e.g., enteric viruses) do not cause chronic diarrhea.[2] Diseases that cause chronic diarrhea generally are not self-limiting, nor do they respond to symptomatic therapy. Specific treatment is needed, which depends on an accurate diagnosis. Determining the etiology of diarrhea, if possible, is based on clinical findings and diagnostic studies, and is key to successful management of chronic diarrhea. In addition, an accurate diagnosis allows a more reliable prognosis to be given to the owner.

◆ GENERAL CAUSES OF CHRONIC DIARRHEA

Diarrhea may be classified according to the anatomic site (small or large intestine), pathophysiology (osmotic diarrhea, secretory diarrhea, exudative diarrhea, and abnormal motility), or etiology.

Normally, the greatest volume of intestinal fluid is absorbed in the small intestine (jejunum). Diarrhea of small-intestinal origin occurs when the volume of fluid entering the colon exceeds the colon's reserve capacity to absorb fluid. The large intestine absorbs less fluid quantitatively than the small intestine, but it removes the remaining fluid very efficiently. Thus, only minor changes in colonic absorptive capacity are needed to cause large-intestinal diarrhea.[1]

Diseases of the small intestine are associated with high-volume diarrhea, weight loss, vomiting, and lethargy (Table 16–1). Appetite often is decreased, although polyphagia is observed occasionally. The frequency of defecation may be increased, but usually not more than 2 or 3 times normal. A typical stool would be a large, pale, soft pile of malodorous, unformed, watery feces. Melena and steatorrhea may be present. (Urgency, tenesmus, fecal mucus, and red blood are absent.) Unabsorbed nutrients that are fermented by intestinal bacteria may cause flatulence and rancid, foul-smelling diarrhea.[2]

Diseases of the large intestine are associated with frequent urges to defecate (greater than 3 times normal frequency), small volumes of feces, mucus, and hematochezia (see Table 16–1). Goblet cells in the colonic mucosa respond to irritation and inflammation by secreting mucus. Total daily fecal output is near normal. Cats make frequent attempts to defecate, often producing little feces, or remain in the squatting position in the litter box for an extended time after defecation. Accidental defecation outside the litter box may result from urgency and inability to retain feces. Severe weight loss, steatorrhea, polyphagia, or vomiting would be rare with diseases of the large intestine.[2] Thus, if there is no weight loss, the underlying disease is of large-intestinal origin. Large-intestinal diseases can cause weight loss in rare cases, but usually there will be obvious signs of colonic involvement (e.g., mucus, hematochezia, or tenesmus) present as well.[3]

Diarrhea can result from a variety of pathophysiologic processes. Four general mechanisms are often described, although 1 or more of these mechanisms may occur simultaneously in cats with diarrhea. These include (1) decreased solute absorption (osmotic diarrhea), (2) hypersecretion of ions (secretory diarrhea), (3) increased permeability (exudative diarrhea), and (4) abnormal motility.[2]

Osmotic diarrhea occurs when osmotically active substances (e.g., unabsorbed solutes) remain in the lumen and hold water with them. Osmotically active solutes usually are malabsorbed carbohydrates (dietary overload or maldigestion/malabsorption) or oral laxatives that are absorbed poorly.[2] Examples of disorders causing osmotic diarrhea include diffuse inflammatory bowel disease and intestinal lymphoma (which cause primary intestinal malabsorption) and hyperthyroidism.

Secretory diarrhea occurs when secretion of fluid and electrolytes into the lumen is increased, independent of changes in mucosal permeability or osmotic gradients generated by osmotically active solutes derived from the diet.[2] Secretion primarily is a function of crypt cells, whereas absorption primarily is a function of the villi. Hypersecretion from hyperplastic intestinal crypt cells can occur after an enteric viral infection that damages the villi. A secretory diarrhea results when hypersecretion

Table 16–1. Differentiation of Chronic Small-Intestinal Diarrhea From Large-Intestinal Diarrhea

Observation	Small-Intestinal Diarrhea	Large-Intestinal Diarrhea
Weight loss	Sometimes	Rare
Blood in feces	Melena (sometimes)	Hematochezia (sometimes)
Mucus in feces	Absent	Often present
Steatorrhea	Sometimes	Absent
Tenesmus	Rare	Sometimes present
Polyphagia	Sometimes	Rare
Frequency of bowel movements	Normal to slightly increased	Usually increased
Volume of feces	Often increased	Normal or often decreased
Vomiting	Sometimes	Rare

overwhelms the diminished absorptive capacity of the diseased villi. Mediators of intestinal hypersecretion (i.e., secretagogues), acting through intracellular second messengers such as cyclic adenosine monophosphate (cAMP) and cyclic guanosine monophosphate (cGMP), stimulate active chloride and bicarbonate secretion by enterocytes, which is accompanied by passive water secretion. This results in net intestinal ion secretion.[1, 2] Bacterial enterotoxins, malabsorbed bile acids, and hydroxy-fatty acids, as well as immune and inflammatory mediators released by cells in the lamina propria, may cause secretory diarrhea.

Diarrhea caused by increased permeability (exudative diarrhea) results from an outpouring of plasma proteins, blood, or mucus from sites of intestinal inflammation, ulceration, or infiltration.[2] Mild inflammation alters tight junctions between intestinal epithelial cells, which allows the back leakage of fluid and ions through these tight junctions into the intestinal lumen. As inflammation intensifies, larger macromolecules such as albumin, globulins, and red blood cells may be lost into the intestinal lumen. With severe inflammation, clinical signs of melena or hematochezia may be noted. Protein-losing enteropathy is rare in cats.[1, 4]

Lastly, derangements of motility that may be associated with diarrhea include reduced peristalsis, which promotes stasis and bacterial overgrowth in the small intestine; accelerated small-intestinal transit such that mucosal contact time for digestion and absorption is inadequate, as in hyperthyroidism; and premature emptying of the colon associated with colonic inflammation and irritability.[2] In the latter, decreased segmental contractions cause less intestinal resistance to the flow of ingesta.[1]

Disorders associated with chronic diarrhea in cats are summarized in (Table 16–2). These include infectious agents (viral enteritis, bacterial enteritis, fungal enteritis, protozoal enteritis, and parasitic enteritis); inflammatory and immune-mediated diseases; metabolic, endocrine, and systemic disorders; neoplastic diseases; anatomic abnormalities; drugs and toxins, and diet-associated disorders.[2]

◆ CLINICAL FINDINGS

History

The first step in categorizing chronic diarrhea is to determine whether it is small or large bowel in origin.[2] This usually is determined by asking the appropriate questions of the owner (Table 16–3). The overall goals are to determine whether diarrhea is (1) acute or chronic, (2) caused by disease of large intestine, small intestine, or both, and (3) part of a more generalized systemic disorder. It also is necessary to gain clues about possible etiologies.

Some cats will have diarrhea that does not fit neatly into a small-intestinal or large-intestinal classification. This may be because the underlying disease process affects both regions simultaneously; for example, inflammatory bowel disease. Also, chronic small-intestinal diarrhea may lead to a low-grade colitis, perhaps from exposure of the colon to malabsorbed toxins (such as fatty acids and bile acids) and to other changes in the colonic microenvironment.[5]

Physical Findings

A thorough physical examination of all body systems should be performed to determine whether a systemic disorder is causing diarrhea. A detailed examination of the eyes should be performed because histoplasmosis and feline immunodeficiency virus (FIV) may affect the anterior or posterior segments of the eye. The neck is palpated for evidence of an enlarged thyroid gland, indicating hyperthyroidism. General inspection also allows an assessment of the cat's attitude, hydration status, and general body condition. Dehydration may be present and caused by diarrheal fluid loss. Depression and weakness may result from electrolyte imbalance and severe debilitation. A dull, unthrifty hair coat results from malabsorption of fatty acids, protein, and vitamins. Pallor (anemia) may be the result of gastrointestinal blood loss, or of anemia of chronic illness or inflammation.[2]

Signs of serious disease (fever, abdominal pain, severe diarrhea, bloody diarrhea, and severe weight loss) should prompt a vigorous work-up and supportive therapy. Fever suggests mucosal damage or transmural inflammatory disease, infection, or neoplasia. Abdominal pain may be localized with gentle palpation. Pain associated with abdominal palpation may result from gastrointestinal inflammation, obstruction, or ischemia, as well as peritonitis. The color of blood can be used to determine whether the diarrhea is small- or large-intestinal in origin. Weight loss may be the result of anorexia, nutrient malassimilation, or protein-losing enteropathy.[1] The combination of chronic diarrhea, weight loss, and increased appetite suggests hyperthyroidism, inflammatory bowel disease, exocrine pancreatic insufficiency (rare), and occasionally lymphoma, as

Table 16–2. Disorders Associated With Chronic Diarrhea in Cats

Viral-Associated Diarrhea

Feline panleukopenia virus
Astrovirus
Enteric coronaviruses
Rotavirus
Feline leukemia virus
Feline infectious peritonitis virus
Feline immunodeficiency virus

Bacterial Diarrhea

Salmonella species
Campylobacter jejuni
Clostridium species
Yersinia species
Bacillus piliformis
Escherichia coli
Mycobacteria

Mycotic Diarrhea

Histoplasma capsulatum
Pythium species
Aspergillus species
Candida albicans

Protozoal Diarrhea

Giardia species
Isospora species
Cryptosporidium species

Parasitic Diarrhea

Ascarids (*Toxocara* species, *Toxascaris leonina*)
Hookworms (*Ancylostoma* species, *Uncinaria* species)
Whipworms (*Trichuris* species)
Strongyloides species
Tapeworms (*Dipylidium caninum*)
Trematodes

Inflammatory and Immune-Mediated Diseases

Lymphocytic-plasmacytic enterocolitis
Eosinophilic enteritis
Neutrophilic colitis
Regional granulomatous enterocolitis
Granulomatous colitis
Histiocytic colitis
Necrotic colitis
Angiopathic colitis with vasculitis and ischemic ulcers

Metabolic, Endocrine, and Systemic Disorders

Hyperthyroidism
Hepatic diseases
Chronic pancreatitis
Exocrine pancreatic insufficiency (rare in cats)
Renal failure (uremia)
Congenital portosystemic shunt

Neoplasia

Intestinal lymphoma
Adenomatous polyps
Intestinal adenocarcinoma
Intestinal mast-cell tumors
Systemic mastocytosis
Other intestinal tumors (e.g., leiomyosarcoma, fibrosarcoma, undifferentiated sarcoma, and leiomyoma)
Extragastrointestinal neoplasia

Anatomic Abnormalities

Short-bowel syndrome
Villous atrophy

Drug-Induced

Nonsteroidal anti-inflammatory agents
Digitalis
Lactulose
Anthelmintics
Antibacterial drugs

Toxin-Induced

Staphylococcal enterotoxin
Metals (lead, arsenic)
Insecticides
House plants

Diet-Associated Disorders (Adverse Reactions to Food)

Dietary indiscretions (hair, bones, plants, string)
Food intolerance (milk, spicy foods, food additives)
Food allergy (hypersensitivity to specific proteins)

some cats with gastrointestinal lymphoma have increased rather than decreased appetites.[4]

The gastrointestinal system also is evaluated serially. Starting with the oral cavity, check for a string foreign body under the tongue, irritant ulcers (caustic agents), chronic stomatitis or gingivitis in a feline leukemia virus (FeLV)– or FIV-infected cat, and icterus, which may indicate hepatic disease (see Chapter 10, Approach to the Icteric Cat). The large and small bowel should be palpated for location, thickness, turgor, presence of fluid or gas, mass lesions, and serosal irregularities. Fluid-distended bowel loops may be palpable with inflammatory disease, obstructive lesions, or ileus causing diarrhea. Neoplasia and inflammatory bowel disease may cause thickened bowel loops. Mesenteric lymph nodes should be assessed for size, location, and consistency; for example, they may be enlarged

with lymphosarcoma, histoplasmosis, or benign inflammation. A rectal examination is not performed routinely as part of the initial examination of an unsedated feline patient, because most cats resist this procedure vigorously, and it rarely provides useful diagnostic information.[6] The fecal material obtained on a thermometer should be examined grossly for foreign material, blood, and mucus, and microscopically for parasites, inflammatory cells, and lipid droplets.[2]

◆ DIAGNOSTIC STUDIES

The data gathered thus far from the history and physical examination should help the clinician decide whether the problem is acute or chronic, and whether the disease is systemic or localized to the

Table 16–3. Questions for Owners of Cats With Chronic Diarrhea

Question	Interpretation
1. Signalment	*Age?* Young cats are prone to dietary, infectious, and parasitic causes of diarrhea. Older cats are more likely to have inflammatory, metabolic, and neoplastic causes of diarrhea.
2. Vaccination status	*Panleukopenia, FeLV protection?*
3. Diet	*Dietary change, food intolerance, food hypersensitivity, food allergy?* Adverse reactions to food are common causes of diarrhea. Recent dietary changes should be noted. Diarrhea that ceases when an animal is not fed suggests osmotic diarrhea.
4. Environment	*Presence of various plants, chemicals, and foreign objects? Health status of other cats in the household?* Outdoor cats are more likely to develop parasitic, toxic, and infectious disorders.
5. Travel history	*Infectious potential or enzootic area (fungal or parasitic diarrhea)?*
6. Current medications	*Drug reaction or toxicity?* Drug therapies that can cause diarrhea should be noted (antibiotics, anti-inflammatory agents, cardiac glycosides).
7. Past medical and surgical problems	*Organ system affected? Recurrence? Response to previous treatment?*
8. Onset and duration of diarrhea	*Acute versus chronic?* Acute diarrheas are abrupt in onset and of short duration, and generally they are self-limiting. Chronic diarrheas persist usually longer than 3 wk and fail to respond to symptomatic therapy.
9. Appearance of diarrhea	*Quantity and quality of the stool (color, consistency, character, presence of blood or mucus)?* Loose-to-watery feces that contains fat droplets, undigested food, melena, and variable colors suggests small intestinal disease. The volume always is increased with small-intestinal disease. Loose-to-semisolid feces containing excess mucus and fresh blood (hematochezia) indicates large-intestinal disease. The volume may be normal to slightly decreased with large-intestinal disease.
10. Description of defecation process	*Tenesmus (straining) and dyschezia (painful defecation)?* These are hallmarks of large-intestinal disease, e.g., inflammatory or obstructive lesions of the colon, rectum, or anus.
11. Frequency of defecation	Frequency is normal to slightly increased with small-bowel disease, but greatly increased with large-bowel disease.
12. Associated physical signs	Vomiting, anorexia, weight loss, and dyschezia may help localize the disorder to a specific part of the gastrointestinal tract. Clinical signs relating to problems in other organs or body systems should be noted, and may suggest a more generalized disease. Vomiting may occur as a consequence of small-intestinal inflammation in some cats with diarrhea. Weight loss may result from decreased caloric intake (anorexia), decreased nutrient assimilation (maldigestion/malabsorption), or excessive caloric loss (protein-losing enteropathy or nephropathy). Weight loss is observed uncommonly with large-bowel disease.

Abbreviation: FeLV, feline leukemia virus.

gastrointestinal tract. Successful management of chronic diarrhea necessitates a thorough diagnostic plan to determine the specific cause of diarrhea (Table 16–4). If anorexia, severe weight loss, frequent vomiting, severe bloody diarrhea, and listless behavior are present, diagnostic efforts should be accelerated. Cats develop hypoproteinemia much less commonly than dogs; hypoproteinemia usually indicates a significant degree of disease in cats (inflammatory bowel disease, alimentary lymphoma, or less commonly, gastrointestinal hemorrhage from ulcerative neoplasia), and intestinal biopsies should be performed early in the work-up, if the cause of hypoproteinemia is likely the gastrointestinal tract.[3] A more conservative, step-by-step approach is indicated if the patient is in good physical condition.

Initial laboratory tests should include a complete blood count, serum biochemistries, and urinalysis primarily to rule out systemic diseases. Certain findings, for example, eosinophilia and panhypoproteinemia, also may be consistent with gastrointestinal disease. Serologic tests for FeLV, FIV, and hyperthyroidism are indicated to rule out infectious

and metabolic etiologies. FeLV may cause diarrhea associated with leukopenia (panleukopenia-like syndrome), lymphoid tumors in the intestinal tract, or secondary immunosuppression allowing other gastrointestinal pathogens to proliferate.[6] Diarrhea is one of the most common clinical signs of FIV infection. Severe leukopenia and secondary infections also result from FIV infection. Diarrhea in feline hyperthyroidism may result from decreased transit time because of adrenergic stimulation or polyphagia leading to osmotic overload.[6]

Multiple, direct fecal smears for protozoa, and fecal flotation examinations for parasite ova should be performed. Negative findings do not rule out parasites; for example, *Giardia*. Gross examination of the feces for mucus, fresh blood, melena, or undigested food may help determine whether malabsorption or maldigestion is occurring. Fecal cytology may be useful for identifying the presence of infectious agents, such as histoplasmosis, or fecal leukocytes with large bowel inflammatory disease. Fecal cultures should be performed for enteropathogenic bacteria such as *Campylobacter* and *Salmonella*

Table 16–4. Diagnostic Studies for Cats With Chronic Diarrhea

Test	Interpretation
CBC	
PCV, Hgb, RBC count	*Anemia:* GI blood loss; depressed erythropoiesis from chronic inflammation, neoplasia, or malnutrition
	Elevated PCV: hemoconcentration from GI fluid loss; hyperthyroidism
	RBC microcytosis: iron deficiency from chronic GI blood loss; congenital portosystemic shunt
	RBC macrocytosis: RBC regeneration; hyperthyroidism; FeLV; nutritional deficiencies (rare)
WBC count	*Eosinophilia:* endoparasitism; eosinophilic enteritis; hypereosinophilic syndrome; mast-cell neoplasia
	Neutrophilia: GI inflammation, necrosis, or neoplasia
	Neutropenia: Panleukopenia virus; FeLV; FIV; endotoxemia or overwhelming sepsis from bowel perforation and peritonitis
	Monocytosis: chronic or granulomatous inflammation
Biochemical Profile	
Serum proteins	*Increased:* dehydration; hyperglobulinemia because of chronic immune stimulation; FIP
	Decreased: protein-losing enteropathy (rare in cats); liver disease; glomerular disease
K+	*Decreased:* GI loss of fluid and electrolytes; polyuria; anorexia
	Increased: hypoadrenocorticism (rare in cats)
BUN	*Increased:* dehydration (prerenal); primary renal failure: GI bleeding (hemorrhage into the GI tract with subsequent catabolism of blood protein can elevate serum urea nitrogen levels disproportionately compared with serum creatinine levels)[11]
	Decreased: liver disease; anorexia
Creatinine	*Increased:* dehydration (prerenal); primary renal failure
ALP	*Increased:* liver disease; cholestasis
GGT	*Increased:* liver disease; cholestasis (GGT may be a more useful indicator of cholestasis in cats because ALP has a short half-life)
ALT	*Increased:* liver disease (primary or secondary degenerative process)
Amylase/lipase	*Increased:* pancreatitis, although normal levels often are found in cats with chronic pancreatitis[12]; mild elevations in enteritis or with azotemia
Calcium	*Decreased:* hypoalbuminemia; pancreatitis
Urinalysis	
Urine specific gravity	*Isosthenuria:* with azotemia implies chronic renal failure
Chemistries	*Proteinuria:* suggests glomerular disease, urinary tract hemorrhage or inflammation
	Bilirubinuria: suggests hepatic disease, bile duct obstruction, or increased RBC destruction
Urine protein-creatinine ratio	Helps to identify more accurately the degree of proteinuria
Cytology	*Cells, casts, bacteria, or crystals:* may support renal disease
Fecal Examination	
Gross examination	Determine fluid consistency; may see melena, fresh blood, or increased mucus
Microscopic examination	Routine fecal flotation for ova (ascarids, hookworms, whipworms, tapeworms, and trematodes) or oocysts (*Isospora*)
	Direct fecal smear or fresh feces mixed with saline for *Giardia* trophozoites or *Strongyloides* species larvae
	Zinc sulfate centrifugation-flotation for *Giardia* cysts[13]
	Sheather's centrifugation-flotation for *Cryptosporidium* oocysts
	Stained fecal smears for fat, leukocytes, and fungi; presence of > 5 clostridial endospores per oil immersion field that have a safety-pin configuration is presumptive evidence for enterotoxigenic *Clostridium perfringens*
Fecal culture (typing of coliforms to identify pathogenic strains)	Culture if indicated for enteropathogenic bacteria (*Salmonella* species, *Campylobacter* species, *Escherichia coli, Yersinia*) or fungi; a heavy and relatively pure growth of a known pathogen or a member of the fecal flora is significant, particularly if a rectal scrape shows corresponding suppurative inflammation[5]
Fecal ELISA for antigen	Positive for *Giardia*-specific antigen (sensitivity?); *Cryptosporidium* fecal ELISA test
Electron microscopy	Virus particle identification for parvovirus, coronavirus, rotavirus, astrovirus
Fecal enterotoxin assay (ELISA or reverse passive latex agglutination test)	Toxin-producing *Clostridium perfringens*

Table continued on following page

Table 16–4. Diagnostic Studies for Cats With Chronic Diarrhea *Continued*

Test	Interpretation
Serum Thyroid Hormone Concentration	T_4 increased: hyperthyroidism
Serology	
FeLV antigen tests (ELISA, IFA)	Positive: FeLV infection
FIV antibody test	Positive: FIV infection
Histoplasmosis	Positive on immunodiffusion and complement fixation for histoplasmosis (sensitivity?)
Serum Bile Acids	Increased: consistent with hepatobiliary disease
Serum Cobalamin/Folate and Trypsin-Like Immunoreactivity	
Folate	Subnormal levels suggest the presence of disease affecting the proximal small intestine
Cobalamin	Subnormal levels are consistent with exocrine pancreatic insufficiency and ileal disease
Serum trypsin-like immunoreactivity assay	Feline-specific assay requires a 12-hr fast and serum sample; <8 μg/L is considered diagnostic for exocrine pancreatic insufficiency (rare in cats)
Radiology	
Survey abdomen	Assess position, size, shape, and density of abdominal viscera May see a GI foreign body, visceral displacement, abdominal mass, peritoneal fluid, etc. A gas-filled dilated bowel greater than 3 rib-widths indicates small-bowel obstruction (e.g., mass, foreign body, or intussusception)
Upper GI barium contrast study (when intestinal obstruction is suspected)	May see delayed gastric emptying consistent with a gastric motility disorder May see filling defect, foreign body, intramural mass, increased bowel-wall thickness, abnormal mucosa, intussusception, ulceration, etc.
Thoracic radiographs	May see metastatic neoplasia in the lungs
Ultrasonography	
Abdominal	May see liver disorders, gallbladder disease, and renal disorders Ultrasound scanning of the GI tract provides an evaluation of peristalsis; wall thickness, diameter, and layering; lesion location; and appearance of luminal contents The sonographic signs of intestinal neoplasia include irregular thickening of the intestinal wall (segmental or diffuse), disruption of the normal layered appearance, irregularity of mucosal or serosal surfaces, and concurrent mesenteric lymphadenopathy[14]
Endoscopy	
Gross examination	May see a foreign body, mucosal hyperemia, hemorrhage, granularity, friability, erosions, ulcers, parasites, mass lesion, obstruction, etc.
Mucosal biopsy	Provides histopathologic diagnosis; inflammatory bowel disease usually is characterized by plasmacytic-lymphocytic mucosal infiltrates, although eosinophilic, suppurative, and granulomatous infiltrates also occur; confirms histoplasmosis Confirms lymphosarcoma and adenocarcinoma[15] *Helicobacter felis* may be identified on histology samples or by their ability to produce large quantities of urease[16]
Duodenal aspirate	May see *Giardia* species
Exfoliative cytology	Useful adjunct to mucosal biopsy for detection of inflammatory bowel disease and alimentary lymphoma[17]
Exploratory Laparotomy	
Gross examination	Visualize all intra-abdominal organs; may see intussusception, neoplasia, GI foreign body, or nothing abnormal
Biopsy	Multiple biopsies should be obtained along the length of the GI tract, even if no lesions are noted on gross inspection; mesenteric lymph nodes also should be biopsied Provides histopathologic diagnosis of inflammatory bowel disease, neoplasia, fungal, *Cryptosporidium,* and mycobacterial enteritis; hepatobiliary disease and chronic pancreatitis

Abbreviations: ALP, alkaline phosphatase; ALT, alanine aminotransferase; BUN, blood urea nitrogen; CBC, complete blood count; ELISA, enzyme-linked immunosorbent assay; FeLV, feline leukemia virus; FIP, feline infectious peritonitis; FIV, feline immunodeficiency virus; GGT, gamma-glutamyl-transferase; GI, gastrointestinal; Hgb, hemoglobin; IFA, indirect fluorescent antibody; K^+, potassium ion; PCV, packed cell volume; RBC, red blood cell; T_4, thyroxine; WBC, white blood cell.

when diarrhea is severe and bloody. If feces is positive for leukocytes, follow-up diagnostic tests should include colonoscopy, fecal assay for clostridial enterotoxin, and fecal cultures.

If the cat can tolerate a delay of several weeks in the diagnostic work-up at this point, then a therapeutic trial is reasonable. Therapeutic trials usually consist of high-fiber diets, hypoallergenic diets, or antibiotics to control clostridial colitis. If a therapeutic trial is performed, it is important to be sure that it is done properly (e.g., long enough, correct dose) so that it will be successful if the animal has the suspected diseases.[3]

Although the diagnosis of exocrine pancreatic insufficiency is easily accomplished by the radioimmunoassay of serum trypsin–like immunoreactivity using a species-specific assay, this disorder is rare in cats.[7] The vast majority of cats with classic signs of exocrine pancreatic insufficiency (polyphagia, weight loss, voluminous pale feces) have underlying small-intestinal disease. Uncommonly, malabsorption may result in subnormal serum folate concentrations. Subnormal serum folate concentrations reflect the presence of disease affecting the proximal small intestine, because specific folate carriers located only in the proximal small intestine transport folate monoglutamate into mucosal cells. Cobalamin malabsorption may result from lesions affecting the intrinsic factor–cobalamin receptors in the distal small intestine. Decreased serum cobalamin appears to be a more common finding in feline intestinal disease, and theoretically could result from exocrine pancreatic insufficiency, ileal disease, small-intestinal bacterial overgrowth, or dietary deficiency.[8] It should be noted that serum folate and cobalamin have very broad control ranges in cats, and that these appear to provide different information than that revealed in dogs.[8] Because healthy cats have relatively high numbers of bacteria in the proximal small intestine, and because these counts do not normally appear to be increased in cats with signs of intestinal disease, small-intestinal bacterial overgrowth may not occur as a clinical syndrome in cats.[8]

Survey abdominal radiographs rarely are rewarding in cats with diarrhea. If vomiting and mass lesions or other gastrointestinal abnormalities are detected on physical examination, a barium contrast upper gastrointestinal study may provide useful information (see Chapter 9, Contrast Radiography for Evaluation of the Gastrointestinal Tract). However, many cases of chronic diarrhea have only minor changes in the intestinal mucosa.

Abdominal ultrasonography is most helpful for examining abdominal parenchymal organs, but may be useful for delineating intestinal mass lesions or mural thickening.[1] The various causes of obstruction can be investigated (e.g., masses, foreign objects, inflammatory disease, intussusception). Thickening of the bowel wall can occur in either inflammatory or neoplastic disease processes. In 1 study, abdominal ultrasonography revealed several intestinal ab-normalities (e.g., poor intestinal wall layer definition, focal thickening) and large mesenteric lymph nodes with hypoechoic changes in 13 of 17 cats with confirmed inflammatory bowel disease.[9] Abdominal ultrasonography may be diagnostic if it reveals lymphadenopathy or intestinal infiltrates that can be aspirated percutaneously.[3]

Thoracic radiographs may be revealing in cats that have absolutely no historic or physical evidence of thoracic disease.[3] Chronic diarrhea occurs in some cats that have *Dirofilaria immitis* infection, and concurrent signs of respiratory distress may or may not be present (see Chapter 33, Heartworm Disease).[6]

Further evaluation includes endoscopic examination and biopsy. If large-bowel signs predominate, colonoscopy and biopsies of the colon, ileum, and cecum with a flexible or rigid colonoscope are recommended. If small-bowel signs predominate, the stomach, duodenum, and occasionally the jejunum can be examined by endoscopy and biopsied. The colon also should be sampled with signs of small-bowel diarrhea, because both small- and large-bowel disease may be present.[3] Endoscopic examination must be thorough, and multiple biopsies should be obtained even if the mucosa appears normal grossly.

Laparotomy is performed when endoscopy is unavailable, or if the diagnosis has not been made after endoscopy. At least 1 full-thickness biopsy specimen should be collected from the stomach, duodenum, jejunum, and ileum. Lymph nodes and other tissues also should be biopsied if they appear abnormal, or if laboratory data suggest pathology in these organs. There is more risk for morbidity and mortality with laparotomy compared with endoscopy, not as many full-thickness biopsies can be obtained as with endoscopic biopsies, and mucosal changes cannot be visualized during surgery as with endoscopy. Thus, it is easier to miss the diseased area, particularly when lesions are spotty.[3]

It is important to note that histologic examination of intestinal biopsies leads to the classification of intestinal diseases by histologic appearance rather than by cause, and this has limitations for effective management.[8] For example, cellular infiltration may represent a nonspecific immunologic response to a variety of intraluminal antigens, including parasites and bacterial pathogens, the resident bacterial flora, and dietary antigens. Or, the response may result from interference with the mucosal barrier or defective mucosal tolerance.[8]

◆ TREATMENT

Cats with chronic diarrhea often have weight loss in addition to biochemical and metabolic derangements. Supportive therapy is indicated, as for acute diarrhea. The underlying cause of diarrhea should be pursued vigorously and treated specifically. This is key to long-term control.

Treatment of diarrhea often involves dietary manipulation, specific anthelmintic therapy for parasite infections, antibacterial drugs for infectious disorders, and anti-inflammatory therapy for small- and large-intestinal inflammatory bowel disease. Some cats with chronic diarrhea may have more than 1 disorder. The rapid resolution of diarrhea is dependent on proper treatment of each underlying problem.[4] In particular, food allergy, parasites, and bacterial pathogens should be identified and treated.[8]

Test diets may be used to determine dietary hypersensitivity or food intolerance (see Chapter 14, The Gastrointestinal Tract and Adverse Reactions to Food). The dietary history is used to determine what the cat has eaten in the past so that a novel single protein source, such as lamb, poultry, or fish, can be chosen.[8] Diagnosis of food allergy is made by feeding an exclusion diet for at least 6 weeks, and observing resolution of clinical signs, with recurrence of signs when the original diet is reintroduced. It is important to continue the diet long enough to be sure that it was the diet that made a difference rather than the cat having a transient improvement related to the cyclical nature of the underlying disease.[3]

High-fiber diets may be beneficial for large-bowel diarrhea.[5] Response to therapy usually can be evaluated after a shorter trial period (2 weeks) compared with that needed to evaluate a hypoallergenic diet.[3]

Although 3 fecal examinations by zinc sulfate centrifugation-flotation at 48-hour intervals can identify most cases of *Giardia* infection, it may be worthwhile to treat for *Giardia* infection with an anti-giardial drug such as metronidazole.[10] Metronidazole administered at 50 mg/kg orally (PO) every (q) 24 hr or 25 mg/kg q 12 hr for 5 to 10 days is effective in most cats. Furazolidone oral suspension (Furoxone, Roberts Pharmaceutical Corp., Eatontown, NJ) at 4 mg/kg PO q 12 hr for 5 days also is effective, and is convenient for cats in its suspension form.[2] Fenbendazole should be considered as empirical treatment if tests are negative.[4] Fenbendazole at 50 mg/kg administered PO for 3 days, repeating in 2 to 3 weeks, is effective against nematodes and *Giardia*.

Alteration of the antigenic challenge from bacteria and bacterial products by administration of oral antibiotics is controversial.[8] Because small-intestinal bacterial overgrowth does not appear to be an important disease in cats, oral antibiotics normally should not be used to treat suspected intestinal disease, unless there are specific indications such as bacterial pathogens. Metronidazole has been used successfully, but it is not clear whether the beneficial effects result from the immunoregulatory action rather than the anaerobic antibacterial activity.

Response to amoxicillin or tylosin (Tylan, Elanco Animal Health) may be one of the best ways to diagnose clostridial colitis presumptively.[3] Tylosin has antibacterial and anti-inflammatory effects. It is administered at 1/16 teaspoon (10 to 40 mg/kg) q 12 hr mixed with food for at least 1 week and preferably 2 weeks before its effectiveness is evaluated.[3]

Sulfasalazine (Azulfidine, Pharmacia and Upjohn) can be helpful in treating inflammatory colitis at a dose of 10 to 15 mg/kg PO q 12 hr for 7 to 10 days. This drug needs to be used with caution in cats because of the potential toxicity of the salicylate moiety.

Corticosteroids and other immunosuppressive agents such as chlorambucil and azathioprine should not be used until the possibility of infectious disease has been ruled out thoroughly; for example, histoplasmosis must be ruled out by colonic biopsies before starting steroid therapy. A histologic diagnosis must show the need for anti-inflammatory therapy (e.g., inflammatory bowel disease). Treatment typically is directed at the cellular infiltrate and involves use of anti-inflammatory and immunosuppressive drugs.[8] Dietary trials, azulfidine, and steroid therapy should have been tried first and should have failed to decrease inflammation before using chlorambucil and azathioprine. Chlorambucil probably is safer in cats than azathioprine (see Chapter 63, Gastrointestinal Lymphoma and Inflammatory Bowel Disease).[3] The typical dose of chlorambucil is 1 mg twice-weekly for cats less than 3 kg, and 2 mg twice-weekly for cats greater than 3 kg. Chlorambucil may cause myelosuppression, and therapy should be monitored.

REFERENCES

1. Jergens AE: Diarrhea. *In* Ettinger SJ, Feldman EC (eds): Textbook of Veterinary Internal Medicine: Diseases of the Dog and Cat, 4th ed. Philadelphia, WB Saunders, 1995, pp. 111–114.
2. Sherding RG: Diseases of the intestines. *In* Sherding RG (ed): The Cat: Diseases and Clinical Management, 2nd ed. New York, Churchill Livingstone, 1994, pp. 1211–1285.
3. Willard M: Clinical manifestations of gastrointestinal disorders. *In* Nelson RW, Couto CG (eds): Small Animal Internal Medicine, 2nd ed. St. Louis, Mosby, 1998, pp. 346–367.
4. Tams TR: Diarrhea. *In* Ettinger SJ, Feldman EC (eds): Textbook of Veterinary Internal Medicine, 5th ed. Philadelphia, WB Saunders, 2000, pp. 121–126.
5. Guilford WG: Approach to clinical problems in gastroenterology. *In* Guilford WG, Center SA, Strombeck DR, et al (eds): Strombeck's Small Animal Gastroenterology. Philadelphia, WB Saunders, 1996, pp. 50–76.
6. Wolf AM: Diarrhea in the cat. Semin Vet Med Surg (Small Anim) 4:212–218, 1989.
7. Steiner JM, Williams DA: Validation of a radioimmunoassay for feline trypsin-like immunoreactivity (FTLI) and serum cobalamin and folate concentrations in cats with exocrine pancreatic insufficiency (EPI). J Vet Intern Med 9:193, 1995.
8. Batt RM, Johnston KL: Feline intestinal disease—Facts and fiction. Proceedings 16th American College of Veterinary Internal Medicine Forum, San Diego, May 22–25, 1998, pp. 532–533.
9. Baez JL, Hendrick MJ, Walker LM, et al: Radiographic, ultrasonographic, and endoscopic findings in cats with inflammatory bowel disease of the stomach and small intestine: 33 cases (1990–1997). J Am Vet Med Assoc 215:349–354, 1999.
10. Leib MS, Matz ME: Diseases of the intestines. *In* Leib MS, Monroe WE (eds): Practical Small Animal Internal Medicine. Philadelphia, WB Saunders, 1997, pp. 685–760.
11. Moore FM: The laboratory and pathologic assessment of vomiting animals. Vet Med 87:796–805, 1992.

12. Hall JA: Diseases of the exocrine pancreas. *In* Morgan RV (ed): Handbook of Small Animal Practice, 3rd ed. Philadelphia, WB Saunders, 1997, pp. 403–416.

13. Reinemeyer CR: Feline gastrointestinal parasites. *In* Kirk RW, Bonagura JD (eds): Current Veterinary Therapy XI. Philadelphia, WB Saunders, 1992, pp. 626–630.

14. Penninck DG: Ultrasonography of the gastrointestinal tract. *In* Nyland TG, Mattoon JS (eds): Veterinary Diagnostic Ultrasound. Philadelphia, WB Saunders, 1995, pp. 125–140.

15. Couto CG: Gastrointestinal neoplasia in dogs and cats. *In* Kirk RW, Bonagura JD (eds): Current Veterinary Therapy XI. Philadelphia, WB Saunders, 1992, pp. 595–601.

16. Fox JC: *Helicobacter*-associated gastric disease in ferrets, dogs, and cats. *In* Bonagura JD, Kirk RW (eds): Current Veterinary Therapy XII. Philadelphia, WB Saunders, 1995, pp. 720–723.

17. Jergens AE, Andreasen CB, Hagemoser WA, et al: Cytologic examination of exfoliative specimens obtained during endoscopy for diagnosis of gastrointestinal tract disease in dogs and cats. J Am Vet Med Assoc 213:1755–1759, 1998.

Endocrine and
Metabolic Diseases

Deborah S. Greco, Editor

◆ Diabetic Neuropathy 139
◆ Diagnosis of Occult Hyperthyroidism 145
◆ Complications of Therapy for Hyperthyroidism 151
◆ Adrenocortical Disease 159
◆ Oral Hypoglycemic Therapy for Type 2 Diabetes
  Mellitus 169
◆ Problems of Diabetic Regulation With Insulin
  Therapy 175
◆ APUDomas: Pheochromocytoma, Insulinoma, and
  Gastrinoma 181

Still-Current Information Found in *Consultations in Feline Internal Medicine 2:*
Adrenal Function Testing (Chapter 17), p. 129
Pathogenesis of Hyperthyroidism (Chapter 18), p. 133
Thyroid Function Testing (Chapter 19), p. 143
Update on Diabetes Mellitus (Chapter 20), p. 155
Acromegaly (Chapter 22), p. 169
Diagnostic Approach to Hyperlipidemia (Chapter 23),
    p. 177

Still-Current Information Found in *Consultations in Feline Internal Medicine 3:*
Pathogenesis of Diabetes Mellitus (Chapter 17), p. 125
Diagnostic and Therapeutic Approach to Insulin Resistance
    (Chapter 18), p. 132
Update on the Medical Management of Hyperthyroidism
    (Chapter 22), p. 155
Endocrine Hypertension (Chapter 23), p. 163
Cutaneous Manifestations of Hyperadrenocorticism (Chap-
    ter 26), p. 191
Thyrotoxic Heart Disease (Chapter 36), p. 279
Hyperthyroidism and the Kidney (Chapter 45), p. 345
Metabolic Encephalopathies (Chapter 49), p. 373
Metastatic Patterns of Feline Neoplasia (Chapter 71), p. 566
Blood Pressure: Population Aspects (Chapter 78), p. 630

Elsewhere in *Consultations in Feline Internal Medicine 4:*
Cytologic Evaluation of Fine-Needle Liver Biopsies (Chap-
    ter 15), p. 118
Clinical Approach to Chronic Diarrhea (Chapter 16), p. 127
Paraneoplastic Alopecia (Chapter 26), p. 196
Cutaneous Xanthomas (Chapter 29), p. 214

Hypertrophic Cardiomyopathy (Chapter 34), p. 261
Systemic Hypertension (Chapter 36), p. 277
Diagnosis and Treatment of Systemic Hypertension (Chapter 47), p. 365
Acquired Myasthenia Gravis and Other Disorders of the Neuromuscular Junction (Chapter 48), p. 374
Management of the Lymphoma Patient With Concurrent Disease (Chapter 64), p. 506
Diagnostic Imaging of Neoplasia (Chapter 70), p. 548

17

◆ Diabetic Neuropathy

Paul A. Cuddon

Peripheral neuropathy is a well-recognized, debilitating complication of feline and human diabetes mellitus. Early recognition and accurate diagnosis of this peripheral nerve disease in cats is an integral part of the successful long-term management of this common feline endocrinopathy.

◆ CURRENT THEORIES ON THE ETIOLOGY AND PATHOGENESIS OF DIABETIC NEUROPATHY

A combination of metabolic and vascular defects has been implicated in the pathogenesis of diabetic neuropathy.[1-3] Proposed metabolic derangements have included altered polyol pathway metabolism with a resultant reduction in nerve myoinositol[4, 5]; decreases in Na^+-K^+-ATPase activity[6, 7]; induced growth factor deficiencies[8, 9]; and nonenzymatic glycosylation of structural proteins in myelin and tubulin with resultant formation of advanced glycosylation end products.[10] Experimental studies in streptozotocin-induced diabetes in rats also have demonstrated a link between imbalances in carnitine metabolism and several metabolic and functional abnormalities associated with diabetic neuropathy.[11] Vascular abnormalities have been implicated as the major cause for increased peripheral nerve oxidative stress.[12-14]

The sorbitol accumulation hypothesis is one of the most popular metabolic theories to explain the pathogenesis of diabetic neuropathy.[4, 5] This polyol pathway consists of 2 consecutive reactions, with free glucose first being reduced to sorbitol by aldose reductase and finally oxidized to free fructose by sorbitol dehydrogenase. In normal nerve, aldose reductase has a very low affinity for its aldose sugar substrate (glucose). Other enzymes (such as hexokinase) have a much higher affinity for glucose, and thus are responsible for glucose metabolism. In diabetic nerve, however, owing to elevated levels of glucose, hexokinase saturation occurs, resulting in higher-level function of aldose reductase with subsequent sorbitol accumulation. Activation of this polyol pathway by hyperglycemia appears essential for depletion of myoinositol, a precursor of the polyphosphoinositides, which are important constituents of plasma membranes.[4, 5] Myoinositol has emerged as a key element in many cellular nerve functions, such as sodium, potassium, and calcium transport and nerve impulse conduction.[6] Myoinositol depletion appears to correlate with reduced conduction velocity in diabetic nerves.[15] Strong support for this theory comes from extensive studies on a rat model of diabetes mellitus based on galactose intoxication.[7] The injury to Schwann cells and myelin in this experimental rat model is remarkably similar to that observed in diabetic cats.[7, 16] Because aldose reductase inhibition has been shown to prevent the reactive and degenerative changes in Schwann cells in galactose intoxication in rats, it has been proposed that the abnormal flux through aldose reductase may be the most likely cause of Schwann cell injury in galactose intoxication, and possibly also in naturally occurring feline diabetic neuropathy.

Much interest also has focused on the role of insulin-like growth factors (IGFs), owing to their neurotrophic actions on sensory, sympathetic, and motor nerves.[8, 17-20] IGFs include IGF-I, more important in the embryonic nervous system, and IGF-II. Endogenous IGF activity is required continually for nerve regeneration and maintenance. Insulin and IGFs increase both α- and β-tubulin mRNAs during neurite growth, and increase the content of tubulin (important in the formation of microtubules necessary for axonal transport).[21] They also increase neurofilament mRNAs, leading to neurofilament production.[22] Loss of insulin activity results in a secondary partial decline in IGF-I activity; an increase in IGF-binding protein-I, resulting in sequestration of IGF-I; and a decline in IGF-I and IGF-II mRNAs in peripheral nerves. In addition, there also is an age-related decline in IGF activity (including the remaining functioning IGF-II).[17] The end result of a decline in both insulin and IGF activity, therefore, is impaired production and axonal transport of tubulins and neurofilaments; diminished microtubule and neurofilament contents; a decrease in axonal diameter; and a decrease in axonal transport.[17] There are species differences in the regulation of IGF genes, which may explain the interspecies variation in the clinical manifestations of diabetic neuropathy.[17] The effect of diabetes mellitus on IGFs in cats currently is unknown.

Increasing evidence points to a significant role for sugar-derived advanced glycation end products (AGEs) in the initial damage to diabetic sensory nerve fibers, as well as impairment of nerve fiber regeneration.[10] Reactive dicarbonyl intermediates formed from sugars react with protein amino groups in diabetes to form AGEs, such as 3-deoxyglucosone and methyglyoxal. Glucose has the slowest rate of glycosylation product formation of any of the naturally occurring sugars. The rate of AGE formation by the intracellular sugars fructose, glucose-6-phosphate, and glyceraldehyde-3-phosphate is considerably faster than the rate for glucose. Therefore, the rate of formation of intracellular AGEs, such as pentosidine, is much more rapid than that in the extracellular compartment. There are 3 general mechanisms by which AGE formation may cause pathologic changes in nerves: (1) extracellular AGEs alter matrix-matrix, matrix-cell, and cell-cell interactions[23, 24]; (2) AGE interactions with cellular receptors, with resultant generation of reactive oxygen species, alter the level of gene expression for a variety of molecules involved in the genesis of vascular and nerve pathology[10, 25]; and (3) rapid intracellular AGE formation can directly alter protein function in neurons by increasing cross-linkage of cytoskeletal protein fractions.[10]

The role of oxidative stress (the vascular hypothesis) has received major attention, and is thought by a number of researchers to be the most logical explanation for the pathogenesis of diabetic neuropathy.[12–14, 26] The basis of this theory is that hyperglycemia results in a reduction in nerve blood flow by altering vasoregulation of nerve microvessels and increasing viscosity.[14] There is an increase in microvascular vasoconstrictor tone and a decrease in vasodilator tone. The vasodilator tone decrease is caused by reduced endothelial activities of nitric oxide, calcitonin gene-related peptide (CGRP), and substance P (SP). Prostacyclin and prostaglandin E_1 generation also is reduced.[14] Insulin administration aggravates hypoxia by increasing arteriovenous shunt flow and reducing nutritive flow. The ensuing endoneurial ischemia and increased nerve microvascular resistance lead to endoneurial hypoxia, resulting in lipid peroxidation and a further reduction in vasomotor tone.[27] This lipid peroxidation is further aggravated by a decrease in nerve growth factor. Lipid peroxidation effects are more severe in nerve root and dorsal root ganglia, because the blood-nerve and perineurial barriers are lower at these sites.[14] Oxidative stress appears to focus its damage on the mitochondrion and its DNA.[28] Mitochondrial damage leads to imbalances in the electron transport chain, resulting in increased superoxide and hydrogen peroxide production, which in turn causes more membrane damage. Nerve cell injury and neuropathy result.

Finally, N-methyl D-aspartate (NMDA) receptors, especially at the nerve root entry zone, may be vitally involved in the pathophysiology of diabetic neuropathy–associated pain syndromes.[14] There appears to be a functional interaction between excitatory amino acids and SP, with activation of NMDA receptors mediating depletion of SP in neuropathic animals.

◆ CLINICAL SIGNS

Diabetes mellitus is a common endocrinopathy in cats, with an incidence of 1 in 400 animals.[29] Most cats (72 per cent) develop diabetes at 7 years of age or older (most are >10 years), and males have a 1.5 to 2 times greater risk of developing diabetes than females.[29] All breeds of cats are at risk of developing diabetes, with little evidence of any breed predisposition. Cats most commonly develop a form of diabetes mellitus that is analogous to human type 2 diabetes, with the main metabolic hallmarks being impaired insulin secretion secondary to pancreatic beta-cell degeneration and insulin resistance in target tissues.[30] Obesity, stress, and intercurrent disease contribute to peripheral insulin resistance. Cats less commonly develop type 1 diabetes secondary to autoimmune destruction of pancreatic β cells. Although there is a higher incidence of type 2 than type 1 diabetes in cats, most cats are insulin-dependent, and eventually will require exogenous insulin therapy.[29] Cats frequently demonstrate significant peripheral nerve involvement associated with either type 1 or type 2 diabetes.[31, 32] Classically, cats show a pelvic limb distal symmetric polyneuropathy, with a plantigrade stance, progressive paraparesis, distal muscle atrophy, and pelvic limb hyporeflexia (Fig. 17–1). Signs may progress to involve the thoracic limbs, with similar neurologic findings noted. Cats with thoracic limb involvement will walk and stand with a palmigrade posture, and have decreased withdrawal and myotatic reflexes (Fig. 17–2).[31, 32] Cranial nerve examination, panniculus reflex, and perineal reflexes remain normal in diabetic neuropathy.[33] The reported clinical incidence of the aforementioned neurologic signs is approximately 8 per cent.[31, 32] The percentage of cats that demonstrate milder degrees of neurologic weakness, however, appears to be much higher.[33] The most frequently observed signs of milder neurologic dysfunction include difficulty in jumping, pelvic limb abduction, distal weakness while standing, inability to retract claws fully (Fig. 17–3), and increased sensitivity to sensory stimuli applied to their feet.[33] Despite specific therapy with either oral hypoglycemic agents or insulin, many cats continue to show some degree of neurologic dysfunction associated with this neuropathy.[33]

◆ DIFFERENTIAL DIAGNOSIS

Any cause of acquired peripheral nerve disease in cats should be considered a differential diagnosis for feline diabetic neuropathy. There is a staggering number of causes of acquired peripheral nerve disease in human beings including metabolic, infectious, immune-mediated, toxic, drug-induced, paraneoplastic, ischemic, and traumatic etiologies; however, very few acquired peripheral neuropathies have been documented conclusively in cats. Spinal lymphosarcoma, most commonly associated with feline leukemia virus infection, could result in a mononeuropathy multiplex owing to incorporation of multiple peripheral nerve roots within the rapidly expanding tumor.[34] This neoplasia has a ten-

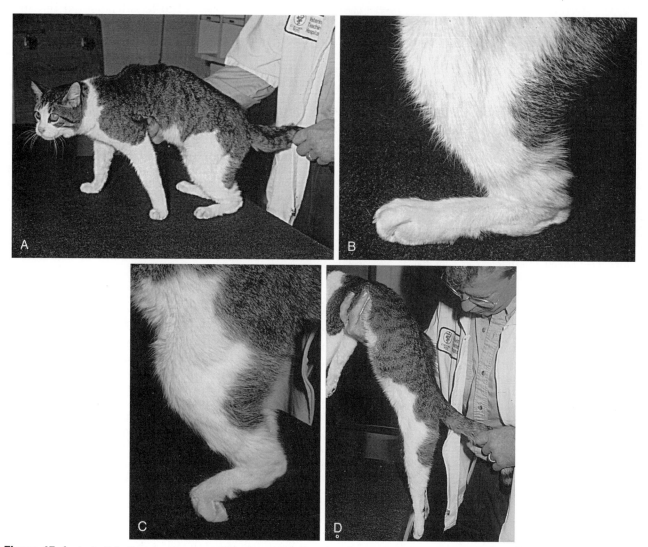

Figure 17–1. *A*, A diabetic cat with severe diabetic neuropathy. Note the marked plantigrade stance in the pelvic limbs. *B*, A close-up view of the plantigrade stance seen in diabetic neuropathy. This is the most commonly recognized sign observed in cats with severe neuropathy. *C* and *D*, Other common neurologic abnormalities seen in cats with diabetic neuropathy—proprioception deficits (C) and decreases in tactile placing (D). These abnormalities are seen much more commonly in the pelvic limbs than in the thoracic limbs.

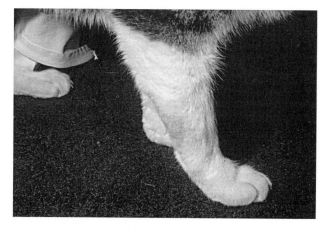

Figure 17–2. A diabetic cat with severe neuropathy, showing the more subtle change of a partial palmigrade stance associated with the thoracic limbs.

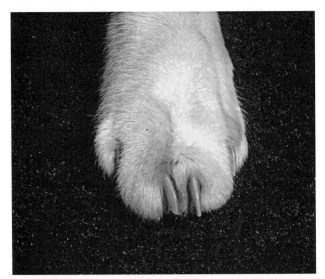

Figure 17–3. Another feature of cats with diabetic neuropathy is an inability to retract their claws completely, especially in the pelvic limbs.

testing also is invaluable in objectively determining the relative success of different potential therapies for this neuropathy. Sixteen diabetic cats, with varying degrees of neurologic dysfunction, that have been studied to date by the author, have all demonstrated significant differences from normal cats in many of the measured parameters assessing both proximal and distal peripheral nerve function.[33] The cats demonstrating the more severe neurologic signs show the more severe electrophysiologic changes, consisting primarily of prominent demyelination at all levels of the motor and sensory peripheral nerves and their corresponding nerve roots (Fig. 17–4). Inconsistent, mild increases in insertional and spontaneous activity in appendicular muscles on electromyography is evidence for the apparent minimum axonopathy associated with this neuropathy. Demyelination in nerves supplying the pelvic limbs appears to be more severe than those of the thoracic limbs.[33]

dency to be multifocal within the vertebral canal, and to spread longitudinally along the epidural space. However, lymphosarcoma usually is accompanied by focal spinal hyperpathia, and would be unlikely to produce bilateral symmetry of lower motor neuron signs, as seen in diabetic neuropathy.[34] Inflammatory polyneuropathies are recognized rarely in cats, and have been reported only sporadically as single case reports.[35, 36] These cats tend to demonstrate more generalized weakness and muscle atrophy, and have additional findings such as whole-body tremors, hyperesthesia, and progression to tetraplegia, compared with cats with diabetic neuropathy.[35, 36] Other more localized syndromes involving only 1 or more peripheral nerves of the pelvic limbs would include ischemic neuromyopathy secondary to arterial thromboembolism of the terminal aortic trifurcation and injection injuries.[37] Other clinical signs such as cold, cyanotic distal pelvic limbs; absent or diminished femoral pulses; painful, firm gastrocnemius muscles; and decreased-to-absent pain sensation distally in the pelvic limbs would aid in differentiation of ischemic neuromyopathy from diabetic neuropathy (see Chapter 39, Aortic Thromboembolism). Injection injuries to the proximal to mid-sciatic nerve, although often resulting in a plantigrade stance and gait, involve only 1 pelvic limb compared with the bilaterally symmetric signs of diabetic neuropathy.[37]

◆ DIAGNOSIS

Electrophysiology

Detailed electrophysiologic studies are essential to understand fully the functional distribution, varying severity, and type of peripheral nerve pathology associated with feline diabetes. Electrophysiologic

Peripheral Nerve and Muscle Biopsy

The most striking histopathologic change on peripheral nerve biopsy in diabetic cats is splitting and ballooning of the myelin sheath at the intraperiod line. Despite the striking myelin defect, most associated axons are normal, except that neurofilament density appears increased in some, suggesting that these axons are shrunken or compressed. Myelin splitting occurs in 4.1 to 20.8 per cent of the total number of myelinated axons in diabetic nerve biopsies, dependent on the severity of the neuropathy. Schwann cell injury in myelinated fibers is characterized by reactive, degenerative, and proliferative changes. Reactive changes include accumulations of pi granules of Reich, lipid droplets, and intermediate cytoplasmic filaments. Degenerative changes range from Schwann cell cytoplasm dissolution at the inner glial loop to demyelination. Mononuclear cells and macrophages filled with myelin debris are present within the neurolemmal tube and surrounding naked or remyelinating axons. Proliferative Schwann cell changes include remyelination and onion bulb formation. These observations highlight the significance of Schwann cell injury in the pathogenesis of feline diabetic neuropathy.[16] Muscle biopsies from the cranial tibial and biceps femoris muscles demonstrate scattered singular, angular, atrophied fibers of both fiber types, consistent with mild denervation. The normal myofiber mosaic pattern is retained without fiber type grouping. Numerous large lipid droplets have been noted within type I myofibers, and may represent disturbances in carnitine and/or mitochondrial oxidative function.[33] These pathologic findings support the electrophysiologic data from the diabetic cats studied thus far by the author, in that the major peripheral nerve abnormality appears to be demyelination and not axonal degeneration. Axonal injury does not appear

NORMAL CAT   **DIABETIC CAT**

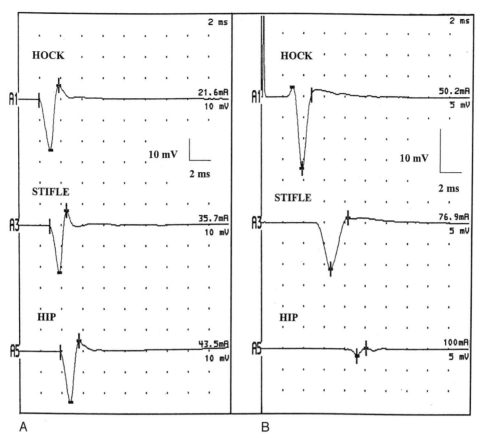

Figure 17–4. Sciatic-tibial nerve motor conduction in a diabetic cat with moderate-to-severe neuropathy (B) compared with a normal cat (A). Note the significant slowing of motor nerve conduction velocities along the entire length of the diabetic nerve (43 and 39 m/ sec) when compared with those of the normal cat (102 and 87 m/sec). This is indicative of demyelination. There also is a marked decrease in compound muscle action potential (CMAP) amplitudes in the diabetic cat (19.66 mV distally; 12.70 mV at the intermediate stimulation site; and 2.05 mV proximally) when compared with the normal cat (31.16 mV distally; 30.08 mV at the intermediate stimulation site; and 29.53 mV proximally). Although the decrease in distal CMAP amplitude in the cat with diabetic neuropathy may indicate mild-to-moderate denervation (as seen also with the electromyogram), the marked sequential CMAP amplitude decrease with more proximal stimulation sites most likely represents multifocal conduction block, a phenomenon seen with severe demyelination.

to be a necessary prerequisite for Schwann cell injury or demyelination.

◆ TREATMENT

At this time, there is no recommended specific therapy to treat the neuropathy associated with feline diabetes mellitus. Early, diligent, and aggressive regulation of serum glucose levels via insulin therapy (either twice-daily neutral protamine Hagedorn [NPH] insulin or once-daily to twice-daily protamine zinc insulin [PZI]), dietary management (high-protein diet with low carbohydrate and fat content), and use of acarbose, an alpha$_1$-glucosidase inhibitor, to decrease intestinal absorption of glucose in obese cats, usually will result in improvement in the associated peripheral neuropathy. The improvement in peripheral nerve function, however, often will take several weeks to months, and often is incomplete.[32, 33] Possible future ancillary therapies to treat the neuropathy specifically may

include aldose-reductase inhibitors and/or IGF replacement.

◆ PREVENTION

Prevention of this complication of feline diabetes mellitus would be the ideal aim in any treatment plan. The main goals of diabetic therapy to prevent the development of neuropathy should be not only to avoid persistent hyperglycemia but also to avoid wide swings in serum glucose levels throughout the day. Success of good glycemic control should be monitored routinely via serum fructosamine levels. The aim is to maintain fructosamine levels as close to the normal range as possible, or if the fructosamine level is high originally, to produce a trend of decreasing serum levels over successive measurement intervals. A trend of increasing fructosamine levels indicates poor glycemic control and appears to be a factor contributing to development of diabetic neuropathy in cats.

REFERENCES

1. Dyck PJ, Thomas PK (eds): Diabetic Neuropathy, 2nd ed. Philadelphia, WB Saunders, 1999.
2. Thomas PK, Tomlinson DR: Diabetic and hypoglycemic neuropathy. *In* Dyck PJ, Thomas PK (eds): Peripheral Neuropathy, 3rd ed. Philadelphia, WB Saunders, 1993, pp. 1219–1250.
3. Llewelyn JG: Diabetic neuropathy. Curr Opin Neurol 8:364–366, 1995.
4. Tomlinson DR: Role of aldose reductase inhibitors in the treatment of diabetic polyneuropathy. *In* Dyck PJ, Thomas PK (eds): Diabetic Neuropathy, 2nd ed. Philadelphia, WB Saunders, 1999, pp. 330–340.
5. Finegold D, Lattimer SA, Nolle S, et al: Polyol pathway activity and myoinositol metabolism: A suggested relationship in the pathogenesis of diabetic neuropathy. Diabetes 32:988–992, 1983.
6. Scarpini E, Bianchi R, Moggio M, et al: Decrease of nerve Na(+),K(+)-ATPase activity in the pathogenesis of human diabetic neuropathy. J Neurol Sci 120:159–167, 1993.
7. Mizisin AP, Calcutt NA: Dose-dependent alterations in nerve polyols and (Na$^+$-K$^+$)-ATPase activity in galactose intoxication. Metabolism 40:1207–1212, 1991.
8. Brownlee M: Advanced glycation end products and diabetic peripheral neuropathy. *In* Dyck PJ, Thomas PK (eds): Diabetic Neuropathy, 2nd ed. Philadelphia, WB Saunders, 1999, pp. 353–358.
9. Thomas PK: Growth factors and diabetic neuropathy. Diabet Med 11:732–739, 1994.
10. Anand P, Terenghi G, Warner G, et al: The role of endogenous nerve growth factor in human diabetic neuropathy. Nat Med 2:703–707, 1996.
11. Ido Y, McHewat J, Chang KC, et al: Neural dysfunction and metabolic imbalances in diabetic rats. Prevention by acetyl-L-carnitine. Diabetes 43:1469–1477, 1994.
12. Stevens MJ, Feldman EL, Greene DA: The aetiology of diabetic neuropathy: The combined roles of metabolic and vascular defects. Diabet Med 12:566–579, 1995.
13. Ward JD: Biochemical and vascular factors in the pathogenesis of diabetic neuropathy. Clin Invest Med 18:267–274, 1995.
14. Low PA, Nickander KK, Scionti L: Role of hypoxia, oxidative stress, and excitatory neurotoxins in diabetic neuropathy. *In* Dyck PJ, Thomas PK (eds): Diabetic Neuropathy, 2nd ed. Philadelphia, WB Saunders, 1999, pp. 317–329.
15. Harati Y: Diabetic peripheral neuropathies. Ann Intern Med 107:546–559, 1987.
16. Mizisin AP, Shelton GD, Wagner S, et al: Myelin splitting, Schwann cell injury and demyelination in feline diabetic neuropathy. Acta Neuropathol 95:171–174, 1998.
17. Ishii DN: Implication of insulin-like growth factors in the pathogenesis of diabetic neuropathy. Brain Res Rev 20:47–67, 1995.
18. Zhuang HX, Snyder CK, Pu SF, et al: Insulin-like growth factors reverse or arrest diabetic neuropathy: Effects on hyperalgesia and impaired nerve regeneration in rats. Exp Neurol 140:198–205, 1996.
19. Ishii DN, Lupien SB: Insulin-like growth factors protect against diabetic neuropathy: Effects on sensory nerve regeneration in rats. J Neurosci Res 40:138–144, 1995.
20. Wuarin L, Guertin DM, Ishii DN: Early reduction in insulin-like growth factor gene expression in diabetic nerve. Exp Neurol 130:106–114, 1994.
21. Fernyhough P, Mill JF, Roberts JL, et al: Stabilization of tubulin mRNAs by insulin and insulin-like growth factor I during neurite formation. Mol Brain Res 6:109–120, 1989.
22. Wang C, Li Y, Wible B, et al: Effects of insulin and insulin-like growth factors on neurofilament mRNA and tubulin mRNA content in human neuroblastoma SH-Y5Y cells. Mol Brain Res 13:289–300, 1992.
23. Kent MJC, Light ND, Bailey AJ: Evidence for glucose-mediated covalent cross-linking of collagen after glycosylation in vitro. Biochem J 225:745–752, 1985.
24. Haitoglou CS, Tsilibary EC, Brownlee M, et al: Altered cellular interactions between endothelial cells and non-enzymatically glycosylated laminin/type IV collagen. J Biol Chem 267:12404–12407, 1992.
25. Yan SD, Schmidt AM, Anderson GM, et al: Enhanced cellular oxidant stress by the interaction of advanced glycation end products with their receptor/binding proteins. J Biol Chem 269:9889–9897, 1994.
26. Ward JD. Abnormal microvasculature in diabetic neuropathy. Eye 7:223–236, 1993.
27. Low PA, Lagerlund TD, McManis PG: Nerve blood flow and oxygen delivery in normal, diabetic, and ischemic neuropathy. Int Rev Neurobiol 13:355–438, 1989.
28. Richter C, Park JW, Ames BN: Normal oxidative damage to mitochondrial and nuclear DNA is extensive. Proc Natl Acad Sci U S A 85:6465–6467, 1988.
29. Lutz TA, Rand JS: Pathogenesis of feline diabetes mellitus. Vet Clin North Am Small Anim Pract 25:527–552, 1995.
30. Feldman EC, Nelson RW: Diabetes mellitus. *In* Feldman EC, Nelson RW (eds). Canine and Feline Endocrinology and Reproduction, 2nd ed. Philadelphia, WB Saunders, 1996, pp. 339–391.
31. Kramek BA, Moise NS, Cooper B, et al: Neuropathy associated with diabetes mellitus in the cat. J Am Vet Med Assoc 184:42–45, 1984.
32. Munana KA: Long-term complications of diabetes mellitus, Part I: Retinopathy, nephropathy, neuropathy. Vet Clin North Am Small Anim Pract 25:715–730, 1995.
33. Cuddon PA. Diabetic neuropathy. *In* Proceedings 17th Annual Vet Med Forum, Chicago, June 10–13, 1999, pp. 650–652.
34. Lane SB, Kornegay JN: Spinal lymphosarcoma. *In* August JR (ed). Consultations in Feline Internal Medicine, vol. 1. Philadelphia, WB Saunders, 1991, pp. 487–490.
35. Lane JR, de Lahunta A: Polyneuritis in a cat. J Am Anim Hosp Assoc 20:1006–1008, 1984.
36. Flecknell PA, Lucke VM: Chronic relapsing polyradiculoneuritis in a cat. Acta Neuropathol 41:81–84, 1978.
37. Cuddon PA: Feline neuromuscular disease. Fel Pract 22:7–13, 1994.

18

◆ Diagnosis of Occult Hyperthyroidism

Mark E. Peterson

The diagnosis of hyperthyroidism in cats usually is straightforward and considered routine by most small-animal clinicians. However, although diagnosis in most cats is not problematic, some cats suspected of having hyperthyroidism may be difficult to diagnose. Many of these cats have early or mild hyperthyroidism and show only mild clinical signs, whereas others appear to have more severe clinical features of hyperthyroidism but also have another obvious (or not so obvious) concurrent disease. The finding of hyperthyroidism concurrent with a nonthyroidal disease is not surprising, given the fact that many of these cats are elderly.

Diagnosis of hyperthyroidism *must* take into account a cat's signalment, history, physical examination findings, and routine laboratory findings, as well as results of specific thyroid function tests. Most cats with hyperthyroidism are middle- to old-aged, with only 5 per cent of cats younger than 10 years of age at time of diagnosis.[1, 2] Common clinical signs observed in hyperthyroid cats include weight loss, hyperactivity, increased appetite, vomiting, diarrhea, polydipsia, and polyuria.[1-5] As hyperthyroidism has become more recognized, veterinarians are diagnosing more cats at an early stage of the disease, in some cases even before owners realize that their cats are ill; such cats with very mild hyperthyroidism may not have any obvious clinical signs or may have only a single sign. In hyperthyroid cats with concurrent disease (e.g., renal disease, hepatic disease, or neoplasia), weight loss usually remains a common clinical sign, but may be accompanied by decreased rather than normal-to-increased appetite. In these cats, depression and weakness also may replace hyperexcitability or restlessness as dominant clinical features.

On physical examination, most (but not all) hyperthyroid cats show evidence of weight loss, hyperexcitability, and tachycardia. Enlargement of one or both thyroid lobes can be detected in 80 to 90 per cent of cats with hyperthyroidism, and this finding is *extremely* important in making the diagnosis.[1-5] Although the thyroid gland usually is not palpable in normal cats, the finding of enlargement of one or both thyroid lobes on physical examination cannot be equated with hyperthyroidism because thyroid enlargement occasionally can be detected in cats without other clinical and laboratory evidence of the disease. Although some of these cats may remain euthyroid (at least for prolonged periods of time), many cats with thyroid gland enlargement eventually develop clinical and biochemical signs of hyperthyroidism as the thyroid nodules continue to grow and begin to oversecrete thyroid hormone.[6-8] Other findings detected commonly on physical examination of hyperthyroid cats include evidence of weight loss, tachycardia, cardiac murmurs, and hyperkinesis.[1-5] These signs may not be pronounced in cats with mild or early hyperthyroidism. In hyperthyroid cats with concurrent disease, other clinical signs caused by the second disease may predominate.

Diagnosis of hyperthyroidism in cats, especially when early and mild or when associated with concurrent nonthyroidal diseases, requires that the veterinarian have a solid understanding of thyroid function and the pituitary-thyroid axis. The understanding of these mechanisms has led to the development and increasing use of provocative thyroid function tests in veterinary medicine. This chapter discusses tests for hyperthyroidism in cats and their clinical applications.

◆ RESTING SERUM THYROID HORMONE CONCENTRATIONS

High basal serum total thyroid hormone concentrations are the biochemical hallmark of hyperthyroidism. Resting serum concentrations of both thyroxine (T_4) and triiodothyronine (T_3) are above the normal range in the majority of cats with hyperthyroidism.[1, 2, 5, 9] However, approximately 25 per cent of hyperthyroid cats have normal serum T_3 values, despite clearly high serum T_4 concentrations,[2] making it evident that determination of serum T_4 is of greater diagnostic value than determination of serum T_3. Some cats with hyperthyroidism (up to 10 per cent of all hyperthyroid cats) have serum concentrations of both T_4 and T_3 that are within the mid- to high-normal range.[2, 10, 11] Because many hyperthyroid cats with normal serum concentrations of T_4 or T_3 have relatively early or mild clinical features of hyperthyroidism, it is likely that the normal thyroid hormone concentrations found in these cats eventually would increase into the thyrotoxic range if the disorder were allowed to progress untreated.

How can a cat develop clinical signs (albeit mild in many cases) of hyperthyroidism when serum thyroid hormone concentrations remain within normal range? The finding of normal serum thyroid hormone concentrations in cats with clinical signs suggestive of hyperthyroidism can be problematic. Two explanations have been proposed to explain the finding of normal serum thyroid hormone concentrations in cats with hyperthyroidism: (1) fluctuation of T_4 and T_3 into and out of the normal range and (2) suppression of high serum T_4 and T_3 concentrations into the normal range because of concurrent nonthyroidal illness.

Thyroid hormone concentrations in cats with hyperthyroidism may fluctuate considerably over time.[12] In cats with thyroid hormone values well above the normal range, this fluctuation does not appear to be of great clinical or diagnostic significance. However, in cats with mild hyperthyroidism, the degree of serum T_4 and T_3 fluctuation that can occur—into the normal range in some cats (Figs. 18–1 and 18–2)—suggests that a diagnosis of hyperthyroidism cannot be excluded on the basis of the finding of a single normal to high-normal serum T_4 or T_3 result alone. In cats with clinical signs consistent with hyperthyroidism (and especially in cats with palpable thyroid nodules), more than 1 serum T_4 determination could be required to confirm a diagnosis. This fluctuation into and out of the normal range may explain, at least in part, the finding of normal or high-normal serum concentrations of T_4 and T_3 in some cats with clinical hyperthyroidism.

In hyperthyroid cats with moderate-to-severe concurrent nonthyroidal illness (e.g., renal disease, diabetes mellitus, systemic neoplasia, primary hepatic disease, other chronic illnesses), mid- to high-normal serum thyroid hormone concentrations may be found at time of initial evaluation (see Fig. 18–2).[10, 11, 13] In cats with extremely severe illnesses (usually leading to the cat's death), low-normal serum thyroid hormone concentrations can even be found. Because severe nonthyroidal illness would be expected to decrease serum thyroid hormone

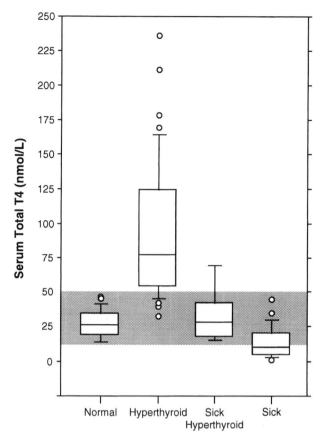

Figure 18–2. Box plots of the serum T_4 concentrations in 25 clinically normal cats, 50 cats with hyperthyroidism, 7 hyperthyroid cats with severe concurrent nonthyroidal disease, and 25 cats with nonthyroidal disease. The *boxes* represent the interquartile range from the 25th to the 75th percentile (the middle one-half of the data). The *horizontal bar* through the *box* is the median. The T-bars represent the main body of data, which in most cases is equal to the range. Outlying data points are represented by *open circles*. To convert serum T_4 concentrations from nmol/L to μg/dl, divide the given values by 12.87.

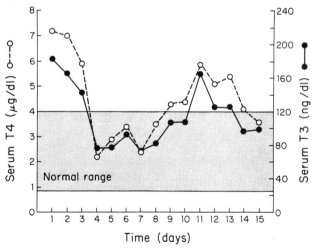

Figure 18–1. Serum thyroxine (T_4) and triiodothyronine (T_3) concentrations determined daily over a 15-day period in a cat with hyperthyroidism. Note the fluctuation into and out of the normal range for both serum T_4 and T_3 values. To convert serum T_4 concentrations from nmol/L to μg/dl, divide the given values by 12.87. To convert serum T_3 concentrations from nmol/L to ng/dl, divide the given values by 0.0154. (From Peterson ME, Graves TK, Cavanagh I: Serum thyroid hormone concentrations fluctuate in cats with hyperthyroidism. J Vet Intern Med 1:142–146, 1987.)

concentrations into the low-to-undetectable range in sick cats without concurrent hyperthyroidism,[11, 13] concomitant hyperthyroidism should be suspected in any middle- to old-aged cat with severe nonthyroidal illness and normal serum T_4 and T_3 concentrations, especially if signs of hyperthyroidism also are present. On stabilization of, or recovery from, the concurrent nonthyroidal disorder, serum thyroid hormone concentrations will increase into the diagnostic thyrotoxic range in these cats with hyperthyroidism.

When the clinician suspects mild hyperthyroidism in a cat but the serum T_4 (and T_3) concentration is not high, the first step always should be to repeat the basal T_4 measurement and rule out nonthyroidal illness. Because there is greater variation in hormone concentrations over a period of days than over a period of hours,[12] the second serum T_4 determination should be made at least 1 to 2 weeks later. If the result is again in the normal to high-normal range and hyperthyroidism is still suspected, determination of a free T_4 concentration (by dialysis) or provocative testing with a T_3 suppression test or thyrotropin-releasing hormone (TRH) stimulation test is recommended.[11, 14–17]

◆ BASAL FREE THYROID HORMONE DETERMINATIONS

Circulating thyroid hormones may be either bound to carrier proteins or free (unbound) in the plasma. Most commercial T_4 and T_3 assays measure total concentrations, both free and protein-bound. Because only the free fraction of thyroid hormone is available for entry into the cells, free T_4 determinations may provide a more consistent assessment of thyroid gland status than total T_4 concentrations.[18, 19] Also, free T_4 concentrations may not be as likely to be influenced by factors such as nonthyroidal illness or drug therapy that may lower total T_4 concentrations falsely.

Free T_4 is determined most accurately by methods that include a dialysis step.[18, 19] In general, non-dialysis techniques for free T_4 determination are less accurate, often underestimate the free T_4 concentration, and offer little, if any, advantage over the measurement of total T_4 concentration.

The finding of a high free T_4 by dialysis is consistent with hyperthyroidism (Fig. 18–3).[11, 20] Occasionally, however, cats with nonthyroidal illness that do not have hyperthyroidism have high free T_4 concentrations for reasons that are unclear (see Fig. 18–3).[11, 20, 21] Therefore, to avoid a misdiagnosis of hyperthyroidism, free T_4 always should be evaluated in conjunction with the total T_4 concentration (as well as the cat's signalment, history, physical examination findings, and routine laboratory findings). In general, the combination of a high free T_4 value with a low total T_4 concentration (<20 nmol/L or <2.5 µg/dl) is indicative of nonthyroidal illness, whereas a high free T_4 value with a high-normal total T_4 concentration (>25 nmol/L or >3.0 µg/dl) is suggestive of hyperthyroidism (see Figs. 18–2 and 18–3).[11, 20]

Free T_4 concentrations are useful in cats with mild or occult hyperthyroidism, in which resting total T_4 concentrations remain in the mid- to high-normal range. The free T_4 concentrations appear to be affected much less by concurrent nonthyroidal illness that may afflict many older cats and, therefore, may reflect true thyroid status more accurately.[11, 20] The finding of a high free T_4 concentration (despite a normal total T_4) in a cat with a consistent history (e.g., weight loss despite good appetite) and physical examination findings (e.g., palpable thyroid nodule) would support the diagnosis of hyperthyroidism. If the thyroid nodule cannot be palpated, however, or if another illness is known to be present, it is recommended to confirm hyperthyroidism with either the T_3 suppression or the TRH stimulation test, which remain the "gold standards" for the diagnosis of occult hyperthyroidism in cats.[14–17]

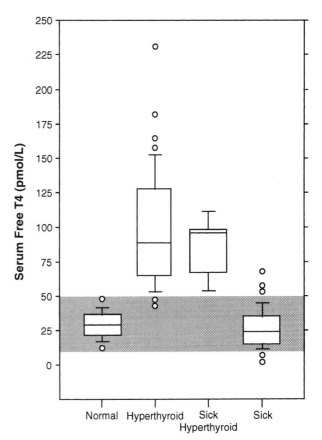

Figure 18–3. Box plots of the serum free T_4 concentrations (by dialysis) in 25 clinically normal cats, 50 cats with hyperthyroidism, 7 hyperthyroid cats with severe concurrent nonthyroidal disease, and 25 cats with nonthyroidal disease. Data are plotted (i.e., box plots) as described in Figure 18–2.

◆ THYROID HORMONE (T_3) SUPPRESSION TEST

Thyroid suppression testing is used to evaluate cats with suspected hyperthyroidism when simpler tests such as basal serum T_4 and T_3 concentrations are nondiagnostic. Inhibition of pituitary thyroid-stimulating hormone (TSH) secretion by high circulating concentrations of thyroid hormone is a characteristic feature of normal pituitary-thyroid regulation.[22] Normally, administration of thyroid hormone decreases TSH secretion; when exogenous T_3 is given to normal cats, this can be detected by a decrease in serum T_4 concentrations. In contrast, when thyroid function is autonomous (i.e., independent of TSH secretion), administration of thyroid hormone has little or no effect on thyroid function because TSH secretion already has been chronically suppressed. This is invariably true with clinical hyperthyroidism.

To perform the T_3 suppression test in cats, a blood sample is drawn for determination of basal serum concentrations of total T_4 and T_3.[14, 15, 17, 20] This blood sample should be centrifuged, and the serum removed and kept refrigerated or frozen. Owners are instructed to administer T_3 orally (liothyronine; Cytomel, Jones Medical Industries, St. Louis) on the following morning at a dosage of 25 μg every (q) 8 hr for 2 days. On the morning of the third day, a seventh 25-μg dose of liothyronine is given, and the cat returned to the veterinary clinic within 2 to 4 hours for serum T_4 and T_3 determinations. Both the basal (day 1) and postliothyronine serum samples should be submitted to the laboratory together to eliminate the effect of interassay variation in hormone concentrations.

When the T_3 suppression test is performed in normal cats, there is a marked fall in serum T_4 concentrations after exogenous T_3 administration (Fig. 18–4). In contrast, when the test is performed in cats with hyperthyroidism, even in cats with only slightly high or high-normal resting serum T_4 concentrations, minimum, if any, suppression of serum T_4 concentrations is seen.

Regarding interpretation of T_3 suppression test results, I find that the absolute serum T_4 concentration after liothyronine administration is the best means of distinguishing hyperthyroid cats from normal cats or those with nonthyroidal disease.[14] Cats with hyperthyroidism have postliothyronine serum T_4 values greater than 20 nmol/liter (~1.5 μg/dl), whereas normal cats and those with nonthyroidal disease have T_4 values less than 20 nmol/liter (see Fig. 18–4B). There may be a great deal of overlap of the per cent decrease in serum T_4 concentrations after liothyronine administration between the 3 groups of cats, but suppression of 50 per cent or more only occurs in cats without hyperthyroidism.

Serum T_3 concentrations, as part of the T_3 suppression test, are not useful in the diagnosis of hyperthyroidism per se. However, these basal and postliothyronine serum T_3 determinations can be used to monitor owner compliance with giving the drug. If inadequate T_4 suppression is found, but serum T_3 values do not increase after treatment with liothyronine, problems with owner compliance should be suspected, and the test result considered questionable.

Overall, the T_3 suppression test is very useful for diagnosis of mild hyperthyroidism in cats, but the disadvantages are that it is a relatively long test (3 days), owners are required to give multiple doses of liothyronine, and cats must swallow the tablets.[14, 15] If the liothyronine is not administered properly, circulating T_3 concentrations will not rise to decrease pituitary TSH secretion, and the serum T_4 value will not be suppressed, even if the pituitary-thyroid axis is normal. Failure of a cat to ingest the liothyronine could result in a false-positive diagnosis of hyperthyroidism in a normal cat or a cat with nonthyroidal disease.

◆ TRH STIMULATION TEST

The TRH stimulation test measures the serum T_4 response to administration of TRH. In clinically normal cats, the administration of TRH causes an increase in TSH secretion and serum T_4 concentrations, whereas in cats with hyperthyroidism, the TSH and serum T_4 response to TRH is blunted or totally absent.[16] The lack of response is because TSH secretion is chronically suppressed to a great extent in cats with hyperthyroidism.

The TRH stimulation test is performed by collecting blood for serum T_4 and T_3 determinations before and 4 hours after intravenous administration of 0.1 mg/kg of TRH (Peninsula Laboratories, Inc., Bel-

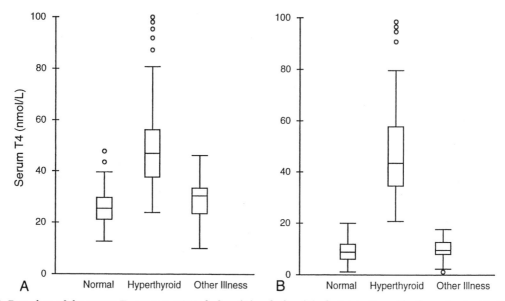

Figure 18–4. Box plots of the serum T_4 concentrations before *(A)* and after *(B)* administration of liothyronine to 44 clinically normal cats, 77 cats with hyperthyroidism, and 22 cats with nonthyroidal disease. Data are plotted (i.e., box plots) as described in Figure 18–2. To convert serum T_4 concentrations from nmol/L to μg/dl, divide the given values by 12.87. (*A* and *B*, From Peterson ME, Graves TK, Gamble DA: Triiodothyronine [T_3] suppression test: An aid in the diagnosis of mild hyperthyroidism in cats. J Vet Intern Med 4:233–238, 1990.)

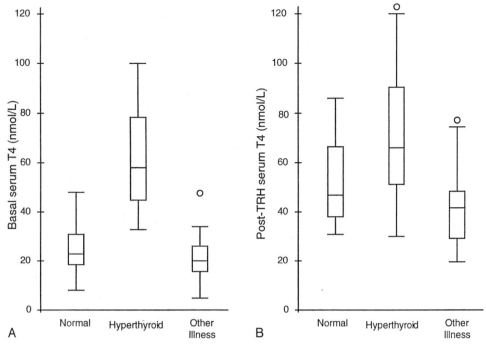

Figure 18–5. Box plots of the serum T_4 concentrations before *(A)* and after *(B)* thyrotropin-releasing hormone (TRH) stimulation in 31 clinically normal cats, 35 cats with hyperthyroidism, and 15 cats with nonthyroidal disease. Data are plotted (i.e., box plots) as described in Figure 18–2. To convert serum T_4 concentrations from nmol/L to μg/dl, divide the given values by 12.87. (*A* and *B*, From Peterson ME, Broussard JD, Gamble DA: Use of the thyrotropin releasing hormone stimulation test to diagnose mild hyperthyroidism in cats. J Vet Intern Med 8:279–286, 1994.)

mont, CA).[16] Cats with mild hyperthyroidism show little, if any, rise in serum T_4 values after administration of TRH, whereas a consistent rise of serum T_4 concentrations (approximately 2-fold increase) occurs after TRH administration in both clinically normal cats and cats with nonthyroidal disease (Fig. 18–5). The serum T_3 response to TRH is less helpful in separating normal from hyperthyroid cats because many normal cats have only a small and inconsistent rise in serum T_3 concentrations after TRH administration. Therefore, although basal T_3 concentration may be helpful in diagnosis of hyperthyroidism in some cats, I do not recommend determining the serum T_3 response as part of the TRH stimulation test.[16]

Regarding interpretation of the TRH stimulation test results, the relative rise (per cent increase) in serum T_4 concentration after administration of TRH is the best (most sensitive) criterion for predicting whether or not cats are hyperthyroid. An increase in serum T_4 of less than 50 per cent is consistent with mild hyperthyroidism, whereas a value of greater than 60 per cent is seen in normal cats and cats with nonthyroidal illness; values between 50 and 60 per cent are equivocal or borderline responses.[16]

Studies have shown a close relationship between the presence (or absence) of suppressed serum T_4 concentrations in response to T_3 suppression and stimulated T_4 values in response to TRH stimulation.[16] Therefore, although the 2 tests evaluate the pituitary-thyroid axis in different ways, my findings indicate that the 2 screening tests provide similar information, and probably can be used interchangeably for diagnosing mild hyperthyroidism in cats.

Advantages of the TRH stimulation test over the T_3 suppression test include the shorter time needed to perform the test (4 hours vs. 3 days) and the fact that the TRH stimulation test is not dependent on the owner's ability to administer oral medication. The major disadvantage of the TRH stimulation test in cats is that side-effects (e.g., salivation, vomiting, tachypnea, and defecation) almost invariably occur immediately after administration of the TRH. It has been reported that TRH evokes these effects in cats via activation of central cholinergic and catecholaminergic mechanisms, as well as by a direct neurotransmitter effect of TRH itself on specific central TRH-binding sites.[23–25] Fortunately, all of the adverse side-effects associated with TRH administration are transient and resolve completely by the end of the 4-hour test period. Therefore, at the discretion of the veterinarian, owners need not be exposed to the occurrence of these side-effects in their cats.

REFERENCES

1. Peterson ME, Kintzer PP, Cavanagh PG, et al: Feline hyperthyroidism: Pretreatment clinical and laboratory evaluation of 131 cases. J Am Vet Med Assoc 183:103–110, 1983.
2. Broussard JD, Peterson ME, Fox PR: Changes in clinical and laboratory findings in cats with hyperthyroidism from 1983 to 1993. J Am Vet Med Assoc 206:302–305, 1995.
3. Peterson ME: Hyperthyroid diseases. *In* Ettinger SJ (ed): Text-

book of Veterinary Internal Medicine: Diseases of the Dog and Cat, 4th ed. Philadelphia, WB Saunders, 1995, pp. 1466–1487.

4. Feldman EC, Nelson RW: Feline hyperthyroidism (thyrotoxicosis). *In* Feldman EC, Nelson RW (eds): Canine and Feline Endocrinology and Reproduction, 2nd ed. Philadelphia, WB Saunders, 1996, pp. 118–166.

5. Thoday KL, Mooney CT: Historical, clinical and laboratory features of 126 hyperthyroid cats. Vet Rec 131:257–264, 1992.

6. Graves TK, Peterson ME: Diagnosis of occult hyperthyroidism in cats. *In* Problems in Veterinary Medicine. Philadelphia, JB Lippincott, 1990, pp. 683–692.

7. Graves TK, Peterson ME: Occult hyperthyroidism in cats. *In* Kirk RW, Bonagura JD (eds): Current Veterinary Therapy XI. Philadelphia, WB Saunders, 1992, pp. 334–337.

8. Peterson ME, Randolph JF, Mooney CT: Endocrine diseases. *In* Sherding RG (ed): The Cat: Diagnosis and Clinical Management, 2nd ed. New York, Churchill Livingstone, 1994, pp. 1404–1506.

9. Peterson ME, Kintzer PP, Hurvitz AI: Methimazole treatment of 262 cats with hyperthyroidism. J Vet Intern Med 2:150–157, 1988.

10. McLoughlin MA, DiBartola SP, Birchard SJ, et al: Influence of systemic nonthyroidal illness on serum concentrations of thyroxine in hyperthyroid cats. J Am Anim Hosp Assoc 29:227–234, 1993.

11. Peterson ME, Melián C, Nichols CE: Measurement of serum concentrations of total and free T$_4$ in hyperthyroid cats and cats with nonthyroidal disease. J Vet Intern Med 12:211, 1998.

12. Peterson ME, Graves TK, Cavanagh I: Serum thyroid hormone concentrations fluctuate in cats with hyperthyroidism. J Vet Intern Med 1987;1:142–146.

13. Peterson ME, Gamble DA: Effect of nonthyroidal illness on serum thyroxine concentrations in cats: 494 cases (1988). J Am Vet Med Assoc 197:1203–1208, 1990.

14. Peterson ME, Graves TK, Gamble DA: Triiodothyronine (T$_3$) suppression test: An aid in the diagnosis of mild hyperthyroidism in cats. J Vet Intern Med 4:233–238, 1990.

15. Refsal KR, Nachreiner RF, Stein BE, et al: Use of the triiodothyronine suppression test for diagnosis of hyperthyroidism in ill cats that have serum concentration of iodothyronines within normal range. J Am Vet Med Assoc 199:1594–1601, 1991.

16. Peterson ME, Broussard JD, Gamble DA: Use of the thyrotropin releasing hormone stimulation test to diagnose mild hyperthyroidism in cats. J Vet Intern Med 8:279–286, 1994.

17. Graves TK, Peterson ME: Diagnostic tests for feline hyperthyroidism. Vet Clin North Am Small Anim Pract 24:567–576, 1994.

18. Ferguson DC: Free thyroid hormone measurements in the diagnosis of thyroid disease. *In* Bonagura JD, Kirk RW (eds): Current Veterinary Therapy XII. Philadelphia, WB Saunders, 1995, pp. 360–364.

19. Kaptein EM: Clinical application of free thyroxine determinations. Clin Lab Med 13:653–672, 1993.

20. Nichols R, Peterson ME: Laboratory diagnosis of hyperthyroidism in cats. Monograph on Hyperthyroidism in Cats. St. Louis, Daniels Pharmaceuticals, 1998, pp. 2–7.

21. Mooney CT, Little JL, Macrae AW: Effect of illness not associated with the thyroid gland on serum total and free thyroxine concentrations in cats. J Am Vet Med Assoc 208:2004–2008, 1996.

22. Utiger RD: Tests of thyroregulatory mechanisms. *In* Ingbar SH, Braverman LE (eds): The Thyroid: A Fundamental and Clinical Text. Philadelphia, JB Lippincott, 1986, pp. 511–523.

23. Holtman JR, Buller AL, Hamosh P, et al: Central respiratory stimulation produced by thyrotropin-releasing hormone in the cat. Peptides 7:207–212, 1986.

24. Beleslin DB, Jovanovic-Micic D, Tomic-Beleslin N: Nature of salivation produced by thyrotropin-releasing hormone (TRH). Brain Res Bull 18:463–465, 1987.

25. Beleslin DB, Jovanovic-Micic D, Samardzic R, et al: Studies of thyrotropin-releasing hormone (TRH)–induced defecation in cats. Pharmacol Biochem Behav 26:639–641, 1987.

19

◆ Complications of Therapy for Hyperthyroidism

Melinda K. Van Vechten

Cats are becoming increasingly important members of many households. Cat owners are providing their pets with routine health care that is greatly improving their longevity, and many cats are living to middle and old age as house pets. Hyperthyroidism, the most common endocrine disorder of older cats, is being diagnosed more frequently. This likely is due to increased clinical suspicion on the part of veterinarians,[1] as well as increased owner awareness of the disease and willingness to care for older pets. Early (mild or occult) hyperthyroidism is recognized as an important clinical syndrome,[2] so that many cats are diagnosed and treated for hyperthyroidism before signs such as cachexia, cardiac disease, and possibly secondary renal disease develop.

Fortunately, a number of excellent therapies are available for treatment of hyperthyroidism. Permanent (curative) modalities include radioiodine therapy and surgical extirpation of abnormal thyroid tissue. Reversible treatment involves long-term medical management with thioureylene drugs such as methimazole or carbimazole, or iodinated contrast agents (calcium ipodate). Ancillary treatments such as beta-receptor blocking agents and stable iodine preparations often are helpful in selected patients. These medical treatments are considered reversible, in that they can be discontinued or dosages lowered in patients that become azotemic when their hyperthyroid state is corrected.

Last, investigational treatments are being developed, such as ultrasound-guided instillation of ethanol into localizable thyroid nodules, and these may prove to be useful additions to the therapeutic armamentarium.

All of the therapies for hyperthyroidism have inherent risks and benefits, as well as logistical concerns that are important to cat owners and that may dictate the choice of therapy as much as medical issues. A large body of clinical experience has been developed since hyperthyroidism began to be diagnosed routinely, but vexatious issues persist: the unmasking of preexisting renal disease and the lack of clinicopathologic data on normal pre- and posttreatment thyroid values for elderly cats.

◆ UNMASKING PREEXISTING RENAL DISEASE

One of the most difficult issues in the treatment of hyperthyroidism is the unmasking of preexisting renal disease. Hyperthyroidism results in increased glomerular filtration rate and increased renal plasma flow,[3] as well as increased cardiac output and blood pressure. These physiologic changes, although detrimental to long-term renal health, may augment renal function in some hyperthyroid cats to the extent that their true renal status is obscured. Evaluation of the true renal status of the hyperthyroid patient also is confounded by clinicopathologic changes that occur with the disease. The poor body condition and loss of muscle mass that are characteristic of hyperthyroidism result in falsely lowered serum creatinine levels,[3] which rise when emaciation is corrected. Conversely, the blood urea nitrogen level may be increased in hyperthyroid cats with normal renal function due to polyphagia and increased protein catabolism.[1] Urine specific gravity, often used as an indication of renal function, also may be falsely lowered in hyperthyroid cats as a result of diuretic effects of thyroid hormone[4] and changes in renal medullary concentrating ability due to thyrotoxic changes in renal blood flow.[5]

Successful treatment of hyperthyroidism by any means and a return to the euthyroid state result in decreased glomerular filtration rate, leading to azotemia in some cats.[3, 6] It is thought that this decline in function represents an unmasking of the cat's true renal function, rather than nephrotoxic effects of treatment. Therefore, it has been recommended that a reversible method of therapy be used as the initial treatment in newly diagnosed cats; thus, if their renal function declines to an unacceptable level, treatment can be discontinued or decreased so that the cat is left mildly hyperthyroid.[5] It is probable that treatments that result in a gradual decrease in serum thyroxine (T_4) values, such as lower initial doses of thioureylene drugs and lower doses of ^{131}I, will result in more gradual changes in renal hemodynamics, allowing better autoregulation.[3] This delicate balance between an "acceptable" level of hyperthyroidism and an "acceptable" level of azotemia may be very difficult if not impossible to achieve in some cats, and treatment should be discontinued.

◆ POSTTREATMENT MONITORING: WHAT IS NORMAL?

Thyroid hormone levels decline with age in human beings,[7] and are suspected to do so as well in cats. One study showed a gradual decrease in T_4 and triiodothyronine (T_3) levels with age in 2 different colonies of healthy research cats, although the values remained within the normal range.[8] It also has been shown that T_4 values in hyperthyroid cats may vary as much as 49 per cent over the course of 24 hours.[9] Cats with mild hyperthyroidism or concurrent nonthyroidal illness may have T_4 values that are within the normal range, or are subnormal[5] (see Chapter 18, Diagnosis of Occult Hyperthyroidism). Clearly, the diagnosis of hyperthyroidism may be difficult in some cats, and a nuclear medicine scan may be required for definitive diagnosis. This begs the question: what is a normal posttreatment T_4 value?

It usually is recommended that cats treated with thioureylene drugs be maintained on dosages that keep their thyroxine levels in the low-normal range.[10] Occasionally, some cats do not thrive with T_4 values in this range, and still may have mild clinical signs. In other cats, it is not possible to find a dosage at which the cat is neither euthyroid nor hyperthyroid, yet the cats seem to flourish with T_4 levels in the subnormal range. Calcium ipodate therapy must be monitored by assessing T_3 levels, and it is recommended that T_3 levels be maintained within the normal range.[11]

Patients treated with permanent therapies (surgery, radioiodine) have a small risk of becoming permanently, clinically hypothyroid. This usually occurs in cats that undergo bilateral thyroidectomy in which all thyroid tissue is removed, and in cats that receive higher doses of radioiodine. It is quite common, however, for cats undergoing these treatments to have subnormal or even undetectable T_4 levels transiently, for weeks to months after their procedure. The vast majority do not have clinical signs of hypothyroidism, even if their T_4 values do not rise into the normal range. It has been postulated that free T_4 levels remain normal in these cats.[5] It also is possible that these cats may compensate with changes in T_3 levels or metabolism, but this has not been proved. More work needs to be done in this area. It is best not to supplement cats with L-thyroxine, regardless of their laboratory values, unless they develop signs of hypothyroidism.

Clinical hypothyroidism usually does not develop until 2 to 4 months after treatment in cats treated with radioiodine. Affected cats usually are very lethargic, become obese, develop very poor-quality hair coats, and may become seborrheic. These cats require lifelong L-thyroxine supplementation, at a dosage that maintains their T_4 in the low-normal range, or at a value that causes correction of the clinical signs.

◆ REVERSIBLE TREATMENT OPTIONS

Therapies that can be decreased or discontinued if objectionable complications occur include medical management with thioureylene drugs and calcium ipodate.

Thioureylene Drugs

Methimazole (Tapazole, Eli Lily) is the most commonly used antithyroid drug in the United States. It is relatively inexpensive, but must be administered at least twice-daily to most hyperthyroid cats.[12] If owners are unable or unwilling to medicate the cat more than once-daily, serum T_4 values should be checked several times over a period of weeks or months just prior to the time the cat is medicated to make sure it is remaining euthyroid. When methimazole treatment is discontinued, the hyperthyroid state usually returns within 48 hours.[5] Methimazole does not affect iodide trapping, and can be used to stabilize surgical or radioiodine candidates without a withdrawal period before a procedure. It has been recommended that all azotemic cats be "test treated"[6] with methimazole until they have been rendered euthyroid for at least several weeks; then their renal function is re-evaluated. Cats that become unacceptably azotemic can receive further treatment at a reduced dose, or their treatment can be discontinued if they develop renal failure. It seems prudent that any cat that may undergo a permanent treatment (radioiodine, surgery) also be rendered euthyroid with methimazole, and its renal function assessed. Cats exhibiting acceptable renal function after several weeks of euthyroidism probably can be treated safely with a permanent modality. Progressive azotemia develops in a few cats, even with careful selection. It is very difficult to know whether this decline in renal function is an unavoidable progression of renal disease caused by hyperthyroidism, a function of senescence, or other factors.

Few complications are seen with short-term methimazole therapy, such as that given to prepare cats for permanent treatment. Cats receiving methimazole as their primary treatment for long-term management are at risk for a host of complications, many of which fortunately are rare or reversible if therapy is discontinued. These side-effects include vomiting, anorexia, lethargy, dermatitis with facial excoriation, bleeding tendencies, hepatopathy, hematologic changes, development of antinuclear antibodies or Coombs' test positivity,[13] and myasthenia gravis.[14]

A conservative dosage protocol for initial therapy with methimazole is well-tolerated by most cats.[6] Treatment is started at 2.5 mg every (q) 12 hr orally (PO) for 2 weeks. A physical examination, serum chemistries, complete blood count, platelet count, and T_4 level are done at the end of this period. If the cat is euthyroid (many mildly hyperthyroid cats may be controlled at this low dose), monitoring is continued as previously discussed every 2 to 4 weeks for the first 3 months of therapy, because this is when most side-effects occur. If the cat remains euthyroid and no untoward complications develop, the cat should be re-examined every 3 to 6 months and the previous tests repeated. It is not uncommon for cats to require upward adjustment of their methimazole dosage over months or years.

Cats that do not become euthyroid after initial dosing may respond to 2.5 mg methimazole q 8 hr PO. Again, monitoring should be done as previously after 2 to 4 weeks of treatment and for the first 3 months of therapy. If the cat remains hyperthyroid, the dosage can be increased by 2.5-mg increments per day every 2 weeks until euthyroidism is achieved. It is rare for cats to require more than 15 mg of methimazole daily.

The most common side-effects of methimazole usage are vomiting, anorexia, and depression. These usually are transient problems, as are mild hematologic changes such as eosinophilia, lymphocytosis, and mild leukopenia. Suspension of treatment usually is not required if these complications occur.

More serious side-effects, such as severe cytopenias, hepatopathy, and dermatologic reactions, require cessation of treatment and appropriate supportive care. Cats that develop facial excoriations may respond to glucocorticoid and H_1-receptor antagonist drugs,[10] and an alternative therapy then should be sought. Patients that develop profound cytopenia usually normalize rapidly after drug therapy is discontinued, but will relapse if the drug is given again. These patients may require blood transfusions, colony-stimulating factor therapy, broad-spectrum bactericidal antibiotic therapy, and other supportive measures until their hematologic picture is normalized. Thrombocytopenia is a fairly common hematologic problem in susceptible cats, but a bleeding diathesis also can develop with normal platelet numbers. The mechanism is unknown, but is probably a platelet function defect.[13] The hepatopathy that can arise with methimazole usage may be severe.[5] Cats should be treated with appropriate supportive care, but recovery may take several weeks.

Cats that are treated with long-term methimazole are at risk for development of positive serum antinuclear antibody titers. This risk is greatest in cats that have been treated with higher doses of methimazole (>15 mg/day) for periods longer than 6 months. No clinical side-effects have been identified in such cats, although a lupus-like syndrome has been reported in human beings.[7] It has been suggested that the lowest possible dose of methimazole that results in euthyroidism be given to help prevent development of positive antinuclear antibody titers.

Certain logistical problems arise with long-term methimazole administration. The medication is bitter-tasting and some patients may strongly resist dosing.[15] The drug can be reformulated into gelatin capsules, or more palatable oral suspensions. If an oral suspension is used, bioavailability and absorption of the medication should be investigated if the patient requires high doses of methimazole. It also is very difficult for some clients to medicate their cats twice- or even once-daily. In these situations, the cat may be staying relatively hyperthyroid over time, and may not thrive. A permanent method of treatment should be sought for any patient that has severe side-effects from methimazole usage, or cannot be medicated reliably.

Methimazole therapy is the easiest and most efficacious treatment for short-term therapy, and some patients tolerate it well and can be managed very effectively over time. Methimazole therapy does not require hospitalization, surgery, anesthesia, or special licensing, as do the permanent forms of treatment. Methimazole therapy also is less expensive initially, although cats that survive 1.5 to 2 years after the initiation of treatment will begin to accrue costs for medical therapy and monitoring greater than those for surgery or radioiodine therapy. Therefore, in patients that are relatively young and healthy other than their hyperthyroidism, a permanent treatment may be more cost-effective in the long term.

Iodinated Contrast Agents

Calcium ipodate is an oral cholecystographic agent that has moderate antithyroid activity. It hinders deiodination of T_4 to the more biologically active T_3, and decreases thyroid hormone secretion by blocking the effects of thyroid-stimulating hormone.[11] The iodide released during the metabolism of ipodate may prevent hormone release from the thyroid gland.[11]

No clinical or clinicopathologic abnormalities were reported in a group of cats treated with 100 to 200 mg calcium ipodate daily.[11] Response to treatment was seen in 8 of 12 cats, and was evidenced by the decline of serum T_3 into the normal range (although T_4 levels were not decreased significantly), increased body weight, and normalization of heart rate. Four of the cats did not respond to the therapy. It seems that mildly affected cats respond best to ipodate therapy, but it may begin to lose effectiveness approximately 3 months after treatment is started. Therefore, it may not be suitable for long-term use in some cats.[5]

Ipodate has not been investigated as a short-term stabilizing agent prior to a permanent therapy, although azotemia was not reported in cats that responded to ipodate therapy. It seems reasonable to use ipodate to prepare patients that cannot tolerate methimazole for thyroidectomy. The effects of ipodate on thyroid iodine-trapping may make it unsuitable as a preparatory agent for radioiodine therapy without a withdrawal period. More work is required in this area.

Ipodate is available only in large quantities. A competent pharmacist must reformulate it into an appropriate size for cats. The medication usually is repackaged into 50- or 100-mg capsules. The medication can be given once-daily, or divided into 2 daily doses.[11]

◆ ANCILLARY THERAPIES

Stable Iodine Preparations

Large doses of stable iodine inhibit thyroid hormone release.[7] This effect usually is transient, and oral stable iodine is not useful for long-term medical management of hyperthyroid patients. Oral iodine therapy reduces the size and vascularity of adenomatous thyroid tissue,[10] and may be useful with or without thioureylene drugs in preparing patients for surgery. It usually is administered at a dose of 30 to 100 mg/day for 10 to 14 days before surgery, as a saturated solution of potassium iodide (100 g potassium iodide per 100 ml solution, yielding 38 mg of iodine/drop)[5] or as Lugol solution. Kelp tablets from natural food stores also can be used, and contain approximately 0.15 mg of iodide per tablet.[10]

Side-effects of oral iodine preparations are mainly anorexia, hypersalivation, and occasional vomiting. It is thought that the objectionable taste of the preparation is the likely cause of these side-effects. Packaging the doses in gelatin capsules or masking it in a strong-tasting vehicle (such as cod-liver oil) largely alleviates these problems.

Abrupt cessation of stable iodine therapy may result in an exacerbation of hyperthyroid signs as the iodine-enriched glands escape from the inhibitory effects of the compound and release additional hormone. Therefore, iodine therapy should be coupled with thioureylene drug therapy, or a permanent treatment such as surgery. Stable iodine administration affects the thyroidal iodine uptake, so oral iodine therapy should be withheld for at least several weeks before radioiodine therapy.

Beta-Adrenergic Blocking Agents

Beta-adrenergic blocking agents may be used to decrease the tachycardia, polypnea, hypertension, hyperactivity, and cardiac arrhythmias seen in many hyperthyroid cats. These drugs do not affect thyroid hormone metabolism or the thyroid gland directly, and are best used in conjunction with thioureylene drugs or calcium ipodate when stabilizing a newly diagnosed patient. They also are used to prepare patients for curative treatment, and are useful in preventing the cardiac arrhythmias seen in many hyperthyroid cats during anesthesia. They may be used to ameliorate hyperthyroid signs in patients that are slow to become euthyroid after radioiodine therapy.[10]

Propranolol (Inderal, Ayerst) is the most commonly used beta-blocking drug. It is a nonselective beta$_1$- and beta$_2$-adrenoceptor blocker, and so must be used cautiously in patients with bronchoconstrictive disease (e.g., feline asthma).[16] Propranolol usually is given at a dose of 2.5 to 5 mg PO q 8 to 12 hr as needed to decrease the heart rate into the normal range,[5] often with thioureylene drugs, calcium ipodate, or stable iodine. Propranolol may act with stable iodine to decrease the vascularity of the gland,[10] and so may be a useful adjunct to surgery when given 3 to 14 days before the procedure. Propranolol also may be given at a dose of 0.1 mg intravenously as needed intraoperatively for management of ventricular arrhythmias.[10]

Atenolol (Tenormin, ICI) is a more selective beta$_1$-blocking drug, and is safer to use in patients with bronchoconstrictive disease.[16] It also has the advantage of requiring only once-daily dosing. It is usually given at 6.25 to 12.5 mg PO per cat daily.

Atenolol and propranolol both must be used with caution in patients with decreased cardiac contractility or bradycardias, and renal or hepatic insufficiency. Both drugs can cause hypo- or hyperglycemia, and should be used carefully with adequate monitoring in diabetic patients.[16]

◆ PERMANENT (CURATIVE) TREATMENT OPTIONS

Radioiodine Therapy

Radioiodine therapy is the treatment of choice for feline hyperthyroidism. It is the safest, least stressful, most specific treatment available, and has an excellent cure rate.[5] It is a particularly useful treatment for cats with bilateral thyroid involvement (approximately 70 per cent of cats),[6] cats with ectopic (noncervical) thyroid tissue, and the rare patient with thyroid carcinoma. No side-effects are seen from the radiation therapy per se, and the treatment is well-tolerated by even the most debilitated, elderly hyperthyroid cat. When patients are pretreated with thioureylene drugs and selected carefully, the risk of unmasking preexisting renal disease is minimum.

Radioiodine therapy is very specific because the thyroid glands are the only tissues in the body that concentrate plasma iodine actively. The glands cannot differentiate between normal dietary iodine (stable iodine, ^{127}I) and radioactive iodine used for therapy (^{131}I). Therefore, radioiodine is concentrated by the active (adenomatous, or rarely, carcinomatous) thyroid tissue, which is destroyed. The normal thyroid tissue is atrophied in the hyperthyroid patient because of lack of stimulation by thyroid-stimulating hormone, does not accumulate radioiodine, and thus is spared. After radioiodine therapy, patients go through a period of subclinical hypothyroidism that is almost always asymptomatic and does not require therapy in the vast majority of patients. During this period, thyroid-stimulating hormone secretion resumes, the atrophied thyroid tissue becomes functional, and the patient then becomes euthyroid.

The radioisotope used in the treatment of hyperthyroidism is ^{131}I. It is available widely as a liquid that can be given as a single subcutaneous injection, eliminating the stress of intravenous catheter placement, and reducing the radiation exposure to workers.[17] Mild sedation is required in only the most fractious of patients; usually the procedure can be performed as simply as a vaccination.

[131]I has a relatively short half-life (8 days), and is both a beta and a gamma emitter. The beta radiation is mainly responsible for the therapeutic effect, and has a very short penetration in tissue (effective range, 50 μm; maximum range, 300 μm). This results in very localized damage to abnormal tissue, and spares atrophied thyroid tissue and the parathyroid glands. Therefore, hypocalcemia does not occur secondary to radioiodine therapy, and permanent hypothyroidism usually occurs only when patients are given very large doses of radioiodine, for example, for ablative therapy for known thyroid carcinomas.

Radioiodine may be given as a fixed dose of 3 to 4 mCi per cat, or the dosage may be estimated for an individual patient based on the T_4 level, the approximate volume of abnormal thyroid tissue, and the severity of the cat's clinical signs. Using this method, doses ranging from 2 to 6 mCi are given, at the clinician's discretion.[5] Sophisticated studies of individual patient thyroid kinetics using a tracer dose of radioiodine to calculate the treatment dose can be done, but have not been shown to increase efficacy.[18] These studies also are time-consuming, expose workers to additional radiation, and may require sedation.

The ideal dose of radioiodine should be such that the largest possible number of patients are rendered euthyroid after 1 injection, and the risk of permanent hypothyroidism is kept to a minimum. In 1 study of 524 cats, 90 per cent of cats were euthyroid at 3 months after treatment, 5 per cent of cats remained hyperthyroid, and 5 per cent were persistently hypothyroid at 4 to 6 months after treatment. Of the persistently hypothyroid cats, approximately 2 per cent required long-term L-thyroxine supplementation (0.05 to 0.15 mg q 12 to 24 hr).[5] Almost all of the cats that remained hyperthyroid were cured after a second treatment. It is thought that some of these cats were resistant to the first treatment because they had very large volumes of functional tissue.

The major disadvantage of radioiodine therapy is its lack of accessibility. Whereas the therapy is simple and relatively stress-free for patients, it does require special licensing, hospitalization facilities, nuclear medicine equipment, and extensive compliance with local and state radiation safety laws. Clinicians handling radioisotopes must observe proper monitoring and safety precautions to prevent self-contamination and health hazards.

Cats treated with radioiodine must be hospitalized for a period of time after treatment, depending on local laws. This hospitalization is done to protect people from radiation exposure, not because the cats require medical care. The hospitalization period varies from cat to cat, and usually is approximately 7 to 10 days for cats treated with typical radioiodine dosages. Cats treated with higher dosages (e.g., for functional thyroid carcinoma) may require longer hospitalization periods. One study showed that 74 per cent of cats treated with radioiodine were euthyroid by the eighth posttreatment day.[19] Therefore, thioureylene drugs are not required after treatment. Cats that are severely symptomatic can be given beta-adrenergic blocking drugs if necessary after treatment until they become euthyroid. The T_4 level, as well as the blood urea nitrogen and creatinine, should be measured at 1 month and 3 months after treatment. If preexisting renal disease is unmasked, appropriate supportive care such as fluid and dietary therapy should be instituted. In patients that develop significant azotemia, blood pressure should be monitored in case antihypertension drugs are required. Patients that are not euthyroid by 3 months after radioiodine therapy probably will require retreatment, although a few patients will become euthyroid as late as 6 months after the procedure.[6] Once patients are rendered euthyroid, owners should be advised to seek a physical examination, blood count, urinalysis, and chemistry profile biannually for their cats, because most patients are elderly and at risk for the development of other health problems.

Owners must obey some safety precautions after their cat is discharged following ^{131}I treatment. These precautions are dictated by state and local laws, and are designed to protect human beings from excessive radiation exposure. These laws usually require keeping the cat strictly indoors for a period of time after treatment (e.g., 2 weeks), spell out the amount of contact time each person should have with the cat daily during this period (10 to 30 minutes per person), and dictate how the cat's waste should be disposed of. If the cat becomes ill during the quarantine period (a very rare occurrence when patients are selected carefully), it should be remembered that contact of veterinary personnel with the cat also should be limited, and special arrangements may be required for hospitalization. Clinical laboratories may decline to accept samples from patients during the quarantine period.

Surgery

Hyperthyroidism is a disease of middle-aged, or more frequently, elderly cats. It is a polysystemic disease, and may cause profound morbidity in many organ systems, resulting in cardiac, renal, hepatic, gastrointestinal, and neuroendocrine dysfunction. Hyperthyroid cats also are typically emaciated and in poor body condition. For these reasons, hyperthyroid cats generally are very poor anesthetic and surgical risks. One study reports a 9 per cent intraoperative and perioperative mortality rate.[20] However, with careful preoperative stabilization and postoperative management, surgical treatment of feline hyperthyroidism can yield very good results. If preoperative technetium scanning could be done to identify patients with bilateral or ectopic thyroid tissue, surgical therapy could be improved greatly.

However, when nuclear scanning facilities are available, treatment with radioiodine usually is chosen.

Thioureylene drugs usually are given for 6 to 12 weeks before surgery, until clinical signs of hyperthyroidism have abated, and weight gain and improvement in the cat's condition are seen.[6] Beta-blocking drugs may be administered if tachycardia or supraventricular arrhythmias persist, or if the patient is hypertensive. Stable iodine may be given for 10 to 14 days before surgery to help decrease vascularity of the thyroid gland.[10] This may be a particularly helpful adjunctive treatment, because thioureylene drugs may cause a bleeding diathesis in some patients, even when platelet counts are normal.[13] The cause of this coagulopathy is unknown, but has been suspected to be caused by a platelet function defect.[21] These cats may bleed excessively from venipuncture sites and during surgery, so the surgeon should be prepared to provide careful hemostasis. This is important to allow identification and preservation of the parathyroid glands.[20]

The fact that approximately 70 per cent of hyperthyroid cats have bilateral disease is a critical issue when selecting patients for thyroidectomy. Two of the most significant complications of thyroidectomy, postsurgical hypocalcemia and failure to become or remain euthyroid, relate directly to the presence or absence of bilateral disease. Also, without a nuclear medicine scan, it may be difficult for a surgeon to decide whether bilateral disease is present at the time of cervical exploration, unless both glands are grossly enlarged. The surgical procedure chosen, either intracapsular or extracapsular removal, also has bearing on the incidence of postsurgical complications. The intracapsular technique may allow greater preservation of the parathyroid glands, and consequently, less risk of postoperative hypocalcemia. However, because it is difficult to remove all thyroid tissue with this technique, a higher rate of relapse after surgery has been reported (8 per cent in one study).[20]

Postsurgical hypocalcemia due to parathyroid gland injury or removal is the most serious side-effect of thyroidectomy. This life-threatening complication usually occurs within 1 to 4 days after surgery, and occurred in 15 per cent of cats when the intracapsular technique was used in one study.[20] Of these cats, 27 per cent required treatment.[20] A technique has been described for autotransplantation of the parathyroid glands that reduces the duration of postoperative hypocalcemia. This procedure does not prevent the development of acute hypocalcemia, so careful postoperative monitoring still must be done.[22]

Patients that undergo bilateral thyroidectomy should have their serum calcium levels checked every day for approximately 7 days after surgery, or until values have stabilized within the normal range.[6] Many patients that undergo unilateral or bilateral thyroidectomy will have subnormal serum calcium levels for several days after surgery. These patients usually do not require therapy. Patients that have clinical signs of hypocalcemia (restlessness, behavior changes, muscle pain or twitching, or seizures) should be treated immediately. Cats that have blood calcium levels below 6.5 mg/dl should be treated even if asymptomatic. Hypoparathyroidism may be permanent if both parathyroid glands are severely damaged or removed. Many cats regain parathyroid function days to months after the procedure. This may be due to repair of damage to the glands, secretion of parathyroid hormone from ectopic sites, or compensatory changes in other calcium-regulating systems.[23]

Treatment for hypocalcemia involves both acute and chronic (maintenance) therapy. Severe acute hypocalcemia is a life-threatening medical emergency. Patients exhibiting signs of hypocalcemia should receive a slow intravenous infusion of calcium to effect. A 10 per cent calcium gluconate solution is given at a dose of 5 to 15 mg/kg over a 10- to 30-minute period, ideally with electrocardiographic monitoring. Bradycardia, premature ventricular contractions, shortening of the Q-T interval, and bradyarrhythmias are indications that the infusion should be stopped briefly and then slowed further.[5]

The duration of action of intravenous bolus calcium replacement is quite short (1 to 12 hours). Maintenance therapy with oral calcium supplementation and vitamin D therapy has an onset of action of about 24 to 96 hours, and should be started as soon as the patient is adequately stable to receive it. In the interim, subcutaneous calcium gluconate is given to prevent recurrence of hypocalcemia. The drug is diluted in an equal volume of saline and given at a dose of 5 to 15 mg/kg q 6 to 8 hr as necessary to maintain the serum calcium levels in the 8 to 9 mg/dl range. Serum calcium is monitored every 48 hours, and if stable, the subcutaneous calcium injections are tapered off over several days.

The aim of oral maintenance therapy is to stabilize the serum calcium levels in the low-normal range. This, hopefully, will allow stimulation of any remaining parathyroid tissue, and recovery of function. If hypercalcemia occurs, maintenance therapy should be adjusted downward, because hypercalcemia may exacerbate occult renal disease, and will prevent stimulation of parathyroid tissue, delaying or preventing return to function.

Maintenance therapy entails administration of oral calcium concurrently with vitamin D. Usually, oral calcium is required only for a few weeks; then dietary calcium provides adequate levels in patients that are eating well. Most cats require calcium supplementation at a dose of approximately 25 to 50 mg/kg/day. Proprietary antacid tablets, such as Tums, are inexpensive and readily available sources for calcium supplementation. One to 2 tablets, crushed and divided into 3 or 4 daily doses, usually suffice.

The ideal source for vitamin D supplementation is reported to be calcitriol (Rocaltrol, Roche Laboratories).[21] This drug has a more rapid onset of action and a shorter duration of action than other vitamin D preparations. Hypercalcemia is the significant toxic effect of vitamin D therapy. Toxicity caused by calcitriol usage can be corrected more easily than with that due to other vitamin preparations, because it is active for 2 to 14 days, versus 7 to 21 days with other products such as dihydrotachysterol (DHT, Roxane). Rocaltrol has been used at a dose of one 0.25-μg capsule PO q 48 hr. After 2 to 3 weeks of therapy, many hypocalcemic cats regain calcium homeostasis, and an attempt can be made to taper them off vitamin D therapy. Serum calcium levels should be monitored closely for several weeks after discontinuation, and vitamin D and possibly calcium therapy resumed if hypocalcemia recurs.

Surgical thyroidectomy also may cause neurologic impairment if the cervical sympathetic trunk or recurrent laryngeal nerves are damaged. This is an infrequent complication, but may result in Horner's syndrome, dysphonia, laryngeal paralysis, and potentially airway dysfunction or obstruction.[21] Patients, particularly those that receive bilateral thyroidectomy, should be monitored carefully after extubation, and during the anesthetic recovery period.

It also has been recommended that cats undergoing bilateral thyroidectomy receive 0.1 to 0.2 mg of L-thyroxine daily to prevent iatrogenic hypothyroidism.[5] Thyroid levels should be checked periodically, and an attempt should be made to wean the cat off supplementation in the weeks or months after surgery.

Ultrasound-Guided Percutaneous Ethanol Injection

Injection of 96 per cent ethanol into tissue causes necrosis and death. Several studies have been done to explore the feasibility and efficacy of percutaneous ethanol injection (PEI) treatment in hyperthyroid cats with both unilateral and bilateral disease.[24, 25] Each cat underwent a nuclear medicine scan to rule out the presence of ectopic thyroid tissue. The cats were anesthetized, and a target dose of ethanol equaling approximately 50 per cent of the volume of the gland was injected. A 10-MHz transducer was used to both locate the abnormal tissue and monitor the ethanol instillation. The cats with unilateral disease became euthyroid within 48 hours of injection, and remained so for the 1-month follow-up period. Of the cats with bilateral disease, 1 died within 12 hours of bilateral injection, possibly due to laryngeal paralysis. Five additional cats were treated by having only the larger of their goiters injected initially. These cats became euthyroid within 72 hours of treatment but 1 cat relapsed within 2 weeks of the first injection. One to 4 additional injections were done to treat the remaining goitrous tissue after the larger nodules were treated in all surviving cats. Hypocalcemia was not identified in any cat. The follow-up period in this study was short, but 4 of 5 cats were still euthyroid several weeks after treatment.

Instillation of a necrotizing substance into tissues can be expected to cause inflammation and local tissue reaction. Cats treated with PEI experienced dysphonia, recurrent gagging and dysphagia, laryngeal paralysis, and Horner's syndrome. These changes were transient, and resolved 4 to 8 weeks after the last injection. The procedure requires general anesthesia, and may need to be repeated multiple times. Unless a nuclear medicine scan is performed, there also is a risk of subjecting patients with ectopic tissue to the procedure. As discussed previously, acute correction of the hyperthyroid state may prevent adequate renal autoregulation, so rapid correction of the hyperthyroid state may not be desirable. As with other potentially permanent forms of treatment, it would seem prudent to render patients euthyroid through medical means and evaluate renal function before proceeding.

Ultrasound-guided PEI requires a highly skilled ultrasonographer and specialized probes. It is crucial that the operator identify placement of the needle and monitor instillation of the ethanol, so as not to damage surrounding normal tissues. In carefully selected patients with unilateral disease, PEI may be superior to surgical treatment, because the side-effects after a single unilateral injection may be minimal. In patients with bilateral disease, side-effects seem to be more serious, and multiple treatments are required. Also, because follow-up times are short, it is unknown whether patients will remain euthyroid for prolonged periods. As with intracapsular thyroidectomy, remnants of viable tissue that remain may regenerate to the extent that hyperthyroidism recurs.[20]

REFERENCES

1. Broussard JD, Peterson ME, Fox PR: Changes in clinical and laboratory findings in cats with hyperthyroidism from 1983 to 1993. J Am Vet Med Assoc 206:302–305, 1995.
2. Refsal KR, Nachreiner RF, Stein BE, et al: Use of the triodothyronine suppression test for diagnosis of hyperthyroidism in ill cats that have serum concentration of iodothyronines within normal range. J Am Vet Med Assoc 199:1594–1601, 1991.
3. Graves TK, Olivier NB, Nachreiner RF, et al: Changes in renal function associated with treatment of hyperthyroidism in cats. Am J Vet Res 55:1745–1749, 1994.
4. Graves TK: Hyperthyroidism and the kidney. In August JR (ed): Consultations in Feline Internal Medicine, vol. 3. Philadelphia, WB Saunders, 1997, pp. 345–348.
5. Peterson ME: Hyperthyroidism. In Ettinger SJ, Feldman EC (eds): Textbook of Veterinary Internal Medicine: Diseases of the Dog and Cat, 5th ed. Philadelphia, WB Saunders, 2000, pp. 1400–1419.
6. Feldman EC, Nelson RW: Feline hyperthyroidism. In Feldman EC, Nelson RW (eds): Canine and Feline Endocrinology and Reproduction, 2nd ed. Philadelphia, WB Saunders, 1996, pp. 118–166.
7. Larsen PR, Davies TF, Hay ID: The thyroid gland. In Williams RH, Wilson JD (eds): Williams Textbook of Endocrinology, 9th ed. Philadelphia, WB Saunders, 1998, pp. 389–515.
8. Skinner ND: Thyroid hormone levels in cats: Colony average and the decrease with age. J Nutr 28:2636S–2638S, 1998.

9. Broome MR, Feldman EC, Turrel JM: Serial determination of thyroxine concentrations in hyperthyroid cats. J Am Vet Med Assoc 192:49–51, 1998.

10. Mooney CT: Update on the medical management of hyperthyroidism. *In* August JR (ed): Consultations in Feline Internal Medicine, vol. 3. Philadelphia, WB Saunders, 1997, pp. 155–162.

11. Murray LAS, Peterson ME: Ipodate treatment of hyperthyroidism in cats. J Am Vet Med Assoc 211:63–67, 1997.

12. Behrend EN: Medical therapy of feline hyperthyroidism. Compend Contin Ed Pract Vet 21:235–244, 1999.

13. Peterson ME, Kintzer PP, Hurvitz AI: Methimazole treatment of 262 cats with hyperthyroidism. J Vet Intern Med 2:150–157, 1988.

14. Shelton GD, Joseph R, Richter K, et al: Acquired myasthenia gravis in hyperthyroid cats on tapazole therapy. J Vet Intern Med 2:120, 1997.

15. Mooney CT, Thoday KL: CVT update: Medical treatment of hyperthyroidism in cats. *In* Bonagura JD (ed): Current Veterinary Therapy XIII: Small Animal Practice. Philadelphia, WB Saunders, 2000, pp. 333–337.

16. Plumb DC: Veterinary Drug Handbook, 2nd ed. Ames, IA, Distributed by Iowa State University Press, 1995.

17. Théon AP, Van Vechten MK, Feldman E: Prospective randomized comparison of intravenous versus subcutaneous administration of radioiodine for treatment of hyperthyroidism in cats. Am J Vet Res 55:1734–1738, 1994.

18. Broome MR, Turrel JM, Hays MT: Predictive value of tracer studies for ^{131}I treatment in hyperthyroid cats. Am J Vet Res 49:193–197, 1988.

19. Meric SM, Hawkins EC, Washabau RJ, et al: Serum thyroxine concentrations after radioactive iodine therapy in cats with hyperthyroidism. J Am Vet Med Assoc 188:1038–1040, 1986.

20. Birchard SJ, Peterson ME, Jacobson A: Surgical treatment of feline hyperthyroidism: Results of 85 cases. J Am Anim Hosp Assoc 20:705–709, 1984.

21. Graves TK: Complications of treatment and concurrent illness associated with hyperthyroidism in cats. *In* Bonagura JD, Kirk RW (eds): Current Veterinary Therapy XII: Small Animal Practice. Philadelphia, WB Saunders, 1995, pp. 369–372.

22. Padgett SL, Tobias KM, Leathers CW, et al: Efficacy of parathyroid gland autotransplantation in maintaining serum calcium concentrations after bilateral thyroparathyroidectomy in cats. J Am Anim Hosp Assoc 34:219–224, 1998.

23. Flanders JA, Harvey HJ, Erb HN: Feline thyroidectomy. A comparison of postoperative hypocalcemia associated with three different surgical techniques. Vet Surg 16:362–366, 1987.

24. Goldstein RE, Long CD, Feldman WJ, et al: Ultrasound guided percutaneous ethanol injection (PEI) for the treatment of 4 cats with unilateral hyperthyroidism. J Vet Intern Med 13:241, 1999.

25. Wells AL, Long CD, Feldman WJ, et al: Ultrasound guided percutaneous ethanol injection (PEI) for the treatment of 6 cats with bilateral hyperthyroidism. J Vet Intern Med 13:242, 1999.

20

◆ Adrenocortical Disease

Ellen N. Behrend
Robert J. Kemppainen

Feline adrenal diseases are uncommon. For example at the University of California at Davis, 34 cats with hyperadrenocorticism (HAC) had been diagnosed over a 10-year period, while over 800 dogs with Cushing's syndrome were examined in the same time span.[1] Despite the scarcity of cases, knowledge of feline adrenal diseases is important. These syndromes can be fatal, and proper recognition is required in order to commence treatment in a timely manner.

◆ HYPERADRENOCORTICISM

Hypercortisolism

(Please note: The information below reflects a summary of the data available on approximately 58 cats. In at least one instance, a few cats were included in 2 reports. Unfortunately, it was not possible to always determine which data pertained to which cats in the reports, so some cats may have been included twice in the numbers in Table 20–1 pertaining to historical and physical examination data. Because this applies to 2 or 3 cats, the data should not be skewed greatly.)

Confirmed, spontaneous HAC (Cushing's syndrome) has been reported in approximately 88 cats since 1975[1–25] and was suspected in 2 others.[26, 27] Of these, 84 per cent (41/49) had pituitary-dependent hyperadrenocorticism (PDH), and the remainder had adrenal tumors (ATs). Histopathology was not available on all cats with PDH. Six were known microadenomas, 7 macroadenomas, and 1 pituitary carcinoma.[3, 5, 10, 11, 14, 17, 23] In 1 case, the adenoma was localized to the pars intermedia.[17] Given the reported paucity of clinical signs that would be expected with a macroadenoma, for example, anorexia, disorientation, it is likely the majority are microadenomas. Of 14 cats with an AT, 7 were benign and 7 malignant.[1, 3, 6, 10, 12, 18, 25] In 1 cat, an adrenal adenoma was removed, and another developed in the contralateral gland over the ensuing 10 months.[10]

Of 42 cats diagnosed with HAC, 19 (45 per cent) were spayed females and 18 (43 per cent) were castrated males. There were also 2 (5 per cent) females and 3 (7 per cent) males whose neuter status was not stated. Of 40 cats, the average age was 10 years, with a reported range of 4.5 to 15 years. The breeds represented included domestic shorthair (11), domestic longhair (3), Siamese (4), Persian (1), Devon rex (1), and Abyssinian (1), and 23 were of mixed breeding.

Polyuria/polydipsia, polyphagia, weight loss, and lethargy were the most common historical findings (see Table 20–1). Because cats receiving exogenous steroids typically are not polyuric and polydipsic,[28–30] whether polydipsia/polyuria in HAC is due to concurrence of diabetes mellitus or to Cushing's syndrome alone was debated previously. However, 4 cats with Cushing's syndrome but not with diabetes mellitus were polyuric/polydipsic.[6, 18, 20] Decreased appetite was noted in 2 cats. In dogs, inappetance in a cushingoid patient is suspicious for the presence of a pituitary macroadenoma.[1] Whether anorexia in a cat with Cushing's syndrome also may signify a large pituitary tumor is unclear. Although 1 anorectic cat had PDH, the size of the mass was unknown[6]; the other cat had a pituitary macroadenoma but also had a pancreatic tumor that may have contributed to the poor appetite.[9]

On physical examination, enlarged abdomen was the most common finding, followed by alopecia (spontaneous) and thin skin (see Table 20–1). Skin changes were a prominent finding, including alopecia, easily torn skin, a rough or dry hair coat, seborrhea, cutaneous hyperpigmentation, and folded pinnae. Besides spontaneous alopecia, failure to regrow hair after clipping also was noted.[23] Easily torn skin may be a dramatic finding, and routine hospital or grooming procedures can cause large wounds. Although overall the reported incidence of easily torn skin is relatively low (26 per cent), 1 report found an incidence of 48 per cent.[31] The presence of infections or abscesses was a historical or physical examination finding in approximately 19 of 47 cats (40 per cent); sites affected included the urinary tract, upper and lower respiratory tract, skin, kidneys, and oral cavity. Urinary tract candidiasis was seen in 1 cat,[16] as well as disseminated candidiasis and toxoplasmosis in another.[17]

On routine bloodwork, a stress leukogram was not a common finding overall (Table 20–2), but lymphopenia was the most consistent change. Hyperglycemia was the most common biochemical change. In early reports, almost 100 per cent of cushingoid cats were diabetic. Although this is no longer true, it appears that the majority (82 per cent) are diabetic. However, even though cortisol can antagonize the actions of insulin, not all diabetic, cushingoid cats are insulin-resistant.[6–8, 10, 23] Elevations in liver enzyme concentrations are relatively common, oc-

Table 20–1. Clinical Findings in Cats With Spontaneous Hyperadrenocorticism[2–20, 23, 25]

Clinical Findings	Number of Cats (%)
Historical Findings	
Polyuria/polydipsia	52/58 (90)
Polyphagia	40/58 (69)
Weight loss	20/58 (34)
Lethargy	18/58 (31)
Weight gain	6/58 (10)
Depression	3/58 (5)
Abnormal gait	3/58 (5)
Constipation	2/58 (3)
Decreased appetite	2/58 (3)
Panting	2/58 (3)
Diarrhea	2/58 (3)
Vomiting	1/58 (2)
Physical Examination Findings	
Enlarged abdomen	41/55 (75)
Alopecia	34/58 (59)
Thin skin	25/55 (45)
Muscle atrophy	24/58 (41)
Rough or dry hair coat	17/55 (31)
Obesity	17/58 (29)
Hepatomegaly	16/55 (29)
Easily torn skin	15/58 (26)
Seborrhea	4/55 (7)
Palpable abdominal mass	3/55 (5)
Cutaneous hyperpigmentation	2/55 (4)
Folded pinnae	1/55 (2)

curring in just under 50 per cent of cases. Like polyuria/polydipsia, this was suspected to be due mainly to diabetes mellitus, but increases may be seen in nondiabetic cushingoid cats.[6] Changes in alkaline phosphatase are not as common as in dogs, because cats are believed not to have a corticosteroid-induced isoenzyme. Hypercholesterolemia also

Table 20–2. Clinicopathologic Results in Cats With Spontaneous Hyperadrenocorticism[2–20, 23, 25]

Test	Number of Cats (%)
Complete Blood Count	
Lymphopenia	23/36 (64)
Eosinopenia	14/36 (39)
Neutrophilia	14/36 (39)
Monocytosis	6/36 (17)
Anemia	4/32 (13)
Leukocytosis	4/33 (12)
Neutropenia	2/36 (6)
Lymphocytosis	1/36 (3)
Biochemical Profile	
Hyperglycemia	49/53 (92)
Diabetes mellitus	47/57 (82)
Elevated alanine aminotransferase	17/34 (50)
Elevated aspartate transaminase	4/9 (44)
Elevated alkaline phosphatase	12/38 (32)
Decreased total thyroxine	3/10 (30)
Elevated blood urea nitrogen	7/32 (22)
Elevated total bilirubin	3/17 (18)
Hypocalcemia	3/24 (13)
Elevated creatinine	3/25 (12)
Hypercalcemia	1/24 (4)

is a common finding, perhaps occurring in as many as 50 per cent of cases.[24, 25]

Abdominal radiography was performed in 29 cats.[6–8, 11–13, 18, 24, 25] Hepatomegaly was the most common finding in 18 out of 23 (78 per cent). In 4 of 5 evaluations of cats with an AT, a mass was identified cranial to the kidneys.[6, 12, 13] In 1 case with PDH, bilateral adrenal calcification was noted.[7] Although this was likely due to the Cushing's disease, adrenal calcification may occur in up to 30 per cent of normal cats.[24] On abdominal ultrasonography, bilaterally enlarged adrenal glands were noted in 11 of 17 cats with PDH.[6–10, 13, 24] In 1 cat, only 1 adrenal gland was visualized, and in another neither was, probably due to the difficulty of imaging feline adrenal glands.[6] Adrenal size was judged to be normal in the rest.[9, 24] All examinations of 4 cats with an AT revealed the tumor, but it also was visible radiographically.[6, 12, 13] Computed tomography has been performed in 11 cats. In 10 cats with PDH, a pituitary tumor was seen in 8 with or without contrast. In 2, bilateral adrenal enlargement was noted as well.[10, 23–25] In a cat with an AT, a right adrenal mass and normal pituitary were seen.[24]

For definitive diagnosis, adrenal function testing must be performed. Please consult the later section on this topic.

For medical therapy, previous reports suggested mitotane (Lysodren) was not as effective in cats as in dogs. In a study of 4 normal cats receiving mitotane (25, 37 or 50 mg/kg divided every [q] 12 hr orally [PO] for 7 days), 2 did not respond and 2 had a progressive decrease in response to adrenocorticotropic hormone (ACTH) stimulation with each increasing dose, but 1 cat suppressed only 44 per cent. One cat also developed signs consistent with drug toxicity.[11] Three cats with Cushing's syndrome did not show any clinical response with doses of 25 mg/kg and/or 50 mg/kg PO for up to 90 days.[1, 13, 25] One report, however, suggested that mitotane therapy may be successful with higher doses and longer induction periods. A cat was treated with mitotane at 25 mg/kg q 24 hr for 18 days with little effect. At 69 days after a dose increase to 37.5 mg/kg daily, there was still minimum effect, but by day 111, the Cushing's syndrome was controlled.[7]

Use of ketoconazole in cats with Cushing's syndrome has been limited. In dogs, a survey of internists and dermatologists found that ketoconazole is not highly effective, as 71.2 per cent believed the drug to be effective in less than 50 per cent of affected dogs.[32] In 1 cat with an adrenocortical carcinoma, ketoconazole caused transient (3.5 months) resolution of polyuria/polydipsia and a reduction in the insulin dose required to control concurrent diabetes mellitus. Interestingly, basal cortisol concentrations decreased during treatment, but adrenocortical response to ACTH stimulation was not altered.[12] Other mechanisms of action of ketoconazole, such as antagonism of glucocorticoid receptors, may account for the clinical improvement, or it may have been coincidental. In 4 other cats, 2 responded to doses of 5 mg/kg q 12 hr for 7 days followed by 10 mg/kg q 12 hr indefinitely, 1 had no response after 2 months, and 1 developed severe thrombocytopenia after 7 days of treatment necessitating withdrawal of therapy.[33]

Metyrapone affects cortisol synthesis through inhibition of 11-β-hydroxylase and has been used in 4 cats with Cushing's syndrome.[8, 21, 25] One cat treated with 65 mg/kg q 8 hr for 6 months improved clinically according to the owner.[25] In 2 cats treated with an unknown dose, 1 had a slight clinical improvement (partial regrowth of hair and slight resolution of polyuria and polydipsia) after 6 months, whereas the other showed no improvement after 1 month.[21] For the fourth cat, toxicity occurred at a dose of 65 mg/kg q 8 hr but the cat was treated successfully at a dose of 65 mg/kg q 12 hr as evidenced by amelioration of clinical signs and decreased ACTH response. After 24 days, therapy was discontinued and adrenalectomy performed.[8]

In 1 cat with a large pituitary mass, cobalt irradiation, with 12 doses over 4 weeks, was performed after the cat failed to respond to mitotane. The cat deteriorated steadily, however, and was euthanatized 1 month after completion of therapy.

Owing to difficulties with medical therapy, unilateral and bilateral adrenalectomy for treatment of AT or PDH, respectively, has been advocated and has been performed 27 times in 26 cats, 20 with PDH[4, 6, 8, 10, 15, 19, 25] and 7 with AT (2 adenocarcinoma, 4 adenoma, 1 unknown).[6, 10, 18, 24, 25] One cat had 2 unilateral adrenalectomies 10 months apart for removal of an adrenal adenoma.[10] Surgical management appears to be effective overall. Survival longer than 1 month was reported in 21 surgeries (78 per cent). Cause of death within the first month in 5 cats, 4 that underwent bilateral adrenalectomy for PDH and 1 with unilateral adrenalectomy for adrenal adenocarcinoma, included a suspected hypoadrenal crisis, suspected renal failure,[6] development of chylothorax secondary to extensive thrombosis of the cranial vena cava, severe pancreatitis and septic peritonitis, and sloughing of large regions of skin.[10] The latter 2 cases were debilitated before surgery, which may have contributed to mortality.[10]

For those cats that lived past the first month postoperatively, reported survival times range from 3 to more than 60 months.[4, 6, 10, 15, 18] Cause of death in 2 that underwent bilateral adrenalectomy was a suspected addisonian crisis due to poor owner compliance with giving prescribed medications.[10] One cat improved for 2 months after bilateral adrenalectomy, and then developed acute signs of circling, wandering aimlessly, and blindness. The cat was euthanatized without necropsy, but an expanding pituitary tumor was suspected.[25] Renal failure was the reason for euthanasia in 2 cats at 3 and 12 months postoperatively. In the latter, regrowth of an adrenocortical carcinoma was noted at necropsy with extensive metastases.[10] Interestingly, although bilateral adrenalectomy is recommended for PDH,

unilateral adrenalectomy in 1 cat with PDH ameliorated clinical signs for at least 3 months.[15]

For cats with extensive morbidity due to Cushing's syndrome, medical therapy for stabilization before surgery may be beneficial if possible.[8] Difficulty arises in choosing a medication owing to varied efficacies. Metyrapone, if available, may be the medication of choice. Treatment of cats during and after surgery relates to the type of surgery. Diabetic cats should receive 50 per cent of their usual insulin dose the morning of surgery. With unilateral or bilateral adrenalectomy, treatment with glucocorticoids during and after surgery is required. In cats with an AT, the contralateral adrenal gland will be atrophied due to constant negative feedback by the tumor on the pituitary decreasing ACTH secretion. At the time of anesthetic induction, a continuous infusion of hydrocortisone (625 μg/kg/hr) should be initiated and should continue for 24 to 48 hours postoperatively. At that time, prednisone (2.5 mg, PO q 12 hr) should be administered.[10] In cats with unilateral surgery, recovery of the unaffected gland with time is expected and glucocorticoid therapy can be withdrawn slowly. Mineralocorticoids are recommended for all cats undergoing bilateral adrenalectomy, beginning when the hydrocortisone infusion is discontinued.[10] Fludrocortisone or desoxycorticosterone pivalate (see later for treatment of hypoadrenocorticism) may be used. Because 3 cats died postoperatively due to a suspected hypoadrenal crisis, the importance of continuing therapy must be communicated to the owner.

Interestingly, in 11 out of 21 cats (52 per cent) in which therapy was tried and long-term follow-up was available, diabetes mellitus resolved with successful treatment of Cushing's syndrome.[6-8, 10, 15, 19] This compares with dogs in which therapy is expected to alleviate insulin resistance, but resolution of the diabetes mellitus is rare. If the diabetes mellitus does not resolve, treatment should decrease daily insulin requirements.[12, 13, 25] Other clinical signs typically resolve 2 to 4 months after control of Cushing's syndrome.

Thus, in summary, HAC should be suspected in cats that are diabetic and have an enlarged abdomen, alopecia, and/or thin skin. Surgery is the therapy of choice—unilateral adrenalectomy for AT and bilateral adrenalectomy for PDH. Metyrapone may be the best medical treatment option. Mitotane may be more effective than previously believed, but extended periods of time may be necessary before an effect is seen.

Hyperprogesteronism

Recently, a progesterone-secreting adrenal mass was reported in a cat with clinical signs of HAC.[34] A 7-year-old cat had a 9-month history of nonpruritic, bilaterally symmetric alopecia that eventually involved the abdomen, flanks, ventral thorax, axilla, inguinal area, and medial and caudal thighs. Polyuria/polydipsia and aggression also were seen eventually. Physical examination revealed alopecia with a greasy unkempt coat and scale elsewhere, comedones at the oral commissures, and thin skin with easily visible blood vessels in the inguinal area. Bruising readily at venipuncture sites was noted on subsequent visits.[34]

Serum glucose was normal initially, but hyperglycemia developed over time. A mild azotemia with inappropriate concentrating ability, glycosuria, hypernatremia, and hypokalemia also were noted. Skin biopsy was consistent with an endocrinopathy. Results of an ACTH stimulation test were consistent with iatrogenic hypoadrenocorticism because the cortisol response to ACTH was blunted, but no history of exogenous glucocorticoid administration existed. The results of a dexamethasone suppression test (0.1 mg/kg) and thyrotropin stimulation test were normal.[34]

Abdominal ultrasonography revealed a left adrenal gland mass. Measurement of sex steroids before and after ACTH stimulation revealed marked hyperprogesteronemia in comparison to a clinically normal cat. Unilateral adrenalectomy was performed, and histopathology was consistent with an adrenocortical carcinoma. The contralateral adrenal gland was not visualized at surgery.[34] Because progesterone can suppress ACTH secretion,[35] the right adrenal gland had presumably atrophied.

Postoperatively, the hyperglycemia and electrolyte abnormalities resolved. After 4 months, an ACTH stimulation test demonstrated resolution of the hyperprogesteronemia, and the hair coat was improving. The cat was receiving 1.25 mg prednisone PO daily. At 1 year after surgery, the cat's hair coat was normal; therapy for chronic renal failure was ongoing.[34] Whether glucocorticoid therapy was continued is unclear. However, it is likely that such therapy could be discontinued with time. Removal of the tumor should have led to restoration of endogenous ACTH secretion and, therefore, adrenal recovery.

Hyperaldosteronism

Three cases of primary hyperaldosteronism have been published since 1983 in a 1-year-old[36] and a 2-year-old spayed female,[37] and in a 10-year-old castrated male cat.[37] Historical complaints and physical examination findings included polydipsia (2 cats), nocturia (1), polyuria (1), generalized weakness, collapse, and anorexia (1), weight loss (1), a pendulous abdomen (1), and blindness (1).[36, 37] Two cats had bilateral retinal detachments and hypertension,[37] but a retinal examination and measurement of blood pressure were not reported in the third.[36] A heart murmur and left anterior fascicular bundle branch block were found in 2 cats and echocardiography showed cardiac hypertrophy.[37] The other cat had a Mobitz type I second-degree atrioventricular block.[36]

Two cats were diagnosed with primary hyper-

aldosteronism on the basis of marked hyperaldosteronemia (at least 6 times higher than normal) in conjunction with hypertension, hypokalemia, inappropriate kaliuresis (urinary fractional excretion of potassium at least 6 times normal), normal plasma renin activity, ultrasonographic confirmation of an adrenal mass, and cytologic and/or histopathologic diagnosis of adrenocortical neoplasia.[37] In the other cat, the diagnosis was made on the basis of serum aldosterone concentration at least 6 times normal in the face of normal serum renin concentration, inappropriate kaliuresis, and hypokalemia.[36] On initial biochemical analysis, hypernatremia, increased serum bicarbonate,[37] and elevated creatine phosphokinase level[36] were noted in 1 cat each. One cat was diabetic,[37] and 1 had glycosuria despite normoglycemia.[36] Serum thyroxine was normal in 2 cats, and a dexamethasone suppression test with 0.1 mg/kg dexamethasone was normal in 1.[37] Two cats had mild renal disease,[37] which could account, at least in part, for the abnormalities in serum potassium and aldosterone.

Unilateral adrenalectomy was performed in 1 cat. Prior therapy with diltiazem and potassium gluconate was partially successful—systemic blood pressure decreased and was intermittently normal, but the cat remained hypokalemic. Histopathology was consistent with adrenocortical tumor, probably a carcinoma. Approximately 2 weeks after surgery, serum potassium normalized, and urinary potassium excretion decreased but was still elevated. Serum aldosterone and hypertension normalized by day 41 postoperatively, but bilateral retinal detachment was found at this recheck, suggesting persistent intermittent hypertension of unknown cause. The cat did well for another year without medication. Necropsy was not permitted, so cause of death or whether the tumor recurred is unknown.

In the other cats, spironolactone and potassium supplementation were prescribed. In 1 cat, this led to normokalemia but hypertension persisted, even with the addition of amlodipine to the treatment regimen. Seven months after diagnosis, the cat was euthanatized after a thromboembolic episode.[37] In the other cat, spironolactone and potassium chloride therapy caused potassium to increase to within or just below the normal range and resolution of clinical signs. The cat was euthanatized 4 months after initial presentation owing to a progressive azotemia of 1 month's duration. On necropsy, the right adrenal gland was enlarged, and the left could not be identified; histopathology of the right gland was consistent with adrenocortical carcinoma. Metastases were found in the liver and pulmonary arterioles.[36] Unfortunately, the glucocorticoid secretory ability of the tumor had never been tested; atrophy of the left adrenal gland suggests some existed.

These cats demonstrate that primary hyperaldosteronism (Conn's syndrome) may be similar in cats and human beings. Clinical signs of hyperaldosteronism typically are nonspecific, and result from potassium depletion.[38] Neuromuscular signs (e.g., weakness, periodic paralysis) and fatigue may be seen,[38] and the elevated creatine phosphokinase noted in 1 cat likely was due to hypokalemic myopathy. Polyuria and nocturia probably result from a hypokalemia-induced renal concentrating defect.[38] Hypertension is due, at least in part, to an increased intravascular fluid volume as a result of sodium and water conservation, and in human beings, hypertensive retinopathy correlates with the severity and duration of the elevated blood pressure.[38] Intracellular potassium depletion also can impair insulin secretion, and cause glucose intolerance or overt diabetes mellitus.[38] Hypokalemia and, if present, hypernatremia are due to the direct effects of aldosterone causing urinary potassium loss and sodium retention.

The hallmark of primary hyperaldosteronism is hypokalemia with an elevated serum aldosterone concentration but a normal or subnormal serum renin; measurement of an elevated serum aldosterone alone is not adequate. In human beings, plasma renin activity is measured after dietary intake of a specific sodium amount. Whether such standardization is necessary in veterinary medicine is unknown, making diagnosis of primary hyperaldosteronism more difficult. The presence of renal failure presents a particular dilemma, because renal failure in and of itself can lead to this constellation of abnormalities. The magnitude of aldosterone elevation may be the key. With primary hyperaldosteronism, serum concentrations were approximately 3000 pg/ml in 2 cats,[37] whereas it was a maximum of 518 pg/ml in azotemic cats.[39] Identification of an AT by radiography or ultrasonography also would be highly suggestive of primary hyperaldosteronism. At the current time, a serum renin assay is not available. Until one is, diagnosis of primary hyperaldosteronism requires that all secondary causes (e.g., states associated with peripheral edema or liver failure) be ruled out.

Two of the 3 feline cases were determined histologically to be an adrenocortical carcinoma; the third also was likely malignant because the tumor invaded the vena cava. Surgical removal would be ideal for treatment of benign or malignant tumors. The role of antineoplastic chemotherapy has yet to be determined. If adrenalectomy is not possible, oral spironolactone and potassium may be administered. Spironolactone is the preferred diuretic because it works by antagonizing aldosterone receptors. A dose of 2 to 4 mg/kg/day has been recommended.[40] Potassium gluconate should be initiated at 2 to 6 mEq/day[40] but the dose may be adjusted as necessary to maintain normokalemia. If blood pressure does not normalize, antihypertensive agents such as amlodipine (6.25 mg/cat/day) may be administered as well.

◆ HYPOADRENOCORTICISM

Naturally occurring hypoadrenocorticism or Addison's disease is a rare endocrinopathy in cats, with

26 confirmed cases[41–47] and 2 suspected cases[48, 49] since 1983. Most cases are idiopathic, but 2 were traumatically induced,[41, 48] and 2 were secondary to lymphoma.[43] Secondary hypoadrenocorticism due to reduced secretion of ACTH usually is a result of treatment with either glucocorticoids or progestins, because such treatment provides a negative feedback to ACTH. Reduced circulating concentrations of ACTH lead to atrophy of the glucocorticoid-secreting zones of the adrenal cortex, while aldosterone secretion is not affected. Withdrawal from treatment with the steroids allows recovery of the adrenal cortex. (Note: In the discussion that follows, the specific term *idiopathic hypoadrenocorticism* refers to 12 confirmed cases of unknown cause, i.e., not due to trauma or lymphoma, for which historical, clinical, and laboratory findings are available.)

In 14 cats for which clinicopathologic data are available, electrolyte abnormalities were found in all, suggesting lack of glucocorticoids and mineralocorticoids; because pituitary failure does not cause aldosterone abnormalities, all 14 cases likely are due to primary adrenal failure. Spontaneous cases of hypoadrenocorticism with selective glucocorticoid deficiency have not been reported in cats. Of 5 idiopathic feline cases that went to necropsy, atrophy was noted in both adrenal glands in all, and lymphocytic infiltration in 2.[42, 44] Lymphocytic infiltration would suggest an immune-mediated basis for idiopathic hypoadrenocorticism, at least in some cats.

For idiopathic hypoadrenocorticism, average age at presentation was approximately 5 to 6 years (range, 1.5 to 14), and all were of mixed breeding; 7 cats were castrated males, and 5 were spayed females.[42, 44] With respect to historical complaints, lethargy was seen in all cats except 1, in which sudden weakness and collapse occurred. Weight loss also is very common, with vomiting, a waxing/waning course, previous therapeutic response, and polyuria/polydipsia being noted less frequently (Table 20–3). Clinical signs may be present for up to 100 days.[42] On physical examination, dehydration, weakness, and hypothermia are seen in the majority of cases. Increased capillary refill time, weak pulses, an inability to rise, a painful abdomen, bradycardia, and cool extremities also have been observed (see Table 20–3).

On routine bloodwork, the most consistent abnormalities, as in dogs, were azotemia with electrolyte changes including hyperkalemia, hyponatremia, hypochloremia, and acidosis (Table 20–4). In 1 cat, hyperkalemia was noted on day 2. Hyperkalemia typically is mild with the highest reported value being 6.2 mEq/L.[42] Hyponatremia ranges from mild to marked. Out of 11 cats for which urine specific gravity was determined at presentation, 7 had inappropriate urine concentration. Whether this represents true renal disease was not mentioned.[42, 43] Hyponatremia itself can cause poor urine concentrating ability, potentially by leading to renal medullary washout. Although the presence of eosinophilia and

Table 20–3. Clinical Findings in Cats With Spontaneous Hypoadrenocorticism[41–44]

Clinical Findings	Number of Cats (%)
Historical Complaints	
Anorexia	14/14 (100)
Lethargy/depression	13/14 (93)
Weight loss	12/14 (86)
Vomiting	5/14 (36)
Waxing/waning course	4/14 (29)
Previous response to therapy	3/14 (21)
Polyuria/polydipsia	3/14 (21)
Sudden collapse/weakness	1/14 (7)
Physical Examination Findings	
Dehydration	12/13 (92)
Weakness	11/13 (85)
Hypothermia	10/13 (77)
Increased capillary refill time	5/13 (38)
Weak pulse	5/13 (38)
Inability to rise	3/13 (23)
Painful abdomen	3/13 (23)
Bradycardia	2/13 (15)
Cool extremities	1/13 (8)

lymphocytosis, that is, lack of a stress leukogram, may be a clue to the presence of hypoadrenocorticism in a sick, stressed cat, they are not common laboratory findings (see Table 20–4). An increased red blood cell count was seen in 2 cats, most likely due to dehydration, and lymphopenia also was seen in 2.

Radiography revealed lung hypoperfusion in 6 of 6 cats,[42, 44] and microcardia in 5.[42] Electrocardiography showed bradycardia in 2 cats, atrial premature contractions in 1,[42] and was normal in 2.[43, 44] No abnormalities typically associated with hyperkalemia such as tall, peaked T waves or diminished P waves were noted, possibly because potassium disturbances were relatively mild.

As in dogs, definitive diagnosis can be made on the basis of an ACTH stimulation test (see

Table 20–4. Clinicopathologic Results in Cats With Spontaneous Hypoadrenocorticism[41–44, 46]*

Test	Number of Cats (%)
Complete Blood Count	
Anemia	4/14 (29)
Lymphocytosis	2/13 (15)
Eosinophilia	1/13 (8)
Biochemistry Profile	
Hyponatremia	15/15 (100)
Hyperkalemia	15/16 (94)
Azotemia	14/15 (93)
Hypochloremia	11/14 (79)
Decreased tCO$_2$	6/14 (43)
Elevated alanine aminotransferase	2/12 (17)
Elevated alkaline phosphatase	1/12 (8)
Increased total bilirubin	1/12 (8)
Increased serum calcium	1/12 (8)

*Includes 2 separate presentations of the same cat.

later).[41–44, 46] Additionally, in 8 cats with idiopathic hypoadrenocorticism in which it was measured, endogenous ACTH concentration was elevated from 10 to 150 times.[42, 44] Increased endogenous ACTH confirms the hypoadrenocorticism in these cases to be due to adrenal failure with lack of negative feedback on the pituitary.

Treatment for a hypoadrenal crisis is directed at expanding fluid volume, supplying exogenous glucocorticoids, and correcting electrolyte abnormalities and acidosis. Fluid replacement is the most important aspect. The fluids should be given intravenously in high volume—40 ml/kg—and 0.9 per cent saline solution is the fluid of choice because it can provide sodium and chloride and is potassium-deficient.[47] However, if normal saline solution is not available, Ringer's or lactated Ringer's is acceptable. These are low in potassium, and their administration will serve to dilute serum concentrations.[47]

For glucocorticoid replacement, prednisolone sodium succinate (4 to 20 mg/kg intravenously [IV][47]) or dexamethasone (0.5 to 1.0 mg/kg IV[22]) may be administered. Prednisolone sodium succinate is the quickest acting, followed by dexamethasone sodium phosphate, and then dexamethasone; if using dexamethasone sodium phosphate, make sure the dose is calculated on the basis of the active ingredient. Because prednisolone cross-reacts with cortisol on most assays, an ACTH stimulation test cannot be performed for 12 hours following its administration. Dexamethasone does not cross-react, so adrenal testing may be performed at any time. The decision of which glucocorticoid to use depends on patient status; because prednisolone sodium succinate is the most rapidly acting, this is the steroid of choice in severe crisis. Adrenal testing then may be performed once the patient is stabilized. Other therapies that may be necessary for treatment of a hypoadrenal crisis include correction of acidosis or hyperkalemia. The reader is referred elsewhere for more in-depth discussion.[45, 47]

Response to therapy appears to be slower for cats than for dogs, and therapy may need to be continued for 3 to 5 days before significant improvement is seen.[22, 42, 47] Once the patient is stabilized, maintenance therapy should be instituted. Only 6 reported cats with idiopathic hypoadrenocorticism have been treated long term.[42] Any combination of a glucocorticoid and mineralocorticoid may be used, but complications of glucocorticoid therapy such as diabetes mellitus may be more likely when injectable glucocorticoids are used.[22] Of 4 cats treated with a combination of fludrocortisone (Florinef, 0.1 mg/cat/day PO) and prednisone (1.25 mg/cat/day PO), 1 cat died suddenly of unknown causes after 47 days and the other 3 cats survived for at least 3 months. Three cats have been treated with a combination of desoxycorticosterone pivalate (DOCP, Percorten-V, 10 to 12.5 mg/cat/q 30 day intramuscularly [IM]) and methylprednisolone acetate, (Depo-Medrol, 10 mg/cat/q 30 day IM). Approximately 50 per cent of dogs receiving Florinef may not require further exogenous glucocorticoids,[47, 50] but whether this is true in cats is unknown. Although some dogs on DOCP have not received glucocorticoid therapy,[51, 52] this practice may not be recommended[47] because DOCP has no glucocorticoid activity, and the patient will always be glucocorticoid-deficient. During times of stress, glucocorticoid requirements increase. On days of planned increased stress, any glucocorticoid dose should be doubled,[47] or if the animal is not receiving any glucocorticoids, prednisone should be administered at a dose of 0.2 to 0.4 mg/kg.

For 6 cats with confirmed, idiopathic hypoadrenocorticism treated long term with either DOCP or Florinef, median survival time was 34 months.[42] In 1 cat with confirmed, traumatically induced hypoadrenocorticism, medication was discontinued eventually owing to adrenal recovery.

◆ EVALUATION OF ADRENAL FUNCTION IN CATS

Tests to evaluate adrenal function in cats are similar to those used in dogs; namely, the ACTH stimulation test, dexamethasone suppression tests, combination test, urine cortisol:creatinine ratio, measurement of endogenous ACTH concentration, and measurement of aldosterone. Interpretation of test results can be difficult for a number of reasons. First, results in cats appear to be more variable than those in dogs. Second, relatively few studies have been published examining the specificity and sensitivity of these tests in suspect cats, possibly because the incidence of adrenal disease is lower in this species.

When collecting samples, the following are our recommendations (Endocrine Diagnostic Service, Auburn University College of Veterinary Medicine).

Sample Handling

Cortisol. Measured in ACTH stimulation and dexamethasone suppression tests. Collect plasma using ethylenediaminetetraacetic acid (EDTA) as anticoagulant. The primary reason for this recommendation is that cortisol preserved in EDTA is more stable than when collected in serum, based on studies using canine blood.[53] Collect blood into EDTA, and centrifuge sample within 15 minutes of collection. Plasma can be shipped to the reference laboratory inside plastic tubes using overnight or second-day delivery without the need for addition of coolant (i.e., frozen gel packs). However, if serum or heparinized plasma is collected, samples should be shipped in an insulated container with cold packs.[53]

Endogenous ACTH. Proper sample handling is critical for this assay. Collect blood into EDTA, mix, and immediately add the protease inhibitor aprotinin (Trasylol, available from many reference laboratories) at 0.1 ml aprotinin (10,000 KIU/ml) to each 2 ml of blood. Mix thoroughly but gently and then centrifuge. Transfer plasma to a plastic storage tube, freeze the plasma if stored for more than 1 day before shipment. Plasma should be mailed to the reference laboratory inside an insulated container with frozen gel packs, using overnight delivery service. Alternatively, if no aprotinin is added, EDTA-plasma can be mailed frozen stored in a plastic tube, providing the sample is packed with a sufficient amount of dry ice.

Urine Cortisol:Creatinine Ratio. Collect urine and centrifuge to clarify. Draw off and save the supernatant; ship it in a plastic tube using an insulated container with frozen gel packs.

Aldosterone. Follow protocol for cortisol as described previously, but ship samples in insulated container with frozen gel packs.

Testing Methods

ACTH Stimulation Test. Collect a pre-ACTH sample for cortisol determination, and then inject synthetic ACTH (cosyntropin [Cortrosyn]) at 0.125 mg/cat IV (this is ½ the content of a vial of Cortrosyn). Collect a single post-ACTH sample 1 hour later for cortisol measurement. Alternatively, collect a sample and inject ACTH gel at 1 IU/kg (0.45 IU/lb) body weight IM, and collect 2 post-ACTH samples, one at 1 hour and another at 2 hours. The use of synthetic ACTH is preferred for this test.

Dexamethasone Suppression Testing. Collect a predexamethasone sample for cortisol determination, then inject dexamethasone or dexamethasone sodium phosphate IV and collect 2 postsamples, one 4 hours and another 8 hours later. If using dexamethasone sodium phosphate, be sure to dose on the basis of the active ingredient. Our laboratory recommends a dexamethasone dose of 0.1 mg/kg for the initial diagnosis of hyperadrenocorticism in cats; this dose is higher than that recommended as a screening test for hyperadrenocorticism in dogs.

Combination Test. Collect a baseline sample for cortisol determination. Inject dexamethasone (0.1 mg/kg IV) and take a postsample 4 hours later. After this collection, perform an ACTH stimulation test as described previously.

Measurement of Aldosterone. If testing for insufficiency, perform the ACTH stimulation test as previously, and collect pre- and post-ACTH plasma samples for measurement of aldosterone. If testing for excess, a single sample is required.

Interpretation of Test Results

For normal values, see Table 20–5.

ACTH Stimulation Test. Causes for low or undetectable pre-ACTH cortisol values with a reduced or

Table 20–5. Normal Values for Adrenal Function Tests

Test	Value
Pre-ACTH cortisol	10–110 nmol/L*
Post-ACTH cortisol	210–330 nmol/L*
Pre-dexamethasone (0.1 mg/kg) cortisol	10–110 nmol/L*
Post-dexamethasone (0.1 mg/kg) cortisol (4 and 8 hr)	<30 nmol/L*
Endogenous ACTH	5–40 pg/ml*
Urinary cortisol:creatinine ratio	<30[57]
Pre-ACTH aldosterone	194–388 pmol/L*†
Post-ACTH aldosterone	277–721 pmol/L†

Abbreviation: ACTH, adrenocorticotropic hormone.
*Note: these are the normals at the Auburn University Endocrine Diagnostic Laboratory; to convert cortisol to μg/dl, divide by 27.6.
†Animal Health Diagnostic Laboratory, Michigan State University.

absent increase in cortisol in response to ACTH include hypoadrenocorticism (primary or secondary) or use of inactive ACTH. We have encountered some types of ACTH gel that lack activity, so synthetic ACTH should be used if possible. Partial adrenocortical insufficiency, based on reduced cortisol response to ACTH and slightly elevated endogenous ACTH concentrations, has been observed in a significant percentage of cats with untreated lymphoma.[54]

As in dogs, an ACTH stimulation test can be used as a screening test for HAC, that is, a test that determines whether Cushing's syndrome is present or not. An elevated post-ACTH cortisol concentration (exaggerated response to ACTH), is consistent with a diagnosis of feline hyperadrenocorticism. In 37 cats with HAC, 48 ACTH stimulation tests were performed, and 39 (81 per cent) were positive.[5, 6, 8–14, 16, 19, 20, 25] Four of these were done as part of a combination test.[8, 11, 12, 14] Interestingly, in 3 cats, 1 test was negative and 1 positive. It should be noted that other reports have not shown as high a sensitivity for the ACTH stimulation test. This likely is due to the retrospective nature of data collection and different test and interpretation protocols used. The ACTH stimulation test has been shown to give exaggerated test results in ill cats with nonadrenal disease as well,[55] so false-positive test results are possible. The ACTH stimulation test cannot be used to differentiate pituitary-dependent disease from adrenocortical tumor.

Dexamethasone Suppression Testing. In dogs, the major use of low-dose dexamethasone suppression testing is to screen for the presence of hyperadrenocorticism; higher doses (0.1 mg/kg) are used in an attempt to differentiate pituitary-dependent hyperadrenocorticism from an adrenocortical tumor. Whereas the recommended dexamethasone doses for use in the low- and high-dose suppression tests have been well-established for use in dogs, they have not been delineated clearly in cats. In 37 cats with HAC, 35 tests (95 per cent) were positive at 8 hours after low-dose dexamethasone (0.01 mg/kg),

that is, suppression was inadequate.[3, 7, 9–11, 13, 20, 22, 23, 25] One result was borderline,[9] and 1 was negative.[25] However, cats with nonadrenal illness also can demonstrate inadequate suppression to a low dose of dexamethasone,[22, 55] and the substantial chance for false-positive results limits usefulness of this dose of dexamethasone in cats. This is of particular concern in cats, because a high proportion also are diabetic. Because most cats with Cushing's syndrome have a positive low-dose dexamethasone suppression test, it may be a good test to use to rule out Cushing's syndrome rather than using it to make a positive diagnosis.[22]

As a consequence, a higher dose of dexamethasone (0.1 mg/kg), which seems to be more reliably suppressive in cats with normal adrenal function, is recommended for screening purposes. In 10 cats with Cushing's syndrome, 8 showed inadequate suppression at 2 to 4 hours,[2, 11, 12, 14, 19, 23] and of 28, 22 (79 per cent) cats showed inadequate suppression at 8 hours.[1, 5, 10, 11, 20, 24] No cat with an AT suppressed.[1, 12, 13, 24] A possible problem associated with use of this dosage of dexamethasone for screening for feline HAC is that it may cause cortisol suppression in some cats with early or mild cases of HAC (i.e., a false-negative test result). All normal cats and cats with nonadrenal illness tested to date have suppressed to a high dose of dexamethasone,[11, 14, 55] but this includes only a small number of cats. Further studies examining the cortisol response to various doses of dexamethasone in normal cats, cats with nonadrenal disease, and cats with documented HAC are needed.

Failure to demonstrate cortisol suppression to 0.1 mg/kg of dexamethasone would be consistent with a diagnosis of HAC, and a higher-dose test (1.0 mg/kg) then could be employed for differentiation. Suppression of plasma cortisol (a decline from baseline by 50 per cent or more) in response to the 1.0 mg/kg dexamethasone would be consistent with pituitary-dependent HAC, in a cat with the disease already confirmed.[1, 13, 23] A suppression to less than 50 per cent of baseline was seen at 2 hours followed by an escape in response to a dexamethasone dose of 1.0 mg/kg given to a cat with PDH.[8] Alternatively, measurement of endogenous ACTH (see later) could be used for the differentiation.

Combination Test. Cats with HAC are expected to have an exaggerated response to ACTH and resistance to dexamethasone suppression at the dose used. However, each part should be interpreted as if the test was done alone with the attendant caveats. The combination test has been used successfully in 7 cats, 6 with PDH and 1 AT, to make a diagnosis of Cushing's syndrome.[8, 11, 12, 14, 19] All 7 cats had an elevated response to ACTH. Two cats with PDH did suppress after the injection of dexamethasone, allowing for diagnosis as well as differentiation. Because most cushingoid cats do not suppress after a high dose of dexamethasone, this test is less likely to provide differentiation than it is in dogs. However, if both limbs of the test are positive—lack of suppression and an increased ACTH response—greater confidence in a diagnosis of HAC would exist.

It has been demonstrated clearly in dogs that nonadrenal illness can alter test results leading to false-positive test results.[56] Therefore, it is important to limit use of the ACTH stimulation and dexamethasone suppression tests to patients whose clinical signs and other laboratory findings support the likelihood of Cushing's syndrome as a diagnosis. Because feline HAC is an infrequent diagnosis, confirmation of the diagnosis is best made by demonstrating either or, preferably, both an exaggerated cortisol response to ACTH and a failure to suppress cortisol normally in response to 0.1 mg/kg dexamethasone.

Endogenous ACTH Measurement. The major use of this test is to differentiate the forms of hypoadrenocorticism and HAC. It should be emphasized that measurement of circulating concentrations of ACTH are of relatively little value as a screening test for the initial diagnosis of either of these disorders. In cats with confirmed hypoadrenocorticism, plasma ACTH concentrations usually are considerably elevated in patients with primary hypoadrenocorticism (Addison's disease). In contrast, ACTH concentrations are in the low-normal to nondetectable range in cats with secondary hypoadrenocorticism. In cats with confirmed HAC, plasma ACTH concentrations should be in the mid-normal to above-normal range (above 15 pg/ml) and low in cats with adrenal tumors (below 10 pg/ml). Levels were consistent with PDH in all 33 cats with pituitary disease in which it was measured,[1, 5, 8, 9, 13, 14, 23-25] and was nondetectable in 3 cats with an AT.[1, 25]

Urinary Cortisol:Creatinine Ratio. Measurement of urinary cortisol:creatinine ratio in cats to evaluate adrenal activity has received relatively little study. The urine cortisol:creatinine ratio was elevated in all 6 cats with PDH in which it was measured.[23] This suggests that measurement of a ratio within the normal range rules out HAC with high likelihood, so that there is a high predictive value when a normal ratio is reported. In contrast, determination of an elevated ratio is likely nondiagnostic for HAC, because cats with nonadrenal illness show elevation in the ratio compared with healthy cats.[57] When an elevated ratio is found in a suspect cat, more definitive screening tests (ACTH stimulation test and/or 0.1 mg/kg dexamethasone suppression test) should be performed.

Aldosterone. The value of measurement of aldosterone (pre- and post-ACTH) is in the diagnosis and differential diagnosis of hypoadrenocorticism. Concentrations of aldosterone are nondetectable or low in cats with primary adrenal failure, but are normal in cats with the secondary form of the disease, that is, ACTH deficiency. This hormone also can be measured to aid in the diagnosis of hyperaldosteronism.

REFERENCES

1. Hyperadrenocorticism (Cushing's syndrome). *In* Feldman EC, Nelson RW: Canine and Feline Endocrinology and Reproduction, 2nd ed. Philadelphia, WB Saunders, 1996, pp. 187–265.
2. Immink WFGA, van Toor AJ, Vos JH, et al: Hyperadrenocorticism in four cats. Vet Q 15:81–85, 1992.
3. Immink WFGA: Four cats with Cushing's syndrome. Tijdschr Diergeneeskd 116:87S–88S, 1991.
4. van Sluijs FJ, Sjollema BE: Adrenalectomy in 36 dogs and 2 cats with hyperadrenocorticism. Tijdschr Diergeneeskd 117:29S, 1992.
5. Furuzawa Y, Une Y, Nomura Y: Pituitary-dependent hyperadrenocorticism in a cat. J Vet Med Sci 54:1201–1203, 1992.
6. Watson PJ, Herrtage ME: Hyperadrenocorticism in 6 cats. J Small Anim Pract 39:175–184, 1998.
7. Schwedes CS: Mitotane (o,p′-DDD) treatment in a cat with hyperadrenocorticism. J Small Anim Pract 38:520–524, 1997.
8. Daley CA, Zerbe CA, Schick RO, et al: Use of metyrapone to treat pituitary-dependent hyperadrenocorticism in a cat with large cutaneous wounds. J Am Vet Med Assoc 202:956–960, 1993.
9. Kipperman BS, Nelson RW, Griffey SM, et al: Diabetes mellitus and exocrine pancreatic neoplasia in two cats with hyperadrenocorticism. J Am Anim Hosp Assoc 28:415–418, 1992.
10. Duesberg CA, Nelson RW, Feldman EC, et al: Adrenalectomy for treatment of hyperadrenocorticism in cats: 10 cases (1988–1992). J Am Vet Med Assoc 207:1066–1070, 1995.
11. Zerbe CA, Nachreiner RF, Dunstan RW, et al: Hyperadrenocorticism in a cat. J Am Vet Med Assoc 190:559–563, 1987.
12. Jones CA, Refsal KR, Stevens BJ, et al: Adrenocortical adenocarcinoma in a cat. J Am Anim Hosp Assoc 28:59–62, 1992.
13. Nelson RW, Feldman EC, Smith MC: Hyperadrenocorticism in cats: Seven cases (1978–1987). J Am Vet Med Assoc 193:245–250, 1988.
14. Peterson ME, Steele P: Pituitary-dependent hyperadrenocorticism in a cat. J Am Vet Med Assoc 189:680–683, 1986.
15. Swift GA, Brown RH: Surgical treatment of Cushing's syndrome in the cat. Vet Rec 99:374–375, 1976.
16. Fox JG, Beatty JO: A case report of complicated diabetes mellitus in a cat. J Am Anim Hosp Assoc 11:129–134, 1975.
17. Gerding PA, Morton LD, Dye JA: Ocular and disseminated candidiasis in an immunosuppressed cat. J Am Vet Med Assoc 204:1635–1638, 1994.
18. Meijer JC, Lubberink AAME, Gruys E: Cushing's syndrome due to adrenocortical adenoma in a cat. Tijdschr Diergeneesk 103:1048–1051, 1978.
19. Drazner FH: Feline hyperadrenocorticism. *In* Drazner FH (ed): Small Animal Endocrinology. New York, Churchill Livingstone, 1987, pp. 263–264.
20. Usher DG: Hyperadrenocorticism in a cat. Can Vet J 32:326, 1991.
21. Peterson ME: Endocrine disorders in cats: Four emerging diseases. Compend Contin Educ Pract Vet 10:1353–1362, 1988.
22. Duesberg CA, Peterson ME: Adrenal disorders in cats. Vet Clin North Am Small Anim Pract 27:321–347, 1997.
23. Goossens MMC, Meyer HP, Voorhout G, et al: Urinary excretion of glucocorticoids in the diagnosis of hyperadrenocorticism in cats. Domest Anim Endocrinol 12:355–362, 1995.
24. Peterson ME, Randolph JF, Mooney CT: Endocrine diseases. *In* Sherding RG (ed): The Cat: Diseases and Clinical Management, 2nd ed. New York, Churchill Livingstone, 1995, pp. 1403–1506.
25. Feldman EC, Nelson RW: Hyperadrenocorticism. *In* Canine and Feline Endocrinology and Reproduction. Philadelphia, WB Saunders, 1987, pp. 137–194.
26. Valentine RW, Silber A: Feline hyperadrenocorticism: A rare case. Feline Pract 24:6–11, 1996.

27. White SD, Carpenter JL, Moore FM, et al: Generalized demodicosis associated with diabetes mellitus in two cats. J Am Vet Med Assoc 191:448–450, 1987.

28. Scott DW, Manning TO, Reimers TJ: Iatrogenic Cushing's syndrome in the cat. Feline Pract 12:30–36, 1982.

29. Scott DW, Kirk RW, Bentinck-Smith J: Some effects of short-term methylprednisolone therapy in normal cats. Cornell Vet 69:104–115, 1979.

30. Greene CE, Carmichael KP, Gratzek A: Iatrogenic hyperadrenocorticism in a cat. Feline Pract 23:7–12, 1995.

31. Helton-Rhodes K, Wallace MS, Baer K: Cutaneous manifestations of feline hyperadrenocorticism. In Tscharner C, Halliwell REW (eds): Advances in Veterinary Dermatology: Proceedings of the First World Congress of Veterinary Dermatology. London, Balliere Tindall, 1993, pp. 391–396.

32. Behrend EN, Kemppainen RJ, Clark TP, et al: Treatment of hyperadrenocorticism in dogs: A survey of internists and dermatologists. J Am Vet Med Assoc 215:938–943, 1999.

33. Nelson RW, Feldman EC: Hyperadrenocorticism. In August JR (ed): Consultations in Feline Internal Medicine, Vol. 1. Philadelphia, WB Saunders, 1991, pp. 267–270.

34. Boord M, Griffin C: Progesterone-secreting adrenal mass in a cat with clinical signs of hyperadrenocorticism. J Am Vet Med Assoc 214:666–669, 1999.

35. Chastain CB, Graham CL, Nichols CE: Adrenocortical suppression in cats given megestrol acetate. Am J Vet Res 42:2029–2035, 1981.

36. Eger CE, Robinson WF, Huxtable CRR: Primary aldosteronism (Conn's syndrome) in a cat: A case report and review of comparative aspects. J Small Anim Pract 24:293–307, 1983.

37. Flood SM, Randolph JF, Gelzer ARM, et al: Primary hyperaldosteronism in 2 cats. J Am Anim Hosp Assoc 35:411–416, 1999.

38. Dluhy RG, Williams GH: Endocrine Hypertension. In Wilson JD, Foster DW, Kronenberg HM, et al (eds): Williams Textbook of Endocrinology, 9th ed. Philadelphia, WB Saunders, pp. 1998, 729–749.

39. Jensen J, Henik R, Brownfield M, et al: Plasma renin activity and angiotensin I and aldosterone concentrations in cats with hypertension associated with chronic renal disease. Am J Vet Res 58:535–540, 1997

40. Ahn A: Hyperaldosteronism in cats. Semin Vet Med Surg (Small Anim) 9:153–157, 1994.

41. Berger SL, Reed JR: Traumatically induced hypoadrenocorticism in a cat. J Am Anim Hosp Assoc 29:337–339, 1993.

42. Peterson ME, Greco DS, Orth DN: Primary hypoadrenocorticism in ten cats. J Vet Intern Med 3:55–58, 1989.

43. Parnell NK, Powell LL, Hohenhaus AE, et al: Hypoadrenocorticism as the primary manifestation of lymphoma in two cats. J Am Vet Med Assoc 214:1208–1211, 1999.

44. Johnessee JS, Peterson ME, Gilbertson SR: Primary hypoadrenocorticism in a cat. J Am Vet Med Assoc 183:881–882, 1983.

45. Hardy RM: Hypoadrenal gland disease. In Ettinger SJ, Feldman EC (eds): Textbook of Veterinary Internal Medicine, 4th ed. Philadelphia, WB Saunders, 1995, pp. 1579–1593.

46. Ballmer-Rusca E: What is your diagnosis? Schweiz Arch Tierheilk 137:65–67, 1995.

47. Feldman EC, Nelson RW: Hypoadrenocorticism (Addison's disease). In Canine and Feline Endocrinology and Reproduction, 2nd ed. Philadelphia, WB Saunders, 1996, pp. 266–306.

48. Brain PH: Trauma-induced hypoadrenocorticism in a cat. Aust Vet Practit 27:178–180, 1997.

49. Mawhinney AD, Rahaley RS, Belford CJ: Primary hypoadrenocorticism in a cat. Aust Vet Practit 19:46–49, 1989.

50. Kintzer PP, Peterson ME: Treatment and long-term follow-up of 205 dogs with hypoadrenocorticism. J Vet Intern Med 11:43–49, 1997.

51. Melian C, Peterson ME: Diagnosis and treatment of naturally occurring hypoadrenocorticism in 42 dogs. J Small Anim Pract 37:268–275, 1996.

52. Lynn RC, Feldman BF, Nelson RW: Efficacy of microcrystalline desoxycorticosterone pivalate for treatment of hypoadrenocorticism in dogs. J Am Vet Med Assoc 202:392–396, 1993.

53. Behrend EN, Kemppainen RJ, Young DW: Effect of storage conditions on cortisol, total thyroxine and free thyroxine concentrations in serum and plasma of dogs. J Am Vet Med Assoc 212:1564–1568, 1995.

54. Farrelly J, Hohenhaus AE, Peterson ME, et al. Evaluation of pituitary-adrenal function in cats with lymphoma. Proceedings 19th Annual Veterinary Cancer Society, Wood's Hole, MA, Nov. 13–16, 1999, p. 33.

55. Zerbe CA, Refsal KR, Peterson ME, et al: Effect of nonadrenal illness on adrenal function in the cat. Am J Vet Res 48:451–454, 1987.

56. Kaplan AJ, Peterson ME, Kemppainen RJ: Effects of disease on the results of diagnostic tests for use in detecting hyperadrenocorticism in dogs. J Am Vet Med Assoc 207:445–451, 1995.

57. Henry CJ, Clark TP, Young DW, et al: Urine cortisol:creatinine ratio in healthy and sick cats. J Vet Intern Med 10:123–126, 1996.

21

◆ Oral Hypoglycemic Therapy for Type 2 Diabetes Mellitus

Deborah S. Greco

◆ ASSESSMENT OF CATS WITH DIABETES MELLITUS

Diabetes mellitus (DM) is one of the most common feline endocrinopathies, affecting 1 in 300 cats.[1] The pathogenesis of type 2 DM in cats has been reviewed previously.[2–4] Diagnosis of DM can be challenging, particularly in the early stages when the cats are non–insulin-dependent. However, once clinical signs of diabetes (polydipsia/polyuria, neuropathy) are observed, many cats still may benefit from alternatives to insulin therapy. In general, the primary abnormalities associated with type 2 DM, such as obesity and insulin resistance, are reversible. Insulin secretory ability, however, may be reversible (glucose toxicity) or irreversible (pancreatic amyloid deposition).[2–4] In cats, the differentiation of insulin-dependent diabetes mellitus (IDDM, type 1) and non–insulin-dependent diabetes mellitus (NIDDM, type 2) is virtually impossible before treatment; therefore, the clinician may have to rely on the response to oral hypoglycemic agents as a guide to whether the cat has sufficient beta-cell function to be managed with these drugs.

Goals of therapy for DM include restoration of normal fasting serum glucose concentrations, normalization of serum fructosamine, and reversal or attenuation of chronic complications such as diabetic neuropathy and nephropathy. As in human beings with type 2 DM, the best approach to diabetic cats is a stepwise progression from dietary management to oral hypoglycemics, and finally to insulin therapy when islet burn-out occurs.

◆ DIET AND EXERCISE

A combination of exercise and diet is the cornerstone of therapy in human beings with type 2 DM. In most diabetic cats, exercise is not a reasonable option. One mechanism by which cats may be encouraged to exercise is by feeding the cat multiple small meals hidden in various places within the house. For example, an obese diabetic cat might be encouraged to jump up on the refrigerator or counter to find small amounts of food and then have to hunt for the rest of the food at the opposite end of the house.

In human diabetics, fiber supplementation is beneficial in the management of the disease. In human beings and dogs, increased amounts of fiber slow the rate of glucose absorption from the intestine, and minimize the postprandial fluctuations in blood glucose. This allows better glycemic control, and correction of obesity; however, the data in cats are less compelling. In the only study of high-fiber diets in cats, 9 of 13 diabetic cats showed significant improvement in glycemic control with consumption of a high-fiber diet.[5] Examples of high-fiber diets include prescription diets w/d and r/d, Science Diet Maintenance Light, Purina OM, and Iams Less Active. Because many cats find high-fiber diets unpalatable, soluble fiber such as psyllium can be mixed into the cat's regular food, and glycemic control still may be enhanced. If the cat's weight is normal at the start of therapy, the diet should be fed at a maintenance level of 60 to 70 kcal/kg/day. If the patient is obese, caloric intake should be limited to 70 to 75 per cent of the energy needs for the cat's optimum weight.

The cat is an obligate carnivore, and as such, is unique among mammals in its insulin response to dietary carbohydrates, protein, and fat. The feline liver exhibits normal hexokinase activity, but glucokinase activity is virtually absent.[6] Glucokinase converts glucose to glycogen for storage in the liver, and is important in "mopping" up excess postprandial glucose. Normal cats in fact are similar to diabetic human beings, because glucokinase levels drop precipitously with persistent hyperglycemia in human beings suffering from type 2 DM. Amino acids, rather than glucose, are the signal for insulin release in cats.[7] In fact, a recent publication demonstrated more effective assessment of insulin reserve in cats using the arginine response test rather than a glucose tolerance test.[8] Another unusual aspect of feline metabolism is the increase in hepatic gluconeogenesis seen after a normal meal. Normal cats maintain essential glucose requirements from gluconeogenic precursors (i.e., amino acids) rather than from dietary carbohydrates. As a result, cats can maintain normal blood glucose concentrations even when deprived of food for over 72 hours[7]; furthermore, feeding has very little effect on blood glucose concentrations in normal cats.[2, 9] In summary, the cat is uniquely adapted to a carnivorous diet (mice), and is not adapted metabolically to ingestion of excess carbohydrate.

When type 2 DM occurs in cats, the metabolic adaptations to a carnivorous diet become even more deleterious, leading to severe protein catabolism; feeding a diet rich in carbohydrates may exacerbate hyperglycemia and protein wasting in these diabetic cats. In fact, in human beings with type 2 DM, the first recommendation is to restrict excess dietary carbohydrates, such as potatoes and bread, and to control obesity by caloric restriction.[10] Furthermore, human beings with type 2 DM have been shown to have improved glycemic control and improvement in nitrogen turnover during weight loss when a low-energy (high-protein) diet was combined with oral hypoglycemic therapy.[11] We therefore propose that a low-carbohydrate, high-protein diet, which is similar in fact to a cat's natural diet (mice), might ameliorate some of the abnormalities associated with DM in cats.

We have found high-protein diets to be beneficial in increasing lean body mass and reducing postprandial hyperglycemia. Caution should be used when high-protein, restricted-carbohydrate diets are used in cats also treated with insulin, because the insulin requirement may decrease. Usually the insulin dose is decreased by 25 per cent in cats given high-protein diets and insulin. On the other hand, high-protein diets and oral hypoglycemic agents appear to be complementary treatments in cats that are underweight.

◆ ORAL HYPOGLYCEMICS

Treatment of NIDDM is aimed at attenuating the physiologic abnormalities of DM by decreasing hepatic glucose output and glucose absorption from the intestine, increasing peripheral insulin sensitivity, and increasing insulin secretion from the pancreas (Fig. 21–1). Oral hypoglycemic agents include the sulfonylureas (glipizide, glyburide, glimepiride), biguanides (metformin), thiazolidinediones (troglitazone), alpha-glucosidase inhibitors (acarbose), and transition metals (chromium, vanadium) (Table 21–1).[12, 13]

Indications for oral hypoglycemic therapy in cats include normal or increased body weight, lack of ketones, probable type 2 diabetes with no underlying disease (pancreatitis, pancreatic tumor), history of diabetogenic medications, and owner's willingness to administer oral medication rather than an injection. Reversal of glucose toxicity using a short course of insulin therapy before or in combination with administration of oral hypoglycemic agents may improve the response to oral hypoglycemic agents.[2] Dietary compliance by the owner is essential to improving the response to oral hypoglycemic agents.

Agents That Inhibit Intestinal Glucose Absorption

The alpha-glucosidase inhibitors impair glucose absorption from the intestine by decreasing fiber digestion, and hence, glucose production from food sources.[12–14] Acarbose is used as initial therapy in obese pre-diabetic human beings suffering from insulin resistance, or as adjunct therapy with sulfonylureas or biguanides to enhance the hypoglycemic effect in patients with type 2 DM. Side-effects include flatulence, loose stool, and diarrhea at high dosages. Acarbose and related compounds are not indicated in patients of low or normal body weight because of the effects of these agents on nutrition. Acarbose may be administered at a dosage of 12.5 to 25 mg/cat orally with meals. Side-effects are more common at the high end of the dosage range, and include semiformed stool, or in some cases, overt diarrhea. The glucose-lowering effect of acarbose alone is mild, with blood glucose concentrations decreasing only into the 250- to 300-mg/dl range. However, acarbose is an excellent agent when combined with insulin or with diet and insulin to improve glycemic control. The author has had good success using acarbose and a low-carbohydrate,

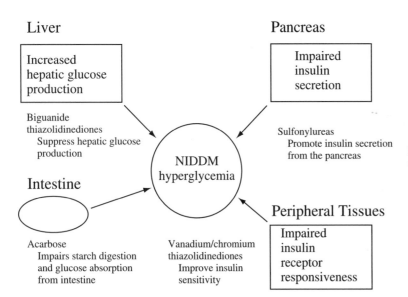

Figure 21–1. Treatment of non–insulin-dependent diabetes mellitus.

Table 21–1. Oral Hypoglycemic Drugs Used in the Treatment of Non–Insulin-Dependent Diabetes Mellitus in Human Beings and Cats

Drug	Dose	Frequency	Side-Effects	Mechanism of Action
Agents That Promote Insulin Release				
Glipizide	2.5–5 mg (C)	q 12 hr	Vomiting, hepatotoxicity, hypoglycemia	Releases insulin, increases insulin receptor sensitivity
Glimepiride (Amaryl)	1–4 mg (H) Unknown (C)	q 24 hr (H) Unknown (C)	Same as above but lower incidence	Releases insulin, increases insulin receptor sensitivity
Agents That Inhibit Hepatic Glucose Production				
Metformin (Glucophage)	500–750 mg (H) 2–10 mg/kg (C)	q 12 hr (H) q 12 hr (C)	Anorexia, vomiting	Inhibits hepatic glucose production
Agents That Impair Glucose Absorption From the Intestine				
Acarbose (Precose)	50 mg (H) 12.5–25 mg (C)	q 8 hr–q 12 hr With meals	Flatulence, soft stool, diarrhea	Inhibits alpha$_1$ glucosidase, impairs glucose absorption from gut
Insulin-Sensitizing Agents				
Troglitazone (Rezulin)*	200–400 mg (H) 25 mg/kg (C)	q 24 hr	Mild decreases in white blood cell, platelet, and hemoglobin counts	Increases insulin receptor sensitivity
Vanadium (Vanadyl Fuel)	½ capsule	q 24 hr in food	Anorexia, vomiting	Increases insulin receptor sensitivity
Chromium picolinate	200 μg/cat	q 24 hr in food		Increases insulin receptor sensitivity

Abbreviations: C, cat; H, human being; q, every.
*Discontinued.

high-protein diet in cats at a dosage of 12.5 mg every (q) 12 hr orally.

Agents That Promote Insulin Release From the Pancreas

The mechanism of action of the sulfonylureas is to increase insulin secretion and improve insulin resistance; however, some of these agents also cause an increase in hepatic glucose output.[12] Sulfonylureas, because of provocation of insulin release, may promote progression of pancreatic amyloidosis. In cats, glipizide has been used to treat DM successfully at a dosage of 2.5 to 5 mg q 12 hr when combined with dietary therapy.[15, 16] The patient is evaluated weekly or every 2 weeks for a period of 2 to 3 months. If the fasting blood glucose decreases to less than 200 mg/dl, the glipizide should be continued at the same dosage and the cat re-evaluated in 3 to 6 months. If the fasting blood glucose remains greater than 200 mg/dl after 2 to 3 months of therapy, and the cat is still symptomatic (polydipsia/polyuria and weight loss), glipizide should be discontinued, and insulin therapy should be instituted. If the blood glucose remains greater than 200 mg/dl, and the cat becomes asymptomatic, the glipizide should be continued indefinitely and the cat should be rechecked in 3 to 6 months.[16] Initial experience with glipizide as an oral hypoglycemic agent

in cats has been disappointing. However, this may be related to patient selection and less-than-ideal diet rather than to overt failure of the drug. Cats with early type 2 DM are most likely to respond to any oral hypoglycemic agent. Side-effects of oral hypoglycemics include severe hypoglycemia (rare in cats), cholestatic hepatitis, and vomiting. Gastrointestinal side-effects, which occur in about 15 per cent of cats treated with glipizide, resolve when the drug is administered with food.[15, 16]

A new sulfonylurea agent, glimepiride (Amaryl), has fewer side-effects than glipizide, and can be dosed once-daily. Initial studies in cats suggest that this may be a viable alternative to glipizide at a dosage of 1 to 2 mg per cat q 24 hr. Again, a combination of sulfonylureas with a low-carbohydrate, high-protein diet has been more successful than dietary fiber therapy in this author's hands.

Agents That Inhibit Hepatic Glucose Output

Metformin belongs to the biguanide group of oral hypoglycemic agents.[12] These agents work by inhibiting hepatic glucose release and by improving peripheral insulin sensitivity.[17, 18] They have been used alone and in conjunction with other oral hypoglycemic agents to treat type 2 DM in human beings.[17] One advantage of the biguanides is that they do not promote insulin release; therefore, there is no potential for hypoglycemia when they are used as a sole agent. Furthermore, the concern about progression of pancreatic amyloid deposition is avoided. Side-effects of the biguanides include lactic acidosis and gastrointestinal signs. Contraindications for metformin therapy in human beings, and presumably in cats, include concurrent renal disease (serum creatinine > 2.1 mg/dl), liver dysfunction, hypoxia, and alcoholism (in human patients). Initial studies using metformin to treat feline NIDDM have been disappointing, because the drug has been associated with severe side-effects. Current research indicates that lower dosages of metformin may be safe, and possibly effective as an oral hypoglycemic in cats.[18] In human beings, combining this drug with a sulfonylurea and diet (carbohydrate restriction) has been the most effective approach.[17]

Agents That Improve Peripheral Insulin Sensitivity

A new class of oral hypoglycemics receiving attention in human medicine is the thiazolidinedione compounds.[19, 20] Thiazolidinediones facilitate insulin-dependent glucose disposal, and inhibit hepatic glucose output by attenuation of gluconeogenesis and glycogenolysis.[19] Troglitazone (Rezulin) increases transcription and translation of proteins necessary for glucose metabolism. Some authors have suggested that use of this drug early in the course of NIDDM may slow the progression of the disease. Side-effects of troglitazone were minimal, and no hypoglycemic reactions have been described. In human beings, improvement in fasting blood glucose, glycosylated hemoglobin, and diabetic complications were noted in all patients, and were significant when compared with placebo.[19] The author has used 200 mg of troglitazone once-daily in cats without observing significant changes in blood glucose regulation or side-effects. However, in human beings, hepatic toxicity (idiosyncratic) has been observed infrequently, and the drug has been discontinued.

Compounds containing the transition metals vanadium and chromium have insulinomimetic properties when administered in the drinking water to mice and rats suffering from experimentally induced DM (type 1 and type 2).[21–24] Current research indicates that transition metals bypass the insulin receptor and activate glucose metabolism within the cell. By acting at a postreceptor site, vanadium/chromium compounds are an ideal treatment for type 2 DM that results from a lack of insulin-receptor responsiveness. Unlike insulin, vanadium and chromium do not lower blood glucose concentrations in normal animals.[21–24] Studies in our laboratory indicate that low doses of oral vanadium decrease blood glucose and serum fructosamine concentrations, and alleviate the signs of diabetes (polydipsia/polyuria) in cats with *early* type 2 DM.[23] Side-effects include anorexia and vomiting initially;

however, most cats showed no ill-effects when vanadium therapy was reinstituted. A recent U.S. Department of Agriculture study of 180 human patients with NIDDM found that administration of 1000 μg of chromium picolinate once-daily resulted in amelioration of the classic signs of DM and normalization of blood levels of hemoglobin A1c.[24] Chromium may be administered at a dosage of 200 μg/cat once-daily as a tablet or capsule, and vanadium is available commercially as Vanadyl Fuel (½ capsule once-daily on food).

◆ COMBINING ORAL HYPOGLYCEMICS WITH INSULIN: CHANGES TO AND FROM INSULIN

Agents that impair glucose absorption from the intestine (acarbose) or increase insulin sensitivity (vanadium, metformin, troglitazone) may be combined with insulin to improve glucose control. In the case of "brittle diabetics" in whom small incremental changes in insulin dose may precipitate hypoglycemia, addition of a drug that enhances the action of insulin may lead to a reduction in the insulin dosage required to attain euglycemia. In human beings, acarbose and metformin are used commonly in conjunction with insulin and other oral hypoglycemics (sulfonylureas) that cause insulin release. Caution should be used in combining any oral hypoglycemic agent with insulin because of the potential for severe or fatal hypoglycemia. Changes from insulin to oral hypoglycemic agents or vice versa may be necessary in some diabetic cats. If a cat is particularly sensitive to insulin or exhibits transient DM because of reversal of "glucose toxicity," a change to an oral hypoglycemic agent should be considered. Conversely, if a cat is being managed with oral hypoglycemic agents and ketosis develops, the oral hypoglycemic agents should be discontinued, and the cat should be treated with insulin.

REFERENCES

1. Panciera DL, Chester BT, Eicker SW, Atkins CE: Epizootiologic patterns of diabetes mellitus in cats. J Am Vet Med Assoc 197:1504–1508, 1990.
2. Rand JS: Management of feline diabetes. Aust Vet Practit 27:68–75, 1997.
3. O'Brien TD, Butler PC, Westermark P, Johnson KH: Islet amyloid polypeptide: A review of its biology and potential roles in the pathogenesis of diabetes mellitus. Vet Pathol 30:317–332, 1993.
4. Lutz TA, Rand JS: A review of new developments in type 2 diabetes mellitus in human beings and cats. Br Vet J 149:527–536, 1993.
5. Nelson RW, Scott-Moncrieff C, DeVries S, et al: Dietary insoluble fiber and glycemic control of diabetic cats (Abstract). J Vet Intern Med 8:165, 1994.
6. Ballard FJ: Glucose utilization in mammalian liver. Comp Biochem Physiol 14:437–443, 1965.
7. Kettlehut IC, Foss MC, Migliorini RH: Glucose homeostasis in a carnivorous animal (cat) and in rats fed a high-protein diet. Am J Physiol 239:R115–R121, 1978.

8. Kitamura T, Yasuda J, Hashimoto A: Acute insulin response to intravenous arginine in nonobese healthy cats. J Vet Intern Med 13:549–556, 1999.

9. Martin GJW, Rand JS: Lack of correlation between food ingestion and blood glucose in diabetic cats. Proceedings 15th ACVIM Forum, 1997, p. 670.

10. Unger RH, Foster DW: Diabetes mellitus. *In* Wilson JD, Foster DW, Kronenberg HM, Larsen PR (eds): Williams Textbook of Endocrinology, 9th ed. Philadelphia, WB Saunders, 1998, pp. 973–1060.

11. Gougeon R, Jones JHP, Styhler K, et al: Effects of oral hypoglycemic agents and diet on protein metabolism in type 2 diabetes. Diabetes Care 23:1–8, 2000.

12. Kahn CR, Shechter Y: Insulin, oral hypoglycemic agents and the pharmacology of the endocrine pancreas. *In* Rall TW, Nies AS, Taylor P (eds): Goodman and Gilman's The Pharmacological Basis of Therapeutics, 8th ed. New York, Pergamon, 1990, pp. 1463–1495.

13. Greco DS: Oral hypoglycemic agents for non–insulin dependent diabetes mellitus in the cat. Semin Vet Med Surg 12:259–262, 1998.

14. Robertson J, Nelson RW, Kass P, et al: Effects of the alpha-glucosidase inhibitor acarbose on postprandial serum glucose and insulin concentration in healthy dogs. Am J Vet Res 60:541–545, 1999.

15. Nelson RW, Feldman EC, Ford SL, Roomer OP: Effect of an orally administered sulfonylurea, glipizide, for treatment of diabetes mellitus in cats. J Am Vet Med Assoc 203:821–825, 1993.

16. Ford S: NIDDM in the cat: Treatment with the oral hypoglycemic medication, glipizide. Vet Clin North Am Small Anim Pract 25:599–615, 1995.

17. DeFronzo RA, Goodman AM: Efficacy of metformin in patients with non–insulin-dependent diabetes mellitus. N Engl J Med 333:541–544, 1995.

18. Michels GM, Boudinot FD, Ferguson DC, et al: Pharmacokinetics of the antihyperglycemic agent metformin in cats. Am J Vet Res 60:738–742, 1999.

19. Saltiel AR, Olefsky JM: Thiazolidinediones in the treatment of insulin resistance and type II diabetes. Diabetes 45:1661–1669, 1996.

20. Berkowitz K, Peters R, Kjos SL, et al: Effect of troglitazone on insulin sensitivity and pancreatic β-cell function in women at high risk for NIDDM. Diabetes 45:1572–1579, 1996.

21. Cam MC, Pederson RA, Brownsey RW, McNeil JH: Long-term effectiveness of oral vanadyl sulphate in streptozotocin-diabetic rats. Diabetologia 36:218–224, 1993.

22. Brichard SM, Pottier AM, Henquin JC: Long-term improvement of glucose homeostasis by vanadate in obese hyperinsulinemic fa/fa rats. Endocrinology 125:2510–2516, 1989.

23. Greco DS: Treatment of type II diabetes mellitus in cats with oral vanadium. Diabetes, May 1997 supplement, #1249.

24. Vincent JB: The biochemistry of chromium. J Nutr 130:715–718, 2000.

22

◆ Problems of Diabetic Regulation With Insulin Therapy

John V. Fondacaro
Deborah S. Greco

Diabetes mellitus (DM) is a common feline disease that typically requires insulin administration for effective medical management. The pathogenesis of the disease has been reviewed thoroughly in *Consultations in Feline Internal Medicine*, vol. 3, Chapter 17, p. 125. DM is a primary disease, or a condition secondary to other illness or drugs. In the latter situation, resolution of the diabetes may occur with treatment of the underlying disease or correction of causative factors. Primary DM in cats usually is the consequence of insulin resistance, and is seen commonly in obese individuals.[1, 2] Early in the course of the disease, feline DM is analogous to non–insulin-dependent diabetes mellitus or type 2 DM in human beings. Because the primary disorder is insulin resistance, some individuals may respond to dietary manipulation or oral hypoglycemic medications early in the course of the disease[3, 4] (see Chapter 21, Oral Hypoglycemic Therapy for Type 2 Diabetes Mellitus). Progression of disease results in the typical clinical signs of polyuria, polydipsia, and weight loss. Persistent hyperglycemia results in glucose toxicity, and progressive amyloid deposition within the pancreas. The result is beta-cell exhaustion and degeneration. This is in contrast to the autoimmune beta-cell destruction that occurs in dogs with type 1 DM, but the outcome may be similar.

Progression of disease occurs commonly in feline DM, and cats most often develop insulin dependence as insulin secretion becomes impaired. The most common scenario encountered by the veterinarian is DM in a cat that has progressed to the point of concurrent insulin resistance and impaired insulin secretion[5, 6]; therefore, the type of diabetes, and the state of insulin dependence, must be considered separately in cats. Furthermore, some cats may fluctuate with regard to their insulin resistance and insulin requirements. Individuals may experience insulin-induced hypoglycemia as insulin resistance is reversed, or as insulin requirements decline with therapy. In some cases, cats may be transiently diabetic.[7] These "brittle" diabetics can be a source of frustration to the veterinarian. It is imperative that clinicians understand the dynamic nature of feline DM, the individual variation in response to therapy, and the importance of monitoring complications of insulin therapy. Because the pathogenesis of feline DM typically results in insulin requirement, it is essential that the owner of a diabetic cat understand these principles, and the commitment of time and money that is often required to manage a diabetic cat successfully. Client communication may reduce the frustration experienced by clinicians and owners faced with this challenging disease.

◆ OWNER/CLIENT FACTORS

Insulin Storage and Administration

Insulin is very sensitive to environmental factors, and improper storage and handling can result in protein degradation and inactivation of insulin. Insulin should be refrigerated, stored in a dark place, and not shaken before administration. The bottle should be rolled gently to form a consistent solution; failure to do so can cause inaccurate dosing. If there is any question regarding the suitability of insulin, a policy of "when in doubt, throw it out" is most prudent. We currently recommend replacing insulin every 2 months. Owner administration of insulin should be witnessed by the clinician, and failure of the cat to respond to insulin with a reduction in blood glucose should prompt an investigation of insulin storage and administration. The most common reason for loss of regulation of diabetes or difficulty in establishing diabetic control in a cat is owner mismanagement at home. The author prefers to shave several areas of the ventral thorax and abdomen to show the owner how to administer insulin. The owner should be instructed to grasp the skin forming a "tent," and insert the needle at a 45-degree angle. Care should be taken not to force the needle through the other side of the skin.

◆ PHARMACOKINETIC FACTORS

Insulin Formulations

The types of insulin currently recommended for use in cats are the long-acting (protamine zinc [PZI] or ultralente) and the intermediate-acting (isophane or lente) insulin preparations. Although once-daily administration of long-acting insulin has been recommended as the initial insulin regimen of choice for cats,[8, 9] better regulation with once-daily long-acting insulin has not been shown.[10] In fact, variability in response to insulin administration appears to be the rule, rather than the exception. Although once-daily administration of ultralente would be most convenient and inexpensive, the authors have not had much success with this therapeutic approach. Twice-daily administration of isophane insulin or PZI is most effective for adequate regulation of diabetic cats in the authors' experience. An absorption kinetic study of neutral protein Hagedorn (NPH) insulin and PZI has shown that most cats with DM require twice-daily injections.[11] Lente insulin was effective in 8 of 12 cats treated with twice-daily injections in 1 study.[9] Most important, the veterinarian must recognize that the response to insulin, and the dosage and schedule required to maintain adequate control, are subject to individual variation. Weekly evaluation of serial blood glucose is recommended initially to determine the most effective plan for a particular patient. Most regimens are determined within 4 to 6 weeks of initial diagnosis.

Poor Insulin Absorption

Absorption of subcutaneously administered insulin is affected by hydration status and local tissue factors. Dehydration results in decreased insulin absorption from the subcutaneous space due to peripheral vasoconstriction. We currently recommend subcutaneous administration of insulin in the lateral thorax, and rotation of injection sites is advised to avoid tissue fibrosis and decreased absorptive capacity. One injection site that should be avoided is the area above the scapula, or the "nape of the neck." This area often is used to administer everything from vaccinations to subcutaneous fluids. It tends to be poorly vascularized, and may contain significant fibrous tissue resulting from previous cat fights, particularly in some intact male cats.

◆ MONITORING INSULIN THERAPY

The adequacy of insulin type, dosage, and duration is best evaluated with serial clinical evaluations, serum fructosamine, and blood glucose curves (see "Update on Diabetes Mellitus," in *Consultations in Feline Internal Medicine,* vol. 2, p. 155). The authors perform weekly blood glucose curves (12 hours for twice-daily insulin administration) until the insulin formulation and dosage are appropriate. Once an acceptable plan is determined, long-term regulation is evaluated by measurement of fructosamine or glycosylated hemoglobin, which reflects the mean blood glucose over the previous 2 to 3 weeks or 2 to 3 months, respectively.[12–14] The authors utilize serum fructosamine (normal < 360 μmol/liter), and consider a cat well-regulated if fructosamine is less than 400 μmol/liter. Moderate control may be reflected by values between 400 to 500 μmol/liter. Fructosamine greater than 500 μmol/liter typically

is associated with persistent clinical signs and the risk of complications of poor regulation such as neuropathy (see Chapter 17, Diabetic Neuropathy). If a loss of adequate regulation is revealed by clinical signs and/or fructosamine evaluations, the following order of consideration is given: (1) potency of insulin and owner administration technique, (2) concurrent illness, and (3) inadequate insulin type, dosage, or duration. Before a repeat glucose curve is performed on a previously well-regulated diabetic that is experiencing difficulties, an investigation of concurrent illnesses recognized to cause insulin antagonism is indicated.

Concurrent Illness

Many illnesses are associated with the release of insulin-antagonistic hormones—for example, glucagon, growth hormone, cortisol, catecholamines, and progesterone. Failure to recognize, treat, and control these concurrent illnesses makes regulation of DM difficult to impossible, depending on the individual circumstances. An investigation of concurrent illness is recommended before starting insulin administration. A typical evaluation includes complete blood count, serum chemistry profile, serum thyroxine, urinalysis, aerobic urine culture, thoracic and abdominal survey radiographs, and abdominal ultrasonography (when available). Owing to the high incidence of concurrent pancreatic disease in cats with DM,[10] ultrasound evaluation of the pancreas is ideal. The incidence of chronic pancreatitis in cats with DM is high[10]; therefore, measurement of serum trypsin-like immunoreactivity may be warranted in some cases. Failure to recognize and treat pancreatitis is a common cause for treatment failure in cats with DM. Confirmed cases of chronic pancreatitis in cats may be responsive to corticosteroids (prednisolone 5–10 mg/cat/day). Corticosteroid use is not indicated in acute pancreatitis. Because cortisol antagonizes insulin, increased doses of insulin may be required to control DM adequately in cats treated with corticosteroids for concurrent pancreatitis. It is the authors' experience that the benefits of corticosteroid administration in cats with concurrent DM and chronic pancreatitis outweigh the disadvantages of insulin antagonism. Concurrent illnesses that commonly antagonize insulin and inhibit diabetic regulation are listed in Table 22–1.

Table 22–1. Concurrent Illnesses That Commonly Antagonize Diabetic Regulation

Urinary tract infection (cystitis, pyelonephritis)
Renal failure
Hepatic disease
Pancreatitis
Hyperthyroidism
Inflammatory bowel disease
Oral disease (stomatitis, indolent ulcers, dental disease)

Table 22–2. Recommended Steps in Work-Up for Diagnosis and Treatment of Insulin Resistance in Cats

Steps	Causes of Insulin Resistance	Procedure or Test	Treatment
Step 1	Glucocorticoids or megestrol acetate administration	History	Discontinue use of drugs
Step 2	Obesity	Physical examination, weight	Diet change (low-calorie, high-fiber)
Step 3	Poor absorption of subcutaneous insulin (long-acting preparation)	Evaluate response to change in insulin type; evaluate serum glucose response to regular insulin administered IV or IM	Change from long-acting insulin to insulin with shorter duration of action; use insulin mixtures (e.g., NPH/regular)
Step 4	Infection, ketoacidosis, or concurrent disease	CBC; serum chemistry profile; urinalysis; urine culture; radiographs; abdominal ultrasound	Appropriate antibiotics; correct ketoacidosis or underlying illness
Step 5	Hyperthyroidism	Serum T_4 concentration	Antithyroid drugs; thyroidectomy; radioiodine
Step 6	Cushing's syndrome	Review clinical signs and physical examination; ACTH stimulation and dexamethasone suppression tests; CT scan	Adrenalectomy; pituitary (cobalt) radiation therapy
Step 7	Acromegaly	Review clinical signs and physical examination; CT scan; measure serum insulin-like growth factor concentration	Pituitary (cobalt) radiation therapy
Step 8	Insulin antibodies	Measure serum insulin concentration 24 hr after last insulin injection; insulin antibody titers (not widely available)	Switch to human insulin (or beef insulin, if available)
Step 9	Clinically undefined insulin resistance	All of the above procedures and tests	Raise insulin dose; change to insulin with shorter duration of action; mix NPH/regular insulin

Abbreviations: ACTH, adrenocorticotropic hormone; CBC, complete blood count; CT, computed tomography; IM, intramuscularly; IV, intravenously; NPH, neutral protamine Hagedorn; T_4, thyroxine.
From Peterson ME: Diagnostic and therapeutic approach to insulin resistance. *In* August JR (ed): Consultations in Feline Internal Medicine, vol. 3. Philadelphia, WB Saunders, 1997.

Insulin Resistance

A state of insulin resistance is suspected when insulin dosage is greater than 1.5 to 2.2 units/kg/dose. A thorough review of insulin resistance is presented in *Consultations in Feline Internal Medicine*, vol. 3, Chapter 18, p. 132. Causes for insulin resistance in cats include poor absorption of subcutaneous insulin, immunologic insulin resistance, infection, ketoacidosis, obesity, acromegaly, hyperadrenocorticism, hyperthyroidism, and drugs (megestrol acetate, corticosteroids).[15] Failure to recognize the insulin-resistant state most often results in poor diabetic regulation. Recommendations for the evaluation of insulin resistance in cats are summarized in Table 22–2.

Update on Immunologic Insulin Resistance (Insulin Antibodies)

The formation of antibody against insulin is an increasing concern since the discontinuation of animal-source insulin. Cat insulin is most similar to beef insulin (differing by only 1 amino acid in structure), and is less similar to pork, dog, or human insulin. Currently, human recombinant insulin is the formulation marketed by nearly all pharmaceutical manufacturers (beef-origin PZI can be obtained from Blue Ridge Pharmaceuticals, OH). In human beings, essentially all patients treated with insulin have antibodies after 3 months of insulin therapy, but the incidence of insulin resistance from anti-

body formation is estimated at 0.01 per cent.[16] In addition to antibody formation due to exogenous insulin administration, insulin antibody formation has been documented in human beings with autoimmune endocrinopathy such as hypothyroidism.[17] Hypoglycemia secondary to inappropriate release of antibody-bound insulin also has been documented, and is thought to be the cause of erratic serum glucose levels and regulation in some individuals.[17] Fortunately, clinical effects from insulin antibody formation are believed to be less common in cats than in dogs at this time. The development of diagnostic tests to detect feline insulin-binding antibody may be helpful in cases of insulin resistance, hypoglycemia, or erratic regulation.

Insulin Overdosage and Hypoglycemia

Overdosage of insulin causes hypoglycemia. The dosage excess can be absolute or relative—for example, decreasing insulin requirement in dynamic DM. The physiologic response to insulin overdose and hypoglycemia is the release of counter-regulatory hormones that antagonize insulin and improve glycemia. If these adaptive mechanisms are overwhelmed, clinical hypoglycemia may occur. Diabetic cats, obese patients in particular, are more predisposed than dogs to insulin overdose and hypoglycemia.[18] Clinical hypoglycemia typically is preceded by signs referable to epinephrine release or central nervous system effects (tachycardia, nervousness, tremor). Cats may experience hypoglycemia without apparent autonomic warning signs (hypoglycemic unawareness).[18] Occasionally, they present comatose without any obvious prior warning. Immediate veterinary attention and the administration of intravenous glucose are critical in these patients.

Posthypoglycemic hyperglycemia (rebound hyperglycemia) has been reported in cats.[19] This effect, also termed the *Somogyi phenomenon*, is believed to be the result of an exuberant response of diabetogenic hormones to hypoglycemia. In human beings, the phenomenon is now considered much less common than previously believed.[16] If a patient does not have glycosuria and hyperglycemia throughout the following day, rebound hyperglycemia likely did not occur.[16] Most cases of documented rebound hyperglycemia in human beings occur in children who typically are suffering from type 1 DM.[16] The occurrence of this phenomenon in cats is in question. Individuals that experience hypoglycemic unawareness would not be expected to experience rebound hyperglycemia, because the defect in hypoglycemic unawareness is a poor counter-regulatory response, and the mechanism of rebound hyperglycemia is an exuberant response. It is the authors' experience that dogs respond to hypoglycemia with an exuberant counter-regulatory response resulting in rebound hyperglycemia. Cats may not have the ability to respond with sufficient counter-regulatory hormone release, which may explain the apparent greater occurrence of clinical hypoglycemia with insulin overdosage in cats.

◆ COMPLICATIONS OF POOR REGULATION

Failure to adequately regulate a diabetic cat results in progressive clinical signs associated with the disease; for example, polyuria, polydypsia, and weight loss. Untreated or poorly regulated diabetic cats that do not develop another disease typically experience anorexia and weight loss, and eventually die from cachexia. Diabetic ketoacidosis occurs when a state of concurrent insulin deficiency and insulin-antagonistic illness exists. This disorder is fatal without therapy, and recovery depends on recognition of concurrent illness and the formulation of an appropriate treatment plan.[20] Nonketotic hyperosmolar coma, a state of severe hyperglycemia (serum glucose > 600 mg/dl), hyperosmolality (serum osmolality > 350 mOsm/liter), and dehydration without evidence of urinary or serum ketones, appears to occur in some cats.[21] These cats typically exhibit neurologic signs, and are predisposed to the development of cerebral edema if rehydration and reduction of serum glucose with insulin are performed too rapidly. The therapeutic protocol is similar to that utilized for diabetic ketoacedosis, but fluid rates and insulin dosage should be reduced to minimize potentially fatal complications.

A long-term complication in poorly regulated diabetics is the development of a plantigrade stance secondary to diabetic neuropathy (see Chapter 17, Diabetic Neuropathy). The exact cause of this abnormality is unknown, but evidence suggests that Schwann cell injury and subsequent demyelination occur.[22] This neuropathy appears to coincide with an irritable disposition, and improvement in regulation can result in improvement in neuropathy and disposition. Cataract formation is not as common in cats as in poorly regulated dogs, and complications commonly seen in human beings (nephropathy, vascular disease, retinopathy) do not appear to occur as frequently in cats.

◆ CONCLUSION

Adequate attention to resolution of clinical signs, improvement in laboratory parameters (fasting blood glucose, fructosamine, glycosylated hemoglobin), and surveillance for the development of concurrent illness are integral to the successful regulation of feline DM. Diabetic cats typically have components of insulin resistance and insufficiency; therefore, insulin is required for the management of most patients. Treatment of DM can result in changing insulin requirements, and the disease has the potential to be quite dynamic. Understanding the pathogenesis of DM, and the measures necessary to control the disease, may reduce the frustration commonly associated with treating this challenging disease. Last, recognition of complications associated with insulin therapy is essential to safe and effective treatment.

REFERENCES

1. Scarlett JM, Donoghue S: Associations between body condition and disease in cats. J Am Vet Med Assoc 212:1725–1731, 1998.
2. Crenshaw KL, Peterson ME: Pretreatment clinical and laboratory evaluation of cats with diabetes mellitus: 104 cases (1992–1994). J Am Vet Med Assoc 209:943–949, 1996.
3. Greco DS: Treatment of non–insulin-dependent diabetes mellitus in cats using oral hypoglycemic agents. In Bonagura JD (ed): Kirk's Current Veterinary Therapy XIII. Philadelphia, WB Saunders, 2000, pp. 354–357.
4. Feldman EC, Nelson RW, Feldman MS: Intensive 50-week evaluation of glipizide administration in 50 cats with previously untreated diabetes mellitus. J Am Vet Med Assoc 210:772–777, 1997.
5. Behrend EN, Clark TP: Pathogenesis of diabetes mellitus. In August JR (ed): Consultations in Feline Internal Medicine, vol. 3. Philadelphia, WB Saunders, 1997, pp. 125–131.
6. Lutz TA, Rand JS: Pathogenesis of feline diabetes mellitus. Vet Clin North Am Small Anim Pract 25:527–552, 1995.
7. Nelson RW, Griffey SM, Feldman EC, Ford SL: Transient clinical diabetes mellitus in cats: 10 cases (1989–1991). J Vet Intern Med 13:28–35, 1999.
8. Feldman EC, Nelson RW: Diabetes mellitus. In Feldman EC, Nelson RW (eds): Canine and Feline Endocrinology and Reproduction, 2nd ed. Philadelphia, WB Saunders, 1996, p. 362.
9. Bertroy EH, Nelson RW, Feldman EC. Effect of lente insulin

for treatment of diabetes mellitus in 12 cats. J Am Vet Med Assoc 206:1729–1731, 1995.

10. Gossens MM, Nelson RW, Feldman EC, Griffey SM: Response of insulin treatment and survival in 104 cats with diabetes mellitus (1985–1995). J Vet Intern Med 12:1–6, 1998.

11. Wallace MS, Peterson ME, Nichols CE: Absorption kinetics of regular, isophane, and protamine zinc insulin in normal cats. Domest Anim Endocrinol 7:509–515, 1990.

12. Reusch CE, Liehs MR, Hoyer M, Vochezer R: Fructosamine. A new parameter for diagnosis and metabolic control in diabetic dogs and cats. J Vet Intern Med 7:177–182, 1993.

13. Elliot DA, Nelson RW, Feldman EC, Neal LA: Glycosylated hemoglobin concentration for assessment of glycemic control in diabetic cats. J Vet Intern Med 11:161–165, 1997.

14. Elliot DA, Nelson RW, Reusch CE, et al: Comparison of serum fructosamine and blood glycosylated hemoglobin concentrations for assessment of glycemic control in cats with diabetes mellitus. J Am Vet Med Assoc 214:1794–1798, 1999.

15. Peterson ME: Diagnostic and therapeutic approach to insulin resistance. *In* August JR (ed): Consultations in Feline Internal Medicine, vol. 3. Philadelphia, WB Saunders, 1997, pp. 132–141.

16. Unger RH, Foster DW: Diabetes mellitus. *In* Wilson JD, Foster DW, Kronenberg HM, Larsen PR (eds): Williams Textbook of Endocrinology, 9th ed. Philadelphia, WB Saunders, 1998, pp. 973–1059.

17. Goldman J, Baldwin D, Rubenstein AH, et al: Characterization of circulating insulin and proinsulin-binding antibodies in autoimmune hypoglycemia. J Clin Invest 63:1050–1059, 1979.

18. Whitley NT, Drobatz KJ, Panciera DL: Insulin overdosage in dogs and cats: 28 cases (1986–1993). J Am Vet Med Assoc 211:326–330, 1997.

19. McMillan FD, Feldman EC: Rebound hyperglycemia following overdosing of insulin in cats with diabetes mellitus. J Am Vet Med Assoc 188:1426–1431, 1986.

20. Bruskiewicz KA, Nelson RW, Feldman EC, Griffey SM: Diabetic ketosis and ketoacidosis in cats: 42 cases (1980–1995). J Am Vet Med Assoc 211:188–192, 1997.

21. Macintire DK: Emergency therapy of diabetic crises: Insulin overdose, diabetic ketoacidosis, and hyperosmolar coma. Vet Clin North Am Small Anim Pract 25:639–641, 1995.

22. Mizisin AP, Shelton GD, Wagner S, et al: Myelin splitting, Schwann cell injury and demyelination in feline diabetic neuropathy. Acta Neuropathol 95:171–174, 1998.

23

◆ APUDomas: Pheochromocytoma, Insulinoma, and Gastrinoma

Deborah S. Greco

◆ APUDOMAS

APUDomas are tumors of endocrine cells that are capable of amine precursor uptake and decarboxylation (APUD) and secretion of peptide hormones. The tumors are named after the hormone they secrete. APUD cells generally are found in the gastrointestinal tract and central nervous system. APUDomas are reported rarely in cats; however, with increased awareness, the practitioner may be able to recognize and treat these unusual feline endocrinopathies. The purpose of this chapter is to describe the clinical syndromes associated with pheochromocytoma, insulinoma, and gastrinoma in cats.

◆ PHEOCHROMOCYTOMA

Pheochromocytomas arise from the chromaffin cells of the adrenal medulla; chromaffin cells are derived embryologically from neural crest cells.[1, 2] Most pheochromocytomas occur in the adrenal medulla; however, some originate in the sympathetic ganglia (paragangliomas) throughout the abdomen.[3, 4] Norepinephrine and epinephrine normally are secreted from the adrenal medulla. In human beings and in dogs, 80 per cent of the catecholamine secreted is epinephrine. Most feline pheochromocytomas, however, secrete norepinephrine predominantly.[2] Pheochromocytomas are very rare in cats.[1–4]

Pathogenesis

Synthesis of norepinephrine and epinephrine begins with the uptake of tyrosine by catecholamine-producing cells. Tyrosine is hydroxylated to dihydroxyphenylalanine (DOPA) by the rate-limiting enzyme tyrosine hydroxylase, which is under negative feedback control from norepinephrine. DOPA is converted to dopamine and then to L-norepinephrine by dopamine beta-hydroxylase. In the adrenal medulla and para-aortic bodies, norepinephrine may be methylated to form epinephrine; however, this does not occur in sympathetic nerve endings.[2] In pheochromocytomas, there is a lack of normal feedback regulating the synthesis and release of catecholamines. This is a result of 1 of 3 possible mechanisms: (1) presence of insensitivity in enzymatic negative feedback; (2) prevention of negative feedback due to sequestration of norepinephrine within cytoplasmic vesicles; or (3) metabolism by the tumor cell of a portion of the catecholamines produced thereby preventing negative feedback inhibition.[2] Degradation of catecholamines occurs via the enzymes catechol-O-methyltransferase (COMT) and monoamine oxidase (MAO) to form vanillylmandelic acid.[2]

Pathophysiology of Clinical Signs

Tissue response to catecholamines is dependent on the number and type of catecholamine receptors present. Adrenergic receptors can be classified as alpha or beta and as subclasses of alpha-1 (postganglionic smooth muscle, glands), alpha-2 (presynaptic membranes, autonomic nerves), beta-1 (cardiac), and beta-2 (smooth muscle and glandular cells).

Physiologic effects of excess catecholamine secretion are variable depending on the size and character of the tumor and whether the predominant catecholamine is norepinephrine (more common) or epinephrine (less common). Hypertension, usually episodic, results from alpha-1–mediated increases in peripheral vascular resistance. Tachyarrhythmias may result from activation of cardiac beta-1 receptors mediated through epinephrine. Weight loss may occur secondary to hypermetabolism caused by excessive catecholamine release. Beta-adrenergic antagonism of insulin resulting in peripheral insulin resistance also may be observed. Gastrointestinal motility is suppressed by adrenergic activation; therefore, constipation may be a clinical sign.

The disease, although rare, tends to occur in middle-aged to older cats, with no gender or breed predilection. Only 5 case reports of pheochromocytoma exist in the literature.[1] Clinical signs develop as a result of the space-occupying nature of the tumor (ascites, edema) or as a result of excessive secretion of catecholamines (hypertension). Signs of hypertension may be constant or paroxysmal, and may be present from days to years before presentation. Common clinical findings related to hypertension include blindness, weakness, and neurologic signs (hyperesthesia). The most common clinical signs of pheochromocytoma in cats are polydipsia, polyuria, lethargy, and anorexia. Less common signs are seizures and intermittent vomiting.

Physical examination findings include lethargy, depression, tachypnea, dyspnea, emaciation, weakness, edema, and ascites. Thoracic auscultation may reveal cardiac arrhythmias, systolic murmurs, and rales. Signs of hypertension may be observed such as epistaxis, hyperemic mucous membranes, and blindness due to ocular bleeding. An abdominal mass and abdominal pain occasionally are detected in patients with large adrenal tumors.

Clinical pathology may reveal a nonregenerative anemia, hemoconcentration, leukocytosis, and mild hyperglycemia. Occasionally, mild uremia, increased liver enzymes, hypoalbuminemia, hypocalcemia, and proteinuria are detected. Radiography may reveal an abdominal mass, calcification of the adrenal mass, heptomegaly, renal displacement, abnormal renal contour, ascites, and enlargement of the caudal venal cava.[1, 2] Thoracic radiographic findings may include generalized cardiomegaly and pulmonary congestion or edema. Ultrasound is superior to radiographs for identification of adrenal masses.[1, 2] Scintigraphic imaging using ^{131}I-metaiodobenzylguanidine, a radioactive isotope taken up selectively by adrenergic cells, has shown promise for the detection and localization of pheochromocytomas.[1, 2] Echocardiography may reveal left ventricular hypertrophy associated with systemic hypertension, and electrocardiographic changes include sinus tachycardia and arrhythmias.

Arterial blood pressure should be measured in cats with clinical evidence of systemic hypertension. Systolic blood pressure greater than 180 mm Hg or diastolic pressure greater than 100 mm Hg in a cat is diagnostic for systemic hypertension. Some cats with pheochromocytoma may not be hypertensive at the time of presentation because of the episodic nature of secretion of some tumors. In a cat with documented hypertension, hyperthyroidism and renal disease should be ruled out first, then a pheochromocytoma should be investigated (see Chapters 36, Systemic Hypertension, and 47, Diagnosis and Treatment of Systemic Hypertension).

Diagnostic Testing

Plasma catecholamine elevation (>1500 pg/ml for norepinephrine, >300 pg/ml for epinephrine) supports a diagnosis of pheochromocytoma; however, proper handling of the sample is crucial to avoid false-negative results.[2] False-positive results may be caused by stress and excitement. Urinary catecholamine and catecholamine metabolite excretion over 24 hours can be measured; however, there is a false-positive rate of 10 to 15 per cent.[1, 2] Sample handling is important in that urine must be acidified (pH < 3). This urine assay has a lower sensitivity (0.42) than that of plasma catecholamines (0.97). The phentolamine test is used in hypertensive patients to evaluate the dependence of hypertension on catecholamine secretion. After a stable arterial blood pressure is obtained, an intravenous bolus of phentolamine is given. Blood pressure is recorded every 30 seconds for the first 3 minutes and every minute thereafter for an additional 7 minutes. The test is positive if the fall in blood pressure is greater than 35 mm Hg systolic and the decline lasts at least 5 minutes. There is a high incidence of false-positive results (other causes of hypertension can result in a positive test), and caution should be used to avoid hypotension.

Surgical Management

Surgical removal of the adrenal tumor is the treatment of choice for pheochromocytomas; however, the surgery is technically demanding and metastasis may have occurred by the time a diagnosis is made.[1–4] Proper anesthetic management is key to successful surgery. Phenoxybenzamine (0.2 to 1.5 mg/kg every [q] 12 hr) is administered for 1 to 2 weeks before surgery.[1, 2] Propranolol is used to control cardiac arrhythmias or tachycardia. However, unopposed beta blockade may lead to severe hypertension. Therefore, beta blockers should never be administered without pretreatment with an alpha-adrenergic–blocking agent. The prognosis for cats with pheochromocytoma is guarded to poor, and usually is determined at the time of surgery, with metastasis carrying a worse prognosis.

◆ INSULINOMA

Insulinomas are the most commonly recognized APUDoma in dogs; however, there are only 3 reported cases of beta-cell neoplasia in cats.[5–10] Insulinoma occurs most frequently as a single entity, but may be part of multiple endocrine neoplasia syndrome type 1 (MEN type 1). Middle-aged to older cats have been reported to develop insulinomas; reported cases included 2 Siamese and 1 female Persian cat.[5–10] Clinical signs are caused by excessive insulin secretion by neoplastic beta cells of the pancreas resulting in decreased serum glucose concentrations. The severity and duration of clinical signs are related to the rate of decline of serum glucose, the duration of hypoglycemia, and the absolute serum glucose concentration. Cortisol, glucagon, epinephrine, and growth hormone are released in response to hypoglycemia. Clinical signs result from neuroglycopenia and increased plasma catecholamines; therefore, signs of hypoglycemia include seizures, weakness, ataxia, collapse, exercise intolerance, muscle fasciculations, shaking, abnormal behavior, attitude changes, polyphagia, and trembling.

Clinical Pathology

Hypoglycemia is observed as the only finding on the serum chemistry profile. Care should be taken to rule out iatrogenic or spurious causes of hypoglycemia such as use of a portable glucose-monitoring device (results can be 25 per cent below the actual value), old test strips, and serum remaining too long on red blood cells without separation. Whipple's triad may be used to increase the suspicion of an insulinoma. The triad is composed of (1) clinical signs after feeding or exercise, (2) serum glucose less than 50 mg/dl at time of clinical signs, and (3) clinical signs relieved by administration of glucose.

The best screening test for an insulinoma is demonstration of excessive serum insulin concentrations when hypoglycemia is present. Serum insulin should be measured when serum glucose is less than 60 mg/dl. In order to document hyperinsulinemia, the feline patient should be fed a normal meal early in the day then fasted for the remainder of the day. Glucose should be monitored at hourly intervals until levels are less than 60 mg/dl. A blood sample then should be obtained for insulin and glucose measurement once the blood glucose is less than 60 mg/dl. The cat then is fed small meals over the next several hours.[10] Insulin concentrations of greater than 20 μU/ml are diagnostic for insulinoma when serum glucose is less than 60 mg/dl. If serum insulin is in the normal range (5 to 20 μU/ml) when serum glucose is less than 60 mg/dl, an insulinoma is probable. In cases in which the insulin concentration is suspicious but not diagnostic for insulinoma, an amended insulin:glucose ratio (AIGR) may be used. An AIGR greater than 30 is diagnostic for an insulinoma.

$$AIGR = \frac{plasma\ insulin\ (\mu U/ml)}{plasma\ glucose\ (mg/dl) - 30} \times 100$$

Only insulin assays that have been validated for use in cats should be used for the diagnosis of insulinoma.[5, 6] Radiographs usually are not helpful in the diagnosis of insulinoma, but ultrasound of the pancreas may document a large pancreatic beta-cell mass and/or metastasis to regional lymph nodes or liver.

Exploratory Surgery

Exploratory surgery often is indicated to determine the location and spread of tumor. The pancreas is visualized and palpated carefully, and if no tumor is found, a hemipancreatectomy is performed.[5, 6, 10] Debulking of the tumors is palliative, and many cats can be managed medically for several months to a year even with metastasis. Dextrose (5 per cent) should be administered intravenously before and during surgery at a rate of at least twice maintenance to ensure good circulation through the pancreatic microvasculature postoperatively. Postsurgical complications include pancreatitis, hypoglycemia (if metastasis is present), and transient diabetes mellitus. Regardless of the extent of surgical manipulation, the clinician should manage the patient as if pancreatitis was present for the first 48 to 72 hours postoperatively; for example, fluid therapy, nothing by mouth, and antiemetics if necessary. First water

and then bland food may be offered on the third day after surgery, provided vomiting is not present.

Medical Management

Emergency medical management of an insulinoma in the veterinary setting consists of intravenous dextrose (5 to 15 ml 50 per cent dextrose diluted 1:4). The owner should be instructed to administer Karo syrup orally to cats that become hypoglycemic at home. Nutritional management of hypoglycemia requires frequent feedings consisting of high-protein canned food and avoidance of semimoist foods that may provoke insulin secretion.

Glucocorticoids may be administered to cats with insulinoma in an effort to antagonize the effects of insulin. Prednisolone (0.55 mg/kg orally [PO] q 12 hr may be effective in controlling signs of hypoglycemia. An increased dosage of 4.4 to 6.6 mg/kg/day may be required to control clinical signs in advanced cases. Diazoxide, a benzothiadiazide diuretic that inhibits insulin secretion and stimulates gluconeogenesis, has been used to treat canine insulinoma. However, the drug is not available currently, and has not been assessed in cats with insulinoma. The prognosis in dogs is guarded to poor; however, only a few cases have been reported in cats. Of the 3 cats with beta-cell carcinomas, survival was highly variable, ranging from 5 weeks to 2 years.[5, 6, 10]

◆ GASTRINOMA

APUD cells that produce gastrin are termed *gastrinomas* and result in a condition called *Zollinger-Ellison syndrome*. Hypergastrinemia from gastrin-secreting tumors can cause gastritis, gastric ulceration, duodenal hyperacidity, intestinal villous atrophy, and esophageal dysfunction from chronic reflux.

Clinical Signs

Gastrinoma is rare, but has been reported in 3 middle-aged to older cats.[5, 6, 10–12] Clinical signs associated with excess gastrin secretion include vomiting, weight loss, anorexia, diarrhea, lethargy, and depression. Polydipsia, melena, abdominal pain, hematemesis, hematochezia, and fever ensue when gastric ulceration occurs. Other conditions associated with hypergastrinemia, gastric hyperacidity, and gastrointestinal ulceration include inflammatory gastritis, uremia, drug-induced ulceration (e.g., nonsteroidal anti-inflammatory drugs or steroids), stress-induced ulceration, hepatic failure, and mast-cell disease.

Laboratory Findings

Results of complete blood count, serum chemistry profile, and urinalysis are normal, or reflect the chronic effects of general disease such as iron-deficiency anemia secondary to gastrointestinal bleeding; increased blood urea nitrogen, and hypoproteinemia secondary to gastrointestinal bleeding; and electrolyte abnormalities associated with chronic vomiting.[5, 6, 10]

Diagnosis

Diagnosis begins with endoscopy accompanied by gastric and duodenal biopsy. Endoscopic biopsy often reveals gastrointestinal ulceration. Histopathologic examination of pancreatic tumors reveals findings consistent with islet-cell tumor; however, immunocytochemical staining may be necessary to provide a specific diagnosis.[9] Histopathologic examination also can reveal metastasis to liver and regional lymph nodes.

Serum gastrin concentrations are normal or high-normal in patients with gastrinoma, and gastric hyperacidity often is observed at endoscopy. Provocative tests of gastrin secretion, when accompanied by an increase in serum gastrin after intravenous calcium gluconate or secretin administration, suggest gastrinoma. Abdominal ultrasound may demonstrate a pancreatic mass, but usually is normal.

Treatment

Owners should be informed that most gastrinomas are malignant and have metastasized by the time of diagnosis. Surgical exploration and excisional biopsy of a pancreatic mass are important both diagnostically and therapeutically, because aggressive medical management can palliate signs for years. Gastric hyperacidity can be treated by histamine$_2$-receptor antagonists, such as famotidine, which decreases acid secretion by gastric parietal cells. Omeprazole, a proton pump inhibitor, is the most potent inhibitor of gastric acid secretion available; unfortunately, it is available in only one pill size, which makes dosing difficult in cats. Sucralfate adheres to ulcerated gastric mucosa, stimulates prostaglandin secretion, and promotes healing by binding pepsin and bile acids; sucralfate and H$_2$ antagonists provide the mainstay of medical treatment of gastrinomas in cats. Although the prognosis for cats with gastrinoma is guarded to poor, patients with gastrinoma have been controlled on medical management for several months.

◆ MULTIPLE ENDOCRINE NEOPLASIA

MEN type 1 or Wermer's syndrome is characterized by parathyroid hyperplasia associated with a pancreatic islet-cell adenoma/carcinoma or adenoma/hyperplasia of the anterior pituitary. MEN type 2 or 2a, Sipple's syndrome, consists of medullary carcinoma of thyroid associated with unilateral or bilateral pheochromocytoma and/or parathyroid hyperplasia. MEN type 3 or 2b, multiple mucosal neuroma syndrome, is an inherited condition encompassing medullary carcinoma of the thyroid associated with pheochromocytoma and/or multiple mucosal neuromas. MEN has not been reported in cats and is very rare in dogs.[2]

REFERENCES

1. Maher ER, McNiel EA: Pheochromocytoma in dogs and cats. Vet Clin North Am Small Anim Pract 27:359–380, 1997.
2. Feldman EC, Nelson RW: Pheochromocytoma and multiple endocrine neoplasia. In Feldman EC, Nelson RW (eds): Canine and Feline Endocrinology and Reproduction, 2nd ed. Philadelphia, WB Saunders, 1996, pp. 306–321.
3. Henry CJ, Brewer WJ, Montgomery RD, et al: Adrenal pheochromocytoma. J Vet Intern Med 7:199–201, 1993.
4. Patnaik AK, Erlandson RA, Lieberman PH, et al: Extra-adrenal pheochromocytoma (paraganglioma) in a cat. J Am Vet Med Assoc 197:104–106, 1990.
5. Feldman EC, Nelson RW: Beta-cell neoplasia, gastrinoma, glucagonoma and other APUDomas. In Feldman ED, Nelson RW (eds): Canine and Feline Endocrinology and Reproduction, 2nd ed. Philadelphia, WB Saunders, 1996, pp. 440–453.
6. Johnson SE: Pancreatic APUDomas. Semin Vet Med Surg (Small Anim) 4:202–207, 1989.
7. McMillan F: Functional pancreatic islet cell tumor in a cat. J Am Anim Hosp Assoc 21:741–743, 1985.
8. O'Brien TD, Norton F, Turner TM, Johnson KH: Pancreatic endocrine tumor in a cat: Clinical, pathological and immuno-histochemical evaluation. J Am Anim Hosp Assoc 26:453–457, 1990.
9. Hawks D, Peterson ME, Hawkins KL, Rosebury WS: Insulin-secreting pancreatic (islet cell) carcinoma in a cat. J Vet Intern Med 6:193–196, 1992.
10. Zerbe CA: Islet cell tumors secreting insulin, pancreatic polypeptide, gastrin, or glucagon. In Kirk RW, Bonagura JD (eds): Current Veterinary Therapy XI. Philadelphia, WB Saunders, 1992, pp. 368–375.
11. Eng J, Du BH, Johnson GF, et al: Cat gastrinoma and the sequence of cat gastrins. Regul Pept 37:9–13, 1992.
12. Middleton DJ, Watson AD: Duodenal ulceration associated with gastrin-secreting pancreatic tumor in a cat. J Am Vet Med Assoc 183:461–463, 1983.

Dermatology

Karen L. Campbell, Editor

◆ Mosquito-Bite Hypersensitivity 186
◆ Photodermatitis 190
◆ Paraneoplastic Alopecia 196
◆ Primary Hereditary Seborrhea Oleosa 202
◆ Bowen's Disease (Multicentric Squamous
  Cell Carcinoma In Situ) 208
◆ Cutaneous Xanthomas 214
◆ Nontuberculous Mycobacterial Diseases 221
◆ What to Do for the Devoted Cat Owner
  Who Is Allergic to His or Her Pet 233

Still-Current Information Found in *Consultations in Feline Internal Medicine 2*:
Diagnostic Approach to the Pruritic Patient (Chapter 25),
    p. 195
Shampoo Therapy in the Management of Dermatoses
    (Chapter 30), p. 227
Antibiotic-Responsive Dermatoses (Chapter 31), p. 233
Use of Lasers in Dermatology (Chapter 32), p. 241
Clinical Applications of Radiotherapy (Chapter 68), p. 553

Still-Current Information Found in *Consultations in Feline Internal Medicine 3*:
Cutaneous Manifestations of Systemic Disease (Chapter 27),
    p. 199
Atopy: Advances in Diagnosis and Management (Chapter
    29), p. 214
Metastatic Patterns of Feline Neoplasia (Chapter 71), p. 566

Elsewhere in *Consultations in Feline Internal Medicine 4*:
Cat Ownership by Immunosuppressed People (Chapter 3),
    p. 18
Oral Hypoglycemic Therapy for Type 2 Diabetes Mellitus
    (Chapter 21), p. 169
Problems of Diabetic Regulation With Insulin Therapy
    (Chapter 22), p. 175
Diagnostic Imaging of Neoplasia (Chapter 70), p. 548

24

◆ Mosquito-Bite Hypersensitivity

Ralf S. Mueller

Mosquito-bite hypersensitivity is associated with a seasonal facial dermatitis in cats.[1] Affected cats exhibit facial pruritus, and develop erythematous papules or plaques over the bridge of the nose and on the pinnae (Figs. 24–1 to 24–3). Other areas of the body also may be involved.

◆ PATHOGENESIS

Mosquito-bite hypersensitivity is a hypersensitivity presumably to antigens in the saliva of mosquitoes.[2, 3] It was first reported as a clinical entity in cats by Wilkinson and Bates.[4] Owing to the seasonal occurrence and the observed remission on hospitalization, the authors initially suspected environmental allergens such as plant pollens to be responsible for the clinical signs.[3] However, Mason and Evans[1] evaluated the syndrome further and demonstrated conclusively that mosquitoes are able to cause clinical signs in affected animals. Cats with classic clinical signs underwent intradermal skin testing, and histopathologic and hematologic evaluation. Four cats with clinical signs improved when kept at home behind insect screening, but flared up when screening was removed. Nonlesional skin of 1 affected cat was exposed to the bites of laboratory-raised mosquito species *(Culex orbostiensis, Aedes multiplex)*, which caused pruritus and skin changes that were clinically and histopathologically similar to the naturally occurring lesions.[1]

Nagata and Ishida[5] reported 26 cats with mosquito-bite hypersensitivity, and studied this syndrome in 5 affected and 3 healthy cats in more detail. Mosquito-bite exposure led to wheal formation after 20 minutes (in 5 of 5 cats), papule formation after 48 hours (in 2 of 5), and eosinophilic dermatitis (in 5 of 5) in the 5 affected cats, and produced transient erythema in the 3 control cats. Intradermal skin testing caused an immediate wheal reaction in 3 of the 5 affected cats, and no reaction in all 3 control cats. Prausnitz-Küstner tests were performed in healthy cats with the serum of 3 affected cats injected intradermally. Twenty-four hours later, these sites were exposed to captured mosquitoes. Mosquito bites caused wheals at 20 minutes on all occasions. The uniform, immediate-type reaction observed indicates the presence of an immediate-type hypersensitivity. Prausnitz-Küstner tests with serum from healthy cats and saline failed to show positive reactions. Neither Prausnitz-Küstner tests nor intradermal tests, but only mos-

quito bites caused a delayed-type papular reaction in the Japanese study.[5]

In human beings, cutaneous reactions to mosquito bites are determined by previous exposure. After an initial nonreactive stage, a delayed reaction may develop. Several months later, an immediate whealing reaction occurs before the delayed reaction. Later, only the immediate reaction is observed, and finally, no reactivity is seen.[6] These changes most likely are due to sensitization and desensitization. In a controlled study with 7 human beings exposed repeatedly to mosquito bites, 4 individuals lost the delayed hypersensitivity during the trial, but despite a decrease in pruritus associated with the immediate reaction, wheal formation was not changed significantly.[1] In cats reported from temperate climates and in those seen in the author's practice in Melbourne and Sydney, Australia, disease recurrence occurs over several years, and desensitization seems to be a slow process, if it occurs at all.

◆ CLINICAL SIGNS

Age, gender, or breed predispositions have not been reported. Mosquito-bite hypersensitivity can occur first in cats as young as 5 months of age and as old as 12 years of age.

In temperate climates, mosquitoes occur in early

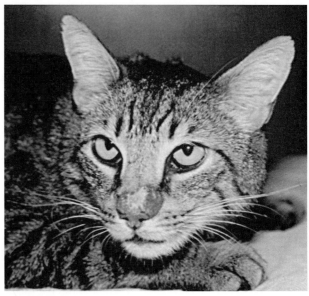

Figure 24–1. Swollen nose in a domestic shorthair cat with mosquito-bite hypersensitivity.

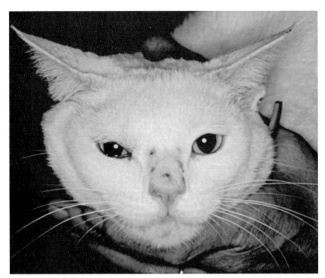

Figure 24–2. Ulceration and crusting of the dorsal muzzle in a 5-year-old domestic shorthair cat with mosquito-bite hypersensitivity.

summer to autumn. Under these climatic conditions, mosquito-bite hypersensitivity is seasonal, and may wax and wane according to varying environmental conditions at any given time. In tropical or subtropical areas, mosquito-bite hypersensitivity may occur year-round.

Exposure to mosquitoes is much greater in cats with access to outdoors, and most cats with mosquito-bite hypersensitivity are outdoor or partially outdoor cats. One publication hypothesizes that darker skin and/or hair color may attract mosquitoes, and predispose cats to the development of disease.[5] However, lighter-colored cats also may be affected. Sweat and lipids seem to be other factors involved in human beings.[7] It is unknown whether these factors play a role in cats.

Commonly affected sites include the lateral (outer) pinnae and the dorsal bridge of the nose (see Figs. 24–1 to 24–3). Lesions may involve the planum nasale in approximately 25 per cent of the

affected cats. Papules are the first lesions observed. Typically, papular lesions progress rapidly to erosions and crusts. Cats sleeping on their sides may develop footpad lesions (Fig. 24–4), whereas cats resting in a crouched position typically do not show signs of pedal disease. Crusting and hyperkeratosis on the margins of the pads are noted most commonly, but papules, erosions, and hyperpigmentation may occur as well. Pruritus varies from mild to marked. Approximately 50 per cent of the cats have a peripheral lymphadenopathy, particularly of the submandibular lymph nodes. Interdigital erosions, paronychia, papules affecting the legs, and indolent ulcer of the lips and hard palate have been reported in some affected patients.

◆ DIFFERENTIAL DIAGNOSIS

Differential diagnostic possibilities include flea-bite hypersensitivity, atopic dermatitis, food adverse reaction, eosinophilic granuloma complex, drug reaction, pemphigus foliaceus, discoid lupus erythematosus, and sun-induced dermatoses such as actinic keratosis and squamous cell carcinoma.

Flea-bite hypersensitivity typically does not affect the nasal bridge, planum nasale, or footpads, rather presenting with a more generalized or truncal dermatitis. Atopic dermatitis also typically does not affect the planum nasale or footpads. However, both atopy and flea-bite hypersensitivity may be seasonal, may respond to symptomatic anti-inflammatory therapy, and possibly may show similar hematologic and histopathologic changes.[8] Some topical insecticides used in intensive flea control may treat

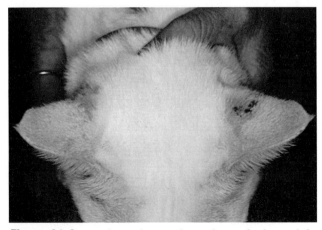

Figure 24–3. Papules and crusted papules at the base of the pinnae in the same cat as shown in Figure 24–2.

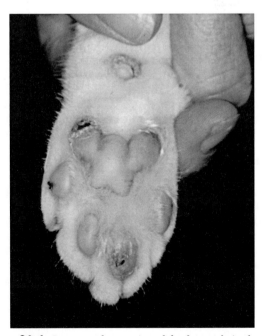

Figure 24–4. Crusts on the margins of the foot pads in the same cat as shown in Figure 24–2.

cats successfully with mosquito-bite hypersensitivity.

Food adverse reaction is a nonseasonal disease, typically characterized by alopecia, and crusting and ulceration of the trunk, head, and neck.[8] Involvement of the footpads and planum nasale is seen rarely.

The *eosinophilic granuloma complex* is the term long used to include eosinophilic plaques, eosinophilic granulomas, and indolent ulcers in cats. The majority of these lesions are a result of hypersensitivities to fleas, environmental allergens, food allergens, and insects including mosquitoes. However, in some cats these lesions are hereditary.[9] Thus, when no hypersensitivity can be documented, a hereditary or idiopathic form of eosinophilic granulomas may be present.

The clinical and histopathologic presentation of drug reactions varies tremendously.[10] Seasonality and medical history are useful differentiating features. Response to drug withdrawal is a further clue. Rechallenge with the suspected drug leads to recurrence of clinical signs, but is rarely performed in veterinary practice.

Autoimmune diseases such as pemphigus foliaceus or discoid lupus erythematosus in cats may present with lesions on face and feet.[8] Typically, the crusts seen in pemphigus affect the medial (inner) aspects of the pinnae, in contrast to the papules on the lateral (outer) pinnae occurring in cats with mosquito-bite hypersensitivity. Seasonal pemphigus foliaceus has been reported in dogs. Discoid lupus erythematosus may be a sun-aggravated disease, and thus initially may be clinically seasonal in some patients with mild clinical signs.[8] Histopathologic features of these autoimmune diseases differentiate them from hypersensitivities.

Sun-induced dermatoses may present with clinical deterioration during summer, and typically affect nonpigmented, sparsely haired skin (see Chapter 25, Photodermatitis). Many cats with mosquito-bite hypersensitivity have dark pinnae and faces. In addition, pedal involvement is very unlikely with actinic keratosis and sun-induced squamous cell carcinoma. Histopathology reliably differentiates sun-induced dermatoses from hypersensitivities.

◆ DIAGNOSIS

A history of seasonal dermatitis in cats with chronic disease is the first clue. Typically, cats with mosquito-bite hypersensitivity have access to outdoors, and show the classic clinical signs of papules and plaques on the bridge of the nose or ear pinnae.

Eosinophilia is present in almost all patients with this disease. Impression smears from eroded lesions reveal numerous eosinophils in the majority of patients. However, blood and lesional eosinophils may be seen in cats with any hypersensitivity, and are not specific for mosquito-bite hypersensitivity.

Hospitalization of affected cats leads to resolution of clinical signs, effectively ruling out autoimmune diseases and adverse reactions to foods.[4] Once returned to their environment, affected cats typically develop clinical signs again within 1 week.

Intradermal skin testing with crude mosquito extract is positive in most affected animals. Details of intradermal skin testing in cats are described elsewhere.[8] A negative test does not rule out mosquito-bite hypersensitivity because it evaluates only immediate-type hypersensitivity and lesions also may result from a delayed hypersensitivity reaction.

Characteristic histopathologic changes of early lesions include acanthosis, spongiosis, eosinophilic epidermitis with microabscesses, and perivascular dermatitis. In later stages, erosions covered by serocellular crusting and collagen degeneration may develop. Eosinophilic furunculosis and focal coagulative epidermal necrosis have been reported.[3, 11, 12] Occasionally, a predominantly neutrophilic and plasmacytic infiltrate may be found in eroded lesions. Biopsy specimens from affected footpads may show a predominantly plasmacytic infiltrate in a small percentage of cases.

◆ TREATMENT

Glucocorticoids will lead to rapid improvement and healing of lesions. Prednisolone is used commonly, and is effective at 0.5 to 1.5 mg/kg orally every (q) 12 hr.[3, 4] The drug is tapered to lower doses or discontinued once the condition is in remission. Alternatives to glucocorticoids or adjunctive therapy in cats with severe clinical signs include antihistamines and fatty acid supplementation.

Antihistamines used in the author's practice and their doses are shown in Table 24–1. In human beings with mosquito-bite hypersensitivity, cetirizine decreased immediate whealing and pruritus as well as delayed reactions and pruritus in a double-blinded, placebo-controlled study.[13] Cetirizine in human beings has significant effects on eosinophil migration.[14] To the author's knowledge, similar studies have not been performed in cats, but the clinical response of cats with eosinophilic skin diseases in general, and with mosquito-bite hypersensitivity specifically, treated with cetirizine has been variable. Other, less expensive antihistamines seem to achieve similar improvement of clinical signs in

Table 24–1. Selected Antihistamines Used in Feline Dermatology

Antihistamine	Dosage
Chlorpheniramine	2–4 mg/cat q 12 hr
Promethazine	10 mg/cat q 12 hr
Hydroxyzine	10 mg/cat q 12 hr
Cyproheptadine	2–4 mg/cat q 12 hr
Loratadine	5–10 mg/cat q 12 hr
Cetirizine	5 mg/cat q 12–24 hr

Abbreviation: q, every.

cats. It is worth noting that some cats responding poorly to glucocorticoids improve significantly on antihistamines. Administration of tablets may be difficult in some patients. Some antihistamines are available in syrup form, but the sweet taste is not always well tolerated. Apothecary pharmacies can assist in formulating tuna-flavored pastes or cod-liver oil mixes incorporating the antihistamines.

Essential fatty acids are available in capsules (which can be pierced and expressed) or liquids that may be mixed with a small portion of food before the main meal. Some cats will tolerate this more readily than capsules or tablets. Eicosapentaenoic acid at 20 mg/kg and gamma-linoleic acid at 50 mg/kg daily are used commonly. Linoleic acid is not an ideal fatty acid supplement for cats owing to their decreased level of delta-6-desaturase.[15]

◆ MANAGEMENT AND PREVENTION

Long-term management of cats with mosquito-bite hypersensitivity may include lifestyle changes, insect repellents, and/or continuous or intermittent symptomatic therapy (e.g., antihistamines, fatty acids, corticosteroids). Keeping a cat indoors permanently will eliminate or decrease the exposure to mosquitoes, and thus minimize the need for symptomatic therapy. For many cats, this is a dramatic and possibly traumatic change. Less extreme and possibly sufficient may be to limit outdoor activities, and keep the cat inside from afternoon to the next morning to avoid times of peak mosquito activity. Feeding cats inside during the afternoon as a regular daily routine facilitates this approach.

Insect repellents are helpful in many patients with mosquito-bite hypersensitivity. Many repellents used in veterinary medicine are licensed for large animals and dogs, but not approved for cats. Pyrethrins are the most commonly used insect repellent in the author's practice, and a pyrethrin spray may be used daily. As most cats dislike being sprayed, a cloth can be wetted and then rubbed gently onto the sparsely haired and affected areas such as the pinnae, nose, and feet. Other repellents recommended in the literature include diethyltoluamide (DEET) and butoxypolypropylene.[8]

Symptomatic therapy with glucocorticoids, antihistamines, and essential fatty acids may be administered intermittently or continuously as needed. The personal and financial background of the owner, the personality and compliance of the patient, the severity of the disease, and the efficacy of the drugs used will determine the medication, dose, and frequency of administration. Even though cats seem to tolerate glucocorticoids better than dogs, care should be taken to minimize long-term administration of these drugs owing to possible long-term side-effects.

REFERENCES

1. Mason KV, Evans AG: Mosquito bite–caused eosinophilic dermatitis in cats. J Am Vet Med Assoc 198:2086–2088, 1991.
2. McKiel JA, West AS: Effects of repeated exposures of hypersensitive humans and laboratory rabbits to mosquito antigens. Can J Zool 39:597–603, 1961.
3. Reunala T, Brummer-Korvenkontio H, Raesaenen L, et al: Passive transfer of cutaneous mosquito bite hypersensitivity by IgE anti-saliva antibodies. J Allergy Clin Immunol 94:902–906, 1994.
4. Wilkinson GT, Bates MJA: A possible further clinical manifestation of the feline eosinophilic granuloma complex. J Am Anim Hosp Assoc 20:325–331, 1984.
5. Nagata M, Ishida T: Cutaneous reactivity to mosquito bites and its antigens in cats. Vet Dermatol 8:19–26, 1997.
6. Melanby K: Man's reaction to mosquito bites. Nature 158:554, 1946.
7. Maibach HI, Skinner WA, Strauss WG, Khan AA: Factors that attract and repel mosquitos in human skin. JAMA 196:263–266, 1966.
8. Scott DW, Miller WH, Griffin CE: Small Animal Dermatology, 5th ed. Philadelphia, WB Saunders, 1995, pp. 484–626.
9. Scott DW, Miller WH, Griffin CE: Small Animal Dermatology, 5th ed. Philadelphia, WB Saunders, 1995, pp. 924–930.
10. Mason KV: Cutaneous drug eruptions. Vet Clin North Am Small Anim Pract 20:1633–1653, 1990.
11. Ihrke PJ, Gross TL: Conference in Dermatology—No 2: Mosquito-bite hypersensitivity in a cat. Vet Dermatol 5:33–36, 1994.
12. Gross TL, Ihrke PJ, Walder E: Veterinary Dermatopathology—A Macroscopic and Microscopic Evaluation of Canine and Feline Skin Disease. St. Louis, Mosby–Year Book, 1992, pp. 210–211.
13. Reunala T, Brummerkorvenkontio H, Karppinen A, et al: Treatment of mosquito bites with cetirizine. Clin Exp Allergy 23:72–75, 1993.
14. Townley RG: Cetirizine: A new H_1 antagonist with antieosinophilic activity in chronic urticaria. J Am Acad Dermatol 25:668–674, 1991.
15. Harvey RG: Essential fatty acids and the cat. Vet Dermatol 4:175–179, 1993.

25

◆ Photodermatitis

Sonya Bettenay

Photodermatitis results from exposure of the skin to solar radiation and can be classified into phototoxic, photoallergic, photosensitive, and miscellaneous categories. *Phototoxicity* is a dose-related reaction that can be seen in all animals. It generally includes the acute (sunburn), chronic (solar dermatitis), and neoplastic (squamous cell carcinoma [SCC]) reactions. Phototoxicity also is implicated with diseases such as lupus erythematosus and pemphigus erythematosus in dogs; these are considered to be aggravated by solar radiation.[1, 2] Although lupus erythematosus and pemphigus erythematosus are seen in cats, photoaggravation has not been reported to date.

Photoallergy is uncommon in domestic animals. It is a response by an animal (or person) to an exogenous chemical that requires participation of the immune system. *Photosensitivity*, in domestic animals, is a term that usually describes phototoxic chemical photosensitivity, and does not involve the immune system. As such, disease can occur with the first exposure to the chemical. In domestic animals, this is associated most commonly with plant alkaloid–induced reactions such as St. John's wort–induced photosensitization in cattle.

In cats, solar-induced phototoxic dermatitis is the relevant clinical entity.

◆ SOLAR RADIATION

Solar radiation, particularly ultraviolet light (UV) such as ultraviolet-A (UVA; 320 to 400 nm) and ultraviolet-B (UVB; 280 to 320 nm), causes a variety of changes in the skin. Ultraviolet-C (200 to 280 nm), although capable of producing tumors in the skin of mice, is totally absorbed by the stratospheric ozone layer. The ultraviolet rays (UVR) cause inflammation, denature proteins and surface antigens on cells, and modify DNA in chromosomes, leading to cell death or mutations. If these mutations lose their proliferation inhibition, overt neoplasia results.

◆ PATHOGENESIS—WHY DOES SOLAR DERMATITIS DEVELOP?

Solar dermatitis occurs when the skin is exposed to the UVR present in solar radiation. A cat's natural protective mechanisms include a dense hair coat and pigmentation. The hair coat protects from UV-induced damage by physical interference; pig-

mented hair also may absorb UVR. Pigmentation protects because the pigment melanin acts as an absorptive agent. Melanin serves as a major defense of the skin against solar rays, and also has an effect in the hair shafts of pigmented coats. Rays that penetrate past the melanin in the hair coat encounter more melanin in the epidermis where it reflects and refracts the solar rays in the stratum corneum. Other epidermal components, such as carotenoids and surface lipids, also may play a role in the absorption and dispersion of solar dermatitis. Nonpigmented (white) skin lacks protection, and is particularly sensitive to solar damage in sparsely haired areas such as the pinnae, periocular skin, and planum nasale of cats. Once the UVR penetrates into the living epidermis, it can induce structural changes in DNA and surface antigen that predispose to cancer. Mutations of the tumor-suppressor gene *p53* were isolated in 9 of 11 cats with pinnal SCC, and in 7 of 14 cats with SCC in other sites such as the nasal planum.[3]

UVB has been implicated in the induction of skin cancers in fair-skinned people[4] and in white-haired cats.[5] It is regarded as the most carcinogenic range of radiation.[6] UVA alone is relatively ineffective in causing radiation-induced erythema, and appears to be 1600 times *less* carcinogenic than UVB. UVB has a direct carcinogenic effect as well as a tumor-promoting effect by interference with cell-mediated immunity. Solar radiation reduces the number of Langerhans cells in the epidermis by up to 50 per cent after a single dose of irradiation. Destruction of Langerhans cells impairs antigen presentation in the epidermis. Indeed, UV radiation is utilized as a research tool when investigating contact allergy[7] because the defective antigen presentation prevents the induction of a normal delayed-type hypersensitivity. Defective antigen presentation also stimulates the production of suppressor T-cells specific for the improperly presented antigen. This may result in suppressor T-cells in UVR-irradiated animals that prevent the rejection of UVR-induced tumors. Non–white-haired cats also present with SCC lesions on nonpigmented, poorly haired areas of the body.[8]

Reductions of stratospheric ozone can be anticipated to allow more solar UVB to reach the earth's surface.[4] UVB rays penetrate deep into the dermis producing inflammation with dilatation of the superficial blood vessels—seen clinically as erythema and swelling/edema. This depth of penetration of UVR predisposes animals to hemangiosarcoma. In human beings, UVB damage to the collagen and elastin of the dermis produces "crow's feet" and wrinkled skin and, more significantly, vascular tumors. In dogs, Whippets have been recognized to be predisposed to cutaneous hemangioma and hemangiosarcoma in the sparsely haired chest, flank, and abdominal skin areas.

◆ CLINICAL SIGNS

The earliest signs of solar radiation damage is a persistent erythema in sparsely haired, nonpigmented skin. Any adjacent pigmented skin is generally unaffected. In cats, the classic affected sites are the nonpigmented (white) and sparsely haired areas such as the ear tips and margins, the perioral and periocular areas, and the planum nasale. Erythema is followed by scaling, alopecia, and a slight thickening of the skin (Fig. 25–1). The lesions may be single or multiple. Comedones may occur in haired skin. A loss of the elastic and collagenous supportive tissue surrounding the hair follicle is thought to be the predisposing factor for the comedones. However, comedones typically are not seen on the pinnae, in periocular areas, and on the planum nasale; as these are the most commonly affected feline sites, comedones are not a major feature of feline solar dermatitis. In more advanced stages, papules, crusted papules, plaques, and crateriform nodules and ulcerations develop, and curling of the ear tips may occur (Figs. 25–2 and 25–3). Ulceration of these areas may occur in the absence of neoplasia. As neoplasia develops, the erythema progresses slowly to larger ulcerative or, in some cases, exophytic lesions. Rarely, nodules and cutaneous horns are seen (Fig. 25–4).

◆ DIAGNOSIS
Examination—Clinical Clues

A careful history and physical examination will suggest the diagnosis. In the early stages, simple

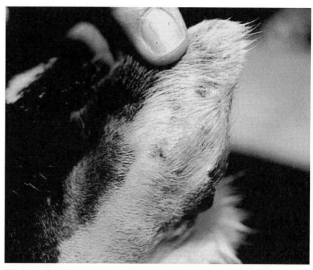

Figure 25–2. Note the erythema along the margins of the ear pinna and the papules and adherent scale-crust. (Courtesy of Dr. Roger Clarke, Australia.)

sunburn occurs. Erythema in nonpigmented sun-exposed skin, with a history of regression with reduced sun exposure and subsequent recurrence on re-exposure, is highly suggestive of solar dermatitis. As the disease progresses to chronic solar dermatitis, the erythema is persistent and accompanied by scaling and crusting. Differential diagnoses of early lesions are few, if one has adjacent, unaffected pig-

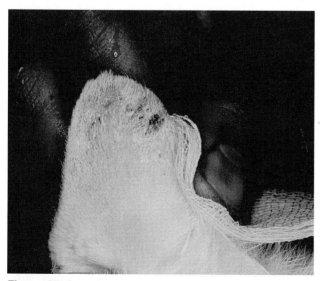

Figure 25–1. Scaling, alopecia, and a slight thickening of the tips of the pinnae are early solar changes.

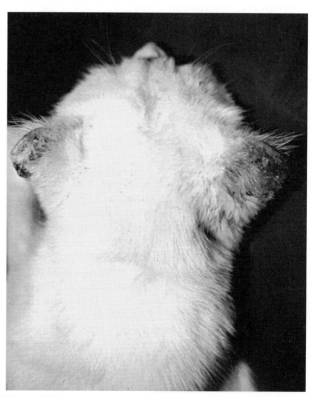

Figure 25–3. Ulceration and curling of the ear tips of a cat with bilateral solar-induced lesions. (Courtesy of Dr. Roger Clarke, Australia.)

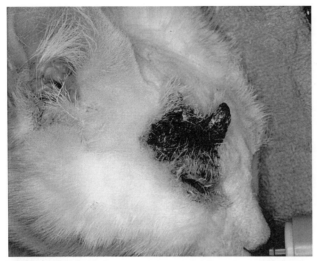

Figure 25–4. This cutaneous horn developed rapidly (within 2 months) in the preauricular area. A large, scaly erythematous patch had been present and apparently static in this area for at least 2 years.

mented skin to compare. In white cats, the anatomic sites and clinical appearance of lesions present for prolonged periods of time are the best clinical clues. The major differential diagnoses for the erythema and scaling include a drug reaction, leishmaniasis, and irritant or contact hypersensitivity. Infectious agents such as sporotrichosis, cryptococcosis, leishmaniasis, and histoplasmosis need to be considered when the plaques and ulcerated lesions are present. Eosinophilic plaque and indolent ulcers, which are generally regarded to have a hypersensitivity etiology, also should be considered. However, the usually lengthy preceding history of chronic erythema and scaling would help to differentiate most of these more acute diseases from solar dermatitis and SCC.

Biopsy

Selection of Lesions and Technique

Diagnosis may be confirmed by biopsy and histopathology. Poor biopsy site selection and technique may hinder a diagnosis. Epidermal changes are the key to diagnosis. It is important to include adjacent normal pigmented skin for comparison. If the adjacent skin is nonpigmented, clinically normal tissue should still be biopsied. If the skin sample submitted contains epidermis that is severely affected by a secondary pyoderma, the diagnostic architectural changes the pathologist seeks may be obscured by inflammatory cells. A 2- to 3-week course of antibiotics is indicated in cases with suspected or confirmed pyoderma. Do not use a sterile scrub technique because the overlying crusts and stratum corneum may harbor clues to the diagnosis. If the sampled skin is ulcerated with no intact adjacent epidermis, the diagnostic part of the biopsy, the epidermis is lost, and the pathologist can report only on the inflammation that underlies the ulcer.

As with all biopsy submissions, the chance of a meaningful result increases if historical and clinical information, as well as a complete list of differential diagnoses, is included with the samples.

Histopathologic Changes

The histopathology report has important implications for treatment and prognosis. Presquamous lesions have a better prognosis, as does carcinoma in situ. Overt SCC presents in different subsets; spindle cell forms are considered to be more aggressive.

Classic histopathologic features of early solar damage include reduced numbers of melanocytes and pigment, "sunburn cells," mild intraepidermal edema, and superficial vascular dilatation. It may be difficult to distinguish early solar dermatitis from lupus erythematosus if the changes at the epidermal junction are pronounced. Epidermal hyperplasia with a perivascular mononuclear infiltrate is the next sequential change. This is a nonspecific change seen with many hypersensitivities. The precancerous pathologic progression includes the presence of dyskeratotic, dysplastic epidermal cells. This is a result of disorderly and imperfect maturation with premature cytoplasmic keratinization.[9] The development of intercellular bridges, a common finding in early SCC in human beings, is relatively uncommon in cats. Desmosomal intercellular bridges appear artifactually as the cells separate during processing.

Unlike SCC, keratoses do not extend into the dermis. A less aggressive form of SCC is referred to as *carcinoma in situ*. In this case, the cells are definitely neoplastic, but have not crossed the basement membrane to the underlying dermis. Anisokaryosis and nuclear hyperchromasia and atypia with prominent nucleoli are cytologic changes associated with true SCC. This accompanies abnormal and jumbled keratinocyte maturation and invasion across the basement membrane. The majority of feline SCCs are well differentiated. In some cases, the cells develop a spindle cell morphology that may be indistinguishable from that of mesenchymal tumors if the continuity with the epidermis is not visible. In this case, immunohistochemical studies may be helpful, using cytokeratins to identify SCC and vimentin to rule out neoplasia of mesenchymal origin.[10]

Moderate dermal scarring is a common feature of solar damage, and solar elastosis may develop in more chronic lesions.

◆ PROGNOSIS

Sunburn, the mildest phototoxic change, will resolve with either no treatment or limited treatment (moisturizers or topical cortisone). Repeated sunburn may proceed to the development of chronic solar dermatitis, which by itself usually is not of any clinical consequence to the cat. However, it predisposes to the development of SCC.

SCC is the most frequent neoplasm in domestic animals to result from chronic solar exposure. Basal cell carcinoma and melanoma, although commonly solar-induced in human beings, rarely are considered to be solar-induced in animals. SCC in domestic animals generally is regarded as being locally invasive and slow to metastasize. However, rapid and aggressive metastatic disease resulting from long-standing (mild) lesions has been observed. In human beings, carcinomas arising from sun-damaged skin have a very low propensity to metastasize, the incidence amounting to only about 0.5 per cent.[11] Even if complete surgical resection of a cancerous lesion is performed in affected cats and the margins are pronounced clear by the pathologist, local adjacent recurrence may occur and has been reported in 23 per cent of cases.[8] In one report, the median disease-free interval after surgery was 19 months.[8] The adjacent skin has received the same amount of solar radiation, and thus has the same potential for malignant transformation, which explains the recurrence after surgical resection.

◆ TREATMENT

Pre–Squamous Cell Carcinoma Lesions

Treatment options vary with the stage of the disease. It is easier to prevent than cure. Early stages of actinic keratosis with no evidence of neoplastic changes may be treated with sunscreens and sun avoidance only. Intense photoprotection is the best preventative, although this is not always possible. Affected cats should be kept indoors between 9:00 AM and 5:00 PM. However, even indoor cats are at risk, especially those that spend significant time near windows, because normal window glass does not totally block UVR.[8] Sunscreen should be used as a daily routine on the nonpigmented, sparsely haired areas to protect these animals against accidental exposure. Waterproof, nonperfumed, "hypoallergenic toddler" sunscreens applied directly before a meal or "cuddle" will dry undisturbed and will maintain their efficacy despite later licking of the affected area. Sunscreens are a good choice for facial and aural lesions. Tattooing is no longer recommended as a preventative treatment. It deposits the pigment into the dermis—below the areas that are most likely to be affected by solar radiation. Tattoos do not protect the epidermis—which is the predominant site for pathogenic effects of UVR—and tattoo ink carries the inherent risk of a foreign-body reaction and sloughing. Vitamins C and E have been touted for human beings as antioxidants that may help to prevent solar damage.

If actinic keratosis is more advanced, medical treatment is indicated. Synthetic retinoids may be helpful, although their use in cats is largely anecdotal. Isotretinoin (13-*cis*-retinoic acid) was reported to be largely ineffective in cats when given at 3 mg/kg every 24 hr for an average of 68 days.[12] However, it has been used with success in human beings.[13] Etretinate, at a dose of 1 to 2 mg/kg orally daily, has been used successfully by the author in some early cases. The currently available product is acitretin (Soriatane). Response, if it is to occur, should be seen within the first 6 weeks of treatment. If there is clinical response, extension of the treatment should continue until complete remission or a leveling of the clinical response. Ongoing maintenance treatment may be required to prevent a relapse. It is important to ensure that there is no secondary infection obscuring assessment in these cases. If successful, therapy can be reduced to alternate days to minimize costs (these drugs are expensive).

Smaller, localized lesions may be treated with cryosurgery and antineoplastic drugs (such as 5-fluorouracil), but the former requires general anesthesia and the latter can cause ulceration of the tongue if licked, and also is neurotoxic in cats. In human beings, "cosmetic skin peeling" is being investigated to help control solar damage, even at the actinic keratosis stage. This is an area yet to be investigated in animals.

It must be remembered that actinic keratosis lesions may transform neoplastically. If medical measures are adopted, any clinical progression is an indication for immediate surgical biopsy and/or resection. If in doubt, biopsy should be performed to ascertain the actual stage of the lesion.

Squamous Cell Carcinoma

Biopsy should be performed early to identify the stage of the lesion. As soon as SCC is identified, appropriate and aggressive therapy should be instituted. There is no place for "watching" such tumors; although they are locally invasive and slow to metastasize, they will progress. In cats with advanced or poorly differentiated lesions, staging should be performed. A comprehensive investigation would include thoracic radiographs, aspirates of the regional lymph nodes, hematology, biochemical profiles, and urinalysis.

Local therapy is the treatment of choice, although access may be technically difficult if the periocular area and nares are involved. When incomplete surgical resection is likely, adjunctive or alternative therapies are employed.

Surgery

Cryosurgery, laser surgery, and excisional surgery all have been used successfully. The technique of choice will depend on the patient, the site affected, the extent of the lesions, the equipment available, and the preference and experience of the surgeon.

Cryosurgery is frequently considered as "one treatment." However, the technique includes the use of liquid nitrogen and nitrous oxide in a variety of application modalities. In a review of cryosurgery involving 102 cats with 163 SCC lesions, there was a remission of 70 per cent of nasal lesions and 100 per cent of ocular and ear tip lesions after a single treatment.[14] Posttreatment remission rates of 78 per cent were obtained after 35 months for 81 per cent of cats with nasal lesions. In this study, treatment was performed using liquid nitrogen with thermocouples to obtain accurate tissue freezing temperatures. Lower remission rates should be expected with standard cryosurgery units, which may not achieve the depth required to eliminate all tumor cells.

Excisional surgery frequently is employed for the planum nasale and eyelids. As with any oncologic surgery, a minimum of 1 to 2 cm from the tumor margin should be obtained wherever possible. With pinnae, this equates practically to "pinnectomy" or resection down to the base of the pinna, and is recommended for all lesions of the pinna, even those involving only the tip. The result is cosmetically acceptable (Fig. 25–5), and has the added bonus that the scar will be protected by the longer hair coat present at the base of the pinna. Although minor excisional resection is frequently successful on the planum nasale without appropriate 1- to 2-cm margins, in some cases the pathology report reveals an incomplete excision. A surgical technique for complete resection of the nasal planum has been described (Fig. 25–6).[15] Once ulceration and invasion of the nasal cartilage occur, these tumors may be refractory to radiation, and are relatively inaccessible for surgery, resulting in a poor prognosis despite the low metastatic rate (Fig. 25–7).

Laser surgery is an alternative treatment modality[16] for areas such as the periocular skin that are inappropriate for cryosurgery (owing to the risk of

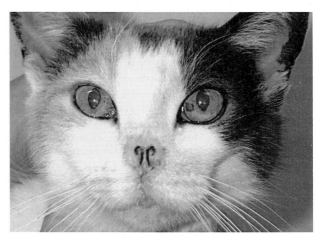

Figure 25–6. Postoperative appearance of a cat with a nasal resection. (Courtesy of Dr. Rod Straw, Australia.)

freezing the cornea) or excision (as the tear film may be affected). As with cryosurgery, the treated tissue cannot be examined for adequate margins. To date, no large-number studies have been published to document the success rate of laser therapy in cats.

Medical and Nonsurgical Therapy

Retinoids are used in the treatment of SCC in human beings.[17] Retinoids are naturally occurring and synthetic compounds with a vitamin A–like activity. They enter the cell as unbound drug and are translocated to the nucleus via cytosolic, retinoic acid–binding protein (CRABP) and cytosolic retinoid-binding protein (CRBP). This leads subsequently to the alteration of RNA, protein, and prostaglandin synthesis; labilization of cell membranes and posttranslational glycolysation; and inhibition of ornithine decarboxylase—which is the key enzyme for cell proliferation and differentiation. Retinoids are

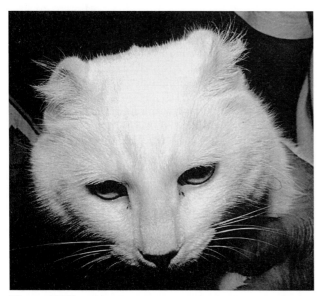

Figure 25–5. Bilateral pinnectomy can give a good cosmetic result. (Courtesy of Dr. Roger Clarke, Australia.)

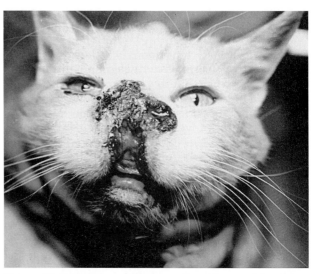

Figure 25–7. End-stage squamous cell carcinoma of the planum and upper lips. This is too advanced for surgical correction. (Courtesy of Dr. Roger Clarke, Australia.)

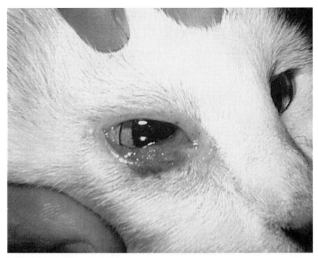

Figure 25–8. Squamous cell carcinoma of the lower eyelid before surgical resection. (Courtesy of Dr. Andrew Turner, Australia.)

teratogenic. Severe defects of the central nervous system, skeleton, thymus, heart, and great vessels have been reported in offspring of treated dams. Etretinate as an adjunctive postoperative agent has been used by the author in sites such as the lower eyelid where surgical resection is difficult and may be incomplete (Fig. 25–8). One such cat was managed with 2 mg/kg every other day and had no recurrence 2 years after the surgery.

Photodynamic therapy is a new treatment modality being explored for feline SCC. It is only applicable for shallow lesions less than 3 to 4 mm thick,[18] and so is most likely to be successful in cases with early SCC in situ. It involves the systemic administration of a photosensitizer that is retained preferentially by tumor tissues; subsequent exposure to light of a certain wavelength results in the formation of cytotoxic free radicals. Photosensitization is the major reported side-effect—treated cats must be kept out of sunlight for at least 2 weeks after therapy. However, facial edema, erythema, and necrosis also have been reported as side-effects.

SCC is reported to respond to radiation therapy, with the 2-year disease-free rates ranging from 37 to 57 per cent.[19] Radiation therapy is not readily available as a therapeutic option in many areas. It requires a general anesthetic, and usually is administered in multiple applications over several weeks.

◆ SUMMARY

Solar-induced phototoxic dermatitis in cats varies from simple erythema to aggressive SCCs. Lesions occur predominantly in sparsely haired, nonpigmented skin, and have a chronic course. Biopsies should be taken for histopathology because treatment recommendations vary based on the stage of the disease. Owners should be advised that close monitoring will be required to treat progressive disease successfully.

REFERENCES

1. Scott DW, Miller WH, Griffin CE: Immunological skin diseases. *In* Muller and Kirk's Small Animal Dermatology; 5th ed. Philadelphia, WB Saunders, 1995, pp. 565–573.
2. Iwasaki T, Maeda Y: The effect of ultraviolet (UV) on the severity of canine pemiphigus erythematosus. Proceedings of the 13th Annual Meeting of the American Academy of Veterinary Dermatology and American College of Veterinary Dermatology, Nashville, April 17–20, 1997.
3. Teifke JP, Lohr CV: Immunohistochemical detection of p53 overexpression in paraffin wax–embedded squamous cell carcinomas in cattle, horses, cats and dogs. J Comp Pathol 114:205–210, 1996.
4. Madronich S, de Gruijl FR: Skin cancer and UV radiation. Nature 366:23, 1993.
5. Dorn CR, Taylor DO, Schneider R: Sunlight exposure and risk of developing cutaneous and oral squamous cell carcinomas in white cats. J Natl Cancer Inst 46:1073–1078, 1997.
6. Kwa RE, Campana K, Moy RL: Biology of cutaneous squamous cell carcinoma. J Am Acad Dermatol 26:1–26, 1992.
7. Granstein RD: Photoimmunology. *In* Fitzpatrick TB, et al (eds): Dermatology in General Medicine, 3rd ed, vol. 1. New York: McGraw-Hill, 1987, pp 1461–1507.
8. Ruslander D, Kaser-Hotz B, Sardinas JC: Cutaneous squamous cell carcinoma in cats. Compend Contin Educ Pract Vet 19:1119–1129, 1997.
9. Yager JA, Wilcock BP: Solid epidermal tumors. *In* Color Atlas and Text of Surgical Pathology of the Dog and Cat. Dermatopathology and Skin Tumors, vol. 1. London, Mosby–Year Book, 1994, pp. 249–256.
10. Gross TL, Ihrke PJ, Walder E: Epidermal tumors. *In* Veterinary Dermatopathology—A Macroscopic and Microscopic Evaluation of Canine and Feline Skin Disease. St. Louis, Mosby–Year Book, 1992, pp. 330–350.
11. Lever WF, Schaumburg-Lever G: Tumors and cysts of the epidermis. *In* Histopathology of the Skin, 7th ed. Philadelphia, JB Lippincott, 1990, p. 552.
12. Evans AG, Madewell BR, Stannard AA: A trial of 13-*cis*-retinoic acid for treatment of squamous cell carcinoma and preneoplastic lesions of the head of cats. Am J Vet Res 46:2553–2557, 1985.
13. Marks R: Treatment of non-melanoma skin cancer and solar keratoses with oral retinoids. *In* Retinoids in Cutaneous Malignancy. Boston, Blackwell Scientific, 1991, p. 102.
14. Clarke RE: Cryosurgical treatment of cutaneous squamous cell carcinoma. Aust Vet Pract 21:148–153, 1991.
15. Withrow SJ, Straw RC: Resection of the nasal planum in nine cats and five dogs. J Am Anim Hosp Assoc 26:219–222, 1990.
16. Beck ER, Hetzel FW: Lasers in veterinary oncology. *In* Kirk RW, Bonagura JD (eds): Kirk's Current Veterinary Therapy XI: Small Animal Practice. Philadelphia, WB Saunders, 1992, pp. 414–418.
17. Lippman SM, Meyskens FL: Treatment of advanced squamous cell carcinoma of the skin with isotretinoin. Ann Intern Med 107:499–501, 1987.
18. Peaston AK, Leach MW, Higgins RJ: Photodynamic therapy for nasal and aural squamous cell carcinoma in cats. J Am Vet Med Assoc 202:1261–1265, 1993.
19. Carlisle CH, Gould S: Response of squamous cell carcinoma of the nose to treatment with x-rays. Vet Radiol 23:186–192, 1982.

26

◆ Paraneoplastic Alopecia

Jennifer L. Matousek
Karen L. Campbell
Carol A. Lichtensteiger

A *paraneoplastic disorder* is defined as a marker for cancer with clinical signs occurring at a site distant to the tumor or its metastases. Paraneoplastic syndromes can affect virtually any organ system, including hematologic, endocrine, neurologic, and dermatologic. For a cutaneous disorder to be classified as a paraneoplastic syndrome, 2 criteria must be satisfied: the dermatosis develops after the tumor, and the dermatosis parallels the activity of the tumor.[1, 2]

Cutaneous syndromes associated with internal malignancy have been well documented in human beings, and recognition of these disorders in veterinary medicine increased during the 1990s. Perhaps the best-known example of a cutaneous paraneoplastic syndrome in animals is hyperadrenocorticism, in which excessive hormone production from a pituitary or adrenal tumor results in thin skin and alopecia. Other examples in dogs include necrolytic migratory erythema associated with pancreatic glucagonomas, and nodular dermatofibrosis associated with renal and uterine tumors. Two paraneoplastic syndromes reported in cats are exfoliative dermatitis associated with thymoma, and paraneoplastic alopecia associated with pancreatic and hepatic tumors.

◆ ETIOPATHOGENESIS

To date, the syndrome of feline paraneoplastic alopecia has only been documented in cats with concurrent pancreatic or bile-duct carcinoma.[3–6] A recent report described a case in which the development of alopecia paralleled the progression of a pancreatic carcinoma.[3] The pathogenesis of the alopecia is unknown, but may be related to a circulating tumor-derived factor. In one case, immunohistochemical staining of a pancreatic carcinoma revealed no abnormalities in insulin, glucagon, somatostatin, or adrenocorticotropic hormone (ACTH) production.[4]

◆ SIGNALMENT

The signalment of cats affected with paraneoplastic alopecia parallels that of pancreatic and cholangiocellular carcinoma, both of which are rare neoplasms affecting older cats.[7, 8] Paraneoplastic alope-

cia typically affects cats 9 to 16 years of age.[3–6] Although a predilection for male cats has been reported with cholangiocellular carcinoma, there is no apparent gender predisposition for paraneoplastic alopecia. This observation may change as more cases are diagnosed.

◆ CLINICAL FEATURES

Cats with paraneoplastic alopecia usually present to the clinician with an acute onset (1 to 2 months) of alopecia and vague constitutional signs such as depression, anorexia, and weight loss. Longer durations of clinical signs (5 to 10 months) also have been reported.[3, 6] Pruritus is not a typical feature of paraneoplastic alopecia, and has been reported in only 2 of 9 cases. One of these cats was no longer pruritic after the resolution of a concurrent *Malassezia* dermatitis.[6]

Hair loss occurs in a ventral pattern along the neck, thorax, and abdomen, and may extend down the medial aspect of the limbs (Figs. 26–1 and 26–2). Alopecia also is seen in the periocular regions and on the dorsal ear pinnae. The fur at the alopecic margins epilates easily. Within the alopecic regions, the skin may be mildly erythematous, with fine scales, and has a characteristic shiny or glistening appearance. The paw pads may be painful and erythematous with crusts and fissures, or may have a shiny, glistening appearance (Fig. 26–3).

Dermatohistopathology characteristically reveals telogenization and atrophy of the hair follicles with varying degrees of epidermal hyperplasia. A superficial perivascular infiltrate also may be present.

◆ DIFFERENTIAL DIAGNOSIS

The differential diagnostic considerations in paraneoplastic alopecia include allergic, infectious, parasitic, endocrine, immune-mediated, drug-induced, neoplastic, and miscellaneous disorders.

Allergic

Feline atopy, food allergy, and flea-bite hypersensitivity present with a variety of clinical signs, including symmetric noninflammatory alopecia. Unlike

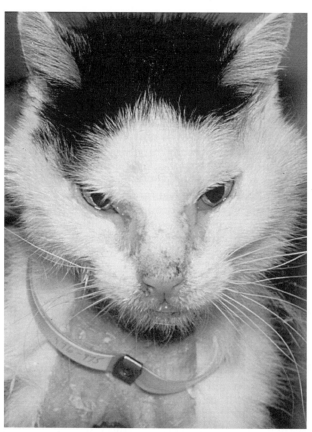

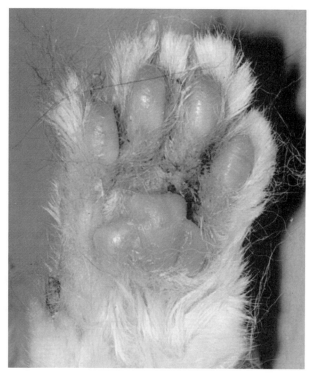

Figure 26–3. Same patient as in Figures 26–1 and 26–2. Erythematous paw pads with fine scales, and alopecia of the medial aspect of the paw.

Figure 26–1. A 15-year-old cat with paraneoplastic alopecia. Alopecia of the periocular area, ventral neck, and thorax extends down the medial aspect of the forelimbs. Note the scales and shiny appearance of the skin.

paraneoplastic alopecia, allergies often begin at a young age (1 to 3 years), and pruritus is a consistent finding. Because many owners are unaware that their cat is overgrooming, a trichogram may be useful to demonstrate damaged hair shafts, which are broken at the distal end instead of tapering to a fine

point. Diagnosis of allergic dermatitis in cats can be challenging, and involves the use of strict flea control, elimination diet trials, and intradermal skin testing. Skin histopathology findings are nonspecific in cats with allergic dermatosis, and include superficial perivascular dermatitis and a slightly hyperplastic epidermis.[9]

Infectious

Dermatophytosis may cause noninflammatory symmetric alopecia with variable pruritus and scale.

Figure 26–2. Alopecia of the ventral abdomen and medial rear limbs (nylon sutures are present from recent skin biopsies). Same patient as in Figure 26–1.

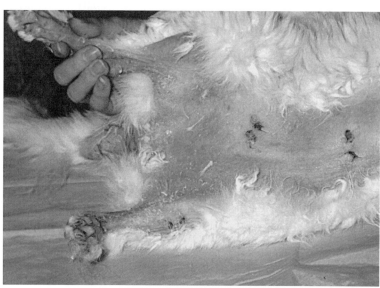

Young cats are affected more commonly than are older cats. The most reliable method for diagnosing dermatophyte infection is fungal culture.[10] Other techniques frequently used include Wood's lamp examination of the hair, potassium hydroxide preparation, and skin histopathology. Histopathology may reveal folliculitis, superficial perivascular to interstitial dermatitis, hyperkeratosis, and fungal organisms within the hair follicle.[10, 11]

Symmetric alopecia has been noted in cats infected with feline leukemia virus (FeLV) or feline immunodeficiency virus (FIV).[12] Currently, it is unknown whether the alopecia is coincidental, caused directly by the viral infection, or a secondary effect. One proposed reason for the alopecia is that it is the result of anagen or telogen defluxion.[13] Pruritus has been reported to be variable in these cats. In one report of giant cell dermatosis in FeLV-infected cats, the animals were pruritic, with alopecia and crusts that primarily affected the face but were generalized in some cases.[14] These authors suggested that FeLV was not a direct cause of the dermatitis, but instead was causing a neoplastic transformation of the keratinocytes.[14] Diagnosis of FeLV and FIV infections can be made from peripheral blood or bone marrow samples.

Parasitic

Parasites such as fleas, lice, *Demodex, Cheyletiella, Notoedres,* and *Otodectes* may cause symmetric alopecia in cats. Most affected cats are young, and pruritus is a common feature. Many techniques are used for the diagnosis of parasitic dermatitis, including physical examination, skin scraping, cellophane-tape preparations, otic cytology, fecal flotation, and response to miticidal therapy.

Endocrine

Feline hyperadrenocorticism is rare and primarily affects middle-aged to older cats[15–17] (see Chapter 20, Adrenocortical Disease). Females appear to be predisposed.[15–17] Dermatologic signs associated with hyperadrenocorticism in cats include thin skin, increased bruising, and an unkempt hair coat with patchy alopecia. Bilaterally symmetric endocrine alopecia is not as common in affected cats as in dogs.[15] Other clinical signs include a pendulous abdomen, polyphagia, polydipsia, and polyuria. The most consistent laboratory abnormalities are hyperglycemia and glucosuria associated with concurrent diabetes mellitus. The diagnosis of hyperadrenocorticism is established using ACTH stimulation and dexamethasone suppression testing. Abdominal ultrasonography also may be useful to demonstrate adrenomegaly or an adrenal mass. Skin histopathology in most cats with hyperadrenocorticism shows a normal epidermis and adnexa; occasionally, there is a decreased amount of dermal collagen.[16–18]

Hyperthyroidism affects middle-aged to older cats, and may cause an unkempt hair coat with alopecia. The pattern of hair loss is not a typical symmetric endocrine alopecia, and is likely caused by overgrooming.[19] Hyperthyroid cats may pull out their fur because of heat intolerance.[19] Many hyperthyroid cats will have palpably enlarged thyroid glands, and a history of weight loss, restlessness, polyphagia, polydipsia, and polyuria. Laboratory abnormalities associated with hyperthyroidism include mild erythrocytosis, azotemia, and elevations in alanine transferase, aspartate transferase, and alkaline phosphatase. Basal total thyroxine (T_4) values usually are elevated. Triiodothyronine (T_3) suppression tests, thyrotropin-releasing hormone stimulation tests, and nuclear scintigraphy may help diagnose borderline or questionable cases (see Chapter 18, Diagnosis of Occult Hyperthyroidism).

Hypothyroidism is rare in cats and more often is congenital rather than acquired. Congenital hypothyroidism causes mental dullness, stunted growth, and retention of the undercoat with loss of primary hairs. Acquired hypothyroidism is usually iatrogenic, although 1 case of naturally occurring lymphocytic thyroiditis has been reported.[20] Alopecia of the ventral abdomen is not common in acquired hypothyroidism, but was observed in a case with lymphocytic thyroiditis. Laboratory abnormalities with hypothyroidism may include nonregenerative anemia, hypercholesterolemia, and low basal total T_4.[21] Thyroid hormone levels should be evaluated within the context of clinical signs and history because some medications and systemic diseases will falsely decrease thyroid hormone concentrations. A definitive diagnosis of feline adult-onset primary hypothyroidism should be based on results of provocative testing with thyroid-stimulating hormone or thyrotropin-releasing hormone.[22]

Immune-Mediated

Alopecia areata is a rare cause of focal or multifocal noninflammatory alopecia in cats. The diagnosis is based on histopathology, which varies at different stages of the disease. Initially, lymphocytes, plasma cells, and histiocytes are arranged in a peribulbar location.[23, 24] Later, telogen hairs may predominate, and follicular atrophy can be present. In chronic cases, hair follicles may be absent.

Systemic lupus erythematosus is a cause of alopecia, scaling, and crusting in cats. Other disorders associated with systemic lupus erythematosus include oral ulceration, conjunctivitis, hemolytic anemia, thrombocytopenia, polyarthritis, myopathy, and glomerulonephritis. The diagnosis of systemic lupus erythematosus is based on a combination of clinical signs, laboratory findings, antinuclear antibody titers, and skin histopathology. The most common histopathologic finding is a lichenoid interface dermatitis with individual basal keratinocyte necrosis.[25]

Drug-Induced

Iatrogenic hyperadrenocorticism is much less common in cats than in dogs. Both corticosteroids and progestogens suppress the adrenal gland, and rarely cause noninflammatory alopecia in cats. Skin histopathology may show decreases in dermal collagen and telogenization of hair follicles, but does not show the "miniaturized" hair follicles characteristic of paraneoplastic alopecia.

Neoplastic

Cutaneous T-cell lymphoma has many different presentations in cats, including pruritus, erythema, alopecia, and nodules. Skin histopathology usually is diagnostic, and reveals atypical lymphocytes with epitheliotropism.

Thymomas have been associated with exfoliative dermatitis in cats. These animals usually are older, and typically have a history of dyspnea, dysphagia, weight loss, anorexia, and lethargy.[26, 27] Cutaneous lesions include generalized scale and erythema, with facial or truncal alopecia. Radiographs and histopathology are helpful in differentiation from paraneoplastic alopecia associated with pancreatic and hepatic tumors. A cranial mediastinal mass may be evident on thoracic radiographs in cats with thymomas (see Chapter 68, Evaluation and Treatment of Cranial Mediastinal Masses). Dermatohistopathology reveals apoptosis of keratinocytes in the stratum basale and stratum spinosum. A mild, primarily lymphocytic interface dermatitis also is present.[26, 27]

Miscellaneous

Necrolytic migratory erythema (NME) is a cutaneous paraneoplastic disorder in dogs and human beings caused by pancreatic glucagonomas. NME also may be associated with liver cirrhosis in some animals. Cutaneous lesions include erosions, crusts, and scale affecting mucocutaneous junctions, paw pads, and areas exposed to increased friction (such as pressure points). The proposed pathogenesis of the cutaneous lesions is that hypoaminoacidemia leads to epidermal necrosis. One case of NME, also known as metabolic epidermal necrosis, has been documented in a cat with pancreatic carcinoma.[28] This cat had alopecia, erythema, and scale in the axillae that extended down the extremities. Stomatitis also was present in this cat, but the mucocutaneous junctions and paw pads were normal. Dermatohistopathology will help to differentiate NME from pancreatic paraneoplastic alopecia. NME has a characteristic "red, white, and blue" pattern of parakeratotic hyperkeratosis, intracellular and intercellular edema in the upper epidermis, and basal cell hyperplasia.[28] Telogenization and atrophy of the hair follicles are not features of NME.

Telogen defluxion may occur after a stressful event or metabolic disease (e.g., pancreatic, hepatic, renal, diabetes mellitus). The hair follicles go into telogen phase synchronously, and alopecia is noted a few months later. Anagen defluxion is much less common in small animals, and leads to hair loss a few days after a disease process causes insult to the anagen hairs. Diagnosis of telogen or anagen defluxions is based on history, microscopic appearance of plucked hairs, and histopathology.

Psychogenic alopecia is caused by overgrooming, which may result from anxiety or stress, or may be an obsessive-compulsive disorder resulting from neurohormonal imbalances. Purebred cats are affected more commonly.[29] The diagnosis is made by eliminating the possibility of other disorders causing symmetric alopecia, such as dermatophytosis, parasites, or allergic dermatitis. Histopathology will differentiate the disorder from paraneoplastic alopecia.

Feline acquired skin fragility syndrome is a rare disorder characterized by thin, friable skin and partial alopecia. Minor trauma to the skin may cause large cutaneous tears. These tears are full thickness, which distinguishes skin fragility syndrome from the epidermal exfoliation associated with feline paraneoplastic alopecia. Acquired skin fragility syndrome is associated most often with diabetes mellitus, spontaneous hyperadrenocorticism, and excessive exogenous corticosteroid or progesterone administration. Diagnosis is based on clinical signs, laboratory testing, and histopathology.

◆ DIAGNOSIS

The ventral alopecia and shiny skin of cats with paraneoplastic alopecia are distinctive and should trigger clinical suspicion of an underlying neoplasia. Skin scrapings, fecal flotation, Wood's lamp examination, potassium hydroxide preparations, and fungal cultures are negative in cats with paraneoplastic alopecia.

A minimum database including a complete blood count and biochemical profile will help to rule out other systemic diseases. Findings in cats with paraneoplastic alopecia have included nonregenerative anemia, leukocytosis, neutrophilia, monocytosis, eosinophilia, and basophilia.[4] Serum chemistry results include hyperproteinemia, hyperglobulinemia, hyperglycemia, hyperbilirubinemia, and increased blood urea nitrogen levels due to concurrent diseases in some cats.[4] To date, all affected cats have had negative FeLV and FIV test results.

Endocrine function testing including a thyroid hormone profile and dexamethasone suppression test is indicated to rule out hyperthyroidism and hyperadrenocorticism. One cat has been reported to have concurrent hyperthyroidism.[6] This cat had an increased basal serum total T_4, lack of T_4 suppression after T_3 administration, and a palpable thyroid slip.[6] An antinuclear antibody test also should be

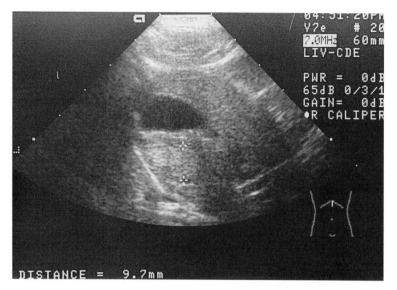

Figure 26–4. An abdominal ultrasound of a 13-year-old male cat with paraneoplastic alopecia due to pancreatic adenocarcinoma. Note the 9.7-mm hyperechoic nodule in the liver, dorsal to the gallbladder.

performed to further evaluate the possibility of systemic lupus erythematosus.

Ultrasonographic evaluation of the abdomen is often valuable, revealing a mass or nodular lesions consistent with neoplasia of the liver or pancreas (Fig. 26–4). Metastatic lesions to the spleen and peritoneum also may be seen. Ultrasound-guided fine-needle aspiration or biopsy of these lesions may be used to confirm the diagnosis. When performed, radiographic examination of the thorax and abdomen has revealed no abnormalities. In some cases, particularly with pancreatic neoplasia, laparoscopy or exploratory laparotomy may be required to identify and biopsy the tumor.

Skin histopathology reveals marked follicular telogenization and atrophy (Fig. 26–5). The periadnexal structures have been reported to be normal or moderately atrophied.[3–6] The presence of "miniaturized" hair follicles is a key diagnostic feature. The epidermis is mildly to moderately acanthotic, and the stratum corneum may be hyperkeratotic or ab-

sent in focal areas. A superficial perivascular infiltrate of mononuclear cells may be present in the dermis.

◆ TREATMENT

Treatment of the underlying neoplasia should result in resolution of the cutaneous signs. Unfortunately, the prognosis for hepatobiliary and pancreatic neoplasia is poor because these tumors are aggressive and frequently have metastasized at the time of diagnosis. Although 2 cats with paraneoplastic alopecia have been reported to survive for 15 and 18 weeks, the majority were euthanized within 1 to 3 days of diagnosis.[3–6] One patient had temporary improvement after surgical removal of the primary pancreatic tumor; however, it relapsed in association with progression of metastatic disease 18 weeks later.[3]

Cholangiocellular carcinoma can occur in 3 different forms in cats: (1) large solitary mass in 1 lobe;

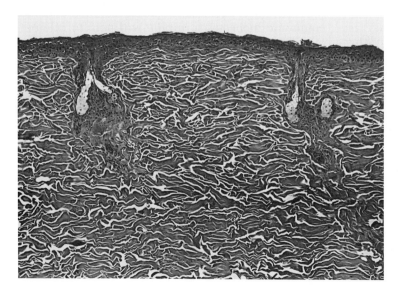

Figure 26–5. Photomicrograph of skin in feline paraneoplastic alopecia depicts mildly acanthotic epidermis and hair follicle atrophy. Hematoxylin and eosin, 100×.

(2) small, discrete nodules in 1 or several lobes; or (3) diffuse infiltration of large areas of the liver. Involvement of more than 1 liver lobe occurs frequently in cats, and metastasis to hepatic lymph nodes, the peritoneum, and lungs is common.[7] This makes complete surgical excision difficult, and chemotherapy generally is ineffective against primary liver tumors.

Pancreatic carcinoma may arise from ductular or acinar cells. Exocrine pancreatic neoplasia is very aggressive in cats, and metastases usually are present at the time of diagnosis. Tumor metastases often involve the duodenal wall, liver, and local lymph nodes. The lungs are affected less commonly. Surgical excision of the tumor and chemotherapy may be palliative, although curative therapies for exocrine pancreatic neoplasia have not been reported.[8]

◆ SUMMARY

Paraneoplastic alopecia is a cutaneous marker for malignant pancreatic and hepatic tumors in cats. The clinical appearance and dermatohistopathologic findings associated with feline paraneoplastic alopecia are unique, and when present, should increase clinical suspicion for concurrent pancreatic or cholangiocellular carcinoma. Recognition of this syndrome is important because these neoplasms often cause nonspecific clinical and laboratory changes, and may be difficult to diagnose. The prognosis is grave, because metastases often are present at the time of diagnosis.

REFERENCES

1. McLean DI, Haynes HA: Cutaneous manifestations of internal malignant disease. In Fitzpatrick TB, Eisen AZ, Wolf K (eds): Dermatology in General Medicine, 4th ed, vol. II. New York, McGraw-Hill, 1993, pp. 2229–2249.
2. McLean DI: Cutaneous paraneoplastic syndromes. Arch Dermatol 122:765–767, 1986.
3. Tasker S, Griffon DJ, Nuttal TJ: Resolution of paraneoplastic alopecia following surgical removal of a pancreatic carcinoma in the cat. J Small Anim Pract 40:16–19, 1999.
4. Pascal-Tenorio A, Olivry T, Gross TL: Paraneoplastic alopecia associated with internal malignancy in the cat. Vet Dermatol 8:47–52, 1997.
5. Brooks DG, Campbell KL, Dennis JS: Pancreatic paraneoplastic alopecia in three cats. J Am Anim Hosp Assoc 30:557–563, 1994.
6. Godfrey DR: A case of feline paraneoplastic alopecia with secondary Malassezia-associated dermatitis. J Small Anim Pract 39:394–396, 1998.
7. Johnson SE: Diseases of the liver. In Ettinger SJ, Feldman EC (eds): Textbook of Veterinary Internal Medicine, 4th ed, vol. 2. Philadelphia, WB Saunders, 1995, pp. 1313–1357.
8. Williams DA: Exocrine pancreatic diseases. In Ettinger SJ, Feldman EC (eds): Textbook of Veterinary Internal Medicine, 4th ed, vol. 2. Philadelphia, WB Saunders, 1995, pp. 1372–1392.
9. Gross TL, Ihrke PJ, Walder EJ: Veterinary Dermatopathology—A Macroscopic and Microscopic Evaluation of Canine and Feline Skin Disease. Chapter 8. St. Louis, Mosby–Year Book, 1992, pp. 114–116.
10. Scott DW, Miller WH, Griffin CE: Fungal skin diseases. In Muller and Kirk's Small Animal Dermatology, 5th ed. Philadelphia, WB Saunders, 1995, pp. 329–391.
11. Gross TL, Ihrke PJ, Walder EJ: Veterinary Dermatopathology—A Macroscopic and Microscopic Evaluation of Canine and Feline Skin Disease. Chapter 15. St. Louis, Mosby–Year Book, 1992, pp. 241–243.
12. Scheidt VJ: Feline symmetrical alopecia. In Birchard SJ, Sherding RG (eds): Saunders Manual of Small Animal Practice. Philadelphia, WB Saunders, 1994, pp. 336–340.
13. Thoday KL: Diagnosis and management of feline symmetric alopecia. In August JR (ed): Consultations in Feline Internal Medicine, vol. 3. Philadelphia, WB Saunders, 1997, pp. 231–245.
14. Gross TL, Clark EG, Hargis AM: Giant cell dermatosis in FeLV-positive cats. Vet Dermatol 4:117–122, 1993.
15. Feldman EC, Nelson RW: Hyperadrenocorticism in cats. In Canine and Feline Endocrinology and Reproduction, 2nd ed. Philadelphia, WB Saunders, 1996, pp. 256–261.
16. Zerbe CA: Feline hyperadrenocorticism. In Kirk RW (ed): Current Veterinary Therapy X. Philadelphia, WB Saunders, 1989, pp. 1038–1042.
17. Helton-Rhodes K: Cutaneous manifestations of hyperadrenocorticism. In August JR (ed): Consultations in Feline Internal Medicine, vol. 3. Philadelphia, WB Saunders, 1997, pp. 191–198.
18. Yager JA, Wilcock BP: Color Atlas of Surgical Pathology of the Dog and Cat, vol. 1. London, Mosby–Year Book, 1994, p. 237.
19. Feldman EC, Nelson RW: Feline hyperthyroidism (thyrotoxicosis). In Canine and Feline Endocrinology and Reproduction, 2nd ed. Philadelphia, WB Saunders, 1996, pp. 118–165.
20. Rand JS, Levine J, Best SJ: Spontaneous adult-onset hypothyroidism in a cat. J Vet Intern Med 7:272–276, 1993.
21. Feldman EC, Nelson RW: Feline hypothyroidism. In Canine and Feline Endocrinology and Reproduction, 2nd ed. Philadelphia, WB Saunders, 1996, pp. 111–115.
22. Peterson ME: Feline hypothyroidism. In Kirk RW (ed): Current Veterinary Therapy X. Philadelphia, WB Saunders, 1989, pp. 1000–1001.
23. Yager JA, Wilcock BP: Color Atlas of Surgical Pathology of the Dog and Cat, vol. 1. London, Mosby–Year Book, 1994, pp. 196–197.
24. Gross TL, Ihrke PJ, Walder EJ: Veterinary Dermatopathology—A Macroscopic and Microscopic Evaluation of Canine and Feline Skin Disease. Chapter 17. St. Louis, Mosby–Year Book, 1992, pp. 291–292.
25. Gross TL, Ihrke PJ, Walder EJ: Veterinary Dermatopathology—A Macroscopic and Microscopic Evaluation of Canine and Feline Skin Disease. Chapter 2. St. Louis, Mosby–Year Book, 1992, pp. 24–46.
26. Carpenter JL, Holzworth J: Thymoma in 11 cats. J Am Vet Med Assoc 181:248–251, 1982.
27. Scott DW, Jager YA, Johnston KM: Exfoliative dermatitis in association with thymoma in three cats. Feline Pract 23(4):8–13, 1995.
28. Patel A, Whitbread TJ, McNeil PE: A case of metabolic epidermal necrosis in a cat. Vet Dermatol 7:221–226, 1996.
29. Scott DW, Miller WH, Griffin CE: Feline psychogenic disorders. In Muller and Kirk's Small Animal Dermatology, 5th ed. Philadelphia, WB Saunders, 1995, pp. 854–857.

27

◆ Primary Hereditary Seborrhea Oleosa

Manon Paradis

Seborrhea is a popular descriptive term that alludes to excessive sebum production.[1] In reality, it is better defined as a chronic skin disease characterized by a defect in cornification with excessive scale formation, occasional excessive greasiness of the skin and hair coat, and sometimes, dermatitis and alopecia.[2, 3] *Cornification defect* and *keratinization defect* are terms often used interchangeably; however, cornification defect is a broader term that encompasses keratinization disorders. Indeed, the cornification process involves 4 distinct cellular events: keratinization, keratohyalin synthesis, formation of the insoluble cornified envelope, and generation of lipid-enriched intercellular domains.[3] Disorders that alter cellular proliferation, differentiation, desquamation, or sebum production are likely to produce some type of seborrhea.[3–5]

Seborrhea can be classified as primary or secondary.[2–5] In most animal species, including cats, seborrhea most frequently is secondary to another underlying cause. Primary seborrhea, which is relatively rare in cats, is an inherited disorder of cornification.[3] Primary hereditary seborrhea oleosa (PHSO) represents the only generalized primary seborrhea reported in cats.[2]

◆ ETIOLOGY AND PATHOGENESIS

PHSO is an incurable genodermatosis of early onset and variable severity, reported in Persian cats.[2] An autosomal recessive mode of inheritance has been demonstrated; however, the actual pathomechanism responsible for this cornification disorder is unknown. It could result from either excessive sebum production or excessive cellular proliferation, or both. Cats of either gender and any color can be affected.

PHSO also has been observed by the author in some lines of Himalayan and exotic breeds. The same mode of inheritance is likely and can be explained logically because these 2 breeds were created from Persian lines. Long hair as well as color-point markings are transmitted through autosomal recessive genes, so multiple genes and associated genetic defects intermix in these 3 breeds. Himalayans are phenotypically and genotypically identical to Persians, with the exception of being homozygous for the color-point autosomal recessive gene. Indeed, they are called *color-point Persians* in many countries. This is also true for the exotic breed. Exotics (which implies short hair in most feline associations) either are heterozygous for the longhair, autosomal recessive gene, or less frequently, are not carriers of the longhair gene. Longhair offsprings produced from a mating of shorthair heterozygote parents are phenotypically and genotypically identical to Persians or Himalayans, being homozygous for the longhair, autosomal recessive gene. Depending on the feline associations in various countries, these cats will be registered either as Persian or as exotic longhair variety.

The worldwide incidence of PHSO in Persians and other related breeds is unknown at present. It seems relatively frequent in Canada, most specifically in Quebec. Breeders claim that initial carrier cats were introduced in Quebec in the 1970s from a specific line in the United States, where the incidence of affected cats still appears surprisingly low. Otherwise, sporadic cases have been reported in various countries including Denmark and New Zealand.[2, 3] It is likely that mildly affected cats are more frequent than thought; however, many cases go undiagnosed, because some affected cats may just be considered lazy and thought not to be grooming themselves properly, whereas others may be diagnosed with idiopathic seborrhea if the owner or attending veterinarian is not aware of PHSO in cats.

◆ CLINICAL SIGNS

PHSO is a genodermatosis with an early onset and variable severity.[2] In severely affected cats, the problem becomes obvious as early as 2 or 3 days of age. Initially, the hair is curly and pasted together, and kittens look dirty, as if the queen did not clean them properly. With time, the whole body becomes scaly and oily, and develops a rancid and unpleasant odor. Generalized accumulation of brownish yellow keratoseborrheic material that adheres to the skin surface and hair coat and comedones may be seen (Figs. 27–1 and 27–2). Ceruminous otitis also is a common finding (Fig. 27–3). Some of the severely affected cats have hair shafts that epilate easily. These severely affected cats leave brownish, greasy stains on furniture, walls, and clothing, making them unacceptable as house pets.

Mildly PHSO-affected cats have similar signs, but these signs are much milder and the problem may go unnoticed until 6 to 8 weeks of age. The whole hair coat appears matted, wavy, unkept, and oily with the same type of keratoseborrheic material, albeit less abundant, that accumulates on the skin surface and at the base of the hair shafts (Fig. 27–4).

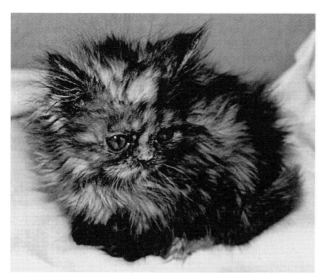

Figure 27–1. Persian kitten moderately affected with primary hereditary seborrhea oleosa (PHSO). Note the matted, dirty, agglutinated hair coat.

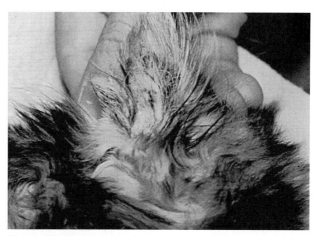

Figure 27–3. Persian moderately affected with PHSO. Note the accumulation of cerumen on the pinna.

Occasionally, the keratoseborrheic material will be more waxy than oily. Accumulation of cerumen can be seen on the concave aspect of the pinnae.

Because many cat breeders are now aware of the disorder, the majority of the severely affected kittens are destroyed shortly after birth by breeders. Cats with mild-to-moderate PHSO are most likely to survive and to be presented to the veterinarian. The majority of these cases come from inexperienced breeders unaware of PHSO. Typically, 1 or 2 kittens per litter are affected by PHSO.

◆ DIFFERENTIAL DIAGNOSIS

Both primary and secondary seborrhea can occur in cats, although the latter is much more frequent[2, 3] (Table 27–1). As is the case for dogs, it is important not to condemn the animal as suffering from primary seborrhea before having ruled out, with appropriate diagnostic tests, secondary causes of cornification disorders.

Primary Seborrhea

Primary seborrhea usually is defined as an inherited disorder of cornification. PHSO apparently represents the only generalized primary seborrhea reported in cats. Feline chin acne and tail seborrhea (stud tail) could represent localized forms of primary seborrhea, not as much in the sense that these disorders are inherited, but rather that underlying, secondary causes are not present. However, because these disorders are seen more often in some lines of cats, a genetic predisposition is possible. Feline chin acne and tail seborrhea are relatively common conditions of cats involving areas that are rich in sebaceous glands. Because of their typical clinical presentations, these rarely present a diagnostic challenge. However, it is imperative that demodicosis,

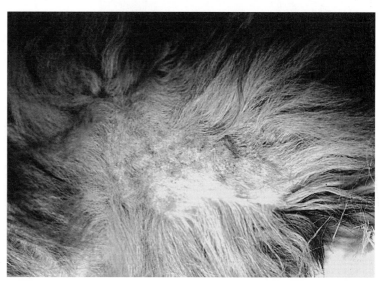

Figure 27–2. Persian moderately affected with PHSO. Note the keratoseborrheic material accumulated on the skin (hairs were shaved for the photograph).

dermatophytosis, and *Malassezia* infection be ruled out as possible underlying or complicating causes.[3, 6, 7]

Secondary Seborrhea

Secondary seborrhea implies that there is an external or internal insult that alters the proliferation, differentiation, or desquamation of the surface and follicular epithelium. Although cats may suffer from many of the same disorders that cause secondary seborrhea in dogs, seborrheic signs are less common in this species. Cats' fastidious grooming habits, which may remove scales quickly, may be partially responsible for this lower incidence.[3] When cats do become seborrheic, they usually have seborrhea sicca with fine white or gray flakes or scales in the coat. When signs are fairly generalized and pruritus is absent, dietary deficiencies, low environmental humidity, endoparasites, ectoparasitic diseases such as cheyletiellosis and pediculosis, diabetes mellitus, hyperthyroidism, and obesity are the primary differential diagnoses.[2, 3] When pruritus is present or when lesions are more localized, demodicosis, cheyletiellosis, dermatophytosis, yeast infections, allergy, and idiopathic facial dermatitis must be considered as possible diagnoses.[2, 3, 6–11]

Secondary seborrhea manifesting as greasy seborrhea is very rare in cats. It has been reported in

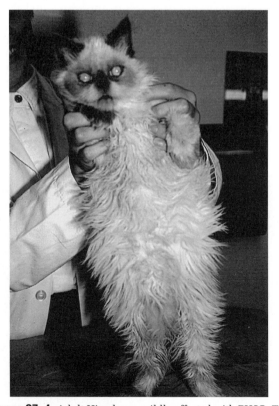

Figure 27–4. Adult Himalayan mildly affected with PHSO. Typical appearance a few days after bathing: the whole hair coat appears matted, wavy, unkempt, and oily.

Table 27–1. Classification of Feline Seborrhea

Primary Seborrhea

Generalized

Primary hereditary seborrhea oleosa

Localized

Tail seborrhea (stud tail)
Feline chin acne

Secondary Seborrhea

Generalized Nonpruritic—Usually Seborrhea Sicca

Low environmental humidity
Dietary deficiency
Endoparasites
Ectoparasites (cheyletiellosis, pediculosis)
Dermatophytosis
Diabetes mellitus
Hyperthyroidism
Overzealous shampooing

Generalized Seborrhea—Usually Oleosa-Type

Associated with chronic hepatic, pancreatic, or intestinal
   diseases
Drug eruption or systemic lupus erythematosus

Localized or Pruritic

Dermatophytosis
Demodicosis
Ectoparasites (cheyletiellosis, pediculosis)
Malassezia dermatitis
Allergy
Idiopathic facial dermatitis (facial seborrhea of Persian cats)

association with severe chronic hepatitis, pancreatic or intestinal diseases, drug eruption, and systemic lupus erythematosus.[3] Whether or not some of those rare, greasy cats with systemic diseases were indeed affected concomitantly with PHSO is not known. Nevertheless, in any case of seborrhea, more so if the seborrhea is dry in nature and late in onset, it is important to try to identify an underlying etiology because spontaneous resolution may result after correction of the cause.

Malassezia Dermatitis

Dermatitis associated with *Malassezia* is rare in cats compared with dogs, in which it is a frequent cause of secondary seborrhea oleosa. Typically, affected cats have a generalized exfoliative erythroderma with excessive greasiness and variable pruritus.[3, 7, 10] A pododermatitis and dark, waxy, greasy erythematous otitis usually are present. Cytology will demonstrate abnormal numbers of *Malassezia* (more than 4 per high-power field) and variable numbers of bacteria.[10] Treatment to remove the yeast with topical or systemic antifungal medications is associated with resolution of clinical signs; however, recurrence is frequent, and occurs soon after cessation of treatment.[10] In PHSO, yeast organisms have not been found to date in the keratoseborrheic material accumulated on the skin or ear canal from cytologic examination, nor have they been identified on histopathologic examination of the skin.

Idiopathic Facial Dermatitis

Idiopathic facial dermatitis (IFD) of Persian cats is a newly recognized entity that differs from PHSO. However, confusion sometimes exists between PHSO and IFD because the latter has been reported as facial seborrhea of Persian cats by some authors,[6] and because the same breeds (Persian, Himalayan, and exotic) are involved.

IFD is characterized as a skin disease that remains confined to the head and neck region.[11] Initially, a black adherent exudate encrusting the lower portions of the hair is observed in the periocular, perioral, and nasal folds and chin regions—hence the colloquial name *dirty face syndrome* or *ectopic feline acne.* Affected skin becomes progressively inflamed, and lesions spread over the face and head. Pruritus, which is mild initially, becomes progressively moderate to severe. Marked erythema, alopecia, and evidence of self-trauma eventually are observed. Ceruminous otitis is seen in approximately 50 per cent of the cases. The initial clinical signs may start at a relatively young age, although, in many instances, it is first noticed in adulthood. Age at onset ranges from 4 months to 4 years (median, 12 months).[11]

The etiopathogenesis of IFD is unknown. In one study, microorganisms isolated included *Malassezia pachydermatis* (6 of 9 patients), *Staphylococcus intermedius* (5 of 10), and gram-negative rods (4 of 10). Peripheral eosinophilia was present in approximately 50 per cent of the cases. Other tests yielding negative or normal results included skin scrapings for ectoparasites, dermatophyte culture, feline leukemia virus/feline immunodeficiency virus assays (9 of 9), elimination diets (8 of 8), and intradermal skin tests (4 of 4). Skin biopsies (9 cases) showed a hyperplastic, superficial, or interface dermatitis with variable numbers of mononuclear cells and polymorphonuclear cells. Neutrophil and eosinophil exocytosis and sebaceous gland hyperplasia were seen.[11] So far, a common etiology has not been identified. An inherited cornification disorder with secondary infection and inflammation could be involved. It has been suggested that after chronic inflammation, apocrine glands become hyperplastic and dilated, with excessive apocrine gland secretion responsible for the changes in color that happen on oxidation. Viral particles such as herpesvirus have been found in affected skin, and apparently some cats were helped with interferon.[11] A combination of genetic factors, long hair, and/or facial folds may be involved.

No satisfactory treatment regimen for IFD has been identified. Although secondary infections with *Malassezia* and gram-negative rods are found in many cases, therapy with antibiotics, antifungal agents, and glucocorticoids, either alone or in combination, given systemically or topically, induce, at best, only partial responses. Topical care such as gentle washing may be recommended; however, black exudate accumulates again 1 to 2 days after washing. Isotretinoin, either oral or topical, and gold salts have been tried in a few cases without significant improvement. Food trials and intradermal skin testing have not been helpful in identifying underlying allergies.[11]

It is unlikely that IFD and PHSO are variants of the same disorder. In contrast with IFD, PHSO has an early onset, the distribution of the lesions is more generalized, and usually the face remains relatively normal, aside from the oily secretion that accumulates on the face and ears in some cats. Cats that are kept alive to adulthood with IFD usually have a relatively mild form, and rarely, if ever, appear to develop secondary infections and pruritus.

◆ DIAGNOSIS OF PHSO

The diagnosis of PHSO is based on history, clinical signs, skin biopsies, and other tests such as skin scrapings, cytology, and fungal culture to rule out parasitic, yeast, or dermatophytic etiologies that could mimic PHSO or contribute to the clinical signs.

Histopathology

Histopathologic examination of skin biopsies from cats with PHSO typically shows a cornification defect, characterized by orthokeratotic hyperkeratosis and sometimes papillomatosis.[2, 3] Sebaceous glands usually are normal in size and appearance, although they sometimes appear hyperplastic. However, this finding has not been evaluated by comparing it with skin biopsies from normal cats of matching sites, breed, and age. A mild perivascular cellular infiltrate usually is present and consists predominantly of lymphocytes. However, the author is aware of a few cases in which the number of mast cells was so significantly increased that the pathologists were tempted to suggest an allergic process in spite of the clinical description typical of PHSO and the absence of pruritus.

◆ CLINICAL MANAGEMENT

PHSO is an incurable disease. Affected cats require a lifelong clinical management program with topical therapy to keep them acceptable as house pets. The intensity of topical care is directly proportional to the severity of the disorder. For example, a mildly affected cat may be controlled with a twice-yearly total-body clipping and monthly baths with antiseborrheic or degreasing shampoo formulations. Moderately and severely affected cats may need monthly total-body clipping and twice-weekly bathing, in spite of which brownish grease stains and spotting on clothes, walls, and furniture may return within 1 or 2 days after bathing.

Conventional medicated shampoo formulated for

seborrhea oleosa with keratolytic, keratoplastic, or degreasing properties containing ingredients such as tar, selenium sulfide, benzoyl peroxide, and pyrithione zinc at first might appear useful topical products to use in PHSO. However, these active ingredients are *not* recommended in cats in most instances, because of their irritant potential and risk of toxicity.[3, 12, 13] Because these products are usually avoided in cats, their potential benefits have not been evaluated in PHSO. Typically, sulfur and salicylic acid shampoo formulations and liquid dishwashing detergents (Joy, Sunlight, Palmolive) have been used to bathe cats with PHSO. Breeders have claimed that hand cleaners with lanolin (which also contain petroleum distillate) applied to the hair coat and washed off 5 minutes later with a liquid dishwashing detergent are the most efficacious way to control the problem. This topical treatment regimen, although time-consuming if performed frequently, appears to be very well tolerated in most cats. Indeed, Persian breeders use this product combination in nonaffected cats as often as once a week for optimum appearance in show cats.

Synthetic retinoids could be valuable systemic therapeutic modalities in PHSO. These drugs have different spectra of action. Isotretinoin (Accutane, Roche) appears to have the best activity in skin diseases in which the hair follicles and sebaceous glands are the primary structures involved; it acts by decreasing the activity of sebaceous glands and normalizing cornification within hair follicles.[3, 14, 15] The primary indication for isotretinoin is severe cystic acne in human beings. Isotretinoin is available in 10-, 20-, and 40-mg capsules. Etretinate (Tegison, Roche) and acitretin (Soriatane, Roche) work by suppressing accelerated cellular kinetics and associated defects in cornification; they have profound beneficial effects in hyperproliferative epidermal disorders such as psoriasis in human beings. Etretinate, which is no longer available commercially, has been replaced by acitretin; this active metabolite of etretinate is less toxic owing to a shorter terminal elimination half-life of 2 days versus 100 days for etretinate.[3]

The therapeutic benefits of retinoids have not been reported in cats with PHSO. Isotretinoin's efficacy has been evaluated by the author only in a 7-year-old spayed female Persian moderately affected with PHSO. For several years, the cat had a total-body clip on a monthly basis and was bathed every 2 weeks with various types of antiseborrheic or degreasing shampoos by its dedicated owners. In addition, the ceruminous otitis was controlled with the use of an ear cleanser preparation (Epi-Otic, Virbac) 3 times weekly. Typically, the hair coat was acceptable for 1 to 2 days after bathing, at which time the cat would invariably leave brownish, greasy secretions on towels that the owners carried around and put on their laps for the cat to lie on. Isotretinoin therapy was initiated at 2 mg/kg (one 10-mg capsule) orally every 48 hr for 2 months, at which time the hair coat remained relatively normal for several days after bathing. At present, the cat is on a maintenance treatment consisting of one 10-mg capsule weekly. Oiliness and brownish secretions, which usually returned within 1 to 2 days after bathing, now remain at a minimum for several weeks, suggesting that isotretinoin can significantly decrease oil and scale formation in these cats. Minimum topical care was otherwise required, making this treatment regimen relatively easy and cheap for this cat, and no adverse reactions were observed.

In spite of the limited data on the use of retinoids in PHSO, isotretinoin should be offered as an option when topical keratolytic, keratoplastic, and degreasing agents have limited effect or require too-frequent applications to be practical for long-term management. Treatment with isotretinoin should be continued for a minimum of 2 months before a determination of efficacy is made. After the disorder has been brought under control, to be more cost-effective, a less frequent administration can be attempted for long-term maintenance. Cats tolerate isotretinoin very well.[3, 14, 15] The incidence of clinical or laboratory side-effects in cats is very low. The most common side-effect seen is anorexia with subsequent weight loss. These side-effects resolve when the dosage is lowered or discontinued. Other side-effects of isotretinoin include conjunctivitis, periocular crusting, vomiting, and diarrhea.[3, 14, 15] Monthly laboratory screenings are suggested when the drug is used over prolonged periods. Retinoids are extremely teratogenic, and appropriate caution should be used for both human beings and animals. There is no information available on the use of etretinate or acitretin for PHSO in cats.

Another systemic therapy that has been evaluated for the treatment of PHSO in cats is a commercial omega-3 and omega-6 fatty acid–containing product (DVM Derm Caps) that was used unsuccessfully in 2 cats.[3] Recently, a Persian breeder and cat groomer claimed that daily yogurt capsules had produced significant improvement within 3 months of initiating the treatment in a few Persians affected with PHSO. Without ever looking normal, coat oiliness apparently remained acceptable for 1 to 2 months without bathing. The oiliness would return within 1 month when yogurt capsule administration was terminated. Although this report is based solely on anecdotal information and there is no scientific explanation supporting its efficacy, it may be worth trying, considering that it is practical, inexpensive, and safe.

◆ PREVENTION

The best way to decrease incidence of PHSO in cats is to avoid breeding affected cats or known carriers. Some breeders have managed to decrease and even eradicate this problem significantly from their catteries. A carrier or preferably a clinically affected cat (i.e., homozygote) is kept in order to perform test breedings with prospective breeding stock. Clinically affected kittens resulting from this mating usually are destroyed, and unaffected siblings should be sterilized. Veterinarians should be aware of PHSO in order to do genetic counseling with the breeders, and advise proper care for the affected kittens.

◆ CONCLUSION

PHSO is an incurable genodermatosis of early onset and variable severity seen in Persian, Himalayan, and exotic breeds of cats. An autosomal recessive mode of inheritance has been demonstrated. Cats of either gender and any color may be affected. In order to make these cats acceptable as house pets, a life-long clinical management program with topical therapy is required. Systemic therapy with isotretinoin or other retinoids also may be of value. Many affected cats are destroyed as kittens by informed breeders.

REFERENCES

1. Plewig G: Seborrheic dermatitis. *In* Fitzpatrick TB, Eisen AZ, Wolff K, et al (eds): Dermatology in General Medicine, 4th ed, vol. I. New York, McGraw-Hill, 1993, pp. 1569–1574.
2. Paradis M, Scott DW: Hereditary primary seborrhea oleosa in Persian cats. Feline Pract 18:17–20, 1990.
3. Scott DW, Miller WH, Griffin CE: Keratinization defects. *In* Muller and Kirk's Small Animal Dermatology, 5th ed., Philadelphia, WB Saunders, 1995, pp. 824–844.
4. Kwochka KW: Keratinization abnormalities: Understanding the mechanisms of scale formation. *In* Ihrke P, Mason IS, White SD (eds): Advances in Veterinary Dermatology, vol. 2. New York, Pergamon, 1993, pp. 91–111.
5. Kwochka KW: Overview of normal keratinization and cutaneous scaling disorders of dogs. *In* Griffin GE, Kwochka KW, MacDonald JM (eds): Current Veterinary Dermatology. The Science and Art of Therapy. St. Louis, Mosby–Year Book, 1993, pp. 167–175.
6. Moriello KA: Scaling and crusting. *In* Moriello KA, Mason IS (eds): Handbook of Small Animal Dermatology. New York, Elsevier Science, 1995, pp. 167–177.
7. Bond R, Howell SA, Haywood PJ, et al: Isolation of *Malassezia sympodialis* and *Malassezia globosa* from healthy pet cats. Vet Rec 141:200–201, 1997.
8. McKeever PJ, Harvey RG: A Color Handbook of Skin Diseases of the Dog and Cat. Ames, IA, Iowa State University Press, 1998, p. 139.
9. Moriello KA, DeBoer DJ: Dermatophytosis: Advances in therapy and control. *In* August JR (ed): Consultations in Feline Internal Medicine, vol. 3. Philadelphia, WB Saunders, 1997, pp. 177–190.
10. Mason KV: *Malassezia pachydermatis*–associated dermatitis. *In* August JR (ed): Consultations in Feline Internal Medicine, vol. 3. Philadelphia, WB Saunders, 1997, pp. 221–223.
11. Bond R, Curtis C, Mason I, et al: An idiopathic facial dermatitis of Persian cats. Vet Dermatol J 11:35–42, 2000.
12. Kwochka KW: Shampoos and moisturizing rinses in veterinary dermatology. *In* Bonagura JM (ed): Kirk's Current Veterinary Therapy XII: Small Animal Practice. Philadelphia, WB Saunders, 1995, pp. 590–595.
13. Kwochka KW: Symptomatic topical therapy of scaling disorders. *In* Griffin GE, Kwochka KW, MacDonald JM (eds): Current Veterinary Dermatology. The Science and Art of Therapy. St. Louis, Mosby–Year Book, 1993, pp. 191–202.
14. Kwochka KW: Retinoids and vitamin A therapy. *In* Griffin GE, Kwochka KW, MacDonald JM (eds): Current Veterinary Dermatology. The Science and Art of Therapy. St. Louis, Mosby–Year Book, 1993, pp. 203–210.
15. Power HT, Ihrke PJ: The use of synthetic retinoids in veterinary medicine. *In* Bonagura JM (ed): Kirk's Current Veterinary Therapy XII: Small Animal Practice. Philadelphia, WB Saunders, 1995, pp. 585–590.

28

◆ Bowen's Disease (Multicentric Squamous Cell Carcinoma In Situ)

Laura B. Stokking
Karen L. Campbell

Bowen's disease in human beings is an in situ form of squamous cell carcinoma. The disease is characterized by solitary or multiple hyperkeratotic crusts to verrucous plaques that occur on the skin, mucous membranes, and nail beds, commonly in sun-exposed areas of skin. The lesions have irregular, but distinct margins, are slow to grow, and do not invade the basement membrane.[1-3] Bowen's disease in cats, also referred to as multicentric squamous cell carcinoma in situ, has been reported with increasing frequency since 1991.[4] The disease is characterized by multifocal hyperkeratotic crusts or plaques. Dysplastic cells are confined to epidermal and follicular infundibular epithelium, and do not penetrate the basement membrane of the epidermis. The feline disease is not associated with sun exposure.[4-8]

Naming of this disease is controversial. Miller and coworkers[7] prefer the name Bowen's disease to multicentric squamous cell carcinoma in situ because the term squamous cell carcinoma connotes invasion and breach of basement membrane. Baer and Helton[6] prefer the term multicentric squamous cell carcinoma in situ because the feline disease differs from human Bowen's disease clinically (most feline cases have multiple lesions) and in proposed etiology (many human cases are associated with solar exposure).

◆ SIGNALMENT

Bowen's disease occurs predominantly in middle-aged to older cats. Ages of affected individuals range from 2 months to 20 years, with a mean of about 11.5 or 12 years.[4-8] No predilections for gender or coat color have been observed.[6-8] Domestic shorthair cats are the most common breed represented, followed by domestic longhair cats. Other breeds diagnosed with Bowen's disease have included Siamese, American shorthair, Himalayan, Persian, and Maine coon.[6-8]

◆ CLINICAL SIGNS

The most common sites of Bowen's disease in cats are the head, neck, shoulders, thoracic limbs, and digits (Figs. 28-1 and 28-2)[9]; less common sites include the ventral abdomen,[9] thighs,[10] and oral mucosae.[4] The lesions may originate in haired or unhaired skin and may become partially alopecic.[6] Le-

sions typically are multifocal[4, 6, 7]; over 30 tumors were reported from a single individual.[4] The thickened and dysplastic epidermal and follicular infundibular epithelium may be elevated or papillated or may form plaques, and may coalesce (Fig. 28-3).[4] An irregular, but distinct, margin surrounds the hyperkeratotic plaques and crusts, which may be pruritic.[4, 6, 7] Crusts form over ulcerated areas. Lesions often bleed and become painful when crusts are removed.[4, 7, 9] Affected areas may be present for months to years before diagnosis.[4-8] In 2 reported studies, lesions were confined to darkly pigmented skin.[6, 7] Pigmented lesions may be mistaken for melanoma or basal cell carcinoma.[7]

◆ HISTOPATHOLOGY

In human beings, histopathologic features of Bowen's disease include acanthosis, large pleomorphic

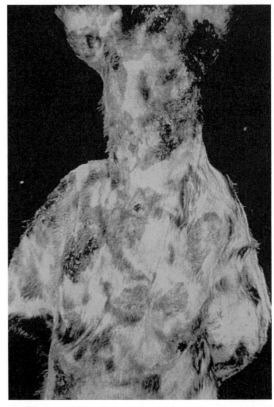

Figure 28–1. Multifocal ulcerative and crusting Bowen's disease lesions over the head, neck, and dorsum of a cat. (Courtesy of Dr. Edward G. Clark, Western College of Veterinary Medicine.)

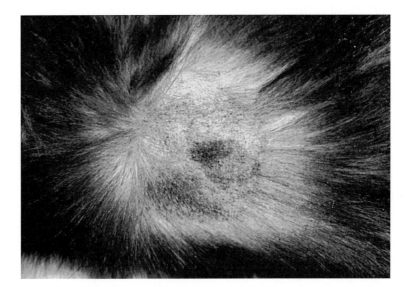

Figure 28–2. Crusts on the dorsum of a cat with Bowen's disease.

nuclei, multinucleated cells, dyskeratotic cells, and abnormal maturation of epidermal epithelial cells.[1, 2, 6] Neoplastic keratinocytes (large, polyhedral, sharply bounded cells with pale eosinophilic cytoplasm) are observed in follicular infundibular epithelium. Clusters of abnormal cells sometimes are present within normal epidermis. Neoplastic cells do not penetrate the basement membrane. Four histologic variants are described: psoriaform (regular acanthosis, thickened rete ridges, parakeratotic hyperkeratosis), atrophic (epidermal thinning, parakeratotic hyperkeratosis), verrucous hyperkeratosis (substantial hyperkeratosis, minor parakeratotic hyperkeratosis, irregular acanthosis), and irregular (variably thickened epidermis without hyperkeratosis).[1, 2, 6] A single lesion can contain more than 1 variant.[6]

In cats, lesions of Bowen's disease are sharply delineated. Epidermal and follicular infundibular epithelia are thickened and disorganized, imparting a "windblown" appearance to the section (Fig. 28–4).[11] Keratinocytes exhibit dyskeratosis, anisocytosis, anisokaryosis, and variable mitotic rates (Fig. 28–5)[7]; mitotic figures are observed throughout the epidermis.[4] As in human beings, clusters of neoplastic cells may occur in normal stratum spinosum.[6] Two histologic variants similar to those in human beings are reported in feline lesions: irregular nonhyperkeratotic and verrucous hyperkeratotic.[6] Focal ulceration is present in some cases, and the epidermis may be covered by a serocellular crust.[7] Suppurative folliculitis and mononuclear perivascular dermatitis have been reported.[7] The basement membrane remains intact.[6, 7, 11]

◆ DIAGNOSIS

Differential diagnoses of Bowen's disease in cats include a multitude of other diseases that produce crusts, ulcers, plaques, and verrucous lesions (Table 28–1).[12] Skin scrapings, cytology, fungal cultures,

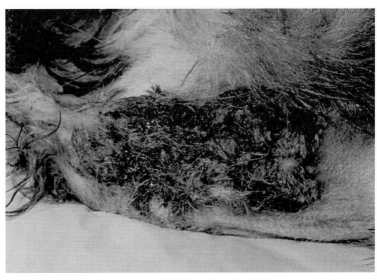

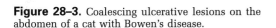
Figure 28–3. Coalescing ulcerative lesions on the abdomen of a cat with Bowen's disease.

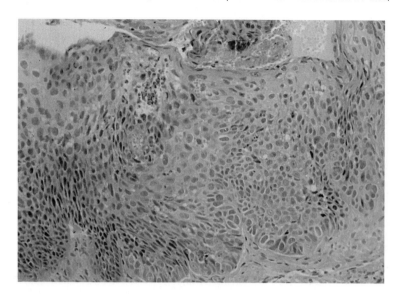

Figure 28–4. Example of the "windblown" appearance of keratinocytes in feline Bowen's disease. ×200. (Courtesy of Dr. Ann M. Hargis, DermatoDiagnostics.)

and histopathology can rule out most differential diagnoses. To diagnose Bowen's disease histopathologically, 3 or more of the following abnormalities should be present: (1) cellular atypia (multinucleate cells; abnormal mitotic figures; giant, pleomorphic, or hyperchromatic nuclei); (2) mitotic cells observed more than 3 cell layers above the basal layer; (3) windblown epidermis; (4) dyskeratosis; and (5) involvement of follicular epithelium.[6, 8, 11] Because Bowen's disease is a carcinoma in situ, the basement membrane should be intact.

Actinic keratosis and Bowen's disease cannot always be distinguished histologically. The distinction between the 2 is thus made generally on the basis of clinical signs.[11] Feline solar or actinic keratosis is most common in poorly pigmented, sparsely haired areas exposed to solar radiation, especially the pinnae, nasal planum, eyelids, and muzzle (see Chapter 25, Photodermatitis).[6, 11] The lesions are generally solitary, but may be multiple. In contrast, lesions of Bowen's disease may occur in haired pigmented areas, may show no association to solar exposure, and usually are multiple.

◆ ETIOLOGY

In human beings, Bowen's disease can result from exposure to sunlight, other forms of radiation, and arsenic. The lesions may be associated with leukoplakia, cutaneous horns, or intraepidermal epithelioma.[1–3, 6] Several authors report a link between Bowen's disease and various types of human papillomavirus, although in situ hybridization and polymerase chain reaction techniques often are required to demonstrate the association.[1, 13, 14] Bowen's disease formerly was thought to be an indication of internal malignancy in human beings; however, this association has been refuted by several studies, particularly in cases of Bowen's disease associated with solar exposure.[15–17]

Invasive squamous cell carcinoma develops in 2

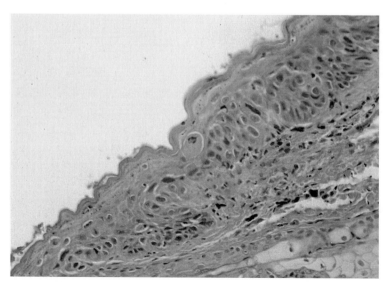

Figure 28–5. Note the disorderly maturation of keratinocytes (dyskeratosis) characteristic of Bowen's disease lesions. ×200. (Courtesy of Dr. Robert W. Dunstan, Texas A&M University.)

Table 28–1. Differential Diagnoses of Bowen's Disease

Crusts

Flea-bite hypersensitivity
Food hypersensitivity
Atopy
Eosinophilic granuloma complex
Dermatophytosis
Notoedres/demodicosis
Actinic keratosis
Sporotrichosis
Mycobacteriosis
Pemphigus
Systemic lupus erythematosus

Plaques/Hyperkeratoses

Eosinophilic plaque
Actinic keratosis
Mast cell tumor
Melanoma
Basal cell tumor or carcinoma
Fibrosarcoma
Cutaneous lymphoma
Papillomavirus

Ulcers

Flea-bite hypersensitivity
Food hypersensitivity
Atopy
Sporotrichosis
Mycobacteriosis
Pemphigus
Systemic lupus erythematosus

to 5 per cent of bowenoid lesions in human beings after several years.[1] Squamous cell carcinoma in situ has been identified in the center or periphery of most invasive squamous cell carcinoma lesions biopsied with wide margins.[18] Reizner and colleagues,[3] however, report only 1 case in which squamous cell carcinoma developed proximal to a bowenoid lesion, and found that the majority of Bowen's disease lesions do not become invasive.

In cats, Bowen's disease is not associated with exposure to solar radiation. Lesions in 12 cats whose exposure to sunlight was limited were present only on pigmented skin. No lesions were observed on white-haired regions of any cat in this study.[6] No association between Bowen's disease and arsenic exposure has been detected in feline cases.[6, 7] A cutaneous horn was reported in a single cat affected by multiple lesions of Bowen's disease.[19]

An infectious etiology for Bowen's disease is supported by reports of spontaneous regression of Bowen's lesions, the development of multicentric as well as solitary lesions, and the association of papillomavirus with Bowen's disease in human beings.[7, 8, 12] No association has been observed between feline leukemia virus (FeLV) or feline immunodeficiency virus (FIV) and Bowen's disease; few cats reported with Bowen's disease were positive for FeLV or FIV. In one study, none of the 14 cats tested for FeLV was positive, and only 1 of 12 tested for FIV was positive.[4] In another study, the 4 cats tested for FeLV were negative, and 2 of 3 cats tested for FIV were

negative.[7] However, 3 of 4 cats with adult-onset demodicosis concurrent with Bowen's disease were FIV-positive.[10] Furthermore, feline Bowen's disease has been reported only since about 1991, whereas FeLV and FIV infections have been recognized since about 1964[20] and 1986,[21] respectively, although antibodies to FIV have been reported from serum collected in 1968.[21] Other studies suggest a possible association between feline papillomavirus and Bowen's disease.[8] Feline papillomavirus infection has been described since 1990.[22–24] Papillomavirus-infected cats exhibit sharply delineated truncal crusts and plaques[22] that are similar to the lesions of Bowen's disease.[7] Le Clerc and associates[8] detected papillomavirus group–specific antigen using immunohistochemical techniques in feline skin near Bowen's disease lesions in 30 of 63 cases, and inferred an etiologic association from the proximity of papillomavirus-infected areas to the Bowen's lesions. More sensitive detection methods, such as in situ hybridization or polymerase chain reaction techniques, may demonstrate a higher percentage of papillomavirus-positive cases in future studies.[8]

Concurrent disease was present in 8 of 15 cats in one study; problems included renal failure, dental disease, hyperthyroidism, and bilateral uveitis.[4] In another study, concurrent disease was identified in 3 of 12 cats (diabetes mellitus, mild azotemia, FeLV infection, demodicosis, mediastinal lymphosarcoma).[6] Rees and Goldschmidt[19] reported a case of multicentric squamous cell carcinoma in situ in a cat that was later diagnosed with a thymoma and a hepatoma.

◆ TREATMENT

The preferred treatment for Bowen's disease in human beings is surgical excision with wide margins; other modalities include laser surgery, cryosurgery, electrodesiccation, radiotherapy, and topical 5-fluorouracil.[1–3] 5-Fluorouracil is neurotoxic in cats.[7] Poor responses have been reported for feline cases treated with alkylating agents, antibiotics, retinoids, and corticosteroids.[4, 6, 7, 10] Miller and coworkers[7] report mixed results from ^{90}Sr plesiotherapy. Plaques on the trunk of 1 cat treated with ^{90}Sr plesiotherapy resolved; however, thicker lesions on the face and pinnae did not, perhaps because of the limited penetration of the beta rays (150 Gy; 2 to 4 mm).[7] In 1 case, lesions improved with no treatment whatsoever.[7] Because lesions typically are multiple in cats, surgical excision, cryosurgery, and laser surgery are not always feasible. We have observed favorable responses to the use of CO_2 laser surgery as a palliative treatment to remove exudative lesions and improve quality of life (Fig. 28–6). After excision or other treatment, new lesions may occur at other sites.[4] Photodynamic therapy has been used to treat human cases in which the presence of multiple or extensive lesions precludes surgical excision.[25] This modality has been effective in treating early

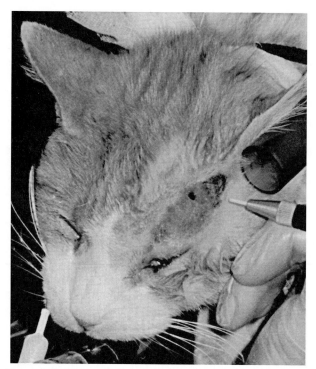

Figure 28–6. Removal of a Bowen disease lesion from the preauricular area of a cat using laser surgery.

cases of invasive squamous cell carcinoma in cats.[26] The photosensitizing agent is taken up preferentially by tumors; thus the modality does not destroy adjacent tissues. Multiple lesions can be treated simultaneously, the therapy can be given in conjunction with other modalities, and treatment can be repeated.[25] Photodynamic therapy can photosensitize the patient for 4 to 6 weeks. The lesions can become painful as neoplastic tissues necrose and slough. Therapy is limited to the upper centimeter of tissue if surface radiation is used as a light source; this can be circumvented by placement of intralesional fiberoptics.[25] One disadvantage of photodynamic therapy in treatment of feline Bowen's disease is that melanin absorbs light, thus preventing activation of the photosensitizer.[25] The modality thus would be less effective in the treatment of pigmented lesions.

Anecdotal reports have mentioned regression of Bowen's disease lesions after treatment of cats with alpha-interferon. Alpha-interferon may prove to be an effective adjunctive therapy for Bowen's disease associated with feline papillomavirus.

◆ SUMMARY

Bowen's disease, or multicentric squamous cell carcinoma in situ, has been reported with increasing frequency in cats.[4] Lesions consist of multifocal hyperkeratotic crusts or plaques that occur typically in the skin of the head, neck, shoulders, thoracic limbs, and digits of middle-aged or older cats. No breed or gender predilections have been reported.[4–9]

Differential diagnoses include the many causes of crusts, ulcers, plaques, and verrucae in cats, most of which can be ruled out by results of skin scrapings, cytology, fungal cultures, and histopathology.[12] Definitive diagnosis of Bowen's disease is made by the identification of 3 or more histopathologic abnormalities, including (1) cellular atypia, (2) mitotic cells more than 3 cell layers above the basal layer, (3) windblown epidermis, (4) dyskeratosis, and (5) follicular epithelial involvement.[6, 8, 11] Dysplastic cells are restricted to epidermal and follicular infundibular epithelium; the basement membrane is intact. Actinic keratosis is histopathologically similar to Bowen's disease; thus the 2 are distinguished on the basis of clinical signs.[11]

The etiology of feline Bowen's disease is unclear. Unlike the human form, feline Bowen's disease is not associated with exposure to sunlight, other forms of radiation, or arsenic.[6, 7] An association between Bowen's disease and feline papillomavirus is supported by immunohistochemical studies.[8]

Excision of Bowen's disease lesions is not always possible in cats because lesions are typically multifocal. Exudative lesions can be removed by CO_2 laser surgery as a palliative therapy. Results of ^{90}Sr plesiotherapy have been mixed.[7] Therapies that may prove beneficial in the future include photodynamic therapy[25] and adjunctive treatment with alpha-interferon.

REFERENCES

1. Cohen PR: Bowen's disease: Squamous cell carcinoma in situ. Am Fam Physician 44:1325–1329, 1991.
2. Kossard S, Rosen R: Cutaneous Bowen's disease. An analysis of 1001 cases according to age, sex, and site. J Am Acad Dermatol 27:406–410, 1992.
3. Reizner GT, Chuang T-Y, Elpern DJ, et al: Bowen's disease (squamous cell carcinoma in situ) in Kauai, Hawaii. J Am Acad Dermatol 31:596–600, 1994.
4. Turrel JM, Gross TL: Multicentric squamous cell carcinoma in situ (Bowen's disease) of cats. Proceedings 11th Annual Conference Veterinary Cancer Society, 1991, p. 84.
5. Rowland P, Affolter V, Suter S, et al: Multifocal intraepidermal dysplasia and carcinoma in situ in four cats. Vet Pathol 29:440, 1992.
6. Baer KE, Helton K: Multicentric squamous cell carcinoma in situ resembling Bowen's disease in cats. Vet Pathol 30:535–543, 1993.
7. Miller WH Jr, Affolter V, Scott DW, et al: Multicentric squamous cell carcinoma in situ resembling Bowen's disease in five cats. Vet Dermatol 3:177–182, 1992.
8. LeClerc SM, Clark EG, Haines DH: Papillomavirus infection in association with feline cutaneous squamous cell carcinoma in situ. 13th Proceedings AAVD/ACVD Meeting, 1997, pp. 125–126.
9. Fox LE: Feline cutaneous and subcutaneous neoplasms. Vet Clin North Am Small Anim Pract 25:961–979, 1995.
10. Guaguère E, Olivry T, Delverdier-Poujade A, et al: *Demodex cati* infestation in association with feline cutaneous squamous cell carcinoma in situ: A report of five cases. Vet Dermatol 10:61–67, 1999.
11. Gross TL, Ihrke PJ, Walder EJ: Veterinary Dermatopathology. St. Louis, Mosby–Year Book, 1992.

12. Scott DW, Miller WH Jr, Griffin CE: Muller and Kirk's Small Animal Dermatology. Philadelphia, WB Saunders, 1995.
13. Deguchi M, Tomioka Y, Mizugaki M, et al: Detection of human papillomavirus type 33 DNA in extragenital Bowen's disease with the polymerase chain reaction. Dermatology 196:292–294, 1998.
14. Kettler AH, Rutledge M, Tschen JA, et al: Detection of human papillomavirus in nongenital Bowen's disease by in situ DNA hybridization. Arch Dermatol 126:777–781, 1990.
15. Arbesman H, Ransohoff DF: Is Bowen's disease a predictor for the development of internal malignancy? JAMA 257:516–518, 1987.
16. Chute CG, Chuang T-Y, Bergstralh EJ, et al: The subsequent risk of internal cancer with Bowen's disease. JAMA 266:816–819, 1991.
17. Braverman IM: Bowen's disease and internal cancer. JAMA 266:842–843, 1991.
18. Guenthner ST, Hurwitz RM, Bucked LJ, et al: Cutaneous squamous cell carcinomas consistently show histologic evidence of in situ changes: A clinicopathologic correlation. J Am Acad Dermatol 41:443–448, 1999.
19. Rees CA, Goldschmidt MH: Cutaneous horn and squamous cell carcinoma in situ (Bowen's disease) in a cat. J Am Anim Hosp Assoc 34:485–486, 1998.
20. Rojko JL, Hardy WD Jr: Feline leukemia virus and other retroviruses. *In* Sherding RG (ed): The Cat: Diseases and Clinical Management. New York, Churchill Livingstone, 1994, pp. 263–432.
21. Macy DW: Feline immunodeficiency virus. *In* Sherding RG (ed): The Cat: Diseases and Clinical Management. New York, Churchill Livingstone, 1994, pp. 433–448.
22. Carney HC, England JJ, Hodgin EC, et al: Papillomavirus infection of aged Persian cats. J Vet Diagn Invest 2:294–299, 1990.
23. Lazando-Alarcón F, Lewis TP II, Clark EG, et al: Persistent papillomavirus infection in a cat. J Am Anim Hosp Assoc 32:392–396, 1996.
24. Egbrink HF, Berrocal A, Bax HAD, et al: Papillomavirus associated skin lesions in a cat seropositive for feline immunodeficiency virus. Vet Microbiol 31:117–125, 1992.
25. Jones CM, Mang T, Cooper M, et al: Photodynamic therapy in the treatment of Bowen's disease. J Am Acad Dermatol 27:979–982, 1992.
26. Peaston AE, Leach MW, Higgins RJ: Photodynamic therapy for nasal and aural squamous cell carcinoma in cats. J Am Vet Med Assoc 202:1261–1265, 1993.

29

◆ Cutaneous Xanthomas

Leslie Henshaw

Cutaneous xanthomas are nodules or infiltrations of the skin that vary in color from yellow (Greek *xanthos*) to brown or red-purple.[1] They result from lipid accumulation in the skin, and most commonly are associated with abnormal serum cholesterol and/or triglyceride levels. Several studies have demonstrated that the lipids in xanthomatous lesions originate from the circulation.[2] Elevated serum lipids, referred to as *hyperlipidemias* or *hyperlipoproteinemias,* either result from primary genetic defects in lipoprotein metabolism or are secondary to other systemic metabolic diseases that interfere with normal lipid metabolism.

In human medicine, cutaneous xanthomas also occur within the cutaneous lesions of patients with various histiocytic disorders. These patients are normolipoproteinemic, and the pathogenesis of lipid accumulation in the skin is unknown.[3] Feline cutaneous histiocytosis is extremely rare, and has not been associated with cutaneous xanthomatous lesions. This chapter therefore deals exclusively with cutaneous xanthomas associated with hyperlipidemia.

◆ LIPOPROTEIN METABOLISM

Cholesterol and triglycerides are essential to many different body functions in widespread tissues. They are hydrophobic and therefore insoluble in the aqueous environment of the plasma. In order to be transported from the sites of absorption and synthesis to the sites of tissue utilization, they are packaged into water-soluble lipid-protein complexes called *lipoproteins.* Lipoproteins contain a hydrophobic core of cholesterol and/or triglycerides with a hydrophilic coat of phospholipids, unesterified cholesterol, and special proteins called *apolipoproteins.* There are 4 main classes of lipoprotein complexes classified by function and by physical characteristics such as size, density, electrophoretic mobility, and lipid and apolipoprotein composition. These include very low density (VLDL), low-density (LDL), and high-density (HDL) lipoproteins, and chylomicrons.

Apolipoproteins are a heterogeneous group of proteins with a variety of functions in lipid metabolism. Some are structural proteins of the lipoprotein complexes, some bind to cell surface receptors to facilitate removal of the lipoprotein complexes from the circulation, and others activate enzymes that promote lipoprotein metabolism. There are 4 main families of apolipoproteins—apolipoprotein (apo)

A, B, C, and E. Variants within each family are designated with numerical subscripts.

Lipoprotein metabolism is complex, and a complete review is beyond the scope of this text. Aspects of lipid metabolism that are pertinent to the pathogenesis of cutaneous xanthomas are discussed with respect to specific diseases. For a more complete discussion of lipoprotein metabolism, readers are referred to an excellent review by Watson and Barrie.[4]

◆ PATHOGENESIS OF PRIMARY HYPERLIPIDEMIA

Primary hyperlipidemias are common in human beings, and are caused by a wide variety of genetic defects in lipoprotein metabolism. These defects are currently classified into 5 syndromes based on serum lipoprotein profiles (Table 29–1). Age of onset and clinical signs also help define the syndromes clinically. Three of these syndromes have been defined further by the discovery of the exact defect in lipoprotein metabolism as well as the underlying genetic mutation. Several cases of feline primary hyperlipidemia have been reported, and similar lipoprotein patterns have been identified in feline and human hyperlipidemias.

The most common and best-characterized feline primary hyperlipidemia is familial hyperchylomicronemia.[5–12] Clinical signs occur in young cats, and include cutaneous xanthomas, lipemia retinalis, splenomegaly, and peripheral neuropathies. Cats with this syndrome have a genetic defect involving the lipoprotein lipase (LPL) gene, which leads to a decrease in LPL activity and a resultant increase in cholesterol and triglyceride levels in the chylomicron fraction.[5, 12] Related cats have been shown to have similar lipoprotein abnormalities, consistent with a hereditary basis for the metabolic defect. Familial hyperchylomicronemia in cats is analogous to type I familial hyperlipidemia in human beings.

Normal fat metabolism begins in the small intestine where dietary triglycerides are digested into monoglycerides, diglycerides, and fatty acids via pancreatic lipase. These fragments then are combined with cholesterol, phospholipids, and bile acids to form mixed micelles. The micelles are absorbed by the enterocytes where re-esterification of the glycerides occurs. The newly formed triglycerides, as well as cholesterol, phospholipids, and apolipoproteins, are packaged into chylomicrons, secreted into the intestinal lacteals, and travel via

Table 29–1. Classification Scheme in Human Familial Hyperlipoproteinemia and Comparative Case Reports in Cats

Type	Specific Metabolic Defect(s)	Lipoprotein Abnormalities	Usual Changes in Lipid Concentrations	Clinical Signs	Reports in Cats
I	Defective LPL or (rarely) presence of LPL inhibitor	CM present and elevated VLDL, LDL, HDL normal or decreased	C normal; TG increased	Prepuberty onset; cutaneous xanthomas, lipemia retinalis, pancreatitis	Yes[5, 12]
IIa and IIb	Defect in both hepatic and peripheral LDL receptor (apo B$_{100}$-receptors)	CM absent; LDL increased; VLDL normal (IIa) or VLDL increased (IIb)	C increased; TG normal (IIa); TG increased (IIb)	Childhood onset; cutaneous and tendinous xanthomas; premature vascular disease	Yes[15]
III	Defect in apo E	VLDL increased with abnormal lipid composition	C increased; TG increased (VLDL C:TG increased)	Adult onset; cutaneous xanthomas, premature vascular disease; often associated with other metabolic disorders	Yes[13]
IV	Not defined	CM absent; VLDL increased; LDL normal	C increased or normal; TG increased (VLDL C:TG variable)	Majority are asymptomatic	None to date
V	Not defined	CM present; VLDL increased	C increased; TG increased (C:TG > 0.34 and < 1.4)	Adult onset, symptoms similar to those of type I	None to date

Abbreviations: [1]apo B$_{100}$, apolipoprotein B$_{100}$; apo C, apolipoprotein C; apo E, apolipoprotein E; C, cholesterol; CM, chylomicron; C:TG, cholesterol-to-triglyceride ratio; HDL, high-density lipoprotein; LDL, low-density lipoprotein; LPL, lipoprotein lipase; TG, triglyceride; VLDL, very low density lipoprotein.

Data from Polano MK: Xanthomatosis and dyslipoproteinemias. *In* Fitzpatrick TB, Eisen AZ, Wolff K, et al (eds): Dermatology in General Medicine, 4th ed. New York, McGraw-Hill, 1994, pp. 1901–1916.

the lymphatics to the thoracic duct where they enter the circulation. As the chylomicrons travel through the blood stream, the triglyceride content is hydrolyzed again into fatty acids and glycerol via LPL located in adipose and striated muscle tissue. These tissues take up the metabolites for energy utilization and storage. The chylomicron remnant then is metabolized by the liver.[4] When LPL is defective, as in feline hyperchylomicronemia, the triglycerides are not removed from the chylomicrons. The chylomicrons subsequently accumulate in the circulation.

A syndrome resembling familial hyperlipoproteinemia type III (FHLP III) of human beings was reported recently in a 3-year-old domestic shorthair cat with multiple cutaneous xanthomas.[13] Both serum cholesterol and triglycerides were elevated. Lipoprotein analysis revealed that the majority of the cholesterol and triglycerides were in the VLDL band. There also was an increased VLDL cholesterol-to-triglyceride ratio. The defect in human FHLP III has been shown to be a mutation in the gene coding for apo E, which results in an apo E that is either partially or completely nonfunctional.[14] During normal fat metabolism, the liver produces triglycerides and cholesterol and incorporates these along with phospholipids and apo B$_{100}$ to form VLDLs. These are secreted into the circulation where they acquire apo E from HDLs. The VLDLs are then acted on by peripheral LPL in the same manner as chylomicrons, causing a reduction in the triglyceride concentration of the VLDL. Because the cholesterol concentration of the VLDL is unchanged, the resultant VLDL remnant has an increased cholesterol-to-triglyceride ratio. Some of these VLDL remnants are removed immediately by the liver via hepatic apo E-receptors.[12] If apo E is dysfunctional, as it is in FHLP III, the remnant cannot bind to its hepatic receptor and fails to be taken up by the

liver.[14] This results in the accumulation of the VLDL remnants that now contain cholesterol and triglycerides in an unusual ratio. On electrophoresis, these fragments migrate near the VLDL position. The lipoprotein profile and clinical signs of the cat in this case report are very similar to those of human patients with FHLP III. A defect in apo E activity of this cat was suspected, but could not be proved because there is currently no method for measuring feline apo E activity.

An 18-month-old Siamese cat was reported to have numerous cutaneous xanthomas associated with primary hypercholesterolemia.[15] Serum cholesterol levels were markedly elevated, whereas triglyceride levels were normal. Lipoprotein electrophoresis revealed the increased cholesterol to be in the LDL band. These findings are similar to those of human familial hyperlipoproteinemia type IIa (FHLP IIa). In this syndrome, there is a defect in both hepatic and peripheral apo B$_{100}$-receptors. Whereas some triglyceride-depleted VLDL remnants are removed quickly from the circulation by the liver via hepatic apo E-receptors, as described previously, other remnants are metabolized by hepatic lipase. This removes even more of the triglycerides, shrinking the VLDL particles to form LDLs that subsequently contain primarily cholesterol. The LDL then is removed from the circulation via apo B$_{100}$-receptors located in a wide variety of tissues such as the liver, ovary, testes, adrenal glands, and many rapidly dividing tissues. When there is a defect in the apo B$_{100}$-receptors, as in FHLP IIa of human beings, these cholesterol-rich LDL particles accumulate in the circulation.[1] Although the exact lipoprotein defect was not determined, the abnormal lipoprotein profile of this case is suggestive of defective apoB$_{100}$ or apoB$_{100}$-receptors similar to that found in FHLP IIa of human beings.

◆ PATHOGENESIS OF SECONDARY HYPERLIPIDEMIAS

Diseases that are known to cause secondary hyperlipidemia in animals include hypothyroidism, hyperadrenocorticism, diabetes mellitus, cholestatic liver disease, nephrotic syndrome, and acute pancreatitis.[16] Although these diseases are commonly encountered causes of secondary hyperlipidemias, reports of cutaneous xanthomas are rare. In cats, cutaneous xanthomas have been reported in association with spontaneous diabetes mellitus,[17] and with megestrol acetate–induced diabetes mellitus.[2] Affected cats had extremely elevated triglyceride levels and a lesser increase in their cholesterol levels, with the majority of these lipids located in the chylomicron and VLDL fractions. Decreased LPL activity was documented in a cat with spontaneous diabetes mellitus. LPL is regulated by nutrients and insulin levels. Insulin levels rise rapidly following carbohydrate or fat intake, and fall during periods of fasting. Insulin causes an increase in the activity of LPL. In the absence of insulin, therefore, LPL activity in adipose tissue is reduced.[17] This results in increased circulating chylomicrons by the same pathomechanism as occurs in LPL-deficient cats with familial hyperchylomicronemia, as described previously. VLDL triglyceride concentration also may be increased in diabetic cats owing to the obesity and high caloric intake often seen in diabetic patients.[18]

◆ PATHOGENESIS OF CUTANEOUS LESIONS

Cutaneous xanthomas are caused by leakage of lipoproteins through capillary walls of the skin. The lipoproteins are phagocytized by dermal histiocytes, producing the characteristic "foam cells." Lesions are most common in areas of trauma, where inflammation and subsequent increased vascular permeability result in leakage of lipoproteins into the dermis.[1, 19]

◆ SIGNALMENT

Feline cutaneous xanthomas resulting from primary hyperlipidemias occur in kittens and young adults. Because these syndromes may be familial, similar clinical findings may occur in related cats. Cats with cutaneous xanthomas owing to secondary metabolic hyperlipidemia would be expected to have the same breed, age, and gender predilections as are found in the underlying metabolic disease.

◆ CLINICAL SIGNS

Cutaneous xanthomas are characterized by multiple white–to–pale yellow or erythematous alopecic papules, plaques, or nodules that primarily involve the dermis but occasionally extend to the subcutaneous tissues (Figs. 29–1 and 29–2). These lesions may be mildly pruritic or painful, and occasionally ulcerate and bleed. Lesions have been reported on the head, distal extremities, trunk, and footpads, and over bony prominences. Noncutaneous signs attributable to the hyperlipidemia include lipemia retinalis, splenomegaly, and peripheral neuropathies. Patients with hyperlipidemia secondary to metabolic disease also have historical and clinical findings consistent with the specific underlying metabolic disease.

◆ DIFFERENTIAL DIAGNOSIS

The differential diagnosis of the cutaneous xanthomatous lesions includes eosinophilic granuloma complex, mycotic granuloma caused by a dermatophyte or subcutaneous or deep fungus, contact dermatitis, atypical mycobacterial infection, and cutaneous neoplasia.

◆ DIAGNOSIS

A diagnosis of cutaneous xanthoma is based on dermatohistopathologic criteria. Punch or wedge biopsies should be obtained from nonulcerated lesions. Histologically, there is nodular-to-diffuse dermal in-

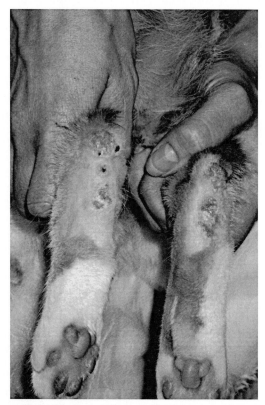

Figure 29–1. Bilateral cutaneous xanthomas on the hocks of a 2-year-old castrated male domestic shorthair cat with primary hyperlipoproteinemia.

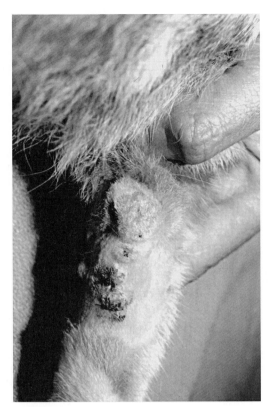

Figure 29–2. Closer view of the lesion on the left hock of the cat in Figure 29–1.

filtration of large macrophages containing abundant, foamy, lipid-filled cytoplasm (Fig. 29–3). Multinucleated histiocytic giant cells also may be present. Small lakes of extracellular, amorphous, pale-staining lipids often are present; these may contain acicular cholesterol clefts. The presence of both intracellular and extracellular lipids can be confirmed by special stains such as oil red O or Sudan IV applied to frozen tissue sections. The epidermis may be moderately hyperplastic, and low numbers of neu-

trophils and lymphocytes may be dispersed throughout the lesion.[20]

Once the diagnosis of cutaneous xanthomas has been made histologically, serum triglyceride and cholesterol levels should be measured after a 16-hour fast. If hyperlipidemia is present, a systematic approach to identify its cause is indicated to initiate appropriate therapy. Historical and clinical findings may indicate the presence of underlying diseases such as diabetes mellitus, hypothyroidism, hyperadrenocorticism, or pancreatitis. The history also may reveal use of drugs known to cause secondary hyperlipidemia, such as progestogens, estrogens, or glucocorticoids. A family history of xanthomas may be present in cases of primary hyperlipidemia.

Hyperlipidemia secondary to metabolic disease is more common than are primary defects in lipid metabolism. Etiologic diagnosis therefore should begin with the process of excluding metabolic diseases known to cause hyperlipidemia. A minimum database consisting of a complete blood count, chemistry profile, and urinalysis is indicated to detect the presence of diabetes mellitus, cholestatic liver disease, or renal diseases. Abdominal ultrasound should be performed to evaluate for acute pancreatitis in patients with a history of abdominal pain, vomiting, or diarrhea. A serum thyroid hormone panel or thyroid-stimulating hormone test is indicated to rule out hypothyroidism. Pituitary-adrenal axis testing with a dexamethasone suppression test or an adrenocorticotropic hormone stimulation test is indicated to rule out hyperadrenocorticism.

If no underlying disease can be identified, the hyperlipidemia should be considered of primary origin. Serum lipoprotein analysis may reveal the nature of the defect in lipid metabolism. In human medicine, this knowledge has led to the provision of more accurate prognoses and has provided for a more rational therapeutic approach.[1] Once a primary hyperlipidemia is suspected, lipoprotein analysis is indicated.

Figure 29–3. "Foamy" appearance of upper dermis is due to lipoproteins within dermal histocytes. Photomicrograph of skin biopsy from the cat in Figures 29–1 and 29–2. Hematoxylin and eosin, ×25.

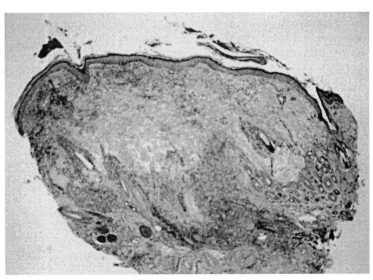

Lipoprotein analysis is performed most often at human laboratories. The distribution of serum lipids and lipoproteins of some species differs from that of human beings. Previous reports have demonstrated that separation techniques used in human laboratories (i.e., ultracentrifugation and selective precipitation) are valid in cats.[21] In addition, human and feline profiles are electrophoretically similar, lipoprotein terminology coincides, and interpretations are directly applicable.[15] If lipoprotein analysis is unavailable or cost-prohibitive, response to dietary therapy (see later) can help to confirm the diagnosis.

In human beings, definitive diagnosis of primary hyperlipidemia relies on identification of the phenotypic or genotypic defect. To date, familial hyperchylomicronemia is the only feline syndrome in which these markers have been identified. The phenotypic marker is a decreased LPL activity that can be measured by an in vivo heparin response test.[6] In this test, serum LPL activity is measured before and after in vivo administration of heparin (40 IU/cat administered intravenously). Heparin acts to release lipase enzymes into the blood. Normal cats have increased LPL activity after heparin administration, whereas LPL-deficient cats do not.[6] The genotypic marker of feline hyperchylomicronemia, a specific DNA defect involving the LPL gene, has been identified.[11] Neither of these tests is readily available at present.

◆ TREATMENT

If an underlying metabolic disorder is present, therapy should be aimed at controlling the specific disease. Plasma lipid concentrations should return to normal after the primary disease is controlled effectively. In the feline patient with hyperlipidemia secondary to spontaneous diabetes mellitus, normolipoproteinemia and resolution of the cutaneous xanthomas occurred within 4 weeks of initiation of insulin therapy.[17] In the cat with diabetes mellitus subsequent to megestrol acetate therapy, the megestrol acetate was discontinued and temporary therapy with insulin instituted. The insulin requirement diminished rapidly and was discontinued after 2 weeks, at which time there were no cutaneous lesions.[2]

Cutaneous xanthomas that result from primary defects in lipoprotein metabolism usually are responsive to dietary therapy. The goal is to restrict caloric intake in patients that are overweight and to reduce the intake of saturated fat and cholesterol. There are many commercially available foods, such as Hill's Feline r/d, that meet these requirements and have resulted in normalization of serum lipid levels and resolution of cutaneous signs. These foods also are typically high in dietary fiber, and although there is no evidence that increased dietary fiber plays a role in the reduction of serum lipid, such an effect is possible and may contribute to the clinical and biochemical improvement seen in these patients.[22] In human medicine, when dietary fat reduction alone fails to lower lipid concentrations adequately, additional therapy with lipid-lowering drugs can be used.[14] This has not been necessary in the affected cats reported to date.

◆ PROGNOSIS

Resolution of clinical signs occurs rapidly once the hyperlipidemia has resolved. The rate and extent of normalization of serum lipid levels depend on the identification of, and the proper therapy for, the cause of the hyperlipidemia.

◆ SUMMARY

Cutaneous xanthomas in cats are a marker for abnormal lipid metabolism. Lesions in young cats are suggestive of familial hyperchylomicronemia; however, it is important to rule out other causes of hyperlipidemia that would be treatable with disease-specific interventions (e.g., insulin for diabetes mellitus, L-thyroxine for hypothyroidism, surgery for adrenal tumor). The cutaneous lesions will regress after normalization of blood lipid concentrations.

REFERENCES

1. Polano MK: Xanthomatosis and dyslipoproteinemias. In Fitzpatrick TB, Eisen AZ, Wolff K, et al (eds): Dermatology in General Medicine, 4th ed. New York, McGraw-Hill, 1994, pp. 1901–1916.
2. Kwochka KW, Short BG: Cutaneous xanthomatosis and diabetes mellitus following long-term therapy with megestrol acetate in a cat. Compend Contin Educ Pract Vet 6:185–192, 1984.
3. Caputo R: Langerhans cell histiocytosis. In Fitzpatrick TB, Eisen AZ, Wolff K, et al (eds): Dermatology in General Medicine, 5th ed. New York, McGraw-Hill, 1999, pp. 1882–1902.
4. Watson TDG, Barrie J: Lipoprotein metabolism and hyperlipidaemia in the dog and cat: A review. J Small Anim Pract 34:479–487, 1993.
5. Bauer JE, Verlander JW: Congenital lipoprotein lipase deficiency in hyperlipemic kitten siblings. Vet Clin Pathol 13:7–11, 1984.
6. Jones BR, Johnstone AC, Cahill JI, Hancock WS: Peripheral neuropathy in cats with inherited primary hyperchylomicronaemia. Vet Rec 119:268–272, 1986.
7. Jones BR, Wallace A, Harding DRK, et al: Occurrence of idiopathic, familial hyperchylomicronaemia in a cat. Vet Rec 112:543–547, 1983.
8. Jones BR, Johnstone AC, Hancock WS, Wallace A: Inherited hyperchylomicronemia in the cat. Feline Pract 16(5):7–12, 1986.
9. Thompson JC, Johnstone AC, Jones BR, Hancock WS: The ultrastructural pathology of five lipoprotein lipase-deficient cats. J Comp Pathol 101:251–262, 1989.
10. Johnstone AC, Jones BR, Thompson JC, Hancock WS: The pathology of an inherited hyperlipoproteinaemia of cats. J Comp Pathol 102:125–137, 1990.
11. Peritz LN, Brunzell JB, Harvey-Clarke C, et al: Characterization of a lipoprotein lipase class III type defect in hypertriglyceridemic cats. Clin Invest Med 13:259–263, 1990.
12. Ginzinger DG, Lewis MES, Ma Y, et al: A mutation in the lipoprotein lipase gene is the molecular basis of chylomicro-

nemia in a colony of domestic cats. J Clin Invest 97:1257–1266, 1996.

13. Henshaw L, Campbell KL, Lichtensteiger CA: Feline primary hyperlipoproteinemia and cutaneous xanthomatosis resembling human type III familial hyperlipoproteinemia. Vet Dermatol (in press).

14. Mahley RW, Rall SC: Type III hyperlipoproteinemia (dysbetalipoproteinemia): The role of apolipoprotein E in normal and abnormal lipoprotein metabolism. *In* Stanbury JB (ed): Metabolic Basis of Inherited Disease, 7th ed. New York, McGraw-Hill, 1995, pp. 1953–1980.

15. Bauer JE: Diet-induced alterations of lipoprotein metabolism. J Am Vet Med Assoc 201:1691–1694, 1992.

16. Whitney MS: Evaluation of hyperlipidemias in dogs and cats. Semin Vet Med Surg Small Anim 7:292–300, 1992.

17. Jones BR, Wallace A, Hancock W, et al: Cutaneous xanthomata associated with diabetes mellitus in a cat. J Small Anim Pract 26:33–41, 1985.

18. Feldman EC, Nelson RW: Canine and Feline Endocrinology and Reproduction, 2nd ed. Philadelphia, WB Saunders, 1996, p. 114.

19. Vitale CB, Ihrke PJ, Gross TL: Diet-induced alterations in lipid metabolism and associated cutaneous xanthoma formation in 5 cats. Adv Vet Dermatol 3:243–249, 1998.

20. Gross TL, Ihrke PJ, Walder EJ (eds): Veterinary Dermatopathology. St. Louis, Mosby–Year Book, 1992, pp. 193–194.

21. Watson TDG, Butterwick RF, McConnell M, Markwell PJ: Development of methods for analyzing plasma lipoprotein concentrations and associated enzyme activities and their use to measure the effects of pregnancy and lactation in cats. Am J Vet Res 56:289–296, 1995.

22. Dimske DS, Buffington CA: Dietary fiber in small animal therapeutics. J Am Vet Med Assoc 199:1142–1146, 1991.

30

◆ Nontuberculous Mycobacterial Diseases

Richard Malik
M. Siobhan Hughes
Daria N. Love

Mycobacteria are gram-positive rods that have as their distinguishing feature a cell wall with outer layers rich in mycolic acids and mycosides. Mycolic acids are long-chain fatty acids found external to the peptidoglycan layer of the cell wall. Mycosides comprise a variety of lipids and related compounds. Together these impart a very thick surface layer to the organism. Lipoarabinomannan is another important lipid that extends from the cytoplasmic membrane to the cell surface and is thought, at least in *Mycobacterium tuberculosis*, to be responsible for many important biologic activities including inhibition and/or stimulation of different classes of cytokines. The lipids of the cell wall of mycobacteria are considered responsible for most of the characteristic features of the genus, including "acid fastness," the ability to withstand drying, as well as the histologic and immunologic features of the disease process within the host.[1, 2]

The name *Mycobacterium* (fungus-bacterium) is a consequence of the hydrophobic nature of the lipid-rich cell wall that gives these organisms the tendency to grow as moldlike pellicles on the surface of liquid medium, and to form stable aerosols when water containing them is disturbed. Historically, mycobacteria have been divided into (1) the *obligate pathogens*, such as *M. tuberculosis*, which do not normally multiply outside vertebrate hosts; (2) *saprophytic mycobacteria*, which have been divided further into the *facultative pathogens* such as *Mycobacterium avium*, *Mycobacterium intracellulare*, and related organisms grouped together as the so-called MAC *(Mycobacterium avium-intracellulare)* complex, which normally exist as saprophytes in the environment, but sporadically cause disease, and (3) those *environmental saprophytes* that almost never cause disease. However, recently, such divisions have been made more complex. *Mycobacterium leprae*, for example, which formerly was considered an obligate pathogen of human beings and armadillos, recently has been proposed to have some yet-to-be-defined environmental niche, whereas a number of formerly nonpathogenic species have been reported to cause significant disease in persons infected with the human immunodeficiency virus or suffering from AIDS.[1–4]

Mycobacteria causing disease in human beings and animals include the tuberculosis bacillus (*M. tuberculosis, M. bovis, M. africanum*, and *M. microti*), *M. leprae* (the cause of human leprosy) and *M. avium* subspecies *paratuberculosis* (the cause of Johne's disease of ruminants). Tuberculosis is acquired principally by inhalation of aerosolized organisms directly or indirectly from an infected host, although ingestion and instillation are less common entry modalities.[1–6] *M. leprae* probably is acquired in a similar manner; colonization of the nasal passages is a common feature in infected individuals. As with many of the other mycobacteria acquired from the environment, infection of the intestinal wall with *M. avium* subspecies *paratuberculosis* follows passage of the lipid-rich organisms through the stomach. Owing to their ability to form stable aerosols, most environmental mycobacteria are able to enter hosts via the respiratory tract or by direct instillation into wounds or abrasions.[1, 7]

M. tuberculosis, M. bovis, and *M. microti* have been isolated from tuberculosis in cats. These diseases have been reviewed recently,[6] and are not covered in great detail here. Classic tuberculosis in cats is caused by *M. bovis* and, occasionally, *M. tuberculosis*. A "new" feline tuberculosis syndrome caused by *M. microti*, a mycobacterium with characteristics intermediate between *M. bovis* and *M. tuberculosis*, has been the subject of considerable recent interest in Europe.[8, 9] Most likely, this disease results from infection with *M. microti* strains inoculated after altercations with voles.[10]

In addition to these well-known agents of disease, many different saprophytic mycobacterial species are capable of producing opportunistic infections in both immunocompetent and immunoparetic cats.[11–13] This group of organisms is the principal subject of this chapter. Although by no means a common cause of disease in feline practice, saprophytic mycobacteria are important "unusual" pathogens.[14] Recent developments in antimicrobial chemotherapy and reconstructive surgery have enabled most mycobacterial infections encountered in cats to be potentially curable, given committed owners and cats with an agreeable disposition.

When mycobacteria give rise to stereotyped clinical syndromes, diagnosis usually is straightforward, providing the opportunity for a successful outcome. Unfortunately, when mycobacteria give rise to "atypical" disease, such as granulomatous pneumonia or disseminated disease with peripheral lymph node and/or internal organ involvement, the clinical picture is suggestive of neoplasia such as lymphoma. Thus, unless appropriate specimens are collected for laboratory examination, animals sometimes may be euthanized on the basis of suspicion of having an untreatable terminal disease. We have adopted a collaborative approach to the diagnosis and management of cats with mycobacteriosis. Our team consists of a group of feline practitioners interested in evaluating these cases, veterinary cytopathologists and microbiologists with a special interest in diseases caused by unusual pathogens, a specialist surgeon interested in novel reconstructive surgical approaches to extensive cutaneous disease, and interested medical colleagues and mycobacteriologists at research institutes, reference laboratories, and human hospitals.

Nontuberculous mycobacteria give rise to a number of different clinical syndromes in feline practice, although sometimes the distinction between the syndromes may become blurred. For purposes of simplicity, the syndromes covered in this review include:

- Mycobacterial panniculitis due to rapidly growing mycobacteria
- Localized or disseminated cutaneous/subcutaneous disease ("feline leprosy–like disease")
- Disseminated mycobacterial infection, with lymph node and/or internal organ involvement
- Miscellaneous localized mycobacterial infections; for example, mycobacterial pneumonia, keratitis

A feature of mycobacterial disease is the associated inflammatory response, which is generally granulomatous or pyogranulomatous, as might be expected for an infection in which antigen-specific cell-mediated immunity is required to activate mononuclear phagocytes to deal effectively with bacteria capable of intracellular survival.[15] Pyogranulomatous inflammation is characteristic of diseases associated with saprophytic mycobacterial infections of human beings or animals, whether associated with the more slowly or poorly growing organisms, such as MAC, *M. marinum, M. xenopi, M. malmoense, M. genavense,* and *M. scrofulaceum,* or the rapidly growing species, such as *M. thermoresistibile, M. fortuitum, M. smegmatis,* and *M. chelonae.* Similar pathology may be seen with diseases associated with other bacteria with high lipid content in their cell walls (such as members of the genera *Corynebacterium, Nocardia,* and *Rhodococcus*) and with some fungal infections. The pathology, however, is clearly distinguishable from that associated with tuberculous mycobacteria in which granulomatous inflammation dominates the cellular response in immunocompetent hosts.[1–3, 5]

Although many other disease processes and agents give rise to (pyo)granulomatous inflammation, mycobacteria should be considered in the differential diagnosis when cytopathology demonstrates mixtures of mononuclear and polymorphonuclear phagocytes and lymphoid cells. The diagnostic laboratory should be requested to perform special stains to demonstrate mycobacteria, including both modified acid-fast stains to demonstrate acid-fast bacilli directly and Romanowsky-type stains (such as DiffQuik) that "negatively" stain the bacilli.[16] Furthermore, material should be collected for mycobacterial culture, which, along with conventional solid-nutrient media (e.g. blood agar), involves using a variety of special media, incubation conditions, and preparatory techniques to maximize the likelihood of isolating causal organisms. It also is prudent to freeze representative tissue from suspect cases, in case molecular analyses such as polymerase chain reaction (PCR) or probe detection systems are contemplated at a later date. These molecular techniques have had a big impact on the clinical management of mycobacterial infections in human patients, because these methods have the potential to provide an etiologic diagnosis more quickly and accurately than culture. Also they can detect infection in cases in which routine mycobacterial culture is negative because of the fastidious nature of disease-producing strains.[17–22]

Application of molecular tools for diagnosis of mycobacterial infections of cats is still in its infancy. However, recent studies have demonstrated the value of molecular approaches for definitive and rapid diagnosis of feline mycobacterioses. Most of these studies were concerned with identification of slow-growing MAC complex species, although molecular detection of mycobacterial species with fastidious growth requirements, such as *M. lepraemurium* and *M. genavense,* also have been reported.[21, 22] In these studies, a variety of molecular techniques were used. *M. avium* was identified in a cat with lymphadenomegaly using PCR, followed by Southern blotting and probing.[23] Culture and biochemical analyses supported the diagnosis, and definitive identification enabled appropriate antimicrobial treatment. Stevenson and colleagues[24] performed a variety of specific PCR amplifications, including an IS901 PCR for *M. avium* strains pathogenic for animals to identify *M. avium* directly in a feline skin granuloma. Culture of acid-fast bacilli from the tissue required 6 weeks, whereas a definitive diagnosis by PCR was made within 48 hours.[24, 25]

Malik and associates[26] performed specific PCR amplifications and DNA probe analyses to identify a mycobacterial species isolated from a feline subcutaneous granuloma. The results of the molecular analyses were conflicting: PCR amplification indicated *M. avium,* and the DNA probe tests excluded this diagnosis, identifying the isolate as a member of the MAC X-cluster. Further molecular analyses by 16S rRNA gene analysis supported the DNA probe diagnosis. This study exemplified the varying discriminatory potential of different molecular methods, and also highlighted potential problems associated with molecular identification of members of the MAC, a group with controversial taxonomy.[25]

In general, the choice of molecular method to be used for diagnosis depends on whether involvement of a particular species is suspected from the clinical and histopathologic observations, whether epidemiologic data such as strain-typing are required, and also on practicalities such as labor intensity, test cost, available expertise in molecular analyses, and result urgency. Specific PCR amplifications, obviating the need for further analyses, can be less labor intensive. However, use of specific PCR amplifications may be of less value if the etiologic agent is unknown. In these cases, PCR amplification of targets such as the 16S rRNA gene, 16S–23S rDNA spacer sequence, rpoB gene and hsp65 gene, which enable mycobacterial species differentiation, may be a more advisable approach.[17–20] This more general approach necessitates further molecular analyses of the PCR product using techniques such as nucleic acid sequencing, restriction fragment length polymorphism, or hybridization with probes, and therefore is more time-consuming and expensive. Rapid diagnosis of zoonotic mycobacterial infections is particularly pertinent whenever pets are considered. Consequently, it is envisaged that molecular techniques will gain more precedence for diagnosis of mycobacterial infections affecting cats in the future, particularly for species that are difficult to culture or that are slow-growing. These techniques also should assist epidemiologic investigation of feline mycobacterial infections—for example, by enabling sources of infection to be traced.

Before discussing specific entities seen clinically in cats, remember that nontuberculous mycobacterial disease should be considered in 2 distinct conceptual categories.

- There are those immunocompetent patients in which some breach in the normal defense mechanisms of the respiratory or alimentary tracts, or integument, allows mycobacteria to enter host tissues and give rise to (relatively) localized disease. In this type of scenario, organisms may be inoculated into an otherwise sterile site (e.g., after disruption of the skin by a penetrating injury or aspiration of abnormal material into the tracheobronchial tree). Likewise, localized gastrointestinal involvement may occur subsequent to ingestion of large numbers of organisms from an environmental source.
- There are cases in which the host has some immunologic defect, typically affecting cell-mediated immunity, that allows saprophytic mycobacteria to produce disseminated disease, often without an obvious breach in integrity of the defense system to account for the site of primary infection. In these cases, it is suspected that organisms colonize some site, such as the gastrointestinal or respiratory tract, and later spread hematogeneously to skin, peripheral or internal lymph nodes, lungs, liver, brain, spleen, and bone marrow—tissues that favor multiplication of mycobacteria.

Some mycobacterial species, such as the rapid growers *M. fortuitum* and *M. smegmatis*, are strongly linked with localized infections in immunocompetent hosts.[12] Other species, such as MAC, can produce either localized disease in an immunocompetent host or disseminated infections in immunodeficient hosts.[11] This distinction is important clinically because cats in the latter category may have identifiable causes of immune compromise, such as inherited immune deficiency, retroviral infection, or history of immunosuppressive therapy, and may be at risk for developing other diseases associated with immune dysfunction subsequent to successful treatment of their mycobacterial infection.

◆ MYCOBACTERIAL PANNICULITIS

Clinical Features

Mycobacterial panniculitis refers to a clinical syndrome characterized by chronic infection of the subcutis and skin of cats with "rapidly growing" saprophytic mycobacteria. Rapidly growing mycobacteria (RGM) are a heterogeneous group of organisms that produce visible colonies on synthetic media within 7 days when cultured at temperatures ranging from 24° to 45°C, depending on the species. They are distributed ubiquitously in nature, and can be isolated commonly from soil and bodies of water. Bacteria in this group of potentially pathogenic saprophytic mycobacteria include *M. fortuitum, M. chelonae, M. smegmatis, M. phlei,* and *M. thermoresistibile.*[12, 27–35]

If introduced through a breach in the integument, saprophytic mycobacteria are capable of replication in mammalian tissues.[14, 30, 31] The preference of certain saprophytic mycobacteria for fat results in their propensity to produce disease in obese individuals, and in tissues rich in lipid, such as the inguinal fat pad,[28, 31–34] and at sites where there have been infusions or injections with oil suspensions.[36, 37] The same phenomenon is observed in human infections—for example, athletes who inject themselves with anabolic steroids suspended in oily vehicles from contaminated multiuse vials, as a complication of lipoid pneumonia,[38] and after augmentation mammoplasty and median sternotomy.[12, 39, 40] Experimental and clinical observations suggest that adipose tissue offers a favorable environment for survival and proliferation of saprophytic mycobacteria, either by providing triglycerides for growth of organisms or by protecting the bacteria from the phagocytic or immune responses of the host.[28, 36, 41]

Initial reports suggested that mycobacterial panniculitis in cats was more common in warm, humid, tropical, and subtropical climates.[30] This appears to be true for human beings where most reported cases in the United States occur in Texas, Florida, and Louisiana.[32] However, cats from a variety of temperate climates have been reported to develop these infections,[34, 42] and the causal organisms have been readily cultivated in temperate soil samples collected from Japan.[43]

In cats, infections tend to start in the inguinal region, usually following environmental contamination of cat-fight injuries, typically associated with raking wounds inflicted with the hind claws. The infection may spread to contiguous subcutaneous tissues of the ventral and lateral abdominal wall and perineum.[30] Penetrating injury by sticks, metallic objects, and vehicular trauma also may give rise to these infections,[28, 40] as can cat- and dog-bite injuries contaminated with soil or dirt. Sometimes infections start in the axillae or flanks and spread into adjacent tissues.

Early in their clinical course, infections may resemble conventional cat-fight abscesses. However, instead of the typical pungent odor and turbid pus, a circumscribed plaque or nodule is apparent at the site of injury. There is progressive thickening of the nearby subcutis, to which the overlying skin becomes adherent. Affected areas become denuded of hair, and numerous punctate fistulas appear, discharging a watery exudate. Fistulas are intermingled with focal purple depressions that correspond to thinning of the epidermis over accumulations of pus. The "lesion" gradually increases in area and depth, and eventually may involve the entire ventral abdomen, adjacent flanks, or limbs (Fig. 30–1). If cats are presented promptly for veterinary attention and the lesion is confused with an anaerobic cat-bite abscess, standard treatment consisting of surgical drainage and administration of a synthetic penicillin typically is followed by wound breakdown and development of a large, nonhealing sinus tract surrounded by indurated, suppurating, granulation tissue (Fig. 30–2).[44, 45]

Some affected cats with severe infections develop constitutional signs. The animals become depressed, pyrexic, and inappetent, and they lose weight, and are reluctant to move. Surprisingly,

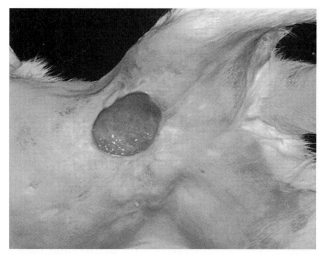

Figure 30–2. Appearance of mycobacterial panniculitis after an unsuccessful attempt at surgical treatment. Resection of tissues infected with mycobacteria often is followed by wound dehiscence, particularly if removal of infected tissues is incomplete, or if antibiotics inactive against mycobacteria are used postoperatively.

other cats remain comparatively well despite extensive pyogranulomatous disease. Usually the problem remains localized to the cutaneous and subcutaneous tissues, as would be expected from an opportunistic infection in an immunocompetent host. Although adjacent structures such as the abdominal wall eventually may be affected, widespread dissemination of the infection to the internal organs and lymph nodes is unusual.[31]

Diagnosis

Cytology

A tentative diagnosis of mycobacteriosis may be confirmed by collection, usually with the cat under sedation or anesthesia, of aspirated pus or deep-tissue samples. This material is used to confirm the diagnosis using appropriately stained cytology specimens, histologic sections, and mycobacterial culture. A histologic diagnosis is unnecessary if appropriate samples for cytology and culture have been procured. In our experience, samples of pus obtained from needle aspirates of affected tissues provide the best laboratory specimens (Fig. 30–3). Biopsies should be triturated in brain-heart infusion broth using a sterile mortar and pestle. Smears prepared from the resulting homogenate or from swabs or aspirates of the purulent exudate should be stained using DiffQuik, Burke's modification of the Gram stain, and a modified acid-fast procedure (decolorizing with 5 per cent sulfuric acid for 3 to 5 minutes). Cytology invariably demonstrates pyogranulomatous inflammation, and it is generally possible to visualize gram-positive and/or acid-fast rods in smears, although an exhaustive search of several smears may be required. Many organisms demonstrate beading. Histologically, there is pyo-

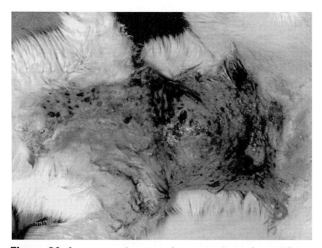

Figure 30–1. A severe, long-standing case of mycobacterial panniculitis in a cat. The infection has spread from the skin and subcutaneous tissues of the inguinal region to the entire ventral abdomen and the integument over the ventral thorax.

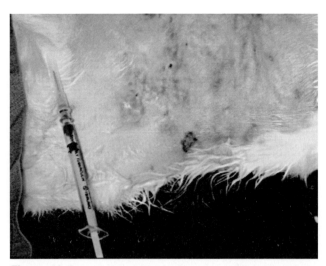

Figure 30–3. Mycobacterial inguinal panniculitis affecting the skin and subcutaneous tissues over the lateral thorax of a cat. This cat had been treated previously for a mycobacterial inguinal panniculitis, but without the benefit of appropriate postoperative antimicrobial therapy. The infection has recurred superficially in adjacent subcutaneous tissues. A sample of purulent fluid obtained from a subcutaneous lesion covered by intact epithelium is visible in the syringe on the left of the photograph—this specimen is ideal for cytology and culture. This cat was treated successfully using ciprofloxacin without the need for further surgery.

granulomatous inflammation of subcutaneous adipose tissue, overlying dermis, and underlying abdominal fascia and musculature. Acid-fast bacteria often are located in lipid vacuoles, and may be hard to find in Ziehl-Neelsen–stained tissue sections.

Bacteriology

Tissue homogenates and pus should be streaked onto duplicate 5 per cent sheep-blood agar plates and a mycobacterial medium such as Lowenstein-Jensen medium or 1 per cent Ogawa egg yolk medium,[46] and incubated aerobically at 37° and 25°C. Moderate-to-heavy growth of pinpoint, smooth or rough (depending on species), nonhemolytic colonies usually is detected after 2 to 3 days on sheep-blood agar at 37°C. When only contaminated specimens are available, tissue homogenates may be treated with 4 per cent sodium hydroxide followed by neutralization with dilute hydrochloric acid before inoculation onto media. Another method that may be used to differentiate RGM selectively from contaminant flora is by primary isolation around antibiotic-sensitivity discs (first-generation cephalosporins or isoxazolyl penicillins) applied to the plate after inoculation; this has become our method of choice for dealing with skin and subcutaneous samples contaminated with staphylococci.[47]

Strain Identification

Species identification can be carried out in a well-equipped veterinary bacteriology laboratory, although often it is more convenient to send the strain

to a mycobacteria reference laboratory after primary isolation.[a, b] Identification takes into account the following phenotypic features: organism morphology in Ziehl-Neelsen–stained smears of growth taken from Lowenstein-Jensen medium, colonial morphology (rough or smooth), pigmentation in the dark and light, degree of acid-fastness, rate of growth at room temperature and 37°C, ability to grow at 42° and 52°C, arylsulphatase activity, iron uptake, p-amino salicylic acid degradation, nitrate reduction, beta-galactosidase activity, acid production from carbohydrates (glucose, inositol, mannitol), utilization of compounds (glucose, fructose, inositol, mannitol, citrate) as the sole carbon source, tolerance to 5 per cent sodium chloride in Lowenstein-Jensen medium, and susceptibility to polymyxin B, tobramycin, and trimethoprim.[47, 48]

Isolates are identified as *M. fortuitum* if they are acid-fast; grow in less than 7 days at 28° and 37°C; produce rough, nonpigmented colonies; produce a positive 3-day arylsulphatase reaction; are positive for iron uptake; reduce nitrate; and are susceptible to polymyxin B but not trimethoprim.[48, 49] *M. fortuitum* strains are divided into biovarieties according to their utilization of mannitol, inositol, and citrate as sole sources of carbon for growth.[48, 50] It is possible to differentiate *M. fortuitum* strains from *M. chelonae* strains based on in vitro susceptibility to polymyxin B (*M. fortuitum* sensitive, *M. chelonae* resistant).[49]

Isolates are identified as *M. smegmatis* if they grow in less than 7 days, grow well at 43°C but not at 52°C, are positive for iron uptake, and have a negative 3-day arylsulphatase reaction. Further, colonies of *M. smegmatis* from clinical material typically are smooth and not immediately pigmented, although a late-developing yellow-to-orange pigmentation is seen in some isolates.[39, 47] Pigment develops in the dark but is enhanced by light. *M. smegmatis* strains have a relatively consistent susceptibility pattern, being resistant to rifampicin and isoniazid, but susceptible to ethambutol, doxycycline, sulfamethoxazole, trimethoprim, gentamicin, and ciprofloxacin.[39] It is possible to differentiate *M. smegmatis* (sensitive) from *M. fortuitum/chelonae* (resistant) using a trimethoprim-susceptibility disc.[47]

Antimicrobial Susceptibility Testing

Minimum inhibitory concentrations (MICs) for ciprofloxacin, gentamicin, trimethoprim, clarithromycin, and doxycycline can be determined easily using the Etest (AB Biodisk, Solna, Sweden) method according to the manufacturer's recommendations. One Etest strip is used for a 90-mm plate containing 20 ml of *Brucella* agar (Difco Laboratories, Detroit, MI).[51, 52] The MIC is read after 72 hours from the

[a]NVSL/USDA, 1800 Dayton Road, Ames, IA 50010.
[b]Centers for Disease Control and Prevention, 1600 Clifton Rd, Atlanta, GA 30333.

scale on the strip, and is the concentration where the elliptical zone of growth inhibition intersects the strip. This methodology is simpler than the "gold standard" of broth microdilution. Antimicrobial susceptibility of clinical isolates also can be determined using disc diffusion methodology based on that of Wallace and coworkers.[53, 54] Typically, isolates are tested against discs containing representative antimicrobials including doxycycline (30 μg), gentamicin (10 μg), ciprofloxacin (5 μg), trimethoprim (5 μg), polymyxin B (300 μg), enrofloxacin (5 μg), and clarithromycin (30 μg). Some antibiotics are included to determine a suitable agent for long-term oral therapy, whereas others (trimethoprim, polymyxin B) are used to provide phenotypic information concerning strains. Suspensions of each organism in saline solution or nutrient broth are inoculated onto sensitivity agar and incubated at 37°C. Results are recorded after incubation for 48 and 72 hours.

Therapy

Our handling of these cases continues to evolve over time according to accumulating clinical experience with a range of infected cats, the availability of new antimicrobial agents, and the development of new surgical procedures. There is a great variation in the severity and extent of lesions in individual patients. The marked variation in disease severity makes it difficult to compare different treatment options.

The most common strategy we have utilized is based on the approach of Malik and colleagues.[42] Treatment commences with either doxycycline or a fluoroquinolone, followed some weeks later by radical surgical excision of infected tissues, with intra- and perioperative intravenous gentamicin. A long period (typically months) of follow-up antimicrobial therapy is prescribed using either doxycycline or a fluoroquinolone. Severe cases benefit from the radical excision technique of Hunt,[55] in which infected tissue is resected en bloc followed by rearrangement of nearby skin to fill the tissue deficits. This strategy has proved to be successful. Gentamicin is administered intraoperatively (2 mg/kg every [q] 8 hr intravenously [IV] or subcutaneously [SQ]) and in the early postoperative period because it is bactericidal, is available in a parenteral form, is inexpensive, and displays good in vitro activity against mycobacterial isolates. Amikacin should be equally effective. Ciprofloxacin and enrofloxacin have comparable efficacy when used postoperatively.

Given the extent and severity of the pathology in many cats, it is understandable that adequate levels of antimicrobial agent may not be achieved throughout all involved tissues, and the best chance for a successful long-term outcome is to remove as much infected tissue as possible after preliminary antimicrobial therapy.[42] Residual foci of infection then can be targeted by the high concentrations of antibiotics achieved during and after surgery. Peri- and postop-

erative antimicrobial therapy is vital to ensure primary-intention healing of the extensive surgical wound. These recommendations are similar to those made for human beings with deep-seated saprophytic mycobacterial infections, in whom antibiotic therapy is used in addition to aggressive surgical débridement.[39, 53, 56] In people, the current recommendation is to pack the infected wound open after surgical intervention,[53] although preference in feline patients is a one-stage procedure including the judicious use of drains because of difficulties in treating an open wound for a prolonged period in a fractious patient.[42]

Some cases treated with doxycycline, enrofloxacin, or ciprofloxacin improve to such an extent that surgery becomes unnecessary. These cases thus can be cured using medical therapy alone, although treatment with oral antimicrobials for periods of up to 6 months is required. As a generalization, cases that resolve without the need for (further) surgical intervention involve a lesser depth of tissues than those cases that eventually require surgery. Successful management of mycobacterial panniculitis using enrofloxacin or clofazimine without surgery has been reported.[34, 57] However, some cases are so severe that only limited improvement can be achieved with antimicrobial therapy alone, and surgical intervention is essential. Because it is not possible to predict with certainty which cases will require operative débridement, our current recommendation is to start empirical therapy using a fluoroquinolone or doxycycline, determine the in vitro susceptibility of the strain to ensure the cat is on appropriate therapy, then reassess the case every 3 to 4 weeks to decide whether continued improvement is occurring, or whether surgery is indicated to effect a cure.

Generally, we have found that there is very good agreement between the in vitro susceptibility results and the in vivo effectiveness of antimicrobials administered at recommended dosages. The Etest method is easily applicable to this group of organisms, and provides quantitative information for selection of optimum drug therapy. However, susceptibility testing using a disc-diffusion method provides very similar information, and is cheaper to use in a general diagnostic laboratory. As a group, *M. smegmatis* strains are generally sensitive to a wide range of antimicrobial agents, whereas *M. fortuitum* strains generally demonstrate resistance to 1 or several agents, and often have higher MICs than those of *M. smegmatis*. *M. chelonae* strains tend to be resistant to all common agents available for oral administration apart from clarithromycin. Clarithromycin is an azalide agent, a macrolide derivative with an extended spectrum of activity and prolonged pharmacokinetics. It has proved to be useful in treating mycobacterial infections in human patients, especially MAC infections, and likewise is useful for many mycobacterial infections in cats. Unfortunately, in our experience, a large proportion of *M. smegmatis* strains are not susceptible to clarithromycin in vitro, and this unpredictable efficacy makes it an unsuitable drug to recommend for empirical therapy. Of the agents suitable for long-term therapy in cats, we consider the fluoroquinolones (ciprofloxacin and enrofloxacin) and doxycycline as the agents of choice for treating these infections, at least in Australia where *M. smegmatis* and *M. fortuitum* strains predominate.

In general, it is necessary to use as high doses as possible of antimicrobial agents when treating mycobacterial infections because affected subcutaneous tissues are not well perfused, and diffusion barriers can prevent blood levels of antimicrobial agents reaching organisms in tissues. Doxycycline is the tetracycline of choice for use in cats, being well tolerated orally, present in a readily available form (Vibravet tablets; Pfizer, Sydney, Australia), and having good lipid solubility. Doxycycline (25 to 50 mg per cat orally q 8 to 12 hr), enrofloxacin (25 to 75 mg per cat orally q 24 hr), and ciprofloxacin (62.5 to 125 mg per cat orally q 12 hr) all have proved effective for monotherapy. In general, treatment commences using the low end of the dose rates given previously, and the dosage is increased slowly (over several weeks) until adverse side-effects (inappetence, vomiting) suggest the need for slight dose reduction.

Based on our Australian experience, one of the fluoroquinolones is recommended for empirical therapy when microbiologic data are lacking, or while susceptibility data are pending. These agents are bactericidal, penetrate well into tissues including fat, and are concentrated in polymorphs and macrophages.[58, 59] Doxycycline may have a cost advantage, and has similar efficacy to enrofloxacin or ciprofloxacin, and thus is equally well-suited to long-term oral therapy. We have had an interesting experience with 2 strains of *M. smegmatis* that were resistant to enrofloxacin and/or ciprofloxacin; both of the cats had been treated with fluoroquinolones before referral and culture, and we suspect that resistance developed during a course of therapy, as has been reported previously for human patients.[60] The propensity of mycobacteria species to develop resistance during treatment is well known, especially for species such as *M. tuberculosis, M. avium,* and *M. leprae,* although this phenomenon has been far less problematic for the RGM.[61] The development of resistance is common for the quinolone agents, probably as a result of selection of preexisting mutants.[58] There is insufficient information to recommend routine combination therapy; however, the possibility of resistance development during monotherapy, especially using fluoroquinolones, should be considered in cases in which the favorable response to therapy does not continue during a course of treatment. The same dilemma is debated in the human literature, where some sources recommend that fluoroquinolones be given in combination with another agent,[50] whereas others consider treatment with a single agent to be appropriate.[61] There has been no evidence of acquired resistance to doxy-

cycline in our experience, and data from human patients indicate that the likelihood of mutational resistance to doxycycline is low. Thus, single-agent therapy with this agent may be employed with a lesser risk of the development of resistance than is found with enrofloxacin or ciprofloxacin.

Antibiotics should be administered for a minimum of 1 or 2 months after the affected tissues look and feel completely normal. Typically, the total duration of therapy is 3 to 6 months.[50] We have not evaluated trimethoprim or sulfamethoxazole/trimethoprim combinations, even though in vitro susceptibility data show many strains are sensitive to both components of the combination. Previous reports, however, concluded that this combination was inferior to doxycycline or a fluoroquinolone for long-term therapy of these deep-seated infections in cats.

In summary, mycobacterial panniculitis is a treatable disease in cats. Diagnosis is straightforward, especially for a practitioner familiar with the syndrome. The prognosis is excellent, even in cases with severe, extensive, and long-standing disease. Treatment involves long courses, typically 3 to 6 months, of antimicrobial agents chosen on the basis of in vitro susceptibility testing, usually combined with extensive surgical débridement and wound reconstruction. Even when surgical intervention is not possible because of financial considerations, long-term, once-daily therapy with doxycycline or enrofloxacin usually will confine the infection sufficiently to enable the cat to lead a normal life.

◆ FELINE LEPROSY–LIKE DISEASE

The term *feline leprosy* refers to a syndrome in which cats develop multiple cutaneous and/or subcutaneous nodules, "classically" about the head and neck, but often over the entire integument. Peripheral lymph node involvement often is observed, and dissemination to spleen, liver, and lungs has been demonstrated at necropsy in some cases.[62–66] This disease entity appears to be most common in New Zealand, the Netherlands, and Western Canada. Cold climates and exposure to rodents have been reported as risk factors in some studies. The disease formerly had been thought to be a result of infection with *M. lepraemurium,* the rat leprosy bacillus. New Zealand and Canadian reports describe histologic features characterized by the presence of small areas of caseation necrosis within a granulomatous inflammatory response. Langerhans giant cells are sometimes seen, and there is a variable infiltrate of lymphocytes, plasma cells, and neutrophils. Some cases present with more pyogranulomatous pathology, perhaps associated with a less-effective immune response. The pathology is characterized by massive infiltration of affected tissues with extremely numerous intracellular acid-fast bacteria, which fail to grow on routine mycobacterial media.

A few investigators have grown *M. lepraemurium* successfully from infected cats,[46, 67] although special media and growth conditions are required. Material from infected cats has been used to transmit disease experimentally to rats and mice.[62, 63, 65]

Work using PCR to amplify the *16S rRNA* gene has suggested that a variety of mycobacteria can give rise to feline leprosy–like disease including *M. lepraemurium, M. avium,* and a novel, fastidious mycobacterium sharing close nucleotide sequence identity with *M. malmoense.*[21] Recently, we have identified this latter "novel" mycobacterial species in biopsy specimens from Australian cats with feline leprosy. Thus feline leprosy is a syndrome rather than a specific infection. A similar situation exists in human mycobacteriology, where the "scrofula syndrome" of localized cervical pyogranulomatous lymphadenitis in children can be caused by a large variety of mycobacteria including *M. scrofulaceum,* MAC, *M. genavense,* and *M. interjectum.*

Clinical Features

The cohort of cats that we recognize clinically as having feline leprosy in Australia have disseminated mycobacterial disease in which there is extensive involvement of the skin and subcutis, and sometimes lymph nodes and internal organs. Contrary to many reports, Australian patients generally are older cats that are presented with numerous subcutaneous nodules affecting a very large proportion of the integument, not just the cranial portion of the cat. In contrast, feline leprosy cases in New Zealand and Western Canada more typically affect young cats (less than 3 years), and have lesions mainly on the head and forelimbs. Whereas many cases in Canada have ulcerated lesions, Australian cases present with nodules that typically are firm, nonpainful, and nonulcerated (Fig. 30–4), and affected cats eventually become constitutionally unwell. Regional lymph nodes sometimes are enlarged, and needle aspirates from them often demonstrate acid-fast bacilli. These features suggest that Australian cases usually are associated with the novel species of mycobacterium, whereas cases from cooler climates typically are due to *M. lepraemurium* infections.

Diagnosis

Diagnosis is straightforward, because needle aspirates and histologic sections contain numerous acid-fast bacilli surrounded by granulomatous inflammation. In DiffQuik-stained smears, mycobacteria can be recognized by their characteristic negative-staining appearance and location within macrophages and giant cells (Fig. 30–5). Acid-fast stains show organisms in smears and tissue sections, typically in enormous numbers (Fig. 30–6). Acid-fast bacteria tend to be arranged in parallel bundles

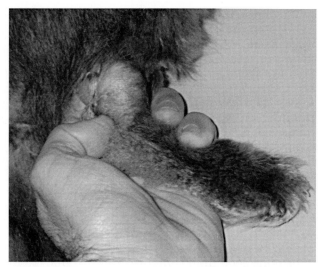

Figure 30–4. Subcutaneous lesion on the hind limb of a cat with feline leprosy–like syndrome. Sequencing of amplicons from 16S rRNA polymerase chain reaction suggested that this case was not caused by *Mycobacterium lepraemurium,* but rather by a "novel" mycobacterial species. This case was treated successfully with combination therapy using clofazimine, clarithromycin, and ciprofloxacin.

within histiocytes and giant cells. Material also should be submitted for culture because occasionally slowly-growing species such as MAC can produce an identical clinical presentation. In the majority of cases, conventional mycobacterial culture is negative owing to the fastidious nature of the organisms, and a mycobacterial etiology can be proved only by using molecular techniques such as PCR amplification and nucleotide sequence determination of gene fragments for mycobacterial species differentiation.[68] Fresh tissue delivered to a mycobacteria reference laboratory with PCR facilities is ideal. PCR can be performed on formalin-fixed paraffin-embedded material, although fixation conditions can cause DNA degradation and may limit the success of the PCR.[69]

Therapy

Too few cases with a documented etiology have been reported to provide accurate guidelines for treatment. The drug clofazimine (at a dose rate of up to 8 mg/kg orally q 24 hr)[70] has the best reported success rate, although it is likely that combination therapy using 2 or more drugs will prove to be a superior approach.[71] Drugs likely to have broad antimycobacterial activity against potential causal organisms include rifampicin, fluoroquinolones, clarithromycin, and clofazimine. We have treated a small number of cases successfully using various combinations of clofazimine (25 to 50 mg per cat orally q 24 to 48 hr), clarithromycin (62.5 mg q 12 hr or q 24 hr), and rifampicin (20 mg/kg q 24 hr). Clofazimine "capsules" can be cut into halves using

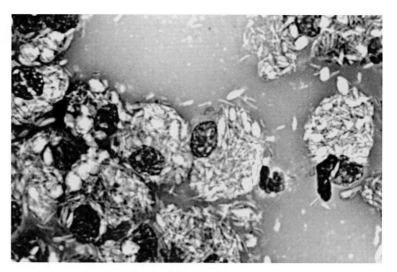

Figure 30–5. DiffQuik-stained smear of an aspirate from a subcutaneous lesion of a cat with feline leprosy–like syndrome. An enormous number of unstained bacilli can be seen as negatively-stained structures within the cytoplasm of macrophages, and free in the extracellular space. Original magnification, ×33.

a scalpel blade while wearing disposable latex gloves, and the 2 portions placed into gelatin capsules to facilitate dosing. Rifampicin is dosed similarly by dividing the contents of a 150-mg capsule, and reformulating in a gelatin capsule. In some cases, we have used 2 antimycobacterial agents, whereas 3 drugs have been used in other cats. Because clofazimine and rifampicin both can produce reversible hepatotoxicity, biochemical monitoring of cats regularly during therapy is mandatory. Vomiting and/or inappetence suggests the need for dosage reduction or temporary discontinuation of therapy. Our experience has been that clarithromycin is the least likely to cause side-effects. Monotherapy with this agent, however, is not recommended be-

cause of the possibility of resistance developing during the course of treatment.

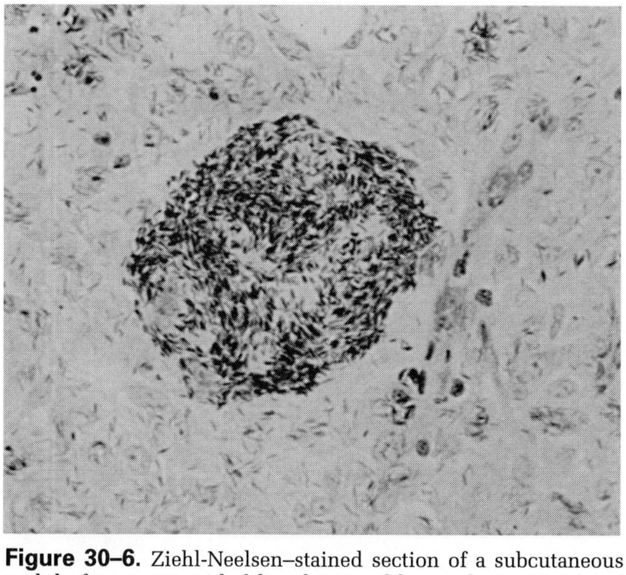

◆ DISSEMINATED MYCOBACTERIAL DISEASE WITH LYMPH NODE AND/OR INTERNAL ORGAN INVOLVEMENT

There have been numerous single case reports in the literature of disseminated nontuberculous mycobacterial infections in cats.[72–78] Some of the recorded cases have been young-adult Siamese cats[76]; we have seen very similar disease in 2 young Abyssinian cats, and the literature also records sporadic disease in mature adult domestic crossbred cats of various ages.

Clinical Features

Affected cats are presented for signs reflecting the particular tissues that are involved, although typically the cats are gravely ill, reflecting widespread disseminated disease with involvement of lymph nodes and organs in either or both body cavities. Sometimes nodular or ulcerative skin lesions are present. Occasionally, a cat may present in good health with apparently localized lymph node involvement. Although surgical excision of the infected node results in temporary resolution of the condition, affected cats may succumb to disseminated disease months later. Most reported cases have been associated with MAC infections, which develop presumably as a result of some subtle immunodeficiency in certain lines of purebred cats. We have recently reported a similar presentation in a feline immunodeficiency virus (FIV)–positive cat that developed a severe disseminated *M. genavense* infection (Fig. 30–7). Circumstantial evidence sup-

Figure 30–6. Ziehl-Neelsen–stained section of a subcutaneous nodule from a cat with feline leprosy–like syndrome. Acid-fast bacilli are present in large numbers in the large giant cell (center of photograph) and macrophages, and free in the extracellular space. Original magnification, ×132.

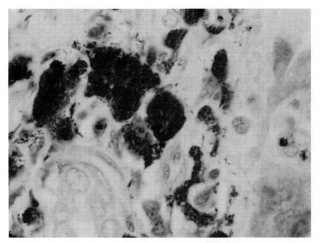

Figure 30–7. Ziehl-Neelsen–stained section of liver from a feline immunodeficiency virus–positive cat with severe, disseminated *Mycobacterium genavense* infection. Kupffer cells are engorged with enormous numbers of acid-fast bacilli. Original magnification, ×330.

ported the notion that mycobacteriosis developed in this cat as a consequence of an AIDS-like state.[22] Considering the high prevalence of FIV infection in countries such as Australia and Japan, it is surprising that more disseminated mycobacterial infections are not encountered in cats with long-standing FIV infection.

Diagnosis

Diagnosis is contingent on obtaining representative samples of tissue for laboratory investigations, typically cytology and culture. The best diagnostic specimen varies from case to case, but would include lymph node aspirates, bronchoalveolar lavage specimens, and portions of abdominal organs obtained at celiotomy. The presence of granulomatous or pyogranulomatous inflammation[79] should alert the cytopathologist to the possibility of a mycobacterial etiology, and the need for special stains and appropriate culture techniques. Organisms usually are not as numerous as in feline leprosy–type specimens, although there are exceptions to this generalization. Because these infections can be caused by very fastidious organisms such as *M. genavense*, collection of appropriate fresh specimens for molecular mycobacteriology also is indicated.

Therapy

We have had the opportunity of treating a small number of these cases, and have had gratifying results in some (but not all) cats using drug combinations similar to those described earlier for the treatment of feline leprosy–like disease. Based on our limited experience and what has been described in the literature, cats with localized lymph node

involvement should be treated with 2 or 3 antimycobacterial agents, even if the affected lymph node has been removed surgically, because they are at risk of developing disseminated disease at a later time.

◆ MISCELLANEOUS LOCALIZED MYCOBACTERIAL INFECTIONS IN IMMUNOCOMPETENT HOSTS

Cats with no detectable immune deficiency may become infected by mycobacteria that gain access to the body through a breach in normal defense mechanisms. Usually, these infections remain localized by a cellular response that is sufficient to prevent more widespread dissemination, but is insufficiently effective to remove the organism from the primary site of infection. Such infections are treated most effectively using surgery and adjunctive antimycobacterial drug therapy, although in some cases medical therapy alone will be successful.[26, 80]

Three infections on which the authors have consulted illustrate the approach to this type of mycobacterial disease. A cat with a localized corneal mycobacterial granuloma was treated by keratectomy after unsuccessful attempts at topical and systemic therapy. *M. intracellulare* was cultured from the resected lesion.[81] Surgical excision was successful, although the lesion recurred 2 years later, necessitating a second keratectomy. Another cat had severe diffuse mycobacterial pneumonia due to *M. thermoresistibile* (Fig. 30–8), and this patient was successfully cured after a long course of combination therapy using clarithromycin, rifampicin, and doxycycline.[82] A third cat being treated with cytotoxic multiagent chemotherapy for lymphoma developed a focal mycobacterial lesion on its nasal bridge. This MAC infection was treated successfully

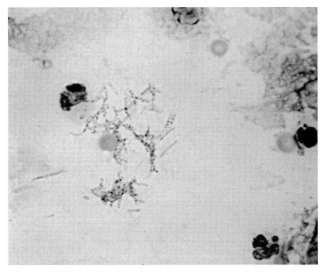

Figure 30–8. Modified acid-fast–stained smear of a lung aspirate from a cat with pneumonia due to *Mycobacterium thermoresistible*. Long, slender, beaded acid–fast bacilli are evident extracellularly in the center of the smear. Original magnification, ×330.

using cytoreductive surgery and follow-up therapy with clofazimine.[26]

◆ PUBLIC HEALTH SIGNIFICANCE

Nontuberculous mycobacteria generally are considered to pose no risk of contagion to other cats or human beings. These organisms are saprophytes found in abundance in a variety of watery environments, and it is unlikely that infected feline patients would secrete enough organisms by any route to pose a threat even to immunosuppressed individuals. In those countries in which tuberculosis is endemic, it is important to differentiate infections attributable to saprophytic mycobacteria from those due to organisms such as *M. tuberculosis* and *M. bovis*, which in contrast pose a significant threat to human beings.

REFERENCES

1. Grange JM: The biology of the genus *Mycobacterium*. J Appl Bacteriol Symp Suppl 81:1S–9S, 1996.
2. Youmans GP: General characteristics of *Mycobacteria*. *In* Youmans GP, Paterson PY, Sommers HM (eds): The Biologic and Clinical Basis of Infectious Diseases, 2nd ed. Philadelphia, WB Saunders, 1980, p. 367.
3. Wolinsky E: Mycobacteria. *In* Davis BD, Dulbecco R, Eisen HN et al (eds): Microbiology. Hagerstown, MD, Harper & Row, 1973, p. 884.
4. Wayne LG, Kubica GP: The mycobacteria. *In* Sneath PHA, Nair NS, Sharpe ME, Holt JG (eds): Bergey's Manual of Systematic Bacteriology, vol. 2. Baltimore, Williams & Wilkins, 1986, pp. 1435–1457.
5. Salyers AA, Whitt DD: Tuberculosis. *In* Bacterial Pathogenesis: A Molecular Approach. Washington, DC, American Society for Microbiology, 1994, pp. 307–319.
6. Greene CE, Gunn-Moore DA: Tuberculous mycobacterial infection. *In* Greene CE (ed): Infectious Diseases of the Dog and Cat, 2nd ed. Philadelphia, WB Saunders, 1998, pp. 313–321.
7. Collins CH, Grange JM, Yates MD: Mycobacteria in water. J Appl Bacteriol 57:193–211, 1984.
8. Huitema H, Jaartsveld FHJ. *Mycobacterium microti* infection in a cat and some pigs. Antonie Van Leeuwenhoek 33:209–212, 1967.
9. Gunn-Moore DA, Jenkins PA, Lucke VM: Feline tuberculosis: A literature review and discussion of 19 cases caused by an unusual mycobacterial variant. Vet Rec 138:53–58, 1996.
10. Kremer K, van Soolingen D, van Embden J, et al: *Mycobacterium microti*: More widespread than previously thought. J Clin Microbiol 36:2793–2794, 1998.
11. Woods GL, Washington JA: Mycobacteria other than *Mycobacterium tuberculosis*. Review of microbiologic and clinical aspects. Rev Inf Dis 9:275–294, 1987.
12. Wallace RJ, Swenson JM, Silcox VA, et al. Spectrum of disease due to rapidly growing Mycobacteria. Rev Infect Dis 5:657–679, 1983.
13. Lotti T, Hautmann G: Atypical mycobacterial infections: A difficult and emerging group of infectious dermatoses. Int J Dermatol 7:499–501, 1993.
14. Pedersen NC: Atypical mycobacteriosis. *In* Pratt PW, Ariello S (eds): Feline Infectious Diseases. Goleta, CA, American Veterinary Publications, 1988, pp. 197–200.
15. Kaufman SHE: Immunity to intracellular bacteria. Annu Rev Immunol 129–163, 1993.
16. Maygarden SJ, Flanders EL: Mycobacteria can be seen as "negative images" in cytology smears from patients with acquired immunodeficiency syndrome. Mod Pathol 2:239–243, 1990.
17. Boddinghaus B, Rogall T, Flohr T, et al: Detection and identification of mycobacteria by amplification of rRNA. J Clin Microbiol 28:1751–1759, 1990.
18. Lappayawichit P, Rienthong S, Rienthong D, et al: Differentiation of *Mycobacterium* species by restriction enzyme analysis of amplified 16S-23S ribosomal DNA spacer sequences. Tuber Lung Dis 77:257–263, 1996.
19. Kim BJ, Lee SH, Lyu MA, et al: Identification of mycobacterial species by comparative sequence analysis of the RNA polymerase gene. J Clin Microbiol 37:1714–1720, 1999.
20. Plikaytis BB, Plikaytis BD, Yakrus MA, et al: Differentiation of slowly growing *Mycobacterium* species, including *Mycobacterium tuberculosis*, by gene amplification and restriction fragment length polymorphism analysis. J Clin Microbiol 30:1815–1822, 1992.
21. Hughes MS, Ball NW, Beck LA, et al: Determination of the etiology of presumptive feline leprosy by 16S rRNA gene analysis. J Clin Microbiol 35:2464–2471, 1997.
22. Hughes MS, Ball NW, Love DN, et al: Disseminated *Mycobacterium genavense* infection in an FIV-positive cat. J Fel Med Surg 1:23–30, 1999.
23. van Dongen AM, Wagenaar JA, Kraus HS, et al: Atypical mycobacteriosis in a cat. Vet Q 18:S47, 1996.
24. Stevenson K, Howie FE, Low JC, et al: Feline skin granuloma associated with *Mycobacterium avium*. Vet Rec 143:109–110, 1998.
25. Ritacco V, Kremer K, van der Laan T, et al: Use of IS901 and IS1245 in RFLP typing of *Mycobacterium avium* complex: Relatedness among serovar reference strains, human and animal isolates. Int J Tuberc Lung Dis 2:242–251, 1998.
26. Malik R, Gabor L, Martin P, et al: Subcutaneous granuloma caused by *Mycobacterium avium* complex infection in a cat. Aust Vet J 76:604–607, 1998.
27. Dewevre PJ, McAllister HA, Schirmer RG, Weinacker A: *Mycobacterium fortuitum* infection in a cat. J Am Anim Hosp Assoc 13:68–70, 1977.
28. Wilkinson GT, Kelly WR, O'Boyle D: Pyogranulomatous panniculitis in cats due to *Mycobacterium smegmatis*. Aust Vet J 58:77–78, 1982.
29. Wilkinson GT, Kelly WR, O'Boyle D: Cutaneous granulomas associated with *Mycobacterium fortuitum* infection in a cat. J Small Anim Pract 19:357–362, 1978.
30. Wilkinson GT, Mason KV: Clinical aspects of mycobacterial infections of the skin. *In* August JR (ed): Consultations in Feline Internal Medicine. Philadelphia, WB Saunders, 1991, pp. 129–136.
31. Kunkle GA, Gulbas NK, Fadok V, et al: Rapidly growing mycobacteria as a cause of cutaneous granulomas: Report of five cases. J Am Anim Hosp Assoc 19:513–521, 1983.
32. White PD, Kowalski JJ: Enrofloxacin-responsive cutaneous atypical mycobacterial infection in two cats. *In* Proceedings of 7th Meeting of the American College of Veterinary Dermatology, Scottsdale, AZ, 1991, p. 95.
33. White SD, Ihrke PJ, Stannard AA, et al: Cutaneous atypical mycobacteriosis in cats. J Am Vet Med Assoc 182:1218–1222, 1983.
34. Studdert VP, Hughes KL: Treatment of opportunistic mycobacterial infections with enrofloxacin in cats. J Am Vet Med Assoc 201:1388–1390, 1992.
35. Willemse T, Groothuis DG, Koeman JP, Beyer EG: *Mycobacterium thermoresistibile*: Extrapulmonary infection in a cat. J Clin Microbiol 21:854–856, 1985.
36. Richardson A: The experimental production of mastitis in sheep by *Mycobacterium smegmatis* and *Mycobacterium fortuitum*. Cornell Vet 61:640–646, 1971.
37. Thomson JR, Mollison N, Matthews KP: An investigation of mastitis due to *S. agalactiae*, *S. uberis* and *M. smegmatis* in a dairy herd. Vet Rec 122:271–274, 1988.
38. Newton JA, Weiss PJ: Aspiration pneumonia caused by *Mycobacterium smegmatis*. Mayo Clin Proc 69:296, 1994.
39. Wallace RJ Jr, Nash DR, Tsukamura M, et al: Human disease due to *Mycobacterium smegmatis*. J Infect Dis 158:52–59, 1988.

40. Newton JA, Weiss PJ, Bowler WA, Oldfield EC: Soft-tissue infection due to *Mycobacterium smegmatis*: Report of two cases. Clin Infect Dis 16:531–533, 1993.
41. Hagan WA, Levine P: The pathogenicity of the saprophytic acid-fast bacilli. J Am Vet Med Assoc 81:723–733, 1982.
42. Malik R, Hunt GB, Goldsmid SE, et al: Diagnosis and treatment of pyogranulomatous panniculitis due to *Mycobacterium smegmatis* in cats. J Small Anim Pract 35:524–530, 1994.
43. Tsukamura M: Properties of *Mycobacterium smegmatis* freshly isolated from soil. Jap J Microbiol 20:355–356, 1976.
44. Monroe WE, August JR, Chickering WR, Sriranganathan N: Atypical mycobacterial infections in cats. Compend Contin Educ Pract Vet 10:1044–1048, 1988.
45. Kunkle GA: Differential diagnosis of nodules and draining tracts in the cat. Vet Int 1:3–9, 1993.
46. Ogawa T, Motomura K: Studies on murine leprosy bacillus. 1. Attempt to cultivate in vitro the Hawaiian strain of *Mycobacterium lepraemurium*. Kitasato Arch Exp Med 43:21–36, 1970.
47. Malik R, Wigney DI, Dawson D, et al: Infection of the subcutis and skin of cats with rapidly-growing mycobacteria: A review of clinical and microbiological findings in 49 cases. J Fel Med Surg 2:35–48, 2000.
48. Silcox VA, Good RC, Floyd MM: Identification of clinically significant *Mycobacterium fortuitum* complex isolates. J Clin Microbiol 14:686–691, 1981.
49. Wallace RJ Jr, Swenson JM, Silcox VA, Good RC: Disk diffusion testing with polymyxin and amikacin for differentiation of *Mycobacterium fortuitum* and *Mycobacterium chelonei*. J Clin Microbiol 16:1003–1006, 1982.
50. Wallace RJ Jr, Brown BA, Silcox VA, et al: Clinical disease, drug susceptibility and biochemical patterns of the unnamed third biovariant complex of *Mycobacterium fortuitum*. J Infect Dis 163:598–603, 1991.
51. Koontz FP, Erwin ME, Barrett MS, Jones RN: Etest for routine clinical antimicrobial susceptibility testing of rapid-growing mycobacteria isolates. Diag Microbiol Infect Dis 19:183–186, 1994.
52. Hoffner S, Klintz L, Olsson-Liljequist B, Bolstrom A: Evaluation of Etest for rapid susceptibility testing of *Mycobacterium chelonae* and *M. fortuitum*. J Clin Microbiol 32:1846–1849, 1994.
53. Wallace RJ Jr, Swenson JM, Silcox VA, Bullen MG: Treatment of nonpulmonary infections due to *Mycobacterium fortuitum* and *Mycobacterium chelonei* on the basis of in vitro susceptibilities. J Infect Dis 152:500–514, 1985.
54. Wallace RJ Jr, Dalovisio JR, Pankey GA: Disk diffusion testing of susceptibility of *Mycobacterium fortuitum* and *Mycobacterium chelonei* to antibacterial agents. Antimicrob Agents Chemother 16:611–614, 1979.
55. Hunt GB: Skin-fold advancement flaps for closing large sternal and inguinal wounds in cats and dogs. Vet Surg 24:172–175, 1995.
56. Plaus WJ, Hermann G: The surgical management of superficial infections caused by atypical mycobacteria. Surgery 110:99–103, 1991.
57. Michaud AJ: The use of clofazimine as treatment for *Mycobacterium fortuitum* in a cat. Fel Pract 22:7–9, 1994.
58. Leysen DC, Haemers A, Pattyn SR: Mycobacteria and the new quinolones. Antimicrob Agents Chemother 33:1–5, 1989.
59. Hooper DC, Wolfson JS: Fluoroquinolone antimicrobial agents. N Engl J Med 324:384–394, 1991.
60. Wallace RJ Jr, Bedsole G, Sumpter G, et al: Activities of ciprofloxacin and ofloxacin against rapidly growing mycobacteria with demonstration of acquired resistance following single drug therapy. Antimicrob Agents Chemother 34:65–70, 1990.
61. Iredell J, Whitby M, Blacklock Z: *Mycobacterium marinum* infection: Epidemiology and presentation in Queensland 1971–1990. Med J Aust 157:596–598, 1992.
62. Lawrence WE, Wickham N: Cat leprosy: Infection by a bacillus resembling *Mycobacterium lepraemurium*. Aust Vet J 39:390–393, 1963.
63. Leiker DA, Poelma FG: On the etiology of cat leprosy. Int J Lepr 42:312–315, 1974.
64. McIntosh DW: Feline leprosy: A review of forty-four cases from Western Canada. Can Vet J 23:291–295, 1982.
65. Schiefer HB, Niddleton DM: Experimental transmission of a feline mycobacterial skin disease (feline leprosy). Vet Pathol 20:460–471, 1983.
66. Thompson EJ, Little PB, Cordes DO: Observations of cat leprosy. N Z Vet J 27:233–235, 1979.
67. Pattyn SR, Portaels F: *In vitro* cultivation and characterization of *Mycobacterium lepraemurium*. Int J Lepr 48:7–14, 1980.
68. Rogall T, Flohr T, Böttger EC: Differentiation of *Mycobacterium* species by direct sequencing of amplified DNA. J Gen Microbiol 136:1915–1920, 1990.
69. Doyle CT, O'Leary JJ. The search for the universal fixative or "magic juice." J Pathol 166:331–332, 1992.
70. Mundell AC: New therapeutic agents in veterinary dermatology. Vet Clin North Am Small Anim Pract 20:1544–1545, 1990.
71. Barrs VR, Martin P, James G, et al: Feline leprosy due to infection with novel mycobacterial species. Aust Vet Pract 29:159–164, 1999.
72. Buergelt CD, Fowler JL, Wright PJ: Disseminated avian tuberculosis in a cat. Calif Vet 10:13–15, 1982.
73. Drolet R: Disseminated tuberculosis caused by *Mycobacterium avium* in a cat. J Am Vet Med Assoc 189:1336–1337, 1986.
74. Evans LM, Caylor KB: Mycobacterial lymphadenitis in a cat. Fel Pract 23:14–17, 1995.
75. Grossman A: Mycobacterial hepatitis associated with long term steroid therapy. Fel Pract 13:37–41, 1983.
76. Jordan HL, Cohn LA, Armstrong PJ: Disseminated *Mycobacterium avium* complex infection in three Siamese cats. J Am Vet Med Assoc 204:90–93, 1994.
77. Latimer KS, Jameson PH, Crowell WA, et al: Disseminated *Mycobacterium avium* complex infection in a cat: Presumptive diagnosis by blood smear examination. Vet Clin Pathol 26:85–89, 1997.
78. Matthews JA, Liggitt HD: Disseminated mycobacteriosis in a cat. J Am Vet Med Assoc 183:701–702, 1983.
79. Farhi DC, Mason UG, Horsburgh CR: Pathologic findings in disseminated *Mycobacterium avium-intracellulare* infection. Am J Clin Pathol 85:67–72, 1986.
80. Kaufman AC, Greene CE, Rakich PM, Weigner DD: Treatment of localized *Mycobacterium avium* complex infection with clofazimine and doxycycline in a cat. J Am Vet Med Assoc 207:457–459, 1995.
81. Deykin AR, Wigney DI, Smith JS, Young BD: Corneal granuloma caused by *Mycobacterium intracellulare* in a cat. Aust Vet Pract 26:23–26, 1996.
82. Foster SF, Martin P, Davis W, et al: Chronic pneumonia caused by *Mycobacterium thermoresistible* in a cat. J Small Anim Pract 40:433–438, 1999.

31

◆ What to Do for the Devoted Cat Owner Who Is Allergic to Her or His Pet

Karen A. Moriello

It has been estimated that 3 to 10 per cent of the general population and 15 to 40 per cent of atopic people are allergic to cats or dogs, with allergy to cats being twice as common as allergy to dogs.[1–3] According to the U.S. Census Bureau, at least half of the homes in the United States have at least 1 dog or cat, and cats are now slightly more common than dogs. Furthermore, 1 out of 3 people allergic to cats lives in a home with 1 or more cats.[4] The high proportion of people with cat allergy still living with their cats is testimony to the strong emotional attachment people have to their pets.

Cat owners with cat allergy sooner or later ask their veterinarian for information on how "to be allergic and still have their cat too." When I am in this situation, I find it useful to ask why they are asking me for information. Cat owners often assume we know not only about diseases of cats but also about diseases in people caused by cats. Sometimes, cat owners may not have consulted with their doctor about possible treatment options because of their fear that they will be told they *must* remove the cat from their home. In other cases, a cat owner might be seeking a "second opinion" from their veterinarian about the necessity of removing the cat from the home. Many clients see their veterinarian more frequently than their allergist or primary care doctor, and may feel more comfortable discussing such a major decision with their veterinarian. In yet other cases, information on how to control cat allergen in the home was not made available to the client by their health care provider. In several cases, I have had allergists refer cat owners to me for instruction on how to bathe their cat, or for reassurance that limiting the access of the cat to certain areas in the home will not be detrimental to the cat. Media coverage of the topic of cat allergy always triggers a barrage of telephone calls, as does the appearance of products that "remove cat allergen." Rather commonly, I have cat owners inquire about the clinical signs of cat allergy and how to "make the cat less allergic," because an intended spouse or roommate is allergic to cats. Finally, I inquire why someone is asking about cat allergy to prevent being drawn into family disputes between couples and roommates over having or keeping a pet cat. Being allergic to cats is often given as the excuse for not wanting to live with someone else's pet cat.

The purpose of this chapter is to provide veterinarians with information on cat allergy and environmental control of cat allergen with the cat in situ.

Patients with cat allergy should be referred to a human allergist for treatment.

◆ Fel d 1: MAJOR CAT ALLERGEN

The term *major allergen* often is used to describe antigens that cause reactions in the majority of patients. *Fel d 1* has been identified as the major allergen of cats responsible for the clinical signs of cat allergy in people. This allergen is the subject of intensive, basic, and clinical research for at least 2 reasons. Cat allergy is one of the most common causes of allergy in people; many of the studies involve treatment trials and methods to remove *Fel d 1* from the environment. Second, because this allergen is responsible for inducing the major part of immunoglobulin (Ig) E antibodies in cat-allergic people, it is a convenient model to study the human immune response to inhalant allergens.

This allergen was first described in 1973 by Ohman and colleagues.[5] Over the next decade, Ohman and coworkers[6] studied the allergen they named *Cat Ag 1* and patients' reactions to cat pelt (fur). Exposure to isolated allergen produced clinical signs of cat allergy in people consistent with symptoms they experienced with natural exposure.[7]

Cat Ag 1 has been renamed *Fel d 1*, has been characterized extensively by protein and immuno-chemical techniques, and more recently has been expressed as a recombinant allergen.[8, 9] This allergen is an approximately 36-kD dimer that is composed of 2 17-kD subunits. Each subunit is composed of 2 different chains (chains 1 and 2). Amino acid sequencing has shown that chain 1 consists of 70 amino acid residues, and chain 2 consists of 92 amino acid residues.

Fel d 1 is present in saliva, pelt, and sebaceous glands of cats.[10] In addition, it is present in a wide variety of internal tissues including brain, muscle, and visceral organs.[10] The original studies by Ohman and associates showed that saliva is a major source of *Fel d 1*, and it was assumed to be deposited on the fur during grooming. However, more recent studies have shown that the primary source of this allergen is the skin. High concentrations of *Fel d 1* are found in the sebaceous glands of hair follicles and, interestingly, anal sac secretions.[11–14] In fact, *Fel d 1* concentrations in anal sac secretions are higher than those reported for cat pelt, body secretions, or tissues. *Fel d 1* concentrations on the skin are under hormonal control; *Fel d 1* concentrations in male cats decreased 1 month after castration.[15] There also is preliminary evidence that secretions may be higher in male cats than in female cats.[16] When concentrations of *Fel d 1* from various parts of the body were measured, the highest concentrations were found on the skin in the intrascapular region.[17] To date, there is no evidence to support claims that one breed of cat is more or less allergenic than another.

The biologic significance of *Fel d 1* is unknown. The close association of *Fel d 1* protein with skin sebaceous glands and anal sacs, all with holocrine function and lipid secretion, suggest a possible physiologic role for *Fel d 1* in the regulation of lipids on the skin and fur.[14] *Fel d 1* also may play a role in gender and species recognition. Further evidence that supports a physiologic role for *Fel d 1* is the finding that there is a *Fel d 1*–like molecule in big cats.[18] In cat-allergic patients, IgE and IgG4 responses were found against a *Fel d 1* equivalent isolated from 7 of 8 members of the Felidae family (ocelot, puma, serval, Siberian tiger, lion, jaguar, and snow leopard).[18]

Finally, it has been shown that the major cat and dog allergens (*Can d 1* and *Can d 2*) have several IgE epitopes in common.[19] These shared epitopes may explain the clinical observation that allergies to cats and dogs often are associated.

◆ CLINICAL ASPECTS OF CAT ALLERGY IN PEOPLE

Clinical Symptoms

The development of cat allergy is associated strongly with the development of atopy in people, but not always. *Atopy* is defined as a familial tendency to produce IgE antibodies to a large number of aeroallergens on exposure. Approximately 20 per cent of the human population in the United States is atopic, and approximately one-seventh of these individuals (3 per cent of total population) have cat allergy.[20, 21] Some individuals with cat allergy are not atopic, yet they have IgE antibody responses to cats.[20, 21]

The clinical manifestations of cat allergy range from local cutaneous reactions to typical rhinoconjunctivitis to severe, life-threatening asthma.[22] Cutaneous reactions range from contact urticaria to an intensely pruritic, maculopapular eruption on the face, neck, and trunk. These reactions usually are associated with respiratory symptoms during airborne exposure. *Allergic rhinitis* is characterized by an inflammatory infiltrate in the nasal mucosa, and is associated with symptoms of sneezing and nasal congestion. Often this disease is complicated by sinusitis, and can contribute to headaches, sleep disturbances, otitis media, nasal polyposis, and exacerbations of asthma. *Allergic conjunctivitis* is characterized by an inflammatory conjunctival infiltrate, associated with pain, itching, and redness of the conjunctiva. *Asthma* is defined as a lung disease with the following characteristics: airway obstruction (or airway narrowing) that is reversible (but not completely in some patients) either spontaneously or with treatment, airway inflammation, and airway hyperresponsiveness to a variety of stimuli.

Other than acute anaphylaxis, the most severe clinical sign associated with cat allergy is asthma, which is present in about 5 per cent of individuals in the United States, and is associated with high economic costs, high morbidity, and possible mortality.[23] Cat allergy is an important risk factor for asthma; exposure to outdoor allergens (e.g., ragweed pollen) is a risk factor for allergic rhinitis, but in most people is not a risk factor for asthma.

Many patients report that symptoms occur almost immediately on exposure. However, in controlled-challenge exposures, both upper and lower respiratory symptoms rarely become clinically significant before 15 to 30 minutes of exposure. In situations in which allergen exposure is low or sensitivity is mild, symptoms may not develop until there have been many days of exposure.

Diagnosis

As with any allergic disease, definitive diagnosis of the offending allergen is a key step in designing a treatment plan. Patient histories of allergic symptoms can be difficult to interpret. In patients experiencing acute symptoms with every visit to a home with a cat, the history may be all that is needed to substantiate a diagnosis. In patients with chronic year-round symptoms, diagnosis is more challenging. Mold, house-dust allergen, and seasonal pollen allergy may complicate the diagnosis. The existence of an allergic threshold also must be considered; people with cat allergy may be more tolerant of symptoms when they are not being challenged by multiple allergens—for example, pollens. Physicians also must consider whether or not historical information is being distorted. In some people, denial is an issue when a beloved pet is involved. Equally important, but hopefully uncommon, is the possibility that some people "embellish" or fabricate clinical symptoms with the purpose of forcing the removal of someone else's pet cat.

The most common diagnostic test is the demonstration of allergen-specific IgE, by either skin testing or in vitro tests.[24] As in animals, there is always the possibility of false-negative and false-positive reactions. The major difficulty with skin testing and in vitro testing, is the quality and standardization of *Fel d 1*. In general, most people with negative skin tests are unlikely to have a positive challenge test, and most people with a positive skin test will react in a 1-hour challenge test.

Challenge testing is becoming less of a research tool and more of a diagnostic tool. Challenge studies may be performed via bronchial, nasal, or conjunctivival provocation, and have been shown to correlate with skin test and in vitro test results.[24] Specially designed challenge rooms, where air flow and cat allergen concentrations can be measured, are being used increasingly as research tools.[25] The major advantage of these rooms is that they can be designed to mimic natural exposure; these rooms are commonly referred to as *cat rooms*, and are furnished with bedroom or living-room furniture. One or more cats are allowed to roam freely in the room with the subject while investigators monitor the development of symptoms and correlate them with airborne exposure concentrations. These challenge-room studies are particularly helpful in treatment trials.

Trials of avoidance also are commonly recommended. These are done by carefully monitoring symptoms on extended vacations or after removal of the cat from the home. There are several disadvantages to avoidance trials. First, if it is done during an extended vacation, the issue of geographic location and its impact on symptoms must be considered. Second, it may take up to 4 to 6 months before allergen concentrations will be reduced significantly in some homes, and in some instances, even this may not be enough. (Given the persistence of cat dander in the environment, individual claims of significant relief after immediate removal of the cat from the home seem somewhat suspect.) The best avoidance trial is to remove the affected individual from the home for an extended period of time and observe whether or not there is a change in symptoms, particularly on return to the home with the cat.[24] Obviously, this is not always possible.

Management

Once a definitive diagnosis of cat allergy has been made, several treatment options are available. Avoidance of any offending allergen is the optimum treatment, but in many situations, this is not possible. Medical management is the second line of treatment, and often is effective. If medical management is not sufficient, immunotherapy is a treatment option. It is important that owners and clinicians understand that it is *not* the responsibility of the veterinarian to recommend or endorse medical treatments for allergic cat owners.

Pharmacologic Treatment of Symptoms

Symptomatic relief of allergic rhinitis involves the use of antihistamines, decongestants, nasal cromolyn, and intranasal glucocorticoids.[24] Symptomatic relief of asthma involves the use of beta-adrenergic agents, cromolyn, and glucocorticoids. These drugs are useful for managing asthmatic attacks, but are not very effective unless used in combination with environmental controls to reduce allergen exposure.

Immunotherapy

Several studies in the literature document the benefit of immunotherapy as a supplemental therapy to manage cat allergy in people, and these have been summarized in a review article.[24] The consensus among the studies is that immunotherapy is efficacious; reactivity as determined by skin tests, inhalation challenge, and conjunctival challenge was reduced by immunotherapy in most studies.[24] It is important to note that it generally is recommended that people undergoing immunotherapy avoid contact with cats. Exposure to 2000 ng/g of cat allergen in settled dust may be associated with clinical symptoms. Concentrations of cat allergen in homes with cats usually are above 50,000 ng/g, and commonly reach 200,000 ng/g.[24] Therefore, the concern is that patients living with pets may be challenged too far above the threshold of response to show any significant benefit from immunotherapy. In a placebo-controlled, double-blinded study conducted in the United Kingdom, immunotherapy provided protection against simulated natural exposure to cats as well as improvement in provocation test thresholds.[26] What was unique in this study was the fact that test groups involved patients who owned cats and those who did not. This suggests that for people unable to avoid exposure to cats, immunotherapy is effective as a supplemental therapy. The general consensus is that immunotherapy alone is only partially effective in modifying clinical signs in people with cat allergy.

Standard immunotherapy involves the administration of increasing doses of *Fel d 1* on a weekly or biweekly basis until a maintenance dose is achieved. The maintenance dose is the highest dose that can be tolerated by the patient. This can take weeks or months. Although there are a variety of protocols, none has proved superior in clinical trials. Oral immunotherapy has not been shown to be effective.[27]

Although successful in modifying the symptoms of cat allergy, compliance by patients is difficult.[28] Part of the reason is cost. Immunotherapy for cat allergy is paid for inconsistently by health insurance. Another major reason for noncompliance is the inconvenience of having to obtain weekly injections at an allergist's office, coupled with a required 30 to 60 minute in-office waiting period postinjection. Unlike the situation in veterinary medicine, in-home administration of allergen is discouraged or not allowed by human allergists. Conversely, patients with cat allergy–induced asthma were found in one study to be the most compliant.[28] One explanation for this is that patients perceived this condition to be more life-threatening, and therefore the treatment was less of an "inconvenience."

◆ COMMENTS REGARDING REMOVAL OF THE CAT

One of the first recommendations for the management of cat allergy is avoidance. From an allergist's perspective, this is a practical recommendation. Avoidance allows for the possibility that the patient may be able to avoid medication or immunotherapy, or at least need less pharmacologic therapy.

In almost all situations, the issue of whether or not to remove the family cat is an emotional one. Except in the case of a child, the decision ultimately is up to the person suffering with the symptoms. In situations in which clinical symptoms are mild, substantial relief may be possible via medications and/or immunotherapy. In addition, the use of some environmental control measures also may augment relief (see later). However, in situations in which exposure is life-threatening or detrimental, there may be no other option.

If the patient is a child, parents need to consider other factors too. Symptoms may be mild and managed with medication, but at what cost? Patients with allergic rhinitis report sleep loss, decreased concentration, and decreased social interaction. Children with allergic rhinitis experience learning impairment because they are absent from school or are fatigued, irritable, or distracted by their symptoms or medications. In addition, there is increasing evidence that chronic asthma and medications can affect sleep, cognition, and learning in school.[29] In the case of children with asthma, it simply may not be possible to keep a pet cat. Wood and Eggleston[24] have stated that "the refusal to remove a pet from the home of a child with severe asthma and documented sensitivity to that pet is tantamount to child abuse." When you consider the best interest of the child, it is difficult to argue with this position.

◆ KEY POINTS ABOUT ENVIRONMENTAL CAT ALLERGEN

- *Fel d 1* is very small (2.5 μm), and is airborne in an undisturbed room.[30] This means that cat allergen is carried on air currents throughout the home. It also can be carried on dust particles. In contrast, house-dust-mite allergen is relatively large (>10 μm in size), and is airborne only when the air is disturbed during dusting, vacuuming, changing linens, and so on, and settles very quickly in an undisturbed room.
- Because cat allergen is so small and so easily dispersed, it is widely prevalent in the environment. Airborne and dust concentrations have been detected in homes and in mattresses where cats have never lived or in newly constructed homes.[31] These concentrations may be clinically significant and capable of sensitizing people.[32] It is believed that cat allergen is carried into these homes by visitors exposed to cats and also may be transmitted via airborne route.
- Upholstered furniture, carpets, curtains, and places where cats sleep are important reservoirs of allergens. The clothing of cat owners also is a reservoir of cat allergen.

- The home is not the only source of exposure to cat allergen. Studies have shown that cat and dog allergen, in clinically significant amounts, is present in schools.[33, 34] In one recent study in Sweden, pet allergens were found to be carried into schools on the clothing of children who owned pets. Cat allergen was even found in the hair samples of children owning cats. In another study, the concentration of dog and cat allergen in settled dust was significantly higher in school classrooms than in homes of families that did not keep pets.[33] Thus, children with asthma and other allergic diseases will be exposed to cat allergen at school by contact with pet owners, even if they avoid pets at home.[34]
- In another study, cat allergen was found to be present in higher concentrations in dust from living rooms than from bedrooms, kitchens, and bathrooms. Levels were higher in homes with poor ventilation and in homes with wall-to-wall carpeting. Higher concentrations of airborne allergen were present in homes with high humidity (relative humidity greater than 45 per cent).[35]
- Cat allergen also may be brought into the home via factory purchases of new furniture. In one study, 15 of 17 new factory-made mattresses were found to contain detectable levels of cat allergen. The longer the mattress was on display, the greater the concentration of cat allergen. Again, the dispersal of cat allergen into the environment can occur via direct and indirect contact with pets and pet owners. High levels of allergen can accumulate, particularly in public places, in a relatively short period of time.[36]

◆ STRATEGIES FOR MANAGING CAT ALLERGY WITH THE CAT IN SITU

Approximately one-third of people with cat allergy live with 1 or more cats.[37] The ability to do so depends on finding a tolerable balance between exposure to major cat allergens and clinical symptoms. The following is a list of suggestions on how to reduce the concentration of cat allergens in house dust or to decrease exposure when interacting with the cat. This information was compiled from reviews of human literature, interviews with clients and veterinarians with cat allergy who live with cats, and my own personal experience with cat allergy. In as many situations as possible, I have suggested practical applications from clinical research studies. It is important to remember that no one "practice" or "treatment" will be uniformly beneficial. The strategies adapted will depend greatly on how symptomatic the cat owner is and how much she or he can tolerate. These suggestions are targeted at limiting direct exposure to cat allergen during play and/or limiting allergen concentrations in the home.

Minimizing Exposure to Cat Allergen During Play or Casual Contact

- *Change clothes after playing with the cat.* Cat dander will adhere to clothing. This is obvious to anyone who owns a cat; cat hair on one's clothes comes with cat ownership. The problem is that cat allergen on clothing can serve as a source of exposure at a later time, particularly if the clothing is not washed immediately. Cat dander also can be "shed" from clothing and contaminate living areas or other public areas where no cats live. Changing clothes after playing with your cat is not always practical or feasible. However, wearing a robe over one's clothing is a simple alternative. Inexpensive, "one-size-fits-all," men's robes are ideal for this. They are large enough to fit comfortably over regular clothing and durable enough to be washed regularly. Cotton-polyester blends are most suitable because cat hairs do not get trapped in the fibers very easily. It may not be possible to change into and out of a robe all day long, but changing clothes or wearing a robe is a reasonable suggestion when you can anticipate times when your cat is going to be on or near your body. In other words, during "cat-lounging" periods such as sitting on your lap when you are reading or watching television.
- *Wash hands after playing with the cat.* Petting your cat is going to result in cat allergen being deposited on your hands. The major source of cat allergen appears to be the skin, particularly the sebaceous glands.[11–14, 17] When concentrations of cat allergen were measured from various areas on the cat's body, the largest amount of cat allergen was found on the dorsal scapular area. Large concentrations of cat allergen also are found in cat anal sac secretions. Cats have large concentrations of sebaceous glands on their face, dorsal back, and proximal one-third of the dorsal tail. Interestingly, these are the areas that are petted most frequently by owners and the areas that cats rub on their owners. Cat allergen is soluble in water. Washing your hands with soap and water is an easy way to remove cat allergen from your hands.
- *Develop a petting or play routine that minimizes contact with areas of large concentrations of sebaceous glands.* The largest concentration of sebaceous glands on a cat is on the face and under the chin, dorsal back, and dorsal tail area. Investigators measuring shed cat allergen did not sample the skin from the face or chin of cats, but had they done so, it is highly likely that these areas would have shed more allergen than other areas they measured. The lowest concentration of cat allergen was on the hair of the ventral abdomen. It is difficult to not want to pet a cat's chin or face or to avoid contact with these areas. The face and chin areas are often rubbed on owners and on other objects of adoration or for territory marking.
- *Wear a face mask.* Inhalation of cat allergen is a major source of exposure. Wearing a face mask when playing with the cat or brushing it will help minimize the inhalation of *Fel d 1*. The face mask should be able to filter out particles less than 2 μg. Surgical masks do not provide adequate protection, but other masks do. Protective masks that filter allergens can be purchased at any store that sells protective masks for industry. Also check hardware stores.
- *Wear protective eyewear.* Eyewear that prevents direct exposure of the conjunctiva to cat allergen may help prevent or minimize the allergic conjunctivitis associated with cat exposure. "Wraparound" sunglasses and protective eyewear for wood-working purchased from hardware stores are options. It also is important to remember *not* to touch your face and eyes until after washing your hands.

Restricting Where the Cat Lives

- *Keep the cat outdoors.* This is a common suggestion from the medical community; however, it is not one that I strongly endorse. In some situations, making the family cat an outdoor cat is a option. Realistically, this is not a solution many cat owners favor, particularly if the cat has been an indoor pet. Any cat living outdoors is at risk for exposure to disease, injury from motor vehicles, attacks from other animals, getting lost or stolen, getting poisoned, or being tormented or tortured by ill-meaning people, and is at the mercy of the weather, just to name a few factors. In addition, outdoor cats have a significantly negative impact on wildlife, even in cities and suburbs. Finally, in many communities, it is illegal to allow cats to roam unsupervised.
- *Limit the cat to a single area of the house.* In some homes, it may be possible to restrict the cat to a limited area of the house. Ideally, this area would be one that is well ventilated and easy to clean. One option would be to create a "cat room" without carpeting, painted with semigloss or glossy paint to allow for easy cleaning, and free of furnishings that will act as dust mops for cat allergen. The rooms can be furnished with plastic patio furniture during visits because this furniture is comfortable and easy to clean. Cat furniture is easy to find. Cat trees can be made easily from logs or tree branches, and paper bags and boxes are wonderful hiding places and can be disposed of rather than cleaned. This suggestion may seem a bit "luxurious" because most people do not have spare rooms. However, I have been amazed at the spare space that can be found when re-homing, euthanizing, and having the cat live outdoors are the only other viable op-

tions. The issue of humane treatment is always a question that I encounter from clients when I suggest a cat room. However, if clients actually consider the amount of direct "quality" time they have with their cat on a day-to-day basis, spending 30 to 60 minutes with them in their cat room is acceptable. Alternatively, in my own home, I allow the cats free roam, and I have a "cat-free room" as a personal sanctuary.

Ideally, the room should be cleaned by someone other than the patient. The furniture should be dusted first and then the floor, and the furnishings vacuumed *before* surfaces are wet-washed. Ventilation to this room should be increased. The use of in-room HEPA (high-efficiency particulate air cleaner) filter air cleaners is debatable.[38] One study found that the levels of airborne *Fel d 1* were significantly reduced when a HEPA air filter was used in the bedroom; however, the study failed to show any correlation to clinical improvement. The investigators did comment that one of the reasons for lack of clinical improvement in symptoms may have been that the study group included severely affected people.[38]

* *Keep the cat out of the bedroom.* This is an almost universal recommendation by allergists. Disturbed sleep is a common problem in people with allergic diseases. Anecdotally, almost all the people with cat allergy said this was a very helpful suggestion.

Making the Cat Less "Allergic"

* *Removal of allergen from the cat.* There is increasing evidence to suggest that the *Fel d 1* has a biologic function in cats. The widespread distribution on the skin and its association with skin lipids suggest some role in regulation of the epidermis. The results of studies on bathing and the removal of cat allergen have been mixed.[39] Some investigators found no significant benefit.[40] One study did document the value of washing cats, and found that it did decrease airborne *Fel d 1*.[17] Whether or not this reduction is associated with any decrease in clinical symptoms is still under debate. However, anecdotal reports from cat owners suggest that for some people, bathing their cat does diminish their symptoms.

Controlled studies have shown that bathing needs to be done at least once a week. The largest amounts of allergen were removed when the cat was immersed in tap water for at least 3 minutes.[17] There have been no controlled studies comparing the efficacy of various shampoos on the removal of cat allergen from the coat. Based on clinical experience with dogs, antiseborrheic shampoos will remove more oils from skin than hypoallergenic cleansing shampoos or plain water. It is reasonable to specu-

late that if cats were washed in mild antiseborrheic shampoos (labeled for use in cats), more cat allergen would be removed. Suggestions:

* Bathe the cat 2 to 3 times per week. None of the published studies bathed cats more than once a week. Given the recent evidence that this allergen is produced in the skin and sebaceous glands, more frequent bathing may be the key to decreasing allergen shedding to tolerable levels.
* Immerse the cat for 3 minutes in water; this time-length was found to be associated with greater removal of allergen. This can be done in a small plastic tub in a kitchen sink. I instruct owners to use the same technique and precautions they would for bathing an infant and do everything possible to *not* make it a frightening experience. Contrary to popular belief, most cats can be acclimated to routine bathing.
* Plain water may be used. Or if desired, use a gentle hypoallergenic shampoo no more than once or twice a week. Predilute the shampoo 1:4 in water before applying it to the hair coat. This will make it easier to rinse the hair coat. The hair coat should be rinsed until it no longer lathers and/or the hair coat "squeaks."
* Wiping a cat with a wet cloth has been advocated as an alternative to bathing the cat. In controlled studies, significant concentrations of allergen were not removed[17]; however, many of my cat-allergic owners report that this is beneficial.
* *Allerpet/c.* There is a commercial product (Allerpet/c, Allerpet, Inc., New York, NY) marketed widely to remove cat allergen from the hair coat and other surfaces; however, its efficacy in controlled studies was questionable.[40] One controlled study found that wiping the cat with this product was no more efficacious than wiping the cat with a dry cloth.[41]
* *Acepromazine.* The lay literature has advocated the use of acepromazine to reduce the shedding of cat allergen. *Research studies have documented conclusively that the use of acepromazine is ineffective as a means to reduce the shedding of cat allergen.*[40]

Changes in Home Furnishings

* *Flooring.* Cat allergen concentrates in rugs, wall-to-wall carpeting, upholstery, and other fabrics. It is very difficult, if not impossible, to remove cat allergen from carpeting. Therefore, it is best to remove carpeting and rugs. Hardwood or vinyl floors are recommended. One company (Allergy Control Products, Inc., Ridgefield, CT) markets a spray that is applied to the carpet before cleaning. It supposedly denatures cat allergen.

- *Furniture.* Furniture that can be wiped and cleaned easily will collect less cat allergen. If possible, furniture should be upholstered in material that can be cleaned easily, for example, leather or equivalent. Small pillows, afghans, and the like should be laundered frequently.
- *Window treatments.* Draperies should be avoided for exactly the same reason as rugs and upholstered furniture—the cat allergen will collect in these materials. Blinds or window shades that can be wiped off and cleaned are an option. Small slatted blinds (i.e., "Venetian" blinds) will collect large amounts of cat allergen. These blinds are very difficult to clean thoroughly. Plastic blinds can be washed at home; there also are commercial companies that specialize in cleaning these blinds.
- *Knick knacks.* Decorative objects that need dusting, are difficult to clean, or collect cat hair are best removed from the home. Curio pieces that cannot be parted with should be kept behind glass doors to minimize their dust-catching potential. Artwork will need to be cleaned and dusted on a regular basis. Wall hangings made of fabric would not be a good decorating choice for someone with cat allergy.

Ventilation Changes in the Home

- *Ventilation.* Many new homes are very "airtight," and there is very little air circulation. House dust and cat allergen concentrations were found to be higher in newer homes with less air circulation, particularly in the winter. Cat allergen is airborne, and the easiest method to increase ventilation in the home and increase air changes per room is to open the windows and increase cross-circulation in the home.
- *Air vents.* Heating and cooling air ducts in the home collect large amounts of dust and dirt. Heat and air conditioning airflow will disperse dusts and particulate matter in the home. These vents should be cleaned on a regular basis; there are commercial companies that clean air vents. Small, disposable, cut-to-fit, air-vent filters are available to help filter out particulate material. These fit inside the air vent grate, and are very cosmetic. Care should be taken to purchase products that filter out particles smaller than 10 μm in diameter.
- *Furnace filters.* Furnace filters should be changed regularly. Once a month is the usual recommendation by companies that manufacture heating and cooling units. During the heating season, furnace filters should be changed 1 to 2 times per month. Disposable furnace filters are recommended. Washable furnace filters are available; however, these are difficult to clean thoroughly.

Allergy Control Products, Inc., specializes in products to help control indoor environmental allergens, and may be a resource for cat owners (1–800–422–DUST).

Clothing and Laundry

- *Clothing and laundry.* Clothing can be a reservoir source in the home for cat allergen. In one study, investigators found that the winter clothing of patients with a cat contained a higher level of allergen than the clothes of patients without pets.[42] In a follow-up study, this group of investigators went on to investigate the effect of washing clothes on cat allergen concentrations. In that study, 22 pieces of cotton fabric were put in the baskets of 22 cats for 1 week. Owners of the cats rotated the cotton to ensure that it was evenly exposed to the napping cats. Investigators found significant concentrations of *Fel d 1* prewashing, and found no appreciable amount of allergen postwashing.[43]

  It is important to note that the fabric used in this study was a tightly woven cotton fabric. This type of material washes easily, and animal hairs do not get caught in the fibers. Removal of allergen may not be similar between various fabrics, particularly loosely woven fibers or fibers in which cat hairs can get embedded. This study suggests that clothing and household furnishings that do not "trap" cat hair and are washable may be beneficial. Another important thing to note in this study is the washing method. These investigators used only plain water. It seems reasonable to assume that the use of a laundry detergent and washing machine will enhance the removal of cat allergen.

Bedroom

- *Bedroom.* The bedroom can be modified and the environment manipulated to minimize a cat-allergic person's exposure to cat allergen. Quite simply, the "cleanest" room is one that is rather Spartan in appearance. The goal is to create a cat-free sleeping environment that can be kept dust-free. Routine weekly cleaning is recommended. Suggestions:
  - Keep the cat out of the bedroom.
  - Remove carpeting and area rugs and replace with vinyl or hardwood floors.
  - Remove drapes and slatted horizontal blinds and replace with shades or vertical blinds that are easier to clean.
  - Paint the walls with a high-quality semigloss paint to make these surfaces easier to clean.
  - Furnish the room with wood furniture; remove any upholstered furniture that may trap dust and cat hair.

◆ Use bed linens made of a tightly woven, machine-washable fabric. This includes sheets, pillow cases, blankets, and comforters.

◆ Do not use decorative pillows on the bed.

◆ Use a mattress and pillow cover designed to keep dust-mite antigen away from allergic patients. These are available commercially from a wide range of companies including Allergy Control Products, Inc. (Ridgefield, CT). This bedding is made of a tightly woven fabric that is machine-washable. The fiber weave allows for air to circulate, but is an effective allergen-proof barrier. These are highly recommended for people with house dust allergy. The pillow cover goes over the pillow and beneath the pillow case. The mattress covers encase the box springs and mattress. The smallest available fabric weave should be used (<4 μm in diameter) because pore size will enlarge with repeated washing.

◆ Wash bed linens weekly.

◆ Increase ventilation in the room. Consider using a HEPA air cleaner. These are most effective after aggressive cleaning of the floor with a HEPA vacuum cleaner.[39]

◆ Keep closet doors closed to minimize exposure to cat allergen on clothing.

◆ Do not keep dirty laundry in the bedroom because this may be a source of allergen exposure or contamination.

Cleaning Procedures

◆ It is important to note that any cleaning procedure will stir up dust and increase *Fel d 1* in the air. If the person doing the cleaning is allergic to cats, that person should wear a mask and/or goggles. Vacuuming should be done before wet cleaning of surfaces.

◆ Walls, windows, and doorway ledges: Any area that collects dust will need to be vacuumed on a weekly or every-other-week basis.

◆ Airborne allergen will collect on the surface of walls. Walls should be cleaned regularly by vacuuming or washing.

◆ Use a high-efficiency filter vacuum cleaner (HEPA). Many of these are available, although very expensive. Water-trapping vacuums can actually produce allergen-containing aerosols. Make sure the hose connections are tight, and change the vacuum cleaner bag biweekly. If possible, use a vacuum system that sends exhaust to the outside of the house through wall-mounted valves (central vacuum units).

◆ Air ducts and vents should be cleaned on a yearly basis by a commercial company.

◆ SUMMARY

Cat allergen is one of the most common environmental allergens of people. The source of major cat allergen *Fel d 1* is the skin. The allergen is ubiquitous in the environment because it can be carried mechanically on the clothes by cat owners. Depending on individual circumstances and severity of clinical signs, it is often possible for cat-allergic clients to keep their cat. However, this will require some compromises and lifestyle changes for both the owner and the cat. The role of the veterinarian is to provide information to clients on how to make some of these changes, particularly those involving the cat. Veterinarians and physicians need to work together increasingly with cat-allergic clients to ensure the best quality of life for both the cat and the owner.

REFERENCES

1. Murray AB, Ferguson AC, Morrison BJ: The frequency and severity of cat allergy vs dog allergy in atopic children. J Allergy Clin Immunol 72:145–149, 1983.
2. Gergen PJ, Turkeltaub PC, Kovar MG: The prevalence of allergic skin test reactivity to eight common aeroallergens in the US population: Results from the second National Health and Nutrition Examination Survey. J Allergy Clin Immunol 80:669–679, 1987.
3. Pollart SM, Chapman MD, Fiocco GP, et al: Epidemiology of acute asthma: IgE antibodies to common inhalant allergens as a risk factor for emergency room visits. J Allergy Clin Immunol 83:875–882, 1989.
4. DeBlay F, Chapman MD, Platts-Mills TAE: Airborne cat allergen (*Fel d 1*). Am Rev Respir Dis 143:1334–1339, 1991.
5. Ohman JL, Lowell FC, Bloch KJ: Allergens of mammalian origin. I. J Allergy Clin Immunol 52:231, 1973.
6. Ohman JL, Lowell FC, Bloch KJ, et al: Allergens of mammalian origin. III. Properties of a major feline allergen. J Immunol 113:1668–1677, 1974.
7. Ohman JL, Lowell FC, Bloch KJ, et al: Allergens of mammalian origin. V. Properties of extracts derived from the domestic cat. Clin Allergy 6:419–428, 1976.
8. Morgenstern JP, Griffith IJ, Brauer AW, et al: Amino acid sequence of *Fel d 1*, the major allergen of the domestic cat: Protein sequence analysis and cDNA cloning. J Allergy Clin Immunol 87:327, 1991.
9. Griffith IJ, Craig S, Pollock J, et al: Expression and genomic structure of the genes encoding FdI, the major allergen of the domestic cat. Gene 113:263–268, 1992.
10. Brown PH, Leiterman K, Ohman JL: Distribution of cat allergen 1 in cat tissues and fluids. Int Arch Allergy Appl Immunol 74:67–70, 1984.
11. Bartholome K, Kissler W, Baer H, et al: Where does cat allergen come from? J Allergy Clin Immunol 76:503–506, 1985.
12. Dabrowski A, Van der Brempt X, Soler M, et al: Cat skin as an important source of *Fel d 1* allergen. J Allergy Clin Immunol 86:462–465, 1990.
13. Charpin C, Mata P, Charpin D, et al: *Fel d 1* allergen distribution in cat fur and skin. J Allergy Clin Immunol 88:77–82, 1991.
14. DeAndrade AD, Birnbaum J, Magalon C, et al: *Fel d 1* levels in cat anal glands. Clin Exp Allergy 26:178–180, 1996.
15. Charpin C, Zielonka T, Charpin D, et al: Effects of castration and testosterone on *Fel d 1* production by sebaceous glands of male cats. II. Morphometric assessment. Clin Exp Allergy 24:1174–1178, 1994.
16. Jali-Colome J, Dornelas de Andrade A, Birnbaum J, et al: Sex differences in *Fel d 1* allergen production. J Allergy Clin Immunol 98:165–168, 1996.
17. Avner DB, Perzanowski MS, Platts-Mills TAE, et al: Evaluation of different techniques for washing cats: Quantitation of allergen removed from the cat and the effect on airborne *Fel d 1*. J Allergy Clin Immunol 100:307–312, 1997.

18. DeGroot H, van Swieten P, Aalberse RC: Evidence for a *Fel d 1*–like molecule in the "big cats" (Felidae species). J Allergy Clin Immunol 86:107–116, 1990.
19. Spitzauer S, Pandjaitan B, Muhl S, et al: Major cat and dog allergens share IgE epitopes. J Allergy Clin Immunol 99:100–105, 1997.
20. Duff AL, Platts-Mills TAE: Allergens and asthma. Pediatr Clin North Am 39:1277–1291, 1992.
21. Gergen PJ, Turkeltaub PC: The association of individual allergen reactivity with respiratory disease in a national sample: Data from the second National Health and Nutrition Examination Survey, 1976–80 (NHANES II). J Allergy Clin Immunol 90:579–588, 1992.
22. Plaut M, Zimmerman EM, Goldstein RA: Health hazards to humans associated with domestic pets. Annu Rev Public Health 17:221–245, 1996.
23. Benson V, Marano MA: Current estimates from the National Health Interview Survey. Vital Health Statistics—Series 10. Data from National Health Survey 189:1–269, 1994.
24. Wood RA, Eggleston PA: Management of allergy to animal danders. Immunol All Clin North Am 12:69–84, 1992.
25. Scherer SH, Wood RA, Eggleston PA: Determinants of airway responsiveness to cat allergen: Comparison of environmental challenge to quantitative nasal and bronchial allergen challenge. J Allergy Clin Immunol 99:798–805, 1997.
26. Varney VA, Edwards J, Tabbah K, et al: Clinical efficacy of specific immunotherapy to cat dander: A double-blind placebo-controlled trial. Clin Exp Allergy 27:860–867, 1997.
27. Oppenheimer J, Areson JG, Nelson HS: Safety and efficacy of oral immunotherapy with standardized cat extract. J Allergy Clin Immunol 93:61–67, 1994.
28. Cohn JR, Pizzi A: Determinants of patient compliance with allergen immunotherapy. J Allergy Clin Immunol 91:734–737, 1993.
29. Simons EFR: Learning impairment and allergic rhinitis. Allergy Asthma Proc 17:185–189, 1996.
30. Luczynska CM, Li Y, Chapman MD, et al: Airborne concentrations and particle size distribution of allergen derived from domestic cats (*Felis domesticus*): Measurements using a cascade impactor, liquid impinger, and a two site monoclonal antibody assay for *Fel d 1*. Am Rev Respir Dis 141:361–367, 1990.
31. Quirce S, Dimich-Ward H, Chan H, et al: Major cat allergen (*Fel d 1*) levels in the homes of patients with asthma and their relationship to sensitization to cat dander. Ann Allergy, Asthma, Immunol 75:325–330, 1995.
32. Bollinger ME, Eggleston PA, Flanagan E, et al: Cat antigen in homes with and without cats may induce allergic symptoms. J Allergy Clin Immunol 97:907–914, 1996.
33. Dybendal T, Elsayed S: Dust from carpeted and smooth floors: Allergens in homes compared with those in schools in Norway. 49:210–216, 1994.
34. Berge M, Munir AK, Dreborg S: Concentrations of cat (*Fel d 1*), dog (*Can f 1*) and mite (*Der f 1* and *Der p 1*) allergens in the clothing and school environment of Swedish school children with and without pets at home. Pediatr Allerg Immunol 9:25–30, 1998.
35. Munir AKM, Bjorksten B, Einarsson R, et al: Cat (*Fel d 1*), dog (*Can f 1*) and cockroach allergens in homes of asthmatic children from three climatic zones in Sweden. Allergy 49:508–516, 1994.
36. Egmar AC, Almqvist C, Lilja EG, et al: Deposition of cat (*Fel d 1*), dog (*Can f 1*), and horse allergen over time in public environments—A model of dispersion. Allergy 53:957–961, 1998.
37. Hayden ML: Environmental control and the management of allergic diseases. Immunol Allergy Clin North Am 19:83–99, 1999.
38. Wood RA, Johnson EF, Van Natta ML, et al: A placebo-controlled trial of a HEPA air cleaner in the treatment of cat allergy. Am J Respir Crit Care Med 158:115–120, 1998.
39. DeBlay F, Chapman MD, Platts-Mills TAE: Airborne cat allergen (*Fel d 1*): Environmental control with the cat in situ. Am Rev Respir Dis 143:1334–1399, 1991.
40. Klucka CV, Ownby DR, Green J, et al: Cat shedding of *Fel d 1* is not reduced by washings, Allerpet-C spray, or acepromazine. J Allergy Clin Immunol 1164–1167, 1995.
41. Perzanowski MS, Wheatley LM, Avner DB, et al: The effectiveness of Allerpet/c in reducing the cat allergen *Fel d 1*. J Allergy Clin Immunol 100:428–430, 1997.
42. D'Amato G, Liccardi G, Fusso M, et al: Clothing as a carrier of cat allergen. J Allergy Clin Immunol 99:577–578, 1997.
43. Liccaardi G, Russo M, Barber D, et al: Washing the clothes of cat owners is a simple method to prevent cat allergen dispersal. J Allergy Clin Immunol 102:143–144, 1998.

Cardiology and Respiratory Disorders

Matthew W. Miller, Editor

◆ Echocardiography 245
◆ Heartworm Disease 253
◆ Hypertrophic Cardiomyopathy 261
◆ Chylothorax 267
◆ Systemic Hypertension 277
◆ Respiratory Therapeutics 283
◆ Holter Monitoring 291
◆ Aortic Thromboembolism 299

Still-Current Information Found in Consultations in Feline Internal Medicine 2:
Hypertrophic Cardiomyopathy (Chapter 34), p. 255
Diagnosis and Management of Dirofilariasis (Chapter 35), p. 267
Pleural Effusion: Physical, Biochemical, and Cytological Characteristics (Chapter 38), p. 287
Chylothorax: Diagnosis and Management (Chapter 39), p. 297
Rational Approaches to the Management of Bronchopulmonary Disease (Chapter 40), p. 309

Still-Current Information Found in Consultations in Feline Internal Medicine 3:
Endocrine Hypertension (Chapter 23), p. 163
Thoracic Radiology (Chapter 33), p. 249
Thyrotoxic Heart Disease (Chapter 36), p. 279
Restrictive Cardiomyopathy (Chapter 37), p. 286
Pulmonary Diagnostics (Chapter 38), p. 292
Bronchial Disease (Chapter 39), p. 303
Blood Pressure: Population Aspects (Chapter 78), p. 630

Elsewhere in Consultations in Feline Internal Medicine 4:
Update on the Diagnosis and Management of Feline Herpesvirus-1 Infections (Chapter 7), p. 51
Clinical Approach to Chronic Diarrhea (Chapter 16), p. 127
Diagnosis of Occult Hyperthyroidism (Chapter 18), p. 145
Complications of Therapy for Hyperthyroidism (Chapter 19), p. 151
Mosquito-Bite Hypersensitivity (Chapter 24), p. 186
Diagnosis and Treatment of Systemic Hypertension (Chapter 47), p. 365
Vascular Disorders (Chapter 52), p. 405
Evaluation and Treatment of Cranial Mediastinal Masses (Chapter 68), p. 533

32

◆ Echocardiography

Matthew W. Miller

Echocardiography is widely used for the diagnosis and management of congenital and acquired cardiac diseases. Whereas a number of different echocardiographic formats are used in clinical practice, each involves reflection of ultrasound from cardiovascular tissues, specialized processing of returned (echoed) signals, and the ultimate display of this information in some recognizable visual or auditory format. Echocardiography has become increasingly sophisticated, and the combined modalities have largely replaced cardiac catheterization and angiocardiography for diagnosis and assessment of cardiac lesions. Although the newest technologies are expensive and limited to referral hospitals and clinics, many practicing veterinarians use, or will soon acquire, echocardiographs. Furthermore, veterinarians who are not yet performing echocardiographic studies often find referral for echocardiography helpful or even essential for establishing a cardiac diagnosis, assessing ventricular function, determining a prognosis, and guiding medical or surgical therapy.

The echocardiographic examination must be placed within a proper clinical perspective. Echocardiography is not a substitute for a careful clinical examination. Cardiac auscultation is still a most cost-effective and expedient examination for identifying serious heart diseases. Echocardiography should be performed, and echocardiograms are best interpreted, by clinicians who understand the pertinent issues and questions regarding specific cardiovascular diseases. Furthermore, a clinician capable of integrating information from all various sources, including the history and physical examination, should direct the clinical assessment and prescribe the treatment plan. These decisions should not be abdicated to any sonographer, unless that individual has a full understanding of the entire clinical situation and has examined the patient physically.

The veterinarian should appreciate the advantages and limitations of an echocardiographic study. A complete echocardiographic study should (1) reveal the pertinent congenital or acquired anatomic lesions (morphologic diagnosis); (2) estimate cardiac chamber size (dilatation and hypertrophy); (3) quantify ventricular systolic function; (4) estimate ventricular diastolic function; (5) evaluate blood flow and valvular function; and (6) assess hemodynamic burden using a variety of imaging and Doppler methods. Properly gathered and interpreted, this information should lead to a definitive cardiac diagnosis and illustrate the hemodynamic consequences of structural and functional cardiac lesions.

◆ IMAGING FORMATS

Two-Dimensional Echocardiography

The most frequently performed and easiest to understand study produces a 2-dimensional echocardiogram (2-DE), which is also called a B-mode (for brightness mode) study or sector scan. These images are the consequence of numerous adjacent lines of B-mode ultrasound. These lines are composed at extraordinary speed to form a slice-of-pie-shaped image displayed within hundreds of "dots" of varying shades of gray, and subsequently displayed in the pixels of the video screen. By updating the image frame—usually at rates between 30 to 60 frames per second—cardiac motion can be appreciated. Newer digital echocardiographs can generate extraordinary frame rates exceeding 150 frames per second. These 2-DE studies typically are viewed in "real time" and are recorded simultaneously onto a videotape or optical disc for subsequent slow-motion replay.

The 2-DE provides substantial anatomic information and serves as the anatomic template for guiding M-mode and Doppler studies. The 2-DE examination also is useful for quantitation of cardiac size and function. Various imaging planes generally are recorded to provide sufficient anatomic detail in 3 dimensions. Image planes may be categorized as long axis (sagittal), short axis (coronal), apical (transducer positioned near the left apex), or angled (specialized or hybrid imaging planes). The specific tomograms used for any given study depend in part on the clinical situation, but most echocardiography laboratories develop standards for specific examinations.[1]

M-Mode Echocardiography

The M-mode echocardiogram is generated by a single line of B-mode ultrasound. The transducer emits a pulse of ultrasound, and then processes echoes reflected from moving cardiac tissues using a very high sampling rate. The echocardiograph updates the depth of the tissues continuously along the line of the ultrasound pulses, and displays the structures as gray-scale dots, which are spaced relative to the static transducer. By sweeping paper (or videotape) along this continuously updated output, a graph of cardiac motion is displayed, showing time (seconds; x-axis) and depth (cm; y-axis).

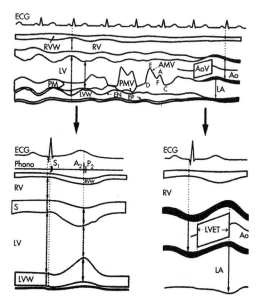

Figure 32–1. Standard electrocardiogram (ECG) M-mode image planes. *Top,* A "sweep" from the apex (left) to the base (right). A₁, Aortic portion of first heart sound; A₂, aortic portion of second heart sound; AMV, anterior mitral valve; Ao, aorta; AoV, aortic valve; EN, endocardium; EP, epicardium; LA, left atrium; LV, left ventricular lumen; LVET, left ventricular ejection time; LVW, left ventricular free wall; P₂, pulmonic portion of second heart sound; Phono, phonocardiogram; PM, papillary muscle; PMV, posterior mitral valve; RV, right ventricular lumen; RVW, right ventricular freewall; S₁, first heart sound. *Bottom,* Expanded versions of *top* images.

Standard M-mode studies of the left ventricle include those recorded between the tips of the ventricular papillary muscles, at the level of the chordae tendineae, across the peak diastolic excursion of the cranioventral (anterior) mitral valve leaflet, and through the aortic valves and left atrium (Fig. 32–1). M-mode studies must be recorded with care to avoid angulation errors and erroneous measures.[2, 3] Recordings should be guided by the 2-DE long- and short-axis images.

Interpretation of the M-mode study requires a preconceived knowledge of normal M-mode echocardiogram images and of cardiac motion at different levels of the heart. Although it is not difficult to comprehend, the graphic nature of this format, and the lack of easily recognizable anatomic landmarks, has diminished its importance. The M-mode study of the left ventricle and the calculation of left ventricular shortening fraction remain a standard for assessing global left ventricular systolic function. However, the clinician should not rely on a single dimensional measure or function index without considering qualifying conditions such as species, breed, body weight, use of tranquilizers, heart rhythm, volume status, mitral valve competency, and global function of the ventricles as seen in 2-DE. These factors must be studied and appreciated to prevent misinterpretation of M-mode–derived values.

The M-mode echocardiogram is useful for quantifying cardiac wall thickness, ventricular luminal size, and left ventricular function. M-mode studies may be combined with contrast echocardiography or color-coded Doppler to detect and time flow events accurately. This modality also is capable of recording high-frequency motion, as with a fluttering valve, which might be missed by the slower sampling rate of a 2-DE study. Normal values for

Table 32–1. Normal Feline Echocardiographic Values*

| Measurement | Source | | | | |
	A (n = 11)	B (n = 25)	C (n = 30)	D† (n = 30)	E† (n = 16)
LVIDd (mm)	15.1 (2.1)	14.8 (2.6)	15.9 (1.9)	14.0 (1.3)	12.8 (1.7)
LVIDs (mm)	6.9 (2.2)	8.8 (2.4)	8.0 (1.4)	8.1 (1.6)	8.3 (1.5)
LVWd (mm)	4.6 (0.5)	3.7 (0.8)	3.3 (0.6)	3.5 (0.5)	3.1 (1.1)
LVWs (mm)	7.8 (1.0)	—	6.8 (0.7)	—	5.5 (8.8)
IVSd (mm)	5.0 (0.7)	4.5 (0.9)	3.1 (0.4)	3.6 (0.8)	—
IVSs (mm)	7.6 (1.2)	—	5.8 (0.6)	—	—
LA (mm)	12.1 (1.8)	7.4 (1.7)	12.3 (1.4)	10.3 (1.4)	9.8 (1.7)
Ao (mm)	9.5 (1.5)	7.5 (1.8)	9.5 (1.1)	9.4 (1.1)	9.4 (1.4)
FS (%)	55.0 (10.2)	41.0 (7.3)	49.8 (5.3)	42.7 (8.1)	34.5 (12.6)
EPSS (mm)	0.4 (0.7)	—	0.2 (0.9)	—	—
Weight (kg)	4.3 (0.5)	4.7 (1.2)	4.1 (1.1)	3.9 (1.2)	—
HR (beats/min)	182 (22)	167 (29)	194 (23)	255 (36)	—

Abbreviations: Ao, aortic root; EPSS, mitral valve E point to septal separation; FS, fractional shortening; HR, heart rate; IVSd, interventricular septum at end-diastole; IVSs, interventricular septum at end-systole; LA, left atrium (systole); LVIDd, left ventricular internal diameter at end-diastole; LVIDs, left ventricular internal diameter at end-systole; LVWd, left ventricular wall at end-diastole; LVWs, left ventricular wall at end-systole.
*Mean value given, ±SD in parenthesis below.
†Data from cats anesthetized with ketamine.
Data from *A,* Moïse NS, Dietze AE, Mezza LE, et al: Echocardiography, electrocardiography, and radiography of cats with dilatation cardiomyopathy, hypertrophic cardiomyopathy, and hyperthyroidism. Am J Vet Res 47:1476–1486, 1986. *B,* Pipers FS, Reef V, Hamlin RL: Echocardiography in the domestic cat. Am J Vet Res 40:882–886, 1979. *C,* Jacobs G, Knight DV: M-mode echocardiographic measurements in nonanesthetized healthy cats: Effects of body weight, heart rate, and other variables. Am J Vet Res 46:1705–1711, 1985. *D,* Fox PR, Bond BR, Peterson ME: Echocardiographic reference values in healthy cats sedated with ketamine hydrochloride. Am J Vet Res 46:1479–1484, 1985. *E,* Soderberg SF, Boon JA, Wingfield WE: M-Mode echocardiography as a diagnostic aid for feline cardiomyopathy. Vet Radiol 24:66–72, 1983.

M-mode measurements in cats under a variety of conditions are listed in Table 32–1.

Contrast Echocardiography

2-DE or M-mode contrast echocardiography is performed to identify abnormal blood flow. The contrast echocardiogram is produced by altering the sonographic appearance of a small portion of the blood pool through the injection of agitated (sonicated) saline or dextrose solution, iodinated contrast media, indocyanine green dye, albumin solution, or carbon dioxide. Following injection of these contrast agents into a peripheral vein, the acoustic impedance of the blood changes as microcavitations develop and act as powerful ultrasonic reflectors. The commonly used contrast agents do not pass through the pulmonary capillaries; therefore, finding echodense contrast within the left side of the heart indicates a right-to-left shunt. For example, with the tetralogy of Fallot, echodense blood can be traced along its path from the right ventricle to the left ventricular outlet.

Doppler Echocardiography

Doppler echocardiography processes returning ultrasound in order to demonstrate the direction and velocity of blood flow during the cardiac cycle.[4] This information is gained by measuring the Doppler frequency shift of returning ultrasound. A number of Doppler examinations have developed, including pulsed-wave examination, continuous-wave examination, and color-coded Doppler echocardiography. Doppler studies are especially useful for assessing heart valves, detecting abnormal blood flow, estimating hemodynamics (blood flow and intravascular pressures), and quantifying ventricular function.[5, 6]

◆ ECHOCARDIOGRAPHIC IMAGING PLANES

A number of imaging planes are used for 2-DE, M-mode, and color Doppler imaging.[7] Color Doppler imaging is often used, when available, to screen for abnormalities of blood flow and to pursue specific abnormalities based on clinical examination. Planes that align blood flow parallel with the interrogating cursor are needed for accurate spectral and continuous-wave Doppler studies (Fig. 32–2; see also Fig. 32–1).

Images From the Right Hemithorax

Examinations usually are performed with long-axis images from the right hemithorax. An intercostal

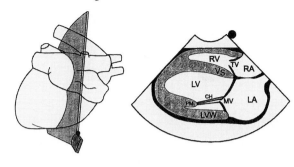

Long-Axis 4-Chamber View

Long-Axis LV Outflow View

Figure 32–2. Long-axis 4-chamber view and long-axis view that optimize for the left ventricular outflow tract. Ao, aorta; CH, chordae tendineae; LA, left atrium; LC, left coronary cusp; LV, left ventricle; LVW, left ventricular free wall; MV, mitral valve; PM, papillary muscle; RA, right atrium; RPA, right pulmonary artery; RV, right ventricle; TV, tricuspid valve; VS, interventricular septum.

(parasternal), 4-chambered, image of the atria and ventricles is recorded first. The cardiac septa, ventricular inlets, atrioventricular valves, and proximal left ventricular outlet are largely perpendicular to the axial beam in these views. Clockwise rotation of the transducer (as the clinician looks down the probe) produces an image of the aortic valve and proximal aorta. Dorsal placement increases the size and availability of the right atrium until lung interference prevents clear imaging. Color Doppler imaging can be used here. Owing to the large angle of incidence between the interrogating beam and normal blood flow in these planes, velocity is underestimated and there is little, if any, signal aliasing of normal flow. Thus, the clinician can more readily distinguish normal flow from high-velocity or turbulent flow patterns. Eccentric high-velocity flow patterns, or "jets," caused by mitral, tricuspid, or aortic valvular regurgitation or left ventricular outflow obstruction, are observed commonly in long-axis planes. Abnormal flow across atrial or ventricular septal defects also may be detected. By placing the transducer more ventrally (apical) and orienting the axial beam more dorsally, the cardiac image becomes vertical and alignment with normal flow is improved. This often yields an image similar to a true human parasternal long-axis image (see Fig. 32–2).

Different *short-axis tomograms* recorded from the right hemithorax at the level of the mitral valve and the aortic valve are then obtained. The typical

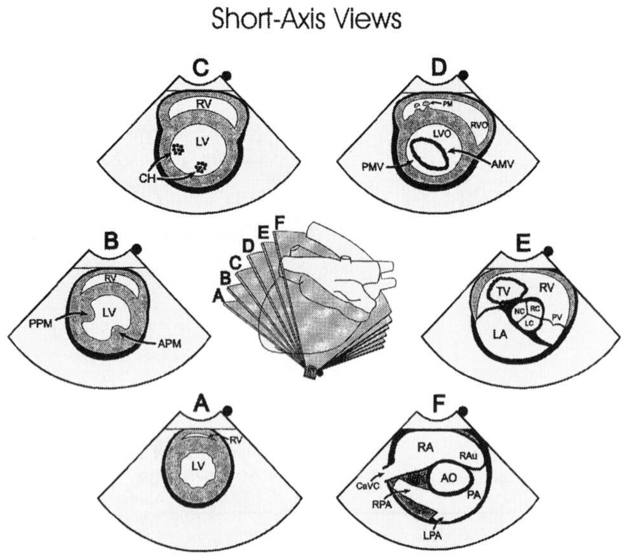

Short-Axis Views

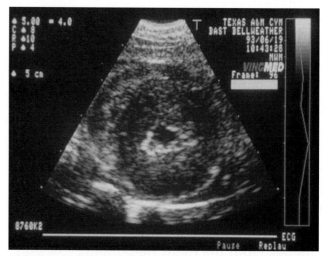

Figure 32–3. *A–F,* Short-axis echo views obtained from right hemithorax. AMV, anterior mitral valve; AO, aorta; APM, anterior papillary muscle; CaVC, caudal vena cava; CH, chordae tendineae; LA, left atrium; LC, left coronary cusp; LPA, left pulmonary artery; LVO, left ventricular outflow; LV, left ventricle; NC, noncoronary cusp; PA, pulmonary artery; PM, papillary muscle; PMV, posterior mitral valve; PPM, posterior papillary muscle; PV, pulmonary valve; RA, right atrium; RAu, right auricle; RC, right coronary cusp; RPA, right pulmonary artery; RV, right ventricle; RVO, right ventricular outflow; TV, tricuspid valve.

positions include the following: low ventricular, papillary muscle level, chordal level, mitral level, aortic/left atrial level (Fig. 32–3). The ventricular images may be used to evaluate circumferential contraction, detect regional wall hypertrophy or motion abnormalities, and measure shortening area. These views also are used to drive the cursor for M-mode studies in the 3 main planes: high papillary/chordal (left ventricle); mitral; aortic/left atrial (see Fig. 32–1).

An angled view of the right atrium, tricuspid valve, right ventricle, right ventricular outlet, and pulmonary artery (in long axis) with bifurcation is the logical extension of the most dorsal images of the left side of the heart (Fig. 32–4). Steep dorsocranial angulation of the transducer produces this image of the right ventricular inlet and outlet tracts. This image also reveals parts of the left atrium, atrial

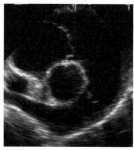

Figure 32–4. Two dimensional angled short-axis image from the right hemithorax used to evaluate the main pulmonary artery and proximal pulmonary artery branches.

septum, and caudal right atrium. At the opposite edge of the sector, the pulmonic valve and main pulmonary artery are visualized in long axis.

◆ THE USE OF ULTRASOUND IN THE DIAGNOSIS OF ACQUIRED HEART DISEASES

Myocardial Disease

Echocardiography allows for rapid, noninvasive identification of myocardial disease and differentiation between hypertrophic, restrictive, and dilated cardiomyopathies. The echocardiographic features of the different forms of cardiomyopathy are summarized in Table 32–2. Image quality and resolution are important for identifying cardiac wall edges, so that septal and ventricular measurements can be made accurately. This is especially important in cats because of their small size. In general, it is easier to measure wall thickness and chamber dimensions using M-mode images; however, the location and level of the M-mode beam are determined optimally using 2-DE.

Hypertrophic cardiomyopathy is characterized by increased septal and left ventricular freewall thickness (Fig. 32–5). A diastolic thickness of these structures greater than 5 to 5.6 mm indicates hypertrophy. Thickened papillary muscles and reduced left ventricular lumen size also are common. In patients with hypertrophic cardiomyopathy, the fractional shortening is normal to increased and the left atrium is often markedly enlarged (Fig. 32–6). With hypertrophic obstructive cardiomyopathy, septal thickness may be greater than the free wall thickness (asymmetric septal hypertrophy), and systolic narrowing of the left ventricular outflow region from the bulging, hypertrophied septum and systolic anterior motion may be seen on M-mode imaging (Fig.

Figure 32–5. Right parasternal short-axis view from a cat with hypertrophic cardiomyopathy. Notice the massive thickening of both the interventricular septum and the left ventricular free wall. Notice also the diminutive left ventricular lumen.

Table 32–2. Echocardiographic Features of the Cardiomyopathies

Cardiac Disorder	Two-Dimensional Echocardiography	M-Mode Echocardiography	Doppler Studies
Feline hypertrophic cardiomyopathy	LA dilatation; LV hypertrophy; hypertrophy may be symmetric and involve the entire ventricle, asymmetric with hypertrophy of the septum or free wall, or focal hypertrophy of the ventricle	Normal-to-decreased LV dimensions; LV hypertrophy; LA dilatation; normal-to-increased shortening fraction; possible systolic anterior motion of the septal mitral valve leaflet	Turbulent, high-velocity systolic signal of mitral regurgitation often recorded in the left atrium; turbulent, high-velocity systolic signal recorded in the LV outlet in cats with obstructive form of hypertrophic cardiomyopathy; ± abnormal isovolumetric relaxation time
Feline restrictive (intermediate cardiomyopathy)	LA dilatation, RA dilatation, ± RV dilatation; mild LV dilatation with variable hypertrophy; hyperechoic subendocardium; regional ventricular wall dysfunction is possible	Normal to mildly decreased LV shortening fraction; LA dilatation; possible regional wall motion abnormalities	Variable; turbulent high-velocity systolic signals of mitral or tricuspid regurgitation may be recorded; restrictive filling pattern (increased E wave, shortened deceleration time; small A-wave)
Dilated cardiomyopathy	LA and LV or generalized cardiac dilatation; global ventricular hypokinesis or marked depression of systolic ventricular free wall contraction and thickening	Ventricular and atrial dilatation; decreased LV shortening fraction is required to establish the diagnosis; increased E-point to septal separation, ± delayed mitral valve closure (B-shoulder) indicates elevated atrial and ventricular diastolic pressures	Turbulent, high-velocity systolic signals of mitral and tricuspid regurgitation are common; decreased aortic velocity and acceleration time; abnormal indices of diastolic ventricular function
Feline hyperthyroidism	Mild-to-moderate LA and LV dilatation; LV hypertrophy; variable RA and RV dilatation; if heart failure, all chambers dilated and pleural effusion	LV hypertrophy; mild-to-moderate LV and LA dilatation; increased LV shortening fraction in most cases; normal-to-decreased shortening fraction if heart failure	Variable: may observe turbulent jets of mitral regurgitation or tricuspid regurgitation; increased aortic velocity may be recorded

Abbreviations: LA, left atrial; LV, left ventricular; RA, right atrial; RV, right ventricular.

32–7). A thrombus is visualized occasionally within the left atrium or auricle in cats with cardiomyopathy (Fig. 32–8).[8]

Dilated cardiomyopathy is characterized by dilatation (eccentric hypertrophy) of the left and, typically, the right heart chambers. Systolic wall and septal motion is poor, causing the left ventricular systolic and diastolic dimensions to be increased; thus, fractional shortening and other indices of myocardial function are reduced. Increased mitral valve E point to septal separation and reduced aortic root motion are common, whereas left ventricular free-wall and septal thicknesses are normal to decreased.[9]

Other forms of cardiomyopathy also occur in cats. Endomyocardial fibrosis and restriction enhances the brightness of the endocardial surface (Fig. 32–9). Excess moderator bands may be visualized as extra echoes toward the left ventricular apex. Left atrial size tends to be greatly increased in cases of restrictive cardiomyopathy.

Valvular Insufficiency

Mitral or tricuspid valve insufficiency results in progressive dilatation of the affected side of the heart. Massive atrial enlargement may develop in patients with chronic valvular regurgitation. Ventricular motion throughout the cardiac cycle is accentuated, especially in mitral insufficiency. The diastolic left (and/or right) ventricular dimension is increased, but systolic dimension is normal until the myocardium itself begins to fail. Therefore, prior to myocardial failure, there is exaggerated septal motion, normal E point–septal separation, and high fractional shortening.

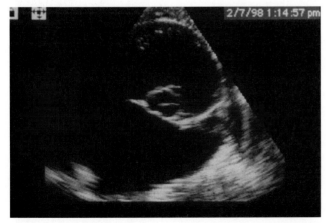

Figure 32–6. Right parasternal short-axis view at the level of the aorta and left atrium. The diameters of the aorta and the left atrium at this level should be about equal. Left atrial enlargement is common to all forms of cardiomyopathy.

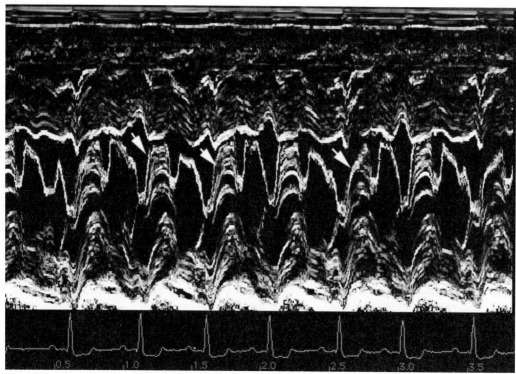

Figure 32–7. M-mode echocardiogram from a cat with hypertrophic obstructive cardiomyopathy. Notice how the anterior mitral leaflet moves toward the interventricular septum in systole *(arrows)*. This is often referred to as *systolic anterior motion*, and is evidence of dynamic outflow tract obstruction. Compare this with the normal mitral valve motion shown in Figure 32–1.

The affected valve cusps are thicker than normal, and may take on a knobby appearance at their edges. With good image resolution, smooth thickening is seen with degenerative disease (endocardiosis); bacterial endocarditis tends to cause rough and irregular vegetative valve lesions. It often is difficult to distinguish between these valve lesions with ultrasound alone, however. Rupture of a chorda tendineae causes part of the valve leaflet to have a flailed or paradoxical motion. Sometimes, the broken chorda itself can be seen.

Aortic insufficiency, whether resulting from infectious endocarditis or congenital malformation, also leads to left ventricular and, possibly, left atrial dilatation. Evidence of a vegetative lesion or rapid diastolic fluttering (as blood leaks back into the ventricle) may be seen while the aortic valve is imaged. A flailed aortic leaflet will prolapse into the ventricular outflow tract during diastole. Also, the regurgi-

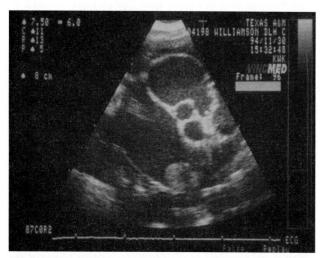

Figure 32–8. Right parasternal short-axis view shows a markedly enlarged left atrium with a thrombus within the lumen. It seems that the larger the left atrium, the more likely a thrombus will form.

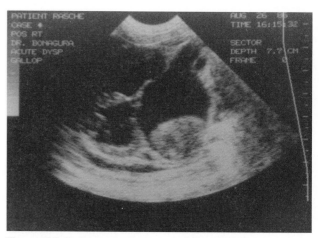

Figure 32–9. Right parasternal short-axis view at the level of the papillary muscles. Note the thinning of the left venticular free wall and the irregularity of the left ventricular lumen. Also note the increased echogenicity of the subendocardial region.

tant jet of blood during diastole may cause the open anterior mitral leaflet to flutter.

Pericardial Diseases

Pericardial effusion can be detected readily using echocardiography. Because fluid is sonolucent, pericardial effusion appears as an echo-free space between the bright parietal pericardium and the epicardium. Pericardial effusion must be differentiated from pleural effusion on the echocardiogram. Evidence of collapsed lung lobes or pleural folds may appear in patients with pleural effusion. Very large amounts of pericardial fluid allow the heart to swing wildly within the pericardial sac. In addition, pericardial effusion of sufficient volume (pressure) to cause cardiac tamponade results in diastolic compression or collapse of the cardiac chambers, especially the right atrium and ventricle. A soft-tissue density mass may be identified in cases of neoplastic pericardial effusion. The usual locations are the right auricle (hemangiosarcoma) and around the ascending aorta (chemodectoma, lymphoma). Tumors of the pericardium itself or the myocardium also may be a cause of pericardial effusion. Sometimes intracardiac masses occur, and are not associated with pericardial effusion. Varying degrees of pericardial effusion are seen commonly in all forms of cardiomyopathy. Most studies suggest the most common cause of pericardial effusion in cats is feline infectious peritonitis.

Heartworm Disease

Some cases of heartworm disease evidence no echocardiographic abnormalities; however, because of the relative size of the host, parasite worms are imaged in as many as 60 to 80 per cent of cases. Therefore, echocardiography is a much more sensitive tool for diagnosing this disease in cats. Worms are identifiable commonly in the main pulmonary artery, and appear as bright dots and closely parallel lines on 2-DE images (see Chapter 33, Heartworm Disease). Infrequently, severe heartworm disease will cause right ventricular enlargement and hypertrophy, with dilatation of the main pulmonary artery. The interventricular septum tends to become "flattened" toward the left ventricle, because of the high right ventricular pressures required to eject blood in the face of pulmonary hypertension.

◆ THE USE OF ULTRASOUND IN THE DIAGNOSIS OF CONGENITAL HEART DISEASES

Echocardiography can help define specific congenital cardiac malformations. Estimation of their severity also may be possible, especially using Doppler imaging. Without Doppler imaging, cardiac catheterization often is necessary for complete diagnosis and quantitation of severity. For a more in-depth discussion of the clinical features of congenital heart disease in cats the reader is referred to Chapter 34, "Congenital Heart Disease," in volume 3 of this series.

Ventricular Outflow Obstruction

Narrowing of the ventricular outlet places a pressure overload on the affected ventricle. The response of the myocardium to this stress is muscular hypertrophy. Thus, with pulmonic stenosis, the right ventricular wall is thicker than normal, and may exceed the left ventricular wall thickness in severe cases. Right ventricular papillary muscles also are prominent. High pressures in the right ventricle tend to push the interventricular septum to the left, causing the left ventricular lumen to appear oval rather than round on the short-axis view. Dilatation of the right ventricle and atrium, and thickening of the right atrial wall, also may be seen. Narrowing at the level of the pulmonic valve with evidence of thickening or asymmetry of the valve leaflets and dilatation of the main pulmonary trunk also are common findings. The pulmonic valve may appear to "dome" toward the pulmonary artery in systole with valvular stenosis.

Stenosis of the aortic valve itself or the presence of a subvalvular fibrous ring causing outflow obstruction is rare in cats. In mild subaortic stenosis, there may be no definitive changes on the echocardiogram. With moderate-to-severe disease, a ridge of tissue below the aortic valve may be evident. Premature closure of the aortic valve and systolic anterior motion of the anterior mitral leaflet may be seen with severe disease. The left ventricular wall is thicker than normal, and dilatation of the ascending aorta (wider than the area of the sinuses of Valsalva) may be visualized. Left atrial enlargement and hypertrophy also may be seen. Doppler echocardiography is helpful for quantitative as well as qualitative assessment of ventricular outflow obstructions.

Cardiac Shunts

Communications between the left and the right sides of the circulation cause volume overload, with subsequent dilatation of the affected cardiac chambers. Intracardiac shunts include ventricular and atrial septal defects; the most common extracardiac shunt is patent ductus arteriosus.

Most ventricular septal defects occur high, in the membranous portion of the septum. Larger defects may be visualized in a plane optimized for viewing the left ventricular outflow tract. The defect usually is located just below the aortic valve, with the septal tricuspid leaflet to the right of the defect. Sometimes echocardiographic "drop-out" occurs at the thin membranous septum, mimicking a ventricular septal defect. Suspected defects should be examined in more than 1 echocardiographic plane. Unless the ventricular septal defect is quite large, causing both ventricles to act as a common chamber, the usual pathophysiology is that of a volume overload to the left heart. Consequently, dilatation of the left ventricle and atrium occurs with significant shunts.

Atrial septal defects usually cause volume overload of the right atrium and ventricle; because left heart pressures normally are higher, blood moves across the shunt from left to right atrium. The thinner region of the fossa ovalis in the atrial septum may be confused with a septal defect, because echocardiographic drop-out also can occur here. Doppler echocardiography often allows identification of smaller intracardiac shunts that cannot be visualized with 2-DE imaging.

The typical (left-to-right shunting) patent ductus arteriosus creates a volume overload on the left heart, with left atrial and ventricular dilatation. Fractional shortening may be normal to decreased, and E point–septal separation often is increased. The actual shunt is difficult to visualize, because it is located between the descending aorta and the pulmonary artery. In some animals, the ductus can be seen using the cranial left parasternal position. Doppler imaging allows identification of this defect, with its turbulent blood flow pattern in the pulmonary artery throughout systole and diastole.

Atrioventricular Valve Dysplasia

Malformation and insufficiency of the mitral or tricuspid valve are 2 of the most common congenital cardiac malformations. This results in dilatation of the associated cardiac chambers, just as it does with acquired valvular insufficiency. Often, chamber dilatation is marked. Abnormally formed papillary muscles and/or chordae tendineae as well as incomplete closure of the valve may be visualized on 2-DE imaging.

Complex Malformations

Tetralogy of Fallot is composed of a large ventricular septal defect and some degree of pulmonic stenosis with a malpositioned aortic root overriding the ventricular septum. Secondary to these malformations, right ventricular hypertrophy and right-to-left shunting of blood across the ventricular septal defect occur. The septal defect, right ventricular hypertrophy, and overriding aorta usually can be appreciated on 2-DE. Use of an echocardiographic contrast study should demonstrate blood flow from the right ventricle into the aorta. Other complex and unusual defects also may be identified using ultrasound.

REFERENCES

1. Feigenbaum H: Echocardiography, 5th ed. Philadelphia, Lea & Febiger, 1994.
2. Jacobs G, Knight DH: Change in M-mode echocardiographic values in cats given ketamine. Am J Vet Res 46:1712–1713, 1985.
3. Fox PR, Bond BR, Peterson ME: Echocardiographic reference values in healthy cats sedated with ketamine hydrochloride. Am J Vet Res 46:1479–1484, 1985.
4. Weyman AE: Principles and Practice of Echocardiography, 1st ed. Philadelphia, Lea & Febiger, 1994.
5. Bonagura JD, Miller MW: Doppler echocardiography. I. Pulsed-wave and continuous-wave examinations. Vet Clin North Am Small Anim Pract 28:1325–1359, 1998.
6. Bonagura JD, Miller MW: Doppler echocardiography. II. Color Doppler imaging. Vet Clin North Am Small Anim Pract 28:1361–1389, 1998.
7. Bonagura JD, Miller MW: Veterinary echocardiography. Echocardiography 6:229–264, 1989.
8. Moïse NS, Dietze AE, Mezza LE, et al: Echocardiography, electrocardiography, and radiography of cats with dilatation cardiomyopathy, hypertrophic cardiomyopathy, and hyperthyroidism. Am J Vet Res 47:1476–1486, 1986.
9. Sisson DD, Knight DH, Helinski C, et al: Plasma taurine concentrations and M-mode echocardiographic measures in healthy cats and in cats with dilated cardiomyopathy. J Vet Intern Med 5:232–238, 1991.

33
◆ Heartworm Disease

Matthew W. Miller

◆ GENERAL INFORMATION

Prevalence studies indicate that cats throughout the world that reside in areas enzootic for heartworm disease in dogs are prone to infection.[1-3] The prevalence in cats seems to parallel the prevalence in dogs in the same area but at a much lower level, with cats having approximately one-tenth the prevalence seen in the unprotected dog population.[4-6] This relative prevalence varies dramatically by region, and may reflect different vector populations with relative prevalence in cats being higher in regions with vectors which are indiscriminate feeders. Indiscriminate feeding vectors are those that will take a blood meal from any source, in contrast to many mosquito species that have very specific host preferences. Aberrant migration of larvae seems to be much more common in cats than in dogs.

The life expectancy of heartworms in cats probably is less than 2 years, compared with approximately 5 years in dogs. The worm burden in cats typically is lower than in dogs, and the worms usually do not attain comparable size in cats. Experimental infections have confirmed the clinical impression that male cats are more susceptible to infection, in terms of both of infection rate (males, 82 per cent; females, 67 per cent) and worm burden (males average 6.3 worms; females average 3.0 worms). The average prepatent period in cats experimentally infected is 8 months, compared with 5.5 to 6 months in dogs. Approximately 50 per cent of experimentally infected cats develop microfilaremia; however, the microfilaremia is usually transient (1 to 2 months) and of low concentration.[7, 8] Clinical studies have estimated that less than 20 per cent of cats have circulating microfilaria at the time of diagnosis.

The majority of the pathologic findings in cats with heartworm disease are restricted to the pulmonary system. Gross pathologic and histopathologic changes are similar to those reported in dogs. Major histologic lesions include villous endarteritis and muscular hypertrophy of the media of the pulmonary arteries. Large muscular arteries associated with bronchi seem to be affected most severely.[9] It should be emphasized that pulmonary artery medial hypertrophy and hyperplasia have been documented in specific-pathogen–free cats; therefore, this lesion in isolation is not pathognomonic for heartworm disease.[10] Focal granulomatous and eosinophilic pneumonia occasionally is present in the pulmonary parenchyma surrounding involved arteries.

◆ EPIDEMIOLOGY

Based on clinical serologic survey data and results of reported retrospective studies, there is no age or breed predisposition to *Dirofilaria immitis* infection or exposure in cats.[11-13] Males have been shown to be more susceptible to infection in some clinical and experimental studies.[7] This gender predisposition has not been supported by serologic surveys; however, these surveys report exposure and not mature infection.[3, 4] A necropsy study from Beaumont, Texas, reported that more males than females harbored adult heartworms, but this difference was statistically insignificant.[14] Interestingly, that study reported that only 50 per cent of the cats in which adult worms were found at necropsy were antibody-positive. Cats that have outdoor exposure are at increased risk of infection, with any exposure to the outdoors increasing the risk of exposure 2-fold.[3] It is important to emphasize that heartworm disease has been diagnosed in cats that, according to the owners, live strictly indoors. Feline leukemia virus infection is not considered to be a predisposing factor. A report describing the results of an animal shelter necropsy study suggested that cats positive for feline immunodeficiency virus (FIV) antibody have a higher incidence of circulating heartworm antibodies than the general population, but do not have a higher incidence of mature infection.[14] This most likely indicates that cats at risk for exposure to FIV also are at higher risk for exposure to heartworm, rather than FIV infection being an independent risk factor.

◆ DIAGNOSIS

Cats may be presented for peracute or chronic signs, or may be completely asymptomatic. The acute syndrome commonly is associated with acute respiratory compromise secondary to severe pulmonary thromboembolism and frequently results in death. Any cat that dies suddenly in an area known to be endemic for heartworm should be evaluated by meticulous necropsy for evidence of *D. immitis* infection. Historical complaints in cats with chronic signs of heartworm disease typically are referable to the cardiopulmonary system (coughing, dyspnea), gastrointestinal system (vomiting unrelated to feeding), but may be quite vague (lethargy, partial anorexia, and weight loss).[15-18] Vomiting and respiratory difficulty seem to be the predominant signs in chronic disease.

Physical examination of cats with heartworm disease frequently is unremarkable. The presence of increased bronchovesicular sounds is one of the more common abnormalities reported, but is a very nonspecific finding. Auscultation of a murmur or gallop rhythm is very unusual in cats with heartworm disease, and should increase the clinician's suspicion of primary and secondary cardiac diseases including idiopathic cardiomyopathy, valvular heart disease, and thyrotoxic or hypertensive heart disease.

◆ CLINICAL PATHOLOGY/ SEROLOGY

Abnormalities detected on routine blood work are fairly nonspecific. Complete blood counts often show a mild nonregenerative anemia and occasionally increased numbers of nucleated red blood cells. Eosinophilia is an inconsistent finding, even on serial samples.[6] Experimentally, peripheral eosinophilia occurs most commonly 4 to 7 months postinfection and intermittently thereafter.[7] If peripheral basophilia is noted in conjunction with eosinophilia, a diagnosis of heartworm disease should be pursued. Hyperglobulinemia is one of the few commonly observed biochemical abnormalities.

Concentration techniques (Difil, Evsco Pharmaceuticals, Buena, NJ; modified Knott's) may be performed in cats suspected of having heartworm disease, but often are of little value because less than 20 per cent of all infections are patent. Even in cats with circulating microfilaria, the low concentration and transient nature of the microfilaremia result in a large number of false-negative test results. The sensitivity of the concentration tests may be improved by performing multiple tests and by using 5 ml of blood for each test rather than the standard 1 ml. Although the concentration tests have a very low sensitivity, a positive test establishes a definitive diagnosis (Table 33–1 and Fig. 33–1).

Several testing methods are available for detection of amicrofilaremic infections. The indirect fluorescent antibody test (IFA) detects host antibodies against microfilarial cuticular and somatic antigens. This test is commercially available only from Antech Labs (Farmingdale, NY; Irvine, CA). Some reports suggest that the IFA test is a highly specific and sensitive indicator of heartworm exposure, detecting some infections as early as 1 to 2 months postinfection.[19] The enzyme-linked immunosorbent

Table 33–1. Establishing a Definitive Diagnosis

Necropsy
Positive antigen test
Positive Difil test
Echocardiography
Worms visualized
Nonselective angiography
Tortuous pulmonary arteries

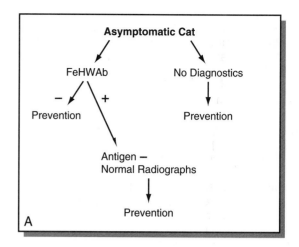

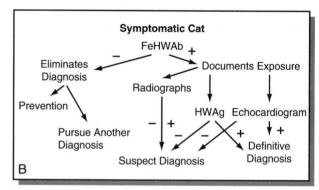

Figure 33–1. Algorithm demonstrates the diagnostic approach to cats suspected of having heartworm (FeHW) disease. The approach varies somewhat, based on the presence *(B)* or absence *(A)* of clinical signs. Although the algorithm would suggest that a negative antibody (Ab) titer eliminates a diagnosis, a small percentage of cats with an adult infection may be antibody-negative. In these situations, additional diagnostic tests may be warranted. HWAg, heartworm antigen.

assay (ELISA) test (Animal Diagnostics [BioClin], St. Louis, MO; Heska Corporation, Fort Collins, CO), which detects antibodies to heartworm antigen, is quite sensitive. The antigen against which the antibody is directed is present in large amounts in the L_4 and L_5 stages, and to a lesser degree, in the L_3 stage. Studies using both tests to evaluate well-characterized feline serum suggest that they are quite specific, even in the presence of heavy intestinal parasitism.[19] A positive antibody test simply documents exposure, whereas a negative test makes a diagnosis of feline heartworm disease less likely. There are, however, some cats with mature heartworm infection (positive ELISA antigen test or documented via necropsy or echocardiography) that have been antibody-negative. This situation was thought to be quite uncommon; however, 1 study suggested this may occur in as many as 50 per cent of adult infections.[13] Antibody-negative cats showing clinical signs typical of heartworm disease, and in which other tests (radiography) support a diagnosis, deserve further evaluation. This additional evaluation might include an echocardiogram, an ELISA antigen test, additional antibody tests (perhaps using an alternative laboratory), and in select cases, nonselective angiography.[20–22] Circulating antibodies typically are detectable within 2 to 4 months of exposure, and the ELISA tests may remain positive for 9 to 12 months, even if a mature infection is not established. An in-house ELISA test marketed by Synbiotics Corporation (Assure/FH) and an immunochromatography format test (SoloStep) marketed by Heska Corporation have been approved by the U.S. Food and Drug Administration and currently are being marketed.[23]

The ELISA tests offered by Heska and Animal Diagnostic laboratories are considered quantitative, with the intensity of the test correlating, to some extent, with the likelihood of mature infection. The results of Heska's test are reported in antibody units per milliliter (AbU/ml). Using these units, a value less than 5 AbU/mL would be considered a negative test, a value greater than 5 but less than 20 AbU/ml would be typical of exposure, whereas a value greater than 20 AbU/ml would be common in cats with a mature infection.[24] It is important to emphasize that these values are guidelines and do not represent definitive categories. The results of the Animal Diagnostics' test is reported as a titer (reported range is 1:70 to >1:5000), with a titer of 1:70 considered positive. The higher the titer, the more likely it represents mature infection. In asymptomatic cats with a titer of less than 1:120, only 1 per cent had a positive antigen test. In symptomatic cats with titers less than 1:120, but greater than 1:70, 28 per cent were antigen-positive. In cats with titers greater than or equal to 1:3000, 78 per cent were antigen-positive.[25] Serial titers may be informative, with increasing AbU concentrations or antibody titers suggesting sustained or ongoing infection. Owing to the nature of the titering system, a titer needs to change by a factor of 4 to be considered significantly different.

The ELISA and immunochromatography tests that detect circulating adult heartworm antigen (HWAg) are the most specific tests currently available to detect mature infections. Although the tests were originally marketed for use in dogs, the methodology allows the tests to be used in any species. The antigen detected is a series of related acidic proteoglycans derived primarily from the uterus of adult female worms. Low worm burdens (less than 3 worms), all-male infections, or immature infections may result in false-negative test results. When evaluating the results of an ELISA or HWAg test in a cat, a negative test result does not rule out dirofilariasis, but a positive test is very strong evidence of heartworm infestation. Several studies (echocardiographic, experimental, and necropsy) suggest that approximately 40 per cent of cats with adult worms are antigen-positive.[13, 15, 26]

◆ RADIOGRAPHY/NONSELECTIVE ANGIOGRAPHY

Thoracic radiography is one of the most useful tests available for the evaluation of suspected *D. immitis*

infection in cats.[15–17] It is important to know not only the radiographic features of dirofilariasis but also the more important differential diagnoses. The most commonly reported radiographic findings in cats with heartworm infection include prominent, enlarged pulmonary arteries that may or may not be notably blunted or tortuous. The caudal lobar arteries usually show the earliest radiographic changes, with the right and left being equally affected. The radiographic changes are best appreciated on the dorsoventral or ventrodorsal views (Fig. 33–2).[27] Evaluation of the pulmonary arteries may be hindered by the presence of significant pulmonary parenchymal disease. Therapy for the pulmonary parenchymal disease may be necessary before diagnostic thoracic radiographs can be obtained. It is uncommon to see significant alterations in cardiac size or shape, and signs of congestive heart failure are quite uncommon. Chylothorax has been described in association with both experimental and natural *D. immitis* infections in cats.[28] Chylous pleural effusion warrants further pursuit of a diagnosis of feline dirofilariasis (see Chapter 35, Chylothorax).

Nonselective angiography may be very helpful in the diagnosis of feline heartworm disease (Table

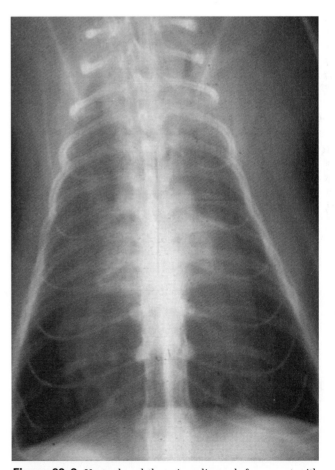

Figure 33–2. Ventrodorsal thoracic radiograph from a cat with heartworm disease. This view often is the best for appreciating subtle enlargement of the caudal lobar arteries. A ratio of greater than 1.6:1 between the width of the pulmonary artery as it crosses the 9th rib and the width of the 9th rib itself is suggestive of important arterial enlargement.

Table 33–2. Nonselective Angiography

1. Mild sedation may be necessary
2. Place large catheter ≥ 20 gauge
   Jugular or cephalic
3. Angiographic contrast (2.2 ml/kg)
   Angioconray
   Renographin
4. Rapid injection (beware vomition)
5. Lateral and/or ventrodorsal radiograph should be taken as soon as the contrast agent is injected

33–2). Nonselective angiography allows critical evaluation of pulmonary arterial size and morphology, even when significant pulmonary parenchymal disease is present. Angiographic abnormalities associated with heartworm disease include enlarged, tortuous pulmonary arteries, pulmonary arterial obstruction, and linear filling defects (Fig. 33–3). Streaming of contrast in the cranial vena cava and right atrium is common, and should not be overinterpreted as a filling defect.[20, 22] Although nonselective angiography may be very informative, its use should be limited to cases in which a definitive diagnosis cannot be established with less invasive means (echocardiography).

◆ ELECTROCARDIOGRAPHY/ ECHOCARDIOGRAPHY

Although evidence of right ventricular enlargement is evident occasionally, the electrocardiogram is normal in most cats with heartworm disease. Significant axis shifts or dysrhythmias should increase the clinician's suspicion of primary cardiac disease.

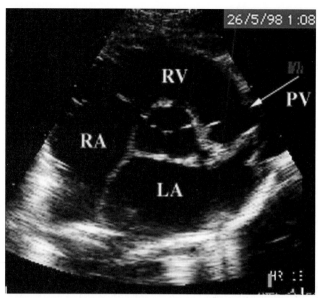

Figure 33–4. Right parasternal short-axis view of the heart. In this view, the right atrium (RA) and right ventricle (RV) can be visualized and interrogated for the presence of heartworms. Worms must be present within the right atrium or right ventricle if transvenous surgical retrieval is being considered. The *arrow* points to the pulmonary valve (PV). LA, left atrium.

Numerous reports and abstracts have documented the diagnostic utility of echocardiography in cats with heartworm disease.[13, 15, 29, 30] Sensitivities ranging from 34 to 100 per cent have been reported, suggesting that worms can be visualized within the cardiac chambers or pulmonary arteries in greater than 50 per cent of cases. It is imperative that adequate visualization be obtained of the entire right heart, bifurcation of the main pulmonary artery, and the proximal portion of the right pulmonary artery. Most worms are seen in the pulmonary arteries and appear as parallel hyperechoic structures typically about 0.7 to 1.2 mm thick and separated by approximately 0.5 to 1.0 mm, most commonly described as resembling a bright "equals (=) sign" (Figs. 33–4 to 33–6). The length, however, is variable, reflecting the angle at which the worms are aligned relative to the echocardiographic imaging plane. Determination of the exact number of worms often is quite difficult. Importantly, echocardiography is very helpful in establishing or refuting a diagnosis of primary cardiac disease.

◆ DIFFERENTIAL DIAGNOSIS

Asthma, cardiomyopathy, pneumonia (bacterial, viral, fungal, or protozoal), pulmonary neoplasia (primary, metastatic) and *Aelurostrongylus abstrusus* and *Paragonimus kellicotti* infections must be considered as possible diagnoses in cats with heartworm disease presented for respiratory signs. The pulmonary parenchymal lesions seen in all these diseases are similar to those seen in heartworm disease, but the pulmonary arterial changes described

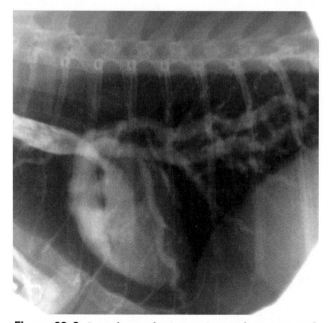

Figure 33–3. Lateral nonselective angiogram from a cat with heartworm disease. Notice the dramatic pulmonary arterial enlargement. Also important is the tortuosity of the pulmonary arteries.

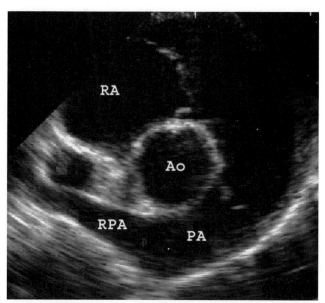

Figure 33–5. Right parasternal short-axis view at the level of the aorta (Ao) and pulmonary artery (PA). This is one of the most useful views with which to detect heartworms in cats. If this view cannot be obtained, the examination should be considered inadequate. RA, right atrium; RPA, right pulmonary artery.

previously are unique to heartworm infection. Cats with primary heart disease and congestive heart failure may have pulmonary artery enlargement, but the arteries are not tortuous or blunted and usually are associated with concurrent pulmonary venous dilatation. When adult worms first reach the pulmonary arteries, they can cause pneumonitis and radiographic signs similar to that seen with asthma. At this stage of the disease, antibody titers most likely would be positive, but an antigen test would be almost invariably negative. These cats often respond

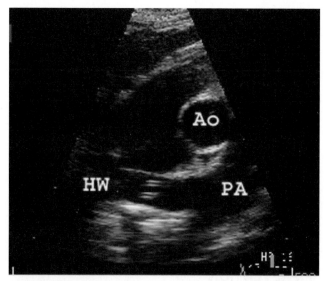

Figure 33–6. Right parasternal short-axis view from a cat with heartworm disease. Notice the parallel hyperechoic linear densities in the lumen of the right pulmonary artery (PA) labeled as heartworms (HW). Ao, aorta.

favorably to corticosteroid administration, as will some cats with asthma, making differentiation of the 2 diseases quite challenging.

◆ TREATMENT

It is the author's opinion that asymptomatic cats with heartworm infection should not receive any form of adulticide therapy. The fact that most cats infected with *D. immitis* are asymptomatic and the lifespan of *D. immitis* in cats is so short, argues against the necessity for adulticide therapy. However, the pulmonary pathology associated with *D. immitis* infection and the possibility of acute death would seem to argue in favor of initiating adulticide therapy following definitive diagnosis. Although many published reports have stated that cats tolerate thiacetarsamide (Caparsolate, Meriel Limited, Iselin, NJ) therapy with minimal renal or hepatic toxicity, these same reports also are quick to point out that cats seem to have severe thromboembolic complications. In an experimental study evaluating the pharmacokinetics of thiacetarsimide in normal cats, 3 of 14 cats developed an idiosyncratic acute respiratory distress syndrome resulting in pulmonary edema, respiratory failure, and death within 1 to 3 hours of the second dose of thiacetarsamide.[31] Subsequent investigations of a similar nature have been unable to reproduce this observation.[31] Few data are available regarding the use of melarsomine dihydrochloride (Immiticide, Meriel Limited, Iselin, NJ) in cats. An abstract reporting the use of melarsomine dihydrochloride (2.5 mg/kg intramuscularly [IM]) in cats with experimental (adult transplant) infection suggested that a single dose reduced the worm burden by approximately 30 per cent (statistically insignificant) without serious complications. Melarsomine dihydrochloride is not approved for use in cats.

Cats presented for cough and/or dyspnea may respond initially to administration of corticosteroids and bronchodilators. The initial prednisolone dose is 1 mg/kg orally (PO) every (q) 12 hr for 10 to 14 days; the dose then is gradually reduced to the minimum dose that will eliminate clinical signs. Theophylline (TheoDur, Schering-Plough, Kenilworth, NJ) may be administered at a dose of 25 mg/kg PO q 24 hr in the evening for the duration of the infection. If clinical signs are not relieved by symptomatic therapy, adulticide therapy may be considered but is not recommended. If adulticide therapy is considered, the American Heartworm Society recommends thiacetarsamide administered at a dose of 2.2 mg/kg intravenously (IV) q 12 hr for 2 days. It generally is accepted that cats have more severe posttherapy thromboembolic complications than dogs, probably due in part to the large size of the worms relative to the cat's pulmonary artery. The clinician should expect a 30 per cent patient mortality rate associated with adulticide therapy and subsequent thromboembolic complications.[6, 13] This high mortality rate may reflect the fact that cats that do not respond to symptomatic therapy may have more severe disease or higher worm burdens, and therefore are at more risk for significant complications. Interestingly, a retrospective report that tried to assess the outcome in treated (adulticide) versus nontreated (only supportive care given) reported no difference in long-term survival.[13]

Supportive care for thromboembolic complications includes corticosteroid administration, oxygen supplementation, and cautious fluid therapy. The thromboembolic complications seem to be most severe approximately 5 to 14 days after adulticide therapy. Although the use of aspirin has been advocated in the treatment of feline dirofilariasis, experimental evidence suggests that even at near-toxic doses, aspirin has little effect on the arteriographic, hemodynamic, and histopathologic abnormalities.[9] Aspirin administration as an adjunctive therapy in heartworm disease is no longer advocated by the American Heartworm Society.

The dismal outcome associated with conventional therapy has prompted several investigators to pursue transthoracic and transvenous approaches for surgical removal of adult heartworms. Brown and Thomas[32] removed adult worms from 5 cats using either a left or a right thoracotomy. Cats with worms located primarily in the right atrium and cavae underwent a right lateral thoracotomy and right atriotomy, whereas cats in which worms were seen only in the pulmonary artery underwent a left lateral thoracotomy and pulmonary arterotomy. Us-

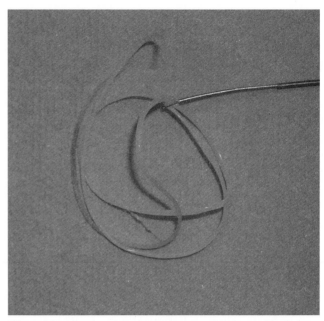

Figure 33–8. Three-pronged grasping forceps shown grasping one heartworm. It is important not to close the forceps completely but rather to attempt to secure the worms gently, then remove them through the venotomy. Crushing or fragmentation of worms during extraction has been associated with sudden death.

ing either a 2.5-mm-diameter 2- to 3-pronged bronchoscopic grasping device (Figs. 33–7 and 33–8) or standard 10-cm-long alligator forceps, Brown and Thomas[32] successfully removed adult worms from 3 of 4 cats. The forceps were manipulated using standard left-sided echocardiographic imaging planes to adjust positioning. Venco and coworkers[33] reported similar results using flexible alligator forceps. As techniques are refined, surgical removal of adult heartworms may become the therapy of choice for symptomatic adult infections. Acute respiratory and cardiovascular failure have been reported during surgical heartworm retrieval, typically following a worm being crushed or fragmented. Pretreatment with corticosteroids and/or antihistamines may reduce the severity of these types of reactions.

Microfilaricide therapy is indicated infrequently because greater than 80 per cent of all feline cases are occult. Dithiazanine iodide may be used at a dose of 6 to 10 mg/kg daily PO for 7 days. Levamisole at a dosage 10 mg/kg daily PO for 7 days should be effective, but may be associated with significant gastrointestinal or central nervous system side-effects. Safety has not been established for either of these compounds. Both ivermectin and milbemycin at the respective preventive doses are effective microfilaricides and should render cats microfilaria-negative after 3 to 12 months of therapy.

◆ PREVENTION

Studies designed to evaluate the tolerance of cats to orally administered ivermectin suggest that cats

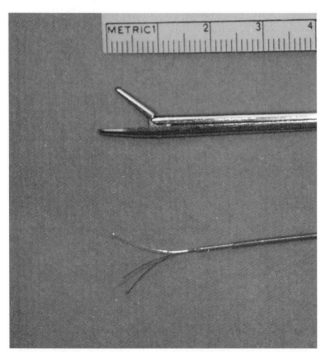

Figure 33–7. The relative sizes of the grasping forceps *(bottom)* and alligator forceps *(top)* are depicted. Subtle manipulation of the stiff alligator forceps is difficult, making the grasping forceps the more useful device. However, despite the small diameter and flexibility of the grasping forceps, manipulation into the pulmonary artery is not possible and should not be attempted.

tolerate dosages of 750 to 1000 μg/kg, and demonstrate signs of ivermectin toxicity (incoordination, mydriasis, hyperactivity) in a dose-dependent manner in doses exceeding 1000 μg/kg. At doses of 24 μg/kg (4 times the dose required for prevention in dogs), ivermectin is 100 per cent effective in preventing development of *D. immitis* in cats when administered 30 or 45 days after inoculation with infective larvae.[34] Heartgard (Meriel Limited, Iselin, NJ) for cats is formulated to provide that dose, has received U.S. Food and Drug Association approval, and is marketed currently. Cats receiving ivermectin at the preventive dose may develop a detectable antibody response to *D. immitis* after exposure, in spite of being protected completely from mature infection. Preliminary data suggest that although antiheartworm antibody is detectable, the intensity of the antibody response is low (<20 AbU/ml), allowing differentiation between simple exposure and infection.[35] Selamectin (Revolution) has received U.S. Food and Drug Administration approval, and is an effective preventive when applied at a dose of 6 mg/kg every 30 days.

Cats also are completely protected against the development of infective larvae of *D. immitis* when milbemycin oxime is administered at the label dose and treatment regimen for dogs (0.5 to 0.99 mg/kg PO q 30 days).[36] Diethylcarbamazine has been administered to cats in endemic areas at the canine dosage (6.6 to 11 mg/kg q 24 hr) without adverse effects; however, the efficacy of such therapy has not been evaluated critically.

◆ ROUTINE TESTING

One common question is whether routine testing is necessary before initiating preventive therapy. Complications associated with administration of monthly preventive therapy to heartworm-positive cats are uncommon, and almost without exception are associated with a high concentration of circulating microfilaria. Because cats very rarely have high levels of circulating microfilaria, the likelihood of complications would be very low. Arguments in favor of routine testing using the antibody test include establishing individual exposure status before dispensing preventive therapy, and establishing information regarding local exposure rates.

REFERENCES

1. Labarthe N, Serrão ML, Melo YF, et al: Heartworm in the state of Rio de Janeiro, Brazil. *In* Knight D (ed): The American Heartworm Society: State of the Heartworm Symposium '98. American Heartworm Society, Batavia, IL, 1998, pp. 67–75.
2. Genchi C, Manfredi MT, Basano FS, et al: Canine and feline heartworm in Europe with special emphasis on Italy. *In* Knight D (ed): The American Heartworm Society: State of the Heartworm Symposium '98. American Heartworm Society, Batavia, IL, 1998, pp. 75–83.
3. Miller MW, Atkins CE, Stemme K, et al: Prevalence of exposure to *Dirofilaria immitis* in cats from multiple areas. *In* Knight D (ed): The American Heartworm Society: State of the Heartworm Symposium '98. American Heartworm Society, Batavia, IL, 1998, pp. 161–167.
4. Wong MM, Pedersen NC, Cullen J: Dirofilariasis in cats. J Am Anim Hosp Assoc 19:855–864, 1983.
5. Elkins AD, Kadel W: Feline heartworm disease and its incidence in western Kentucky. Comp Small Anim 10:585–590, 1988.
6. Dillon R: Feline dirofilariasis. Vet Clin North Am Small Anim Pract 14:1185–1199, 1984.
7. Donahoe JM: Experimental infection of cats with dirofilaria immitis. J Parasitol 61:599–605, 1975.
8. McCall JW, Dzimianski MT, McTier TL, et al: Dirofilariasis in domestic cats: Biology of experimental heartworm infections in cats. *In* Soll MD (ed): Proceedings of the Heartworm Symposium '92. American Heartworm Society, Batavia, IL, 1994, pp. 71–80.
9. Rawlings CA, Farrell RL, Mahood RM: Morphologic changes in the lungs of cats experimentally infected with *Dirofilaria immitis*. J Vet Intern Med 4:292–299, 1990.
10. Rogers WA, Bishop SP, Rohovsky MW: Pulmonary artery medial hypertrophy and hyperplasia in conventional and specific-pathogen–free cats. Am J Vet Res 32:767–774, 1971.
11. Miller MW, Zoran DL, Relford RL, et al: Seroprevalence of antibodies to *Dirofilaria immitis* in asymptomatic cats in the Bryan/College Station area of Texas. *In* Knight D (ed): The American Heartworm Society: State of the Heartworm Symposium '98. American Heartworm Society, Batavia, IL, 1998, pp. 159–161.
12. Dillon AR, Brawner WR, Robertson CK, et al: Feline heartworm disease: Correlations of clinical signs, serology, and other diagnostics: Results of a multicenter study. *In* Knight D (ed): The American Heartworm Society: State of the Heartworm Symposium '98. American Heartworm Society, Batavia, IL, 1998, pp. 153–159.
13. Atkins CE, DeFrancesco TC, Coats JR, et al: Feline heartworm disease: The North Carolina experience. *In* Knight D (ed): The American Heartworm Society: State of the Heartworm Symposium '98. American Heartworm Society, Batavia, IL, 1998, pp. 123–127.
14. Nelson CT, Young TS: Incidence of *Dirofilaria immitis* in shelter cats from Southeast Texas. *In* Knight D (ed): The American Heartworm Society: State of the Heartworm Symposium '98. American Heartworm Society, Batavia, IL, 1998, pp. 63–67.
15. Atkins CE, DeFrancesco TC, Miller MW, et al: Prevalence of heartworm infection in cats with signs of cardiorespiratory abnormalities. J Am Vet Med Assoc 212:517–520, 1998.
16. Sisson D: A definitive approach to heartworm disease in cats. Vet Forum 22:40–48, 1998.
17. Calvert CA, Mandell CP: Diagnosis and management of feline heartworm disease. J Am Vet Med Assoc 180:550–552, 1982.
18. Hawkins EC: Feline heartworm disease. Kal Kan Forum 8:1–7, 1989.
19. McCall JW, Guerrero J, Supakorndej P, et al: Evaluation of the accuracy of antigen and antibody tests for detection of heartworm infection in cats. *In* Knight D (ed): The American Heartworm Society: State of the Heartworm Symposium '98. American Heartworm Society, Batavia, IL, 1998, pp. 127–135.
20. Green BJ, Lord PF, Grieve RB: Occult feline dirofilariasis confirmed by angiography and serology. J Am Anim Hosp Assoc 19:847–854, 1983.
21. Donahoe JM, Kneller SK, Lewis RE: In vivo pulmonary arteriography in cats infected with *Dirofilaria immitis*. J Vet Radiol Soc 17:147–151, 1976.
22. Rawlings CA: Pulmonary arteriography and hemodynamics during feline heartworm disease. J Vet Intern Med 4:285–291, 1990.
23. Bestul KJ, McCall JW, Supakorndej N, et al: Evaluation of the ASSURE/FH assay for the detection of feline heartworm antibody. *In* Knight D (ed): The American Heartworm Society: State of the Heartworm Symposium '98. American Heartworm Society, Batavia, IL, 1998, pp. 179–187.

24. Piché CA, Radecki SV, Donoghue AR: Results of antibody and antigen testing for feline heartworm infection at HESKA® Veterinary Diagnostic Laboratories. *In* Knight D (ed): The American Heartworm Society: State of the Heartworm Symposium '98. American Heartworm Society, Batavia, IL, 1998, pp. 139–145.

25. Watkins BF, Toro M: Results found using the Animal Diagnostics' heartworm antibody test. *In* Knight D (ed): The American Heartworm Society: State of the Heartworm Symposium '98. American Heartworm Society, Batavia, IL, 1998, pp. 145–153.

26. Genchi C, Kramer L, Venco L, et al: Comparison of antibody and antigen testing with echocardiography for the detection of heartworm (*Dirofilaria immitis*) in cats. *In* Knight D (ed): The American Heartworm Society: State of the Heartworm Symposium '98. American Heartworm Society, Batavia, IL, 1998, pp. 173–179.

27. Schafer M, Berry CR: Cardiac and pulmonary artery mensuration in feline heartworm disease. Vet Radiol Ultrasound 36:499–505, 1995.

28. Birchard SJ, Bilbrey SA: Chylothorax associated with dirofilariasis in a cat. J Am Vet Med Assoc 197:507–509, 1990.

29. DeFrancesco TC, Atkins CE: Utility of echocardiography for the diagnosis of feline heartworm disease. *In* Knight D (ed): The American Heartworm Society: State of the Heartworm Symposium '98. American Heartworm Society, Batavia, IL, 1998, pp. 103–107.

30. Venco L, Morini S, Ferrari E, et al: Technique for identifying heartworms in cats by 2D echocardiography. *In* Knight D (ed): The American Heartworm Society: State of the Heartworm Symposium '98. American Heartworm Society, Batavia, IL, 1998, pp. 97–103.

31. Turner JL, Lees GE, Brown SA, et al: Thiacetarsamide in healthy cats: Clinical and pathological observations. J Am Anim Hosp Assoc 27:275–280, 1991.

32. Brown WA, Thomas WP: Surgical treatment of feline heartworm disease [Abstract]. Proceedings 16th ACVIM Forum 1998, p. 88.

33. Venco L, Borgarelli M, Ferrari E, et al: Surgical removal of heartworms from naturally infected cats. *In* Knight D (ed): The American Heartworm Society: State of the Heartworm Symposium '98. American Heartworm Society, Batavia, IL, 1998, pp. 241–247.

34. Paul AJ, Acre KE, Todd KS, et al: Filaricide therapy in domestic cats: Efficacy of ivermectin against *Dirofilaria immitis* in cats 30 and 45 days post-infection. *In* Soll MD (ed): Proceedings of the Heartworm Symposium '92. American Heartworm Society, Batavia, IL, 1994, pp. 117–120.

35. Donoghue AR, Piché CA, Radecki SV, et al: Effect of prophylaxis on heartworm antibody levels in cats receiving trickle experimental infections of *Dirofilaria immitis*. *In* Knight D (ed): The American Heartworm Society: State of the Heartworm Symposium '98. American Heartworm Society, Batavia, IL, 1998, pp. 135–139.

36. Stewart VA, Hepler DI, Grieve RB: Efficacy of milbemycin oxime in chemoprophylaxis of dirofilariasis in cats. Am J Vet Res 53:2274–2277, 1992.

34

◆ Hypertrophic Cardiomyopathy

Kathryn M. Meurs
Alan W. Spier

Hypertrophic cardiomyopathy (HCM) is a primary heart muscle disease characterized by increased wall thickness and ventricular mass in the absence of an underlying cause of hypertrophy (e.g., hyperthyroidism, systemic hypertension, aortic valve stenosis).[1] HCM is the most common form of acquired heart disease in cats.[2, 3] Both the clinical presentation and the clinical progression of this disease are variable. The classic presentation of a cat affected with HCM is a male, middle-aged cat; however, the disease is observed commonly in both male and female cats ranging from less than 1 year to greater than 16 years of age. Although breed predispositions have been suggested, the most commonly affected breed appears to be the domestic shorthair.[2, 4, 5] The myocardial hypertrophy affects the left ventricle predominantly, and the hypertrophy can be either symmetric (i.e., affect both the interventricular septum [IVS] and the left ventricular free wall [LVFW]) or asymmetric (IVS or LVFW hypertrophy). Although the disease typically is progressive, some cats appear to have fairly static, mild disease for years, some die suddenly, presumably from arrhythmias or embolic episodes, whereas others appear to progress steadily into congestive heart failure. These variations someday may be explained by different etiologies of the disease, but at this time the etiology, although suspected to be familial, largely is unknown.

◆ PATHOLOGY

HCM is characterized by thickening of the ventricular walls and an attendant increase in ventricular mass. Post-mortem measurements of wall thickness are often inaccurate, because of the degree of post-mortem myocardial contracture frequently observed.[6] Therefore, pathologic evaluation of the heart should include a heart weight:body weight ratio to document an increased ventricular mass. The normal heart weight:body weight ratio is 3 to 5 g/kg, whereas cats with HCM typically have ratios exceeding 6.0 g/kg.[4, 6, 7] Hypertrophy of the LVFW, IVS, papillary muscles, and left atrial wall may be observed. Interestingly, the hypertrophy may be symmetric or asymmetric, predominantly affecting either the LVFW or the IVS. If the asymmetric hypertrophy affects the IVS, the hypertrophy often occurs in the anterior portion of the septum, causing partial obstruction of the left ventricular outflow tract.[7]

Histopathologic findings typically include enlarged myocytes with large, rectangular, hyperchromatic nuclei. The muscle bundles may be separated by increased interstitial connective tissue and fibrosis. Disorganization of the muscle cells (myofiber disarray) may be observed. However, this finding is inconsistent, and has been reported in 44 to 100 per cent of the cats evaluated in various studies.[4, 6, 7] Abnormal intramural coronary arteries with thickened walls and narrowed lumens are reported occasionally.[4, 6]

◆ ETIOLOGY

In the majority of cases, the etiology of feline HCM is unknown. There is substantial evidence that the disease is inherited in an autosomal dominant pattern in at least 2 breeds, the Maine coon cat and the American shorthair.[6, 8] Anecdotal information exists regarding families of affected ragdoll, rex, and British shorthair cats, suggesting that HCM also may be inherited in these breeds. It is reasonable to advise owners of affected breeding cats not to breed those animals and to screen closely related family members carefully. Unfortunately, the most commonly affected patient is a domestic shorthair cat without familial history of disease.

◆ PATHOPHYSIOLOGY

The development of clinical signs is related to a cascade of events begining with left ventricular hypertrophy. The hypertrophy of the LVFW and the IVS causes diastolic dysfunction by physical and functional obstruction of the left ventricle, impairing diastolic filling. As the walls hypertrophy, they become stiffer, preventing normal relaxation and contributing to diastolic dysfunction. In some cases, the anterior mitral valve leaflet becomes displaced during systole and is pulled into the left ventricular outflow tract. This causes variable degrees of outflow obstruction and substantial mitral valve insufficiency. This phenomenon is referred to as systolic anterior motion of the mitral valve (SAM). The left ventricular diastolic dysfunction and the mitral valve insufficiency cause stretching and dilatation of the left atrium and increased left atrial pressure. Eventually, this increase in left atrial pressures causes increased pulmonary venous pressures, pulmonary venous congestion, pulmonary edema, and the development of left heart failure. In cats, pulmonary hypertension and right heart failure are believed to develop commonly secondarily to chronic left heart failure. Therefore, in many cases, clinical manifestations of biventricular heart failure are observed.

Cardiac output frequently is decreased because the small left ventricular lumen size and decreased diastolic filling decrease the available stroke volume. If the IVS is hypertrophied asymmetrically, obstruction of the left ventricular outflow tract can occur. This pattern of hypertrophy has been referred to as hypertrophic obstructive cardiomyopathy. The presence of SAM is a marker for HOCM and contributes to obstruction of the left ventricular outflow tract. All of these factors may lead to a low output state, resulting in decreased perfusion.

Cats with HCM are at risk of developing atrial thrombi that may release emboli that obstruct the distal aortic trifurcation, renal arteries, mesenteric arteries, or cerebral vessels.[5] The pathogenesis of these atrial thrombi is poorly understood, but atrial dilatation and hyperaggregability of platelets have been shown to be important factors in their development.[5, 9]

Finally, focal areas of myocardial ischemia may develop when the hypertrophic myocardium is not supplied adequately by the existing coronary circulation. These areas of ischemia may serve as a site for the development of ventricular arrhythmias that may cause syncope or sudden death.

◆ CLINICAL SIGNS

The clinical presentation of cats with HCM is varied. The initial diagnosis is commonly made when an asymptomatic cat presents for routine evaluation and a heart murmur or gallop is ausculted. Alternatively, the initial diagnosis may be made when the cat is presented for sudden onset of hindlimb paralysis due to a saddle thrombus, or dyspnea with the development of congestive heart failure.

Physical examination findings may include a systolic heart murmur or gallop rhythm, ausculted loudest over the sternum or left apex. An arrhythmia may be detected. In one study, 55 per cent of cats with HCM were asymptomatic and were diagnosed based on suspicion of the disease after detection of auscultatory abnormalities.[2] Affected cats may have elevated heart rates, due either to a sinus tachycardia or to other forms of tachyarrhythmias. However, many affected cats, even those in heart failure, have heart rates below 200 bpm.[2] In severe cases, in which congestive heart failure has developed, tachypnea or dyspnea may be observed at rest. Although pulmonary edema is a common development in cats with severe HCM, auscultation of crackles is rare. Cats with advanced left heart failure are at risk of developing pulmonary hypertension, right heart failure, and pleural effusion. Therefore,

cats with cardiac disease that present with dyspnea or tachypnea should be evaluated closely for both pulmonary edema and pleural effusion.

Cats suffering an embolic event typically present with bilateral hindlimb paresis with diminished or nonexistent femoral pulses. Affected legs are often firm and very painful on palpation. Nailbeds may be cyanotic. Less commonly, a thrombus may affect only 1 leg, including the front leg.

◆ RADIOLOGY

HCM commonly is a progressive disease, and radiographic findings are dependent on the stage of progression. If the animal is diagnosed in the early stages, the radiographs may be within normal limits, because the hypertrophy is concentric and may not yet be apparent radiographically. As the disease progresses, left ventricular and left atrial enlargement, pulmonary venous congestion, pulmonary edema, and pleural effusion may be evident (Figs. 34–1 and 34–2).

◆ ELECTROCARDIOGRAPHY

Pathologic changes in the myocardium and associated conduction tissue are noted in cats with HCM. Within the conduction system, these changes are noted primarily in the atrioventricular node and bundle branches, with the sinoatrial node affected uncommonly.[10] Conduction disturbances, such as sinus bradycardia, atrioventricular block, and bundle branch block—most notably left anterior fascicular block—may be observed (Fig. 34–3). Ischemia, cardiac enlargement, and myocardial fibrosis may predispose to atrial fibrillation, and atrial and ventricular premature complexes (VPCs). Cardiac arrhythmias, manifesting as bradyarrhythmias, tachyarrhythmias, or conduction disturbances, occurred in about 30 per cent of cats in one study.[11] In addition to the identification of rhythm disturbances, electrocardiography also may be used to identify chamber enlargement. Electrocardiographic evidence of chamber enlargement has been documented as a common finding.[11] However, in cats, electrocardiographic identification of atrial and ventricular enlargement is poor, because little correlation seems to exist between electrocardiographic findings and echocardiographic and radiographic abnormalities.[12]

Cats affected with HCM can die suddenly, and continuous evaluation of cardiac rhythm is becoming an increasingly important aspect of patient management. In addition to routine electrocardiographic assessment, the use of ambulatory (Holter) monitoring of affected cats has gained in popularity (see Chapter 38, Holter Monitoring). Holter monitoring may provide a means to detect occult cardiac arrhythmias, which may serve to identify cats at risk for arrhythmic deaths or to identify hemodynami-

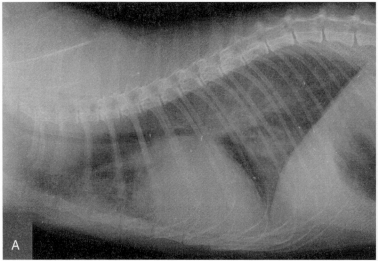

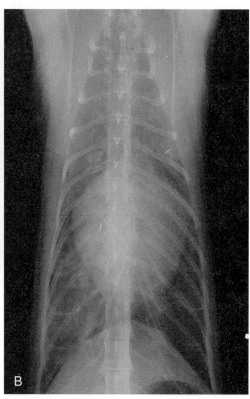

Figure 34–1. Lateral *(A)* and ventrodorsal *(B)* radiographic views of a cat with advanced hypertrophic cardiomyopathy (HCM). Note left ventricular and left atrial enlargement, pulmonary venous congestion, and pulmonary edema.

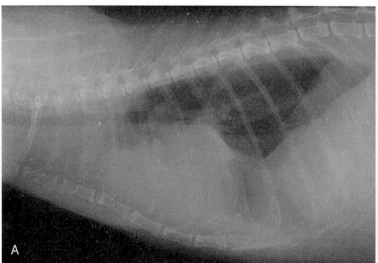

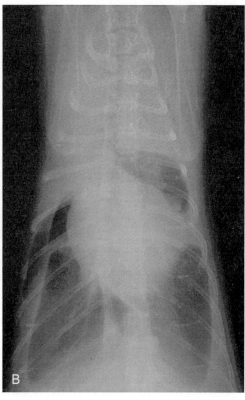

Figure 34–2. Lateral *(A)* and ventrodorsal *(B)* radiographic views of a cat with advanced HCM. Note the pleural effusion and prominent left side *(B)*.

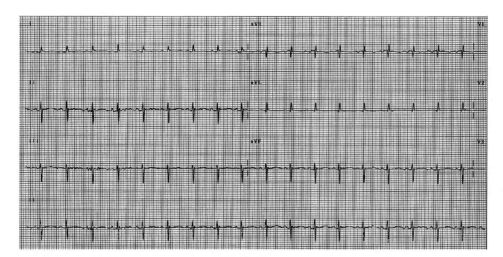

Figure 34–3. An electrocardiogram from a 4-year-old male castrated cat with HCM at a paper speed of 50 mm/sec. The heart rate is 214 bpm. The complexes are of normal height and duration, but there is a prominent, deep S wave in leads II, III, and AVF but not in lead I. This is a pattern that is consistent with a left anterior fascicular block (axis, −53 degrees).

cally important arrhythmias.[13] When interpreting the results of a Holter monitor, it should be remembered that very little information about Holter monitoring of normal cats exists. One investigation disclosed the presence of ventricular premature ectopic beats in normal cats, especially in cats older than 8 years of age. The number of VPCs was not very high; 19 of 20 normal cats had less than 60 VPCs/24 hr. Supraventricular premature complexes were uncommon.[14] Therefore, the observation of a small number of VPCs may be a normal finding in some cats.

◆ ECHOCARDIOGRAPHY

Echocardiography currently is the most sensitive method for the diagnosis of HCM (see Chapter 32, Echocardiography). Because HCM is now the most common form of acquired heart disease in cats, patients with heart murmurs, gallops, or auscultable arrhythmias should be evaluated by echocardiography to determine whether HCM is present. Echocardiography should be performed in right lateral recumbency. Evaluation should include both a 2-dimensional and an M-mode study, to avoid missing asymmetric areas of hypertrophy. The recommended criterion for diagnosis is demonstration of LVFW or IVS thickness greater than 6 mm at maximal diastole using M-mode and 2-dimensional measurements.[13, 15] The location and distribution of the hypertrophy are quite variable. It would appear that asymmetric hypertrophy of either the IVS or the LVFW occurs more frequently than diffuse symmetric hypertrophy.[4, 15]

Although ventricular function should be evaluated, most cases have fractional shortening values within normal range (30 to 60 per cent). A small percentage of cats with HCM have been observed to have abnormally low fractional shortening values. It has been suggested that this may be a natural progression of some cases of HCM; however, it also is possible that these cats may have a slightly different form of the disease, or one caused by a different etiology. Those cats with diminished fractional shortening appear to have a poorer prognosis.[15]

In some cases, the distal tip of the anterior mitral valve can be observed to make contact with the IVS during midsystole. This is the echocardiographic manifestation of SAM. This finding may be observed on a long-axis view of the left ventricle, but often is easier to see in the M-mode view of the mitral valve. Continuous-wave Doppler may be used to determine the degree of obstruction caused by SAM.

Left atrial enlargement is observed frequently. Left atrial size measurements may be obtained either from a short axis 2-dimensional view at the base of the heart or from the right parasternal long-axis projection, with the beam oriented to measure left atrial size. The ratio of left atrial size to aortic root diameter probably is more accurate than measurement of left atrial size alone. Most normal cats will have a left atrial:aortic root ratio less than or equal to 1.3.

◆ CLINICAL PATHOLOGY

There are no classic hematologic or chemistry abnormalities associated with HCM. In advanced cases in which cardiac output is significantly reduced, elevations in blood urea nitrogen and creatinine may be observed. If biventricular failure has occurred resulting in hepatic venous congestion, mild elevations in liver enzymes may exist.

◆ DIFFERENTIAL DIAGNOSIS

Ventricular hypertrophy can be the result of several other disease processes. HCM is a primary heart muscle disease, and the diagnosis should be made only after ruling out other causes of ventricular hypertrophy. The most common cause of secondary left ventricular hypertrophy (LVH) is hyperthyroidism. Thyroid hormone levels should be evaluated in all cats with LVH that are in the at-risk age group. Systemic hypertension (see Chapter 36, Systemic

Hypertension, and 47, Diagnosis and Treatment of Systemic Hypertension) can lead to the development of hypertrophy; however, it usually is very mild.[16] It is very uncommon for systemic hypertension to lead to the development of severe hypertrophy and congestive heart failure; however, it is important to evaluate blood pressure in all cats with LVH. Aortic stenosis can cause LVH secondary to increased left ventricular systolic pressures. This is fairly uncommon in cats, but should be considered in cats with a left basilar systolic heart murmur, especially if the murmur had been present since a young age.

◆ THERAPY

Therapy for affected cats is directed toward palliation of clinical signs. There are no known treatments for successful reduction of myocardial hypertrophy in cats. Efforts in human medicine have included both surgical and chemical ablation of muscle tissue.[17, 18] Treatment for the affected cat typically is directed toward 2 goals: control of heart rate to allow for maximum passive diastolic filling, and improved diastolic relaxation (lusitropy). Two commonly used classes of drugs for the treatment of HCM are beta blockers (atenolol, propranolol) and calcium channel blockers (diltiazem). The decision to choose a beta blocker preferentially over a calcium channel blocker, or vice versa, rarely is a clear-cut choice, and often is based on personal experience. Esmolol, a short-acting intravenous beta blocker, reduced the degree of outflow tract obstruction and heart rate in 6 cats with hypertrophic obstructive cardiomyopathy.[19] Therefore, beta blockers may be indicated in cats with this form of the disease. Some authors believe that calcium channel blockers have a stronger lusitropic effect than beta blockers in human beings, although significant clinical evidence is lacking.[20] One feline study suggested beneficial effects when cats with HCM were given diltiazem, a calcium channel blocker at 7.5 mg/cat, orally (PO) every (q) 8 hr.[21] It should be emphasized, however, that large controlled therapeutic studies do not exist for cats with HCM, and there is little evidence that one class of drug is substantially better than the other.

Two beta blockers are used commonly in cats with HCM, propranolol and atenolol. The more selective nature of atenolol and the ability to dose less frequently than with propranolol has made atenolol a more attractive option. Although atenolol originally was believed to be appropriate at once-daily dosing, pharmacologic studies have demonstrated that beta blockade did not last 24 hours. Therefore, the current recommendations are for a dose of 3 mg/kg PO q 12 hr.[22]

Diltiazem HCL is the calcium channel blocker used most commonly in affected cats. Unfortunately, serum concentrations of diltiazem HCL are only in the therapeutic range for approximately 8 hours after oral administration.[23] The inconvenience of dosing a medication 3 times daily may be alleviated by using one of the longer-acting diltiazem products. Diltiazem CD at 10 mg/kg PO q 24 hr has been shown to be a reasonable option. This product is dispensed in a 180-mg capsule containing smaller capsules that can be divided for administration.

Therapy for congestive heart failure should be initiated as needed. Thoracocentesis should be performed if pleural fluid is present. Lasix and oxygen therapy should be given if necessary. The use of angiotensin converting enzyme inhibitors for therapy of heart failure in the cat with HCM has not been well studied; however, one study did show that enalapril appeared to be well tolerated at 1.25 to 2.5 mg/cat PO q 24 hr. Side-effects such as azotemia, hyperkalemia, and hypotension were not observed.[3]

◆ SADDLE THROMBUS

Treatment for the cat with a saddle thrombus requires attention to both the embolic episode and the cardiovascular status. It is important to keep the cat quiet and as comfortable as possible. Treatment for congestive heart failure should be initiated if needed. Treatment for pain may include a combination of butorphanol tartrate and acepromazine. Heparin should be given at 220 IU/kg intravenously (IV) initially to prevent additional clots from forming and then 100 to 200 IU/kg subcutaneously (SQ) q 8 hr. Retrospective studies suggest that at least 50 per cent of cats with an embolic event secondary to HCM will have a second embolic episode within 12 months.[24]

The severity of the consequences of thromboembolic episodes and the likelihood of recurrent embolic events have created an interest in prophylactic use of anticoagulants. Aspirin frequently is given as a prophylactic treatment when left atrial enlargement is diagnosed, or after the first embolic episode occurs. A dose of 25 mg/kg inhibits platelet aggregation for 3 to 5 days in cats.[25, 26] The current recommendation is 1 baby aspirin (81 mg) q 72 hr. Although this dose has been shown to decrease platelet aggregation, it has never been demonstrated to decrease the risk of a second embolic episode. Owing to the significant risk of a second embolic episode, some investigators have attempted to use different anticoagulants, including warfarin (Coumadin). Unfortunately, the risk of re-embolization for cats on warfarin therapy has been shown to be at least 40 per cent, and the use of warfarin (see Chapter 39, Aortic Thromboembolism) is associated with the risk of spontaneous hemorrhage.[24]

◆ PROGNOSIS

The prognosis for cats affected with HCM is quite variable, with several factors being important in disease outcome. Perhaps the most important indicator for prognosis is the presence or absence of clinical signs associated with disease. Cats that present with no clinical signs, whose evidence of cardiovascular disease is limited to physical findings such as a heart murmur and/or gallop rhythm, have a better survival rate than cats that present with clinical signs such as congestive heart failure or thromboembolism. In one study, median survival for all cats affected with HCM was 732 days.[2] However, in cats with no clinical signs, median survival was over 5 years, whereas cats with CHF and thromboembolism had median survival times of 92 and 61 days, respectively.[2] Six months after diagnosis, 60 per cent of cats with congestive heart failure and all cats with thromboembolism were dead.[2] Survival of cats with thromboembolic disease has been reported to be somewhat better (average of 11 months) by other investigators.[5] Prognosis for cats that survive a thromboembolic episode depends on the severity of the embolic event, the severity of the underlying cardiac disease, the presence or absence of congestive heart failure, and whether abdominal organ involvement has occurred (generally a very poor prognostic sign). It should be noted that a high percentage of cats with embolic episodes are euthanized owing to the severity of the cats' underlying disease process, making it difficult to estimate survival time accurately.

Heart rate, left atrial size, and degree of IVS hypertrophy all have been suggested as additional prognostic indicators.[2, 4, 5, 15] Cats that had heart rates greater than or equal to 200 bpm at initial presentation had worse long-term survival times than cats that presented with heart rates less than 200 bpm. Median survival times for cats with heart rates less than 200 bpm were over 5 years, and cats with heart rates above 200 bpm had median survival times of 152 days.[2] Cats with left atrial enlargement and cats with severe IVS hypertrophy also have a poorer prognosis.[4, 5, 15]

REFERENCES

1. Davies MJ, McKenna WJ. Hypertrophic cardiomyopathy—Pathology and pathogenesis. Histopathology 26:493, 1997.
2. Atkins CE, Gallo AM, Kurzman ID, et al: Risk factors, clinical signs, and survival in cats with a clinical diagnosis of idiopathic hypertrophic cardiomyopathy: 74 cases (1985–1989). J Am Vet Med Assoc 201:613, 1992.
3. Rush JE, Freeman LM, Brown DJ, et al: The use of enalapril in the treatment of feline hypertrophic cardiomyopathy. J Am Anim Hosp Assoc 34:38, 1998.
4. Fox PR, Liu S-K, Maron BJ: Echocardiographic assessment of spontaneously occurring feline hypertrophic cardiomyopathy: An animal model of human disease. Circulation 92:2645, 1995.
5. Laste N, Harpster N: A retrospective study of 100 cases of feline distal aortic thromboembolism: 1977–1993. J Am Anim Hosp Assoc 31:492, 1995.
6. Kittleson, MD, Meurs, KM, Munro, MJ, et al: Familial hypertrophic cardiomyopathy in Maine coon cats: An animal model of human disease. Circulation 99:3172, 1999.
7. Liu S-K: Pathology of feline heart diseases. Vet Clin North Am Small Anim Pract 7:323, 1977.
8. Meurs KM, Kittleson MD, Towbin JA, et al: Familial systolic anterior motion of the mitral valve and/or hypertrophic cardiomyopathy is apparently inherited as an autosomal dominant trait in American shorthair cats [Abstract]. J Vet Intern Med 11:138, 1997.
9. Helenski CA, Ross JN: Platelet aggregation in feline cardiomyopathy. J Vet Intern Med 1:24, 1987.
10. Liu S-K, Tilley LP, Tashjian RJ: Lesions of the conduction system in the cat with cardiomyopathy. Recent Adv Stud Cardiac Struct Metab 10:681, 1975.
11. Liu S-K, Tilley L: Animal models of primary myocardial diseases. Yale J Biol Med 53:191, 1980.
12. Moïse NS, Dietze AE, Mezza LE, et al: Echocardiography, electrocardiography, and radiography of cats with dilatation cardiomyopathy, hypertrophic cardiomyopathy, and hyperthyroidism. Am J Vet Res 47:1476, 1986.
13. Goodwin JK, Lombard CW, Ginex DD: Results of continuous ambulatory electrocardiography in a cat with hypertrophic cardiomyopathy. J Am Vet Med Assoc 200:1352, 1992.
14. Ware WA: Twenty-four-hour ambulatory electrocardiography in normal cats. J Vet Intern Med 13:175, 1999.
15. Peterson E, Moïse NS, Brown CA, et al: Heterogeneity of hypertrophy in feline hypertrophic heart disease. J Vet Intern Med 7:183, 1993.
16. Nelson OL, Riedesel EA, Ware WA: Echocardiographic and radiographic changes associated with systemic hypertension in cats [Abstract]. J Vet Intern Med 13:246, 1999.
17. Kofflard MJ, van Herwerden LA, Waldstein DJ, et al: Initial results of combined anterior mitral leaflet extension and myectomy in patients with obstructive hypertrophic cardiomyopathy. J Am Coll Cardiol 28:197, 1996.
18. Faber L, Seggewiss H, Gleichmann U: Percutaneous transluminal septal myocardial ablation in hypertrophic obstructive cardiomyopathy. Circulation 98:2415, 1998.
19. Bonagura JD, Stepien RL, Lehmkuhl LB: Acute effects of esmolol on left ventricular outflow obstruction in cats with hypertrophic cardiomyopathy: A doppler-echocardiographic study [Abstract]. J Vet Intern Med 9:878, 1991.
20. Betocchi S, Piscione F, Losi M-A, et al: Effects of diltiazem on left ventricular systolic and diastolic function in hypertrophic cardiomyopathy. Am J Cardiol 78:451–457, 1996.
21. Bright JM, Golden AL, Gompf RE, et al: Evaluation of the calcium channel–blocking agents diltiazem and verapamil for treatment of feline hypertrophic cardiomyopathy. J Vet Intern Med 5:272, 1991.
22. Quinones M, Dyer DC, Ware WA, Mehvar R. Pharmacokinetics of atenolol in clinically normal cats. Am J Vet Res 57:1050, 1996.
23. Johnson LM, Atkins CE, Keene BW, et al: Pharmacokinetic and pharmacodynamic properties of conventional and CD-formulated diltiazem in cats. J Vet Intern Med 10:316, 1996.
24. Harpster NK, Baty CJ: Warfarin therapy of the cat at risk of thromboembolism. In Bonagura JD (ed): Current Veterinary Therapy XII. Philadelphia, WB Saunders, 1995, p. 868.
25. Greene CE: Effects of aspirin and propanolol on feline platelet aggregation. Am J Vet Res 46:1820, 1985.
26. Allen DG, Johnstone IB, Crane S: Effects of aspirin and propanolol alone and in combination on hemostatic determinants in the healthy cat. Am J Vet Res 46:660, 1985.

35

◆ Chylothorax

Theresa W. Fossum

Chylous effusions, particularly chylothorax, are reported frequently in cats.[1] *Chyle* is the term used to denote lymphatic fluid arising from the intestine and therefore containing a high quantity of fat. Chyle normally is transported to the venous system by a network of lymphatics in the mesentery (intestinal trunk). These lymphatics arborize in the cisterna chyli, a large dilated sac that lies adjacent to the aorta at L1–L4. The thoracic duct is the cranial continuation of the cisterna chyli, and is generally said to begin between the crura of the diaphragm.[2] In cats, the thoracic duct lies between the aorta and the azygous vein on the left side of the thorax, and terminates in the venous system of the neck (left external jugular vein or jugulosubclavian angle).[3]

The initial report of chylothorax in the veterinary literature appeared in 1958, and described the surgical treatment of 3 dogs and 1 cat.[4] Although the surgery has been refined since this early report, our ability to treat many patients has been hindered by a lack of understanding of the etiology of this disease. Appropriate management of cats with chylous effusions depends on critical evaluation of the fluid and a thorough understanding of underlying causes.

Regardless of the etiology, chylothorax is a potentially devastating disease. The basal rate of lymph flow in the thoracic duct of dogs has been estimated to be 2 ml/kg/hr[5, 6]; it is probably similar for cats. This rate varies depending on diet, being greatest after a high-fat meal. Sixty to 70 per cent of all ingested fats are conveyed to the blood stream by way of the thoracic duct, and the thoracic duct also is the main pathway for protein transport from the capillary spaces to the venous system. Consequently, chylothorax results in both compromised respiration and debilitation because of loss of large amounts of proteins, fats, fat-soluble vitamins, and lymphocytes into the pleural cavity. Electrolyte abnormalities may occur in patients with chylothorax; hyperkalemia and hyponatremia have been noted in dogs with both experimental and spontaneous chylothorax undergoing multiple thoracenteses.[7]

Chylous fluid usually is a white or pinkish, opaque fluid in which a cream layer will form when left to stand (Figs. 35–1 and 35–2 and Table 35–1). Although chylous effusions are classified routinely as exudates, the physical characteristics of the fluid may be consistent with a modified transudate (protein content >2.5 gm/dl but <4.0 gm/dl, and total nucleated cell count of >1000 but <7000 cells/μl).[1] The protein content is variable, and often measured inaccurately owing to changes in the refractive index by the high lipid content of the fluid. Cytolog-

ically, the fluid consists primarily of small lymphocytes or neutrophils, with lesser numbers of lipid-laden macrophages (Fig. 35–3). Chronic chylous effusions may contain lower numbers of small lymphocytes if the body is unable to compensate for the continued loss of lymphocytes into the fluid. Nondegenerative neutrophils often predominate with prolonged loss of lymphocytes, particularly if multiple therapeutic thoracocenteses have induced inflammation. Degenerative neutrophils associated with microbial contamination are uncommon due to the bacteriostatic effect of lecithin and fatty acids, but infection may occur iatrogenically with repeated aspirations. When centrifuged, chylous fluid will not clear (versus an exudate with a high cellular content, such as a pyothorax), and chylomicrons usually can be seen on smears.

Although chylous effusions have a characteristic appearance, the physical characteristics of chylous effusions and other exudative effusions may be sim-

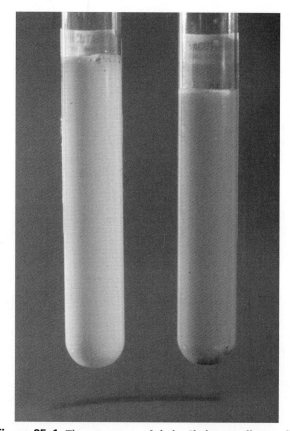

Figure 35–1. The appearance of chyle. Chyle typically is milky white (left tube), but may be red or pink if contaminated with blood (right tube).

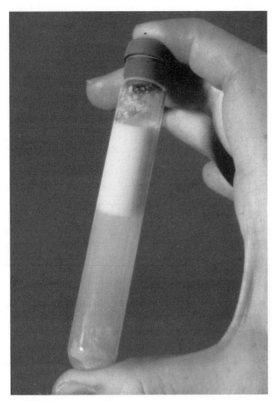

Figure 35–2. The appearance of chyle when it is left to stand. Note that a cream layer has formed in the tube. Fluid analysis should be performed only on fluid that is well-mixed.

Table 35–1. Characteristics of Feline Chylous Effusions

Color	White or pink (occasionally red)
Clarity	Opaque, remains opaque when centrifuged
Specific gravity	1.019–1.050 (avg., 1.032)
Total protein (g/dl)	2.6–10.3 (avg., 5.0)
Chylomicrons	Present
Total WBC/μl	1650–24,420 (avg., 7987)
Predominant cell type	Lymphocytes or neutrophils
Triglyceride content	>Serum
Cholesterol content	≤Serum
Sudanophilic fat globules	Present
Ether clearance test	Clears

Abbreviation: WBC, white blood cells.
Modified from Surgery of the lower respiratory system: Pleural cavity and diaphragm. *In* Fossum TW (ed): Small Animal Surgery. St. Louis, Mosby, 1997, Tables 27–8 and 27–9.

ilar. Additionally, the appearance and cell populations of chylous effusions may be altered by diet and chronicity. To help determine whether a pleural effusion is truly chylous, several tests may be performed, including comparison of fluid and serum triglyceride levels, Sudan III stain for lipid droplets, and ether clearance test. The most diagnostic test is comparison of serum and fluid triglyceride levels.[8] True chylous effusions are those in which the pleural fluid triglyceride is greater than the serum triglyceride. True chylous effusions have been re-

ported in association with many diseases in cats, including right heart failure due to numerous causes, including cardiomyopathy,[9] congenital cardiac disease, and heartworm infection[10, 11]; mediastinal masses[1, 12]; and pericardial effusion. Because appearance and triglyceride content of the fluid are affected by dietary fat intake, chylous effusions in anorexic animals may not appear white, and may have lower than expected triglyceride concentrations. Pleural fluid samples should be submitted after feeding in such animals.

Both the Sudan III staining and the ether clearance tests are crude estimates of fat content.[13] Staining the fluid with Sudan III to evaluate for the presence of lipid droplets may be diagnostic for chylous effusion, but the absence of fat droplets does not rule out chylothorax. Feeding a high-fat meal 2 hours before collecting fluid for Sudan III is recommended to help decrease the number of false-negative results. The ether clearance test is based on the solubility of chylomicrons in ether. Equal volumes of ether and pleural fluid are mixed after alkalinization of the pleural fluid with 1 to 2 drops of sodium hydroxide. If the fluid is chyle, the chylomicrons will dissolve and the fluid will clear. Because the

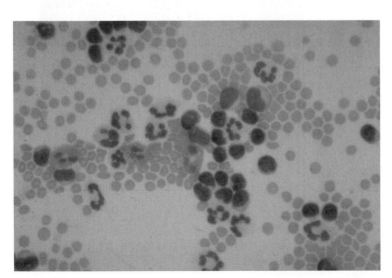

Figure 35–3. Typical cytologic appearance of a chylous effusion. Note that both nondegenerative neutrophils and lymphocytes are present. 40×.

ether clearance test also is a crude test and is often difficult to interpret, it should be used only as an ancillary aid to diagnosis.

◆ SIGNALMENT

Although a gender predisposition to chylothorax has not been identified in the veterinary literature, both age and breed appear to be predisposing factors.[1] Purebred cats were overrepresented in one study population (particularly Siamese cats), suggesting that they may have a congenital predisposition to chylothorax, similar to that seen in Afghan hounds.[1, 14] The etiology of such a predisposition in both species, if genuine, is unknown. In the former study, purebred cats also appeared to have a higher probability of survival than did mixed-breed cats, which may signify differences in the etiology or pathophysiology of this disease in the 2 groups.

Chylothorax may affect cats of any age; however, in one study, older cats were more likely to develop chylothorax than were younger cats.[1] This finding was believed to be indicative of an association between chylothorax and neoplasia in some cats.

◆ CLINICAL SIGNS

Clinical signs associated with chylothorax vary depending on the underlying etiology, rapidity of fluid accumulation, and volume of fluid. Most cats do not exhibit clinical signs until there is significant impairment of ventilation; hence, pleural effusion first may be suspected by the veterinarian on careful thoracic auscultation. Muffled heart sounds, absence of lung sounds ventrally, and increased bronchovesicular sounds dorsally may be noted, before the presence of obvious clinical signs.

The most common presenting clinical sign in cats with chylothorax is dyspnea. The owners often report that the animal has had rapid heavy breathing, exercise intolerance, and lethargy for months and may have been treated for nonspecific respiratory problems without improvement before the diagnosis. The dyspnea in cats with chylothorax, as in other types of pleural effusion, usually is marked by a forceful inspiration with what appears to be a delayed expiration, as though the cat is "holding its breath." Interestingly, many of the owners report that the first abnormality they noted was coughing. Coughing, although not typically associated with pleural effusion of noncardiac origin, appears to be a common finding in chylothorax. It is the author's belief that the cough is not a causative agent in the development of the chylothorax, but rather is a result of irritation caused by the effusion, or is related to the underlying disease process (such as cardiomyopathy or thoracic neoplasia).

On physical examination, increased bronchovesicular sounds heard dorsally and absence of lung sounds ventrally (usually bilaterally, but occasionally unilaterally), weight loss, and tachycardia may be noted. Most cats with chylothorax present with a normal body temperature, unless extremely excited or severely depressed. Cats with elevated temperatures should be evaluated for the presence of pyothorax, rather than chylothorax. If the cat has had previous thoracenteses, secondary bacterial infections of the chyle may be superimposed. Although chyle generally is thought to be bacteriostatic, the author is aware of several cats with chylothorax that developed pyothorax after multiple thoracenteses or surgical intervention. Additional findings in patients with chylothorax may include depression, anorexia, weight loss, pale mucous membranes, arrhythmias, murmurs, ascites, and pericardial effusion.

◆ DIAGNOSIS

If the cat is not overtly dyspneic, thoracic radiographs should be taken to confirm the diagnosis of pleural fluid (Figs. 35–4 and 35–5). During radiographic procedures, minimizing manipulation and stress by performing dorsoventral (rather than ventrodorsal) views, and standing lateral views may be necessary to prevent further compromise of respiration. Supplementing oxygen by face mask during the procedure also may be beneficial. In the severely dyspneic cat, it is best to remove fluid by needle

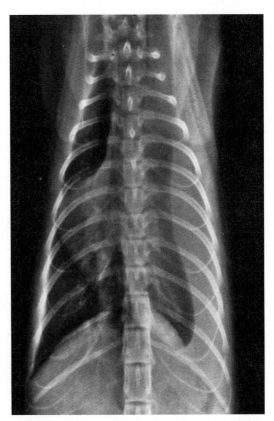

Figure 35–4. Dorsoventral thoracic radiograph of a cat with unilateral chylothorax. Unilateral effusions typically occur with exudative effusions such as pyothorax and chylothorax.

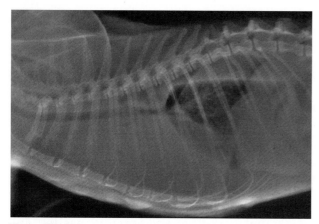

Figure 35–5. Lateral thoracic radiograph of a cat with chylothorax. Note the dorsal elevation of the trachea. A mediastinal mass was suspected based on these radiographs, and was confirmed by fine-needle aspiration of the cranial mediastinal area.

thoracentesis before taking radiographs. A small-gauge (21 or 23) butterfly system (Butterfly catheter, Abbotts Hospital Inc., North Chicago, IL) works well. Removal of even small amounts of pleural effusion may greatly improve the cat's ability to ventilate. Large amounts of pleural effusion may interfere with normal movement of the diaphragm and chest wall. Inversion of the diaphragm, as occurs with massive pleural effusion, may cause it to move paradoxically with respiration. Thus, removal of small amounts of pleural effusion, if associated with the diaphragm returning toward normal contour, may cause significant relief of dyspnea. Animals that remain dyspneic after removal of pleural fluid should be suspected of having underlying pulmonary parenchymal or pleural disease, such as fibrosing pleuritis.

Fluid recovered should be placed in an ethylenediaminetetraacetic acid (EDTA) tube for cytologic examination. Placing the fluid in an EDTA tube rather than a "clot-tube" will allow cell counts to be performed. Triglyceride concentrations should be determined on both the pleural fluid and the serum for comparison (see earlier). Fluid also should be submitted for culture and sensitivity.

The presence of pleural fluid often will prevent satisfactory visualization of the structures of the thoracic cavity on radiography. Adequate visualization of the entire thorax is necessary to rule out anterior mediastinal masses, such as lymphosarcoma or thymoma. If ultrasonographic capabilities are present, they should be performed before removing large quantities of fluid because the fluid acts as an "acoustic window" enhancing visualization of thoracic structures. Chylous fluid in the thoracic cavity may be free or encapsulated. When encapsulated, the fluid is confined by fibrinous adhesions, and its distribution is not affected by gravity.

Fibrosing pleuritis is a condition that has been associated with chylothorax in cats.[15, 16] Although the cause of the fibrosis is unknown, it apparently can develop subsequent to any prolonged exudative

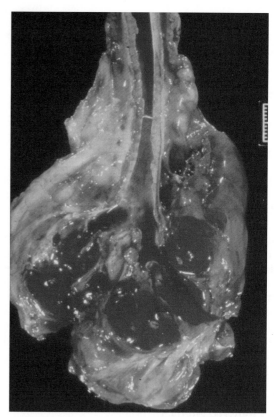

Figure 35–6. The lungs of a cat with fibrosing pleuritis associated with chylothorax. Note the thickened pleura and the rounded appearance of the lung lobes.

(chylothorax, pyothorax) or blood-stained (hemothorax) effusion. In patients with fibrosing pleuritis, the pleura is thickened by diffuse fibrous tissue that restricts normal pulmonary expansion (Figs. 35–6 and 35–7). Animals with fibrosing pleuritis may be misdiagnosed as having large amounts of pleural effusion, when in fact the pleural effusion is minimal. Diagnosis of fibrosing pleuritis is difficult. The atelectatic lobes may be confused with metastatic or

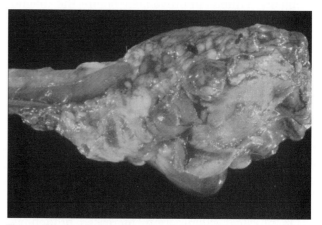

Figure 35–7. Lateral view of lungs of a cat with chronic chylothorax. Note the severe atelectasis and rounded appearance of the cranial lung lobes.

primary pulmonary neoplasia, lung lobe torsion, or hilar lymphadenopathy. Radiographic evidence of pulmonary parenchyma that fails to re-expand after removal of pleural fluid should be considered possible evidence of atelectasis with associated fibrosis. Fibrosing pleuritis also should be considered in animals with persistent dyspnea, but with minimal pleural fluid. In human beings, computed tomography occasionally is helpful in differentiating pleural fibrosis from other abnormalities, such as neoplasia.[17, 18]

◆ ETIOLOGY

Chylothorax previously was thought to be due to thoracic-duct rupture secondary to trauma; however, this is now known to be a rare cause of chylothorax in animals. Other causes include mediastinal lymphosarcoma,[12] cardiomyopathy[9] (particularly secondary to hyperthyroidism), pericardial effusion, congenital cardiac abnormalities, and heartworm infection.[10, 11] In a majority of cats, despite extensive diagnostic work-ups, the underlying etiology is undetermined (idiopathic chylothorax).[1] Because the treatment of this disease varies considerably depending on the underlying etiology, it is imperative that the clinician identify concurrent disease processes before instituting definitive therapy (Table 35–2).

Any disease that results in high venous pressures may cause chylothorax; cardiomyopathy, pericardial effusion, congenital cardiac abnormalities, and heartworm disease have been associated with chylothorax in cats. Thus, a complete cardiac work-up is

Table 35–2. Checklist for Managing Cats With Chylothorax

Thoracentesis
Fluid analysis
  Triglyceride concentrations (compare with serum concentrations)
  Cytologic examination
  Culture and sensitivity
  ±Ether clearance test
Perform as necessary to relieve dyspnea

Radiology
Lateral and ventrodorsal (or dorsoventral) views

Ultrasonography
Evaluate for the presence of mediastinal masses
Assess cardiac function and structure

Blood Work
Complete blood count
Biochemical profile, including serum triglyceride concentrations
Heartworm test (occult)
FeLV antigen and FIV antibody tests

Abbreviations: FeLV, feline leukemia virus; FIV, feline immunodeficiency virus.

warranted in all cats with confirmed chylothorax. Treatment of cats with cardiomyopathy and chylothorax should be based primarily on palliation when necessary with thoracentesis, and improving cardiac output and decreasing venous pressures with appropriate drug therapy. Although heartworm infection is uncommon in cats (see Chapter 33, Heartworm Disease), experimental infection with *Dirofilaria immitis* results in chylothorax in a small number of cases.[10] Naturally occurring heartworm disease also has been associated with chylothorax in a cat.[11] It is recommended that cats with chylothorax be screened for heartworm infection. If pericardial effusion is diagnosed, the underlying etiology should be determined and pericardiectomy performed, if indicated.

If an anterior mediastinal mass is identified, a fine-needle aspirate may be performed to determine the tumor or tissue type (see Chapter 68, Evaluation and Treatment of Cranial Mediastinal Masses). Specific therapy (i.e., radiation therapy, chemotherapy, antifungal therapy, surgery) then should be instituted according to findings. In these animals, the chylous effusion probably is secondary to compression of the cranial vena cava by the mass, and shrinkage of the mass may result in resolution of the pleural fluid. For prognostic purposes, it is prudent to assess feline leukemia virus and feline immunodeficiency virus status in affected cats. Traumatic chylothorax probably occurs more commonly in animals with chylothorax than would be expected based on reported cases. However, in most of these animals the thoracic duct heals spontaneously.

When no obvious underlying disorder can be found, the term *idiopathic* chylothorax is used. Unfortunately, treatment of cats with idiopathic chylothorax is difficult because no highly effective treatment exists. Until the etiology of chylothorax in these patients is understood, therapy will remain palliative and less than optimal in many instances. One possibility is that these animals have increased volumes of lymph being transported through the thoracic duct. These increased flows may occur secondary to abnormal right-sided venous pressures that cause much of the lymph, which normally would be transported from the liver into the venous system, to be shunted into the lymphatic system. Possibly, minimally elevated venous pressures, in association with other unknown factors, may be sufficient to elevate lymphatic flows substantially through the thoracic duct.

◆ MEDICAL MANAGEMENT

Because the surgical options for treating this condition require a high level of expertise to be successful, and because the condition may resolve spontaneously with time, many cats are initially treated medically. This involves feeding a low-fat diet, performing needle thoracentesis as needed to relieve dyspnea (not on a regular basis), and supplementing the cat with a benzopyrone such as Rutin (The Solgar Vitamin Co., Lynbrook, NY; 50 to 100 mg/kg orally [PO] every [q] 8 hr). Owners should be warned of the potential development and grave prognosis associated with severe fibrosing pleuritis in cats with chronic chylothorax. If medical management is being attempted, it is important to provide for the patient's nutritional and metabolic needs until the effusion resolves spontaneously. Generally, meeting the animal's caloric needs by feeding a low-fat diet or a homemade diet is adequate (Table 35–3). Supplementing the diet with low- or medium-chain triglycerides is no longer advised because cats find these supplements to be unpalatable and their efficacy is questionable.

◆ SURGICAL OPTIONS

Surgical intervention may be warranted in patients that do not have underlying disease and in which medical management becomes impractical, such as in cats that require thoracentesis more frequently than once weekly, or those in which repeat thoracentesis fails to relieve the dyspnea. Surgical options in cases uncomplicated by severe fibrosing pleuritis include mesenteric lymphangiography and thoracic-duct ligation, subtotal pericardiectomy,

Table 35–3. Feline Homemade Low-Fat Diet

Ingredient	Amount*
Cooked white rice	3⅔ c
Stewed chicken	½ lb
Dicalcium phosphate†	1½ tsp
GNC Ca-Mg (600 mg Ca/tab)‡	1½ tablets
Morton Lite Salt	1 tsp
Taurine tablets (500 mg taurine/tab)§	3 tablets
Zinc (50 mg zinc/tab)‖	½ tablet
Feline Pet Tab	3 tablets
Radiant Valley Natural Selenium (100 μg Se/tab)¶	½ tablet
Nature Made Balanced B-50 Complex**	½ tablet
GNC Choline (250 mg choline/tab)‡	1 tablet

Directions: Cook the rice without salt. Boil the chicken and skim off the fat. Crush the tablets to a fine powder. Combine all ingredients and mix well. Refrigerate unused portions.

*Calculations based on average published nutrient content of each ingredient indicate that this diet meets or exceeds the nutrient requirements for adult maintenance cats published by the Association of American Feed Control Officials. This recipe makes about 2¼ lb of food that contains 1293 kcals of metabolizable energy.
†Dicalcium phosphate 18.5% phosphorus, 22–24% calcium, available at farm supply and feed stores.
‡General Nutrition Corporation, Pittsburgh, PA; available at GNC Nutrition Centers.
§Taurine tablets can be purchased at most health food stores and cooperatives as 500-mg and 1000-mg tablets.
‖Available at many supermarkets.
¶Perrigo Company, Allegan, MI; available at many supermarkets or health food stores.
**Nature Made Nutritional Products, Los Angeles, CA; available at many supermarkets.
From Fossum TW (ed): Small Animal Surgery. St. Louis, Mosby, 1997.

passive pleuroperitoneal shunting, active pleuroperitoneal or pleurovenous shunting, and pleurodesis. Of these, only thoracic-duct ligation and pericardiectomy are recommended by the author.

Thoracic-Duct Ligation With Mesenteric Lymphangiography

Thoracic-duct ligation is performed in cats from a left lateral intercostal thoracotomy or transdiaphragmatically. The mechanism by which thoracic-duct ligation is purported to work is that after thoracic-duct ligation, abdominal lymphaticovenous anastomoses form for the transport of chyle to the venous system. Therefore, chyle bypasses the thoracic duct and the effusion resolves. Unfortunately, thoracic-duct ligation results in complete resolution of pleural effusion in only 50 per cent of dogs operated[19]; in cats, the success rate is even less (<40 per cent).[1, 20] Advantages of thoracic-duct ligation are that if it is successful, it results in complete resolution of pleural fluid (as compared with palliative procedures, described later), and may prevent fibrosing pleuritis from developing. The disadvantages include a long operative time, which is problematic in debilitated cats; there is a high incidence of continued or recurrent chylous or nonchylous (from pulmonary lymphatics) effusions; and mesenteric lymphangiography is often difficult to perform in cats. Without mesenteric lymphangiography, complete ligation of the thoracic duct cannot be ensured; however, an experimental paper assessing lymphangiography in cats suggested that this technique may not be uniformly successful in verifying complete ligation of the thoracic duct.[21] Additionally, some animals may form collateral lymphatics past the site of the ligature and thus re-establish thoracic duct flow. If chyle flow is directed into the diaphragmatic lymphatics, chylothorax may continue or recur.

For lymphangiography, food is withheld 12 hours before surgery. Either the left side of the thorax and left abdomen, or just the abdomen if a midline celiotomy is being performed, is prepared for aseptic surgery. If a thoracic approach to the thoracic duct is being used, a left paracostal incision is made to exteriorize the cecum. Once the cecum has been exteriorized, a lymph node adjacent to the cecum is located. A small volume (0.1 to 0.2 ml) of methylene blue (USP 1%, American Quinine, Shirley, NY) may be injected into the lymph node to increase visualization of lymphatics. Repeated doses of methylene blue should be avoided owing to the risk of inducing a Heinz body anemia or renal failure. Careful dissection of the mesentery near this node allows large lymphatic vessels to be visualized and cannulated with a 22-gauge over-the-needle catheter (Surflo, The Burrows Co., Wheeling, IL).[22] Cannulation of this lymphatic is more difficult in cats than in dogs, because cats have more fat in their mesentery, and their lymphatics are significantly smaller. Two sutures (3-0 silk) are placed in the mesentery and used to secure the catheter and an attached piece of extension tubing in place (the ends of the suture can be looped over the hub of the extension tubing). An additional suture may be placed around the extension tubing and through a segment of intestine to prevent dislodgment of the catheter. A 3-way stopcock is attached to the end of the extension tubing and a water-soluble contrast agent such as Renovist (ER Squibb & Sons, Princeton, NJ) is injected at a dosage of 1 ml/kg diluted with 0.5 ml/kg of saline solution. A lateral thoracic radiograph is taken while the last milliliter is being injected. This lymphangiogram may be used to identify the number and location of branches of the thoracic duct that need to be ligated, and it can be repeated after ligation to determine whether or not complete ligation of the thoracic duct was performed. It also will help determine the extent of lymphangiectasia present in the cranial thorax (Fig. 35–8).

The thoracic duct is approached in cats through a left caudal intercostal thoracotomy (8th, 9th, or 10th intercostal space), or via an incision in the left diaphragm. Once the duct has been located, hemostatic clips (Hemoclip [medium], Edward Weck and Co., Inc., Research Triangle Park, NC) may be used to ligate it. The advantage of using hemoclips is that they may be used as a reference point on subsequent radiographs if further ligation is necessary. However, the author prefers also to place a nonabsorbable suture, such as silk, on the duct. Visualization of the thoracic duct may be aided by injecting methylene blue into the lymphatic catheter (Fig. 35–9). If a catheter was not placed, the dye can be injected into a mesenteric lymph node.

Pericardiectomy

Thickening of the pleura and pericardium occurs in patients with chylothorax. Although the role of the

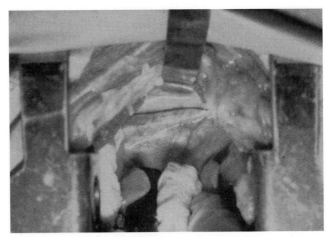

Figure 35–9. Identification of the thoracic duct may be aided by injecting methylene blue into the lymphatic catheter or directly into a mesenteric lymph node.

thickened pericardium in this disease is not well understood, it has been the observation of the author that some cats benefit from pericardiectomy. If the thickened pericardium causes even a slight elevation in venous pressures, the thoracic duct may respond to this as an obstruction with resultant formation of numerous lymphatics in the cranial thorax. These lymphatics may likely leak transmurally. Although experimental at this point, the author has had some success with pericardiectomy as the sole treatment of cats with chylothorax. Further studies and additional experience are necessary to recommend this technique in affected animals, however, it looks promising as sole therapy or as adjunctive therapy to thoracic-duct ligation in animals with chylothorax.

Other Treatments

Passive pleuroperitoneal shunting has been recommended as treatment of chylothorax in cats, but this technique is no longer recommended by the author. The goal of placing a fenestrated Silastic sheet in the diaphragm was to allow drainage of the chylous fluid into the abdomen where the fluid could be reabsorbed by visceral and peritoneal lymphatics, thereby alleviating the respiratory distress and need for subsequent thoracentesis (Fig. 35–10).[23] The author has not found this technique to be effective, and chronic irritation of the sheeting may be associated with neoplastic transformation of tissues.[24]

Active pleuroperitoneal or pleurovenous shunting has been recommended for the treatment of chylothorax in dogs and cats, and may be a reasonable consideration in patients in which all other therapies have failed. Commercially made shunt catheters (Hakim-Cordis ventricular-peritoneal shunt system, Cordis Corp., Miami, FL; Denver double valve peritoneous shunt, Denver Biomaterials, Inc., Evergreen, CO) are available and may be used to pump fluid from the thorax to the abdomen.[25–27] The cathe-

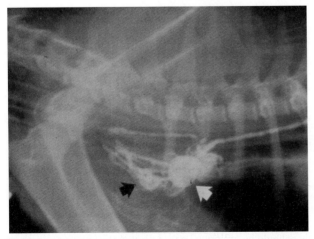

Figure 35–8. Lymphangiogram performed in a cat with chylothorax and thoracic lymphangiectasia. Note the multiple, dilated lymphatics near the entrance of the thoracic duct *(arrows)* into the venous system.

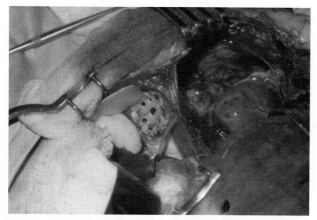

Figure 35–10. Silastic sheeting used for passive pleuroperitoneal drainage in a cat with chylothorax. The sheeting is sutured to a defect created in the diaphragm. This technique no longer is recommended by the author.

ter is placed with the patient under general anesthesia. A vertical incision is made over the middle of the 5th, 6th, or 7th rib. A purse-string suture is placed in the skin at this site, and following the placement of fenestrations in the venous end of the

shunt catheter, the catheter is inserted bluntly into the pleural space. A tunnel is created by blunt dissection under the external abdominal oblique muscle, and the pump chamber is pulled through the tunnel. The efferent end of the catheter then is placed into the abdominal cavity through a preplaced purse-string suture and incision located just caudal to the costal arch. The shunt must be placed with the pump chamber directly overlying a rib, so that the chamber can be compressed effectively (Fig. 35–11). Advantages of pleurovenous or pleuroperitoneal shunting of chyle are that it may allow more complete drainage of the thorax than that achieved with passive peritoneal drainage. Pleurovenous shunting overcomes problems with inadequate peritoneal absorption that may occur with pleuroperitoneal shunting. Disadvantages are that the shunts are expensive, they may occlude easily with fibrin, some animals will not tolerate compression of the pump chamber, and the shunts require a high degree of owner compliance and dedication. Additionally, thrombosis, venous occlusion, sepsis, and electrolyte abnormalities have been reported in human beings.[28–32]

Pleurodesis is the formation of generalized adhe

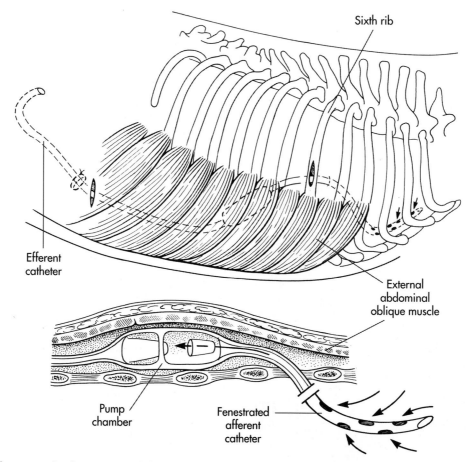

Figure 35–11. Placement of a pleuroperitoneal shunt. The pump chamber should be positioned over a rib so that it can be compressed manually. (From Surgery of the lower respiratory system: Pleural cavity and diaphragm. *In* Fossum TW [ed]: Small Animal Surgery. St. Louis, Mosby, 1997.)

sions between the visceral and the parietal pleura. Adhesions may occur spontaneously in association with pleural effusion, or in some species, they can be induced following instillation of an irritating substance into the pleural cavity.[33, 34] This technique has been recommended for the treatment of chylothorax in dogs and cats, but is not recommended by the author. In order for pleurodesis to occur, the lungs must be able to contact the body wall; however, many animals with chronic chylothorax have some thickening of their visceral pleura that prohibits normal lung expansion (see discussion of fibrosing pleuritis earlier in this chapter). Neither mechanical (surgical) pleurodesis nor talc administration resulted in pleurodesis in experimental dogs; however, thickening of the pleura did occur in some animals.[34] Chemical or surgical pleurodesis is unlikely to be successful in cats with chylothorax.

◆ SUMMARY

Chylothorax is a complex disease with many identified underlying causes, including cardiac disease, mediastinal masses, heartworm disease, and trauma. Management of this disease should be directed at identifying the cause, if possible, and treating the underlying disorder. In cats with idiopathic chylothorax, medical management is recommended initially because the condition may resolve spontaneously. Owners should be aware of the potential development of fibrosing pleuritis in affected cats. When medical management is impractical or unsuccessful, surgical intervention may be considered. Surgical options include mesenteric lymphangiography and thoracic-duct ligation, pericardiectomy, passive pleuroperitoneal shunting, active pleuroperitoneal or pleurovenous shunting, and pleurodesis. Of these, the first 2 are recommended by the author. Until the etiology of the effusion in cats with idiopathic chylothorax is understood, the treatment success rate will be less than ideal. Future research needs to be directed at determining the pathophysiologic mechanisms underlying this disease in cats.

REFERENCES

1. Fossum TW, Forrester SD, Swenson CL, et al: Chylothorax in cats: 37 cases (1969–1989). J Am Vet Med Assoc 198:672–678, 1991.
2. Evans HE, Christensen GC: Miller's Anatomy of the Dog. Philadelphia, WB Saunders, 1979, pp. 803–806.
3. Lindsay FEF: The cisterna chyli and thoracic duct of the cat. J Anat 117:403–412, 1974.
4. Patterson DF, Munson TO: Traumatic chylothorax in small animals treated by ligation of the thoracic duct. J Am Vet Med Assoc 133:452–458, 1958.
5. Haider M, Schad H, Mendler N: Thoracic duct lymph and PEEP studies in anaesthetized dogs. II. Effect of a thoracic duct fistula on the development of a hyponcotic-hydrostatic pulmonary oedema. Intensive Care Med 13:278–283, 1987.
6. Schad H, Brechtelsbauer H: Thoracic duct lymph flow and composition in conscious dogs and the influence of anaesthesia and passive limb movement. Pflugers Arch 371:25–31, 1977.
7. Willard MD, Fossum TW, Torrance A, et al: Hyponatremia and hyperkalemia associated with idiopathic or experimentally induced chylothorax in four dogs. J Am Vet Med Assoc 199:353–358, 1991.
8. Fossum TW, Jacobs RM, Birchard SJ: Evaluation of cholesterol and triglyceride concentrations in differentiating chylous and nonchylous pleural effusions in dogs and cats. J Am Vet Med Assoc 188:49–51, 1986.
9. Birchard SJ, Ware WA, Fossum TW, et al: Chylothorax associated with congestive cardiomyopathy in a cat. J Am Vet Med Assoc 189:1462–1464, 1986.
10. Donahoe JM, Kneller SK, Thompson PE: Chylothorax subsequent to infection of cats with Dirofilaria immitis. J Am Vet Med Assoc 11:1107–1110, 1974.
11. Birchard SJ, Bilbrey SA: Chylothorax associated with dirofilariasis in a cat. J Am Vet Med Assoc 197:507–509, 1990.
12. Forrester SD, Fossum TW, Rogers KS: Diagnosis and treatment of chylothorax associated with lymphoblastic lymphosarcoma in four cats. J Am Vet Med Assoc 198:291–294, 1991.
13. Willard MD: Fluid accumulation disorders. In Willard MD, Tvedten H, Turnwald GH (eds): Small Animal Clinical Diagnosis by Laboratory Methods. Philadelphia, WB Saunders, 1989, pp. 229–242.
14. Suter PF, Greene RW: Chylothorax in a dog with abnormal termination of the thoracic duct. J Am Vet Med Assoc 159:302–308, 1971.
15. Fossum TW, Evering WN, Miller MW, et al: Severe bilateral fibrosing pleuritis associated with chronic chylothorax in 5 cats and 2 dogs. J Am Vet Med Assoc 201:317–324, 1992.
16. Glennon JC, Flanders JA, Rothwell JT, et al: Constrictive pleuritis with chylothorax in a cat: A case report. J Am Anim Hosp Assoc 23:539–542, 1987.
17. Rosenstock L, Hudson LD: The pleural manifestations of asbestos exposure. Occup Med 2:383–407, 1987.
18. Schabel SI: Imaging of pleural infections. Semin Respir Infect 3:298–307, 1988.
19. Birchard SJ, Smeak DD, Fossum TW: Results of thoracic duct ligation in dogs with chylothorax. J Am Vet Med Assoc 193:68–71, 1988.
20. Harpster NK. Chylothorax. In Kirk RW (ed): Current Veterinary Therapy IX. Philadelphia, WB Saunders, 1986, pp. 295–303.
21. Martin RA, Leighton D, Richards S, et al: Transdiaphragmatic approach to thoracic duct ligation in the cat. Vet Surg 17:22–26, 1988.
22. Kagan KG, Breznock EM: Variations in the canine thoracic duct system and the effects of surgical occlusion demonstrated by rapid aqueous lymphography, using an intestinal lymphatic trunk. Am J Vet Res 40:948–958, 1979.
23. Peterson SL, Pion PD, Breznock EM: Passive pleuroperitoneal drainage for management of chylothorax in two cats. J Am Anim Hosp Assoc 25:569–572, 1989.
24. Fossum TW: Gastric neoplasia associated with Silastic sheeting placement for the treatment of chylothorax in a cat. (in press).
25. Willauer CC, Breznock EM: Pleurovenous shunting technique for treatment of chylothorax in three dogs. J Am Vet Med Assoc 191:1106–1109, 1987.
26. Smeak DD, Gallagher L, Birchard SJ, et al: Management of intractable pleural effusion in a dog with a pleuroperitoneal shunt. Vet Surg 16:212–216, 1987.
27. Donner GS: Use of the pleuroperitoneal shunt for the management of persistent chylothorax in a cat. J Am Anim Hosp Assoc 252:619–622, 1989.
28. Vacek JL, Wolfe MW, Hightower BM, et al: Right heart pseudotumor simulated by ascitic pseudocyst: An unusual complication of peritoneovenous shunting. Chest 91:138–139, 1987.
29. Holm A, Rutsky EA, Aldrete JS: Short- and long-term effectiveness, morbidity, and mortality of peritoneovenous shunt

inserted to treat massive refractory ascites of nephrogenic origin: Analysis of 14 cases. Am Surg 55:645–652, 1989.

30. Smith RE, Nostrant TT, Eckhauser FE, et al: Patient selection and survival after peritoneovenous shunting for nonmalignant ascites. Am J Gastroenterol 79:659–662, 1984.

31. Moskovitz M: The peritoneovenous shunt: Expectations and reality. Am J Gastroenterol 85:917–929, 1990.

32. Fildes J, Narvaez GP, Baig KA, et al: Pulmonary tumor embolization after peritoneovenous shunting for malignant ascites. Cancer 61:1973–1976, 1988.

33. Birchard SJ, Fossum TW, Gallagher L: Pleurodesis. In Kirk RW, (ed): Current Veterinary Therapy X. Philadelphia, WB Saunders, 1989, pp. 405–408.

34. Jerram RM, Fossum T, Berridge B, et al: The efficacy of mechanical abrasion and talc slurry as methods of pleurodesis in normal dogs. Vet Surg 28:322–332, 1999.

36

◆ Systemic Hypertension

Patti S. Snyder
Kirsten L. Cooke

Systemic hypertension is a condition diagnosed uncommonly in cats (see also Chapter 47, Diagnosis and Treatment of Systemic Hypertension). Whether this is due to infrequent occurrence or to lack of documentation is not known. Unlike in human patients, primary (essential) hypertension is thought to be rare in cats, and most cases of hypertension in this species are secondary to other diseases. However, there are no studies evaluating blood pressure in large populations of healthy and ill cats, and most published reports focus on changes in blood pressure in cats with specific diseases (e.g., renal failure).

◆ ETIOLOGY/PATHOGENESIS

Maintenance of blood pressure is dependent on cardiac output and systemic vascular resistance; if either of these parameters increases and other conditions remain constant, blood pressure rises. The mechanisms responsible for the elevated blood pressure depend on the cause.

Renal disease and hyperthyroidism are thought to be the most common causes of systemic hypertension in cats.[1] Studies of cats with chronic renal failure have demonstrated mean systolic blood pressures of 146 ± 25, 168 ± 26, 202 ± 25, and 219 ± 43 mm Hg using various indirect measurement techniques.[1–4] Eighty-seven per cent of hyperthyroid cats had elevated systolic or systolic and diastolic pressures (mean 167 ± 29 mm Hg) when compared with an age-matched control population.[1]

Other potential causes of hypertension in cats that are not well-documented include hyperadrenocorticism, pheochromocytoma, mineralocorticoid-secreting tumor, and primary (essential) hypertension.[5, 6] It has been postulated that age has an effect on systemic blood pressure. This has been confirmed recently by a study showing a significant increase in systemic blood pressure in healthy cats older than 11 years of age compared with healthy cats less than 11 years of age (158 to 179 versus 123 to 127 mm Hg, respectively).[2]

Blood volume, cardiac output, and peripheral vascular resistance are the primary factors involved in maintenance of normal blood pressure. These factors can be affected by the sympathetic and parasympathetic nervous systems, the renin-angiotensin-aldosterone system (RAAS), antidiuretic hormone, and endothelins.[5]

Hypertension Secondary to Renal Failure

Although a number of theories have been postulated, the exact mechanism by which renal failure leads to hypertension is not known. Activation of the RAAS secondary to decreased renal blood flow or localized renal ischemia may contribute to hypertension. Release of renin from the juxtaglomerular apparatus occurs in response to decreased renal blood flow, intrarenal hypotension, or decreased delivery of sodium and chloride to the distal tubule. Renin stimulates the production of angiotensin I, which is converted subsequently to angiotensin II. Angiotensin II causes vasoconstriction, increasing peripheral vascular resistance and resulting in increased blood pressure. Additionally, angiotensin II stimulates adrenocortical secretion of aldosterone causing retention of sodium and fluid and increasing blood volume. Plasma renin activity, angiotensin II, and aldosterone concentrations have been evaluated in cats with chronic renal disease.[3] Plasma renin activity levels were increased in some cats with renal disease, but normal or decreased in others. Aldosterone concentrations were increased in cats with renal disease compared with healthy controls, but angiotensin II concentration did not differ significantly between the 2 groups.[3]

A second proposed mechanism suggests that diseased kidneys may be unable to excrete adequate amounts of sodium and water, leading to expansion of extracellular fluid volume.[1] Jensen and others, however, showed that fractional excretion of sodium was decreased in some cats with chronic renal failure but increased or normal in others.[3] This suggests that abnormal sodium excretion is unlikely to be the sole cause of systemic hypertension in cats with chronic renal failure. It also has been suggested that diseased kidneys may not produce sufficient quantities of vasodilatory substances such as prostaglandins.[1, 7]

Finally, activation of the RAAS may stimulate the production of endothelin 1 (ET-1), a potent vasoconstrictor expressed in vascular endothelial cells and vascular smooth muscle.[8] ET-1 levels have been evaluated in healthy dogs and in dogs with congestive heart failure, renal failure, diabetes mellitus, and hyperadrenocorticism; there was no significant difference in ET-1 levels between healthy and ill dogs.[9] However, detection of ET-1 may be difficult, owing to its rapid removal from circulation.[8] To our knowledge, endothelin levels have not been evaluated in cats.

Hypertension Secondary to Hyperthyroidism

Hyperthyroidism in human beings increases the number and sensitivity of beta receptors in the myocardium, causing an increased responsiveness to a normal degree of sympathetic stimulation. This also may be true of the beta receptors on the juxtaglomerular apparatus that, when stimulated, have been shown to increase renin secretion in human hyperthyroid patients. Additionally, activation of a thyroid hormone–specific adenylate cyclase–cyclic adenosine monophosphate system leads to increased heart rate, stroke volume, and cardiac output.[7, 10] Increasing cardiac output increases systolic arterial pressure, unless the aorta can stretch to accommodate the additional load. However, hyperthyroidism is a disease of older cats, and because the aorta may be less distensible, it may be less able to compensate for the increase in cardiac output and stroke volume, thereby leading to an increase in blood pressure.[5]

Arteriolar Response to Hypertension

The initial arteriolar response to hypertension is vasoconstriction, an attempt to protect adjacent capillary beds from exposure to high pressure. The arterioles then may go on to develop medial hypertrophy and arteriosclerosis.[11] These changes eventually can lead to ischemia, infarction, and/or increased vascular permeability.

◆ CLINICAL SIGNS

Clinical signs of hypertension, when present, most often are attributable to tissues with a rich arteriolar supply including ophthalmic, cardiovascular, renal, and cerebrovascular tissues. Retinal detachment and acute blindness are the most common presenting complaints for cats with systemic hypertension. In one study, 80 per cent of hypertensive cats were presented for evaluation of blindness.[4] Polyuria, polydipsia, and weight loss may be present if the hypertension is secondary to either renal failure or hyperthyroidism. Central nervous system signs may include seizures, posterior paresis, nystagmus, and sudden death.

◆ EXAMINATION FINDINGS
Ophthalmic

Fundic examination may show varying degrees of retinal detachment in addition to tortuous retinal vessels, retinal hemorrhage, and retinal edema.[11a] Autoregulatory arteriolar constriction leads to ischemia and retinal degeneration. Hemorrhage also may occur into the vitreous and lead to development of glaucoma.[7, 12] Retinal detachment is reported to carry a poor prognosis for return of vision.[6, 13] However, in our experience, a significant number of these cats appear to regain some if not all of their vision. A study currently is being conducted at the University of Florida to evaluate retinal function in hypertensive cats with retinal detachment and subsequent reattachment.

Cardiac

Because the heart pumps against increased pressure in hypertensive patients, it is expected that some degree of cardiac remodeling will occur. Eighty-one per cent of cats in one study had radiographic, echocardiographic, or necropsy findings of cardiomegaly.[4] Of the cats that were necropsied, all had left ventricular hypertrophy and concentric coronary arterial hypertrophy/hyperplasia.[4] However, it is unusual to find severe left ventricular hypertrophy with systemic hypertension as the sole cause. Left atrial diameter is either normal or only slightly increased. In some instances, the hypertrophy may be restricted to the interventricular septum. Other cardiac abnormalities can include systolic murmurs (42 per cent of cats in one study), gallop rhythms, and occasional ventricular or atrial premature complexes.[4]

Renal

In one retrospective study of hypertensive cats, some form of renal pathology was present in all 24 cats studied, with azotemia occurring in 83 per cent and bilaterally small kidneys in 48 per cent.[4] Isosthenuria also may be seen; however, proteinuria is rare.[1, 4] Because chronic renal failure can cause systemic hypertension, it may be difficult, if not impossible, to determine whether renal changes are a cause or an effect of the hypertension in an individual patient. However, uncontrolled hypertension most likely contributes to progression of renal damage.[11]

Central Nervous System

Seizures, cerebrovascular accidents, and/or dementia have been reported in human patients with systemic hypertension. Reports of specific neurologic signs in cats are rare. However, one study reported signs suggestive of neurologic involvement in 11 of 24 cats with hypertension.[4] These signs included seizures, acute collapse or death, intermittent paresis/paralysis of 1 or both pelvic limbs, nystagmus, and decorticate posturing of 1 or both forelegs. Clinical signs were reported to begin when hypertension was not controlled.[4]

Table 36–1. Signs of Systemic Hypertension

Body System	Common Clinical Signs
Cardiac	Systolic murmur, cardiac gallop
Ocular	Blindness, bullous retinopathy, retinal edema/serous exudates, intra- and pre-retinal/vitreal hemorrhage, retinal detachment, hyphema
Nervous	Seizures, paresis, disorientation, ataxia, circling, nystagmus[12, 13]

◆ DIFFERENTIAL DIAGNOSIS

With the exception of the ocular abnormalities, the signs of systemic hypertension in cats are often so vague (Table 36–1) that the attending veterinarian must have a high index of suspicion or must measure blood pressure routinely before a diagnosis of hypertension is made.

The ocular abnormalities reported in hypertensive cats may resemble those found with coagulopathies, hyperviscosity, systemic infection, or paraneoplastic disorders.[13] Individual case reports of retinal hemorrhage and detachment subsequent to ethylene glycol intoxication and megestrol acetate administration also have been documented. However, blood pressure was not measured in these cats, so the possibility exists that these lesions may have been related to systemic hypertension.[14, 15] Hypertensive retinopathy is seen less commonly in hypertensive cats with hyperthyroidism, compared with hypertensive cats with chronic renal failure.[12, 16]

Systolic cardiac murmurs and cardiac gallop sounds are found frequently in most types of feline heart disease (such as hypertrophic cardiomyopathy, dilated cardiomyopathy, unclassified forms of cardiomyopathy, restrictive cardiomyopathy, and thyrotoxic heart disease) including hypertensive heart disease. Tachycardia and congestive heart failure are uncommon in cats with essential hypertension or hypertension secondary to renal failure.[4, 7]

Polyuria and polydipsia may be seen in cats with renal insufficiency, hyperthyroidism, and diabetes mellitus. Renal insufficiency may be due to degenerative, infectious, immune-mediated, or neoplastic causes. It is important to remember that hyperthyroidism and renal insufficiency may occur concurrently, and that hyperthyroidism with its coexistent increase in cardiac output may mask azotemia (see Chapter 19, Complications of Therapy for Hyperthyroidism).

Neurologic signs may be persistent or transient, and localized or generalized.[4, 16] Because the neurologic signs observed suggest either brain or spinal-cord involvement, infectious, inflammatory, toxic, or traumatic processes, neoplasia, and disc protrusion could result in similar findings. Spinal pain has not been described as a feature of the neurologic abnormalities that occur secondary to systemic hypertension. Nystagmus has been reported in 2 hypertensive cats, but the type of nystagmus was not characterized.[4]

Once systemic hypertension has been documented, determining the underlying cause is paramount. Chronic renal failure and hyperthyroidism are the most common diseases causing hypertension in cats.[1, 4] There are isolated case reports of hypertension in an anemic cat, and in a cat fed a high-salt diet.[13, 17] Finally, in some cases, an underlying cause for the hypertension is not identified. Whether these represent examples of primary (essential) hypertension or simply that the underlying cause was not discovered is not known. Hyperadrenocorticism and pheochromocytoma have been reported to be associated with systemic hypertension in dogs.[18–20] Both conditions have been identified in cats; however, there are no published clinical reports of concurrent hypertension in cats with these diseases.

◆ DIAGNOSIS

Unlike our colleagues in the field of human medicine, veterinarians studying systemic hypertension have not formed a consensus as to the normal blood pressure range for cats. The majority agree, however, that systolic blood pressure (measured indirectly) in excess of 170 mm Hg should be considered suspect, especially in cats with clinical signs of systemic hypertension.[7, 21] There is less agreement about the normal range for diastolic and mean blood pressure. Most investigators concede that an important "white-coat" effect occurs when blood pressure is measured.[22] In a recent study of cats with experimentally induced renal insufficiency implanted with radiotelemetric devices, systolic blood pressure was 22.3 ± 0.9 mm Hg higher in an examination room compared with the average daily systolic blood pressure measurement.[22] Steps should be taken to minimize this white-coat effect, and blood pressure measurements always should be interpreted in light of the patient's clinical signs and the circumstances surrounding the recording of blood pressure. Measuring blood pressure in the presence of the owner, after acclimatization to the surroundings but before examining the patient and with the least restraint possible, may help minimize the white-coat effect. In addition, several measurements should be taken at each visit and averaged in an attempt to minimize the effect of a single high or low reading. Because sedative agents will affect blood pressure, measurements should be obtained in the awake animal, and any elevation in blood pressure should be substantiated by performing multiple measurements before antihypertensive medication is initiated.

Blood pressure may be measured directly by arterial puncture with a needle or by catheterization of a peripheral artery. Whereas this method is considered the "gold standard," it is fraught with problems and used rarely in clinical patients. The restraint necessary to position the cat for arterial puncture and the pain from insertion of the needle or catheter are associated with sympathetic discharge and subsequent blood pressure elevation. Long-term peripheral arterial cannulation (e.g., radiotelemetric devices) has not been reported in client-owned cats. Less invasive indirect blood pressure devices are relied on most often.

Three indirect methods of blood pressure determination (Doppler flowmeter, oscillometric device, and a photoplethysmograph) have been compared with direct blood pressure measurement over a wide range of blood pressures in anesthetized cats.[23, 24] Binns and others[23] found the Doppler and the photoplethysmographic methods were the most accurate overall when compared against direct blood pressure determination. However, frequent repositioning of the instrument was necessary with the photoplethysmographic device. Equipment used most often to measure blood pressure indirectly in cats detects arterial blood flow (Doppler ultrasonic flowmeter), or cuff oscillations created by a change in pulse pressure (oscillometric device).[25, 26] Whereas the oscillometric device determines systolic, diastolic, and mean blood pressure, the Doppler flowmeter device only determines systolic blood pressure reliably. The diastolic blood pressure may be estimated when the pitch of the Doppler flowmeter's sound changes.[27] Familiarity with equipment, proper selection of the cuff, and placement of the cuff and probe are important in obtaining reliable and repeatable recordings. It is the authors' experience and that of others, that the oscillometric devices do not work consistently in awake cats.[7, 23]

The finding of a normal blood pressure in an awake cat substantially reduces the likelihood that systemic hypertension is present. However, in a clinical trial conducted by 1 of the authors, 1 untreated hypertensive cat with chronic renal failure, hypertensive retinopathy, and daily systolic blood pressures averaging 205 mm Hg had a systolic blood pressure at or below 140 mm Hg 17.5 per cent of the times when blood pressures were recorded.[21]

Because systemic hypertension in cats often occurs as a sequela to a primary disease process such as renal disease or hyperthyroidism, hypertensive cats should be evaluated for these diseases. This allows the clinician to tailor the therapeutic approach to the patient. A serum biochemical panel, urinalysis, and serum thyroxine (T_4) test should be performed in all cats with systemic hypertension. If the T_4 test is normal but hyperthyroidism is still suspected, additional testing, such as nuclear scintigraphy or the triiodothyronine (T_3) suppression test, may be indicated (see Chapter 18, Diagnosis of Occult Hyperthyroidism). In cats, the degree of azotemia or elevation in T_4 has not correlated with the severity of hypertension.[1, 21]

Although cardiomegaly has been seen radiographically in some cats with systemic hypertension, the finding is not specific enough to establish a diagnosis of hypertensive heart disease. Thoracic radiographs should be used primarily to exclude other differential diagnoses. Electrocardiograms usually are normal but may demonstrate a left anterior fascicular block pattern (deep S waves in leads II, III, and aVF). Left ventricular enlargement patterns and supraventricular and ventricular premature complexes are seen in only a small number of hypertensive cats. Echocardiography provides the best means by which to evaluate the hypertensive cat with abnormal cardiac auscultation. The most common findings are increased interventricular septal and/or left ventricular free wall thickness; substantial increases in left atrial size are rare. Because these findings may mimic those of hypertrophic cardiomyopathy and thyrotoxic heart disease, systemic hypertension should be considered in the differential diagnoses of any cat with left ventricular concentric hypertrophy. A common misconception exists that hypertension occurs secondarily to cardiac disease in cats. The cardiac changes that are seen are the result rather than the cause of the hypertension. The aortic diameter also has been reported to be increased in hypertensive cats, compared with normotensive cats of similar age.[28]

◆ TREATMENT

Treatment should focus initially on controlling the underlying cause of the hypertension. Hyperthyroid cats symptomatic for hypertension should be treated simultaneously for hyperthyroidism and systemic hypertension. Once the hyperthyroidism is controlled, antihypertensive therapy may be discontinued in many instances. In contrast, cats with renal disease and concurrent systemic hypertension usually require antihypertensive medication indefinitely.

A cause for the hypertension cannot be identified readily in some patients. In these cases, specific antihypertensive therapy usually is necessary. Because hypertension has been reported to occur with corticosteroid use in dogs and human beings, discontinuation of corticosteroids is recommended if possible in cats with hypertension. Although a cause-and-effect relationship cannot be established, it is interesting to note that, of all the medications being given to cats when their hypertension is diagnosed, corticosteroids were the most common (Snyder PS, personal observation, 1999). This also was found in a retrospective study of 24 cats with hypertension.[4]

The urgency of correcting hypertension depends on clinical presentation and the severity of the hypertension. Abrupt declines in blood pressure can lead to cerebral hypoperfusion because of the adaptations of the cerebral vasculature to long-standing hypertension.[29] This can compromise cerebral perfusion, placing the patient at risk for the development of neurologic signs. For this reason, emergency use of intravenous antihypertensive agents to lower blood pressure rapidly is recommended rarely in companion animals.

Although gradual sodium restriction is advocated in hypertensive patients, the authors have not found this alone to be effective in controlling blood pressure. Discontinuation of or reduction in parenteral fluid supplementation (NaCl or lactated Ringer's solution) is advised unless deemed absolutely necessary. Weight reduction is recommended in obese animals, although the direct link between obesity and hypertension is not strong in veterinary patients.

Diuretics such as furosemide have not been reliably effective antihypertensive agents in cats.[4] The angiotensin-converting enzyme inhibitor enalapril (0.25 to 0.5 mg/kg every [q] 12 to 24 hr) and the beta-adrenergic blocking agent propranolol (2.5 to 5 mg/cat q 8 to 12 hr) have been used alone and together with mixed results.[30] Atenolol (6.25 to 12.5 mg/cat q 12 to 24 hr) also has been substituted for propranolol. In some instances, phenoxybenzamine (2.5 to 7.5 mg/cat q 8 to 12 hr), an alpha-adrenergic blocking agent, has been used successfully alone or in combination with enalapril and propranolol.

The authors recommend the calcium channel blocker amlodipine (Norvasc, 0.625 to 1.25 mg/cat q 24 hr) as an effective single-agent antihypertensive medication.[21, 30] Amlodipine has been used in many cats with renal disease and hyperthyroidism to control hypertension. Although overall there was no effect of amlodipine administration on renal parameters, there are isolated reports of worsening azotemia in amlodipine-treated cats with concurrent renal disease (Snyder PS, personal observation, 1999).[21, 30] Other treatments that have been suggested include the angiotensin-converting enzyme inhibitors benazepril (0.25 to 1 mg/kg q 24 hr), and lisinopril (0.25 to 0.5 mg/kg q 24 hr).[31]

The use of an endothelin-receptor antagonist in human beings with essential hypertension has been reported recently. In a randomized, double-blinded study, patients receiving the endothelin-receptor antagonist bosentan had a significant reduction in blood pressure. Additionally, administration of the endothelin-receptor antagonist did not result in activation of either the sympathetic nervous system or the RAAS.[32] There are no reports of the use of this drug in veterinary patients.

Because antihypertensive medication will be given indefinitely to most affected cats, every attempt should be made to minimize the number of medications administered and the dosing frequency to improve owner and patient compliance.

MANAGEMENT AND CONTROL

In all instances, frequent monitoring of the cat's blood pressure and clinical status is imperative. Until adequate blood pressure control is achieved (systolic blood pressure measured indirectly < 170 mm Hg), weekly to bimonthly monitoring of blood pressure is recommended. Measurements should be obtained at various times of the dosing schedule to ensure continuous blood pressure control. The authors observed a decline in blood pressure after 1 dose of amlodipine, and blood pressures were controlled in most cats after 1 week of amlodipine therapy.[21]

Serum urea nitrogen and creatinine concentrations should be monitored weekly in cats with concurrent renal disease until blood pressure and drug dosage are stable. Once blood pressure is stable, re-evaluation of the patient should occur every 2 to 4 months or as dictated by the patient's clinical status. Prognosis is determined by the underlying disease process and ability to control the hypertension adequately.

After instituting erythropoietin therapy in anemic cats, blood pressures should be followed closely, because increases in blood pressure have been reported in some azotemic dogs receiving erythropoietin.[33]

PREVENTION

There is strong evidence of an association between elevated systemic arterial blood pressure and development or progression of chronic renal failure in human beings.[34, 35] At this time, no such relationship has been identified in dogs or cats with naturally occurring renal disease. Researchers have suggested that normalization of blood pressure slows progression of renal disease if intrarenal as well as systemic blood pressure is lowered.[36] Angiotensin-converting enzyme inhibitors appear to be renoprotective. There also is evidence that the newer calcium channel blockers, such as amlodipine, may have a renoprotective effect.[36, 37] This research is based on experimental models, and may not be true in naturally occurring renal disease in companion animals.

PATHOLOGIC FINDINGS

Arteriosclerosis is the principal pathologic finding in cats with systemic hypertension.[38] It is characterized by muscular hyperplasia, medial hypertrophy, and intimal hyalinization of arterioles. Arteriolar fibrinoid necrosis is less consistent. Microscopic changes are expected to be evident throughout the systemic arterial system. Additionally, gross abnormalities including ventricular hypertrophy and retinal hemorrhage or detachment may be apparent. Renal lesions, interstitial fibrosis, glomerulonecrosis, and sclerosis may be found.

Differentiating cause from effect with respect to the renal changes seen in hypertensive, azotemic cats is a frustrating clinical dilemma. Mesangial-cell proliferation and glomerulosclerosis often are present in the kidneys of cats with systemic hypertension and azotemia. However, these changes are seen less commonly in normotensive cats with chronic renal failure, leading some investigators to interpret these findings as being the result rather than the cause of hypertension.[4]

Resolution of retinopathy, cardiac hypertrophy, and neurologic signs depends on many factors, including the severity and chronicity of the abnormality and the ability to control hypertension.

REFERENCES

1. Kobayashi DL, Peterson ME, Graves TK, et al: Hypertension in cats with chronic renal failure or hyperthyroidism. J Vet Intern Med 4:58–62, 1990.
2. Bodey AR, Sansom J: Epidemiological study of blood pressure in domestic cats. J Small Anim Pract 39:567–573, 1998.
3. Jensen JL, Henik RA, Brownfield M, et al: Plasma renin activity and angiotensin I and aldosterone concentrations in cats with hypertension associated with chronic renal disease. Am J Vet Res 58:535–540, 1997.
4. Littman MP: Spontaneous systemic hypertension in 24 cats. J Vet Intern Med 8:79–86, 1994.
5. Kienle RD, Kittleson MD: Pulmonary arterial and systemic arterial hypertension. In Kittleson MD, Kienle RD (eds): Small Animal Cardiovascular Medicine. St. Louis, Mosby, 1998, pp. 433–448.
6. Henik RA: Systemic hypertension and its management. Vet Clin North Am Small Anim Pract 27:1355–1372, 1997.
7. Henik RA: Diagnosis and treatment of feline systemic hypertension. Compend Contin Educ Pract Vet 19:163–179, 1997.
8. Turk JR: Physiologic and pathophysiologic effects of endothelin: Implications in cardiopulmonary disease. J Am Vet Med Assoc 212:265–270, 1998.
9. Vollmar AM, Preusser U, Gerbes AL, et al: Endothelin concentration in plasma of healthy dogs and dogs with congestive heart failure, renal failure, diabetes mellitus and hyperadrenocorticism. J Vet Intern Med 9:105–111, 1995.
10. Feldman EC, Nelson RW: Feline hyperthyroidism (thyrotoxicosis). In Feldman EC, Nelson RW (eds): Canine and Feline Endocrinology and Reproduction. Philadelphia, WB Saunders, 1996, pp. 118–166.
11. Labato MA, Ross LA: Diagnosis and management of hypertension. In August JR (ed): Consultations in Feline Internal Medicine, vol. 1. Philadelphia, WB Saunders, 1991, pp. 301–308.
11a. Maggio F, DeFrancesco TC, Atkins CE, et al: Ocular lesions associated with systemic hypertension in cats: 69 cases (1985–1998). J Am Vet Med Assoc 217:695–702, 2000.
12. Stiles J, Polzin DJ, Bistner SI: The prevalence of retinopathy in cats with systemic hypertension and chronic renal failure or hyperthyroidism. J Am Anim Hosp Assoc 30:564–572, 1994.
13. Morgan RV: Systemic hypertension in four cats: Ocular and medical findings. J Am Anim Hosp Assoc 22:615–621, 1986.
14. Herrtage ME, Barnett KC, Macdougall DF: Diabetic retinopathy in a cat with megestrol acetate–induced diabetes. J Small Anim Pract 26:595–601, 1985.
15. Barclay SM, Riis RC: Retinal detachment and reattachment associated with ethylene glycol intoxication in a cat. J Am Anim Hosp Assoc 15:719–724, 1979.
16. Sansom J, Barnett KC, Dunn KA, et al: Ocular disease associated with hypertension in 16 cats. J Small Anim Pract 35:604–611, 1994.
17. Turner JL, Brogdon JD, Lees GE, et al: Idiopathic hypertension in a cat with secondary hypertensive retinopathy associated with a high-salt diet. J Am Anim Hosp Assoc 26:647–651, 1990.
18. Gilson SD, Withrow SJ, Wheeler SL, et al: Pheochromocytoma in 50 dogs. J Vet Intern Med 8:228–232, 1994.
19. Barthez PY, Marks SL, Woo J, et al: Pheochromocytoma in dogs: 61 cases (1984–1995). J Vet Intern Med 11:272–278, 1997.
20. Ortega TM, Feldman EC, Nelson RW, et al: Systemic arterial blood pressure and urine protein/creatinine ratio in dogs with hyperadrenocorticism. J Am Vet Med Assoc 209:1724–1729, 1996.
21. Snyder PS: Amlodipine: A randomized, blinded clinical trial in 9 cats with systemic hypertension. J Vet Intern Med 12:157–162, 1998.
22. Belew AM, Barlett T, Brown SA: Evaluation of the white-coat effect in cats. J Vet Intern Med 13:134–142, 1999.
23. Binns SH, Sisson DD, Buoscio DA, et al: Doppler ultrasonographic, oscillometric sphygmomanometric, and photoplethysmographic techniques for noninvasive blood pressure measurement in anesthetized cats. J Vet Intern Med 9:405–414, 1995.
24. Caulkett NA, Cantwell SL, Houston DM: A comparison of indirect blood pressure monitoring techniques in the anesthetized cat. Vet Surg 27:370–377, 1998.
25. Grandy JL, Dunlop CI, Hodgson DS, et al: Evaluation of the Doppler ultrasonic method of measuring systolic arterial blood pressure in cats. Am J Vet Res 53:1166–1169, 1992.
26. Grosenbaugh DA, Muir WW: Blood pressure monitoring. Vet Med 93:48–59, 1998.
27. Kazamias TM, Gander MP, Franklin DL, et al: Blood pressure measurement with Doppler ultrasonic flowmeter. J Appl Physiol 30:585–588, 1971.
28. Nelson OL, Riedesel EA, Ware WA: Echocardiographic and radiographic changes associated with systemic hypertension in cats. Proceedings 17th ACVIM Forum, 17:712, 1999.
29. Conen D, Bertel O, Dubach UC: Cerebral blood flow and calcium antagonists in hypertension. J Hypertens Suppl 5:S75–S80, 1987.
30. Henik RA, Snyder PS: Treatment of systemic hypertension in cats with amlodipine besylate. J Am Anim Hosp Assoc 33:226–234, 1997.
31. King JN, Humbert-Droz E, Maurer M: Pharmacokinetics of benazepril and inhibition of plasma ACE activity in cats. Proceedings 14th ACVIM Forum, 14:745, 1996.
32. Krum H, Viskoper RJ, Lacourciere Y, et al: The effect of an endothelin-receptor antagonist, bosentan, on blood pressure in patients with essential hypertension. Bosentan Hypertension Investigators. N Engl J Med 338:784–790, 1998.
33. Cowgill LD, James KM, Levy JK, et al: Use of recombinant human erythropoietin for management of anemia in dogs and cats with renal failure. J Am Vet Med Assoc 212:521–528, 1998.
34. Epstein M: Hypertension as a risk factor for progression of chronic renal disease. Blood Press Suppl 1:23–28, 1994.
35. Tolins JP, Raij L: Antihypertensive therapy and the progression of chronic renal disease. Are there renoprotective drugs? Semin Nephrol 11:538–548, 1991.
36. Salvetti A, Giovannetti R, Arrighi P, et al: What effect does blood pressure control have on the progression toward renal failure? Am J Kidney Dis 21:10–15, 1993.
37. Epstein M: Calcium antagonists and renal hemodynamics: Implications for renal protection. Clin Invest Med 14:590–595, 1991.
38. Mohr FC, Carpenter JL: Arteriolosclerosis in a cat. Vet Pathol 24:466–469, 1987.

37

◆ Respiratory Therapeutics*

Lynelle R. Johnson

Successful treatment of respiratory disorders depends on appropriate pharmacologic therapy directed at a specific etiologic agent or physiologic response. Dosages of certain drugs have been well established for use in dogs or human beings; however, it is difficult to extrapolate use of these dosing regimens to cats because of unique metabolism in the feline species. Fortunately, studies that establish safe and effective drug therapy for treatment of feline diseases continue to be produced, providing the practicing veterinarian with current updates on pharmacologic therapy in cats.

◆ ANTIBACTERIAL THERAPY

Bacterial infection can occur in the upper or lower respiratory tract of cats. Knowledge of the normal flora inhabiting different locations within the respiratory tract, and of the species most likely to become pathogenic, aids in determining appropriate antibiotic therapy. Various bacteria can be recovered from airways of healthy cats,[1, 2] although only cats with pulmonary disease have had *Mycoplasma* isolated from lower airways[2] (Table 37–1). Normal oropharyngeal flora and *Mycoplasma* can act as opportunistic invaders after viral damage to epithelium of the upper respiratory tract, and in these cases, large numbers of bacterial colonies are found in association with inflammatory cells. These bacteria also may infect the lower respiratory tract in association with local or systemic disease, such as with megaesophagus or when a bronchial foreign body is present. *Bordetella* can act as a primary pathogen of the respiratory tract, resulting in serious disease in young kittens.

In cats with viral upper respiratory disease, flora of the upper respiratory tract (*Staphylococcus, Streptococcus, Pasteurella, Bordetella,* and anaerobes) may overwhelm local defenses and colonize the nasal cavity, leading to clinical signs of sneezing and mucopurulent nasal discharge. Antibiotics are administered commonly to cats or kittens with acute upper respiratory infection for 1 to 2 weeks to reduce bacterial numbers and decrease bacterial invasion of epithelium damaged by viral infection. Fortunately, many commonly encountered bacterial strains remain susceptible to amoxicillin–clavulanic acid. A recent European study found that a new fluoroquinolone (marbofloxacin at 2 mg/kg orally

[PO] every [q] 24 hr for 5 days) and amoxicillin–clavulanic acid had equal clinical efficacy in cats with acute upper respiratory infection.[3] Given the potential for development of bacterial resistance against quinolones and equal efficacy of an alternative drug, quinolones are not recommended as first-line treatment of acute infections, and amoxicillin–clavulanic acid remains a viable option. Penicillin derivatives are less efficacious against *Bordetella*, and are ineffective against *Mycoplasma*, a cell wall–deficient bacterium. If infection with these organisms is documented, use of a fluoroquinolone or doxycycline would be more appropriate. Cartilage deformities seen in puppies treated with high doses of enrofloxacin have not been reported in kittens. (*Editor's note:* Recent reports of retinopathy following high-dose administration of enrofloxacin to cats suggest that caution should be exercised in the use of this drug at higher-than-recommended dosages.)

Chronic upper respiratory disease typically is characterized by infection of bone, the presence of devitalized tissue with reduced blood supply, and accumulation of inflammatory products. Bacterial culture of nasal tissue may be helpful in choosing an appropriate antibiotic, because long-term antibiotic therapy (>6 weeks) is anticipated. Fluoroquinolones are a rational antibiotic choice in some cases, because these drugs have excellent efficacy against most gram-negative bacteria and *Mycoplasma*. Higher doses often are required for successful treatment of *Pseudomonas* infections. Most fluoroquinolones lack efficacy against *Streptococcus/Enterococcus* species and anaerobic organisms, although extended-spectrum drugs are being investigated currently (e.g., premafloxacin). For cats with underlying osteomyelitis or suspected anaerobic infection, a drug such as clindamycin could be more effective in controlling clinical signs, because this drug reportedly penetrates bone tissue. At standard doses,

Table 37–1. Bacteria Isolated From Airway Samples of Healthy Cats

Acinetobacter	*Klebsiella*
Bordetella	*Pasteurella*
Corynebacterium	*Staphylococcus*
Enterobacter	α-Streptococci
Flavobacterium	

Adapted from Dye JA, McKiernan BC, Rozanski EA, et al: Bronchopulmonary disease in the cat: Historical, physical, radiographic, clinicopathologic, and pulmonary functional evaluation of 24 affected and 15 healthy cats. J Vet Intern Med 10:385–400, 1996.

*This work was supported by the National Institutes of Health Grant HL–03856.

clindamycin has not been associated with biochemical abnormalities, vomiting, or loose/watery stools.

Lower respiratory tract infections require 2 to 6 weeks of antibiotic treatment, and long-term therapy should be determined by results of bacterial culture and susceptibility testing. *Mycoplasma* appears able to cause primary lower respiratory tract infection in cats,[4] and it is important to remember that this organism requires special culturing techniques (consult your laboratory). Initial antibiotic choices for respiratory infections must consider the likely species involved and known resistance patterns of commonly encountered bacteria (Table 37–2). Anaerobic bacteria often are found in culture samples taken from various sites in the body, and frequently these sites are coinfected with aerobic bacteria, particularly enteric organisms and *Pasteurella* species.[5] The incidence of anaerobic infections in lower respiratory disease of cats is unknown, although positive anaerobic cultures have been obtained in dogs with respiratory infection. Therefore, appropriate therapy for bacterial respiratory infections often requires antibiotics directed at gram-negative and gram-positive aerobes, anaerobes, and *Mycoplasma* organisms. Rational choices for broad-spectrum therapy of newly diagnosed infections (before final culture results are available) would include enrofloxacin and amoxicillin, clindamycin and enrofloxacin, and gentamicin in combination with a penicillin or cephalosporin derivative. *Bacteroides* species are relatively resistant to clindamycin therapy,[5] and metronidazole and chloramphenicol would be better choices when infection with this anaerobe is documented. Chloramphenicol has excellent efficacy against a number of organisms commonly implicated in respiratory infection; however, use of this drug may be associated with central nervous system depression, anorexia, vomiting, or bone marrow suppression.

A new class of antibiotics (azalides) commonly used in human medicine has efficacy against gram-positive and gram-negative organisms. These drugs have the advantage of producing high and prolonged tissue levels, typically resulting in enhanced bacterial killing. Recent studies in cats showed variability in drug half-life, but relatively high bioavailability (58 per cent) and sustained accumulation of drug in tissues after a single oral dose of 5.4 mg/kg.[6] The efficacy of azithromycin in feline respiratory diseases is not yet known; however, its pharmacokinetic properties and pulmonary penetration could prove valuable in treatment of respiratory infections. An empirical dosage of 5 to 10 mg/kg PO q 24 hr for 3 to 5 days has been suggested. Doxycycline is effective against a number of respiratory organisms, including *Yersinia pestis*, the agent of bubonic, pneumonic, and septicemic plague. *Mycoplasma* species also appear to be susceptible to doxycycline therapy.[4] Speakman and colleagues[7] found that the majority of feline *Bordetella* infections were susceptible to treatment with tetracycline, doxycycline, and enrofloxacin, with intermediate sensitivity to amoxicillin–clavulanic acid. Resistance of *Bordetella* to trimethoprim and ampicillin is common.[7]

◆ ANTIFUNGAL THERAPY

Fungal infection of the respiratory tract most commonly involves *Cryptococcus neoformans* in the nasal cavity (see Chapter 6, Cryptococcosis: New Perspectives on Etiology, Pathogenesis, Diagnosis, and Clinical Management) and *Histoplasma capsulatum* or *Blastomyces dermatitidis* in the lungs. Cryptococcosis is best treated with imidazole therapy, although prolonged therapy (4 to 12 months) should be anticipated. Imidazoles (ketoconazole, itraconazole, fluconazole) are fungistatic agents that inhibit P450 enzymes involved in synthesis of ergosterol, a key component of the fungal cell wall. Newer imidazoles have greater specificity for fungal P450 enzymes over mammalian forms, and are associated with fewer side-effects. Ketoconazole (Nizoral, Janssen Pharmaceuticals Inc.) is dosed at 50 to 100 mg/cat/day PO, but it has relatively poor efficacy against most fungal organisms, and is associated with significant side-effects such as anorexia and gastrointestinal upset. Itraconazole (Sporanox, Janssen Pharmaceuticals Inc.) is a newer imidazole available in 100-mg capsules containing small pellets of drug, and as a solution (5 mg/ml). Itraconazole reportedly is efficacious in approximately 50 per cent of nasal cryptococcosis cases. The standard dose recommendation is 5 to 10 mg/kg PO q 12 to 24 hr for the capsules and 1.25 to 1.5 mg/kg for the oral solution.[8] Itraconazole is excreted by the liver, and side-effects of therapy include hepatic toxicity and anorexia. Toxicity can be reduced and bioavailability improved by giving itraconazole with a meal, because absorption is improved in an acid environment. Therapeutic efficacy should be determined 2 to 3 weeks after initiating therapy, when most cats will have reached steady-state drug levels.[8] In a study from Australia (see Chapter 6, Cryptococcosis: New Perspectives on Etiology, Pathogenesis, Diagnosis, and Clinical Management), fluconazole (Diflucan, Roerig/Pfizer US Pharmaceutical Group) at a dose of 25 to 100 mg/cat orally q 12 hr resulted in cure of nasal cryptococcosis in 97 per cent of cats, despite disseminated disease or the presence of feline immunodeficiency virus in 28 per cent of cases.[9] It is unclear whether fluconazole is as effective in treating cases of cryptococcosis in the United States; however, it is considered the drug of choice for nasal cryptococcosis by some investigators because of its ability to penetrate the blood-brain barrier. The drug is available in 50-, 100-, and 200-mg tablets. Some cats may develop mild anorexia throughout treatment. Fluconazole is excreted renally, and a reduced dosage is recommended for cats with renal insufficiency. Therapy for cryptococcosis generally is continued for 4 weeks beyond clinical remission of disease or until the latex agglutination titer to capsular antigen is substantially reduced;

Table 37–2. Common Antibiotic Choices for Respiratory Infections With Select Microorganisms

Organism	First-Line Antibiotics	Dosage	Alternate Antibiotics	Dosage
Bordetella	Doxycycline Tetracycline Enrofloxacin	2.5–5 mg/kg PO q 12 hr 15–20 mg/kg PO q 12 hr 2.5–5 mg/kg PO q 12 hr	Amoxicillin–clavulanic acid	62.5 mg/cat PO q 12 hr
Escherichia coli	Enrofloxacin Ceftiofur Amikacin Gentamicin	2.5–5 mg/kg PO q 12 hr 2.2–4.4 mg/kg SQ q 12–24 hr 5–10 mg/kg IV, IM, SQ q 8 hr 2–4 mg/kg IV, IM, SQ q 8 hr	Chloramphenicol Trimethoprim/sulfonamide	50 mg/cat PO q 12 hr 15 mg/kg PO q 12 hr
Klebsiella	Enrofloxacin Amikacin Ceftiofur Amoxicillin–clavulanic acid	2.5–5 mg/kg PO q 12 hr 5–10 mg/kg IV, IM, SQ q 8 hr 2.2–4.4 mg/kg SQ q 12–24 hr 62.5 mg/cat PO q 12 hr	Trimethoprim/sulfonamide Gentamicin	15 mg/kg PO q 12 hr 2–4 mg/kg IV, IM, SQ q 8 hr
Pseudomonas	Enrofloxacin Carbenicillin Amikacin	2.5–5 mg/kg PO q 12 hr 10–15 mg/kg PO, IV q 8 hr 5–10 mg/kg IV, IM, SQ q 8 hr	Cephalosporin and gentamicin	
Pasteurella	Amoxicillin–clavulanic acid Cephalexin Trimethoprim/sulfonamide	62.5 mg/cat PO q 12 hr 10–30 mg/kg PO q 8–12 hr 15–30 mg/kg PO q 12 hr	Erythromycin Tetracycline Chloramphenicol	10–20 mg/kg PO q 8–12 hr 15–20 mg/kg PO q 12 hr 50 mg/cat PO q 12 hr
Yersinia pestis	Doxycycline	2.5–5 mg/kg PO q 12 hr		
Streptococcus	Amoxicillin–clavulanic acid Ampicillin	62.5 mg/cat PO q 12 hr 10–20 mg/kg IV, IM, SQ q 6 hr	Cephalexin Erythromycin	10–30 mg/kg PO q 8–12 hr 10–20 mg/kg PO q 8–12 hr
Staphylococcus	Methicillin Cloxacillin	20 mg/kg IM, IV q 6 hr 20–40 mg/kg PO q 8 hr	Cephalexin Clindamycin	10–30 mg/kg PO q 8–12 hr 5.5–11 mg/kg PO q 12–24 hr
Mycoplasma	Doxycycline	2.5–5 mg/kg PO q 12 hr	Chloramphenicol	50 mg/cat PO q 12 hr
Anaerobes	Metronidazole Clindamycin Chloramphenicol	10–25 mg/kg PO daily 5.5–11 mg/kg PO q 12–24 hr 50 mg/cat PO q 12 hr	Cefoxitin	30 mg/kg IV q 8 hr

Abbreviations: IM, intramuscularly; IV, intravenously; PO, orally; q, every; SQ, subcutaneously.

285

however, disease recurrence has been noted with either protocol.

Deep-seated mycotic infection of the lower respiratory tract can be treated with intravenous infusion of amphotericin B, a fungicidal drug; however, the protocol requires intravenous saline diuresis to limit nephrotoxicity, frequent monitoring of renal function, and prolonged use of jugular catheters. Cats likely are more sensitive to this drug than are dogs. Respiratory infection with histoplasmosis and blastomycosis can resolve after treatment with itraconazole or fluconazole at 5 to 10 mg/kg PO q 12 hr. Treatment should be continued for 2 months or longer to achieve cure.

◆ ANTI-INFLAMMATORY THERAPY

Anti-inflammatory drugs provide primary therapy for feline bronchial disease, an inflammatory airway disorder characterized by reversible bronchoconstriction, smooth-muscle-cell hypertrophy, and hypertrophy of mucous glands. Corticosteroids are indicated when airway infection with bacteria or parasites has been ruled out. Initial drug dosages range from 0.5 to 1.0 mg/kg prednisolone PO q 12 to 24 hr for 1 to 2 weeks. The dosage is decreased slowly, and the interval increased to allow alternate-day therapy whenever possible. Many cats require life-long or intermittent treatment with prednisolone, and fortunately, this drug is well-tolerated in the majority of cats.

Some cats do not respond adequately to steroid therapy alone, and may require addition of a bronchodilator (see later) or additional/alternative anti-inflammatory therapy. Most of the information gained about the pathogenesis of feline asthma and potential treatment modalities has been obtained from an experimental model of asthma in cats using antigen sensitization to induce airway hyper-responsiveness.[10–13] In vitro studies from this model have shown that cyproheptadine (Periactin, Merial), a serotonin receptor antagonist, reduces smooth-muscle contraction in response to potassium chloride or antigen in isolated airways.[10] This suggests that serotonin blockade could provide a means for reducing small-airway constriction in cats with bronchial disease. Use of cyproheptadine in combination with steroids, or as sole therapy in cats that cannot tolerate steroids, may be helpful in controlling signs associated with bronchoconstriction and airway inflammation. Cyproheptadine is characterized by high oral bioavailability; however, this may vary significantly among cats, resulting in requirements for once-daily to 3-times-daily dosing in different individuals.[14] Higher doses may be associated with excitability and aggression. Effective plasma levels for serotonin-receptor antagonism have not been established, although typically 1 to 2 mg/cat PO q 12 hr is used for initial therapy. Steady-state plasma concentrations may not be achieved for 1 to

5 days; therefore, the drug should be given continuously for several days to assess efficacy.[14]

Cyclosporine (Sandimmune, Novartis Pharma AG) is an inhibitor of interleukin-2 production and T-cell activation. This drug acts by blocking the immune cascade that leads to production of cytokines and activation of immune cells, and has proved beneficial in reducing airway inflammation in human asthmatics and in rat and cat models of asthma. In cats with experimentally induced airway disease, treatment with cyclosporine during the antigen-sensitization process prevented induction of airway hyper-reactivity and lessened histologic remodeling associated with antigen exposure.[11] However, cyclosporine had no effect on the early-phase asthmatic reaction, and did not inhibit mast-cell degranulation in this model,[12] despite attenuation of the late-phase asthmatic response. Thus, it appears less likely that this drug would limit acute bronchoconstrictive episodes, although it may lessen signs associated with chronic airway inflammation. In experimental studies, cyclosporine was dosed at 10 mg/kg PO q 12 hr, and dosing was adjusted through biweekly blood levels to maintain trough levels of 500 to 1000 ng/ml.[12] Plasma samples (collected in ethylenediaminetetraacetic acid [EDTA]) must be monitored weekly at the start of therapy, then monthly throughout treatment because of the potential for changes in drug metabolism over time. In human beings, drug interactions have been reported with antibiotics, antifungals, antiarrhythmics, and anticonvulsants. Side-effects of cyclosporine in cats include soft stool and complications associated with immunosuppression. The variable pharmacokinetics of this drug and requirement to obtain frequent drug levels may limit its use.

In antigen-sensitized cats, use of an inhibitor of 5-lipoxygenase failed to attenuate airway smooth muscle contraction in vitro, suggesting that leukotriene metabolites of this enzyme do not play a role in smooth-muscle contraction in experimentally induced airway hyper-responsiveness.[10] Also, in a recent report, cats with naturally occurring bronchial disease had similar urinary excretion of a leukotriene metabolite (leukotriene E_4), as did normal cats or cats with lower urinary tract disease.[15] Therefore, although drugs that block receptors for leukotriene D_4 or inhibit metabolic generation of leukotrienes are useful in some forms of human asthma, data are not available to support use of these drugs in feline patients. In addition, although histamine may be released during mast-cell degranulation in the early asthmatic response, antihistamines are not recommended for anti-inflammatory treatment in cats because histamine receptors in the feline airway mediate both bronchoconstriction and bronchodilatation.

Cats that have been antigen-sensitized are hyper-responsive to acetylcholine,[13] suggesting that airway inflammation may result in increased muscarinic receptors on airway smooth muscle or decreased degradation of acetylcholine. Cats with naturally occurring bronchial disease also are hyper-responsive to acetycholine[1]; however, use of muscarinic receptor–blocking drugs has not been investigated for therapeutic use. Airway hyper-responsiveness likely is due to complex interactions among several neural pathways in feline airways, and defining useful adjunctive therapy will require further study.

◆ ANTIVIRAL THERAPY

Viruses (feline herpesvirus-1 [FHV-1], calicivirus) have been implicated as major etiologic agents of feline upper respiratory disease complex (see Chapter 7, Update on the Diagnosis and Management of Feline Herpesvirus-1 Infections), and feline infectious peritonitis can lead to lower respiratory tract disease. In clinical syndromes, disease may result from viral infection or from the host's response to the virus. Many respiratory manifestations of feline infectious peritonitis virus infection are related to the host's immune response and subsequent vasculitis, making it difficult to determine whether antiviral therapy is warranted in these cases. Similarly, clinical signs in viral upper respiratory infection may be due to direct cytopathic effects mediated by the virus or to the host's response to infection. Unknown features of viral pathogenesis and the role of active infection in clinical disease make it difficult to determine specific indications for antiviral therapy.

Efficacy of antiviral agents in clinical feline respiratory diseases has not been established; however, pharmacokinetics have been studied for some drugs. Acyclovir (Zovirax, Glaxo Wellcome) at a dose of 50 mg/kg resulted in plasma drug levels well below the effective dose needed to inhibit FHV-1 replication by 50 per cent.[16] In addition to developing ineffective plasma levels, this dose of acyclovir may result in life-threatening toxicity in some cats. Although valacyclovir, a prodrug of acyclovir, can produce effective plasma levels,[16] this also leads to significant nephrotoxicity and bone marrow toxicity, and should not be used in cats. Human alpha-interferon has been investigated for use in treatment of viral diseases because of its broad spectrum of activity against many viruses and its immunomodulatory effects. Whereas interferon (1×10^6 units/kg subcutaneously) administered to cats before challenge with FHV-1 can reduce clinical signs, efficacy of continued therapy with high-dose interferon appears to be limited by the production of neutralizing antibodies. Acyclovir and human alpha-interferon appear to exert synergistic activity against FHV-1 in vitro, although efficacy in vivo has not been determined. Additional therapy under investigation for ocular complications of FHV-1 is the use of dietary supplementation with the amino acid lysine. Lysine competes with arginine in protein synthesis by FHV-1, and inhibition of synthetic activity may decrease replication of the virus.

Despite the lack of proven efficacy, antiviral therapy could be considered in cats or kittens severely affected by an upper respiratory infection that is presumed to be viral in origin. Antiviral therapy may reduce viral shedding, decrease clinical signs, or hasten resolution of disease. Specific combinations of drugs must be tailored to the individual patient and to the situation. To the author's knowledge, low-dose oral interferon (30 units PO daily for 7 days, administered every other week) has not been shown to result in production of neutralizing antibodies, and can be used relatively safely in cats and kittens. This drug can be formulated inexpensively from a concentrated human recombinant interferon. The human product (Roferon, Roche Laboratories) is sold in 3-million-unit vials. Dilution in 1 liter of sterile saline solution results in a 3000-unit/ml solution that can be frozen in 1-ml aliquots and stored for several months. One unit thawed and added to 100 ml of sterile saline solution provides a solution of 30 units/ml that can be refrigerated (1 month) for later use, and is administered easily to cats or kittens with viral disease. Interferon can be administered in combination with acyclovir and standard antibacterial therapy in hopes of achieving synergistic effects on viral killing, along with reduction in bacterial colonization of respiratory epithelium. Acyclovir is available in a 200-mg/ml suspension that is easy to dose to kittens and cats; however, animals on this drug must be monitored closely. Treatment with oral lysine (250 mg PO q 12 to 24 hr) also might be helpful in cats with upper respiratory disease. It is unclear whether cats with chronic rhinitis suffer exacerbations of disease mediated by viral replication that also might be amenable to antiviral therapy; however, trial therapy with antiviral medication and lysine in addition to antimicrobial therapy might be warranted in certain cases.

◆ BRONCHODILATOR THERAPY

Bronchodilators are useful as adjunct therapy in treating airway and parenchymal disorders in cats. Generally, these drugs are used in combination with corticosteroids for inflammatory lung disease or with antibiotics for infectious lung disease. Two main classes of bronchodilators are used in veterinary medicine: methylxanthine derivatives and beta$_2$ agonists.

The molecular mechanism of bronchodilatation in response to methylxanthine derivatives (aminophylline, theophylline) remains unknown. In clinically relevant plasma levels, methylxanthine drugs antagonize adenosine receptors on airway smooth muscle, and they may cause some inhibition of phosphodiesterase activity, resulting in increased cyclic adenosine monophosphate in smooth-muscle cells and airway relaxation. Additional cellular effects include alterations in intracellular calcium and stimulation of catecholamine release. In addition to bronchodilatation, theophylline has been reported to be beneficial in treatment of human lung diseases through suppression of airway inflammation and hyper-responsiveness, increased diaphragmatic contractility, and decreased microvascular permeability.

Pharmacokinetic studies performed in cats have identified 2 sustained-release theophylline products useful for management of lung disease in the species. Slo-bid Gyrocaps (Rhone-Poulenc-Rorer) and Theo-Dur Tablets (Key Pharmaceuticals/Schering Plough) at a dosage of 25 mg/kg q 24 hr in the evening reliably produce plasma concentrations approaching the human therapeutic range of 5 to 20 μg/ml. This dosage is higher than that recommended for aminophylline, because sustained-release formulations have decreased drug absorption that allows once-daily dosing, yet they achieve adequate plasma levels. Although generic sustained-release theophylline products are bioequivalent in human beings, similar studies have not been performed in cats, and generic substitutions are not recommended. In human medicine, theophylline metabolism is influenced by smoke in the environment, high fiber in the diet, congestive heart failure, liver disease, and use of many different classes of drugs, such as antibiotics, anticonvulsants, and antiarrhythmics (Table 37–3). A drug interaction between theophylline and enrofloxacin has been confirmed in dogs, and theophylline should be used cautiously in cats on other medications. In human beings, theophylline can antagonize the sedative effects of propofol.

Beta$_2$ agonists such as terbutaline and albuterol provide more rapid and profound bronchodilatation by binding to airway smooth-muscle-cell receptors and activating adenylate cyclase to increase cyclic adenosine monophosphate, resulting in direct smooth-muscle relaxation. Therefore, this class of drug likely is superior to theophylline in alleviating signs associated with acute bronchospasm. Terbutaline (0.01 mg/kg, intravenously or subcutaneously) results in a reduction in airway resistance in some cats with reversible airway obstruction,[1] and cats with dyspnea or increased expiratory effort due to bronchoconstriction or pneumonia can benefit from administration of terbutaline. Pharmacokinetic studies in cats indicate that an oral dosage of 0.625 mg/cat produces plasma concentrations 10 times the therapeutic range for bronchodilatation in human

beings.[17] This dosage administered orally twice-daily appears effective in reducing clinical signs in some cats with airway or lung disease, and is not associated with significant side-effects. Terbutaline also improves diaphragmatic contractility, and may allow reduction of the dosage of corticosteroid required for control of clinical signs in cats with bronchial disease.

Adverse-effects seen either with methylxanthines or with beta agonists include nervousness or hyper-excitability, tachycardia, and gastrointestinal upset. Central nervous system toxicity with use of methylxanthines likely is mediated through adenosine antagonism. Side-effects associated with beta agonists probably are due to cross-stimulation of beta$_1$ receptors resulting in tachycardia and hypotension. Relatively high doses are required for toxicity, and cats appear to exhibit side-effects less often than dogs. Combined use of theophylline and beta$_2$ agonists can result in more potent bronchodilatation, because methylxanthines inhibit metabolism of cyclic adenosine monophosphate and prolong its effect. However, adverse effects are more common with combined use of bronchodilators, and this type of therapy rarely is warranted in veterinary medicine.

Aerosolized therapy with bronchodilators is used commonly in human medicine, and most studies suggest that nebulized bronchodilators are more efficacious than intravenously administered drugs, despite the fact that only 5 to 10 per cent of the drug is likely to reach the lower airways. Aerosolized bronchodilators may result in more uniform and peripheral distribution of pulmonary gases; however, this therapy has not been assessed in cats. Cats with acute bronchoconstriction may be less likely to tolerate aerosol therapy, and drug may be absorbed poorly if significant inflammatory debris or mucus is present within the airway. However, cats that do not tolerate oral medication probably would benefit from aerosolized bronchodilator therapy, and this therapy should be considered for certain cases.

◆ VACCINES

Intranasal vaccines against calicivirus and FHV-1 (a bivalent vaccine); calicivirus, panleukopenia, and FHV-1 (a trivalent vaccine); and *Bordetella bronchiseptica* currently are available for use in prevention of upper respiratory disease. These vaccines induce secretory immunoglobulin (Ig) A antibody responses through activation of B cells in nasal-associated lymphoid tissue. Experimental studies in rats have shown that lymphocyte trafficking results in transfer of IgA-committed B cells to other mucosal effector sites, and leads to systemic IgG antibody responses.[18] Intranasal vaccines provide rapid effective immunity, they can be used in place of subcutaneous injections, and they circumvent interference by maternal antibodies. Any type of vaccination against upper respiratory diseases reduces the severity of disease, but does not prevent infection or

Table 37–3. Reported Drug Interactions for Theophylline in Human Medicine

Agents That May Increase Plasma Theophylline	Agents That May Decrease Plasma Theophylline
Beta blockers	Beta agonists
Calcium channel blockers	Ketoconazole
Cimetidine	Barbiturates
Loop diuretics	Loop diuretics
Corticosteroids	
Macrolides	
Mexitil	
Fluoroquinolones	
Thyroid hormones	
Thiabendazole	

abolish shedding. Therefore, viral infection may still result in induction of the carrier state. The *Bordetella* vaccine appears to be useful in limiting spread of disease in high-volume catteries, and in shelters where many cats are kept in closely confined areas.

◆ SUPPORTIVE CARE

Oxygen therapy should be employed in cats presenting with respiratory distress. Usually, an oxygen cage or tent is most advantageous because it provides a low-stress environment in addition to oxygen supplementation. Cats may struggle against oxygen administered through a face mask, and residual odors from anesthetic gases can worsen the animal's distress. Nasal oxygen can be used for continuous oxygen therapy, although it should not be employed in cats with chronic rhinitis. A soft, 6-French rubber catheter is lightly coated with anesthetic gel, and passed through the ventral nasal meatus into the nasopharynx. Oxygen administration at a flow of 0.5 to 1.0 liter/minute should improve oxygenation.

Cats with any type of respiratory disease benefit from therapy designed to hydrate respiratory secretions and enhance removal of mucus. Adequate systemic hydration should be ensured for all cases through intravenous, subcutaneous, or oral administration of fluids. In cats with airway disease or pneumonia, nebulization therapy is used to create small water particles that hydrate lower airways. Jet nebulizers (driven by flow of air or oxygen) or ultrasonic nebulizers (driven by a piezoelectric crystal) are preferred for creating particles small enough to penetrate the lower airway (2–5 μm in diameter). Affordable air compressors for jet nebulization are available through hospital supply companies, and nebulizer units may be obtained from several companies. Sterile saline solution (4–6 ml) is used most commonly in nebulization therapy, because antibiotics and bronchodilators often are administered more easily and reliably via oral or parenteral routes. Nebulization can result in bronchoconstriction or excessive stimulation of cough receptors, and systemic administration of a bronchodilator before local therapy can limit induction of excessive airway reflexes. Typically, aerosol therapy is followed by chest coupage, induction of a cough, gentle exercise, or other types of physical therapy to facilitate clearance of respiratory secretions. Coupage is performed less easily in cats than in dogs; however, removal of excess respiratory fluid should be encouraged. Cats with nasal disease also benefit from hydration of the respiratory tract. Airway humidification or instillation of saline nasal drops is adequate in these cases because particle size is not important for ensuring nasal deposition of fluid. Nasal secretions are made more fluid by this therapy, and stimulation of sneezing enhances removal of excess mucus. Young kittens may learn to tolerate this therapy more easily than older cats, and local treatment certainly is limited by the cat's aversion to this maneuver.

Cough suppressants are rarely if ever used in cats. Nasal decongestants also are rarely indicated because of the possibility of rebound nasal congestion after use of alpha-adrenergic vasoconstrictors. Although early viral infection is characterized by serous nasal discharge, infection typically leads to mucopurulent discharge, and decongestants are unlikely to be beneficial at this stage.

◆ CONCLUSION

Respiratory therapy must be based on knowledge of the etiologic agent and the likely pathogenesis of disease. The mechanisms of drug action, biologic behavior of organisms involved, and bacterial susceptibility testing will guide therapy; however, successful management of disease requires individualization of treatment.

REFERENCES

1. Dye JA, McKiernan BC, Rozanski EA, et al: Bronchopulmonary disease in the cat: Historical, physical, radiographic, clinicopathologic, and pulmonary functional evaluation of 24 affected and 15 healthy cats. J Vet Intern Med 10:385–400, 1996.
2. Randolph JF, Moïse NS, Scarlett JM, et al: Prevalence of mycoplasmal and ureaplasmal recovery from tracheobronchial lavages and of *Mycoplasma* recovery from pharyngeal swabs in cats with and without pulmonary disease. Am J Vet Res 54:897–900, 1993.
3. Dossin O, Gruet P, Thomas E: Comparative field evaluation of marbofloxacin tablets in the treatment of feline upper respiratory tract infections. J Small Anim Pract 39:286–289, 1998.
4. Foster SF, Barrs VR, Martin P, Malik R: Pneumonia associated with *Mycoplasma* spp in three cats. Aust Vet J 76:460–463, 1998.
5. Jang SS, Breher JE, Dabaco LA, et al: Organisms isolated from dogs and cats with anaerobic infections and susceptibility to selected antimicrobial agents. J Am Vet Med Assoc 210:1610–1614, 1997.
6. Hunter RP, Lunch MJ, Ericson JF, et al: Pharmacokinetics, oral bioavailability, and tissue distribution of azithromycin in cats. J Vet Pharmacol Ther 18:38–46, 1995.
7. Speakman AJ, Binns SH, Dawson S, et al: Antimicrobial susceptibility of *Bordetella bronchiseptica* isolates from cats and a comparison of the agar dilution and E-test methods. Vet Microbiol 54:63–72, 1997.
8. Boothe DM, Herring I, Calvin J, et al: Itraconazole disposition after single oral and intravenous and multiple oral dosing in healthy cats. Am J Vet Res 58:872–877, 1997.
9. Malik R, Wigney DI, Muir DB, et al: Cryptococcosis in cats: Clinical and mycological assessment of 29 cases and evaluation of treatment using orally administered fluconazole. J Med Vet Mycol 30:133–144, 1992.
10. Padrid PA, Mitchell RW, Ndukwu IM, et al: Cyproheptadine-induced attenuation of type-1 immediate-hypersensitivity reactions of airway smooth muscle from immune-sensitized cats. Am J Vet Res 56:109–115, 1995.
11. Padrid PA, Cozzi P, Left AR: Cyclosporine A inhibits airway reactivity and remodeling after chronic antigen challenge in cats. Am J Respir Crit Care Med 154:1812–1818, 1996.
12. Mitchell RW, Cozzi P, Ndukwu MI, et al: Differential effects of cyclosporine A after acute antigen challenge in sensitized cats *in vivo* and *ex vivo*. Br J Pharmacol 123:1198–1204, 1998.
13. Mitchell RW, Ndukwu IM, Leff AR, Padrid PA: Muscarinic

hyper-responsiveness of antigen-sensitized feline airway smooth muscle *in vitro*. Am J Vet Res 58:672–676, 1997.

14. Norris CR, Boothe DM, Esparza T, et al: Disposition of cyproheptadine in cats after intravenous or oral administration of a single dose. Am J Vet Res 59:79–81, 1998.

15. Mellema MS, Gershwin LJ, Norris CR: Urinary leukotriene E4 levels in cats with allergic bronchitis (Abstract). Proceedings of the 17th Annual ACVIM Forum, Chicago, June 10–13, 1999.

16. Owens JG, Nasisse MP, Tadepalli SM, Dorman DC: Pharmacokinetics of acyclovir in the cat. J Vet Pharmacol Ther 19:490–499, 1996.

17. McKiernan BC, Dye JA, Powell M, et al: Terbutaline pharmacokinetics in cats. Proceedings of the 9th Annual ACVIM Forum, New Orleans, May 1991, p. 877.

18. Lathers DMR, Gill RF, Montgomery PC: Inductive pathways leading to rat tear IgA antibody responses. Invest Ophthalmol Vis Sci 39:1005–1011, 1998.

38
◆ Holter Monitoring

Wendy A. Ware

Holter monitoring is a form of continuous ambulatory electrocardiography. The typical recording period is 24 hours, although shorter or longer times may be used. Such prolonged and continuous electrocardiographic (ECG) recording provides a practical, noninvasive means of documenting the complexity and frequency of cardiac rhythm disturbances, as well as correlating their occurrence with clinical signs. In human beings, Holter monitoring is used not only to detect cardiac arrhythmias but also to determine the effectiveness of antiarrhythmic therapy, identify ST-segment changes accompanying ischemia, and evaluate other parameters during normal daily activities. In clinical veterinary medicine, Holter monitoring has been used most commonly in dogs, especially to evaluate those patients with syncope or episodic weakness thought to be caused by intermittent arrhythmias, and to assess the effectiveness of antiarrhythmic drug therapy.[1-6] It also is used to screen for ventricular arrhythmias associated with subclinical cardiomyopathy of boxers and Doberman pinschers.[7-9] Standard ECG recordings, because of their short time duration, do not detect even frequent arrhythmias consistently,[10] and they are likely to result in over- or underestimation of the severity of any identified rhythm disturbance. Furthermore, because there is naturally wide fluctuation in the occurrence of cardiac arrhythmias over time, intermittent ECG strips cannot evaluate the effectiveness of antiarrhythmic therapy accurately. Studies in human beings suggest that a decrease of up to 90 per cent in the occurrence of ventricular premature beats over a 24-hour recording period is necessary to confidently conclude antiarrhythmic drug efficacy.[11-13] Holter monitoring can be useful in cats also, although the small size and rapid heart rates of cats present additional logistical and interpretation challenges.

◆ EQUIPMENT

Holter monitors are small, battery-powered analogue tape (cassettes or, less commonly, reel-to-reel) or digital recorders. Most analogue units weigh about a pound or less with tape, battery, lead wires, and case included. Preferably, at least 2 ECG channels (leads) are recorded simultaneously; this allows more accurate differentiation of abnormal beats from artifact than does a single ECG channel. An internal clock records time, so that ECG events can be correlated with the time of day or night. Most Holter recorders also have an "event" button that, when pushed, records a signal allowing correlation of clinical signs (e.g., weakness or syncope) with concurrent ECG events. Although the usual ECG recording period is 24 hours, monitoring for 2 or 3 days can be accomplished by replacing the tape and battery every 24 hours. The recorded tape is digitized and analyzed using a computer-scanning process; control and editing of the analysis by a skilled technician are important for accuracy of the final report. Commercial Holter scanning services are used commonly in human medicine; some of these provide a Holter monitor and tape analysis for veterinary use. It is preferable that the Holter technician be experienced in evaluating recordings from animals. LabCorp Ambulatory Monitoring Services (Burlington, NC [800] 289–4358) is 1 commercial service that has had experience interpreting veterinary Holter recordings, especially from dogs and cats. Holter monitoring also is available at many university veterinary teaching hospitals and cardiology referral practices. Other types of long-term ECG monitoring include small "event" recorders and radiotelemetry. Event recorders must be activated by the patient (or owner) before they begin recording, and therefore are often impractical for animals, although some are arrhythmia-activated.

◆ HOLTER MONITOR ATTACHMENT

The electrodes are applied to the chest wall, and the recorder is either attached directly to the cat's back or placed in a cage with the animal. With direct attachment, the cat may be sent home, and a normal daily routine encouraged. Although the size of the recording device may interfere somewhat with activity, many cats appear to tolerate wearing the recorder fairly well. In a study of 20 normal cats,[14] almost all animals tolerated the directly attached recorder fairly well after an initial adjustment period, although many appeared to have reduced activity over the 24-hour period. Only 1 older cat was clearly upset for the duration of the recording period. Some cats displayed fairly normal activity, including jumping up onto furniture. But clinical judgment must be used in deciding whether to attach a Holter monitor directly to an ill cat or one of high-strung temperament; cage confinement with the recorder placed nearby may be more appropriate, especially if the cat shows evidence of cardiac decompensation or other distress, or is of very small size (e.g., ≤3 kg).

The hook-up procedure used by the author is outlined here; other specific instructions provided by the Holter scanning service should be followed as directed. Supplies are listed in Table 38–1. The Holter recorder is prepared by inserting a fresh battery, checking the internal clock, and resetting if necessary to the correct (military) time. Directions for setting the clock should be provided with the recorder. The lead wires should be plugged firmly into the appropriate insertion points on the back of the recorder. Generally the gain setting inside the recorder is set at "×1.0." The cassette tape is prepared by removing the plastic tape "stopper," if present, and taking up any slack in the tape. The cassette is labeled with the names of the patient and doctor, date of hook-up, start time of the recording, and any other information requested by the scanning service. The tape then is placed into the recorder. When the recorder lid is closed, the tape should turn slowly. The recorder lid may be left open until other hook-up preparations are complete.

The recording leads usually are oriented transversely across the heart (e.g., left mid/dorsal to right ventral thorax, and right mid/dorsal to left ventral thorax). A ground electrode also may be used, depending on the monitor type. Electrodes are oriented circumferentially around the chest just behind the front legs, but allowing enough space behind the forelimbs so that movement is not inhibited. The electrodes will be fairly close together because of the small size of the thorax. Shaving the hair at the electrode sites will provide better skin contact. In cats, shaving a U-shaped strip from mid–left thorax down ventrally across the sternum and up to the mid- to upper right thorax is recommended, rather than a small patch for each electrode (Fig. 38–1). This facilitates rapid attachment of the adhesive electrode pads without getting hair caught on them. Furthermore, when hair on the ventral body wall is removed, removal of the bandaged electrodes is faster and better tolerated by the cat. Holter hook-up kits supplied by commercial scanning services usually include a razor, but it is not necessary to further shave the electrode sites.

The skin at the electrode sites is cleansed with

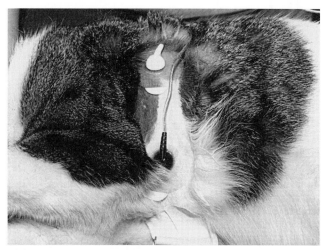

Figure 38–1. A U-shaped strip of hair is clipped behind the forelimbs and across the sternum for easier attachment of electrode pads.

Nolvasan (Fort Dodge Laboratories, Fort Dodge, IA) or similar agent followed by alcohol wipes to remove dirt, loose hair, and excess oil. The hair surrounding the electrode sites should be kept dry. The electrode attachment sites then are scrubbed with an alcohol preparation pad containing pumice (generally supplied with the hook-up kit) and allowed to dry. While the skin is drying, the electrodes and lead wires are prepared. A small dab of ECG contact gel or paste is placed on the pre-gelled sponge in the center of each electrode to enhance skin contact; it is best to avoid getting gel on the sticky adhesive part. A lead wire is snapped onto each electrode, and the electrode gently set back onto its plastic backing until needed (Fig. 38–2). Although the electrode patches may be attached to their skin sites before the wires are attached, I have found that the pressure and/or skin pinch needed to snap the lead wire connector to the "button" on the electrode patch is often annoying and disruptive to cats. Before the actual hook-up, the bandaging materials needed to attach the electrodes and recorder also are prepared. I use 4 strips of adhesive tape a little longer than the dorsoventral length of the thorax, and two 12-inch strips of Elastikon (Johnson & Johnson Medical Inc., Arlington, TX). A roll of 2-inch Elastikon and a roll of Vetrap (3M Animal Care Products, St Paul, MN) also should be readily at hand. The cover of the recorder should be closed, and the turning motion of the tape verified, if this has not been done already. The recorder then is placed in its case.

During electrode attachment, it is important to have the cat standing or held still, and to work quickly until the bandage is secure. The electrode patches as well as adhesive tape may not stick well to the skin and hair coat, especially if these are moist, but the covering bandage stabilizes the electrodes well, and subsequent removal of the apparatus is much easier with this method. Strips of Elastikon may be used instead of adhesive tape; however,

Table 38–1. Supplies Used for Holter Monitor Attachment

Holter recorder and patient cables
Fresh 9-volt battery
Cassette (or other) tape
Pre-gelled silver/silver chloride electrodes
Clippers
Skin cleansing scrub
Alcohol preparation pads with pumice
1″ Adhesive tape
2″ Elastikon
2″ or 3″ Vetrap
Bandage scissors
ECG contact gel or paste
Patient diary

Abbreviation: ECG, electrocardiographic.

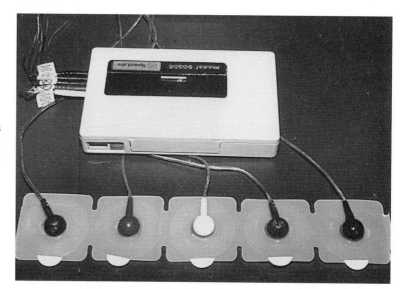

Figure 38–2. The Holter lead wires have been snapped onto the adhesive electrode pads, and a small amount of electrocardiographic (ECG) paste has been applied to the pre-gelled electrode surfaces underneath before placement on the cat.

removal of the bandage is much more difficult. For each side of the chest, each electrode and attached wire is stuck to the appropriate (see instructions supplied with the recorder) prepared skin site while the skin is gently held taut. It is more convenient to attach the dorsalmost electrode first and work ventrally, while orienting the lead wires straight dorsally. The electrodes are stabilized by placing a strip of adhesive tape from dorsal to ventral over the front edges and another over the back edges of the electrode patches (Fig. 38–3). The wires should be directed dorsally. With the lead wires gathered at the top of the back, the electrode patches, lead wires, and adhesive tape strips are covered with 2-inch Elastikon to encircle the thorax. A minimum amount of hair is included in the Elastikon wrap. The wires should exit the Elastikon wrap all together on top of the animal.

If the monitor is to be attached directly to the cat, the excess wire is coiled and the recorder is placed on top (Fig. 38–4). The 12-inch strips of Elastikon are used to secure the recorder case on top of the wire coil and to the Elastikon strip that covers the electrodes. The chest is wrapped with Vetrap to cover the electrode areas, all exposed wire, and recorder, making sure the event button on the recorder is accessible (Fig. 38–5). The Holter monitor will tend to slide toward one side of the chest during the recording period, but this should not reduce the recording's quality.

If direct attachment of the recorder to the patient would cause undue stress, the animal should be placed in a cage with the recorder nearby. A light wrap (e.g., Vetrap) also can be used to further protect the electrode sites (Fig. 38–6), and may be wound around the lead wires to keep them together. The animal should be observed closely to prevent entanglement in or chewing of the wires.

A "patient activity diary" including name, date, and time the recording was started is used to record the cat's activity at different times of the day along with any clinical signs. If clinical signs are observed, the event button on the recorder should be pushed and the time noted in the diary. If possible, the cat is sent home, and normal activity encouraged during the recording period. Although most animals do not chew at the bandage, they should be watched for this activity. If syncope or episodic weakness is the reason for monitoring, activities or circumstances that have been associated with that event should be pursued. At the end of the recording period, the monitor is removed easily by separating the bandage digitally from underlying skin ventrally, carefully cutting the bandage along the sternum, then peeling it up both sides of the chest.

A request form provided by the scanning service and a copy of the patient diary are mailed with the tape to be analyzed. It is helpful to ask for a "full-disclosure" printout (Fig. 38–7) on this form and note any other special instructions. Because of the high heart rates in cats, it may be necessary to ana-

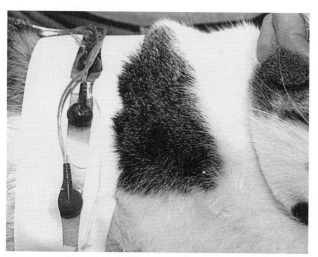

Figure 38–3. Strips of adhesive tape are placed over the front and back edges of the electrode pads to help stabilize them during the hook-up procedure.

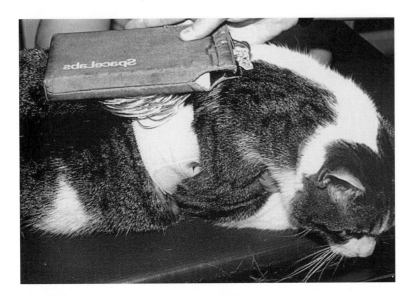

Figure 38–4. An adhesive elastic bandage (e.g., Elastikon) has been wrapped around the thorax to cover and secure the electrodes. Excess lead wire has been coiled over the cat's back, and the Holter recorder, within its case, is placed on top. Additional Elastikon is used to secure the recorder to the underlying Elastikon wrap.

lyze the tape in two 12-hour segments if the ECG data exceed the scanning service's computer memory capacity (LabCorp is familiar with this procedure). The upper and lower limits of normal heart rate used by the scanning service for cats should be ascertained.

◆ THE HOLTER REPORT

The report from the Holter monitoring service indicates the hook-up time, duration of recording, and quality of the recording. Information about hourly minimum, maximum, and average heart rates, as well as over the entire scanning period, is included. Episodes of "tachycardia" or "bradycardia" also are listed, based on the upper and lower limits of normal heart rate as set by the scanning technician for the species. Computer algorithms are used to classify and group normal and abnormal QRS complexes, with the scanning technician making necessary modifications. Ectopic beats are identified by variations in configuration and/or timing. The report

also contains representative ECG strips that illustrate abnormal and normal rhythms during the recording period (Fig. 38–8).

Critical evaluation of the Holter report by the requesting veterinarian is important because interpretation errors can occur, especially if the Holter technician is unfamiliar with animal ECGs. The rapid heart rates and small QRS complexes of cats also increase the challenge of interpreting Holter recordings. A source of interpretation error that is less common in cats than in dogs is marked sinus arrhythmia; faster cycles may be identified mistakenly as atrial premature complexes, sinus pauses may be called *dropped beats*, and baseline tremor with sinus arrhythmia may be misinterpreted as atrial fibrillation. Frequent ectopic beats or complex arrhythmias may be misinterpreted and/or miscounted, especially at fast heart rates. All selected ECG strips included with the report as well as the

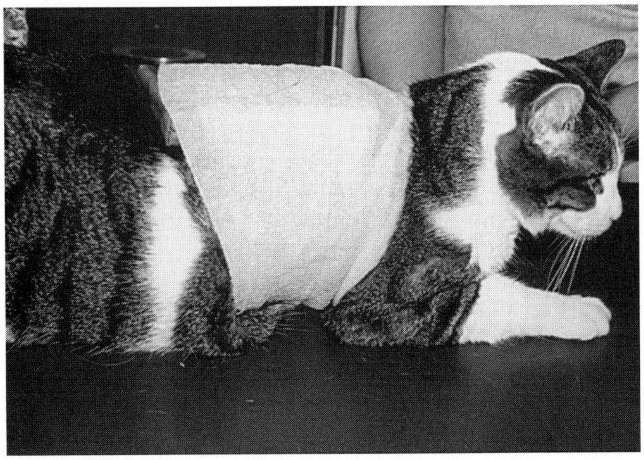

Figure 38–5. Vetrap, or similar self-adhesive elastic wrap, is used to cover the entire apparatus.

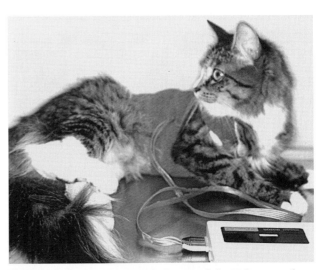

Figure 38–6. When direct attachment of the Holter recorder to the cat is not desired, the electrodes are secured and covered as described previously, but the monitor is placed in or on top of the cat's cage. (Courtesy of Dr. Philip R. Fox.)

06:09 am

06:13 am

Figure 38–7. A portion of the full-disclosure printout from a normal cat shows sinus arrhythmia. Two ECG channels of opposite polarity are printed at 20 minutes of time per page. The time of day is indicated along the left margin.

summary data should be examined carefully. In addition, the full-disclosure printout should be scanned visually and compared with the selected ECG strips. The full-disclosure printout also should be evaluated closely at the times of clinical signs, as noted in the patient diary. The Holter technician may be able to answer questions that arise, and can enlarge other segments of the full-disclosure recording if needed. Input from a veterinary cardiologist regarding interpretation of the recording also may be advisable.

◆ HEART RATE AND RHYTHM VARIATIONS IN CATS

In normal cats, heart rates vary widely over 24 hours. Heart rates ranging from 68 to 294 bpm were observed in a recent study.[14] Regular sinus rhythm was predominant in recordings from normal cats; however, periods of mild-to-moderate sinus arrhythmia frequently were evident at lower heart rates in most cats, especially during the early morning hours. Second-degree atrioventricular block was al-

most never observed.[14] Average heart rates in individual cats ranged from 114 to 202 bpm. The mean 24-hour average heart rate was not different between younger cats (157.6 ± 5.7 bpm; average, 2.5 years old) and older cats (156.3 ± 6.4 bpm; average, 10.4 years old). But females (of all ages together) had higher average heart rates over the 24-hour period compared with males (167 ± 5.8 and 147 ± 4.4 bpm, respectively). Minimum heart rates also were higher in females. The overall range of heart rates for females was 95 to 292 bpm, and for males was 68 to 294 bpm.[14] The total duration of time the heart rate exceeded 240 bpm (defined as tachycardia) for both younger and older cats ranged from 0 to 144 minutes with a mean of 19.4 ± 7.2 minutes. There were no differences between the means for age groups or genders. Duration of bradycardia (heart rate of less than 99 bpm) ranged from 0 to 475.3 minutes throughout the 24 hours, but the median time was 0 seconds. The heart rate never fell below 99 bpm in 14 cats; 9 of these were females. Although 1 cat with a consistently lower heart rate had "bradycardia" for a total of almost 8 hours, the next longest total duration was 0.7 minute. Maximum

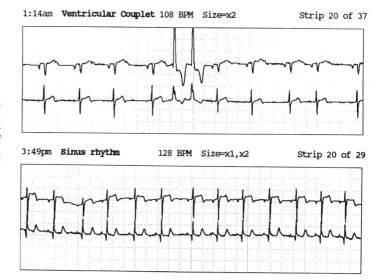

Figure 38–8. Two of the representative ECG samples from a commercial Holter report on an American shorthair cat with hypertrophic obstructive cardiomyopathy are shown. Each strip is marked with the time of day, rhythm interpretation, and heart rate. In this cat, a pair of ventricular premature beats occurred at 1:14 A.M. The underlying rhythm in both strips is sinus arrhythmia.

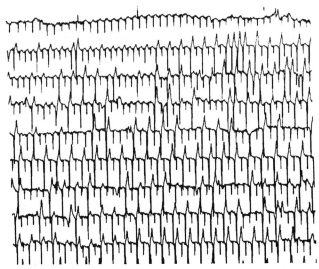

Figure 38–9. A portion of the full-disclosure printout from a British shorthair cat with hypertrophic cardiomyopathy indicates frequent ventricular premature beats, with several ventricular couplets and a short paroxysm of ventricular tachycardia.

heart rates between 250 and 295 bpm were common, and were not different between age groups or genders.

Mean heart rates of 182 (range, 142 to 222) bpm[15] and 197 (range, 160 to 240) bpm[16] have been reported from routine electrocardiograms in awake, normal cats; but rates from normal cats taken at home late at night by the owner were lower (mean 118, range 80 to 160 bpm), illustrating the importance of psychological stress on heart rate response.[15] Based on average heart rates, the technique of Holter monitoring in the home environment with an attached recorder appears to produce comparatively less stress overall than in-hospital electrocardiography, while providing a much longer observation time. Nevertheless, some degree of sustained stress from the attached monitor was likely, as average heart rates during the night in this study were higher than late-night owner observations.[14, 15] Similar mean 24-hour average heart rates were found in

hospitalized normal cats,[17] but mean minimum heart rate was higher (117 ± 15 bpm) and maximum heart rate was lower (241 ± 21 bpm).

Diurnal variation in heart rate occurs. A rise in hourly average, minimum, and maximum heart rates has been observed in the midafternoon through about 9:00 P.M. Rates were lowest just after midnight.[14] The acceleration in heart rates seen during the late afternoon and into the night probably reflects increased activity, consistent with the nocturnal nature of cats. Hourly average and minimum heart rates were about 20 bpm higher in females than in males. There were no gender differences in hourly maximum heart rates.[14]

Low numbers of ventricular premature beats occur in normal cats. In 1 study,[14] the total number of ventricular ectopic beats ranged from 0 to 59, excluding 1 cat with an accelerated idioventricular rhythm. Younger cats had fewer ectopic beats than those in older cats (3.8 ± 0.9 and 18.7 ± 7.2, respectively).[14] Occasional pairs were seen, and 1 older cat had 2 short runs of ventricular tachycardia. Multiform configuration was seen in 5 younger and 7 older cats. From 0 to 50 single ventricular extrasystoles were noted in a Holter study of hospitalized normal cats,[17] although the distribution of ventricular premature beats between older and younger cats was not reported. Supraventricular premature complexes are uncommon, but occur more frequently in older cats.[14, 17] These studies suggest that occasional ventricular (and supraventricular) ectopic activity is common in healthy young cats, and the number of ventricular extrasystoles increases with age, as in human beings.[18, 19] But as in dogs, it is still unclear how many premature beats can be considered "normal" in cats. Holter recordings from cats with hypertrophic cardiomyopathy (personal observations)[17, 20] or myocardial failure[17] have documented variably frequent multiform premature ventricular complexes as well as paroxysmal ventricular tachycardia (Fig. 38–9), although some cardiomyopathic cats have had no more frequent ventricular premature complexes observed than normal cats. Conversely, bradycardia followed by asystole was seen

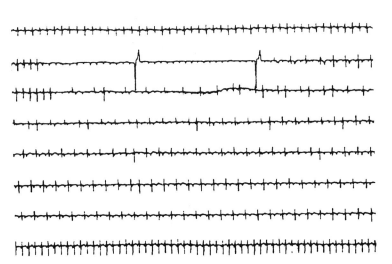

Figure 38–10. Holter monitoring demonstrated the cause of syncope in a 14-year-old domestic shorthair cat that had third-degree atrioventricular (AV) block with an apparently stable ventricular escape rhythm at about 100 bpm on routine electrocardiogram. This portion of the full-disclosure report shows sinus rhythm with normal AV conduction on the *top line*. Complete AV block developed during the initial part of the *second line* (only negative P-waves are seen); 2 ventricular escape complexes finally occurred after greater than 5 and 6 seconds, respectively, followed by a more regular escape rhythm. Lines 3 to 8 show periods of normally conducted sinus rhythm as well as complete AV block with a ventricular escape rhythm at about 90 bpm. (Courtesy of Dr. O. Lynne Nelson.)

in 5 cats with cardiomyopathy that died during Holter monitoring.[17]

Correlation of the activities noted in the patient diary (especially with regard to any signs of weakness, lethargy, or syncope) with the heart rate and rhythm obviously is important in view of the wide heart rate range and the rhythm variations observed in normal animals. Patients with clinically significant sinus or atrioventricular nodal conduction disease may not be able to increase heart rate commensurate with what is required for the activity level. Inappropriate sinus bradycardia, prolonged sinus pauses, and frequent atrioventricular nodal conduction failure are likely to provoke clinical signs (Fig. 38–10). Likewise, large numbers of ventricular premature complexes and the presence of paroxysmal ventricular tachycardia are of concern.

REFERENCES

1. Moïse NS, DeFrancesco T: Twenty-four hour ambulatory electrocardiography (Holter monitoring). *In* Bonagura JD (ed): Kirk's Current Veterinary Therapy XII. Philadelphia, WB Saunders, 1995, pp. 792–799.
2. Goodwin JK: Holter monitoring and cardiac event recording. Vet Clin North Am Small Anim Pract 28:1391–1407, 1998.
3. Miller RH, Lehmkuhl LB, Bonagura JD, et al: Retrospective analysis of the clinical utility of ambulatory electrocardiographic (Holter) recordings in syncopal dogs: 44 cases (1991–1995). J Vet Intern Med 13:111–122, 1999.
4. Miller MS, Calvert CA: Special methods for analyzing arrhythmias. *In* Tilley LP (ed): Essentials of Canine and Feline Electrocardiography, 3rd ed. Philadelphia, Lea & Febiger, 1992, pp. 289–319.
5. Rush JE, Keene BW: ECG of the month. J Am Vet Med Assoc 194:52, 1989.
6. Calvert CA, Jacobs GJ, Pickus CW: Bradycardia-associated episodic weakness, syncope, and aborted sudden death in cardiomyopathic Doberman pinschers. J Vet Intern Med 10:88–93, 1996.
7. Calvert CA: Diagnosis and management of ventricular tachyarrhythmias in Doberman pinschers with cardiomyopathy. *In* Bonagura JD (ed): Kirk's Current Veterinary Therapy XII. Philadelphia, WB Saunders, 1995, pp. 799–806.
8. Goodwin JK, Cattiny G: Further characterization of boxer cardiomyopathy. Proceedings of the 13th ACVIM Forum, Lake Buena Vista, FL, 1995, pp. 300–302.
9. Calvert CA, Hall G, Jacobs G, et al: Clinical and pathologic findings in Doberman pinschers with occult cardiomyopathy that died suddenly or developed congestive heart failure: 54 cases (1984–1991). J Am Vet Med Assoc 210:505–511, 1997.
10. Marino DJ, Matthiesen DT, Fox PR, et al: Ventricular arrhythmias in dogs undergoing splenectomy: A prospective study. Vet Surg 23:101–106, 1994.
11. Morganroth J, Michelson EL, Horowitz LN, et al: Limitations of routine long-term electrocardiographic monitoring to assess ventricular ectopic frequency. Circulation 58:408–414, 1978.
12. Winkle RA: Antiarrhythmic drug effect mimicked by spontaneous variability of ventricular ectopic activity. Circulation 57:1116–1121, 1978.
13. Raeder EA, Hohnloser SH, Graboys TB, et al: Spontaneous variability and circadian distribution of ectopic activity in patients with malignant ventricular arrhythmias. J Am Coll Cardiol 12:656–661, 1988.
14. Ware WA: Twenty-four-hour ambulatory electrocardiography in normal cats. J Vet Intern Med 13:175–180, 1999.
15. Hamlin RL: Heart rate of the cat. J Am Anim Hosp Assoc 25:284–286, 1989.
16. Gompf RE, Tilley LP: Comparison of lateral and sternal recumbent positions for electrocardiography of the cat. Am J Vet Res 40:1483–1486, 1979.
17. Fox PR, Moïse NS, Price RA, et al: Analysis of continuous ECG (Holter) monitoring in normal cats and cardiomyopathic cats in congestive heart failure (Abstract). J Vet Intern Med 12:199, 1998.
18. Takada H, Mikawa T, Murayama M, et al: Range of ventricular ectopic complexes in healthy subjects studied with repeated ambulatory electrocardiographic recordings. Am J Cardiol 63:184–186, 1989.
19. Rossi A: Twenty-four-hour electrocardiographic study in the active very elderly. Cardiology 74:159–166, 1987.
20. Goodwin JK, Lombard CW, Ginex DD: Results of continuous ambulatory electrocardiography in a cat with hypertrophic cardiomyopathy. J Am Vet Med Assoc 200:1352–1354, 1992.

39

◆ Aortic Thromboembolism

Catherine J. Baty

◆ ETIOLOGY

Aortic thromboembolism (ATE) is the term commonly applied to the localization of a blood clot within the aorta when there is reason to believe that the clot originated somewhere upstream in the vascular tree or left side of the heart. In some cases, the term *systemic embolization* may be more appropriate in that thrombi are not strictly limited to the aorta, but may occur in various arterial branches off the aorta, for example, the renal or brachial arteries. Cats presenting with ATE are most often found to have some form of cardiomyopathy, an acknowledged risk factor for the development of intracardiac thrombus and subsequent embolization. For this reason, even when an intracardiac thrombus is not detected, clinicians generally assume that the aortic thrombus originated in the affected heart. Rarely, cats present with ATE with no evidence of heart disease, and other etiologies including systemic disease resulting in hypercoagulable states, primary coagulopathies, vascular disease, and trauma must be investigated. An underlying cause sometimes is not identified.

◆ EPIDEMIOLOGY

Investigations of ATE for the most part have been limited to retrospective studies of cats treated at large referral centers, and therefore may not reflect the full spectrum of disease. Most surveys have been conducted by cardiologists or cardiovascular pathologists so there has been a bias to report feline ATE associated with heart disease. One study done in the 1970s provides the broadest perspective of the potential significance of ATE in a population of over 1500 routinely necropsied cats.[1] Of these, it was found that 112 cats (7.2 per cent) had acquired heart disease leading to congestive heart failure: 10 per cent of these cats had atrial thrombi, 41 per cent had aortic thromboemboli, and 21 per cent with atrial thrombi had systemic thromboemboli. At the time of this study, cardiomyopathies were not classified as they are today, but it is evident from the pathologic descriptions that hypertrophic and dilated cardiomyopathy were well represented in this population.

The largest population of ATE cases is summarized in a retrospective study restricted to cats with distal ATE (defined by clinical signs of loss or significant decrease of 1 or both femoral pulses and other supportive signs consistent with acute arterial occlusion): 100 cases gleaned from medical records from a 17-year period.[2] The resultant profile of cats suffering distal ATE was not compared with the normal hospital population, but male cats were affected more often (67 per cent total, 63 per cent neutered) than females (32 per cent total, 31 per cent spayed) with a mean age of 7.7 years (median, 10.5 years). Most cats were domestic varieties. The dramatic finding was that for nearly 90 per cent of cases, the ATE episode was the first indication of possible heart disease. Hypertrophic cardiomyopathy (HCM) is the most commonly diagnosed feline heart disease, and is often suspected to be the underlying risk factor in cats presenting with ATE without previously diagnosed heart disease; and in this study, it was found to be the most common underlying disease (diagnosed in 58 per cent of cats). This actually may be an underestimate of the prevalence of HCM in cats with ATE, because some of the cats diagnosed with a restrictive (6 per cent) or an intermediate form of feline cardiomyopathy (27 per cent) may have end-stage HCM when remodelling, dilatation, and systolic failure occur. Only 2 cases of dilated cardiomyopathy were identified. No congenital heart disease was reported among the 63 cats studied echocardiographically.

Most recently, a retrospective case series of 44 cats with distal ATE was described from a hospital population in England.[3] In this population, neutered male cats predominated (75 per cent), with a mean age of 8.7 years, with preexisting heart disease noted in 23 per cent of cases and heart failure in 51 per cent. No characterization of the underlying heart disease was provided.

Surveys of cats with HCM also provide useful perspective on the epidemiology of cats with ATE. One retrospective study of a university hospital population summarized 74 cases of HCM; 9 cats (12 per cent) had systemic arterial embolization.[4] Another retrospective study that did not specifically exclude cats with hyperthyroidism or systemic hypertension found that 13 per cent of the cats with HCM experienced thromboembolism.[5] A necropsy-based study of 51 cats with HCM reported ATE in 41 per cent of the cats.[6] It is unclear exactly how arterial embolization was diagnosed in the clinical studies, but post-mortem examination was not discussed in one study,[5] and occurred in only 9 of 74 cases in the other.[4] The average lengths of patient follow-up in the clinical series were not provided, but the studies encompassed admissions over 5 or 4 years. Clinical diagnosis and a relatively short average patient follow-up might be expected to minimize the estimate of prevalence of ATE in HCM cats.

◆ PATHOGENESIS

Experimental research in the 1970s showed that simple ligation of the distal aorta in normal cats would not induce the clinical signs associated with ATE; induction of a thrombus also was required.[7, 8] These studies showed that the thrombus might be induced experimentally by a variety of agents (e.g., bovine thrombin, autologous blood mixed with glass beads, blood, and 5-hydroxytryptamine) and supported the theory that vasoactive agents associated with the thrombus contributed to the rear limb paresis or paralysis observed in cats with ATE.[7-11] Pretreatment with aspirin or cyproheptadine (a 5-hydroxytryptamine antagonist) showed some benefit in these experimental models by lessening the severity of clinical signs or showing relatively improved collateral circulation.[9, 10]

Despite early insight into the sequelae of the thrombus once it is lodged in the distal aorta, many important questions about the initiating factors and superimposed risk factors of ATE are unanswered. What makes cats with various forms of cardiomyopathy develop ATE, but relatively few cats with thyrotoxic heart disease develop ATE? Is impaired left ventricular function an important risk factor for thromboembolism in cats as it is in human beings? Do thrombi usually originate in the left atrium, and is an enlarged left atrium an important risk factor for ATE? Why do most clots apparently lodge in the distal aorta? The acute presentation of these patients coupled with their cardiovascular instability and poor survival (including euthanasia based on poor prognosis) makes the thorough and systematic study of these patients particularly challenging.

Virchow's century-old trinity for predisposition to thrombosis—disturbances in blood flow, vascular surface, or coagulation—still holds true but may be interpreted slightly differently in light of recent genetic and molecular biologic research. Hemostatic control apparently is exerted differently in different regions of the vascular tree and can be modified by local factors.[12] What has been interpreted as a systemic hypercoagulable state may in fact not be—but rather serves only to increase the risk of thrombosis in a given vascular bed. For example, in human beings, normal levels of proteins C and S and antithrombin III appear relatively unimportant in maintaining an anticoagulant state in coronary vessels, but critical in preventing deep venous thrombosis in the legs.[13] Whereas there is evidence of different hemostatic control in different vascular beds in human beings and gene-targeted mice, there are no comparable data to date in cats.[12] Such regional differences might prove to be a factor favoring distal aortic embolization in cats.

Hypercoagulable conditions have not been investigated extensively in cats with ATE. Disseminated intravascular coagulation has been described in some cats with thromboembolism, whereas elevated levels of antithrombin III were measured in a small group of cats with cardiomyopathy secondary to hyperthyroidism.[14, 15] No evaluation for hemostatic genetic determinants that may predispose to hypercoagulation or arterial thrombosis has been published in cats. In human beings, there is strong evidence of the contribution of various hemostatic genetic factors to venous thrombosis, but the genetic determinants leading to arterial thrombosis, although suspected, are less clear.[16]

The relative hyperaggregability of feline platelets, as compared with other species, has been hypothesized to explain the apparent increased risk of thrombosis in cats. A small experimental study evaluated cats with cardiomyopathy (HCM and dilated cardiomyopathy), and found that their platelets aggregated in response to relatively lower levels of adenosine diphosphate (ADP) than normal cats.[17] Another factor that might contribute to platelet hyperaggregability relative to other species is the relatively large size of feline platelets.[18] However, results in clinical trials in human patients with atrial fibrillation showing greater benefit with prophylactic warfarin than aspirin has lent support to the theory that stasis-related thrombi are important to subsequent thromboembolization.[19-21] Stasis contributes to low shear rates, which lead to deposition of fibrin and activation of coagulation processes.[19, 20] Platelet activation is thought to be more important in arterial mural thrombosis or where there is an endocardial or endothelial nidus for thrombus formation.[20, 21] Whereas aspirin prophylaxis appears disappointing in cats with ATE, it has not been compared systematically with warfarin or other anticoagulants, and so a parallel argument cannot be made.

Most clinicians assume that the source of the thrombus in feline ATE usually is the left atrium, even though intra-atrial thrombi are not observed frequently antemortem. In a necropsy-based study, atrial (both right and left) thrombi were found in 21 per cent of 46 cats with systemic thromboembolism.[1] The advent of transesophageal echocardiography has substantially enhanced the detection of thrombi in the left atrium and left auricular appendage in human patients; however, this technique is not generally available in veterinary medicine, and indeed may not hold similar promise in cats. Several investigators have proposed that left atrial enlargement is a risk factor for ATE, and some data support this claim. Of 58 cats evaluated echocardiographically in the large retrospective study of cats with distal ATE, only 3 were reported to have normal left atrial dimension.[2] However, this observation is confounded by the study population, which were more likely to have enlarged left atrial dimensions than normal cats. Another small study compared left atrial size in cats with cardiomyopathy and congestive heart failure with those in cats with cardiomyopathy, congestive heart failure, and thromboembolism, and found significantly larger left atria in the group with thromboembolism.[22] Whereas an enlarged left atrium has been considered a risk factor in human beings for stroke or embolization, impaired left ventricular function is considered to be a more powerful predictor of embolic risk.[20, 23]

◆ CLINICAL SIGNS

Whereas the hallmarks of acute arterial occlusion are classically described as the 5 Ps—pulselessness, pain, pallor, paresis, poikilothermia—the presenting signs may vary substantially depending on the location of the thrombus and whether the cat is suffering from concurrent heart failure. Signs also will vary according to the extent of arterial occlusion; cats with only partial arterial obstruction may present only with a complaint of lameness. The classic feline patient with distal ATE will have posterior paralysis or paresis, firm cold rear limbs, pale footpads, with pale or cyanotic nail beds, and very weak or no palpable femoral pulses. The cats usually cry spontaneously and more with manipulation of the affected limbs. Neurologic findings vary, but usually tail movement and anal sphincter tone are preserved.

Many cats with underlying heart disease have abnormalities detectable by auscultation; at least 60 per cent of cats with distal ATE were reported to have a murmur, gallop, or arrhythmia.[2] Tachypnea and dyspnea also are observed commonly, reflecting the pain and cardiovascular impairment of these patients. Electrocardiographic abnormalities are common, although no one arrhythmia or pattern can be judged as diagnostic for ATE, because different forms of cardiomyopathy and variable electrolyte abnormalities may be contributory.

◆ DIFFERENTIAL DIAGNOSIS

Because the actual location of the thrombus will determine many of the clinical signs observed, it also will affect the range of differential diagnoses. Cats with impairment of renal perfusion may not be suspected initially of ATE, but rather of causes of acute renal failure. Forelimb lameness due to trauma often is the primary differential diagnosis in cats with a proximal thrombus involving a brachial artery. However, most cats present with a distal ATE, and frequently without overt concurrent heart disease. Owners who have not observed the cat just before the thromboembolic episode often assume that the cat has broken its back, but if there is complete arterial occlusion, as there is in most cases, loss of regional pulses direct the clinician to rule out ATE.

Clinicians sometimes may suspect a primary neurologic disorder if there has been only partial arterial occlusion or time for reperfusion. Reasonable neurologic differential diagnoses in these cases may include such conditions as intervertebral disc extrusion, spinal masses, trauma, myasthenia gravis, diabetic neuropathy, and foreign body.[23, 24] Despite no overt signs of heart disease, most cats with ATE and neurologic signs will have some discrete signs of cardiac disease. Conscientious physical examination often will reward the clinician with a murmur, gallop, or arrhythmia. This combination of neurologic and cardiac abnormalities should cause clinicians to seriously consider ATE, even if regional pulses are not overtly abnormal.

◆ DIAGNOSIS

Cats suffering from acute obstruction of the distal aorta often have pathognomonic physical examination findings coupled with cardiovascular instability; in these circumstances, a definitive diagnosis sometimes is not pursued. Especially in instances in which the cat is in concurrent heart failure, definitive diagnostics may be delayed until the patient is judged more stable and can be manipulated more readily once its pain is controlled and respiratory distress is eased. Because most cats will present acutely without previously diagnosed underlying disease and because cardiomyopathy is usually the primary differential diagnosis, echocardiography often is performed as soon as possible to allow optimum treatment of the acute respiratory and cardiovascular signs.

Echocardiography also can be used to investigate the cardiac chambers for thrombi and spontaneous echo contrast. Spontaneous echo contrast or, informally, "smoke" is believed to result from blood stasis and underlying rouleaux formation of red blood cells.[25, 26] Smokelike echoes are seen to curl through a cardiac chamber, and are distinct from background noise that may be induced by high gain settings. Whereas this phenomenon is not well-documented in veterinary literature, it can be observed in some cats with ATE and enlarged left atria. Some data suggest that erythrocytes of cats may be relatively hyperaggregable as compared with other species besides the horse.[27] It seems somewhat surprising then that spontaneous echo contrast is not reported more commonly in cats with ATE. Data in people support a high association between the presence of smoke and intracardiac thrombi, but there are insufficient data to evaluate this association in cats.[19, 25, 28] Interestingly, smoke may not be as good a predictor of subsequent systemic embolization in human beings as are history of previous embolization, and left atrial thrombi that are mobile or large.[20, 28]

Other forms of imaging such as thoracic or abdominal radiographs (if a foreign body or neoplasm is suspected), angiography, and Doppler ultrasound of the aorta, are often used. Some clinicians will only pursue a definitive diagnosis aggressively with angiography or a nuclear perfusion study when no obvious risk factor is identified for the apparent embolic episode. Documentation of partial arterial obstruction may be challenging, especially in cases in which the embolic episode may have occurred some time ago and in which there now are palpable pulses and persistence of neurologic signs. In such cases in which pulses are difficult to palpate or hard to compare between 2 limbs, a Doppler device for measurement of systolic blood pressure may be useful. Some clinicians advocate the use of a nail-clip test to confirm the lack of normal blood flow. Cats with partial arterial obstruction tend to be more stable, so angiography or nuclear perfusion scanning may be appropriate to help confirm neurologic impairment secondary to ischemia.

A baseline coagulation profile including platelet count may be drawn routinely at the time of admission to screen for any preexisting coagulopathy that would predispose to thromboembolism and prepare for any subsequent anticoagulation therapy.[14, 29] Baseline chemistries also are useful, especially because they may provide the first indication of impairment of renal vascular supply as well as being supportive of the diagnosis. The most common laboratory abnormalities include elevated aspartate aminotransferase and alanine aminotransferase, hyperglycemia, azotemia, and hypocalcemia.[2] Whereas atherosclerotic change has been reported rarely in cats, it is interesting that hypercholesterolemia also was reported in 30 per cent of cases.[2, 30]

◆ TREATMENT

Acute conventional treatment of ATE should address 3 issues: minimization of further clot enlargement by immediate heparinization; stabilization of any cardiovascular impairment; and control of pain. Given the potential benefit of aspirin in cats with experimentally induced ATE, it may be recommended to have the owner administer an aspirin (81 mg) as soon as possible in circumstances where ATE is even suspected.[10] Injections should be avoided in the region of impaired perfusion to prevent potential problems with uptake or subsequent necrosis. Blood can be drawn for baseline coagulation profile and platelet count in most cases, but immediate heparinization is appropriate in acute cases with classic signs. Heparin initially may be administered intravenously (IV) with a loading dose of 200 U/kg; subsequently a dose of 100 U/kg subcutaneously (SQ) every (q) 6 to 8 hr is adjusted to achieve a goal of 1.5 to 2.0 times baseline activated partial thromboplastin time (aPTT). Patients frequently are in substantial pain associated with the ischemia, and may be treated with an analgesic such as butorphanol tartrate at 0.1 to 0.4 mg/kg IV q 2 to 5 hr as needed. If the cat is in concurrent heart failure, it should be treated appropriately based on its underlying condition; for cats with HCM, it may be desirable theoretically to avoid propranolol because of its potential vasoconstrictive effect. Cats

with underlying cardiac disease, but not presenting in failure, should be monitored closely for signs of failure developing during hospitalization. Some clinicians recommend the use of acepromazine maleate (0.03 mg/kg SQ) for its vasodilatory effect and potentially as an anxiolytic; others feel that it simply contributes to hypotension and should be avoided. It should be understood that these are only conventional therapies, and have not been proved in the setting of feline ATE to be more or less efficacious than others.

Whereas thrombolytic agents hold an important place in the armamentarium of human cardiologists treating patients with acute arterial occlusion, they have not yet gained similar status for veterinarians treating cats with ATE. There are real economic considerations, depending on which thrombolytic agent is chosen, and these are complicated further by needing to have the drug available on an emergency basis. Unfortunately, these agents have been found to be difficult to use in cats. Whereas use of thrombolytic agents may result in early reperfusion, management of the systemic sequelae of reperfusion, such as severe acidosis and hyperkalemia, is challenging.[31, 32] Although there are minimal published data on ATE cases treated with thrombolytic agents, one group with previous experience using streptokinase reported an acute mortality rate of 50 per cent during therapy with recombinant tissue plasminogen activator (rt-PA).[32] Over 70 per cent of the deaths were attributed to hyperkalemia, whereas 14 per cent were attributed to heart failure. Meaningful estimates of survival in acute ATE are difficult to obtain because of the substantial number of cats euthanized without treatment, and the number euthanized in the first 24 to 48 hours after a definitive diagnosis is made, and any underlying heart disease identified. Some cats die acutely while being treated due to complications of the ATE, especially if there is renal arterial compromise, or from heart failure. In the retrospective case series of 100 cats with ATE, about 30 per cent died during initial hospitalization and 35 per cent were euthanized in this same period.[2] The cats in this series were treated conservatively with supportive care to prevent additional thromboembolization and to allow time for the development of collateral circulation; hyperkalemia was only reported in 1 of 53 cases with laboratory data available. There may be particular instances in which the use of thrombolytics is preferred, possibly in cases of renal arterial thrombosis, but such agents may be best used by experienced clinicians with the ability to provide extensive monitoring and aggressive supportive therapy to carry a patient through the likely complications associated with reperfusion.

Other treatments for acute arterial obstruction have not been well documented in cats. There is some justifiable reluctance to treat the occlusion aggressively if there is underlying cardiomyopathy and risk of recurrence. A case report described a paraplegic cat with signs consistent with ATE that had a foreign body and several thrombi occluding its distal aorta; no underlying cardiac disease was identified.[23] Aortotomy was performed successfully to remove the BB and thrombi, and the cat ultimately recovered with minimal tarsal impairment. In human beings with acute leg ischemia, if the involved vessel is judged to be normal (no atherosclerosis or underlying vascular disease), immediate heparization and emergency embolectomy generally are indicated.[21] Percutaneous clot aspiration or thrombolysis tend to be used in more distal-limb emboli. Whereas some cardiologists apparently have attempted balloon embolectomy in cats, no details have been reported.

◆ MANAGEMENT

Initially bed rest and protection from direct heat or mechanical trauma are important if there is paraplegia or paraparesis. Supportive care, such as routine physical therapy of affected limbs, should be tailored to the individual circumstances of the patient. In some cases with substantial ischemic damage, surgical débridement may be necessary to control excessive ischemic necrosis. The use of external coaptation splints has been described in the literature for management of gait abnormalities.[23] It may be appropriate to optimize a patient's cardiovascular medications after survival of an acute ATE episode.

◆ PREVENTION

Given the high mortality and intensive acute and chronic management of cats suffering ATE, prevention is a logical and potentially cost-effective approach to this disease. Ideally, elimination of important underlying risk factors should be pursued. The best actual example of this scenario is treatment of dilated cardiomyopathy associated with taurine deficiency. In rare instances of valvular endocarditis, antimicrobial therapy may reduce the risk of thromboembolism. If a paraneoplastic syndrome contributes to a hypercoagulable state, treatment of the neoplasm may be possible. Similarly, treatment of a systemic disease contributing to disseminated intravascular coagulation likely would reduce the risk of ATE. However, in most cases in which HCM cardiomyopathy is the only known risk factor, prophylaxis currently involves antiplatelet or anticoagulant drugs. Whereas we try to optimize these nonspecific therapies, we should continue to strive to investigate and identify other risk factors in affected cats that may be amenable to treatment. So-called environmental factors (e.g., in human beings: hypertension, age, diabetes mellitus) should be considered. Some investigators have begun to investigate the possible association of hyperhomocysteinemia and cardiomyopathy or ATE.[22, 33] Impaired left ventricular function should be investigated as a risk

factor for ATE because of its importance in human beings and its reported association with poor survival in cats with HCM.[5]

Conventional Therapy

Low-dose aspirin therapy is used commonly for prophylaxis for ATE in cats diagnosed with cardiomyopathy. Aspirin usually is prescribed at 25 mg/kg orally (PO) q 72 hr.[34, 35] This particular dosage schedule has been devised theoretically to provide inhibition of platelet aggregation by inhibiting thromboxane A_2 while allowing some production of prostacyclin by vascular endothelium. Although there is no clinical trial that evaluates the efficacy of aspirin to decrease the occurrence/recurrence of ATE in cats, there are short-term experimental studies supportive of some beneficial effects of aspirin therapy.[10, 34, 35] More recently, an acute evaluation of in vitro and in vivo aspirin to modify platelet aggregation or capillary bleeding time in normal cats found little if any inhibition of platelet aggregation in the in vivo system and no change in capillary bleeding time.[35] Unfortunately, in a clinical setting, it is clear that cats on aspirin therapy often embolize or re-embolize.[2, 36] This observation is consistent with the variable efficacy of aspirin prophylaxis in various forms of arterial thromboembolic disease in human beings.[20]

Warfarin Prophylaxis

Ample precedence for prophylactic warfarin therapy in ATE is provided in human medical literature.[20, 25, 37, 38] In human beings, atrial fibrillation is the most common cardiac disorder predisposing to systemic embolization. Several randomized prospective clinical studies in human patients with nonrheumatic atrial fibrillation have demonstrated the benefit of warfarin over placebo or aspirin to decrease the incidence of stroke or systemic embolization.[20, 37, 38] No published study has evaluated the use of anticoagulants in human patients with HCM, but warfarin is recommended in individuals with atrial fibrillation and HCM because of the high incidence of embolic events and the demonstrated benefit of warfarin in atrial fibrillation. Routine use of warfarin in human beings with dilated cardiomyopathy without atrial fibrillation recently has become more controversial. Whereas severe left ventricular dysfunction in human beings has long been an acknowledged risk factor for intracardiac thrombosis, some data suggest that systemic embolization in these patients is not a significant cause of mortality.[25]

Veterinary experience with warfarin is limited, although some veterinarians use and recommend warfarin especially in instances in which cats suffer an embolic episode while on aspirin therapy. Some cardiologists resort to warfarin treatment for patients they believe to be at particularly high risk of embolization: cats in which the left atrium is large, for example, a left atrium:aortic ratio of 2.0 or greater.[39] As with aspirin therapy, cats have been documented to embolize while being treated with warfarin.[2] Although some cardiologists believe that warfarin is more efficacious than aspirin in preventing ATE, there is no randomized prospective study supporting this conclusion. Given the lack of definitive evidence of the benefit of warfarin over placebo or aspirin, coupled with the well-documented risk of hemorrhage and challenges of monitoring chronic warfarin therapy, veterinarians must be very cautious in their selection of patients (and clients) for warfarin therapy.[39] Warfarin therapy often is restricted to use in indoor cats, to minimize traumatic incidences and to ensure adequate patient supervision. Unlike many prescribed prophylactic therapies, the use of warfarin requires extensive client education before deciding to initiate therapy, and it will continue to require conscientious and regular client contact and support. Warfarin therapy requires substantial patience from all parties involved.

Warfarin inhibits the vitamin K–dependent clotting factors (II, VII, IX, X) and anticoagulant proteins C and S. The difference in half-lives among these procoagulants and anticoagulants results in the transient hypercoagulable state documented in human beings when warfarin therapy is first initiated. The actual antithrombotic effect of warfarin is attributable to decreases in Factors IX and X, which do not occur for 4 to 6 days in human patients. Thus, patients may be hypercoagulable for the first 3 or 4 days of treatment when the anticoagulant protein C level is low while the concentrations of Factors IX and X are still unaffected. This is why heparin and warfarin therapies are overlapped in patients at risk of thromboembolism. Some veterinarians manage feline patients in a similar manner, although there is no published investigation of this suspected transient hypercoagulable state in cats treated with warfarin.

Historically, warfarin dosages for cats at risk of ATE were extrapolated from human guidelines and adjusted to result in a 1-stage prothrombin time (PT) of 1.3 to 1.6 times normal. However, because of the variability of commercial thromboplastin used in the PT assay, it is now recommended that PTs be standardized using the international normalization ratio (INR).[37, 40] This ratio expresses the PT as though it was determined using the international reference preparation of standardized human brain thromboplastin. In this way, PTs and thus warfarin dosages can be compared directly from laboratory to laboratory and study to study. This has been found to be particularly important when comparing anticoagulant treatments used in Europe to those in North America because of the significant difference in the sensitivity of thromboplastins used.

$$INR = (\text{patient PT divided by control PT})^{ISI}$$

The ISI is the international sensitivity index of the thromboplastin used in the PT assay and reflects the responsiveness of a given thromboplastin to reduction of vitamin K–dependent coagulation factors as compared with that of the international reference preparation. Manufacturers of thromboplastin determine the ISI of each batch produced, and this information is provided to the user. Clinical human laboratories routinely calculate INRs, and veterinary laboratories can be requested to do the same. Extrapolating from human data, the recommended INR for prophylactic warfarin for feline ATE is 2.0 to 3.0. The usual dosage is 0.5 mg (per cat) warfarin sodium (Coumadin) PO q 24 hr; in small cats, it may be preferable to start with a lower dose of 0.25 mg q 24 hr.

There appears to be substantial individual variation in a cat's anticoagulation response to a given dose of warfarin, as there is in human beings, and cats must be monitored closely by owners and by laboratory tests (PT/INR) when warfarin therapy is initiated.[39] Usually, after the first 2 weeks of treatment, the frequency of monitoring can be decreased gradually until a regular interval of 6 to 8 weeks is achieved. The smallest tablet size of warfarin sodium is 1 mg, and thus it can be difficult to manipulate the dose accurately if 0.5 mg once-daily is too much and 0.25 mg is too little. Some clinicians manipulate the dose given to the patient over a full week using a 2-dose scheme, e.g., 0.5 mg on Monday, Wednesday, Friday, Sunday and 0.25 mg on Tuesday, Thursday, and Saturday. If the dose is close to therapeutic range, changes of one-seventh of the week's dose are recommended.

Drug interactions with warfarin are abundant, and changes in medications warrant increased monitoring of INR/PT. Concomitant use of drugs having anticoagulant or antiplatelet effects (e.g., aspirin, nonsteroidal anti-inflammatory drugs) should be used with extreme caution. Veterinarians should remember that major hemorrhage is a risk with warfarin therapy even within therapeutic range; one human study found that 45 per cent of patients suffering major hemorrhage had a PT ratio less than or equal to 2.0.[41] Clients should be instructed specifically how to monitor for signs of bleeding in cats receiving warfarin.

Low-Molecular-Weight Heparins

Low-molecular-weight heparins (LMWHs) offer the prospect of anticoagulation without the relatively frequent laboratory monitoring needed with warfarin. LMWHs are administered subcutaneously like standard unfractionated heparin (UFH), but there is reason to believe that they may be appropriately dosed on a once-daily basis in cats.[41]

The efficacy of LMWHs for both acute management and prophylaxis of thrombosis has been documented in human beings for a variety of different disease conditions.[42-44] However, very recent data suggest that LMWHs may be less efficacious in the treatment or prevention of arterial (stroke) compared with venous thromboembolism. The very limited need for any laboratory monitoring in human beings is because LMWHs produce a predictable anticoagulation response.[42–45] The smaller molecules of LMWHs have less ability to inhibit thrombin than those of UFH and therefore exert negligible effect on the aPTT. LMWHs also do not undergo much of the nonspecific protein-binding suffered by UFH.

Investigators at Tufts University recently evaluated the use of dalteparin (Fragmin) in normal cats.[43] A dose of 100 U/kg SQ q 24 hr was recommended based on monitoring of antifactor-Xa activity and aPTT. However, no assessment of efficacy was made. Given the more predictable anticoagulant effect of LMWHs, one might expect to have less hemorrhagic complications than with UFH or warfarin, but there are no currently available data on this risk in cats. One potentially important consideration in cats at risk for thromboembolism is that LMWHs have much less inhibitory effect on collagen-induced platelet activity than UFH.[43] If cats are indeed at a greater risk of thrombosis than other species due to their relatively hyperaggregable platelets, then antiplatelet therapy may be needed in combination with LMWHs.

REFERENCES

1. Liu SK: Acquired cardiac lesions leading to congestive heart failure in the cat. Am J Vet Res 31:2071–2088, 1970.
2. Laste NJ, Harpster NK: A retrospective study of 100 cases of feline distal aortic thromboembolism: 1977–1993. J Am Anim Hosp Assoc 31:492–500, 1995.
3. Schoeman JP: Feline distal aortic thromboembolism: A review of 44 cases (1990–1998). [Abstract]. Ninth European Society of Veterinary Internal Medicine Congress, 1999. J Vet Intern Med 14:242, 2000.
4. Atkins CE, Gallo AM, Kurman ID, et al: Risk factors, clinical signs, and survival in cats with a clinical diagnosis of idiopathic hypertrophic cardiomyopathy: 74 cases (1985–1989). J Am Vet Med Assoc 201:613–618, 1992.
5. Peterson EN, Moïse NS, Brown CA, et al: Heterogeneity of hypertrophy in feline hypertrophic heart disease. J Vet Intern Med 7:183–189, 1993.
6. Liu SK, Maron BJ, Tilley LP: Feline hypertrophic cardiomyopathy: Gross anatomic and quantitative histologic features. Am J Pathol 102:388–395, 1981.
7. Imhoff RK: Production of aortic occlusion resembling acute aortic embolism syndrome in cats. Nature 192:979–980, 1961.
8. Butler HC: An investigation into the relationship of an aortic embolus to posterior paralysis in the cat. J Small Anim Pract 12:141–158, 1971.
9. Olmstead ML, Butler HC: Five-hydroxytryptamine antagonists and feline aortic embolism. J Small Anim Pract 18:247–259, 1977.
10. Schaub RG, Gates KA, Roberts RE: Effect of aspirin on collateral blood flow after experimental thrombosis of the feline aorta. Am J Vet Res 43:1647–1650, 1982.
11. Loots M, De Clerck F: 5-Hydroxytryptamine dominates over thromboxane A$_2$ in reducing collateral blood flow by activated platelets. Am J Physiol 265:H158–164, 1993.
12. Rosenberg RD, Aird WC: Vascular-bed–specific hemostasis and hypercoagulable states. N Engl J Med 340:1555–1564, 1999.
13. Thomas DP, Roberts HR: Hypercoagulability in venous and arterial thrombosis. Ann Intern Med 126:707–711, 1997.
14. Fox PR, Dodds WJ: Coagulopathies observed with spontaneous aortic thromboembolism in cardiomyopathic cats [Abstract]. Proceedings American College Veterinary Internal Medicine Annual Forum, 1982, p. 82.
15. Welles EG, Boudreaux MK, Crager CS, et al: Platelet function and antithrombin, plasminogen, and fibrinolytic activities in cats with heart disease. Am J Vet Res 55:619–627, 1994.
16. Lane DA, Grant PJ: Role of hemostatic gene polymorphisms in venous and arterial thrombotic disease. Blood 95:1517–1532, 2000.
17. Helenski CA, Ross JN: Platelet aggregation in feline cardiomyopathy. J Vet Intern Med 1:24–28, 1987.
18. Weiser MG, Kociba GJ: Platelet concentration and platelet volume distribution in healthy cats. Am J Vet Res 45:518–522, 1982.
19. Ezekowitz MD, Cohen IS, Gornick CC: The left atrium. In Ezekowitz MD (ed): Systemic Cardiac Embolism. New York, Marcel Dekker, 1994.
20. Halperin JL, Petersen P: Thrombosis in the cardiac chamber: Ventricular dysfunction and atrial fibrillation. In Verstraete M, Fuster V, Topol EJ (eds): Cardiovascular Thrombosis: Thrombocardiology and Thromboneurology, 2nd ed. Philadelphia, Lippincott Raven, 1998, pp. 415–438.
21. Verhaeghe R, Bounameaux H: Peripheral arterial occlusion: Thromboembolism and antithrombotic therapy. In Verstraete M, Fuster V, Topol EJ (eds): Cardiovascular Thrombosis: Thrombocardiology and Thromboneurology, 2nd ed. Philadelphia, Lippincott Raven, 1998, pp. 631–656.
22. Hohenhaus AE, Simantov R, Fox PR, et al: Evaluation of plasma homocysteine concentrations in cardiomyopathic cats with congestive heart failure and aortic thromboembolism. J Vet Intern Med 13:249, 1999.
23. Whigham HM, Ellison GW, Graham J: Aortic foreign body resulting in ischemic neuromyopathy and development of collateral circulation in a cat. J Am Vet Med Assoc 213:829–832, 1998.
24. Flanders JA: Feline aortic thromboembolism. Compend Contin Educ Pract Vet 8:473–478, 1986.
25. Ezekowitz MD: The left ventricle. In Ezekowitz MD (ed): Systemic Cardiac Embolism. New York, Marcel Dekker, 1994.
26. Wang XF, Liu L, Cheng TO, et al: The relationship between intracardiovascular smoke-like echo and erythrocyte formation. Am Heart J 124:961–965, 1992.
27. Ohta K, Gotoh F, Tomita M, et al: Animal species differences in erythrocyte aggregability. Am J Physiol 262:H1009–H1012, 1992.
28. Leung DY, Davidson PM, Cranney GB, et al: Thromboembolic risks of left atrial thrombus detected by transesophageal echocardiogram. Am J Cardiol 79:626–629, 1997.
29. Hogan DF, Dhaliwal RS, Sisson DD, et al: Paraneoplastic thrombocytosis-induced systemic thromboembolism in a cat. J Am Anim Hosp Assoc 35:483–486, 1999.
30. Ginzinger DG, Wilson JE, Redenbach D, et al: Diet-induced atherosclerosis in the domestic cat. Lab Invest 77:409–419, 1999.
31. Pion PD: Feline aortic thromboemboli and the potential utility of thrombolytic therapy with tissue plasminogen activator. Vet Clin North Am Small Anim Pract 18:79–86, 1988.
32. Pion PD, Kittleson MD, Peterson SL, et al: Thrombolysis with recombinant tissue-type plasminogen activator (rt-PA) in feline aortic thromboembolism: Clinical and experimental data [Abstract]. Proceedings of the American College of Veterinary Internal Medicine, Annual Forum, 1987, p. 925.
33. McMichael M, Freeman L, Selhul J, et al: Cats with cardiomyopathy have low B vitamins [Abstract]. J Vet Intern Med 13:247, 1999.
34. Greene CE: Effects of aspirin and propranolol on feline platelet aggregation. Am J Vet Res 46:1820–1823, 1985.
35. Allen DG, Johnstone IB, Crane S: Effects of aspirin and propranolol alone and in combination on hemostatic determinants in the healthy cat. Am J Vet Res 46:660–663, 1985.
36. Hart S, Sommer B, Kietzmann M, et al: Effect of acetylsalicylic acid on platelet aggregation and capillary bleeding time

in healthy cats. DTW Dtsch Tierarztl Wochenschr 102:476–480, 1995.

37. Fox PR: Evidence for or against efficacy of beta-blockers and aspirin for the management of feline cardiomyopathies. Vet Clin North Am Small Anim Pract 21:1011–1022, 1991.

38. Hirsch J, Dalen JE, Deykin D, et al: Oral anticoagulants. Mechanism of action, clinical effectiveness, optimal therapeutic range. Chest 102(Suppl 4):312S–320S, 1992.

39. Ezekowitz MD, Bridgers SL, James KE, et al: Warfarin in the prevention of stroke associated with nonrheumatic atrial fibrillation. N Engl J Med 327:1406–1412, 1992.

40. Baty CJ, Harpster NK: Warfarin therapy of the cat at risk of thromboembolism. *In* Bonagura J (ed): Current Veterinary Therapy XII. Philadelphia, WB Saunders, 1995, pp. 868–873.

41. Smith RE: The INR: A perspective. Semin Thromb Hemost 23:547–549, 1997.

42. Petitti DB, Strom BL, Melmon KL: Prothrombin time ratio and other factors associated with bleeding in patients treated with warfarin. J Clin Epidemiol 42:759–764, 1989.

43. Goodman JS, Rozanski EA, Brown D, et al: The effects of low-molecular-weight heparin on hematologic and coagulation parameters in normal cats [Abstract]. J Vet Intern Med 13:268, 1999.

44. Turpie AGG: Pharmacology of the low-molecular-weight heparins. Am Heart J 135:S329–S335, 1998.

45. Harenberg J, Huhle G, Piazolo L, et al: Long-term anticoagulation of outpatients with adverse events to oral anticoagulants using low-molecular-weight heparin. Semin Thromb Hemost 23:167–172, 1997.

Urinary System

Stephen P. DiBartola, Editor

◆ Lily Nephrotoxicity 308
◆ Idiopathic Hypercalcemia 311
◆ New Treatments in the Medical
  Management of Interstitial Cystitis 315
◆ Renal Transplantation in the Management
  of Chronic Renal Failure 319
◆ Medical Management of Chronic Renal Failure 328
◆ Use of Hemodialysis in Chronic Renal Failure 337
◆ Calcium Oxalate Urolithiasis 352
◆ Diagnosis and Treatment of Systemic
  Hypertension 365

Still-Current Information Found in *Consultations in Feline Internal Medicine 2*:

Diagnostic Approach to Disorders of Calcium Homeostasis (Chapter 21), p. 161

Management of Anemia Associated With Renal Failure (Chapter 43), p. 331

Renal Transplantation: Patient Selection and Postoperative Care (Chapter 44), p. 339

Calcium Oxalate Urolithiasis: Cause, Detection, and Control (Chapter 45), p. 343

Feline Lower Urinary Tract Disease: Relationships Between Crystalluria, Urinary Tract Infections, and Host Factors (Chapter 46), p. 351

Still-Current Information Found in *Consultations in Feline Internal Medicine 3*:

Update on the Medical Management of Hyperthyroidism (Chapter 22), p. 155

Endocrine Hypertension (Chapter 23), p. 163

Bladder Neoplasia: Difficulties in Diagnosis and Treatment (Chapter 41), p. 319

Medical Management of Chronic Renal Failure in Cats: Current Guidelines (Chapter 42), p. 325

Changing Demographics of Feline Urolithiasis: Perspectives From the Minnesota Urolith Center (Chapter 46), p. 349

Nonobstructive Lower Urinary Tract Disease (Chapter 47), p. 361

Blood Pressure: Population Aspects (Chapter 78), p. 630

Elsewhere in *Consultations in Feline Internal Medicine 4*:

Diagnosis of Occult Hyperthyroidism (Chapter 18), p. 145

Complications of Therapy for Hyperthyroidism (Chapter 19), p. 151

Systemic Hypertension (Chapter 36), p. 277

Transfusion Medicine (Chapter 58), p. 461

Evaluation and Treatment of Cranial Mediastinal Masses (Chapter 68), p. 533

Cognitive Dysfunction in Geriatric Cats (Chapter 74), p. 583

40
◆ Lily Nephrotoxicity

Jeffrey O. Hall

◆ ETIOLOGY

Since the first report of toxicity,[1] it has been found that cats are uniquely sensitive to the nephrotoxic syndrome caused by ingestion of species from both the *Lilium* and the *Hemerocallis* genera of plants.[2–6] Both of these plant genera are widely used ornamental plants that provide access to housecats in the form of flower arrangements and potted plants. Plants in these genera that have been associated with nephrotoxicity in cats include Easter lily *(Lilium longiflorum),* tiger lily *(L. tigrinum),* Japanese show lily *(L. hybridum),* rubrum lily *(L. rubrum),* numerous *Lilium* hybrids, and day lilies *(Hemerocallis* species). The quantity of plant material necessary for toxicity is relatively small, and ingestion of as few as 2 leaves has been lethal. Based on the data available, ingestion of any *Lilium* species or *Hemerocallis* species plants should be considered potentially toxic to cats, and exposure should be prevented. Ingestion of leaves or flowers from either genus results in an acute, severe nephrotoxic syndrome that culminates in anuric renal failure. To date, the toxic principle of these plants has not been identified.

◆ EPIDEMIOLOGY

Nephrotoxicity has been observed only in cats, with no age or breed predilection. Even with large quantities of plant ingestion, no toxic effects were identified in rats or rabbits. Furthermore, dogs that ingested large quantities of plant material developed only mild, short-term gastrointestinal upset.

◆ PATHOGENESIS

The exact mechanism of renal tubular damage is not known, but the overall syndrome requires 2 distinct components. The first component is ingestion of the plant material. This portion of the syndrome initiates polyuric renal failure, resulting in dehydration. The dehydration component is essential for development of the anuric renal failure associated with the toxicity of these plants. Thus, prevention of dehydration is a critical factor in the management of affected cats.

◆ CLINICAL SIGNS

The clinical signs associated with lily toxicosis generally are associated with the gastrointestinal and renal effects.[1–4] The typical clinical signs follow a fairly consistent onset and duration (Table 40–1). Initially, the syndrome consists of vomiting, lethargy, and anorexia. Most cats do not eat or drink throughout the course of the disease. Frequently, when the initial vomiting ends, both owners and veterinarians mistakenly think that the affected cat is recovering from a mild gastric upset. However, in most cases, these cats eventually progress into the life-threatening portion of the syndrome—anuric renal failure. Experimentally, polyuria occurred as early as 12 hours postingestion, causing affected cats to become dehydrated. Dehydration is a critical part of the syndrome, and is required for the affected cat to progress into the anuric phase of the disease. Once anuria has developed, the clinical signs resemble those of any other cause of acute renal failure. Lily poisoning generally results in death of the affected cat by 3 to 7 days postingestion, usually as a result of complications of anuric renal failure.

◆ CLINICAL PATHOLOGY

The hemogram and serum biochemistry results may assist in the diagnosis of lily poisoning, but these results do not differ greatly from those that occur with other causes of acute renal failure. The only change observed in the hemogram is the presence of a stress leukogram. Serum biochemistry abnormalities generally include moderate-to-severe increases in blood urea nitrogen, creatinine, phosphorus, and potassium concentrations. In addition, aspartate transaminase, alanine transaminase, and alkaline phosphatase concentrations may be increased late in the syndrome. The most prominent

Table 40–1. Onset and Duration of Common Clinical Signs That Occur With Lily Poisoning in Cats

Clinical Sign	Onset	Duration From Onset
Vomiting	0–3 hr	4–6 hr
Salivation	0–3 hr	4–6 hr
Anorexia	0–3 hr	Throughout syndrome
Lethargy	0–3 hr	Throughout syndrome
Polyuria	12–30 hr	12–24 hr
Dehydration	18–30 hr	Until corrected
Vomiting recurs	30–72 hr	Through remainder of syndrome
Anuria	24–48 hr	Through remainder of syndrome
Weakness	36–72 hr	Through remainder of syndrome
Recumbency	48–72 hr	Through remainder of syndrome
Death	3–7 day	

finding is a dramatic, disproportionate increase in serum creatinine concentration. In most cases, by the time the cat is identified as being anuric, the serum creatinine concentration is 15 to 20 mg/dl. In some cases, serum creatinine concentrations greater than 30 mg/dl have been observed. Several cases of lily toxicosis have been identified by using these exceedingly high serum creatinine concentrations as a prompt to question owners about potential plant exposure and to subsequently verify lily ingestion.

Urinalysis provides direct evidence of renal damage before serum chemistry changes occur. Urine from affected cats generally contains high concentrations of glucose and protein. In addition, the urine often is isosthenuric. Large numbers of renal tubular epithelial casts are present, and early in the syndrome they often contain enough cellular detail that the nuclei of the epithelial cells still can be identified. Later in the syndrome, the casts are better described as granular, because they likely have been retained in the bladder and have begun to degenerate. It is important to note that poisoning by these plants does not cause crystalluria.

◆ DIAGNOSIS

At the present time, the toxic principle in the lily has not been identified, making analytic diagnosis impossible. Diagnosis of this condition rests not only with the verification that one of these plant species has been ingested but also with compatible clinical signs and clinicopathologic abnormalities. Even with post-mortem examination, verification of plant exposure and appropriate clinical and laboratory findings still are necessary to arrive at a tentative diagnosis of lily poisoning.

◆ TREATMENT

Successful treatment requires early intervention with gastrointestinal decontamination and fluid therapy. In most instances, affected cats have vomited before presentation, but if cats are observed to ingest the plant material, decontamination via induction of vomiting should be initiated. In both cases (i.e., cats that already have vomited on their own and those in which vomiting has been induced), activated charcoal with a cathartic should be given in an attempt to minimize further systemic exposure to the plant toxin(s).

In addition to decontamination, fluid therapy must be initiated before development of anuria. Dehydration is a critical factor in the development of anuric renal failure. Initiating fluid diuresis with normal saline solution at 2 to 3 times maintenance requirements within 24 hours of exposure has prevented the occurrence of anuric renal failure in all cases to date. Fluid diuresis should be maintained for a period of 24 hours. Additional cases have occurred in which development of anuria was prevented with fluid diuresis that was initiated more than 24 hours after exposure, but before development of anuria. Several drugs commonly used to initiate urine production have been unsuccessful in anuric lily-poisoned cats, including dopamine, furosemide, hypertonic dextrose, thiazides, and mannitol.

Once anuria has developed, the only possible means of treatment is the use of peritoneal dialysis or hemodialysis. The author is aware of 2 cases in which peritoneal dialysis for 10 to 14 days resulted in return of renal function. The recommendation for this treatment was supported by evidence of early renal tubular repair and intact basement membranes from instances in which cats died of lily poisoning. Thus, dialysis should be a potentially effective method of treatment in cats that already have developed anuria. Appropriate protocols and dialysate solutions must be used (see Chapter 45, Use of Hemodialysis in Chronic Renal Failure).

◆ PATHOLOGIC FINDINGS

Gross pathologic findings are limited to systemic congestion and renal lesions. Mild-to-severe pulmonary and hepatic congestion are common. In most cases, the kidneys are swollen, and there is abundant perirenal edema. The stomach and small intestine commonly are empty.

Histopathologic findings corroborate the pulmonary, hepatic, and renal lesions. Vascular congestion is prominent in the lungs and liver. Occasionally, there is mild hepatocellular swelling adjacent to the central vein. The most prominent lesion is moderate-to-severe, diffuse acute renal tubular necrosis. In the moderately severe cases, the lesions often are limited to the proximal tubular segments, but in the severe cases, tubular necrosis occurs in the distal tubules and collecting ducts. Renal tubular basement membranes are intact, and mitotic figures often are present among the renal tubular cells. Large numbers of granular and hyaline casts are present in the collecting ducts.

◆ CONCLUSIONS

With the data currently available, all plants of the *Lilium* and *Hemerocallis* genera should be considered toxic to cats. Ingestion of several species of these 2 genera by cats causes acute nephrotoxicity resulting in anuric renal failure. Successful management of lily poisoning requires intervention with gastric decontamination and fluid diuresis early in the course of the disease. Fluid therapy must be initiated before development of anuria. Once anuria develops, peritoneal dialysis or hemodialysis is the only effective means of treatment.

REFERENCES

1. Hall JO: Are Easter lilies toxic to cats? NAPINet Report, vol. 3, no. 2. July 16, 1990, p. 1.

2. National Animal Poison Control Center (NAPCC) Computerized Case Database. University of Illinois College of Veterinary Medicine, 1987–1992.

3. Gathers TM: Acute renal failure in a cat: Was it tiger lily? NAPINet Report, vol. 3, no. 2. February 1, 1991, p. 2.

4. Hall JO: Nephrotoxicity of Easter lily *(Lilium longiflorum)* when ingested by the cat (abstract). Proceedings of the Annual Meeting of the American College of Veterinary Internal Medicine, San Diego, May 28–31, 1992.

5. Mullaney TP, Slanker MR, Poppenga RH: Easter lily associated nephrotoxicity in cats (abstract). North Central Conference of Veterinary Laboratory Diagnosticians, Madison, WI, July 16–17, 1993.

6. Carson TL, Sanderson TP, Halbur PG: Acute nephrotoxicosis in cats following ingestion of lily *(Lilium* sp.) (abstract). Proceedings of the Annual Meeting of the American Association of Veterinary Laboratory Diagnosticians, Grand Rapids, MI, Oct. 29–Nov. 1, 1994, vol. 37, p. 43.

41

◆ Idiopathic Hypercalcemia

Angela M. Midkiff
Dennis J. Chew
John F. Randolph
Sharon A. Center
Stephen P. DiBartola

Hypercalcemia in cats may be associated with malignant neoplasia, renal failure, primary hyperparathyroidism, hypoadrenocorticism, or the ingestion of cholecalciferol-containing rodenticides. Tumors associated with hypercalcemia in cats include lymphosarcoma, squamous cell carcinoma, and multiple myeloma. Hypercalcemia has been considered less common in cats than in dogs, and until recently, hypercalcemia was detected infrequently in cats. Since about 1990, however, veterinarians and veterinary diagnostic laboratories increasingly have recognized unexplained hypercalcemia as an incidental finding on the serum biochemical profiles of cats. In some recent reports, hypercalcemia in cats has been associated with calcium oxalate urolithiasis. This chapter summarizes the clinical and laboratory findings in cats with *idiopathic hypercalcemia*, defined as abnormally high serum total or ionized calcium concentration, the cause of which remains unknown after extensive medical evaluation to rule out known causes of hypercalcemia.

◆ PATHOGENESIS

The pathogenesis of idiopathic hypercalcemia in cats at present is unknown. A few affected cats have had azotemia that preceded development of hypercalcemia, and azotemia has been diagnosed concurrently in some cats with hypercalcemia; however, the majority of cats with idiopathic hypercalcemia are not azotemic at the onset of hypercalcemia, and a few cats have developed azotemia after becoming hypercalcemic. These features suggest that renal disease is not the cause of hypercalcemia in affected cats, but the possibility remains that some cats with idiopathic hypercalcemia may develop progressive renal disease and failure as a consequence of hypercalcemia. The relationship between idiopathic hypercalcemia and renal disease in cats requires further study.

In some recent reports, hypercalcemia has been reported in cats with oxalate urolithiasis,[1–3] and results reported from the University of Minnesota Urolith Center indicate that mild hypercalcemia (11.5 to 13.5 mg/dl) has been observed in 35 per cent of cats with calcium oxalate uroliths.[4] In a series of case reports, 5 cats with hypercalcemia and calcium oxalate urolithiasis presented for evaluation of lower urinary tract signs (e.g., pollakiuria, hematuria), and either had been fed acidifying diets (Hill's Prescription Diet c/d, Hill's Prescription Diet s/d) or had received urinary acidifiers (*d,l*-methionine).[1] In a case-control study of 84 cats, feeding of a urine-acidifying diet was the factor most highly associated with development of calcium oxalate urolithiasis.[5] Most cats with idiopathic hypercalcemia have a history of having been fed an acidifying diet.

One hypothesis about the relationship between hypercalcemia and calcium oxalate urolithiasis in cats is that feeding magnesium-restricted, acidifying diets for the control of struvite urolithiasis is associated with increased bone turnover of calcium and hypercalciuria as a consequence of chronic metabolic acidosis. Dietary acidification and metabolic acidosis may promote skeletal mobilization of calcium and increase renal excretion of calcium.[6] In adult cats, dietary acidification causes chronic metabolic acidosis, increased serum ionized calcium concentration, increased bone resorption of calcium, and hypercalciuria.[7, 8]

Taken together, these findings suggest that dietary acidification may predispose cats to hypercalcemia, hypercalciuria, and calcium oxalate urolithiasis. Many cats are fed acidifying diets, and presumably relatively few develop hypercalcemia and calcium oxalate urolithiasis. Consequently, other factors, such as hyperabsorption of calcium or oxalate from the gastrointestinal tract, or renal tubular dysfunction characterized by hypercalciuria or hyperoxaluria, may contribute to development of hypercalcemia and calcium oxalate urolithiasis in a susceptible subpopulation of cats. The presence of promoters of calcium oxalate crystal growth, or a deficiency of crystal growth inhibitors, also could contribute to the development of calcium oxalate crystal growth in susceptible cats.

◆ CLINICAL SIGNS
Signalment

In a retrospective study of cats with idiopathic hypercalcemia presented to the Ohio State University

Veterinary Teaching Hospital, the Cornell University College of Veterinary Medicine, and selected private practices, affected cats ranged in age from less than 2 years to greater than 13 years at presentation. Both male and female cats were affected, and no gender predilection was identified. Forty per cent of affected cats were longhaired.

Historical Findings

Common initial presenting complaints for cats with idiopathic hypercalcemia include vomiting, weight loss, anorexia, and lethargy. Dysuria, hematuria, pollakiuria, stranguria, and inappropriate urination also occur frequently, usually as a result of concurrent calcium oxalate urolithiasis. Polyuria and polydipsia also have been reported.

Physical Examination Findings

The majority of affected cats have kidneys that seem normal on abdominal palpation, but some have small kidneys that are firm or irregular in shape. Urethral obstruction or cystic calculi sometimes are identified in affected cats that also have calcium oxalate urolithiasis. The remainder of the physical examination usually is unremarkable.

◆ DIAGNOSIS
Laboratory Findings

Hypercalcemia most often is discovered fortuitously on serum biochemical profiles performed in an attempt to diagnose the cause of the presenting clinical signs (e.g., vomiting, weight loss, lethargy, anorexia). On serum biochemistry, either the serum total calcium concentration or the serum ionized calcium concentration, or both, may be abnormally high. In cats with idiopathic hypercalcemia, serum parathyroid hormone (PTH) concentrations are low or in the low-normal range (0 to 2.5 pmol/L), and it is not unusual for affected cats to have serum PTH concentrations of zero. Serum parathyroid hormone–related polypeptide (PTHrP) usually is undetectable. Serum 25-hydroxycholecalciferol (vitamin D_3) concentrations are normal in affected cats, as are serum phosphorus and albumin concentrations. Serum creatinine and blood urea nitrogen concentrations are normal in most affected cats at presentation. Venous blood gas analysis may indicate the presence of metabolic acidosis. The hemograms in affected cats have been normal.

Crystalluria and hematuria often are observed on urine sediment examination in cats with idiopathic hypercalcemia. The observed crystals may be calcium oxalate or struvite. Mild-to-moderate proteinuria also is common, and urine pH usually is in the acidic range. Urinary fractional excretion of calcium

in cats with idiopathic hypercalcemia may be abnormally high. Values above 1 per cent have been observed in affected cats, whereas urinary fractional excretion of calcium in normal cats is below 0.2 per cent.[9, 10] This finding supports the presence of hypercalciuria in some cats with idiopathic hypercalcemia.

Radiographs of the abdomen of cats with idiopathic hypercalcemia frequently identify radiopaque renal, ureteral, or cystic calculi. Small kidneys also are observed in some affected cats. Abdominal ultrasonography confirms these radiographic findings, and may identify irregular kidneys, nephrocalcinosis, or renal pelvic dilatation in some affected cats. Thoracic radiographs are normal in most cats with idiopathic hypercalcemia. Ultrasonography of the neck has disclosed normal parathyroid glands in affected cats in which this procedure has been performed.

Cats with idiopathic hypercalcemia have been negative for feline leukemia virus and feline immunodeficiency virus on enzyme-linked immunosorbent assay (ELISA) testing, and bone marrow aspirates that have been performed in some affected cats in an attempt to identify neoplasia have been cytologically normal. The parathyroid glands have been normal both grossly and histologically in cats with idiopathic hypercalcemia that have undergone exploratory surgery of the neck in attempts to identify parathyroid adenomas as the cause for the observed hypercalcemia. In such cats, serum calcium concentrations transiently return to normal after subtotal parathyroidectomy, but abnormally high serum total or ionized calcium concentrations recur within 7 days of surgery.

◆ DIFFERENTIAL DIAGNOSIS

Malignant tumors are thought to be the most common cause of hypercalcemia in cats, and those tumors associated with hypercalcemia include lymphosarcoma,[11–15] squamous cell carcinoma,[16, 17] and multiple myeloma.[18] Neoplasms are not evident on physical examination of cats with idiopathic hypercalcemia. Abdominal and thoracic radiography, abdominal ultrasonography, and bone marrow aspirates also fail to disclose evidence of neoplasia. In addition, serum concentrations of PTHrP are low or undetectable in cats with idiopathic hypercalcemia, whereas increased PTHrP concentrations would be expected in at least some cats with malignancy-associated hypercalcemia. Many cats with idiopathic hypercalcemia have survived for more than 7 years after diagnosis, making neoplasia an unlikely cause of hypercalcemia in affected cats.

Renal failure, resulting in renal secondary hyperparathyroidism, is another cause of hypercalcemia in cats. Mild hypercalcemia has been reported in 11.5 per cent of cats with chronic renal failure, with the highest serum total calcium concentration being 12.7 mg/dl.[19] Cats with renal secondary hyperparathyroidism have abnormally high serum or plasma PTH concentrations, whereas cats with idiopathic hypercalcemia have low-to-normal PTH concentrations (0 to 2.5 pmol/L). In a study of 13 cats treated for chronic renal failure, mean plasma PTH concentration before dietary phosphorus restriction was 137.8 pg/ml, and the lowest PTH concentration observed was 40.0 pg/ml.[20]

Primary hyperparathyroidism[21–23] results in abnormally high or occasionally normal serum or plasma PTH concentrations. Most affected cats also have palpable cervical masses. Physical examination, ultrasonography, and surgical exploration of the neck of cats with idiopathic hypercalcemia have not disclosed parathyroid tumors. Also, hypercalcemia generally recurs within a few days of surgery in cats with idiopathic hypercalcemia that have undergone subtotal parathyroidectomy, making primary hyperparathyroidism an unlikely cause of the observed hypercalcemia.

Hypoadrenocorticism is a rare cause of hypercalcemia in cats.[24] Although adrenocorticotropic hormone stimulation tests are not performed routinely in cats with idiopathic hypercalcemia, affected cats do not have the typical clinical or laboratory features of hypoadrenocorticism. Laboratory findings in cats with hypoadrenocorticism include hyponatremia, hyperkalemia, and hypochloremia, findings that have not been observed in cats with idiopathic hypercalcemia.

Hypercalcemia has been reported in cats that have ingested cholecalciferol-containing rodenticides, resulting in hypervitaminosis D and hyperphosphatemia.[25, 26] Cats with idiopathic hypercalcemia have no history of rodenticide ingestion, and have normal serum vitamin D_3 and phosphorus concentrations, making this diagnosis unlikely.

◆ TREATMENT

Treatment of cats with idiopathic hypercalcemia consists of dietary modification, orally administered glucocorticoids, or both. Discontinuation of acidifying diets and the feeding of a low-fat, high-fiber diet have been used in an attempt to reduce the availability of calcium for intestinal absorption. It is speculated that increased binding of intestinal calcium and altered intestinal transit time may reduce gastrointestinal absorption of calcium. In one report, feeding of a diet low in fat and high in fiber (Hill's Prescription Diet w/d) was associated with resolution of hypercalcemia in 5 cats with calcium oxalate urolithiasis.[1] This beneficial effect was observed despite the fact that Hill's Prescription Diet w/d has reduced magnesium content, and calcium and phosphorus content similar to that of acidifying diets, and produces acidic urine. Minimum to no response was noted in the cats with idiopathic hypercalcemia that we treated by similar dietary modification. The reason for these different results is unknown.

Corticosteroids promote reduction of serum calcium concentration by reducing bone resorption, decreasing intestinal absorption of calcium, and increasing renal excretion of calcium.[27] Corticosteroids may be beneficial in animals with lymphosarcoma, multiple myeloma, thymoma, hypoadrenocorticism, hypervitaminosis D, hypervitaminosis A, or granulomatous disease, but typically have little effect in those cats with hypercalcemia of other cause.[28] Most cats with idiopathic hypercalcemia treated with orally administered corticosteroids (prednisone, 5 to 12.5 mg/day) demonstrated a partial or complete reduction in serum total or ionized calcium concentration to within the normal range during treatment. The potential for exacerbation of hypercalciuria and calcium oxalate urolithiasis is of concern, however, given the likelihood of increased renal excretion of calcium.

Further assessment of idiopathic hypercalcemia in cats will require balance studies that evaluate dietary intake, bone resorption, intestinal absorption, and fecal and urinary excretion of calcium. Alkali therapy also should be considered to assess the role of dietary acidification and subclinical metabolic acidosis in cats with idiopathic hypercalcemia. Treatment with bisphosphonates may elucidate the role of bone resorption.

REFERENCES

1. McClain HM, Barsanti JA, Bartges JW: Hypercalcemia and calcium oxalate urolithiasis in cats: A report of five cases. J Am Anim Hosp Assoc 35:297–301, 1999.
2. Kyles AE, Stone EA, Gookin J, et al: Diagnosis and surgical management of obstructive ureteral calculi in cats: 11 cases (1993–1996). J Am Vet Med Assoc 213:1150–1156, 1998.
3. Savary KCM, Price GS, Vaden SL: Hypercalcemia in cats: A retrospective study of 71 cases (1991–1997). J Vet Intern Med (In press).
4. Osborne CA, Lulich JP, Thumchai R, et al: Feline urolithiasis: Etiology and pathophysiology. Vet Clin North Am Small Anim Pract 26:217–232, 1996.
5. Kirk CA, Ling GV, Franti CE, et al: Evaluation of factors associated with development of calcium oxalate urolithiasis in cats. J Am Vet Med Assoc 207:1429–1434, 1995.
6. Zerwekh JE, Pak CY: Mechanisms of hypercalciuria. Pathobiol Annu 12:185–201, 1982.
7. Ching SV, Norrdin RW, Fettman MJ, et al: Trabecular bone remodeling and bone mineral density in the adult cat during chronic dietary acidification with ammonium chloride. J Bone Min Res 5:547–556, 1990.
8. Ching SV, Fettman MJ, Hamar DW, et al: The effect of chronic dietary acidification using ammonium chloride on acid-base and mineral metabolism in the adult cat. J Nutrit 119:902–915, 1989.
9. Hoskins JD, Turnwald GH, Kearney MT, et al: Quantitative urinalysis in kittens from four to thirty weeks after birth. Am J Vet Res 52:1295–1299, 1991.
10. Finco DR, Brown SA, Barsanti JA, et al: Reliability of using random urine samples for "spot" determination of fractional excretion of electrolytes in cats. Am J Vet Res 58:1184–1187, 1997.
11. McMillan FD: Hypercalcemia associated with lymphoid neoplasia in two cats. Feline Pract 15:31–35, 1985.
12. Dust A, Norris AM, Valli VEO: Cutaneous lymphosarcoma with IgG monoclonal gammopathy, serum hyperviscosity and hypercalcemia in a cat. Can Vet J 23:235–239, 1982.
13. Engelman RW, Tyler RD, Good RA, et al: Hypercalcemia in

cats with feline-leukemia-virus–associated leukemia-lymphoma. Cancer 56:777–781, 1985.

14. Zenoble RD, Rowland GN: Hypercalcemia and proliferative, myelosclerotic bone reaction associated with feline leukovirus infection in a cat. J Am Vet Med Assoc 175:591–595, 1979.

15. Chew DJ, Schaer M, Liu SK, et al: Pseudohyperparathyroidism in a cat. J Am Anim Hosp Assoc 11:46–52, 1975.

16. Klausner JS, Bell FW, Hayden DW, et al: Hypercalcemia in two cats with squamous cell carcinomas. J Am Vet Med Assoc 196:103–105, 1990.

17. Hutson CA, Willauer CC, Walder EJ, et al: Treatment of mandibular squamous cell carcinoma in cats by use of mandibulectomy and radiotherapy: Seven cases (1987–1989). J Am Vet Med Assoc 201:777–781, 1992.

18. Sheafor SE, Gamblin RM, Couto CG: Hypercalcemia in two cats with multiple myeloma. J Am Anim Hosp Assoc 32:503–508, 1996.

19. DiBartola SP, Rutgers HC, Zack PM, et al: Clinicopathologic findings associated with chronic renal disease in cats: 74 cases (1973–1984). J Am Vet Med Assoc 190:1196–1202, 1987.

20. Barber PJ, Rawlings JM, Markwell PJ, et al: Effect of dietary phosphate restriction on renal secondary hyperparathyroidism in the cat. J Small Anim Pract 40:62–70, 1999.

21. den Hertog E, Goossens MM, van der Linde-Sipman JS, et al: Primary hyperparathyroidism in two cats. Vet Q 19:81–84, 1997.

22. Marquez GA, Klausner JS, Osborne CA: Calcium oxalate urolithiasis in a cat with a functional parathyroid adenocarcinoma. J Am Vet Med Assoc 206:817–819, 1995.

23. Kallet AJ, Richter KP, Feldman EC, et al: Primary hyperparathyroidism in cats: Seven cases (1984–1989). J Am Vet Med Assoc 199:1767–1771, 1991.

24. Peterson ME, Greco DS, Orth DN: Primary hypoadrenocorticism in ten cats. J Vet Intern Med 3:55–58, 1989.

25. Peterson EN, Kirby R, Sommer M, et al: Cholecalciferol rodenticide intoxication in a cat. J Am Vet Med Assoc 199:904–906, 1991.

26. Moore FM, Kudisch M, Richter K, et al: Hypercalcemia associated with rodenticide poisoning in three cats. J Am Vet Med Assoc 193:1099–1100, 1988.

27. Mahgoub A, Hirsch PF, Munson PL: Calcium-lowering action of glucocorticoids in adrenalectomized-parathyroidectomized rats. Specificity and relative potency of natural and synthetic glucocorticoids. Endocrine 6:279–283, 1997.

28. Rosol TJ, Chew DJ, Nagode LA, et al: Disorders of calcium. *In* DiBartola SP (ed): Fluid Therapy in Small Animal Practice, 2nd ed. Philadelphia, WB Saunders, 2000, pp. 108–162.

42

◆ New Treatments in the Medical Management of Feline Interstitial Cystitis

C. A. Tony Buffington
Dennis J. Chew

Feline interstitial cystitis (FIC) is one of the most common chronic lower urinary tract disorders of cats.[1] FIC is characterized by signs of chronic irritative voiding (e.g., dysuria, hematuria, pollakiuria, inappropriate urination, or some combination of these signs), sterile and cytologically negative urine, and cystoscopic observation of submucosal petechial hemorrhages. The diagnosis of FIC is made only when all 3 of these features are documented, and attempts to find an alternative cause for the clinical signs fail. FIC is a diagnosis of exclusion, and this definition must be considered provisional. It currently is not known whether FIC is a specific disease, or whether it represents different diseases that cause similar signs. The term *idiopathic cystitis* describes cats with clinical signs of irritative voiding that have sterile and cytologically negative urine in which appropriate diagnostic procedures other than cystoscopy (e.g., ultrasonography, plain and contrast radiography) have not identified an alternative cause. Idiopathic cystitis may be acute or chronic, whereas FIC by definition is a chronic process. Although cats with FIC are a subset of cats with idiopathic cystitis, we presume that our recommendations pertain to both groups. We prefer to add the adjective *feline* to interstitial cystitis because interstitial cystitis also occurs in human beings,[2] and species differences in etiology may exist.

◆ COURSE OF DISEASE

In 50 to 70 per cent of cats examined for an initial episode of irritative voiding, clinical signs resolve within 5 to 7 days regardless of treatment. The remainder of cats will continue to display signs indefinitely, either continuously or intermittently. Urethral obstruction may develop in some males as a result of the inflammatory process within the bladder and urethra.[3] Whether FIC is a self-limiting disease or a chronic disorder with acute attacks remains to be determined. Some affected cats have a striking increase in severity of clinical signs that appears to be associated with increases in environmental stressors. Such episodes are referred to as *flares*. In other cats with FIC, however, the waxing and waning of clinical signs occur in the absence of apparent changes in the "load" of stressors.

◆ TREATMENT

Overview

The underlying cause of FIC is unknown, and few controlled clinical trials have been reported. Consequently, treatment recommendations necessarily must be tentative. Results from controlled clinical trials should be used to guide future treatment recommendations, but few such studies have been performed. Depending on the severity and chronicity of the disease, some combination of educational, dietary, and pharmacologic recommendations usually is offered to owners. These include explanation of normal cat behaviors and activities that might provide stress reduction for their cat, a discussion of feeding and litter-box management, and how to clean any soiled areas in the household. Once these changes have been instituted successfully, modifications in diet, increased water intake, provision of pain relief, and drug therapy are considered if signs recur. Patients with FIC appear unusually susceptible to alterations in their environment, including abrupt diet changes, and any modifications should be instituted cautiously. Increasing water intake to dilute urine and increase frequency of urination may be an important part of treatment. One mechanism for this benefit may be the dilution of noxious components of urine that gain access to the bladder wall as a result of increased bladder permeability.

Stress Management

FIC may result when a "sensitive" cat lives in a "provocative" environment, and stressors that activate clinical signs often are identified. Activation of the sympathetic nervous system in affected cats appears to be important in the modulation of inflammation and pain by a variety of mechanisms. We believe that stress is very important in the development of flares in cats with FIC, and may be important in precipitating the first episode of signs in susceptible animals. Unfortunately, stress is difficult to quantitate. A detailed history is necessary to expose stressors in a cat's life, which may include changes in the environment, weather, activity, use of the litter pan, food intake, owner work schedule, additions or subtractions from the household population of human beings or animals, and other factors.[4] Regimens to reduce stress may prove essential in the management of FIC. To reduce the impact of environmental stressors, we recommend that the patient be provided places to hide, and opportunities to express the natural predatory behavior of cats. These opportunities may include climbing posts and toys that can be chased and caught. Many other behavioral strategies can be considered.[5, 6] Additionally, pilot studies are under way to determine whether facial pheromones (Feliway, Abbott Laboratories) can reduce stress in this patient population. If so, this approach also might prove useful to modulate the animal's perception of its environment.

Diet

Some diet modifications may reduce the risk of recurrence of lower urinary tract signs related to FIC. Struvite crystals do not appear to damage normal urothelium, and heroic efforts to reduce struvite crystalluria are not warranted. Moreover, efforts to acidify the urine have no known value in the treatment of cats not suffering from struvite urolithiasis. Pending future improvements in understanding of the etiology of FIC, dietary treatment recommendations include consideration of the constancy, consistency, and composition of the diet.

Constancy

Our clinical experience suggests that diet change can result in recurrence of signs of irritative voiding in some patients. Moreover, with the advent of many similarly formulated veterinary and commercial foods marketed for use in cats with lower urinary tract disease, signs sometimes recur when cats are switched from one to another of these foods. These observations suggest that diet change may result in recurrence of signs. Pending further study of this hypothesis, limiting the frequency of diet changes in this group of patients may be prudent.

Consistency

Cats with idiopathic cystitis are significantly more likely to eat dry food exclusively.[1] Recently, we reported that lower urinary tract signs recurred in only 11 per cent of cats with FIC during a year of feeding the canned formulation of a veterinary food[a] designed to result in production of acidic urine.[7] Recurrence occurred in 39 per cent of cats fed the dry form of the food, suggesting that both constancy and consistency (dry versus canned) may be important, although the reasons for this effect remain to be determined. Both diets contained similar potential renal solute loads, and resulted in similar urine pH. Interestingly, the urine specific gravity of

cats fed the dry form averaged 1.050, whereas that of those fed the canned diet averaged 1.030. It appears that the canned form protected nearly 90 per cent of cats against recurrence of lower urinary tract signs for up to 1 year, constancy of diet protected about 60 per cent, and signs recurred in 10 per cent of cats despite the diet change.

Composition

In addition to the canned diet, diet-related decreases in urine magnesium or increases in urine calcium, potassium, or hydrogen ion concentrations all might increase activity of sensory nerve fibers in the urothelium.[8] Unfortunately, most of these effects have been identified only by using in vitro experimental systems. The effects of urine electrolyte composition on lower urinary tract signs have not been studied adequately, but may be important in treatment of some patients.

Cats suffering from FIC seem to benefit from provision of a single-product, canned diet, if such a feeding plan is not too stressful to the cat or the owner. Some cats will not eat canned foods, and in our practice, many owners are reluctant to feed canned foods owing to the lack of convenience compared with dry foods. The issues surrounding stress, diet change, and disease currently are controversial, and further investigation of these relationships is needed.

Amitriptyline

Amitriptyline is a tricyclic antidepressant and analgesic with both serotonin and norepinephrine re-uptake inhibition in the central nervous system; however, norepinephrine re-uptake inhibition predominates. Moreover, its beneficial effects do not seem to be related to serotonin, because antidepressants that selectively inhibit serotonin re-uptake are not effective in treatment of interstitial cystitis in human beings.[9] Although the full range of its actions is not known, the beneficial effects are not attributable primarily to its antidepressant actions.[9] The beneficial effects of amitriptyline on pain in human beings appear to be independent of its effect on depression, developing at much lower dosages than those required to improve depression.[10] Potential beneficial effects of amitriptyline include decreased noradrenergic outflow from the central nervous system[9, 11] (possibly by an alpha$_2$-mediated mechanism[12]), induction of endogenous opioid release,[13] and inhibition of H$_1$-receptors and release of histamine from mast cells (demonstrated in vitro).[11, 14] Activation of mast cells and release of secretory granules may contribute to the vasodilatation and inflammation observed in the bladder of some cats with FIC.[3] Although tricyclic antidepressants exerted no effect on acute pain in clinically normal cats during tail-flick studies,[15] amitriptyline inhibited segmental transmission of wide dynamic range

---

[a]Waltham Veterinary Diet Feline Control pHormula (dry) and Waltham Veterinary Diet Feline Control pHormula in Gel (canned), Waltham USA, Inc., Vernon, CA.

and nociceptive neurons in the feline trigeminal nucleus,[16, 17] which could explain some of its analgesic effects. Amitriptyline also exerts some anticholinergic effects, which might reduce detrusor contractions and increase bladder capacity.

We recently reported the beneficial effects of amitriptyline treatment in 15 cats with severe recurrent FIC.[18] Failure during this study was defined as the recurrence of any lower urinary tract sign during 12 months of treatment. Amitriptyline at 2 mg/kg orally every (q) 24 hr (usually at the owner's bedtime) successfully eliminated clinical signs of FIC in 73 per cent of the cats for the first 6 months, and in 60 per cent of cats studied for the entire 12 months. Despite clinical remission, cystoscopic abnormalities persisted in all cats at the 6- and 12-month evaluations. Weight gain, somnolence, decreased grooming, and transient cystic calculi were observed in some cats.

We consider amitriptyline for treatment of FIC only when other "standard" therapies have failed (i.e., client education about feeding and litter-box management, stress reduction, and methods to increase water intake). There is no good argument to use amitriptyline in cats with acute signs of irritative voiding because spontaneous resolution of clinical signs often occurs within a few days, whereas it may take weeks for amitriptyline to exert a maximum effect.

Further studies of amitriptyline for safety and efficacy during treatment of FIC are needed, but amitriptyline has been used safely in cats by animal behaviorists for many years. Hemograms and serum biochemistry remained normal throughout treatment in our series. Amitriptyline has its place in the control of signs of lower urinary tract disease associated with FIC, but it is not an ideal drug because the lesions of cystitis are still apparent cystoscopically during treatment, and undesirable side-effects occurred in some cats. It is conceivable that lower doses of amitriptyline may be effective when given in combination with other drugs. Effective doses of amitriptyline range from 2.5 mg to 12.5 mg orally q 24 hr, and the dosage should be titrated to effect. We used a standardized dose of 10 mg per cat in our clinical study, but we usually start at 5 mg daily and increase the dose if needed every 2 to 4 weeks to a maximum of 12.5 mg daily. Caution should be used in administering amitriptyline to cats with known cardiac disease or arrhythmia, but problems are encountered infrequently at the low doses used to treat inflammation.

Glycosaminoglycans

Some human patients with interstitial cystitis appear to have a quantitative or qualitative defect in the glycosaminoglycan (GAG) layer lining the urothelium.[19] Cats with FIC excrete fewer GAGs and have greater bladder permeability, even during quiescent periods, than do normal cats. Decreased GAG excretion could permit urine to penetrate the urothelium and induce inflammation.[20] A defective GAG layer or damaged urothelium[21] also could permit constituents of the urine, such as protons and other ions, to come into contact with the axons of sensory fibers innervating the bladder. This effect could result in local release of neurotransmitters that either initiate or perpetuate neurogenic inflammation, or could send impulses signaling pain to the central nervous system. Alternatively, alterations in the GAG layer could be a result of local inflammation.[22] The possibility of qualitative defects in GAG excretion in cats with FIC has not yet been explored, but has been suggested in human beings with interstitial cystitis.

An orally administered GAG (pentosan polysulfate sodium, Elmiron) that is excreted into urine has been available for treatment of women with interstitial cystitis in the United States since 1996. Pentosan polysulfate is a semisynthetic polysaccharide derived from birch bark. The assumption underlying GAG therapy is that GAG is excreted into the urine in a concentration high enough to allow it to "coat" the defective urothelium and decrease urothelial permeability. This effect may be specific to only some GAGs, as there appear to be differences among the various GAGs in their relative efficacy in producing this effect.[23] GAGs also can exert analgesic and anti-inflammatory effects,[24] and may inhibit histamine release from mast cells.[25] A double-blind placebo-controlled multicenter study of pentosan polysulfate treatment of FIC has been concluded recently in the United States.

Prospects for the Future

Although 2 controlled therapeutic studies recently were published, one demonstrating the benefit of a canned diet[7] and the other of amitriptyline,[18] there are many unproven treatments for FIC. Clinical results are variable and inconsistent, and results of prospective, randomized, controlled clinical studies are lacking. Moreover, although some reports of "lack of effect" in placebo-controlled studies of treatments in cats have appeared, they generally have used too few cats to achieve sufficient statistical power to be convincing. Additionally, safety questions remain regarding some treatments. Despite these limitations, the renewed efforts to understand this disease that have resulted from recognition of its similarities with interstitial cystitis in human beings[26] already have provided 2 new effective therapies for some cats with FIC, and suggest that more may become available in the near future.

REFERENCES

1. Buffington CA, Chew DJ, Kendall MS, et al: Clinical evaluation of cats with nonobstructive urinary tract diseases. J Am Vet Med Assoc 210:46–50, 1997.
2. Sant GR: Interstitial Cystitis. Philadelphia, Lippincott-Raven, 1997.

3. Buffington CA, Chew DJ, DiBartola SP: Interstitial cystitis in cats. Vet Clin North Am Small Anim Pract 26:317–326, 1996.
4. Jones B, Sanson RL, Morris RS: Elucidating the risk factors of feline urologic syndrome. N Z Vet J 45:100–108, 1997.
5. Bohnenkamp G: From the Cat's Point of View. San Francisco, Perfect Paws, 1991.
6. Overall KL: Clinical Behavioral Medicine for Small Animals. St. Louis: Mosby, 1997.
7. Markwell PJ, Buffington CAT, Chew DJ, et al: Clinical evaluation of commercially available urinary acidification diets in the management of idiopathic cystitis in cats. J Am Vet Med Assoc 214:361–365, 1999.
8. Maggi CA, Lecci A, Abelli L, et al: The role of capsaicin-sensitive afferents in the genesis of vesical pain and inflammation. *In* Vecchiet L, Albe-Fessard D, Lindblom U (eds): New Trends in Referred Pain and Hyperalgesia. Amsterdam, Elsevier Science, pp. 161–175, 1993.
9. Max MB, Lynch SA, Muir J, et al: Effects of desipramine, amitriptyline, and fluoxetine on pain in diabetic neuropathy. N Engl J Med 326:1250–1256, 1992.
10. Max M, Culnane M, Schafer S, et al: Amitriptyline relieves diabetic neuropathy pain in patients with normal or depressed mood. Neurology 37:589–596, 1987.
11. Hanno PM: Amitriptyline in the treatment of interstitial cystitis. Urol Clin North Am 21:89–91, 1994.
12. Gray AM, Pache DM, Sewell RDE: Do alpha$_2$-adrenoceptors play an integral role in the antinociceptive mechanism of action of antidepressant compounds? Eur J Pharmacol 378:161–168, 1999.
13. Gray AM, Spencer PSJ, Sewell RDE: The involvement of the opioidergic system in the antinociceptive mechanism of action of antidepressant compounds. Br J Pharmacol 124:669–674, 1998.
14. Theoharides TC: The mast cell: A neuroimmunoendocrine master player. Int J Tissue React 18:1–21, 1996.
15. Sharav Y, Singer E, Schmidt E, et al: The analgesic effect of amitriptyline on chronic facial pain. Pain 31:199–209, 1987.
16. Fromm GH, Glass JD: The effect of tricyclic antidepressants on corticofugal inhibition of the spinal trigeminal nucleus. Electroencephalog Clin Neurophysiol 43:637–645, 1977.
17. Fromm GH, Nakata M, Kondo T: Differential action of amitriptyline on neurons in the trigeminal nucleus. Neurology 41:1932–1936, 1991.
18. Chew DJ, Buffington CAT, Kendall MS, et al: Amitriptyline treatment for idiopathic cystitis in cats (15 cases 1994–1996). J Am Vet Med Assoc 213:1282–1286, 1998.
19. Hurst RE, Roy JB, Parsons CL: The role of glycosaminoglycans in normal bladder physiology and the pathophysiology of interstitial cystitis. *In* Sant GR (ed): Interstitial Cystitis. Philadelphia, Lippincott-Raven, pp. 93–100, 1997.
20. Parsons CL: The therapeutic role of sulfated polysaccharides in the urinary bladder. Urol Clin North Am 21:93–100, 1994.
21. Lavelle JP, Meyers SA, Ruiz WG, et al: Urothelial pathophysiological changes in feline interstitial cystitis: A human interstitial cystitis model. Am J Physiol 278:F540–F553, 2000.
22. Baggio B, Gambaro G, Cicerello E, et al: Urinary excretion of glycosaminoglycans in urological disease. Clin Biochem 20:449–450, 1987.
23. Nickel JC, Downey J, Morales A, et al: Relative efficacy of various exogenous glycosaminoglycans in providing a bladder surface permeability barrier. J Urol 160:612–614, 1998.
24. Saliba MJ Jr: The effects and uses of heparin in the care of burns that improves treatment and enhances the quality of life. Acta Chir Plast 39:13–16, 1997.
25. Patra PB, Hesse L, Boucher W, et al: Chondroitin sulfate (CS) inhibits mast cell secretion. FASEB J 13:A149, 1999.
26. Buffington CAT, Chew DJ, Woodworth BE: Feline interstitial cystitis. J Am Vet Med Assoc 215:682–687, 1999.

43

◆ Renal Transplantation in the Management of Chronic Renal Failure

Kyle G. Mathews

Although the first experimental feline renal transplant was performed in 1907, it was not until the introduction of the immunosuppressive drug cyclosporin A (CyA; now, cyclosporine) in the 1980s that renal transplantation was performed in cats as a treatment for chronic renal failure (CRF).[1] Feline renal transplantation as a treatment for CRF was first performed at the University of California School of Veterinary Medicine in 1987.[2] Since that time, over 150 cats have received renal allografts at transplantation units around the country. Feline renal transplantation units have increased in number since about 1995 (Table 43–1). This has resulted in an increase in the amount of information published on this subject, and hopefully will continue to improve our ability to manage transplant recipients successfully postoperatively. In 1992, long-term results of the first 23 cases were reported.[3] For those initial 23 cats, ureteral obstruction was a common complication, no deaths were attributed to renal allograft rejection, and the longest survival time was 31 months. Since that report, changes in operative technique essentially have eliminated ureteral obstruction as a postoperative complication, survival times have increased, hypertension-related seizure activity has been identified as a major cause of post-operative morbidity, and rejection and immunosuppression-related complications have been identified as contributors to mortality after discharge.[4]

◆ THE RECIPIENT

It is not possible to predict how long a given cat will survive with medically managed CRF, and the optimum time to perform a renal transplant is based on the individual animal's response to therapy. The appropriate diagnostic evaluation and management of cats with CRF is covered in Chapter 44, Medical Management of Chronic Renal Failure. As noted, a variety of medical treatment options exists, depending on the physical and biochemical abnormalities that are present. Some of these treatment options include protein-restricted diets, subcutaneous fluid administration, phosphate binders, erythropoietin, and antihypertensive medications (e.g., amlodipine) (see Chapters 36, Systemic Hypertension, and 47, Diagnosis and Treatment of Systemic Hypertension). A chemistry panel, hematocrit and body weight should be evaluated on a regular basis (usually monthly) so that medical management can be adjusted, and so that failure of medical therapy can be detected early. I consider transplantation to be an option when a rising serum creatinine concentration is detected despite increasingly aggressive medical management. If worsening azotemia is identified before the cat becomes uremic and has stopped eating, the cat is a better surgical candidate.

If a transplant candidate has lost 10 per cent or more of its body weight, and does not respond to appetite stimulation (cyproheptadine, lorazepam, or diazepam), H_2 receptor antagonists, and treatment of uremic stomatitis if present, placement of a percutaneous endoscopic gastrostomy (PEG) tube and caloric supplementation is recommended until the cat shows a positive response before scheduling the procedure. The dietary management of feline transplant recipients recommended in this chapter is based on clinical experience, and studies evaluating the response to dietary manipulation in the pre- and postoperative periods need to be performed. If the recommendation that all cats with 10 per cent or more loss of body weight receive nutritional supplementation were applied to historical cases, the majority of feline recipients would have had PEG tubes placed before transplantation. Preoperative caloric requirements can be estimated using the formula:

Table 43–1. Active Feline Renal Transplantation Programs in the United States

University of California–Davis, School of Veterinary Medicine, Davis, CA
Contact: Dr. Clare R. Gregory

North Carolina State University, College of Veterinary Medicine, Raleigh, NC
Contact: Dr. Kyle G. Mathews

University of Florida, College of Veterinary Medicine, Gainesville, FL
Contact: Dr. Gary Ellison

University of Pennsylvania, School of Veterinary Medicine, Philadelphia, PA
Contact: Dr. Lillian Aronson

Cornell University, College of Veterinary Medicine, Ithaca, NY
Contact: Dr. James A. Flanders

University of Wisconsin, School of Veterinary Medicine, Madison, WI
Contact: Dr. Jonathan F. McAnulty

Michigan State University, College of Veterinary Medicine, Lansing, MI
Contact: Dr. Richard Walshaw

Michigan Veterinary Specialists, Southfield, MI
Contact: Dr. Dan A. Degner

$$IER \text{ (kcal ME)} = (1.2 \times 70\{BW_{kg}\}^{0.75}) \text{ or}$$
$$(BW_{kg} \times 30) + 70$$

where IER is illness energy requirements, ME is metabolizable energy, and BW is body weight. The cat should be offered a commercially available CRF diet (e.g., Hill's Feline k/d). The addition of arginine (250 mg/cat, every [q] 12 hr) to the diet also may be beneficial in maintaining amino acid and acid-base homeostasis. (Jackson M, personal communication, 2000).

Many factors should be considered before evaluating the cat's suitability as a potential renal recipient. The initial cost of the diagnostic evaluation, surgical procedure, and postoperative care of both the recipient and the donor must be taken into consideration. The typical cost for a renal transplant recipient will be thousands of dollars. In addition, the costs of repeated veterinary visits, blood sampling, and treatment of potential complications must be considered by the owner before making the decision. The owner, referring veterinarian, and referral surgeon also must consider the well-being of the donor cat. Is the owner willing to accept the responsibility of caring for an additional cat? I consider adoption of the donor by the owner of the recipient mandatory regardless of outcome. The majority of owners view the donor as a lifesaver and a welcomed member of the household. The upper age limit for a transplant candidate has not been defined, but 16 years of age has been used as a subjective upper limit in the past. The risks to the geriatric candidate must be weighed against the potentially reduced benefit of transplantation as the cat nears the end of its normal life expectancy. Finally, if there is any question as to the owner's ability to give oral medications to the cat, he or she should demonstrate this ability before referral to a transplantation unit. Obviously, a fractious cat that cannot be medicated is not considered a candidate for transplantation.

When it is clear that the owner has considered all of the socioeconomic factors associated with feline renal transplantation, evaluation of the cat as a potential transplant recipient may proceed. Transplant candidates are evaluated for evidence of cardiomyopathy (echocardiography), infectious diseases (feline leukemia virus/feline immunodeficiency virus serology, urinalysis, and urine culture), and neoplasia (abdominal ultrasonography, thoracic radiographs). Positive findings on any of these tests eliminates the cat as a candidate. If there is evidence on ultrasonographic examination of renomegaly consistent with lymphosarcoma, a fine-needle aspirate or percutaneous biopsy of the kidney is warranted as long as consideration is given to possible coagulopathy associated with the renal disease.[5]

One report indicated that hyperthyroidism was the second most common concurrent disease in cats with CRF.[6] Therefore, evaluation of the transplant candidate for hyperthyroidism should be considered, especially if the cat is hypertensive or if echocardiographic changes consistent with hyperthyroidism are identified.[7] Treatment of hyperthyroidism may result in worsening of the renal failure in some instances owing to a decrease in glomerular filtration rate.[8]

Toxoplasma gondii titers also should be evaluated. Transplant candidates that are seropositive for *T. gondii* should be monitored after transplantation for rising antibody titers so that early treatment can be initiated.[9] Other options include eliminating transplantation as a consideration or administering cyclosporine (Neoral, Sandoz Pharmaceuticals Corp., East Hanover, NJ) for several months with serial evaluation of titers before surgery. Candidates with rising titers then could be treated appropriately, immunosuppressive therapy could be withdrawn, and transplantation could be eliminated as an option.

Any cat with a prior history of urinary tract infection should be given a cyclosporine challenge several weeks before the procedure. Cyclosporine is given for 2 weeks at the same dosage (noted later) used to immunosuppress the recipient. Urine then is collected by cystocentesis and cultured. Cats that develop a urinary tract infection while on cyclosporine are given appropriate antibiotic therapy based on sensitivity results for a minimum of 2 weeks. If a second urine culture is positive after having withdrawn the antibiotic, the cat is not considered a candidate for transplantation because of the risk of developing pyelonephritis or early allograft rejection. We now start all of our transplant candidates on cyclosporine 2 weeks before surgery and re-evaluate a urinalysis. This allows us to identify occult infections before referral. Furthermore, the absorption and metabolism of cyclosporine vary greatly from cat to cat, and postoperative peaks and troughs in cyclosporine concentration occur when the drug is started just before surgery. Therefore, identification of the dosage necessary to maintain stable blood concentrations of cyclosporine may hasten the cat's recovery from surgery. A stable and effective cyclosporine concentration in the postoperative period reduces the potential for cyclosporine nephrotoxicity and rejection, and should limit the postoperative hospital stay. It is too early to tell whether this procedure will result in adverse effects, such as delayed graft function, in some cats.

Cyclosporine is derived from the fungus *Tolypocladium inflatum*. Cyclosporine has many actions including diminished interleukin-2 transcription and production by T-helper lymphocytes, and inhibition of lymphocyte responsiveness to interleukin-2.[10, 11] As a result, a coordinated immunologic response to the allograft can not be mounted. The improved absorbability of a microencapsulated formulation of cyclosporine (Neoral) has decreased the dosage requirement from 7 mg/kg orally q 12 hr with Sandimmune (Sandimmune Oral Solution, Sandoz Pharmaceuticals Corp., East Hanover, NJ) to approximately 3 mg/kg q 12 hr orally with Neoral. Cyclosporine is metabolized by both hepatic and intestinal cytochrome P-450 enzyme systems.[12] There is considerable variability among cats in its metabolism and in the dosage required to prevent allograft rejection. Competitive inhibition of cyclosporine metabolism has been noted for a variety of drugs including calcium channel blockers, angiotensin-converting enzyme inhibitors, antibiotics (e.g., erythromycin), and antifungal azoles.[12–14] Marked reduction in the amount of drug needed to maintain adequate cyclosporine concentrations has been seen in a cat treated orally with itraconazole for a systemic fungal infection after transplantation. The effect of orally administered ketoconazole on cyclosporine metabolism in cats was investigated recently.[15] This report showed significantly increased cyclosporine concentrations and decreased cyclosporine clearance when ketoconazole was given in conjunction with cyclosporine. In addition, 6 cats were given ketoconazole (10 mg/kg orally q 24 hr) starting the day after transplantation. Cyclosporine administration was simultaneously decreased from twice to once daily. Four cats were managed successfully on this protocol for a mean duration of 585 days. One other cat required twice-daily cyclosporine, but at a 60 per cent reduction in the required dose. The convenience and potential cost savings associated with this protocol must be weighed against the potential for adverse reactions to ketoconazole.

◆ THE DONOR

Donors are healthy young adult cats usually from shelter and laboratory sources, and should be of similar size or larger than the recipient. Occasionally, the owner of the recipient will have a suitable donor in the household. Tissue-typing and leukocyte crossmatching have not been used in cats to evaluate the suitability (histocompatability) of renal donors. Instead, red cell crossmatching (blood transfusion compatibility) has been found to be adequate. Histocompatible donors would be difficult to locate for most cats in CRF because related potential donors rarely are available.

Cats that match the recipient then are screened for organic and infectious disease by complete blood count, chemistry panel, and urinalysis. A recent study suggests that cats that are seropositive for *Toxoplasma gondii* should not be used as donors for seronegative recipients.[9] If no abnormalities are found, renal morphology is evaluated by excretory urography and abdominal ultrasonography. Findings suggestive of previous or subclinical renal disease (e.g., dilatation of the renal pelves, mineralization, abnormal renal shape) eliminate the cat as a donor. One center also performs nuclear scintigraphy and calculates the glomerular filtration rate and relative contribution of each kidney for both the donor and the recipient preoperatively. This allows identification and rejection of potential donors that have abnormalities in renal function. In addition,

scintigraphic follow-up of the allograft likely will yield valuable information (Ellison G, personal communication, 1999).

In many situations, the donor cat had been scheduled for euthanasia, and donation has resulted in lifesaving adoption into a caring environment. Follow-up on 16 donors 24 to 67 months postoperatively has been reported.[16] The median age of the donors at the time of surgery was 34 months. Fifteen of the donors were clinically normal at re-examination. Serum creatinine concentrations for these 15 cats increased from a mean of 1.36 to 1.71 mg/dl, but remained within the reference range. One cat was diagnosed with chronic renal insufficiency 52 months postoperatively at the age of 8 years. One cat had a single episode of acute renal insufficiency owing to presumptive pyelonephritis 20 months postoperatively at the age of 29 months. The development of chronic renal insufficiency in 1 of 16 (6.3 per cent) cats in this small study is similar to the previously reported prevalence of 5 per cent in 7- to 10-year-old cats.[17] Although the effect of uninephrectomy on donors has not been evaluated after they become geriatric, conversations with the owners of adopted donors have not identified any widespread clinical problems.

◆ PREOPERATIVE MANAGEMENT OF THE RECIPIENT

Preoperative management includes subcutaneous or intravenous fluid replacement as needed. Nutritional supplementation was discussed previously. Blood transfusions are administered if necessary to achieve a packed cell volume of 30 per cent or more before surgery. I prefer to have a jugular catheter placed the day before surgery to simplify anesthetic induction and allow monitoring of central venous pressure postoperatively. In the past, microemulsified cyclosporine has been administered orally at 3.0 mg/kg q 12 hr beginning 24 to 36 hours preoperatively. As noted previously, I now start the recipient on this dosage of cyclosporine 2 weeks preoperatively. Prednisolone, 0.25 to 0.5 mg/kg q 12 hr is administered orally starting the day of surgery. Trough whole-blood cyclosporine concentrations are determined by either high-performance liquid chromatography (HPLC) or immunoassay (see Monitoring). Blood samples are collected in ethylenediaminetetraacetic acid (EDTA) 12 hours after the previous evening's dose. Additional cyclosporine trough concentrations are determined at approximately 3-day intervals during the perioperative period. Both the donor and the recipient receive prophylactic antibiotics (e.g., ampicillin 25 mg/kg intravenously [IV]) immediately before surgery.

◆ ANESTHETIC MANAGEMENT AND SURGICAL PROCEDURE

The anesthetic protocol has remained relatively unchanged from that described for the first 23 cats, but important changes in the surgical procedure have taken place.[1, 4] After the cat is premedicated with atropine sulfate (0.01 to 0.04 mg/kg subcutaneously [SC]) and oxymorphone (0.05 mg/kg SC), the cat is masked or box-induced, intubated, and maintained on isoflurane inhalant and oxygen. In addition to balanced electrolyte solutions administered via a cephalic venous catheter, whole blood is administered at 5 to 10 ml/kg/hr to maintain the packed cell volume at 30 per cent or higher. Mannitol is administered IV at 1 g/kg over 30 minutes at completion of the ureteral anastomosis. The same dosage of mannitol is given to the donor immediately before harvesting the kidney.

Once the surgical team has isolated the donor kidney, the recipient is brought into the operating room. Abnormalities in the renal vasculature that preclude transplantation occur infrequently, but delaying induction of the recipient until the renal vessels of the donor have been inspected is suggested. Delaying induction of the recipient also shortens the recipient's anesthetic time and the potential for development of marked hypothermia. The left kidney of the donor is preferred because the increased length of the renal vein on this side improves visibility during venous anastomosis. Once the renal vasculature has been inspected, the vessels are cleaned of all adventitia, and the ureter is isolated along its entire length. Monopolar electrocoagulation is not utilized near the vessels and the ureter to avoid damage to these structures. Regional vessels are either ligated or cauterized with a battery-operated electrocautery unit or by bipolar coagulation. To assist the surgeons in making appropriate-sized windows in the recipient aorta and vena cava, foil templates are made that match the diameter of the renal vessels.

At this point in the procedure, a second surgical support team should have the recipient in the operating room and prepared for surgery. The surgeons pack off the abdomen of the donor with warm, moist laparotomy sponges and proceed to prepare the recipient vessels for anastomosis. Placement of the kidney in the inguinal fossa and anastomosis of the donor renal artery and vein to the recipient external iliac artery (end-to-end) and vein (end-to-side) are performed at some centers. Either standard suture techniques or microvascular anastomotic coupling devices (Microvascular Anastomotic System, Medical Companies Alliance, Bessemer, AL) may be employed. Others now anastomose the renal vessels directly to the abdominal aorta and vena cava in an end-to-side manner because of concern with hindlimb ischemia associated with the inguinal fossa method.[4] In addition, the aorta and vena cava caudal to the native left kidney are easier to visualize and less vessel preparation is required, thus decreasing anesthetic and surgery time for the recipient.[18]

Once the adventitia of the recipient vessels has been removed, they are crossclamped, and appropriate-sized windows are created in the side wall of each vessel. Crossclamping of these vessels has not

resulted in ischemic problems to date. The vessels are flushed with heparinized saline solution, and sutures are placed at each end of either the venous or the arterial window. The recipient bed now is ready to receive the allograft. The surgeons retrieve the kidney from the donor, and immediately proceed with the microvascular anastomosis. A third surgeon then enters the room to close and help recover the donor.

The artery and vein of the allograft are flushed with chilled heparinized saline solution after being removed from the donor in an attempt to decrease warm ischemic damage to the graft. Some surgeons prefer to stage the procedures by harvesting the allograft in the morning and completing the transplantation in the afternoon. Perfusion of the allograft with a preservation solution is required when the procedure is staged.[19] All anastomoses are performed with the aid of an operating microscope. The vein of the left donor kidney is sutured to the caudal vena cava in an end-to-side manner (simple continuous-suture pattern). An end-to-side anastomosis of the renal artery and abdominal aorta then is performed (simple continuous- or interrupted-suture pattern). Suture materials vary in size from 7-0 to 10-0 (waxed silk, nylon, or Vascufil [Monofilament polybutester coated with polytribolate. Davis & Geck, Inc., Manati, PR]) for the venous, and 8-0 to 10-0 (nylon or Vascufil) for the arterial anastomoses. The venous and then the arterial clamps are removed, and the anastomotic sites are inspected for hemorrhage.

After the allograft is reperfused, a ventral midline cystotomy is performed. The dorsal wall of the bladder is penetrated with a fine pair of hemostatic forceps, and the distal end of the donor ureter is grasped and pulled into the lumen of the bladder. Previous use of a simple ureteral drop-in technique resulted in a 32 per cent rate of ureteral obstruction postoperatively.[4] The inflammatory effects of urine on the exposed periureteral tissues presumably caused granuloma formation at the end of the ureter. Failure of the serum creatinine concentration to decrease or an increase after initial improvement, warrants ultrasonographic examination of the ureter as noted later. Obstruction occurred an average of 10 days postoperatively. Since switching to a mucosal apposition technique, ureteral obstruction caused by granuloma formation has not been reported.[20] After the distal end is amputated the ureter is spatulated and the periureteral fat removed. Accurate apposition of the ureteral mucosa to the urinary bladder mucosa is performed with multiple 8-0 to 10-0 simple interrupted nylon sutures. Placing a piece of 5-0 monofilament suture material in the lumen of the ureter as a temporary marker enhances visualization.

After the cystotomy is closed (Fig. 43–1), the donor kidney is secured to the abdominal wall by placing it in a peritoneal pocket (incision through the peritoneum and transversus abdominis muscle) with sutures running from the renal capsule to the abdominal musculature. Simple placement of su-

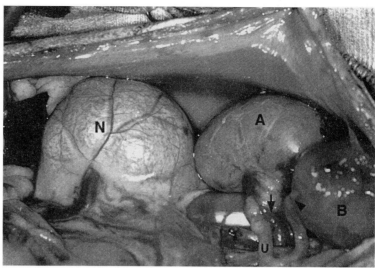

Figure 43–1. The renal allograft (A) as it appears immediately after cystostomy closure and before nephropexy. The cat's head is to the left. Left native kidney (N). Allograft ureter (U) as it enters *(arrowhead)* the dorsocranial wall of the urinary bladder (B). Donor vein *(arrow)* courses toward the abdominal vena cava. (Courtesy of Dr. Lillian Aronson, University of Pennsylvania, School of Veterinary Medicine.)

tures from the renal capsule to the body wall is inadequate in this location. Increased mobility of the allograft in this location compared with the inguinal fossa may predispose a simple nephropexy to failure with subsequent torsion of the vascular pedicle and ischemic necrosis of the kidney. After nephropexy, a biopsy of one of the native kidneys is performed, and a PEG tube is placed if not already present. Routine abdominal closure then is performed.

Measures taken to maintain normothermia before, during, and after the procedure include wringing out scrub sponges before use to keep each cat as dry as possible during aseptic preparation of the surgical site, limiting abdominal lavage with warm sterile saline solution, placing a diaper under the cat to collect excess lavage fluid, placing a heating pad under and over the cranial aspect of the cat during the procedure, and finally, drying the cat postoperatively with a hand-held blow dryer.

◆ POSTOPERATIVE MANAGEMENT OF THE RECIPIENT

Postoperatively, the recipient is given a balanced electrolyte solution during the first 24 hours and then weaned off intravenous fluids gradually depending on the cat's hydration status and water intake. Intravenous antibiotics (e.g., cefazolin, 22 mg/kg IV q 8 hr) typically are administered for as long as an intravenous catheter is in place as a precaution against immunosuppression-related catheter infections. Antibiotics (e.g., amoxicillin/clavulanate potassium, 62.5 mg q 12 hr) are administered orally or via the PEG tube after intravenous catheters have been removed. Owing to the risk of infectious complications with the PEG tube, I prefer to keep the recipient on oral antibiotics until after tube removal.

Venous blood gases, electrolytes, blood glucose

concentration, hematocrit, total solids, and urine specific gravity on voided urine typically are evaluated every 6 to 8 hours initially. Central venous pressure is monitored intermittently, and is maintained between 0 and 10 cm H_2O. Electrolyte replacement and fluid rate adjustments are performed as needed. Blood transfusions are given as needed to maintain the packed cell volume at 30 per cent or higher. The frequency of monitoring laboratory parameters gradually is reduced, so that the recipient typically is transferred out of the intensive care unit and into a renal transplant isolation ward 3 to 5 days postoperatively.

Fluid and caloric supplementation is given via the PEG tube as needed during the remainder of the hospital stay. Anorexia in the immediate postoperative period is common. This may be due to a combination of factors including stress, altered gastric motility, and residual effects of uremia including nausea and gastritis.[21] Studies in human beings have shown that the catabolic state induced by CRF and posttransplantation recovery results in a negative nitrogen balance and continued loss of muscle mass in the postoperative period. These adverse events can be reversed with a high-protein diet after transplantation.[22] Based on these findings, a recovery diet should be considered postoperatively for feline transplant recipients (e.g., Hill's Feline p/d). Diet changes should be made gradually (e.g., 25:75 recovery/CRF diet for 2 days, 50:50 for 2 days, 75:25 for 2 days, and full feeding of recovery diet on day 7) (Jackson M, personal communication, 2000). A longer transition period may be needed for cats with continued increases in blood urea nitrogen, creatinine and phosphorus concentrations after transplantation. Before each gastrostomy feeding, the volume of residual food and fluid in the stomach should be assessed, and if excessive, the feeding should be skipped, and the administration of prokinetic agents such as metoclopramide should be considered. H_2-receptor antagonists and sucralfate also are used routinely in the postoperative period. Cimetidine interferes with cyclosporine metabolism in human beings.[23] It is not known whether there is a clinically relevant interaction between cimetidine or other H_2-receptor antagonists and cyclosporine in cats. As a precaution, the frequency of monitoring cyclosporine concentrations may need to be increased. Once it is clear that the cat is eating and drinking sufficient amounts to meet its caloric and fluid requirements, supplementation via the PEG tube is discontinued gradually.

Sixteen of 66 cases (24 per cent) in one report developed postoperative central nervous system (CNS) complications.[4] Fourteen of the 16 cases (88 per cent) with CNS complications developed postoperative seizure activity. Seven of those 14 (50 per cent) died, experienced cardiac arrest subsequent to, or were euthanized as a result of seizure activity. The median time of onset of seizure activity was 24 hours postoperatively. Another report showed no difference between affected and unaffected cats with respect to preoperative serum creatinine, blood urea nitrogen, or blood cholesterol concentrations or intraoperative blood pressure.[24] In addition, there were no differences between groups in postoperative serum electrolyte concentrations, osmolality, or serum glucose concentration. Cyclosporine-mediated effects do not appear to be primarily responsible for these complications in feline renal transplant recipients. Withholding cyclosporine until the postoperative period failed to diminish the frequency of CNS complications (Mathews KG, Gregory CR, clinical experience, 1997). CNS complications may be linked to the development of hypertension postoperatively. Attempts to decrease postoperative hypertensive crises by pretreating transplant recipients with propranolol orally and treating them with IV or SC hydralazine or acepromazine as needed has decreased the frequency and severity of seizures.[25] Of 34 cats evaluated, 21 (64 per cent) developed and were treated for hypertension postoperatively. Postoperative neurologic complications were seen in 4/32 cats (12 per cent). Seizures were observed in only 1 cat, 3 cats developed other CNS complications (e.g., blindness, ataxia, stupor), and all of the affected cats survived. This represents a significant decrease in seizure activity, but the frequency of other CNS complications was not altered significantly. Hypertension was observed preoperatively in only 4 of 26 (15 per cent) of cats evaluated. One of these 4 cats seizured pre- and postoperatively, and another became obtunded during the postoperative period.

Direct arterial pressure monitoring would be ideal in the postoperative period because this approach would minimize increases in blood pressure due to stress associated with handling the recipient. Although placement of a catheter in the dorsal pedal artery for monitoring arterial pressure would be ideal, concerns regarding potential lack of collateral circulation in cats have prompted indirect blood pressure monitoring with a Doppler unit (Ultrasonic Doppler Flow Detector, Parks Medical, Inc., Aloha,

OR). The Doppler crystal is placed on either the tail or the dorsal metatarsus. Systolic pressure is measured and recorded every 30 minutes initially. The frequency of monitoring is decreased gradually over the first 48 hours as the risk of postoperative seizure activity diminishes. Hydralazine (0.5 mg/kg IV or SC) or acepromazine (0.025 to 0.05 mg/kg IV) typically is given if the systolic pressure exceeds 160 mm Hg, and analgesics (e.g., oxymorphone 0.05 mg/kg IV) already have been given. Indirect blood pressure measurement with the Doppler unit placed on the palmar aspect of the paw in anesthetized cats is a better measure of the mean rather than the systolic arterial pressure.[26] As noted, some surgeons also prefer to start transplant recipients on the beta antagonist propranolol (5 mg/cat orally q 12 hr) preoperatively to decrease the likelihood of rebound tachycardia if hydralazine is needed postoperatively. If the cat is refractory to injectable antihypertensive therapy, administration of the calcium channel blocker amlodipine (0.625 mg/cat orally q 24 hr) should be considered. Cyclosporine monitoring may need to be intensified in this situation because calcium channel blockers also may interfere with cyclosporine metabolism.

The average hospital stay for the recipient is 2 weeks. Cats are discharged when serum creatinine concentrations decrease to normal or nearly normal and the cyclosporine concentrations have reached a plateau so that frequent dose adjustments are unlikely to be necessary. Ultrasonographic examination of the transplanted kidney and ureter is performed to evaluate for evidence of hydronephrosis or hydroureter if ureteral obstruction is suspected based on failure of the serum creatinine concentration to decrease toward normal within the first 3 to 5 days, or due to increasing serum creatinine concentration and decreased urine specific gravity after initial postoperative improvement. If the ultrasound unit has Doppler capability, renal blood flow also is assessed. If evidence of ureteral obstruction is found, the cat is anesthetized and the ureter reimplanted into the urinary bladder. If evidence of ureteral obstruction is not found and renal blood flow is present, a presumptive diagnosis of acute allograft rejection is made, a blood sample is drawn and submitted for determination of cyclosporine concentration, and the cat is started on antirejection therapy.

Antirejection therapy in cats consists of IV cyclosporine (Sandimmune [cyclosporine concentrate for injection], 50 mg/ml, 6.6 mg/kg q 6 hr IV) and prednisolone sodium succinate (Solu-Delta Cortef, Pharmacia and Upjohn Co., Kalamazoo, MI) (10 mg/kg IV q 12 hr). Each milliliter of the IV solution is diluted with 20 to 100 ml of 5 per cent dextrose or 0.9 per cent NaCl (but not lactated Ringer solution). If given rapidly, the patient will vomit. I calculate the cat's fluid requirement of 1.5 to 2 times maintenance in milliliters per hour, multiply by 6 hours to determine the volume of fluids to which the cyclosporine should be added, draw up this volume of fluid in a 60-ml syringe or buretrol, add the cyclosporine, and administer as a constant-rate infusion with a syringe pump or other fluid-delivery system. Once the cyclosporine infusion is complete, the cat is continued on IV fluids as needed. Diagnosis of allograft rejection is considered definitive if serum creatinine concentration returns toward normal after therapy, or if biopsy of the allograft confirms rejection. Antirejection therapy is discontinued and oral prednisolone therapy reinstated when the serum creatinine concentration decreases to normal or prerejection concentration. IV cyclosporine has been given on a daily basis until serum creatinine concentration decreases. A single IV bolus of cyclosporine while waiting for the cyclosporine concentration results, followed by appropriate adjustments in the oral dose to maintain the cyclosporine trough concentration in the therapeutic range may be sufficient. If steroid pulses fail to rescue a failing renal allograft in a human patient, other treatments such as monoclonal antilymphocyte antibody therapy are attempted.[27] Similar rescue protocols have not been evaluated in cats.

Recently, the scintigraphic, sonographic, and histologic changes that occur in the feline kidney after autotransplantation were described.[28] Histologic changes including hemorrhage, necrosis, and inflammation generally were mild. Glomerular filtration rate as measured by ^{99m}Tc pentetate scintigraphy decreased 42 per cent after autotransplantation and still was reduced 23 per cent 28 days after surgery. Renal size increased postoperatively, but consistent changes in the resistive index as calculated from arcuate artery flow velocity were not identified. These ultrasonographic findings were confirmed in another recent study after bilateral nephrectomy and autotransplantation of a single kidney.[29] Similar studies after allotransplantation have been performed on human recipients, and need to be performed on feline recipients to evaluate the utility of these tests in determining the cause and appropriate treatment of renal transplant complications in cats.[30]

◆ LONG-TERM CARE

At discharge, the owners are supplied with both oral and IV cyclosporine (for emergency use) and multiple copies of explicit instructions on home and emergency care. They are asked to give a copy to their regular veterinarian, and to the local after-hours emergency clinic, so that it is readily available if treatment for rejection is required. The closest veterinarian with an ultrasound unit should be identified, so that ultrasonographic examination of the transplanted kidney may be performed as needed. The transplant patient will need to receive cyclosporine and prednisolone twice a day indefinitely. Some transplant units gradually diminish and eliminate the prednisolone. I ask the owners to develop a routine and adhere to it as closely as

possible. Major changes in this schedule, especially missing doses, put the recipient at risk for rejection. If the cat vomits within 1 hour of receiving the medications, redosing is suggested.

During the first several weeks, the recipient's 12-hour trough cyclosporine concentrations are monitored once to twice weekly to ensure that the correct dose is being administered. This monitoring process is diminished gradually if the cat is doing well (stable creatinine and cyclosporine concentrations). Serum creatinine concentration, hematocrit, total solids, and body weight are checked at each visit. Blood collected in EDTA is submitted to the appropriate laboratory for analysis of cyclosporine concentration. The clinician at the transplantation unit then discusses all current laboratory results with the referring veterinarian and owner, so that appropriate dose adjustments and a coordinated treatment plan can be made. The PEG tube is removed after 2 to 4 weeks if the recipient has adjusted to its home situation, is eating well, is adequately hydrated, and the owner is having little difficulty medicating the cat.

The initial target 12-hour trough cyclosporine concentration in feline renal allograft recipients as assayed with high-performance liquid chromatography (HPLC) is approximately 500 ng/ml. Mono- and polyclonal antibody tests also are available for measuring cyclosporine concentrations, and have replaced the more cumbersome, time-consuming HPLC assay at many laboratories. These tests measure both the parent compound and the cyclosporine metabolites, and therefore the target range for cyclosporine concentrations is higher.[10] In our laboratory, a monoclonal whole-blood fluorescent polarization immunoassay (TDx/TDxFLx Cyclosporine Monoclonal Whole Blood Assay, Abbott Laboratories, Abbott Park, IL) has been used and has given results that generally are twice as high as those obtained by HPLC. One study showed that TDx values were approximately 3.5 times higher than those obtained by HPLC in human renal transplant patients, with considerable interindividual variability.[31] Another study recently compared the 2 assays in cats after renal transplantation, and concluded that each cat initially should have both tests performed so that the conversion factor from TDx to HPLC results can be individualized.[32] The authors further recommended re-evaluating cyclosporine concentrations intermittently by both methods.[32]

Acute rejection of the new kidney can occur at any time, but is most common within the first 2 months after surgery. Rejection is the recognition (afferent phase) of foreign feline leukocyte antigens and subsequent destruction of the graft (efferent phase) by humoral and cell-mediated mechanisms, and the activation of cascading enzyme systems (e.g., coagulation). The end result of untreated rejection is graft necrosis. Biopsy of a kidney experiencing rejection will reveal lymphoplasmacytic infiltration of the graft. Cats that are rejecting a kidney often act lethargic and are anorexic, but may look normal with rejection detected only by increasing serum creatinine concentration. Consequently, periodic blood sampling is critical. If the owner believes the cat may be going through a rejection episode, she or he is urged to call the transplantation unit and their veterinarian immediately. Ultrasonographic examination of the kidney is performed as noted previously to look for evidence of ureteral obstruction. If the ultrasound unit has Doppler capabilities, renal blood flow also is assessed. If the ureter does not appear to be obstructed, and there is no evidence of renal torsion or thrombosis, blood samples are drawn and therapy for rejection is instituted as described previously. Waiting for laboratory results may lead to irreversible damage to the kidney. Treatment is modified when the results return.

◆ RESULTS

The morbidity and mortality of the first 66 cats to receive renal allografts at the University of California during the years 1987 to 1996 have been reported.[4] By the following year, an additional 20 cats were transplanted, and the descriptive statistics updated as outlined later. Further updates will certainly follow because more than 100 cats have now been transplanted at U.C. Davis. As of July 1997, 66 (77 per cent) of the first 86 cats that received kidney transplants at U.C. Davis had survived to be discharged from the hospital. The mean age of these cats was 7.8 years (range, 1 to 16 years). Chronic interstitial nephritis (37 cats), ethylene glycol nephrotoxicity (11), and polycystic kidneys (8) were the most common diagnoses.

Of the 20 in-hospital deaths, 7 (35 per cent) were due to seizures or seizure-related complications (see previously). Transient pelvic limb lameness or paresis occurred in 9 of 81 cats (11 per cent), and 1 cat developed hindlimb ischemia requiring amputation when the allograft was anastomosed to the external iliac vessels. Anastomosis directly to the aorta and vena cava has eliminated this postoperative complication as noted previously.

Sixty-five of the 66 discharged cats were available for follow-up. Twenty-seven of 65 (42 per cent) were still alive 1 to 87 months after discharge (mean, 21 months, median, 14 months). Thirty-eight cats had died or were euthanized 1 to 74 months (mean, 13 months; median, 9 months) postoperatively. The 1-year survival rate was 51 per cent. The most common causes of death after discharge from the hospital were recurrence of renal failure caused by allograft dysfunction (15), infectious complications (7), and neoplasia (5) (possibly associated with immunosuppression). Of the 15 cats that died or were euthanized owing to allograft dysfunction, 9 were thought to have experienced allograft rejection, 3 were undiagnosed, 2 cats had allografts that never functioned well and the owners declined a second surgery, and 1 cat developed oxalate nephrosis.[33] There were 21 confirmed episodes of allograft rejection in 17 cats. Ten rejection episodes were confirmed by biopsy of the allograft, and 11 by recovery of serum creatinine concentration after treatment for rejection.

Of the first 86 cats to receive renal transplants at U.C. Davis, 65 were discharged from the hospital and available for follow-up. Nine of these 65 cats (14 per cent) developed neoplasia 2 to 28 months postoperatively (mean, 12 months). The most common neoplasm diagnosed was lymphosarcoma in 4 cats (2 gastric, 1 jejunal, 1 multicentric). After transplantation and associated immunosuppression, human patients are at increased risk for certain types of neoplasia. Decreased immune surveillance, chronic antigenic stimulation from the allograft, and activation of latent oncogenic viruses in some instances may predispose recipients to development of neoplasia. Squamous cell carcinoma is one of the most common forms, especially in countries where recipients are exposed to higher levels of ultraviolet light. In Australia, one report found a 63 per cent probability of developing neoplasia if the recipient survived 20 years posttransplantation.[34] Excluding skin tumors, the 4 to 7 per cent incidence of cancer in human transplant recipients is roughly 100 times greater than that observed in age-matched controls.[35, 36] Of nonskin malignancies, lymphoma, genitourinary, and gastrointestinal neoplasia are among the most common forms. The high (14 per cent) frequency of neoplasia in the cats described previously seems to indicate an increased risk of neoplasia in feline transplant recipients as well. Further study, including comparisons to age-matched controls, is needed.

◆ CONCLUSION

Renal transplantation is a viable alternative for cats in renal failure that have failed, or are beginning to fail, conventional medical management. The owners must be made aware of the morbidity and mortality associated with this procedure, as well as the cost, and the need for daily home nursing care for the remainder of their pet's life. Ongoing research into the causes of posttransplantation complications has resulted in a decrease in morbidity and an increase in postoperative survival times. Further research on preoperative management, postoperative monitoring, and detection and treatment of allograft rejection likely will result in further improvements.

REFERENCES

1. Carrel A: Transplantation in mass of the kidneys. J Exp Med 10:98–140, 1908.
2. Gregory CR, Gourley IM, Taylor NJ, et al: Preliminary results of clinical renal allograft transplantation in the dog and cat. J Vet Intern Med 1:53–60, 1987.
3. Gregory CR, Gourley IM, Kochin EJ, et al: Renal transplantation for treatment of end-stage renal failure in cats. J Am Vet Med Assoc 201:285–291, 1992.
4. Mathews KG, Gregory CR: Renal transplants in cats: 66 cases (1987–1996). J Am Vet Med Assoc 211:1432–1436, 1997.

5. Harris CL, Krawiec DR: The pathophysiology of uremic bleeding. Compend Cont Educ Pract Vet 12:1294–1298, 1990.
6. Krawiec DR, Gelberg HB: Chronic renal disease in cats. *In* Kirk RW (ed): Current Veterinary Therapy X. Philadelphia, WB Saunders, 1989, pp. 1170–1173.
7. Kobayashi DL, Peterson ME, Graves TK, et al: Hypertension in cats with chronic renal failure or hyperthyroidism. J Vet Intern Med 4:58–62, 1990.
8. Graves TK: Hyperthyroidism and the kidney. *In* August JR (ed): Consultations in Feline Internal Medicine, Vol. 3. Philadelphia, WB Saunders, 1997, pp. 345–348.
9. Bernsteen L, Gregory CR, Aronson LR, et al: Acute toxoplasmosis following renal transplantation in 3 cats and a dog. J Am Vet Med Assoc 215:1123–1126, 1999.
10. Vaden SL: Cyclosporine and tacrolimus. Semin Vet Med Surg Small Anim 12:161–166, 1997.
11. Morris PJ: Cyclosporine. *In* Morris PJ (ed): Kidney Transplantation: Principles and Practice, 4th ed. Philadelphia, WB Saunders, 1994, pp. 179–201.
12. Watkins PB: The role of cytochromes P-450 in cyclosporine metabolism. J Am Acad Dermatol 23:1301–1309, 1990.
13. Gomez DY, Wacher VJ, Tomlanovich SJ, et al: The effects of ketoconazole on the intestinal metabolism and bioavailability of cyclosporine. Clin Pharmacol Ther 58:15–19, 1995.
14. Baciewicz AM, Baciewicz FA: Cyclosporine pharmacokinetic drug interactions. Am J Surg 157:264–271, 1989.
15. McAnulty JF, Lensmeyer GL: The effects of ketoconazole on the pharmacokinetics of cyclosporine A in cats. Vet Surg 28:448–455, 1999.
16. Lirtzman RA, Gregory CR: Long-term renal and hematologic effects of uninephrectomy in healthy feline kidney donors. J Am Vet Med Assoc 207:1044–1047, 1995.
17. Polzin DJ, Osborne CA, Adams LG, et al: Medical management of feline chronic renal failure. *In* Kirk RW (ed): Current Veterinary Therapy XI. Philadelphia, WB Saunders, 1992, pp. 848–853.
18. Bernsteen L, Gregory CR, Pollard RE, et al: Comparison of two surgical techniques for renal transplantation in cats. Vet Surg 28:417–420, 1999.
19. McAnulty JF: Hypothermic storage of feline kidneys for transplantation: Successful ex vivo storage up to 7 hours. Vet Surg 27:312–320, 1998.
20. Gregory CR, Lirtzman RA, Kochin EJ, et al: A mucosal apposition technique for ureteroneocystostomy after renal transplantation in cats. Vet Surg 25:13–17, 1996.
21. Goldstein RE, Marks SL, Kass PH, et al: Gastrin concentrations in plasma of cats with chronic renal failure. J Am Vet Med Assoc 213:826–828, 1998.
22. Whittier FC, Evans DH, Dutton S, et al: Nutrition in renal transplantation. Am J Kidney Dis 6:405–411, 1985.
23. D'Souza MJ, Pollock SH, Solomon HM: Cyclosporine-cimetidine interaction. Drug Metab Dispos 16:57–59, 1988.
24. Gregory CR, Mathews KG, Aronson LR, et al: Central nervous system disorders after renal transplantation in cats. Vet Surg 26:386–392, 1997.
25. Kyles AE, Gregory CR, Wooldridge JD, et al: Management of hypertension controls postoperative neurologic disorders after renal transplantation in cats. Vet Surg 28:436–441, 1999.
26. Caulkett NA, Cantwell SL, Houston DM: A comparison of indirect blood pressure monitoring techniques in the anesthetized cat. Vet Surg 27:370–377, 1998.
27. Powelson JA, Cosimi AB: Antilymphocyte globulin and monoclonal antibodies. *In* Morris PJ (ed): Kidney Transplantation: Principles and Practice, 4th ed. Philadelphia, WB Saunders, 1994, pp. 215–232.
28. Newell SM, Ellison GW, Graham JP, et al: Scintigraphic, sonographic, and histologic evaluation of renal autotransplantation in cats. Am J Vet Res 60:775–779, 1999.
29. Pollard R, Nyland TG, Bernsteen L, et al: Ultrasonographic evaluation of renal autografts in normal cats. Vet Radiol Ultrasound 40:380–385, 1999.
30. Delaney V, Ling BN, Campbell WG: Comparison of fine-needle aspiration biopsy, Doppler ultrasound, and radionuclide scintigraphy in the diagnosis of acute allograft dysfunction in renal transplant recipients: Sensitivity, specificity, and cost analysis. Nephron 63:263–272, 1993.
31. Schroeder TJ, Brunson ME, Pesce AJ, et al: A comparison of the clinical utility of the radioimmunoassay, high-performance liquid chromatography, and TDx cyclosporine assays in outpatient renal transplant recipients. Transplantation 47:262–266, 1989.
32. McAnulty JF, Lensmeyer GL: Comparison of high performance liquid chromatography for measurement of cyclosporine A blood concentrations after feline kidney transplantation. Vet Surg 27:589–595, 1998.
33. Gregory CR, Olander HJ, Kochin EJ, et al: Oxalate nephrosis and renal sclerosis after renal transplantation in a cat. Vet Surg 22:221–224, 1993.
34. Sheil AGR: *In* Disney APS (ed): XIV Report of the Australia and New Zealand Combined Dialysis and Transplant Registry. Woodville, Australia, The Queen Elizabeth Hospital, 1991, p. 100.
35. Sheil AGR: Cancer in dialysis and transplant patients. *In* Morris PJ (ed): Kidney Transplantation: Principles and Practice, 4th ed. Philadelphia, WB Saunders, 1994, pp. 390–400.
36. Penn I: Incidence of malignancies in transplant recipients. Transplant Proc 7:323–326, 1975.

44

◆ Medical Management of Chronic Renal Failure

Katherine M. James

◆ SELECTED DIAGNOSTIC CONSIDERATIONS

Early detection of chronic renal failure (CRF) in cats improves the chance for long-term survival because feline CRF often is slowly progressive. One tool for early diagnosis is to recommend annual urine specific gravity (USG) checks for all cats. Normal cats have concentrated urine (>1.040). A cat with a USG less than 1.040 should be considered suspect. If USG is less than 1.040, urinalysis, serum biochemistry, and (for older cats) serum thyroxine concentration are indicated. Another early detection tool is to record weights at all visits. Weight loss often is the first and only sign of CRF in cats. Many cats with CRF have normal kidney size on abdominal palpation.

When interpreting laboratory data, remember that certain results within the reference range or at the upper or lower limits of normal are diagnostically interesting. The clinician should understand the physiologic basis of the laboratory tests performed and not merely the normal range of expected values. For example, serum creatinine concentration depends on muscle mass and testosterone-induced tubular secretion. A serum creatinine concentration of 2.0 mg/dl may be within a laboratory's normal range and be normal for a young cat, but may reflect mild azotemia in a geriatric cat. It also is important to know which tests are subject to in vitro errors. For example, serum total carbon dioxide (TCO_2) may be falsely low, suggesting acidosis, if the sample is not maintained anaerobically. It also is critical to note trends. For example, a packed cell volume (PCV) of 30 per cent may be within the normal range, but in a cat that has had a stable PCV of 35 per cent for the preceding year, it may represent anemia.

When azotemia is identified, the first step in the diagnostic process is to localize it as prerenal, primary renal, or postrenal. In distinguishing prerenal from primary renal azotemia in cats, USG values between 1.006 and 1.030 suggest primary renal disease unless other causes of reduced urine concentrating ability (e.g., hyperthyroidism, diabetes mellitus) are present. Primary renal azotemia also is probable, but not certain, when the USG is between 1.030 and 1.040. When azotemia is of prerenal origin, a USG of greater than 1.040 is expected. Although oliguria is expected in most cases of postrenal azotemia, it is important to rule out ureteral obstruction superimposed on chronic renal disease. Postrenal azotemia potentially is reversible, and abdominal ultrasonography to rule out ureteral ob-

struction should be considered for all cats experiencing a uremic crisis. The differentiation between acute renal failure and CRF is based largely on historical (e.g., chronic weight loss, polyuria, polydipsia, reduced appetite), physical (poor body condition, reduced kidney size, renal osteodystrophy), and laboratory (nonregenerative anemia) findings indicative of chronic disease.

The diagnostic evaluation of cats suspected of having CRF includes a complete blood count, serum chemistry panel, and urinalysis. A serum thyroxine concentration is included for older cats. The USG should be determined, whenever possible, before fluid therapy. Even if the patient remains dehydrated after intravenous fluids have been given, the USG loses its diagnostic validity. After CRF has been confirmed, the problem-specific database should include blood pressure, fundic examination, abdominal radiographs, and urine culture. Abdominal ultrasonography also may be helpful, and is indicated especially whenever unilateral or bilateral renomegaly is present. If the cat was clinically ill and dehydrated at the time of initial diagnosis, new baseline data for renal function tests and electrolyte concentrations should be obtained after rehydration and diuresis to better formulate the treatment plan for at-home care.

◆ MONITORING

The management of CRF should be viewed from the outset as an ongoing endeavor. The first step in formulating a monitoring plan individualized for each patient is to determine the level of commitment of the owner. Never make assumptions about the level of nursing care a particular owner is willing to do at home. Include in the discussion the impact of veterinary visits and medications on the cat's quality of life and the costs of the monitoring and supplies for the owner. A successful CRF management plan is customized for each owner and patient.

When blood is drawn for the purpose of monitoring, the minimum volume of blood that is needed should be taken, especially if sampling is being done frequently. CRF cats have diminished red blood cell regenerative capacity, and sampling can contribute to iron deficiency and anemia. I routinely monitor and chart blood urea nitrogen (BUN), creatinine, BUN:creatinine ratio, sodium, potassium, TCO_2, phosphorus, ionized calcium, PCV, and total solids. Also at each recheck visit, the systolic blood

Table 44–1. Topics to Cover in Client Education in Chronic Renal Failure

Nature of CRF

CRF is an irreversible and progressive disease. The treatment plan is designed to both delay progression and mitigate the consequences of failing kidneys.

Cats with CRF are less tolerant of other illnesses because they are prone to dehydration. Most problems that arise require prompt attention.

Resources

Written owner education handouts about medications, side-effects, and how to administer subcutaneous fluids should be provided.

Although online resources can be very valuable, it is important to be a smart user of the Internet. There is no online substitute for a good doctor-owner-patient relationship. (*The Feline Chronic Renal Failure Information Center*—http://www.best.com/~lynxpt/)

Interested owners should be provided with copies of laboratory data and flow sheets. A discussion should include which values are being monitored and the target values.

Fluid Therapy

Demonstrate how to administer fluids and where on the body they may be given.

Suggest the owner try multiple sizes of needles because different cats prefer different sizes. Mention that some cats prefer to have the fluids warmed before administration.

The owner should try to associate the administration of fluids with something the cat enjoys.

Medications

Specify clearly which medications may be given at the same time (including together in the same gel capsule) and which should be given at separate times.

Specify which medications should be given in or with food and which can be compounded differently (such as into a flavored liquid).

For some patients that are particularly difficult to medicate orally, offer parenteral options. Many owners giving subcutaneous fluids prefer this option.

Diet

Have available all CRF foods that you believe are of good quality. Give owners as many options as possible.

Emphasize that gradual changes are acceptable for cats that resist dietary intervention.

Explain which foods are best if the owner needs to "cheat" to get the cat to eat enough.

Know something of the ingredients and nutrient profiles of the special diets you recommend. Many owners read pet food labels and will ask for explanations.

Common Complications

Constipation is common in older cats, and may be a sign of dehydration.

Cats with CRF produce large volumes of diluted urine and often need several litter boxes to prevent house-soiling accidents.

Intensive support measures such as feeding tubes and renal transplantation should be discussed long before these decisions must be made.

Abbreviation: CRF, chronic renal failure.

pressure should be determined and a fundic examination performed. Serum iron and ferritin determinations are recommended in CRF patients with anemia or a history of blood loss, or in those cats for which erythropoietin (EPO) therapy is contemplated. Serum parathyroid hormone (PTH) concentrations may be determined occasionally for monitoring patients on calcitriol therapy. Urine cultures should be performed intermittently even if clinical signs of lower urinary tract disease are absent. Although hematuria, pyuria, bacteriuria, and clinical signs of lower urinary tract disease prompt evaluation for urinary tract infection, none of these findings is pathognomonic for bacterial infection. Urine cultures should be performed to verify urinary tract infection when any of these signs are present.

Feline CRF is a chronic disease, and can be very stressful to owners. Nevertheless, the owner performs most of the treatments and is a critical member of the "medical team." A comprehensive approach to owner education is essential for CRF management (Table 44–1).

◆ MINIMIZING AZOTEMIA

The BUN concentration is a useful surrogate marker for the uremic toxins that cause CRF patients to feel ill. Most cats with CRF generally behave as if they feel well when the BUN is less than 60 mg/dl, al-

though this varies somewhat from patient to patient. When the BUN concentration is higher than 100 mg/dl, more severe clinical signs of CRF, including anorexia, vomiting, and uremic gastritis, occur with increased frequency. The observation that a lower BUN concentration seems to correlate with a patient that feels well and lacks systemic signs of illness is one of the reasons for recommending protein-restricted diets. It is generally believed that products of protein metabolism are clinically important uremic toxins.

Recently, the use of indigestible carbohydrates (e.g., nonfermentable fiber, fermentable fiber, fermentable oligosaccharides) has been advocated to increase intestinal clearance of urea and guanidino compounds. The use of lactulose (a nonabsorbed disaccharide) for this purpose has shown some promise in clinical trials in human beings with pre-dialysis CRF, but the side-effect of diarrhea precluded its use in many patients.[1, 2] The rationale for using lactulose is that with low-fiber diets, colonic bacteria ordinarily use unabsorbed proteins from the small intestine (including endogenous proteins such as trypsin, amylase, lipase, and proteins from sloughed epithelial cells) to sustain their growth. When increased indigestible carbohydrates are present to stimulate growth of colonic bacteria, those sources of nitrogen may be insufficient, and blood urea and other nitrogenous substances become an important, readily available source of nitrogen to sustain rapid bacterial growth. Thus, increases in indigestible carbohydrates in the diet result in urea transfer to the gut and its incorporation into bacterial proteins.[3] Whether lactulose or other indigestible fibers can be used in cats at dosages sufficient to lower serum concentrations of urea and other nitrogenous compounds, without causing side-effects, is unknown.

Achieving the best possible BUN:creatinine ratio is an important therapeutic goal. A BUN:creatinine ratio of no more than 10 to 15 is a desirable goal for patients on protein-restricted diets, especially when the cat is on subcutaneous fluid therapy. Charting the patient's BUN:creatinine ratio over the course of therapy allows changes to be recognized, which can signal a correctable problem (e.g., dehydration, gastrointestinal bleeding, loss of dietary compliance).

◆ MAINTAINING ADEQUATE TOTAL-BODY POTASSIUM

Cats with CRF are prone to the development of hypokalemia. I try to maintain serum potassium concentration in the upper half of the laboratory normal range because serum potassium concentration may be preserved when total-body potassium is low. Factors that may promote hypokalemia should be identified and eliminated. Such dietary factors include diets with high protein or acid content or low potassium or magnesium content. Other factors that may contribute to hypokalemia include muscle wasting, overzealous use of subcutaneous fluids, or use of drugs that promote kaliuresis, such as furosemide and glucocorticoids.

Dietary modification alone may be sufficient to increase serum potassium concentration to the upper half of the normal range in cats that do not have overt hypokalemia. Patients with overt hypokalemia, or those in which dietary modification alone is inadequate, should receive potassium supplementation. Cats undergoing intravenous fluid diuresis for a uremic crisis should have their fluids supplemented with potassium, and such cats should be monitored closely. Oral administration is preferred for supplementation in cats with stable CRF. Parenteral therapy with subcutaneous fluids is reserved for cats that cannot or will not accept oral therapy. Potassium may be administered orally as potassium gluconate in tablet, gel, or powder form and placed in food (Tumil-K, JPI-Jones Animal Health, Inc.). When concurrent acidosis is present ($TCO_2 < 17$ mEq/liter), potassium citrate solution or tablets (Polycitra-K, Baker Norton Pharmaceuticals, Inc.; Urocit-K, Mission Pharmacol Co.) are preferred because of the alkalinizing action of citrate. Potassium chloride generally should be avoided because it is not palatable and may promote acidosis. Depending on the size of the cat and severity of the hypokalemia, starting doses of potassium are between 2 and 4 mEq per cat per day divided into 2 or 3 doses. Dosage thereafter should be adjusted based on serum potassium concentration. Most cats require continued therapy at a dosage of 1 to 4 mEq/day to maintain serum potassium concentration in the upper half of the normal range. Hyperkalemia is an uncommon consequence of even advanced CRF in cats. In most cases, it is iatrogenic and associated with overzealous potassium supplementation or the use of angiotensin-converting enzyme inhibitors.

◆ MAINTAINING OPTIMUM CALCIUM AND PHOSPHORUS BALANCE

Prevention of hyperphosphatemia can retard the progression of CRF in many species, including cats.[4, 5] Hyperphosphatemia leads to hyperparathyroidism, which then leads to deposition of calcium salts in the kidney (i.e., nephrocalcinosis). PTH increases calcium channel activity and intracellular calcium content, which in turn is thought to promote nephrocalcinosis. Thus, dietary phosphate restriction has been a mainstay of CRF therapy for many years. In general, dietary phosphorus restriction has been achieved with the same diets that restrict dietary protein. Now that dietary protein restriction is not being advocated as early in the course of CRF, adequate control of serum phosphorus concentration may require earlier use of intestinal phosphorus binders. Aluminum-based phosphate binders are not used routinely in human beings on dialysis because of concern about aluminum accumulation in tissues. This complication has not been demonstrated in cats; thus, aluminum-containing phosphate binders are used more commonly than calcium-containing agents, because of the risk of hypercalcemia with the latter compounds. Intestinal phosphorus-binding agents of either type should be administered with food when possible. In acutely ill animals that are not eating, aluminum-containing intestinal phosphorus binders still can be advantageous in lowering serum phosphorus concentration by binding phosphorus in saliva, intestinal juices, and bile. Calcium-containing formulations should be given only with food to minimize the risk of hypercalcemia.

I prefer aluminum carbonate (Basalgel, Wyeth) because the capsules can be opened and the powder hidden in food, usually without a marked effect on palatability. Most cats require 125 to 250 mg per day divided into multiple feedings. Aluminum hydroxide, available as a liquid or tablet, is another option. Calcium carbonate (90 to 150 mg/kg/day) or calcium acetate (60 to 90 mg/kg/day) may be used in cats in which serum calcium concentration is monitored routinely. For all intestinal phosphorus binders, dosages should be adjusted with the goal of keeping serum phosphorus concentration at approximately 4 mg/dl. One potential side-effect of intestinal phosphorus binders is constipation. In general, the addition of a stool-softening agent such as lactulose will correct the problem for most patients, and the phosphorus-binding agent need not be discontinued.

Calcitriol synthesis is decreased in CRF owing to nephron loss and decreased 1α-hydroxylase enzyme activity, and also is inhibited by increased phosphorus concentration. In CRF, especially when hyperphosphatemia is present, calcitriol concentrations are low and insufficient to stimulate adequate intestinal calcium absorption. This effect leads to hypocalcemia, which further stimulates PTH production in an attempt to return serum calcium concentration to normal. Supplementation with calcitriol will interrupt this cycle and mitigate secondary renal hyperparathyroidism. In addition to inhibiting the development of nephrocalcinosis, calcitriol also may inhibit the development of glomerulosclerosis, and thereby delay progression of renal disease.[6] No randomized clinical trials of calcitriol therapy have been reported in naturally occurring CRF in dogs or cats. My own clinical experience and that of others suggest that calcitriol therapy improves quality of life and can slow progression of renal failure in these patients.[7] However, patient selection for calcitriol therapy is very important. Calcitriol should be used only in those patients being followed closely and in those with serum phosphorus concentrations consistently less than 6 mg/dl (preferably near 4 mg/dl). Calcitriol is a very potent agent and may cause hypercalcemia. When serum phosphorus concentration also is high, nephrocalcinosis can occur with devastating and potentially irreversible effects on the kidney. The recommended therapeutic dosage for calcitriol is 2.5 to 3.5 ng/kg/day.[7, 8] Currently, I recommend calcitriol therapy in appropriate patients as soon as CRF is detected. Preferably, patients receiving calcitriol should be monitored by measuring serum ionized calcium concentration rather than serum total calcium concentration whenever possible. Patients initially are monitored once every 1 to 2 weeks, and this interval is increased if serum calcium and phosphorus concentrations are stable and within normal limits.

◆ TREATING METABOLIC ACIDOSIS

The prevalence of metabolic acidosis in cats with CRF is unknown and may be affected by trends in the acidification of commercial maintenance diets for cats. In one retrospective case series, approximately 80 per cent of cats with CRF had metabolic acidosis based on venous blood pH and bicarbonate concentrations.[9] Urine pH is an insensitive predictor of acidosis. Acidosis should be monitored with serum TCO_2 concentration. This test has been removed from the chemistry panel at some laboratories because it is prone to in vitro errors. When blood collection tubes are not fully filled or are left exposed to air while awaiting analysis, the vacuum or air above the tube will draw carbon dioxide out of the serum. This falsely lowers the measured concentrations, and may result in the incorrect conclusion that the patient has metabolic acidosis.[10] Acidosis appears to be common in cats with CRF, and it is important that TCO_2 concentration, like ionized calcium concentration, be included on the chemistry panel of cats with CRF.

Although they are not well studied, the consequences of chronic metabolic acidosis in cats with CRF may include negative calcium balance and bone demineralization, negative potassium balance and hypokalemia, taurine depletion, protein malnutrition, and possibly progression of CRF.[11] Correction of even mild metabolic acidosis is important for CRF cats, especially those on protein-restricted diets. When acid-base status is normal, adaptive reductions in skeletal muscle protein degradation protect patients on low-protein diets from losses in lean body mass. When even mild acidosis is present in human beings and rats, these adaptive responses are overridden and lean body mass declines. Based on my own clinical observations in feline patients with CRF, correction of acidosis may be more effective than the addition of anabolic steroids for the maintenance of lean body mass in cats with CRF.

Depending on the laboratory, serum TCO_2 concentrations less than or equal to 17 mEq/liter are an indication for alkalinization therapy. Oral sodium bicarbonate has been the most commonly used alkalinizing agent, but it does not appear to be well absorbed or palatable when used by this route. Cats with CRF are prone to potassium depletion, and potassium citrate is the preferred oral alkali replacement therapy except for patients with hyperkalemia. A starting dosage of 0.3 to 0.5 mEq/kg every [q] 12 hr is recommended. The dosage of potassium citrate is adjusted to maintain serum TCO_2 concentration between 18 and 22 mEq/liter. Doses of potassium citrate that correct hypokalemia may exceed the citrate dose required to correct acidosis.

◆ PREVENTING AND TREATING ANEMIA

Progressive, hypoproliferative, normocytic, normochromic anemia is common in cats with advanced CRF. Many of the clinical signs of moderate-to-advanced CRF may be attributed in part to anemia. Such signs include fatigue, lethargy, weakness, lack of interest in social interactions, inappetence, and weight loss.[12] Although the EPO deficiency that accompanies CRF is the primary cause of anemia, there may be many contributory factors that when eliminated will delay the development of clinically significant anemia until the advanced stages of CRF (Table 44-2).

The development of an assay for serum ferritin concentration in cats will improve the ability to distinguish true iron deficiency from other causes of low serum iron concentration. This test also will improve our understanding of the prevalence of iron deficiency in cats with CRF. Iron deficiency is

Table 44–2. Management of Anemia in Chronic Renal Failure

Factors That Contribute to Anemia in Chronic Renal Failure	Therapy
Decreased erythropoietin production owing to reduced renal mass	Human recombinant erythropoietin, anabolic steroids
Decreased red blood cell life span	Control secondary renal hyperparathyroidism
Uremic inhibitors of erythropoiesis	Control secondary renal hyperparathyroidism and azotemia
Extrarenal blood loss	
Uremic gastritis	Control azotemia, H_2 blockers
Blood sampling	Avoid excessive sampling
Nutritional deficiencies	
B vitamins	Supplement, especially during diuresis
Iron	Supplement
Calorie malnutrition	Improve intake, avoid excessive restriction of protein
Marrow fibrosis	None; end-stage lesion

Adapted from James K: Feline non-regenerative anemias—Diagnostic approach and treatment. Proceedings 17th Annual Veterinary Medical Forum, American College of Veterinary Internal Medicine, Chicago, June 10–13, 1999, pp. 545–547.

thought to be relatively common, affecting approximately 25 per cent of cats with CRF (James KM, unpublished observations). The cause of iron deficiency in CRF is unknown, but chronic blood loss (e.g., uremic gastritis, repeated blood sampling) probably is important. I routinely supplement feline CRF patients with oral iron in the hope of preventing iron deficiency. Orally administered iron can irritate the gastrointestinal tract, and very low dose supplementation is used (ferrous sulfate 1 mg/cat/day). For cats with documented mild iron deficiency, and for which EPO therapy is not yet indicated, higher dosages of iron are used (ferrous sulfate 10 to 15 mg/cat/day). In cats with severe iron deficiency, iron initially is administered parenterally (iron dextran, 50 mg/cat intramuscularly [IM]). Iron-deficient patients that do not tolerate oral iron supplementation or those that are beginning EPO therapy also may require parenteral therapy. Such patients should be started simultaneously on low-dose oral iron supplementation.

Because it is difficult to detect, chronic gastrointestinal blood loss probably is an underrecognized contributor to anemia in CRF. In some cases, a higher BUN:creatinine ratio than expected for a given diet can alert the clinician to the possibility of gastrointestinal bleeding. As discussed previously in the section on anorexia and vomiting, cats with serum creatinine concentrations greater than 3.0 mg/dl can be assumed to be at risk for hypergastrinemia and uremic gastritis.[8, 13] H_2-receptor antagonist therapy routinely is recommended for such patients to prevent nausea, vomiting, and gastrointestinal blood loss.

The peripheral blood smears of CRF cats should be evaluated for the presence of Heinz bodies. When Heinz bodies are present, an evaluation for oxidant compounds in the diet should be initiated. Anemia of chronic inflammatory disease is perhaps the contributor to anemia in CRF that is most difficult to identify, localize, and correct. A low serum iron concentration without low serum ferritin concentration may be present. A persistent, unexplained neutrophilia also may be observed. Such patients often require diagnostic re-evaluation to identify the site of inflammation or infection. The use of antibiotics without localizing and verifying infection is discouraged.

EPO therapy should be considered when all other potential causes of anemia have been corrected, and the anemia remains severe enough to impact quality of life negatively. Such cats are expected to have serum creatinine concentrations greater than 5 mg/dl. At present, only recombinant human erythropoietin (rHuEPO) is available for clinical patients. Therapy is delayed for most cats until the PCV is between 12 and 19 per cent because of the problem with anti-rHuEPO antibodies. The initial starting dosage of rHuEPO is 50 to 150 units/kg 3 times weekly. The PCV is monitored weekly until a target PCV of 30 to 35 per cent is achieved. Downward adjustments in the dosage should be made to avoid overshooting the target if correction of the anemia is made in less than 2 months. To avoid potentiating hypertension, initial daily therapy is considered only for those patients with severe anemia (PCV < 15 per cent). Once the target PCV is reached, maintenance dosages of 50 U/kg 2 to 3 times weekly will be sufficient for most patients, but there is considerable variation among patients. Animals on maintenance therapy should have their PCV monitored monthly initially, and eventually no less frequently than every 2 months to allow for dosage adjustments. The prevalence of anti-rHuEPO antibody induction is approximately 33 per cent of cats during the first 5 months of treatment.[14] No commercial test for anti-EPO antibodies is available. There is no evidence to suggest that intermittent dosing (i.e., treating with rHuEPO until anemia is corrected and then discontinuing the drug until anemia recurs) lessens the risk of antibody development. Another alternative management technique is to correct the anemia with rHuEPO, and then attempt to maintain the PCV with the use of anabolic steroids. I have not evaluated this approach owing to the side-effects of anabolic steroids and the advanced nature of the renal failure in cats requiring rHuEPO to correct their anemia. Canine recombinant EPO may be available for evaluation in cats in the future.

◆ MANAGING APPETITE AND GASTROINTESTINAL COMPLICATIONS

Although decreased appetite and vomiting are common consequences of uremia, they are amenable to therapy, and are rare in stable, well-managed CRF cats. Appetite stimulants (e.g., cyproheptadine, diazepam, progesterone, anabolic steroids) rarely are needed. I have not used any of these compounds in the management of CRF in cats in several years. Cats with serum creatinine concentrations less than 5 to 6 mg/dl should not experience nausea and are expected to eat, provided all the contributory factors presented in Table 44–3 are addressed. Debilitated cats with severe CRF or those being considered for transplantation will benefit most from placement of an esophageal or gastric feeding tube so that adequate nutrition can be provided. The best approach when confronted with the anorexic CRF patient is to systematically evaluate and address all factors that contribute to anorexia (see Table 44–3).

The possibility of uremic gastritis should be considered whenever anorexia or vomiting is present. Of human CRF patients on dialysis, approximately 50 per cent have endoscopically detectable gastritis and 17 per cent have overt gastrointestinal bleeding.[15] Famotidine is the preferred H_2-receptor antagonist for cats with CRF. The precise dosage of famotidine for cats with CRF is not known because it is largely eliminated unchanged by renal excretion. Its renal elimination in human beings decreases proportionally with creatinine clearance.[16] In human beings, the dosage is decreased by 50 per cent in moderate renal failure and by 75 per cent in severe renal failure. I currently use a starting dose of 2.5

mg/cat q 48 hr for most feline CRF patients. When antiemetics are needed in more advanced CRF, metoclopramide may be used, but it decreases the oral bioavailability of H_2-receptor antagonists, and oral administration of these medications should be separated by at least 1 hour (Mandelker L, personal communication). Cats with stable, well-controlled CRF that have persistent vomiting should be evaluated for other causes of their persistent gastrointestinal signs.

Constipation is not an uncommon complication of CRF in older cats, and it probably is multifactorial. Common contributing factors include dehydration, intestinal phosphorus-binding agents, inadequate dietary fiber, decreased gastrointestinal motility due to uremia, and megacolon. The onset of constipation may herald the need for subcutaneous fluid therapy in some cats. Many constipated CRF cats seem to benefit from supplemental lactulose. Cisapride is of benefit in megacolon, and dosage adjustment is not required for moderate renal failure.[17]

◆ MAINTAINING HYDRATION STATUS

Supplemental fluid therapy, usually given subcutaneously, is used to prevent dehydration in cats that have insufficient fluid intake from food and water to keep up with urinary losses. A common misconception is that ongoing subcutaneous fluid therapy is used in CRF to promote diuresis, but this is not correct. Diuresis is not, in a long-term sense, a substitute for dialysis. Diuresis improves renal function tests acutely because it augments the glomerular filtration rate (GFR). There is some evidence to suggest that when this is done chronically, it promotes progression of CRF. Artificially augmented GFR for a given degree of renal disease makes the kidney work harder because more energy is expended reabsorbing sodium.[18] Diuresis also increases single-nephron GFR and promotes glomerular hyperfiltration, which may promote progression. Short-term diuresis lowers uremic toxin concentrations in the blood and improves the patient's clinical status during acute decompensation. Chronic subcutaneous fluid therapy is aimed solely at prevention of chronic dehydration. How much fluid to give in any given patient is at best an educated guess. I typically use 100 ml of lactated Ringer's solution per day. Very large cats, or those with advanced disease, may require higher volumes. So as not to induce marked fluctuations in fluid intake from day to day, daily dosing regimens are preferred to every other day whenever the owner's schedule permits daily treatment. The subcutaneous route generally is safe and forgiving for fluid administration, but sodium and fluid overload are possible in patients with cardiac disease. Lactated Ringer's solution is preferred for chronic fluid therapy in CRF because of the added buffer and the potentially adverse effect of 0.9 per

Table 44–3. Factors Contributing to Decreased Appetite and Weight Loss in Cats With Chronic Renal Failure

Factors That Contribute to Anorexia in Chronic Renal Failure	Therapy
Uremic gastritis and associated nausea	Manage azotemia, H_2-receptor antagonists
Uremic toxins—effect on chemoreceptor trigger zone	Administer metoclopramide
Dehydration	Supplement fluids
Drug-associated anorexia and nausea	Avoid unnecessary medications
	Avoid empirical use of antibiotics
Anemia	Address all contributing factors (see Table 44–2)
Impaired taste and smell	Use fresh, warm food
Hypokalemia	Supplement potassium
Hyperparathyroidism	Control hyperphosphatemia; calcitriol
Acidosis	Institute alkalinization therapy
Food-associated factors	
Palatability	Provide numerous diet choices
Force-feeding	Employ a feeding tube
Food aversion	Do not feed therapeutic diets when patient is hospitalized for uremic crisis
Stomatitis	Manage azotemia; topical treatment; sucralfate suspension
B vitamin deficiency	Supplement B vitamins

cent NaCl on hypertension. Hypernatremia is an uncommon consequence of chronic isotonic fluid administration, but serum sodium concentration should be monitored in cats on chronic subcutaneous fluid therapy. The sodium content of lactated Ringer's solution may be too high for patients with hypertension or those prone to congestive heart failure.

For cats that are intolerant of oral alkalinizing agents, acidosis may be treated by adding sodium bicarbonate to the fluids. Lactated Ringer's solution and sodium bicarbonate are incompatible at concentrations of bicarbonate above 40 mEq/liter. Concentrations of 4 to 8 mEq/liter do not appear to cause precipitation. At concentrations between 8 and 40 mEq/liter, the risk of formation of insoluble precipitates exists and probably is dependent on temperature. Because of this concern, I supplement subcutaneous fluids with bicarbonate only at concentrations below 8 mEq/liter and only for patients intolerant of oral alkalinization. I generally start with doses of 0.5 to 1 mEq/day. Potassium also can be included in the fluid prescription for those cats intolerant of oral supplementation. Parenteral potassium supplementation should be implemented conservatively because of the risk of hyperkalemia. I do not exceed a dose of 10 mEq/liter of potassium in subcutaneous fluids for patients with CRF unless serum potassium concentration is monitored carefully.

◆ MANAGING ARTERIAL HYPERTENSION

Estimates of the prevalence of systemic hypertension in cats with CRF vary, ranging from 29 to 69 per cent.[11, 19-21] A recent study in which a systolic arterial blood pressure of greater than 175 mm Hg was used to define hypertension showed a prevalence of 29 per cent.[21] Other investigators have used an upper limit of 160 mm Hg to define hypertension.[11, 20]

Little is known about the long-term consequences of untreated arterial hypertension in cats, and specifically in cats with CRF. Numerous complications of untreated hypertension have been reported in cats in addition to ocular abnormalities (e.g., retinal hemorrhage, retinal detachment). These include left ventricular hypertrophy and dysfunction, ventricular arrhythmias, thromboembolic disease, seizures, and ataxia.[22] Although the incidence of these complications is unknown and the impact of untreated hypertension on the progression of renal disease is difficult to quantify, the common occurrence of devastating ocular complications suggests that treatment of hypertension is warranted.

Management of systemic hypertension is complicated by difficulties in monitoring blood pressure in cats (see Chapters 36, Systemic Hypertension, and 47, Diagnosis and Treatment of Systemic Hypertension). Although Doppler units are relatively easy to use, it is difficult to assess the contribution of visit-associated stress. Most cats adapt to having their blood pressure taken, and I do most blood pressure determinations in the examination room as part of the physical examination, with the owner as an assistant. Consistency of cuff size and placement is important, as is following trends from visit to visit. I institute therapy when systolic pressure is greater than 200 mm Hg, or reproducibly greater than 160 mm Hg, or when compatible ocular signs (reduced pupillary light reflexes, papilledema, retinal arterial tortuosity, retinal hemorrhage, retinal detachment, hyphema, uveitis, glaucoma) are present.

Vasodilators, specifically calcium channel antagonists and angiotensin-converting enzyme (ACE) inhibitors, have become the mainstays of antihypertensive therapy in cats with CRF (see Chapters 36, Systemic Hypertension, and 47, Diagnosis and Treatment of Systemic Hypertension).[23] At this time, which drug class is preferred seems to be a matter of clinician preference and experience. The recommended dose for the long-acting calcium channel antagonist amlodipine besylate is 0.625 mg/cat/day. Amlodipine appears to be well tolerated at this dose, and reported side-effects are uncommon. Benazepril is becoming the ACE inhibitor of choice for CRF because dosage adjustments are not required. The recommended dosage of benazepril is 0.25 to 0.5 mg/kg q 12 hr to q 24 hr. A low dosage should be used initially, and may be increased as needed if the drug is well tolerated.[23] Amlodipine and benazepril may be used in combination for refractory hypertension, although this appears to be uncommon in cats.

How to treat cats whose temperament precludes reliable blood pressure monitoring is a difficult question. Based on clinical experience with amlodipine, it appears that conservative lowering of arterial blood pressure in nonhypertensive CRF cats causes them no adverse consequences. For patients assessed as being at higher risk of hypertension, such as geriatric cats with long-standing CRF, cautious use of antihypertensive agents may be considered in the absence of blood pressure monitoring. ACE inhibitors such as benazepril have the added benefit of lowering glomerular capillary pressure in addition to systemic arterial pressure, which may be of some benefit in delaying progression of CRF.[24] Patients on ACE inhibitors require regular monitoring of serum electrolyte and creatinine concentrations to ensure that they do not develop hyperkalemia or decreased GFR.

◆ DIETARY MANAGEMENT

There is no evidence in cats with CRF that dietary protein restriction delays disease progression independent of the effects of phosphorus restriction. Protein restriction as needed to maintain BUN less than 60 to 75 mg/dl is recommended because metabolites from protein breakdown are uremic toxins, as discussed earlier. Whether protein should be restricted earlier in CRF is unknown. Low-protein diets also are low-phosphorus diets, and they have the advantage of delaying the need to add phosphorus binders to the treatment regimen. Diet acceptance also may be an issue. It may be more difficult to get the cat to accept a diet change once CRF has advanced to the extent that BUN is increased sufficiently to warrant protein restriction. The impact of early protein restriction on body condition, quality of life, and long-term survival is unknown. Cats typically find diets higher in protein more palatable, which may improve overall nutrient intake. However, excess calorie intake itself may promote progression of CRF in cats.[8]

Dietary lipids also may play a role in the progression of renal disease. Diets with high concentrations of omega-6 fatty acids caused renal damage and increased mortality in remnant kidney models in dogs compared with diets high in omega-3 fatty acids. The impact of both the absolute amount of dietary lipids and the ratio of omega-6 to omega-3 fatty acids is an area that requires further study before specific recommendations can be made.[25]

Whether cats with CRF benefit from routine supplementation of water-soluble vitamins is unknown. Supplementation of water-soluble vitamins may be warranted in cats whose diets consist primarily of foods intended for human beings. The entire ingredient list of the cat's diet should be evaluated, and vitamin or iron supplements containing vitamins D or A should be avoided. I have seen CRF cats on iron supplements containing vitamin D that became hypercalcemic.

◆ URINARY TRACT INFECTION

Urinary tract infection, though rare in younger cats, is relatively common in cats with CRF, especially in females.[26] Urine culture and sensitivity should be employed in the management of urinary tract infections in CRF cats. An attempt should be made to distinguish pyelonephritis from lower urinary tract infections, especially in cats without dysuria. Renal ultrasonography can provide evidence of pyelonephritis, but the diuresis that accompanies fluid therapy can itself cause mild pyelectasia. Many antibiotics cause anorexia, vomiting, or diarrhea, especially in cats with CRF. For this reason, antibiotics should not be used presumptively when urinary tract infection merely is suspected but not confirmed. Pyelonephritis is difficult to diagnose with certainty, and it is crucial to distinguish relapsing urinary tract infection from ascending infection. If pyelonephritis is considered likely, 4 to 6 weeks of continuous antibiotic therapy is recommended. Urine cultures should be performed when the patient is on antibiotics to ensure that the urine has been sterilized.

◆ GENERAL CONSIDERATIONS IN DRUG THERAPY

Most treatments for the biochemical aberrations of CRF lack fixed dosages. Dosages of potassium, iron supplements, phosphate binders, alkalinizing agents, EPO, and subcutaneous fluids are adjusted to the individual patient's need based on monitored parameters.

Many drugs are excreted by the kidney and require dosage or dose interval adjustments. Guidelines provided for human beings or dogs often must be followed when selecting drug dosages for cats with CRF because specific recommendations for cats may be unavailable. Based on information for human beings, drugs that require dosage adjustment in CRF include beta-lactam antibiotics, enrofloxacin, trimethoprim/sulfamethoxazole, aminoglycosides, enalapril, digoxin, and furosemide.

REFERENCES

1. Miura M, Nomoto Y, Sakai H: Short term effect of lactulose therapy in patients with chronic renal failure. Tokai J Exp Clin Med 14:29–34, 1989.
2. Vogt B, Frey FJ: Lactulose and renal failure. Scand J Gastroenterol 32 (Suppl 222):100–101, 1997.
3. Younes H, Demigne C, Behr SR, et al: A blend of dietary fibers increases urea disposal in the large intestine and lowers urinary nitrogen excretion in rats fed a low protein diet. Nutr Biochem 7:474–480, 1996.
4. Ross LA, Finco DR, Crowell WA: Effect of dietary phosphorus restriction on the kidneys of cats with reduced renal mass. Am J Vet Res 43:1023–1026, 1982.
5. Finco DR, Brown SA, Crowell WA, et al: Effects of dietary phosphorus and protein on dogs with chronic renal failure. Am J Vet Res 53:2264–2271, 1992.
6. Schwarz U, Amann K, Orth SR, et al: Effect of 1,25 (OH)$_2$ vitamin D$_3$ on glomerulosclerosis in subtotally nephrectomized rats. Kidney Int 53:1696–1705, 1998.
7. Nagode LA, Chew DJ, Podell M: Benefits of calcitriol therapy and serum phosphorus control in dogs and cats with chronic renal failure. Vet Clin North Am Small Anim Pract 26:1293–1330, 1996.
8. Adams LG, Polzin DJ, Osborne CA, et al: Effects of dietary protein and calorie restriction in clinically normal cats and in cats with surgically induced chronic renal failure. Am J Vet Res 54:1653–1662, 1993.
9. Lulich J, Osborne C, O'Brien T, et al: Feline renal failure: Questions, answers, questions. Compend Contin Educ Pract Vet 14:127–153, 1992.
10. James KM, Polzin DJ, Osborne CA, et al: Effects of sample handling on total carbon dioxide concentrations in canine and feline serum and blood. Am J Vet Res 58:343–347, 1997.
11. Polzin D, Osborne C, Bartges J, et al: Chronic renal failure. In Ettinger S, Feldman E (eds): Textbook of Veterinary Internal Medicine, 4th ed. Philadelphia, WB Saunders, 1995, pp. 1734–1760.
12. Cowgill LD, James KM, Levy JL, et al: Use of recombinant human erythropoietin for management of anemia in dogs and cats with renal failure. J Am Vet Med Assoc 212:521–528, 1998.
13. Goldstein RE, Marks SL, Kass PK, et al: Gastrin concentrations in plasma of cats with chronic renal failure. J Am Vet Med Assoc 213:826–828, 1998.
14. Polzin DJ, Osborne CA, James KM. Medical management of chronic renal failure in cats: Current guidelines. In August JR (ed): Consultations in Feline Internal Medicine, vol. 3. Philadelphia, WB Saunders, 1997, pp. 325–336.
15. Kang JY: The gastrointestinal tract in uremia. Dig Dis Sci 38:257–268, 1993.
16. Echizen H, Ishizaki T: Clinical pharmacokinetics of famotidine. Clin Pharmacokinet 21:178–194, 1991.
17. FitzSimons H: Pharm Profile: Cisapride. Compend Contin Educ Pract Vet 20:324–326, 1999.

18. Nath KA, Croatt AJ, Hostetter TH: Oxygen consumption and oxidant stress in surviving nephrons. Am J Physiol 258:F1354–F1362, 1990.

19. Kobayashi DL, Peterson M, Graves TK, et al: Hypertension in cats with chronic renal failure or hyperthyroidism. J Vet Intern Med 4:58–62, 1990.

20. Stiles J, Polzin D, Bistner S: The prevalence of retinopathy in cats with systemic hypertension and chronic renal failure or hyperthyroidism. J Am Anim Hosp Assoc 30:564–572, 1994.

21. Elliot J, Rawlings JM, Markwell PJ, et al: Incidence of hypertension in cats with naturally occurring chronic renal failure (Abstract). Proceedings 17th Annual Veterinary Medical Forum, American College of Veterinary Internal Medicine, Chicago, June 10–13, 1999, p. 717.

22. Bright J: Feline hypertension: Therapeutic strategies. Proceedings 17th Annual Veterinary Medical Forum, American College of Veterinary Internal Medicine, Chicago, June 10–13, 1999, pp. 134–135.

23. Brown SA: Systemic hypertension in renal disease. Proceedings 17th Annual Veterinary Medical Forum, American College of Veterinary Internal Medicine, Chicago, June 10–13, 1999, pp. 36–37.

24. Brown SA, Brown CA, Jacobs G, et al: Hemodynamic effects of angiotensin converting enzyme inhibition (benazepril) in cats with chronic renal insufficiency (Abstract). Proceedings 17th Annual Veterinary Medical Forum, American College of Veterinary Internal Medicine, Chicago, June 10–13, 1999, p. 716.

25. Finco DR, Brown SA, Barsanti JA: Divergent views on dietary management of renal failure: The Georgia experience. Proceedings 17th Annual Veterinary Medical Forum, American College of Veterinary Internal Medicine, Chicago, June 10–13, 1999, pp. 31–33.

26. Barber PJ, Rawlings JM, Markwell PJ, et al: Incidence and prevalence of bacterial urinary tract infections in cats with chronic renal failure (Abstract). Proceedings 17th Annual Veterinary Medical Forum, American College of Veterinary Internal Medicine, Chicago, June 10–13, 1999, p. 717.

45

◆ Use of Hemodialysis in Chronic Renal Failure

Denise A. Elliott
Larry D. Cowgill

Chronic renal failure (CRF) ensues from the irreversible loss of the metabolic, endocrine, and excretory capacities of the kidney. Although commonly considered an illness of older cats, CRF may occur at any age, and is considered a leading cause of death in cats. The etiology of CRF is multifactorial, but replacement of functional nephrons by nonfunctional scar tissue and inflammatory infiltrates is a unifying feature. The onset of renal failure tends to be insidious as renal function generally declines over a period of months to years. The uremic syndrome manifests itself when residual renal mass is less than 25 per cent of normal, and compensatory changes fail to meet the metabolic and excretory needs of the body. Tailored supportive medical therapy has been the mainstay of management for CRF for decades[1] (see Chapter 44, Medical Management of Chronic Renal Failure). The goals of medical management are to reduce the renal workload; alleviate the clinical signs and biochemical consequences of uremic intoxication; minimize disturbances in fluid, electrolyte, vitamin, mineral, and acid-base balance; and slow progression of the disease. Despite appropriate tailoring of the therapy to the patient's condition, CRF typically is dynamic and progressive, and eventually leads to end-stage renal failure. Dietary and conventional medical therapy generally become poorly accepted or ineffective when serum creatinine concentration exceeds 6 mg/dl and blood urea nitrogen (BUN) concentration exceeds 90 mg/dl. At this point, owners are frustrated with the poor quality of life of their cat, and euthanasia often is the ultimate outcome.

Renal replacement therapy should be instituted when the clinical consequences and morbidity of CRF no longer can be alleviated by conservative medical therapy (Table 45–1). For approximately 300,000 people in the United States affected with end-stage renal failure, modalities of renal replacement therapy include renal transplantation, peritoneal dialysis, and hemodialysis.[2] Eighty-five per cent of human patients receive hemodialysis as their initial renal replacement therapy, and 28 per cent ultimately receive renal transplantation.[2] Renal transplantation is a viable procedure for cats with severe end-stage renal disease[3] (see Chapter 43, Renal Transplantation in the Management of Chronic Renal Failure). However, many candidates for transplantation have overt nutritional deficiencies, anemia, and other metabolic disorders that pose substantial risk for anesthesia and successful transplantation surgery.

Peritoneal dialysis utilizes an indwelling catheter to instill dialysate into the abdominal cavity. The peritoneum serves as the dialyzing membrane to remove uremic toxins. Although peritoneal dialysis has been performed in cats, technical difficulties and complications have prevented its development as a practical renal replacement therapy for cats with end-stage renal disease.[4]

Hemodialysis utilizes an extracorporeal circulation of the patient's blood to exchange solute through an artificial kidney (hemodialyzer or dialyzer).[5] The advent of human neonatal dialysis equipment and delivery systems has allowed hemodialysis to be technically feasible for cats with severe uremia.[6, 7] Preoperative hemodialysis is used to improve the medical condition of renal transplant recipients, and may be required while a suitable donor is located, especially for cats with type B blood. Comorbid conditions including inflammatory bowel disease, cardiac insufficiency, feline leukemia virus infection, feline immunodeficiency virus infection, urinary tract infections, uncontrolled hyperthyroidism, and neoplasia preclude renal transplantation owing to risks of postoperative complications or renal graft rejection. For these patients, indefinite intermittent hemodialysis (2 or 3 times weekly) may be the only option to provide good-quality life.

The objective of chronic intermittent hemodialysis is to promote an improved quality of life by ameliorating the azotemia, fluid, electrolyte, and acid-base abnormalities, as well as systemic hypertension. Frequently, intermittent hemodialysis may be prescribed for a finite period of time to allow the family to accept the terminal condition of their pet. Hemodialysis also is indicated in the postoperative period of renal transplantation complicated by delayed graft function, acute rejection, or acute pyelonephritis in the graft in order to maintain the cat until the episode has resolved.

Table 45–1. Indications for Chronic Intermittent Hemodialysis

Refractory azotemia (BUN > 90 mg/dl, creatinine > 6 mg/dl)
Intractable uremic signs
Preoperative conditioning for renal transplantation
Postoperative delayed graft function
Acute renal graft rejection
Acute exacerbations of chronic renal failure

Abbreviation: BUN, blood urea nitrogen.

◆ PRINCIPLES OF HEMODIALYSIS

Hemodialysis is performed using a hemodialyzer (artificial kidney), a hemodialysis machine (dialysis delivery system), and blood tubing (extracorporeal circuit). These components contain separate blood and dialysate circuits (Fig. 45–1). In the blood circuit, blood is pumped through an input ("arterial") line from the patient to the hemodialyzer. Blood passes through capillary tubes located in the hemodialyzer, and is returned to the patient under positive pressure via an output ("venous") tubing. The dialysate circuit is a single-pass system in which concentrated dialysate and bicarbonate solutions are diluted with highly purified water and pumped in a counter-current direction through the hemodialyzer between the capillary tubes containing the patient's blood. Spent dialysate then is discarded into a drain. The job of the hemodialyzer, dialysate, and dialysis machine is to take over many of the complex tasks that the failed kidneys can no longer perform.

The blood and dialysate are separated in the hemodialyzer by a thin semipermeable membrane perforated with pores or diffusion channels (Fig. 45–2). Water and low-molecular-weight solutes (e.g., urea, creatinine) can pass readily through the membrane by either diffusion or ultrafiltration (convection), but the movement of larger solutes, plasma proteins, and the cellular components of blood is restricted by the size of the membrane pores.[8]

The rate of solute diffusion is dependent on the solute concentration gradient established between the blood and the dialysate, the kinetic motion of the solutes, and the permeability of the semipermeable membrane. Membrane permeability is determined by its thickness, surface area, and the number, size, and shape of the pores or diffusion channels.[9] Resistance to solute movement will be high if the membrane is thick, if the number of pores is small, or if the pores are narrow. Low-molecular-weight uremic toxins such as urea and creatinine diffuse from the region of higher concentration (blood) to the region of lower concentration (dialysate). Conversely, depleted solutes such as bicarbonate can be replenished by movement from a higher concentration in dialysate to a lower concentration in blood. The solute concentrations on both sides of the semipermeable membrane will equalize, and the concentration gradient will be abolished if adequate time is allowed. At filtration equilibrium, there is no further change in composition of either the blood or the dialysate.[10] Filtration equilibrium is prevented to maximize diffusion of uremic solutes during hemodialysis by continuously replenishing blood and dialysate to maintain the diffusion gradients. Filtration equilibrium is exploited to preserve vital electrolytes by formulating dialysate so that concentrations of these electrolytes in the dialysate correspond to concentrations in plasma. Unstirred layers of fluid may develop on either side of the semipermeable membrane and slow net solute movement. The design of the hemodialyzer and optimization of dialysate and blood flow rate collectively dissipate the unstirred layer to facilitate solute movement.

Convective transport associated with ultrafiltration is the second mechanism of solute movement across semipermeable membranes. *Ultrafiltration* refers to the directed movement of water through the membrane along hydrostatic or osmotic pressure gradients.[11] Diffusible solutes in the ultrafiltered water are swept through the membrane by solvent drag, independent of their concentration gradient across the membrane. The transmembrane pressure required for ultrafiltration is established by a positive pressure created by the blood pump in the blood compartment of the hemodialyzer, and by a negative pressure produced by a vacuum pump in the dialysate compartment. Ultrafiltration is opposed by plasma oncotic pressure, and a minimum transmembrane pressure of 25 mm Hg is required for ultrafiltration to occur.[9] The hydraulic permeability of the hemodialyzer to water is determined similarly by the thickness and pore size of the semipermeable membrane and defined by an ultrafiltration coefficient (K_{uf}), expressed as the milliliters of water transferred per hour per millimeter of mercury of transmembrane pressure. The rate of ultrafiltration (and convective transfer of solute) is controlled by adjusting the transmembrane hydrostatic pressure gradient across the blood and dialysate compartments and selection of a hemodialyzer with an appropriate K_{uf}. Convective transport contributes significantly to net solute removal, and facilitates removal of large solutes with poor diffusibility.

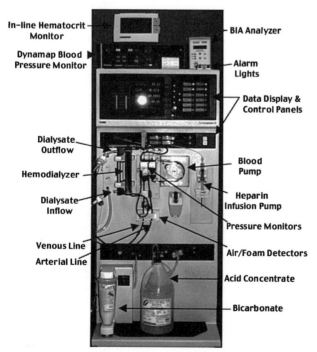

In-line Hematocrit Monitor
Dynamap Blood Pressure Monitor
BIA Analyzer
Alarm Lights
Data Display & Control Panels
Dialysate Outflow
Hemodialyzer
Dialysate Inflow
Blood Pump
Heparin Infusion Pump
Pressure Monitors
Venous Line
Arterial Line
Air/Foam Detectors
Acid Concentrate
Bicarbonate

Figure 45–1. Arrangement of the hemodialysis delivery system. BIA, bioelectrical impedance analyzer.

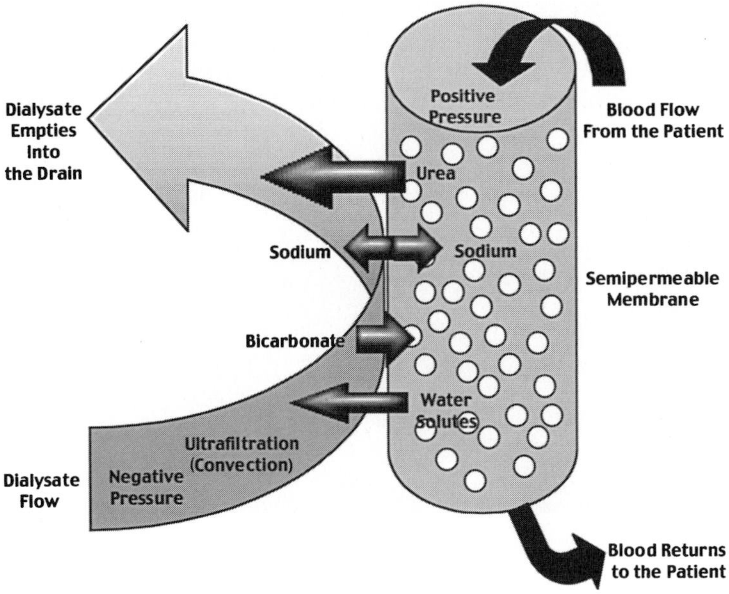

Figure 45–2. Principles of diffusion and ultrafiltration (convection) across a semipermeable membrane. The blood and dialysate flow in opposite (countercurrent) directions. Uremic toxins such as urea diffuse down a concentration gradient from blood into the dialysate. Depleted solutes such as bicarbonate diffuse from the higher concentration in dialysate to replenish blood. Vital electrolytes such as sodium are preserved by filtration equilibrium. Water is driven into dialysate via a hydrostatic transmembrane pressure gradient, and diffusible solutes are transferred convectively into dialysate by the process of solvent drag.

◆ HEMODIALYSIS EQUIPMENT

Hemodialysis is a technically demanding procedure that requires an extensive array of sophisticated delivery equipment to perform, monitor, and ensure the integrity and safety of the dialysis procedure and clinical trends in critically ill patients (Table 45–2).[5]

The regular and reproducible delivery of large volumes of blood from the body to the hemodialyzer is paramount for successful hemodialysis. In human patients with CRF, vascular access most commonly is accomplished by surgical anastomosis of a peripheral artery (usually the radial artery) with a peripheral vein (cephalic vein) to form arteriovenous fistulas (created from native vessels) or grafts (constructed from synthetic vascular materials).[12, 13] Percutaneous needles provide access during the hemodialysis procedure. Neither arteriovenous fistulas nor grafts have been used for routine dialysis in cats. Rather, long-term high-volume vascular access is achieved most commonly with transcutaneous silicone double-lumen neonatal dialysis catheters (Pediatric Hemo-Cath [diameter, 8 French; length, 18 cm], Medcomp, Inc., Harleysville, PA) (Fig. 45–3). The catheter is inserted into the external jugular vein surgically and advanced to the right atrium or cranial vena cava (Fig. 45–4). The extravascular portion of the catheter is tunneled subcutaneously to exit the skin in the cranial cervical area of the neck, and contains a Dacron cuff to help stabilize its position, prevent accidental displacement from the vessel, and impair extension of local cutaneous infection (Fig. 45–5). Frequently, the jugular vein in cats is smaller than the neonatal catheter, and surgical placement can be technically demanding. The recently developed twin-lumen Tesio Catheter (Medcomp Tesio-Cath with Cuff [diameter, 7 French pediatric; arterial, 29 cm; venous, 32 cm], Bio-Flex Tesio Catheter, Medcomp, Inc., Harleysville, PA) may be advantageous compared with double-lumen designs for prolonged access by providing reduced thrombogenicity, enhanced flow characteristics, reduced recirculation, reduced susceptibility to infection, and more flexible replacement (Fig. 45–6).[14, 15] Between hemodialysis sessions, each lumen of the catheter is filled with 500 to 1000 units/ml of heparin (Heparin Sodium Injection, Organon, Inc., West Orange, NJ) to prevent intraluminal thrombosis. Aspirin (Bayer Children's Aspirin, Bayer Corporation, Morristown, NJ) is administered at 1 to 5 mg/kg every (q) 48 hr to reduce intravascular thrombosis. Strict asepsis and proper catheter maintenance are mandatory to prevent physical damage, occlusion, and infection, and to ensure adequate blood flow. Dialysis catheters are the "lifeline" for dialysis patients, and are reserved exclusively for dialysis. They should be handled only by trained dialysis personnel to pre-

Table 45–2. Hemodialysis Equipment Required to Ensure Safe, Adequate, and Efficient Hemodialysis

Specifically trained, dedicated staff
High-volume vascular access
Hemodialyzer
Extracorporeal blood circuit
Dialysis delivery system
  Bicarbonate proportioning system
  Sodium modeling
  Volumetric ultrafiltration control
Ultrapure water
Indirect blood pressure monitor
  Indirect oscillometry
  Indirect Doppler
Coagulation monitor
  Activated clotting time
  Partial thromboplastin time
Electrocardiogram
Accurate body weight scale
In-line hematocrit monitor
Pulse oximeter
Multifrequency bioimpedance spectrophotometer

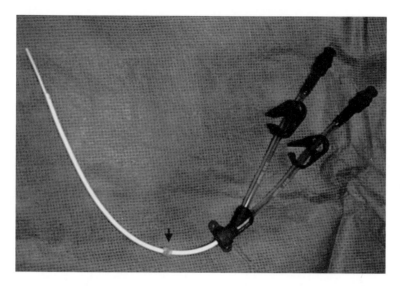

Figure 45–3. Transcutaneous silicone double-lumen neonatal hemodialysis catheter (Pediatric Hemo-Cath [diameter, 8 Fr.; length, 18 cm], Medcomp, Inc., Harleysville, PA) utilized to provide high-volume vascular access. The subcutaneous Dacron cuff (*arrowhead*) stabilizes the catheter and impairs extension of local cutaneous infection.

vent inadvertent injection of the heparin lock or bacterial contamination.

Hemodialyzers are classified according to their physical design (hollow fiber or parallel plate) and membrane characteristics (composition, surface area, hydraulic permeability, biocompatibility, and priming volume).[9, 16] Hollow-fiber hemodialyzers are composed of bundles of hollow capillary tubes (analogous to soda straws) through which blood flows, while dialysate solution flows on the outside of the capillary in a direction counter-current to blood (Fig. 45–7). Hollow-fiber designs provide a large surface area:blood volume ratio and low blood flow resistance, and the thinness and porosity of the capillary wall promote efficient solute diffusion and strength to accommodate high transmembrane pressures for ultrafiltration. Membrane composition determines the effectiveness of diffusive and convective transfer of solutes and water, and biocompatibility for

patient safety and comfort. Synthetic polymer membranes (polyacrylonitrile, polysulfon, polymethylmethacrylate) have high permeability and hydraulic characteristics, and are considered to be extremely biocompatible.[16] These characteristics permit shortening of dialysis treatment times, but these materials are relatively expensive and require multiple reuses to be cost-effective.[16] Conventional (cellulosic) hemodialyzer membranes are made of chemically modified cellulose (cuprophan, regenerated cellulose, cellulose acetate, cellulose triacetate, hemophan).[16] They are relatively inexpensive, have good diffusion characteristics for low-molecular-weight solutes and lower ultrafiltration coefficients, and are more bioreactive than synthetic membrane hemodialyzers.[16] Cellulosic (hemophan) hollow-fiber hemodialyzers (COBE Centrysystem 100 HG Hollow Fiber Dialyzer, COBE Laboratories, Inc., Lakewood, CO) with a surface area between 0.2 and 0.3 m² and a priming volume of less

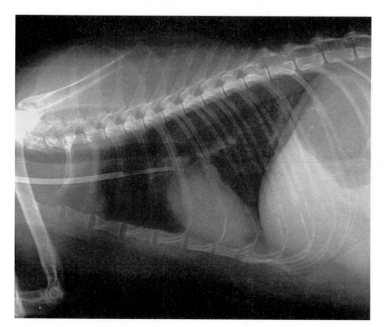

Figure 45–4. Lateral thoracic radiograph of a cat illustrates a transcutaneous double-lumen catheter placed in the external jugular vein advanced to the position of the right atrium.

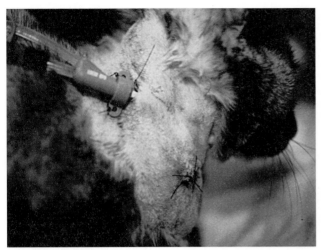

Figure 45–5. Correct positioning of a transcutaneous double-lumen neonatal dialysis catheter (Pediatric Hemo-Cath [diameter, 8 Fr.; length, 18 cm], Medcomp, Inc., Harleysville, PA) in the cranial cervical area of the neck.

than 20 ml, are selected for hemodialysis in cats owing to their low cost, disposability, adequate solute removal, ultrafiltration characteristics, and improved biocompatibility compared with other cellulosic materials.[5, 17–22]

The extracorporeal blood circuit carries the patient's blood from the hemodialysis catheter to the hemodialyzer and back to the catheter. It includes the arterial blood line, blood pump segment, heparin infusion pump, hemodialyzer, venous blood line, saline infusion line, and monitors for blood flow, blood pressure, blood leaks, clots, air, and foam (Fig. 45–8). To minimize the risks of hypotension and hypovolemia during the dialysis session, the extracorporeal circuit should contain less than 10 per cent of the patient's blood volume.[23] The inclusive volume of the available neonatal blood circuits (COBE Centrysystem C3 Pediatric Low Volume Cartridge Set, COBE Laboratories, Inc., Lakewood, CO) is approximately 60 ml, which depending on body weight, can represent 17 to 33 per cent of a cat's blood volume. Hence, to dialyze cats

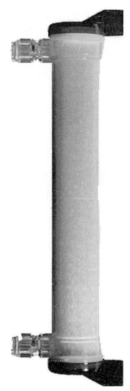

Figure 45–7. Neonatal cellulosic (hemophan) hollow-fiber hemodialyzer shows the arterial and venous blood and dialysate ports used for feline hemodialysis.

safely, the extracorporeal circuit must be primed with compatible blood or volume expanders (3 to 6 per cent dextran 70 [6 per cent Gentran 70, Baxter Healthcare Corporation, Deerfield, IL]).[7]

The modern hemodialysis machine (Centrysystem 3 Dialysis Delivery Systems, COBE Laboratories, Inc., Lakewood, CO) is a complex, microprocessor-controlled unit that formulates and delivers dialysate, controls blood flow in the extracorporeal circuit, delivers anticoagulant, regulates ultrafiltration, and monitors the integrity and safety of the entire dialysis process. A variable-ratio dialysate-proportioning system mixes concentrated solute so-

Figure 45–6. Lateral thoracic radiograph of a cat illustrates a transcutaneous Tesio twin single-lumen dialysis catheter (Medcomp Tesio-Cath with Cuff [7-Fr. pediatric; arterial = 29 cm; venous = 32 cm], Bio-Flex Tesio Catheter, Medcomp, Inc., Harleysville, PA) placed in the external jugular veins and advanced to the position of the right atrium. The twin vascular segments minimize infection and thrombosis.

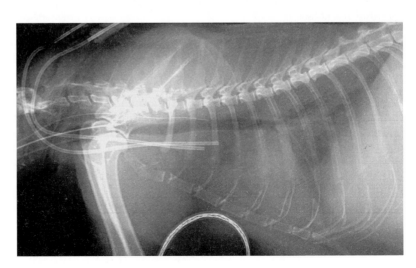

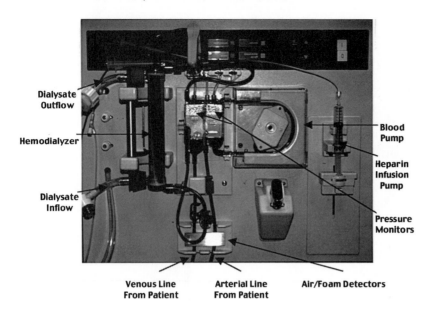

Figure 45–8. Extracorporeal blood path and neonatal cellulosic (hemophan) hollow-fiber hemodialyzer used for feline hemodialysis.

lution, concentrated bicarbonate solution, and highly purified water to generate the appropriate composition of the dialysate solution. Sophisticated proportioning systems permit continuous adjustment and modeling of dialysate sodium and bicarbonate concentrations throughout the hemodialysis treatment. The proportioning system also monitors the composition of the dialysate by measuring its conductivity, pH, temperature, flow rate, and pressure to ensure that it remains safe for the patient. Internal alarms are activated if alterations in any of these variables are detected, and the dialysate is diverted (bypassed) away from the hemodialyzer to protect the patient until the abnormality is corrected. Dialysate solutions containing acetate as the buffer circumvent the requirement for separate proportioning systems for solutes and bicarbonate; however, the associated high acetate loads have been associated with nausea, vomiting, fatigue, hypoxemia, hypoventilation, vasodilatation, reduced myocardial contractility, hypotension, and hemodynamic instability.[24, 25] These complications have not been associated with bicarbonate-based dialysis. Consequently, bicarbonate dialysate is recommended for cats.[5]

Precise volumetric ultrafiltration control systems are essential to regulate the rate and volume of ultrafiltration during dialysis so that subtle or undetected fluctuations in transmembrane pressure do not induce volume depletion or hypotension. The desired volume or rate of ultrafiltration is programmed at the start of the dialysis session, and fluid removal is regulated automatically and accurately by the dialysis delivery system throughout the treatment.

Heparin therapy is required to prevent blood clotting in the hemodialyzer and extracorporeal circuit. The dialysis machine can be programmed for bolus injections of heparin in addition to constant-rate infusions. A separate automated device (Automated Coagulation Timer, HemoTec, Inc., Englewood, CO) is required to measure activated clotting time to determine the initial dose of heparin to anticoagulate the patient (the heparin prime), and to regulate ongoing heparin requirements during treatment so that both spontaneous patient bleeding and clotting in the hemodialyzer are avoided.

Many cats are predisposed to hemodynamic instability, especially when undergoing ultrafiltration. Hypotension and hypovolemia can be avoided by regular monitoring of blood pressure using indirect Doppler or oscillometric blood pressure monitors. Changes in intravascular volume can be evaluated with in-line blood volume–profiling equipment (Crit-Line, In-Line Diagnostics, Inc., Riverdale, UT) that monitors hematocrit and oxygen saturation simultaneously during the treatment.[26, 27] Instantaneous alterations in total-body water and intracellular and extracellular fluid volume can be monitored using a bioimpedance spectrometer (Hydra ECF-ICF Bio-Impedance Analyzer, Xitron Technologies, Inc., San Diego, CA).[28–32]

The average cat may drink 50 to 300 ml of water per day. In contrast, a thin semipermeable membrane separates a hemodialysis patient's blood from approximately 150 liters of dialysate per hemodialysis session. The sheer magnitude of this exposure suggests that even minute quantities of water-treatment chemicals (fluorine, chloramine), contaminants, or impurities such as bacteria, viruses, endotoxins, metals, or chemicals constitute a formidable risk to dialysis patients. Therefore, the water used to generate dialysate must be processed carefully with a series of water-treatment devices (particulate filters, carbon sorbents for organic solutes, water softeners to reduce excessive minerals, deionization beds to remove inorganic cations and anions, and reverse osmosis to remove residual contaminants) to be chemically pure. Furthermore, the plumbing system must remain free from bacterial and chemical contaminants to guarantee that the purified water is not altered in route to the dialysis machine. Routine water monitoring and microbial testing of the water-treatment system is required to validate water safety.[33]

◆ HEMODIALYSIS PRESCRIPTION

The factors to consider in the prescription of hemodialysis include the severity of the uremia, the frequency of hemodialysis sessions, and the choice of hemodialyzer, extracorporeal circuit, dialysate composition, dialysate flow rate, blood flow rate, dialysis treatment time, heparin dosage, priming solution, ultrafiltration rate, and ultrafiltration volume (Table 45–3). The prescription should be formulated to reduce the azotemia maximally during each hemodialysis session, and to promote a predialysis BUN less than 90 mg/dl, a postdialysis BUN less than 10 mg/dl, and a time-averaged BUN less than 60 mg/dl over the interdialysis interval (see Efficacy and Outcome). Severely uremic cats (i.e., BUN > 100 mg/dl) should be managed initially with an acute dialysis prescription specifically to reduce the intensity of the treatment, and to prevent an excessive rate of urea clearance and dysequilibrium syndrome (see Complications).[5]

Twice-weekly dialysis will benefit cats with serum creatinine concentrations between 5 and 8 mg/dl. Three treatments per week are used for patients with serum creatinine concentrations greater than 8 mg/dl. There are no indications for once-weekly dialysis treatments because such patients can be managed with aggressive medical therapy. Neonatal low-volume hemodialyzers and extracorporeal circuits are utilized to minimize extravascular volume depletion. Three per cent dextran 70 is used as the priming solution to minimize the risk of a hemodynamic crisis. Depending on the predialysis activated clotting time, heparin is administered at 50 to 100 U/kg, and is continued as a constant-rate infusion of 200 to 1200 U/hr to maintain an activated clotting time between 150 and 200 seconds. The constant-rate infusion is terminated 30 minutes before completion of the hemodialysis session to prevent excessive or prolonged bleeding after dialysis. Protamine sulfate (1 mg/100 U of estimated residual heparin) can be administered to antagonize heparin if bleeding persists after discontinuation of dialysis.

The typical dialysate composition is sodium 150 mmol/l, potassium 3.0 mmol/liter, chloride 112 to 122 mmol/liter, calcium 3.0 mmol/liter, magnesium 1.0 mmol/liter, and dextrose 200 mg/dl (3-K Renalyte Rx Acid Concentrate for Bicarbonate Dialysis, COBE Laboratories, Inc., Lakewood, CO). Potassium-free dialysate (K-Free Renalyte Rx Acid Concentrate for Bicarbonate Dialysis, COBE Laboratories, Inc., Lakewood, CO) is indicated for cats with persistent predialysis hyperkalemia (serum potassium concentrations between 6 and 9 mEq/liter). Sodium modeling using a sodium concentration of 160 mmol/liter for the initial 20 per cent of the dialysis session, 155 mmol/liter for the next 40 per cent of the session and 150 mmol/liter for the remainder of the session is recommended to minimize dialysis dysequilibrium and hypotension while facilitating ultrafiltration.[34] Alternatively, dialysate with a sodium concentration lower than that of plasma may be employed if sodium removal is needed for control of hypertension. The dialysate can be formulated with bicarbonate concentrations ranging from 25 to 35 mmol/liter. Typically, a dialysate bicarbonate concentration of 30 mmol/liter will produce a postdialysis serum bicarbonate concentration of approximately 25 mmol/liter. Higher dialysate bicarbonate concentrations have been associated with relentless panting throughout the hemodialysis treatment. The dialysate sodium and bicarbonate concentration may be adjusted during the dialysis treatment. Dialysate flow conventionally is 500 ml/min.

Blood flow rate and dialysis time largely determine the efficiency of the hemodialysis treatment. An extracorporeal blood flow rate of 10 to 20 ml/kg/min and dialysis time of 240 minutes typically achieve a urea reduction ratio (URR) of greater than 0.9 (see Efficacy and Outcome). Blood flow rate is increased slowly over the first 30 minutes of the dialysis session to avoid dialysis-related hypotension or nausea.

Patients with end-stage renal disease may develop fluid overload if ingestion of sodium and water exceeds renal excretory capacity. An assessment of the volume of fluid to remove to achieve ideal dry body weight and the rate of ultrafiltration is necessary (Table 45–4). Consideration also should be given to compensate for fluids, blood, or plasma administered during the dialysis session.

◆ CONCURRENT MEDICAL THERAPY

Animals supported with chronic hemodialysis must be supplemented with conservative medical therapy to manage the anemia, hypertension, nutritional deficiencies, electrolyte abnormalities, and acid-base

Table 45–3. The Hemodialysis Prescription

Hemodialyzer type and lot number
Extracorporeal circuit type and lot number
Extracorporeal prime
  Saline
  Dextran 70
Dialysate
  Sodium concentration
  Bicarbonate concentration
  Potassium concentration
  Temperature
  Flow rate
Heparin prime
Treatment time
Ultrafiltration volume
Blood flow rate
Liters of blood to be processed

Table 45–4. Clinical Manifestations of Hypervolemia

Increase in historical weight
Increased skin turgor
Chemosis
Serous nasal discharge
Edema, ascites, pleural effusion
Strong pulses
Venous engorgement, jugular pulses
Elevated central venous pressure
Tachycardia
Tachypnea/dyspnea
Increased breath sounds, crackles, or wheezes on thoracic auscultation
Systemic hypertension
Hemodilution (decreased hematocrit and plasma proteins)

disturbances characteristic of the uremic syndrome (Table 45–5).[1] Nutritional assessment and institution of nutritional support are crucial because dialysis only partially alleviates uremic anorexia. Protein calorie malnutrition, primarily due to poor food intake, is common in dialysis patients. Practical measures to improve food intake include using highly odoriferous foods, warming the food before feeding, and stimulating eating by positive reinforcement by petting and stroking the cat. Appetite stimulants such as the benzodiazepine derivatives or serotonin antagonists may be administered judiciously. Effective dietary management of cats reluctant to eat appropriate amounts of food ad libitum may be facilitated by the placement of enteral feeding devices such as percutaneous endoscopic gastrostomy (PEG) tubes (Fig. 45–9). Enteral feeding of caloric and protein requirements is achieved by the administration of blended commercial prescription diets or formulated liquid diets through the PEG tube (Table 45–6). Furthermore, PEG tubes may be utilized to facilitate

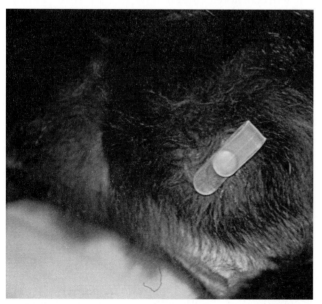

Figure 45–9. Correct placement of an 18-Fr., 1.2-cm low-profile gastrostomy tube (Applied Medical Technologies, Cleveland, OH) in a cat. The device had been placed 3 months previously. Note the hair regrowth and lack of inflammation around the stoma site.

administration of medications and additional fluids for patients with persistent negative fluid balance. Nutritional status and body composition should be evaluated routinely by consecutive body weight measurements, body condition scoring, and multi-frequency bioelectrical impedance analysis to record sequential changes in body cell mass, fat free mass, and per cent body fat.[35–37] Serial assessment of nutritional status and body composition will enable identification of patients that would benefit from a more aggressive therapeutic approach.

◆ COMPLICATIONS

A variety of complications including intradialytic cardiovascular instability, malnutrition, and vascular access problems confound the course of many hemodialysis patients (Table 45–7).[7] A thorough understanding of the pathophysiology of dialysis-related complications, coupled with innovative technological developments and specifically trained dedicated personnel, will minimize the risk of adverse events and ensure safe, adequate, and efficient hemodialysis.

Cardiovascular Instability

Cardiovascular instability with hypotension or hypovolemia is a common phenomenon during hemodialysis.[7] Important causes include the relatively large volume of the extracorporeal circuit, ultrafiltration-induced volume depletion, and extracellular volume depletion resulting from osmolar shifts. Priming the extracorporeal circuit with colloids such as dextran 70 helps to support intravascular volume. Excessive or rapid ultrafiltration of fluid depletes the vascular compartment faster than it can be replenished from the extravascular reserves, thereby inciting hypovolemia and hypotension. Furthermore, rapid removal of plasma solutes in the early stages of dialysis treatment diminishes intravascular volume and opposes vascular refilling from the extravascular space. Therefore, preservation of plasma osmolality during dialysis is fundamental to preventing dialysis hypotension. Dialysate sodium profiling allows initially higher plasma sodium concentrations to alleviate the osmotic drain and to promote vascular refilling from the interstitial space.[38] Sodium overload is avoided by proportionally lowering the dialysate sodium concentrations during the hemodialysis session. Intradialytic hypotension and hypovolemia may be minimized by monitoring heart rate and blood pressure every 15 to 30 minutes, and continually assessing blood and extracellular fluid volume with an in-line hematocrit monitor and bioelectrical impedance analyzer. Modern dialysis delivery systems that provide precise volumetric ultrafiltration control, sodium modeling, and bicarbonate-based dialysate are imperative to ensure safe and efficient dialysis. Most hypotensive events are treated successfully by re-

Table 45–5. Therapeutic Agents Used in the Management of Chronic Renal Failure*

Uremic Complication	Conventional Dose
Gastrointestinal	
Chlorhexidine (CHX-Guard VRx Products)	Oral rinse q 6–8 hr
Cimetidine† (Tagamet, Smith Kline Beecham)	5–10 mg/kg PO, IM, IV q 6–8 hr
Ranitidine† (Zantac, Glaxo)	0.5–2.0 mg/kg PO, IV q 8–12 hr
Famotidine† (Pepcid, Merck Sharp Dohme)	0.5–1.0 mg/kg PO, IM, IV q 12–24 hr
Omeprazole (Prilosec, Merck Sharp Dohme)	0.5–1.0 mg/kg PO q 24 hr
Sucralfate† (Carafate, Marion)	0.25–0.5 g PO q 8–12 hr
Misoprostol (Cytotec, Searle)	1–5 μg/kg PO q 6–12 hr
Metoclopramide† (Regulan, Robins)	0.1–0.5 mg/kg PO, IM, SQ q 6–8 hr
Chlorpromazine (Thorazine, Smith Kline Beecham)	0.2–0.5 mg/kg PO, IM, SQ q 6–8 hr
Prochlorperazine (Compazine, Smith Kline Beecham)	0.1–0.5 mg/kg PO, IM, SQ q 8–12 hr
Acepromazine (PromAce, Fort Dodge)	0.01–0.05 mg/kg PO, IM, SQ q 8–12 hr
Cisapride (Propulsid, Jansen Pharmaceutica, Inc.)	0.1–0.5 mg/kg PO q 8–12 hr
Hypertension	
Amlodipine (Norvasc, Pfizer)	0.625–1.25 mg/cat PO q 12–24 hr
Atenolol† (Tenormin, ICI)	2 mg/kg PO q 24 hr
Diltiazem (Cardizem, Marion-Merrel Dow)	1.0–2.25 mg/kg PO q 8–12 hr
Enalapril† (Enocard, Merck)	0.25–0.5 mg/kg PO q 12–24 hr
Furosemide (Lasix, Hoechst)	0.5–2.0 mg/kg PO q 8–24 hr
Hydralazine† (Apresoline, Ciba)	1–2 mg/cat PO q 12 hr
Lisinopril† (Prinivil, Merck Sharp Dohme)	0.4–2.0 mg/kg PO q 24 hr
Prazosin (Minipress, Pfizer)	0.25–1.0 mg/kg PO q 8–12 hr
Propranolol (Inderal, Ayerst)	2.5–5.0 mg/kg PO q 8–12 hr
Anemia	
Erythropoietin (Epogen, Amgen)	100 U/kg SQ 1–3 times per wk
Ferrous sulfate (Fer-In-Sol, Mead Johnson)	50–100 mg/day PO
Iron dextran (Ferrextran, Fort Dodge)	10 mg/kg monthly
Metabolic Acidosis	
Sodium bicarbonate (generic)	30–90 mg/kg PO q 12 hr
Hypokalemia	
Potassium gluconate (Tumil-K, Daniels)	2–6 mEq/cat PO q 12–24 hr
Hyperphosphatemia	
Aluminum hydroxide/carbonate/oxide	30–90 mg/kg PO q 12–24 hr
Renal Osteodystrophy	
Calcitriol (Rocaltrol, Roche)	1.5–6.0 ng/kg PO q 24 hr
Appetite Stimulants	
Cyproheptadine (Periactin, Merck)	2–4 mg/cat PO q 12 hr
Oxazepam (Serax, Wyeth-Ayerst)	2 mg/cat PO q 12 hr

Abbreviations: IM, intramuscularly; IV, intravenously; PO, by mouth; q, every; SQ, subcutaneously.
*Most of these drugs have not been approved for use in cats.
†Agent undergoes renal excretion, and the dosage must be adjusted accordingly to prevent toxicity.

Table 45–6. Composition of Selected Commercial Feline Modified Protein Formulations

Product	Caloric Content	Nutrients (% of total kcal)		
		Protein	*Fat*	*Carbohydrate*
k/d Canned (Hill's)	562 kcal/can	23	50	28
k/d Dry (Hill's)	498 kcal/cup	22	43	35
CNM NF-Formula Canned (Ralston-Purina)	234 kcal/can	22	54	24
CNM NF-Formula Dry (Ralston-Purina)	398 kcal/cup	27	25	47
Waltham Feline Low Protein Canned	250 kcal/can	21	73	6
Waltham Feline Low Protein Dry	385 kcal/cup	22	50	28
Renalcare (Abbott) 260 mOsm/kg	0.84 kcal/ml	22	57	21

ducing the rate of ultrafiltration, administering intravenous saline solution to refill vascular volume transiently while fluid from the extracellular space is mobilized, or both.

Neurologic Complications

Neurologic complications in the dialysis patient may be a consequence of advanced uremia and its associated metabolic abnormalities, or may arise from the dialysis procedure itself. Advanced uremia often is associated with diffuse, nonspecific alterations of cerebral cortical and peripheral neuromuscular functions termed *uremic encephalopathy*. Signs such as fatigue, lethargy, impaired mentation, altered behavior, confusion, stupor, tremors, seizures, muscular cramps, muscle weakness, myoclonus, hypotonic peripheral reflexes, and peripheral neuropathies generally are seen before the initiation of dialysis. Although no single pathogenic mechanism or toxin has been identified, uremic encephalopathy generally improves with amelioration of azotemia.

Rapid correction of severe azotemia (BUN > 120 mg/dl) and metabolic acidosis may be accompanied by an acute metabolic encephalopathy called *dialysis dysequilibrium syndrome*. Disproportionate clearance of urea from blood as compared with cerebrospinal fluid generates an osmotic gradient that drives water into the central nervous system.[39] Concurrently, a carbon dioxide gradient is established between plasma and cerebrospinal fluid, precipitating paradoxical cerebral acidosis that exacerbates the osmotic gradient by the in situ induction of idiogenic osmoles. The consequent osmotic imbalance initiates tissue swelling and cerebral edema. Clinical signs may develop during the dialysis session or up to 24 hours after hemodialysis, and include tremors, restlessness, disorientation, vocalization, amaurosis, seizures, and coma. Many cats, however, lapse acutely into a coma without prodromal warnings. Death may result from respiratory arrest, cerebral herniation and compression, and cerebellar herniation of the brain stem. Treatment includes slowing or discontinuing hemodialysis, administering mannitol (25% Mannitol Injection USP, Abbott Laboratories, North Chicago, IL) (0.5 to 1.0 g/kg IV) to increase plasma osmolality and reduce brain swelling, diazepam (Diazepam Injection, USP, Schein Pharmaceutical, Inc., Norham Park, NJ) to control seizures, and ventilatory support until cerebral edema resolves. The hemodialysis prescription of patients considered to be at risk for dysequilibrium syndrome should be formulated specifically to reduce the rate of solute removal by using lower blood and dialysate flow rates, reversing dialysate flow in the hemodialyzer to dissipate the countercurrent concentration gradients, and lowering the dialysate bicarbonate concentration.[5] Prophylactic mannitol also can be administered at 0.5 to 1.0 g/kg intravenously. Important differential diagnoses for acute neurologic dysfunction during or immediately

Table 45–7. Complications of Hemodialysis

Hypotension/Hypovolemia
Ultrafiltration
Decrease in plasma osmolality
Bioincompatibility
Bleeding
Electrolyte abnormalities (hypokalemia, hyperkalemia, hypercalcemia)
Acetate dialysate
Sepsis
Cardiovascular disease

Neurologic
Dialysis disequilibrium
Uremic encephalopathy

Respiratory
Hypoxemia
Hypoventilation
Pulmonary thromboembolism
Uremic pneumonitis

Hematologic
Transient leukopenia/thrombocytopenia
Anemia

Gastrointestinal
Anorexia, nausea, vomiting

Technical
Inappropriate dialysate composition
Blood pump–induced hemolysis
Undetected ultrafiltration
Air embolism
Blood leakage into dialysate
Extracorporeal blood leakage or clotting
Water contamination

Vascular Access
Positional blood flow interference
Thrombosis
Catheter-related infection

after dialysis include cerebral hemorrhage and cerebral thromboembolism (see later).

Respiratory Complications

Respiratory complications encountered in hemodialysis patients include pulmonary edema, pleural effusion, and intradialytic dyspnea. In the absence of cardiac disease, excessive interdialytic fluid gain is the most common cause of pulmonary edema and pleural effusion (Fig. 45–10). An idiopathic pleural effusion, however, may develop without concomitant overhydration, apparently due to uremia-induced alterations in capillary permeability. Overhydration is managed most appropriately by ultrafiltration to achieve dry body weight, coupled with strict attention to interdialytic fluid management. Water used to blend commercial diets for enteral feeding often is the culprit in interdialytic fluid gain, and every effort must be made to minimize this volume. Idiopathic pleural effusion may require intermittent thoracentesis to alleviate clini-

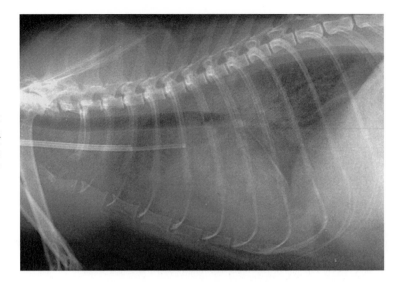

Figure 45–10. Lateral thoracic radiograph of a cat illustrates moderate bilateral pleural effusion and an interstitial pattern in the perihilar region indicative of pulmonary edema. A double-lumen neonatal dialysis catheter is present in the external jugular vein, terminating at the level of the right atrium.

cal signs, in addition to increasing the dose of dialysis to ameliorate the uremic syndrome.

Intradialytic dyspnea may be a consequence of hypoxemia, hypoventilation, pulmonary thromboembolism, or uremic pneumonitis. Dialysis-associated hypoxemia is a biocompatibility reaction in which the alternate complement pathway is activated after contact with the hemodialyzer membrane. Activated complement induces sequestration of neutrophils in the pulmonary capillaries, thus interfering with oxygen diffusion. The hypoxemia generally is mild, but it may be deleterious in patients with concurrent anemia, pulmonary disease, or cardiovascular disease. Hypoxemia develops within 30 to 60 minutes of the start of dialysis, and resolves within 120 minutes after the treatment is discontinued.[40] Administering supplemental oxygen during the hemodialysis session and ensuring adequate oxygen-carrying capacity will minimize hypoxemia. Dialysate with an acetate buffer exacerbates hypoxemia by causing hypoventilation secondary to loss of carbon dioxide into dialysate. This effect is not seen with bicarbonate-based dialysate.[40] *Uremic pneumonitis* refers to a high-protein pulmonary edema that presumably is a consequence of uremic toxins damaging alveoli and increasing capillary permeability.[41] Supplemental oxygenation or mechanical ventilation may be necessary when the injury is severe. Uremic pneumonitis improves with amelioration of azotemia.

Hematologic Complications

Hematologic complications include leukopenia, thrombocytopenia, and anemia. Leukopenia and thrombocytopenia are common, transient, and clinically insignificant consequences of biocompatibility reactions with the hemodialyzer membrane that occur during dialysis.[42] Dialysis-related blood loss may occur from clotting in the hemodialyzer, repeated diagnostic blood sampling, or bleeding from excessive heparinization and platelet dysfunction.

Hemolysis also may occur during the hemodialysis procedure as a result of improper adjustment of the blood pump, excessive pressures in the extracorporeal circuit, dialysate contamination (e.g., copper, aluminum, zinc, nitrates, formaldehyde), dialysate overheating, or dialysate hypotonicity. Periodic blood transfusions may be required to supplement routine treatment with recombinant human erythropoietin (Epogen, Amgen, Inc., Thousand Oaks, CA).

Intradialytic Anorexia, Nausea, and Vomiting

Intradialytic anorexia, nausea, and vomiting are a consequence of hypotension, biocompatibility reactions, dialysis dysequilibrium syndrome, or contaminants in the dialysate. Patient discomfort may be minimized by the use of slow blood flow rates at the start of dialysis treatment with gradual increases to the prescribed rate.

Technical Complications

Technical complications include malfunctions in the dialysate circuit (incorrect composition, incorrect temperature, impure water) or the blood circuit (blood pump hemolysis, undetected ultrafiltration, air embolism, blood leakage into the dialysate, blood losses from leaks, or clotting in the extracorporeal path). These complications are eliminated by employing modern dialysis equipment containing intrinsic safeguards and internal sensors. Temptations to initiate a hemodialysis program with obsolete, discarded, or surplus equipment based on outdated technology should be abandoned solely on the basis of the inherent technical risks.

Vascular Access

Vascular access undoubtedly is the most predictable, problematic, and serious source of dialysis-

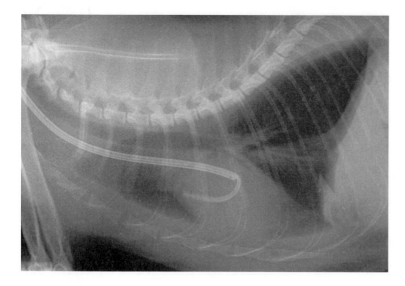

Figure 45–11. Lateral thoracic radiograph of a cat illustrates malpositioning of a transcutaneous double-lumen hemodialysis catheter. Note that the catheter has been advanced past the preferred location (tip of the right atrium), and the catheter tip has folded back on itself in the region of the right atrium.

related complications. Problems that may occur with cuffed tunneled dialysis catheters include placement difficulties, flow impediments, and infectious complications. Strict attention to the initial placement and tip-positioning of hemodialysis catheters will help avoid positional interference with blood flow precipitated by intermittent contact with the right atrium or vena cava (Fig. 45–11). Positional problems may be managed by reducing the blood pump speed temporarily, and by manipulating catheter position by either altering the position of the cat or applying mild traction to the catheter. If these techniques do not afford adequate blood flow, the catheter and extracorporeal blood line connections can be reversed. Habitual flow-related problems necessitate catheter replacement.

Thrombosis

Thrombosis remains the most common and frustrating complication of hemodialysis catheter management (Fig. 45–12). Thrombi impede extracorporeal blood flow and reduce the adequacy of dialysis. Thrombi may develop from the adsorption of thrombin to the catheter, from inadequate interdialytic filling with heparin, or because of an underlying hypercoagulable state. Thrombi may be mural (attached to the wall of the vessel or right atrium), intraluminal, or attached to the tip of the catheter, or may form a sheath around the entire length of the catheter (fibrin sheath thrombus). Intraluminal clots can be managed by thromboaspiration, disruption with a J-tipped guide wire, or instillation of urokinase or streptokinase in volumes sufficient to fill the catheter lumen followed by aspiration after a 30-minute dwell time. Fibrin sheaths, catheter tip clots, and clots in the vascular space or the right atrium are more common and difficult to correct. Attempts to dissolve mural thrombi with fibrinolytic agents or to dislodge the thrombi with J-tipped guide wires generally have been unsuccessful, ne-

cessitating catheter removal and replacement in an alternate vessel. Pulmonary thromboembolism with acute respiratory distress is a serious, but infrequent, complication of dislodged mural thrombi (Fig. 45–13).

Infectious Complications

Infectious complications associated with hemodialysis catheters include bacteremia, sepsis, subcutaneous tunnel infection, Dacron cuff infection, and exit-site infection. Infection typically results from the migration of microorganisms through the catheter insertion site and down the outer surface of the catheter, or from contamination of the catheter lumen during the hemodialysis procedure. Meticulous care of both the catheter and the catheter exit site is necessary to limit the risk of infection. The catheter exit site and catheter ports should be scrubbed with antiseptic soap (Exidine-4 Scrub Solution, Baxter Healthcare Corporation, Deerfield, IL), and a disin-

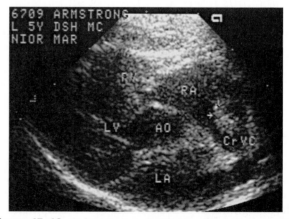

Figure 45–12. Right parasternal oblique cardiac ultrasound image demonstrates a large thrombus (*arrows*) adherent to the right atrium (RA) in a cat with a transcutaneous hemodialysis catheter. AO, aorta; CrVC, cranial vena cava; LA, left atrium; LV, left ventricle; RV, right ventricle.

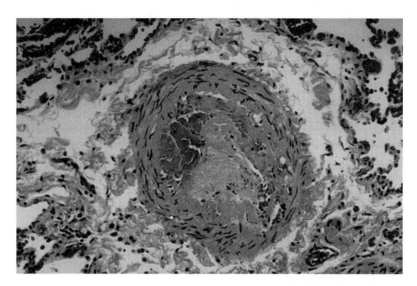

Figure 45–13. Histopathology from a cross section of pulmonary parenchyma from a cat with acute respiratory distress illustrates an acute arterial thrombus (×250).

fectant soaked dressing (0.2 per cent chlorhexidine solution [chlorhexidine diacetate {Nolvasan Solution, Fort Dodge Laboratories, Inc., Fort Dodge, IA}]) should be applied at each dialysis session. Bacterial culture and sensitivity testing is indicated if fever, erythema, pain, or exudate from the catheter exit site are observed. Infections should be managed aggressively with antibiotics and disinfectant-soaked dressings until the inflammation is resolved. If the fever or bacteremia is not resolved within 48 to 72 hours, the catheter should be removed and the Dacron cuff and catheter tip cultured. A new catheter should be placed in an alternate vessel.

◆ EFFICACY

Apart from prolonging survival, the major aim of chronic intermittent hemodialysis is to reduce patient morbidity and improve the quality of life. Several methods have been developed to standardize the assessment of dialysis adequacy, and to permit serial evaluation of dialysis efficiency in human beings. Central to these strategies has been the concept of Kt/V, which describes the dose of dialysis as the hemodialyzer clearance of urea (K) times the duration of dialysis (t) divided by the urea distribution volume (V).[43] Gotch and Sargent[43] described Kt/V as calculated from predialysis and postdialysis BUN and the next predialysis BUN through urea kinetic modeling, a mathematical description of the generation and removal of urea from hemodialysis patients. This approach has been modified by Daugirdas[44] to a formula that uses predialysis and postdialysis BUN concentrations, predialysis and postdialysis body weights, and the duration of dialysis to calculate single-pool or double-pool Kt/V. Kt/V is an index of dialysis adequacy: The higher the Kt/V, the greater the dose of dialysis and efficacy of the dialysis treatment. Values less than 1.0 have been associated with higher rates of treatment failure, morbidity, and mortality.[45, 46]

The URR is a simpler method to evaluate dialysis adequacy. The URR is the change in BUN (predialysis BUN minus postdialysis BUN) divided by the predialysis BUN. The URR is highly correlated with Kt/V, and both URR and Kt/V show an inverse correlation with mortality.[47] Typically, a URR of 0.85 to 0.95 is obtained in cats on standard hemodialysis treatment schedules.[7]

A third method to evaluate dialysis adequacy is the time-average urea concentration (TAC), which reflects the effective exposure of the patient to urea over successive dialysis treatments.[48] TAC is influenced by the individual dialysis treatment, the dialysis schedule, and nondialysis influences on urea metabolism. The higher the TAC, the greater the toxicity and clinical expression of uremia. The dialysis prescription should be formulated to achieve a predialysis BUN less than 90 mg/dl and a TAC of 60 mg/dl or less over the week (Fig. 45–14).

◆ OUTCOME

Hemodialysis and renal transplantation remain the only treatment options available for cats with end-stage renal disease not amenable to conservative medical management. Although there are stringent criteria for selecting patients for renal transplantation, there are no absolute contraindications for the institution of hemodialysis. The purpose of hemodialytic therapy is multifaceted. For many clients, the rationale is to support the cat while pursuing renal transplantation. For cats precluded from transplantation, the goal is to enable good quality of life; in other cases, finite periods of hemodialysis will allow the family to accept the terminal condition of their pet. Since the inception of hemodialysis treatments in 1994, 31 cats with end-stage renal disease have received 221 treatments. Of the 31 cats that started maintenance hemodialysis therapy, 65 per cent died or were euthanized, 15 per cent underwent renal transplantation, and 20 per cent recov-

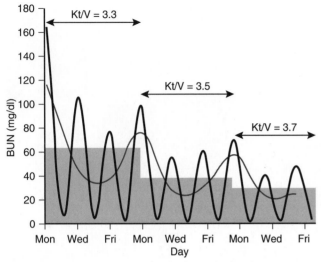

Figure 45–14. Effects of thrice-weekly hemodialysis treatments (4 hr) on blood urea nitrogen (BUN) concentrations (*black curve*) and weekly time-average urea concentration (TAC; *shaded area*) in a 7-year-old 3.6-kg cat with end-stage renal disease prior to renal transplantation. The *lighter curve* is the day-by-day TAC. The average BUN before initiation of hemodialysis was 249 mg/dl. Average predialysis BUN, TAC, the effective urea exposure, and weekly dialysis dose (Kt/V) are shown for 3 dialysis prescriptions. Increasing the Kt/V from 3.3 to 3.7 caused a progressive reduction in predialysis BUN and TAC. Kt/V, hemodialyzer clearance of urea (K) times the duration of dialysis (t) divided by the urea distribution volume (V).

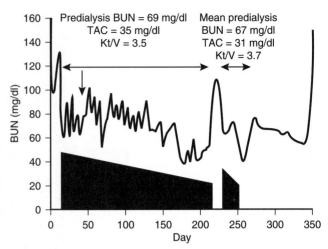

Figure 45–15. Predialysis blood urea nitrogen (BUN) concentrations (*curve*), time-average urea concentrations (TAC; *shaded area*), and average dialysis dose (Kt/V) in a 12-year-old cat undergoing long-term hemodialysis. This cat was managed with conventional medical therapy for chronic pyelonephritis for 155 days before presentation (average BUN, 120 to 170 mg/dl). Hemodialysis was initiated on day 15 after presentation, and performed thrice-weekly for the first 30 days of treatment and twice-weekly (*vertical arrow*) until day 202. The average Kt/V during the first 57 hemodialysis treatments was 3.2; however, there was a gradual reduction in the TAC or effective urea exposure mediated by improvement in residual renal function. Conventional medical management was reinstituted from day 202 until day 216, and from day 248 to day 336, inclusive. Hemodialysis was reinstated between day 216 and day 248 because of acute decompensation. With few exceptions, the BUN remained less than 90 mg/dl. This cat survived nearly 12 months on intermittent hemodialysis with good quality of life. Death was due to cardiac failure secondary to restrictive cardiomyopathy.

ered sufficient renal function to be removed from dialytic therapy (acute exacerbation of underlying CRF). Hemodialysis-related complications (dysequilibrium syndrome or acute respiratory distress and pulmonary thromboembolism) accounted for 45 per cent of all mortality. Forty per cent of cats died or were euthanized owing to comorbid disease (cardiovascular failure, pulmonary edema, diabetes mellitus, hepatic dysfunction). The remaining 15 per cent of cats were withdrawn from hemodialysis on exclusion from renal transplantation. The mean patient survival was 25 days, which is remarkable in light of the severity of uremic syndrome at presentation (mean BUN concentration, 196 mg/dl; mean creatinine concentration, 13.3 mg/dl). It is important to note, however, that some patients have survived for almost a year on maintenance hemodialysis (Fig. 45–15).

◆ CONCLUSIONS

The advent of sophisticated dialysis delivery systems and neonatal dialysis delivery equipment has permitted hemodialysis to be an effective treatment modality for cats with end-stage renal disease. The institution of dialysis should not be based merely on the level of low-molecular-weight solute clearance, but rather on the overall clinical tolerance of the patient to advanced uremia. Important criteria to assess include nutritional status, acid-base and calcium-phosphate equilibria, adequate control of

blood pressure, and comorbid conditions. Many factors influence the choice of hemodialysis including distance to a hemodialysis center, education, and socioeconomic parameters. Future trends may be influenced by increased awareness and acceptance of dialysis as an effective renal replacement therapy, increased demand by owners, and expansion and availability of companion-animal hemodialysis units (Table 45–8).

Table 45–8. Regional Hemodialysis Referral Centers

Companion Animal Hemodialysis Unit
Veterinary Medical Teaching Hospital
University of California–Davis
Davis, CA 95616
Phone: 530–752–1393

The Animal Medical Center
510 E. 62nd Street
New York, NY 10021
Phone: 212–838–8100

Veterinary Referral Associates, Inc.
15021 Dufief Mill Road
Gaithersburg, MD 20878
Phone: 301–340–3224

Veterinary Clinical Center
Michigan State University
East Lansing, MI 48824
Phone: 517–347–5034

REFERENCES

1. Polzin D, Osborne C, Bartges J, et al: Chronic renal failure. *In* Ettinger SJ, Feldman EC (eds): Textbook of Veterinary Internal Medicine: Diseases of the Dog and Cat, 4th ed. Philadelphia, WB Saunders, 1995, pp. 1734–1760.
2. U.S. Renal Data System. Bethesda, MD, National Institutes of Health, National Institute of Diabetes and Digestive and Kidney Disease, April 1999.
3. Mathews KG, Gregory CR: Renal transplants in cats: 66 cases (1987–1996). J Am Vet Med Assoc 211:1432–1436, 1997.
4. Crisp MS, Chew DJ, DiBartola SP, et al: Peritoneal dialysis in dogs and cats: 27 cases (1976–1987). J Am Vet Med Assoc 195:1262–1266, 1989.
5. Cowgill LD, Elliott DA: Hemodialysis. *In* DiBartola SP (ed): Fluid Therapy in Small Animal Practice, 2nd ed. Philadelphia, WB Saunders, 2000, pp. 528–547.
6. Cowgill LD, Langston CE: Role of hemodialysis in the management of dogs and cats with renal failure. Vet Clin North Am Small Anim Pract 26:1347–1378, 1996.
7. Langston CE, Cowgill LD, Spano JA: Applications and outcome of hemodialysis in cats: A review of 29 cases. J Vet Intern Med 11:348–355, 1997.
8. Sargent JA, Gotch FA: Principles and biophysics of dialysis. *In* Maher JF (ed): Replacement of Renal Function by Dialysis, 3rd ed. Dordrecht, The Netherlands, Kluwer Academic, 1989, pp. 87–143.
9. Mujais SK, Schmidt B: Operating characteristics of hollow fiber dialyzers. *In* Nissenson AR, Fine RN, Gentile DE (eds): Clinical Dialysis, 3rd ed. Norwalk, CT, Appleton & Lange, 1995, pp. 77–92.
10. Van Stone JC, Daugirdas JT: Physiological principles. *In* Daugirdas JT, Ing TS (eds): Handbook of Dialysis, 2nd ed. Boston, Little, Brown, 1994, pp. 13–29.
11. Henderson LW: Biophysics of ultrafiltration and hemofiltration. *In* Maher JF (ed): Replacement of Renal Function by Dialysis, 3rd ed. Dordrecht, The Netherlands, Kluwer Academic, 1989, pp. 300–326.
12. Brescia MJ, Cimino JE, Appel K, et al: Chronic hemodialysis using venipuncture and a surgically created arteriovenous fistula. N Engl J Med 275:1089–1092, 1989.
13. Berkoben MS, Schwab SJ: Vascular access for hemodialysis. *In* Nissenson AR, Fine RN, Gentile DE (eds): Clinical Dialysis, 3rd ed. Norwalk, CT, Appleton & Lange, 1995, pp. 26–45.
14. Tesio F, De Baz H, Panarello G, et al: Double catheterization of the internal jugular vein for hemodialysis: Indications, techniques, and clinical results. Artif Organs 18:301–304, 1994.
15. Prabhu PN, Kerns SR, Sabatelli FW, et al: Long-term performance and complications of the Tesio twin catheter system for hemodialysis. Am J Kidney Dis 30:213–218, 1997.
16. Hoenich N, Woffindin C, Ward MK: Dialyzers. *In* Maher JF (ed): Replacement of Renal Function by Dialysis, 3rd ed. Dordrecht, The Netherlands, Kluwer Academic, 1989, pp. 144–180.
17. Ward RA, Schaefer RM, Falkenhagen D, et al: Biocompatibility of a new high-permeability modified cellulose membrane for haemodialysis. Nephrol Dial Transplant 8:47–53, 1993.
18. Falkenhagen D, Bosch T, Brown GS, et al: A clinical study on different cellulosic dialysis membranes. Nephrol Dial Transplant 2:537–545, 1987.
19. Cases A, Reverter JC, Escolar G, et al: In vivo evaluation of platelet activation by different cellulosic membranes. Artif Organs 21:330–334, 1997.
20. Hoenich NA, Woffindin C, Mathews JN, et al: Biocompatibility of membranes used in the treatment of renal failure. Biomaterials 16:587–592, 1995.
21. Schaefer RM, Horl WH, Kokot K, et al: Enhanced biocompatibility with a new cellulosic membrane: Cuprophan versus hemophan. Blood Purif 5:262–267, 1987.
22. Lucchi L, Bonucchi D, Acerbi MA, et al: Improved biocompatibility by modified cellulosic membranes: The case of hemophan. Artif Organs 13:417–421, 1989.
23. Fine RN, Tejani A: Dialysis in infants and children. *In* Daug-

24. irdas JT, Ing TS (eds): Handbook of Dialysis, 2nd ed. Boston, Little, Brown, 1994, pp. 553–568.
24. Ward RA: Acid-base homeostasis in dialysis patients. *In* Nissenson AR, Fine RN, Gentile DE (eds): Clinical Dialysis, 3rd ed. Norwalk, CT, Appleton & Lange, 1995, pp. 495–517.
25. Ledebo I: Bicarbonate in high-efficiency hemodialysis. Cont Issues Nephr 27:9–25, 1993.
26. Steuer RR, Harris DH, Conis JM: A new optical technique for monitoring hematocrit and circulating blood volume: Its application in renal dialysis. Dialysis Transplant 22:260–265, 1993.
27. Steuer RR, Leypoldt JK, Cheung AK, et al: Reducing symptoms during hemodialysis by continuously monitoring the hematocrit. Am J Kidney Dis 27:525–532, 1996.
28. De Lorenzo A, Andreoli A, Matthie J, et al: Predicting body cell mass with bioimpedance by using theoretical methods: A technological review. J Appl Physiol 82:1542–1558, 1997.
29. Matthie J, Zarowitz B, De Lorenzo A, et al: Analytic assessment of the various bioimpedance methods used to estimate body water. J Appl Physiol 84:1801–1816, 1998.
30. Jabara AE, Mehta RL: Determination of fluid shifts during chronic hemodialysis using bioimpedance spectroscopy and an in-line hematocrit monitor. ASAIO J 41:M682–M687, 1995.
31. Jaffrin MY, Maasrani M, Boudailliez B, et al: Extracellular and intracellular fluid volume monitoring during dialysis by multifrequency impedancemetry. ASAIO J 42:M533–M538, 1996.
32. Fisch BJ, Spiegel DM: Assessment of excess fluid distribution in chronic hemodialysis patients using bioimpedance spectroscopy. Kidney Int 49:1105–1109, 1996.
33. Vlchek DL, Burrows-Hudson S: Quality assurance guidelines for hemodialysis devices. DHHS Publication FDA 91-4161 Washington, DC: U.S. Government Printing Office, 1991.
34. Stewart WK: The composition of dialysis fluid. *In* Maher JF (ed): Replacement of Renal Function by Dialysis, 3rd ed. Dordrecht, The Netherlands, Kluwer Academic, 1989, pp. 199–217.
35. Munday HS: Assessment of body composition in cats and dogs. Int J Obes 18:S14–S21, 1994.
36. Elliott DA, Cowgill LD: Body composition analysis in uremic dogs: Methods and clinical significance. *In* Proceedings ACVIM Forum. San Diego, May 22–25, 1998, pp. 661–663.
37. Pencharz PB, Azcue M: Use of bioelectrical impedance analysis measurements in the clinical management of malnutrition. Am J Clin Nutr 64:485S–488S, 1996.
38. Stewart WK, Fleming LW: Blood pressure control during maintenance haemodialysis with isonatric (high sodium) dialysate. Postgrad Med J 50:260–264, 1974.
39. Arieff AI: Dialysis disequilibrium syndrome: Current concepts on pathogenesis and prevention (Editorial). Kidney Int 45:629–635, 1994.
40. DeBroe MJ: Haemodialysis-induced hypoxaemia. Nephrol Dial Transplant 9:173–175, 1994.
41. Grassi V, Malerba M, Boni E, et al: Uremic lung. Contrib Nephrol 106:36–42, 1994.
42. Levett DL, Woffindin C, Bird AG, et al: Complement activation in haemodialysis: A comparison of new and re-used dialysers. Int J Artif Organs 9:97–104, 1986.
43. Gotch FA, Sargent JA: A mechanistic analysis of the National Cooperative Dialysis Study (NCDS). Kidney Int 28:526–534, 1985.
44. Daugirdas JT: Simplified equations for monitoring Kt/V, PCRn, eKtV, and ePCRn. Adv Ren Replace Ther 2:295–304, 1995.
45. Held PJ, Blagg CR, Liska DW, et al: The dose of hemodialysis according to dialysis prescription in Europe and the United States. Kidney Int 38:S16, 1992.
46. Collins AJ, Ma JZ, Umen A, et al: Urea index and other predictors of hemodialysis in patient survival. Am J Kidney Dis 23:272–282, 1994.
47. Held PJ, Port FK, Wolfe RA, et al: The dose of hemodialysis and patient mortality. Kidney Int 50:550–556, 1996.
48. Depner TA: Urea modeling: Introduction. *In* Prescribing Hemodialysis: A Guide to Urea Modeling. Boston, Kluwer Academic, 1991, pp. 39–64.

46

◆ Calcium Oxalate Urolithiasis

Joseph W. Bartges

Calcium oxalate urolith formation is not a specific disease, but results from underlying disorders that promote precipitation of calcium oxalate in urine. Calcium oxalate is the most common mineral component found in uroliths occurring in cats, although struvite remains the most common mineral component of urethral matrix-crystalline plugs.

◆ EPIDEMIOLOGY

In the early 1980s, 88 per cent of feline uroliths submitted to the Minnesota Urolith Center for analysis were composed of struvite (magnesium ammonium phosphate hexahydrate). By 1989, the frequency of struvite uroliths had declined to 70 per cent. By 1991, it was 64 per cent, and by 1996, it was 48 per cent. During the same period, the percentage of feline calcium oxalate uroliths increased. Five per cent of feline uroliths submitted in 1984 were calcium oxalate, whereas 40 per cent submitted in 1996 were calcium oxalate (Fig. 46–1). These trends suggest a disproportionate increase in the prevalence of calcium oxalate uroliths compared with other urolith types.[1] Furthermore, the majority of nephroliths occurring in cats are composed of calcium salts, and calcium oxalate is most common.

◆ ETIOPATHOGENESIS

Mechanisms of Urolith Formation

Overview

Urolith formation, dissolution, and prevention involves complex physical processes. Major factors include: (1) supersaturation resulting in crystal formation, (2) effects of inhibitors of crystallization and inhibitors of crystal aggregation and growth, (3) crystalloid complexors, (4) effects of promoters of crystal aggregation and growth, and (5) effects of noncrystalline matrix.[2, 3] A sequence of events leading to urolith formation is illustrated in Figure 46–2.

Concept of Urine Saturation

An important driving force behind urolith formation is supersaturation of urine with calculogenic substances.[2] This concept can be illustrated with table salt (NaCl) and deionized water. When a salt is added to a solvent (such as NaCl in water), it dissolves in the solvent. The solution is said to be *undersaturated* because water contains such a low concentration of NaCl that if more NaCl is added, it will dissolve. As more NaCl is added, a concentration is reached beyond which further dissolution of NaCl is not possible (Fig. 46–3). At this point, water

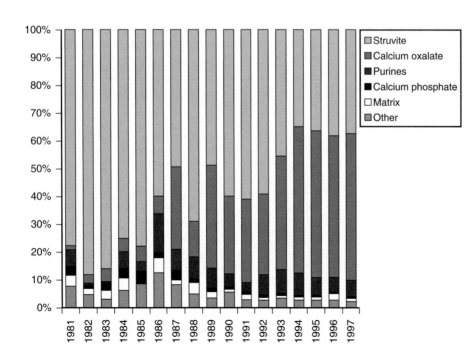

Figure 46–1. Changing trends in mineral composition of feline uroliths submitted to the Minnesota Urolith Center. (Modified from Osborne CA, Kruger JM, Lulich JP, et al: Feline lower urinary tract diseases. *In* Ettinger SJ, Feldman EC [eds]: Textbook of Veterinary Internal Medicine, 5th ed. Philadelphia, WB Saunders, 2000, pp. 1710–1746.)

(solvent) is said to be *saturated* with NaCl. If additional NaCl is added to the water, it will form crystals unless the temperature and/or pH is changed. The concentration at which saturation is reached and crystallization begins is called the *thermodynamic solubility product* (Fig. 46–4; see also Fig. 46–3). The thermodynamic solubility product is a constant at which pure crystals of NaCl form in pure water.

Urine, however, is a more complex solution than pure water. Urine contains ions and proteins that interact with and potentially complex with calcium and oxalic acid so as to allow them to remain in solution. This explains why calcium and oxalic acid in urine do not normally precipitate to form calcium oxalate crystals. Compared with water, urine normally is *supersaturated* with respect to calcium and oxalic acid. Energy is required to maintain this state of calcium and oxalic acid solubility, and urine must constantly "struggle" to maintain calcium and oxalic acid in solution. Thus, urine is described as being *metastable,* implying varying degrees of

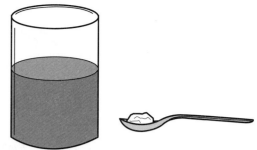

1 tsp of salt dissolves completely (water is *undersaturated* with respect to salt)

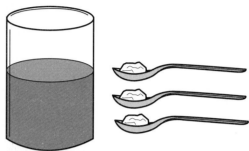

3 tsp of salt dissolves completely, but any additional salt will result in precipitation (water is *saturated* with respect to salt)

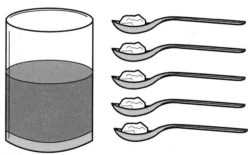

5 tsp of salt does not dissolve completely and results in precipitation (water is *supersaturated* with respect to salt)

Figure 46–3. States of saturation illustrated by adding salt to water.

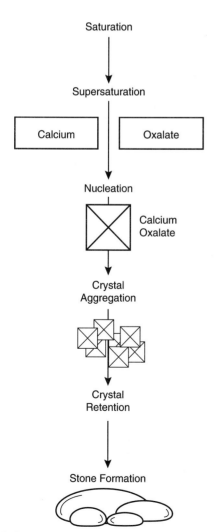

Figure 46–2. Sequence of events leading to calcium oxalate urolith formation.

instability with respect to the potential for calcium oxalate crystals to form (see Fig. 46–4). In this metastable state, new calcium oxalate crystals will not precipitate, but if already present, crystals can be maintained and even may grow in size. If the concentration of calcium and oxalic acid is increased, a threshold eventually is reached at which urine cannot hold more calcium and oxalic acid in solution. The urine concentration at which this occurs is the *thermodynamic formation product* of calcium oxalate. Above the thermodynamic formation product, urine is *oversaturated* and unstable with respect to calcium and oxalic acid. Thus, calcium oxalate crystals will precipitate spontaneously, grow in size, and aggregate together.

Why is conceptual understanding of these interrelated concepts of clinical importance? The answer is that uroliths (e.g., struvite) may be dissolved by medical treatment that changes urine from a state of oversaturation or metastability to a state of undersat-

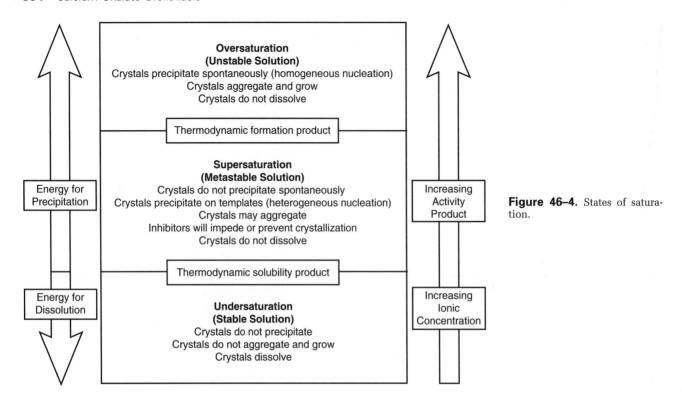

Figure 46–4. States of saturation.

uration with the components of minerals in the uroliths. Medical therapy used to prevent urolith formation must be designed to create a state of undersaturation (or at least metastability) as long as there is no mechanism for heterogeneous nucleation present (see Fig. 46–4).

Calcium Oxalate Crystallization and Urolith Formation

Overview

Calcium oxalate urolith formation occurs when urine is oversaturated with calcium and oxalate.[4] Additional risk factors for urolith formation include breed, gender, age, and diet. Once initiation of urolith formation has occurred, the nidus must be retained within the urinary tract, and conditions must favor continued precipitation of minerals to promote growth of uroliths. Therefore, for calcium oxalate to form, urine must be oversaturated with calcium and oxalic acid, and certain conditions (e.g., aciduria) must be present. Alterations in the balance between urine concentrations of calculogenic substances (calcium and oxalic acid) and crystallization inhibitors (citrate, phosphorus, magnesium, sodium, or potassium) have been associated with initiation and growth of calcium oxalate uroliths. In addition to these alterations in activities of ions, high-molecular-weight proteins occurring in urine, such as nephrocalcin, uropontin, and Tamm-Horsfall mucoprotein, have an influence on calcium oxalate formation.[5] The role of these macromolecular and ionic inhibitors of calcium oxalate formation has not been studied in cats.

Few studies have been performed concerning calcium oxalate uroliths in cats. Risk of struvite and calcium oxalate formation is inversely related in cats depending on age. Young non–urolith-forming cats apparently have higher struvite and lower calcium oxalate urine saturation, and older cats apparently have lower struvite and higher calcium oxalate urine saturation.[6] In non–urolith-forming young adult cats, urine saturation is in the metastable range for calcium oxalate (Bartges JW, personal observation, College of Veterinary Medicine, The University of Tennessee, 1999).

Etiologic Risk Factors

Hypercalciuria

Excessive urinary excretion of calcium is a significant contributor to calcium oxalate formation in human beings and dogs. In human beings, however, 24-hour urinary excretion of calcium is normal in some calcium oxalate urolith-formers, and in some non–urolith-forming human beings, 24-hour urinary excretion of calcium is increased.[7] Hypercalciuria is thought to be a risk factor, but not necessarily the cause of calcium oxalate urolith formation in human beings.

Calcium homeostasis is achieved through actions of parathyroid hormone (PTH) and 1,25-dihydroxycholecalciferol (1,25-vitamin D) on bone, intestine, and kidney. When serum ionized calcium concentration decreases, PTH and 1,25-vitamin D activities increase, resulting in mobilization of calcium from bone, increased absorption of calcium from intestine, and increased reabsorption of calcium by renal tubules. Conversely, high serum ionized calcium concentration suppresses release of PTH and production of 1,25-vitamin D, resulting in decreased bone mobilization of calcium, decreased intestinal absorption of calcium, and increased urinary excretion of calcium. Therefore, hypercalciuria can result from excessive intestinal absorption of calcium (gastrointestinal hyperabsorption), impaired renal reabsorption of calcium (renal leak), or excessive skeletal mobilization of calcium (resorptive). In miniature schnauzers, gastrointestinal hyperabsorption appears to occur most commonly, although renal leak hypercalciuria also has been observed.[8]

Consumption by cats of diets supplemented with the urinary acidifier ammonium chloride has been associated with increased urinary calcium excretion.[9] Additionally, consumption by human beings of diets containing high amounts of animal protein results in increased urinary calcium excretion. These factors result in metabolic acidosis. Metabolic acidosis promotes hypercalciuria by promoting bone turnover (release of calcium with buffers from bone), increasing serum ionized calcium concentration leading to increased urinary calcium excretion, and decreasing renal tubular reabsorption of calcium. In dogs, hypercalciuria resulting from ammonium chloride administration was decreased by bicarbonate administration.[10] In cats, magnesium supplementation was associated with increased urinary calcium excretion, and diets containing magnesium chloride, which promotes aciduria, were associated with greater urinary calcium excretion than that found in diets supplemented with magnesium oxide, which promotes alkaluria.[11] Magnesium may increase blood ionized calcium concentration while suppressing PTH release.

Although excessive dietary intake of calcium may result in hypercalciuria, studies in human beings refute this hypothesis. Apparently, dietary calcium may bind to dietary oxalic acid, resulting in calcium oxalate formation in the lumen of the gastrointestinal tract thereby preventing absorption of calcium and oxalate. Hypercalciuria also may occur with administration of loop diuretics, glucocorticoids, urinary acidifiers, and vitamin D or C.

Hyperoxaluria

Oxalic acid is a metabolic end-product of ascorbic acid and several amino acids, such as glycine and serine, derived from dietary sources. Oxalic acid forms soluble salts with sodium and potassium ions, but a relatively insoluble salt with calcium ions. Therefore, increased urinary excretion of oxalic acid may promote calcium oxalate formation. Hyperoxaluria has been observed in kittens consuming diets deficient in vitamin B_6 (<1 mg/kg of diet).[12] Hyperoxaluria also has been recognized in a group of related cats with reduced quantities of hepatic D-glycerate dehydrogenase, an enzyme involved in metabolism of oxalic acid precursors (primary hyperoxaluria type II).[13] Hyperoxaluria also has been

associated with defective peroxisomal alanine-glyoxylate aminotransferase activity (primary hyperoxaluria type I) and intestinal disease in human beings (enteric hyperoxaluria). These disorders have not been evaluated in cats.

Altered Inhibitors and Promoters of Calcium Oxalate Crystal Formation

Urine is a complex solution containing many substances that may inhibit or promote crystal formation and growth. Some inhibitors, such as citrate, magnesium, and pyrophosphate, form soluble salts with calcium or oxalic acid and thereby reduce the availability of calcium or oxalic acid for precipitation. Other inhibitors are macromolecular proteins, such as Tamm-Horsfall glycoprotein and nephrocalcin, which interfere with the ability of calcium and oxalic acid to combine thereby minimizing crystal formation and growth. Other urinary substances, such as uric acid, may promote calcium oxalate formation by blocking inhibitors of crystallization, whereas others, such as calcium phosphate crystals or extraluminal suture material from a previous cystotomy, may serve as templates for heterogeneous crystal nucleation. The role, if any, of these crystallization inhibitors and promoters has not been evaluated in cats, but such studies are under way.

◆ CLINICAL SIGNS

Clinical signs observed with urolithiasis depend on the location of uroliths, underlying disease processes, and sequelae related to presence of uroliths. More than 95 per cent of calcium oxalate uroliths that occur in cats form in the lower urinary tract, and approximately 2.5 per cent of calcium oxalate uroliths form in the upper urinary tract.[14] Cats with calcium oxalate urocystoliths may exhibit inappropriate urination, stranguria, pollakiuria, and hematuria. If uroliths become lodged in the urethra, anuria may be noted. Calcium oxalate nephroliths may be associated with abdominal pain, hematuria, or uremia if uroliths are bilateral and cause ureteral obstruction. In some cats, clinical signs are not present.

◆ DIFFERENTIAL DIAGNOSIS

Clinical signs of calcium oxalate uroliths that occur in the lower urinary tract are similar to those of other lower urinary tract diseases. In cats less than 10 years of age, idiopathic feline lower urinary tract disease occurs in 55 to 70 per cent of cats with lower urinary tract signs, urolithiasis occurs in 10 to 20 per cent, urethral plugs in 20 per cent, and bacterial urinary tract infection in 1 to 2 per cent.[15, 16] However, in cats older than 10 years, bacterial urinary tract infection may occur in up to 45 per cent of those with lower urinary tract signs, urolithiasis in 10 to 20 per cent, idiopathic feline lower urinary tract disease in 5 per cent, and urethral plugs in 5 per cent. The majority of uroliths occurring in older cats are composed of calcium oxalate.[17]

◆ DIAGNOSIS

Patient Signalment

Calcium oxalate urolith formation occurs in many breeds of cats, but Himalayans and Persians appear to be at greater risk. In dogs and human beings, males are more commonly affected with calcium oxalate uroliths than are females, but the incidence is approximately equal in cats. The male-to-female ratio of calcium urolith formation is 3.5:1.0 in human beings,[18] 2.7:1.0 in dogs,[19] and 1.4:1.0 in cats.[20] Although cats of any age may form calcium oxalate uroliths, most affected cats are older than 4 years. The median age of calcium oxalate urolith detection is 5 years in affected cats.

Urinalysis

Two types of calcium oxalate crystals have been recognized in urine: calcium oxalate dihydrate (Fig. 46–5) and calcium oxalate monohydrate. Detection of calcium oxalate crystals indicates that urine is supersaturated with calcium oxalate, and if persistent, represents an increased risk for calcium oxalate urolith formation. However, calcium oxalate crystalluria is present in less than 50 per cent of cases at the time of diagnosis of urolithiasis.

Although urine pH is an important determinant of struvite, urate, and cystine solubility, it has minimum influence on calcium oxalate solubility between pH values of 5.0 and 7.5. Nevertheless, acid-uria usually is present at the time of calcium oxalate urolith detection. Aciduria may represent a risk factor for calcium oxalate formation because acidemia promotes mobilization of carbonate and phosphorus from bone to buffer the acid load. Mobilization of bone results in mobilization of calcium, which may result in hypercalciuria.

Another risk factor for urolith formation is highly concentrated urine. Cats can achieve urine specific gravities in excess of 1.065, indicating a marked ability to produce concentrated urine. Highly concentrated urine may result in increased urinary concentrations of calcium or oxalic acid, which increases the risk for urolith formation. Many cats with calcium oxalate uroliths have urine specific gravity values greater than 1.040 unless there is some impairment of renal function or concentrating ability.

Serum Biochemical Analysis

In most cats, results of serum biochemical analysis including calcium concentration are normal. However, in approximately 33 per cent of cats with calcium oxalate uroliths, hypercalcemia in the range of 11.0 to 14.0 mg/dl occurs. Although hyperparathyroidism, hypervitaminosis D, and malignant neoplasia may result in hypercalcemia, they are diagnosed rarely in cats with calcium oxalate uroliths. If calcium oxalate uroliths result in urethral obstruction or bilateral ureteral obstruction, serum biochemical changes consistent with postrenal uremia may be present.

Imaging Characteristics

Calcium oxalate uroliths may be located anywhere in the urinary tract, and may be observed to occur

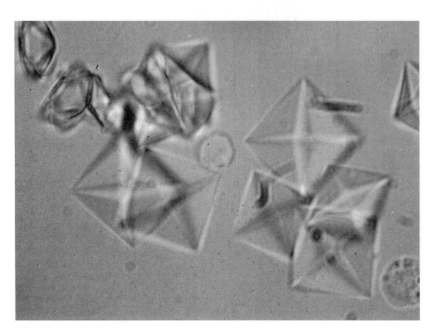

Figure 46–5. Photomicrograph of calcium oxalate dihydrate crystals in urine sediment of an adult male cat. Original magnification, ×160.

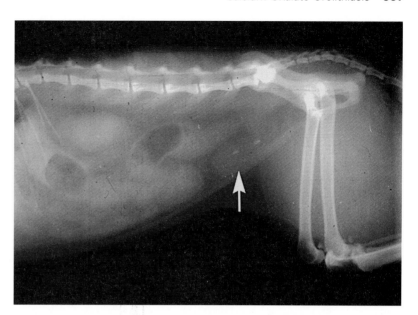

Figure 46–6. Lateral abdominal radiograph of a 9-year-old male cat with 2 uroliths in the urinary bladder (*arrow*). The urocystoliths were composed of 90 per cent calcium oxalate dihydrate and 10 per cent calcium oxalate monohydrate.

in both the upper and the lower urinary tract at the same time, but they are located most commonly in the urinary bladder.[20] Analysis of uroliths submitted to the Minnesota Urolith Center revealed that a higher percentage of nephroliths were composed of calcium oxalate (40.6 per cent, n = 101) compared with uroliths from the lower urinary tract (23.7 per cent, n = 2667).[21]

Calcium oxalate uroliths tend to have radiographic density similar to that of bone and therefore are radiodense relative to soft tissue by survey abdominal radiography (Fig. 46–6). Calcium oxalate uroliths may be single or multiple and vary from less than 1 mm to several centimeters in diameter. Uroliths composed primarily of calcium oxalate monohydrate tend to be round or elliptical and have a smooth surface (Fig. 46–7). Uroliths composed primarily of calcium oxalate dihydrate or a combination of calcium oxalate dihydrate and monohydrate tend to be round or ovoid and have an irregular surface (Fig. 46–8).

Contrast radiography usually is not necessary to identify calcium oxalate uroliths because of their radiodensity, but contrast radiography may be beneficial in assessing the consequences of urolithiasis. Excretory urography may be performed to determine whether a renal mineral density is located in the pelvis or ureter or whether ureteral obstruction is present (Fig. 46–9), and contrast urethrography may be used to determine whether the urolith is located in the urethral lumen.

Abdominal ultrasonography also may be used to determine location of calcium oxalate uroliths, but it cannot be used to aid in estimation of mineral composition (Fig. 46–10). Ureteral obstruction may be diagnosed by ultrasonography if renal pelvic dilatation or proximal ureteral dilatation is present.

Endocrine Testing

In the few cats with calcium oxalate uroliths that have been evaluated, hyperparathyroidism and hy-

pervitaminosis D were not present[22] despite hypercalcemia occurring in approximately 33 per cent of affected cats.[20] In cats that have persistent hypercalcemia, serum PTH concentrations should be determined (see Chapter 41, Idiopathic Hypercalcemia).

Urine Chemistry Analysis

There is a paucity of information concerning urinary concentrations of calculogenic substances in cats. In studies performed in our laboratory, non–urolith-forming cats excrete 0.2 to 0.7 mg/kg/day of calcium. This is similar to what has been reported in clinically healthy beagles.[8] No data have been published in calcium oxalate urolith-forming cats, but such studies are under way. Collection of 24-

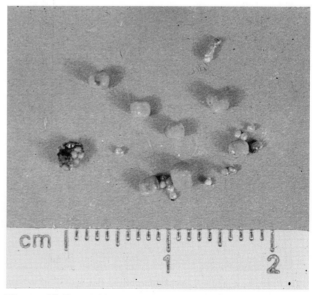

Figure 46–7. Urocystoliths composed of 100 per cent calcium oxalate monohydrate removed from a 7-year-old male cat.

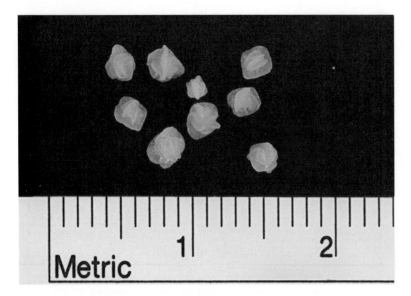

Figure 46–8. Urocystoliths composed of 100 per cent calcium oxalate dihydrate removed from a 12-year-old male cat.

hour or optimally 48-hour urine samples is preferred to urine metabolite–to–urine creatinine ratios or fractional excretions of urinary metabolites because these values have been determined to be unreliable.

Tests of Urine Saturation

Preliminary evaluation of clinically healthy cats in our laboratory has revealed that urinary activity product ratios for calcium oxalate (APR$_{caox}$), a measure of urinary saturation with calcium oxalate, are in the metastable range (APR$_{caox}$ = 1.5 to 3.0). Urine in the metastable range is oversaturated with calcium oxalate, but crystals do not form spontaneously or precipitate, presumably owing to the presence of crystallization inhibitors. In the few cats with naturally-occurring calcium oxalate uroliths that we have evaluated, APR$_{caox}$ was greater than 5.0. Additional studies are under way.

Analysis of Voided or Retrieved Uroliths

Quantitative analysis of uroliths voided during micturition or retrieved via voiding urohydropropul-

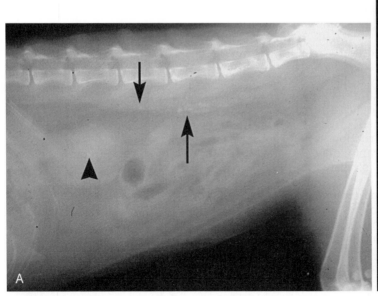
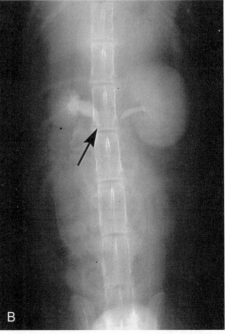

Figure 46–9. *A,* Survey lateral abdominal radiograph of a 7-year-old male cat with uroliths in the right ureter (*arrows*) and a urolith in the right kidney (*arrowhead*). *B,* Ventrodorsal abdominal radiograph obtained 10 minutes after injection of radiopaque contrast agent into the cat. The proximal right ureter and right renal pelvis are dilated owing to obstruction by ureteroliths (*arrow*). Also, the right kidney is small. The mineral composition of the ureteroliths was 95 per cent calcium oxalate dihydrate and 5 per cent calcium oxalate monohydrate.

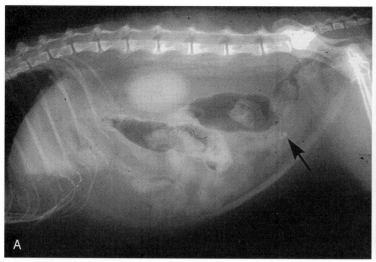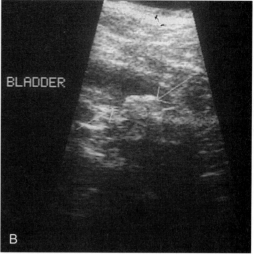

Figure 46–10. *A,* Survey lateral abdominal radiograph of a 13-year-old female cat with a urolith in the urinary bladder (*arrow*). *B,* Ultrasonographic image of the urocystolith (*arrow*) described in *A.* The urocystolith was composed of 85 per cent calcium oxalate dihydrate and 15 per cent calcium oxalate monohydrate.

sion, urinary catheterization, or cystotomy provides the most information about the mineral composition of uroliths. When compared with quantitative analysis, qualitative analysis agreed in only 43 per cent of cases. Consequently, quantitative analysis is preferred.

◆ TREATMENT
Urocystoliths and Urethroliths

Medical protocols that will promote dissolution of calcium oxalate uroliths in cats are not currently available, and uroliths must be removed physically. If urethral obstruction is present, uroliths should be retropulsed into the urinary bladder. Voiding urohydropropulsion or catheterization may retrieve uroliths that have a diameter smaller than the smallest luminal diameter of the urethra. Typically, uroliths smaller than approximately 5 mm in female cats and 1 mm in male cats can be retrieved. For larger uroliths, a cystotomy must be performed. After surgery, abdominal radiography should be performed to ensure that all uroliths have been removed. Calcium oxalate urocystoliths may be removed incompletely in approximately 20 per cent of cases undergoing cystotomy.[20] Occasionally, urethroliths cannot be retropulsed into the bladder because of the irregular surface contour of calcium oxalate uroliths. If located in the distal penile urethra, a perineal urethrostomy should be considered. If uroliths are not causing clinical signs and surgery is not an option, measures may be taken to prevent further increase in size or number (see Prevention).

Nephroliths and Ureteroliths

Nephroliths and ureteroliths commonly are composed of calcium oxalate. Calcium oxalate uroliths

cannot be dissolved using medical protocols, and surgical removal is the only option if the urolith must be removed. Lithotripsy has been used in dogs, but data from a small number of cats indicate that use of extracorporeal shock wave lithotripsy (using a Dornier HM-3 lithotriptor) is not effective and may be associated with complications.[23] Therefore, lithotripsy is not recommended in cats at this time. Frequently, nephroliths or renal mineral densities are observed incidentally on survey abdominal radiographs. In animals that are hematuric or have renal failure or nonspecific abdominal pain, nephroliths or ureteroliths may be the cause. The decision to remove a nephrolith or ureterolith should be made carefully, because of the difficulty associated with ureteral surgery in cats and the long-term renal damage induced by nephrotomy. Upper urinary tract uroliths should be removed if they are causing obstruction resulting in diminished renal function, if they are associated with severe hematuria, pain, or persistent bacterial infection, or if they are increasing in size and damaging renal tissue. If none of these conditions is present, a reasonable alternative approach may be to use preventive measures to minimize an increase in size or number of uroliths (see Prevention). Monitoring may be accomplished by performing abdominal radiography every 3 to 6 months. If uroliths increase in size or number, or cause pain, hematuria, infection, or obstruction, they should be removed surgically, hopefully to prevent loss of the affected kidney.

◆ PREVENTION

After surgical or nonsurgical removal of uroliths, medical protocols should be considered to minimize urolith recurrence or to prevent further growth of uroliths remaining in the urinary tract (Fig. 46–11). No studies have been performed to evaluate the

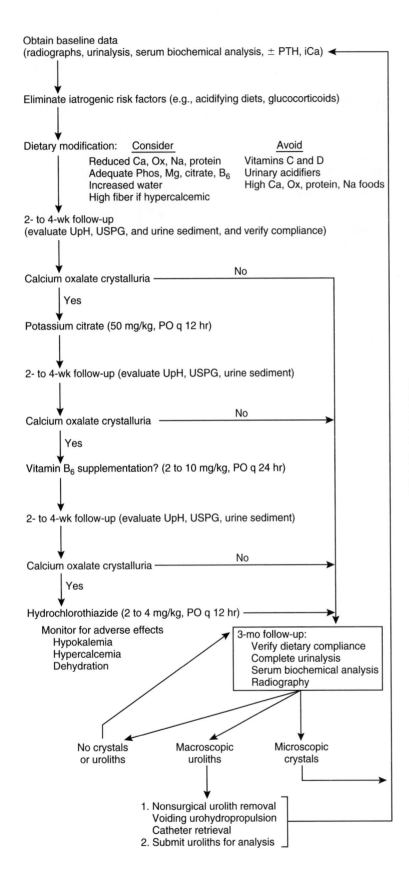

Obtain baseline data
(radiographs, urinalysis, serum biochemical analysis, ± PTH, iCa)

Eliminate iatrogenic risk factors (e.g., acidifying diets, glucocorticoids)

Dietary modification: Consider   Avoid
                        Reduced Ca, Ox, Na, protein   Vitamins C and D
                        Adequate Phos, Mg, citrate, B₆   Urinary acidifiers
                        Increased water   High Ca, Ox, protein, Na foods
                        High fiber if hypercalcemic

2- to 4-wk follow-up
(evaluate UpH, USPG, and urine sediment, and verify compliance)

Calcium oxalate crystalluria ———————————— No

Yes

Potassium citrate (50 mg/kg, PO q 12 hr)

2- to 4-wk follow-up (evaluate UpH, USPG, urine sediment)

Calcium oxalate crystalluria ———————————— No

Yes

Vitamin B₆ supplementation? (2 to 10 mg/kg, PO q 24 hr)

2- to 4-wk follow-up (evaluate UpH, USPG, urine sediment)

Calcium oxalate crystalluria ———————————— No

Yes

Hydrochlorothiazide (2 to 4 mg/kg, PO q 12 hr) ————————

Monitor for adverse effects
    Hypokalemia
    Hypercalcemia
    Dehydration

3-mo follow-up:
    Verify dietary compliance
    Complete urinalysis
    Serum biochemical analysis
    Radiography

No crystals   Macroscopic   Microscopic
or uroliths   uroliths   crystals

1. Nonsurgical urolith removal
   Voiding urohydropropulsion
   Catheter retrieval
2. Submit uroliths for analysis

Figure 46–11. Algorithm for managing feline calcium oxalate uroliths. B₆, vitamin B₆; Ca, calcium; iCa, ionized calcium; Mg, magnesium; Na, sodium; Ox, oxalate; Phos, phosphorus; PO, by mouth; PTH, parathyroid hormone concentration; q, every; UpH, urine pH; USPG, urine specific gravity. (Modified from Lulich JP, Osborne CA, Felice LJ: Calcium oxalate urolithiasis: Cause, detection, and control. *In* August JR [ed]: Consultations in Feline Internal Medicine, vol. 2. Philadelphia, WB Saunders, 1994, pp. 343–349.)

likelihood of recurrence of calcium oxalate uroliths in cats. However, many cats that are evaluated have a history of recurrent urolithiasis, and it is likely that calcium oxalate uroliths are as likely to be recurrent in cats as they are in dogs and human beings.

In cats with hypercalcemia, the cause of hypercalcemia should be investigated and corrected if possible (see Chapter 41, Idiopathic Hypercalcemia). Potential but uncommon causes of hypercalcemia in cats with calcium oxalate uroliths include primary hyperparathyroidism, chronic vitamin D toxicity, neoplasia (thymoma, multiple myeloma, lymphosarcoma, squamous cell carcinoma), and chronic granulomatous disease associated with systemic mycotic infections.

Dietary Considerations

Goals of dietary prevention include reducing calcium concentrations in urine, reducing oxalic acid concentrations in urine, promoting high concentration and activity of inhibitors of calcium oxalate crystal growth and aggregation in urine, and maintaining dilute urine.

Calcium and Oxalic Acid

Although reduction of urine calcium and oxalic acid concentrations by reduction of dietary calcium and oxalic acid appears logical, it is not without potential harm. Reducing consumption of only one of these constituents may increase the availability and absorption of the other from the intestinal tract, resulting in increased urinary excretion. Therefore, to be effective, both calcium and oxalic acid should be reduced. Although excessive consumption of calcium and oxalic acid should be avoided, the general consensus is that restricting dietary calcium is unwarranted, unless gastrointestinal hyperabsorption of calcium has been documented. Even then, only moderate restriction is advised.

Sodium

Consumption of large amounts of sodium may augment renal calcium excretion in dogs and human beings. Although not evaluated in cats, dietary sodium restriction appears warranted. Orally administered sodium chloride or use of loop diuretics, which promote renal sodium excretion, for diuresis also should be avoided because they may increase urinary calcium excretion and increase the risk of calcium oxalate urolith formation.

Phosphorus

Dietary phosphorus should not be restricted in cats with calcium oxalate urolithiasis because reduction in dietary phosphorus may be associated with activation of vitamin D, which promotes intestinal calcium absorption and increases urinary calcium excretion. Additionally, pyrophosphate is an inhibitor of calcium oxalate urolith formation. If calcium oxalate urolithiasis is associated with hypophosphatemia and normal calcium concentration, oral phosphorus supplementation may be considered. Caution should be used, however, because excessive dietary phosphorus may predispose to formation of calcium phosphate uroliths. Whether this occurs in cats is unknown.

Magnesium

Urinary magnesium is an inhibitor of calcium oxalate crystal formation. Magnesium may bind oxalic acid, thereby preventing it from combining with calcium to form calcium oxalate. Many diets formulated to minimize recurrence of struvite (magnesium ammonium phosphate hexahydrate) are reduced in magnesium. It appears logical that magnesium should not be restricted in diets that are consumed by cats with calcium oxalate urolithiasis. Supplemental magnesium has been used to minimize recurrence of calcium oxalate uroliths in human beings, but supplemental magnesium may increase the risk of struvite formation. At this time, the risks and benefits of magnesium supplementation to cats with calcium oxalate urolithiasis have not been evaluated, and magnesium supplementation is not advised.

Protein

Consumption of high amounts of animal protein by human beings is associated with an increased risk of calcium oxalate formation. Dietary protein of animal origin may increase urinary calcium and oxalic acid excretion, decrease urinary citrate excretion, and promote bone mobilization in order to buffer the acid intake from metabolism of animal protein that in turn results in increased urinary calcium excretion. Cats are obligatory carnivores, and the effectiveness and safety of dietary protein restriction in the management of calcium oxalate urolithiasis are unknown in this species.

Acidifying Diets

Solubility of calcium oxalate in urine is influenced minimally by pH, but epidemiologic studies have identified aciduria as a risk factor for calcium oxalate formation in cats.[1] Persistent aciduria may be associated with low-grade metabolic acidosis, which promotes bone mobilization and increases urinary excretion of calcium. Administration of ammonium chloride to healthy cats resulted in increased urinary calcium excretion.[9] In 5 cats with hypercalcemia and calcium oxalate uroliths, discontinuation of acidifying diets or urinary acidifiers was associated with normalization of serum calcium concentration.[22] Therefore, feeding an acidifying diet or administering urinary acidifiers is discouraged. A reasonable goal in cats that have had calcium oxalate uroliths is to induce a urine pH of 6.5 to 7.5.

Vitamins B₆, C, and D

Excessive amounts of vitamin D (which promotes intestinal absorption of calcium) and vitamin C (which is a precursor of oxalic acid) should be avoided. Furthermore, vitamin C is a weak urinary acidifier, which may increase the likelihood of urolith recurrence. The diet should be adequately fortified with vitamin B₆, because vitamin B₆ deficiency promotes endogenous production and subsequent urinary excretion of oxalic acid.[12]

Fiber

Increased dietary fiber intake is associated with decreasing risk of calcium oxalate recurrence in some human beings. Certain types of fiber decrease calcium absorption from the gastrointestinal tract, which may decrease urinary calcium excretion. Also, higher-fiber diets tend to be less acidifying. In 5 cats with idiopathic hypercalcemia and calcium oxalate uroliths, feeding a high-fiber diet resulted in normalization of serum calcium concentrations.[22] However, the safety and efficacy of increased fiber intake are unproved at this time.

Water

Increasing urine volume is a mainstay of preventive therapy for calcium oxalate urolithiasis in human beings. By increasing urine volume, concentrations of calculogenic minerals may be reduced, but increasing urine volume may decrease the concentrations of inhibitors. Despite this potential problem, increasing urine volume appears to be a logical recommendation. This may be accomplished by feeding canned formulated diets or by adding water to dry formulated diets. Sodium chloride should not be added to the diet in an effort to stimulate thirst because the increased dietary sodium may increase urinary calcium excretion.

Available Diets

At the time of writing, there are 3 diets that are formulated and marketed for prevention of calcium oxalate uroliths in cats (Table 46–1). These diets contain potassium citrate (as an alkalinizing agent and as a source of citrate) and induce a urine pH of approximately 7.0. None has been tested in cats that form calcium oxalate uroliths, but consumption of c/d^oxl (Hill's Pet Nutrition, Inc.) and S/O pH Control Formula (Waltham, England) by healthy cats results in low urine saturation with calcium oxalate. Clinical trials are under way. I have had some success in reducing mild hypercalcemia in some calcium oxalate urolith-forming cats by feeding a high-fiber diet (Prescription diet w/d, Hill's Pet Nutrition, Inc.,

Topeka, KS) and administering potassium citrate (see later).

Pharmacologic Treatment

Occasionally, dietary management is not sufficient to control calcium oxalate crystalluria or urolithiasis. Several pharmacologic agents have been used in human beings and dogs, and may be of benefit in cats with difficult-to-control calcium oxalate uroliths.

Citrate

Citric acid inhibits calcium oxalate crystal formation because it forms a soluble salt with calcium. Some human beings with abnormally low urinary concentration of citric acid are at risk for calcium oxalate urolith formation. Oral potassium citrate may be beneficial in managing calcium oxalate uroliths because of its alkalinizing effects, in addition to potentially increasing urinary citric acid concentration. In dogs, chronic metabolic acidosis inhibits renal tubular reabsorption of calcium, whereas metabolic alkalosis enhances tubular reabsorption of calcium.[24] Potassium citrate is preferred to sodium bicarbonate or sodium citrate because oral administration of sodium may increase urinary calcium excretion. Potassium citrate is administered at a starting dosage of approximately 50 mg/kg orally (PO) every (q) 12 hr. Dosage is titrated by monitoring urine pH with the goal of obtaining values between 7.0 and 7.5.

Vitamin B₆

Vitamin B₆ increases transamination of glyoxylate, a precursor of oxalic acid, to glycine. Experimentally induced vitamin B₆ deficiency resulted in renal precipitation of calcium oxalate and hyperoxaluria in kittens,[12] but a naturally occurring form of this syndrome has not been observed. In cats consuming diets deficient in vitamin B₆, additional vitamin B₆ was associated with decreased oxalic acid excretion, but the ability of supplemental vitamin B₆ to reduce urinary oxalic acid excretion in cats with calcium oxalate urolithiasis is unknown. Vitamin B₆ supplementation is inexpensive and safe, and therefore it may be considered in cats with difficult-to-manage calcium oxalate uroliths. A dosage of 2 to 10 mg/kg PO q 24 hr may be used.

Thiazide Diuretics

Thiazide diuretics are recommended to reduce recurrence of calcium-containing uroliths in human beings because of the ability of these agents to reduce urinary calcium excretion. The exact mechanism by which thiazide diuretics achieve this effect is unknown. Studies in rats revealed that thiazide diuretics directly stimulated distal renal tubular re-

Table 46–1. Comparison of Diets Formulated for Prevention of Calcium Oxalate Urolithiasis

Component	c/d^{oxl}Dry*†	c/d^{oxl} Canned*†	pH/O Dry†	pH/O Canned†	S/O Dry‡	S/O Canned‡
Moisture						
As fed (%)	8	75	10	78	12	85
Protein						
As fed (%)	31.8	10.4	32.4	10.6	33.8	7.8
Dry matter (%)	34.6	43.3	36.0	48.3	38.5	52.0
g/100 kcal ME	8.5	9.9	7.7	9.2	8.8	7.5
Fat						
As fed (%)	15.0	5.2	16.5	6.9	18.2	8.4
Dry matter (%)	16.3	21.7	18.3	31.2	20.7	56.0
g/100 kcal ME	4.0	5.0	3.9	5.9	4.7	8.0
Fiber						
As fed (%)	0.7	0.5	1.7	0.2	2.0	0.3
Dry matter (%)	0.8	2.1	1.9	1.0	2.3	2.0
g/100 kcal ME	0.2	0.5	0.4	0.2	0.5	0.2
Sodium						
As fed (%)	0.34	0.14	0.44	0.11	0.85	0.22
Dry matter (%)	0.37	0.60	0.49	0.5	0.97	1.47
g/100 kcal ME	0.09	0.14	1.04	0.99	0.22	0.21
Calcium						
As fed (%)	0.80	0.15	1.01	0.27	0.65	0.18
Dry matter (%)	0.87	0.63	1.12	1.23	0.74	1.20
g/100 kcal ME	0.21	0.15	0.24	0.23	0.17	0.17
Phosphorus						
As fed (%)	0.62	0.12	0.87	0.20	0.81	0.22
Dry matter (%)	0.67	0.51	0.97	0.91	0.92	1.47
g/100 kcal ME	0.16	0.12	0.21	0.17	0.21	0.21
Magnesium						
As fed (%)	0.05	0.01	0.08	0.03	0.06	0.02
Dry matter (%)	0.05	0.06	0.09	0.14	0.07	0.13
g/100 kcal ME	0.01	0.01	0.02	0.02	0.02	0.02

Key: As fed, percentage of nutrient in product after moisture is removed; g/100 kcal ME, nutrient intake for every 100 kcal of metabolizable energy consumed.
*c/d^{oxl}, nutrient information for diets as of March 1999. Diet is manufactured by Hill's Pet Nutrition, Inc., Topeka, KS.
†pH/O, nutrient information for diets as of January 1999. Diet is manufactured by Iams Company, Dayton, OH.
‡S/O, nutrient information for diets as of August 1999. Diet is manufactured by Waltham, Waltham-on-the-Wolds, England.

absorption of calcium.[25] The hypocalciuric response to thiazide diuretics was blocked when volume depletion was prevented by sodium chloride administration in human beings, and the hypothesis has been proposed that thiazide diuretics promote mild extravascular volume contraction and thereby promote proximal tubular reabsorption of several solutes, including sodium and calcium. Hydrochlorothiazide diuretics may be beneficial in minimizing urinary calcium excretion in human beings and dogs (2 to 4 mg/kg PO q 12 hr),[19] but they have not been evaluated in cats. Thiazide diuretic administration may be associated with adverse effects such as dehydration, hypokalemia, and hypercalcemia. Consequently, their use cannot be recommended until additional studies are performed.

Other Agents

Other agents have been used for management of calcium oxalate uroliths in human beings. Allopuri-nol has been used to minimize heterogeneous nucleation of calcium oxalate on uric acid crystals, but this appears to occur rarely in cats. Sodium cellulose phosphate binds calcium in the intestinal tract limiting its absorption, but the mechanism of calcium oxalate formation including enteric hyperoxaluria in cats is unknown. Orthophosphate may minimize urinary calcium excretion. None of these agents has been evaluated in cats.

REFERENCES

1. Osborne CA, Lulich JP, Thumchai R, et al: Feline urolithiasis. Etiology and pathophysiology. Vet Clin North Am Small Anim Pract 26:217–232, 1996.
2. Coe FL, Parks JH, Asplin JR: The pathogenesis and treatment of kidney stones. N Engl J Med 327:1141–1152, 1992.
3. Brown C, Purich D: Physical-chemical processes in kidney stone formation. *In* Coe F, Favus M (eds): Disorders of Bone and Mineral Metabolism. New York, Raven, 1992, pp. 613–624.

4. Bartges JW, Osborne CA, Lulich JP, et al: Methods for evaluating treatment of uroliths. Vet Clin North Am Small Anim Pract 29:45–58, 1999.

5. Balaji KC, Menon M: Mechanism of stone formation. Urol Clin North Am 24:1–11, 1997.

6. Smith BHE, Moodie SJ, Wensley S, et al: Differences in urinary pH and relative supersaturation values between senior and young adult cats. 15th ACVIM Forum. Orlando, FL, 1997, p. 674.

7. Wilson DM: Clinical and laboratory evaluation of renal stone patients. Endocrinol Metab Clin North Am 19:773–803, 1990.

8. Lulich JP, Osborne CA, Nagode LA, et al: Evaluation of urine and serum metabolites in miniature schnauzers with calcium oxalate urolithiasis. Am J Vet Res 52:1583–1590, 1991.

9. Ching SV, Fettman MJ, Hamar DW, et al: The effect of chronic dietary acidification using ammonium chloride on acid-base and mineral metabolism in the adult cat. J Nutr 119:902–915, 1989.

10. Sutton RA, Wong NL, Dirks J: Effects of metabolic acidosis and alkalosis on sodium and calcium transport in the dog kidney. Kidney Int 15:520–533, 1979.

11. Buffington CA, Rogers QR, Morris JG: Effect of diet on struvite activity product in feline urine. Am J Vet Res 51:2025–2030, 1990.

12. Bai SC, Sampson DA, Morris JG, et al: Vitamin B_6 requirement of growing kittens. J Nutr 119:1020–1027, 1989.

13. McKerrell RE, Blakemore WF, Heath MF, et al: Primary hyperoxaluria (l-glyceric aciduria) in the cat: A newly recognized inherited disease. Vet Rec 125:31–34, 1989.

14. Osborne CA, Kruger JM, Lulich JP, et al: Disorders of the feline lower urinary tract. In Osborne CA, Finco DR (eds): Canine and Feline Nephrology and Urology. Baltimore, Williams & Wilkins, 1995, pp. 625–680.

15. Kruger JM, Osborne CA, Goyal SM, et al: Clinical evaluation of cats with lower urinary tract disease. J Am Vet Med Assoc 199:211–216, 1991.

16. Buffington CA, Chew DJ, Kendall MS, et al: Clinical evaluation of cats with nonobstructive urinary tract disease. J Am Vet Med Assoc 210:46–50, 1997.

17. Bartges JW: Dietary management of lower urinary tract disease in cats. World Veterinary Association Small Animal Congress, Buenos Aires, Argentina, 1998.

18. Robertson WG: Urinary tract calculi. In Nordin BEC, Need AG, Morris HA (eds): Metabolic Bone and Stone Disease. Edinburgh, Churchill Livingstone, 1993, pp. 249–311.

19. Lulich JP, Osborne CA, Bartges JW, et al: Canine lower urinary tract disorders. In Ettinger SJ, Feldman EC (eds): Textbook of Veterinary Internal Medicine, 4th ed. Philadelphia, WB Saunders, 1995, pp. 1833–1861.

20. Osborne CA, Kruger JM, Lulich JP, et al: Feline lower urinary tract diseases. In Ettinger SJ, Feldman EC (eds): Textbook of Veterinary Internal Medicine, 4th ed. Philadelphia: WB Saunders, 1995, pp. 1805–1832.

21. Lulich JP, Osborne CA, Felice LJ: Calcium oxalate urolithiasis: Cause, detection, and control. In August JR (ed): Consultations in Feline Internal Medicine, vol. 2. Philadelphia, WB Saunders, 1994, pp. 343–349.

22. McClain HM, Barsanti JA, Bartges JW: Hypercalcemia and calcium oxalate urolithiasis in cats: A report of five cases. J Am Anim Hosp Assoc 35:297–301, 1999.

23. Adams LG, Senior DF: Electrohydraulic and extracorporeal shock-wave lithotripsy. Vet Clin North Am Small Anim Pract 29:293–302, 1999.

24. Osborne CA, Lulich JP, Thumchai R, et al: Diagnosis, medical treatment, and prognosis of feline urolithiasis. Vet Clin North Am Small Anim Pract 26:589–627, 1996.

25. Costanzo LS, Windhater EE: Calcium and sodium transport by distal convoluted tubules of the rat. Am J Physiol 235:F492–F506, 1978.

47

◆ Diagnosis and Treatment of Systemic Hypertension

Scott A. Brown

High systemic arterial blood pressure, referred to as *systemic hypertension*, is a frequent complication of 2 common feline diseases: chronic renal failure and hyperthyroidism.[1–13] Systemic hypertension has been associated with ocular pathology, chronic renal failure, neurologic complications, and cardiovascular changes. A thorough understanding of the consequences, diagnosis, and management of systemic hypertension is essential to the proper management of feline patients.

◆ PATHOGENESIS

Primary or essential hypertension apparently is rare in cats, and systemic hypertension in veterinary practice nearly always will be associated with another disease or condition. Systemic arterial pressure is determined as the product of cardiac output times peripheral vascular resistance, and any disease that enhances cardiac output or systemic vasoconstriction could produce systemic hypertension. The genesis of systemic hypertension has not been well studied in cats. However, the causes of systemic hypertension are likely to be inappropriate sodium and water retention enhancing cardiac output in chronic renal failure, or increased blood volume and heart rate enhancing cardiac output in hyperthyroidism.

◆ EPIDEMIOLOGY

The prevalence of systemic hypertension in cats is not known. Published reports indicate that high systemic arterial blood pressure often is present in cats with chronic renal failure or hyperthyroidism.[1–16] Although other metabolic and endocrine diseases may be associated with systemic hypertension in cats, these clearly are the 2 most common disease conditions associated with increased systemic arterial blood pressure. Other clinical findings and risk factors (Table 47–1) may be used to identify those cats most likely to have increased systemic arterial blood pressure. Although advanced age is not a risk factor by itself, the high prevalence of chronic renal disease and hyperthyroidism, both of which may be present in their early form in the absence of clinical or laboratory signs, makes it reasonable to screen elderly cats routinely for the presence of systemic hypertension.

◆ CLINICAL SIGNS

Systemic hypertension is an insidious abnormality. It is a condition that may or may not produce clinical findings suggestive of its presence (see Table 47–1), and often is present for a long time in the absence of any observable consequences. Thus, hypertensive signs often are nonspecific, and may require months to years to develop. Indeed, lesions may never be apparent in some affected cats. Acute ocular and neurologic changes associated with systemic hypertension in cats seem to behave as if they are threshold phenomena occurring suddenly after a nonremarkable clinical course.

There is a clear association between ocular injury and marked systemic hypertension in cats. Findings associated with hypertensive injury to the eye include intraocular hemorrhage, retinal detachment or atrophy, retinal edema, perivasculitis, retinal vessel tortuosity, and glaucoma.[3–5, 9, 10] Ocular lesions are observed most frequently in markedly hypertensive cats with systolic blood pressures exceeding 200 mm Hg.

Other complications of systemic hypertension, such as progressive renal injury or cardiac hypertrophic failure, are linked to high blood pressure in cats, but the cause-and-effect nature of this association remains poorly understood. The kidney is susceptible to hypertensive injury, but preglomerular arterioles usually constrict whenever blood pressure is increased, protecting the renal glomerulus from

Table 47–1. Observations Suggestive of Systemic Hypertension

Risk Factors

Renal azotemia or glomerular disease
Hyperthyroidism
>10 yr of age (?)
Markedly obese
Hypercortisolism
Pheochromocytoma
Hyperaldosteronism

Clinical Findings

Blindness (particularly of sudden onset)
Intraocular vascular abnormality
Polyuria, polydipsia
Unexplained proteinuria
Tachycardia
Cardiac failure (?)
Acute onset of neurologic abnormalities of unexplained cause

Table 47–2. Minimum Database for Cats Suspected of Having Systemic Hypertension

Blood pressure measurement
Ocular examination (including thorough fundic examination)
Serum creatinine and blood urea nitrogen determinations
Urinalysis and urine protein-to-creatinine ratio

hypertensive injury. In dogs and cats with renal insufficiency, these preglomerular arterioles are dilated[17, 18] and poorly responsive to changes in blood pressure.[19] Thus the increased blood pressure is transmitted directly to the glomerular capillary bed. This causes an increase in glomerular capillary pressure, referred to as *glomerular hypertension*, which may produce glomerular damage and a progressive decrease in renal function, unless hypertension is treated effectively.

Tachycardia is not a common finding with hypertension, although some primary diseases that lead to secondary hypertension, such as hyperthyroidism, may produce an increased heart rate. However, because the heart is working against increased arterial pressure (i.e., afterload), left ventricular hypertrophy and secondary valvular insufficiency may be observed. Left ventricular hypertrophy may regress with antihypertensive treatment.

Signs consistent with cerebrovascular hemorrhage (e.g., head tilt, lethargy, seizures) have been seen clinically in cats with uncontrolled hypertension, and often are associated with a poor prognosis. Rarely, cats suffering from severe systemic hypertension (systolic blood pressure > 300 mm Hg) develop a syndrome of progressive stupor, head pressing, or seizures, which resolves rapidly with effective antihypertensive therapy. This syndrome probably is due to cerebral edema caused by high intracapillary hydrostatic pressure.

◆ DIAGNOSIS

In the simplest sense, the diagnosis of systemic hypertension requires measurement of systemic arterial blood pressure. Therefore, reliable measurement of blood pressure is required both to establish a diagnosis of systemic hypertension and to properly evaluate the efficacy of antihypertensive therapy. However, blood pressure is difficult to measure in cats, and the interpretation of blood pressure results must incorporate a thorough clinical assessment of the patient, including the collection of a minimum database (Table 47–2). With regard to the measurement protocol, there are considerations related to choice of equipment, cuff choice and placement, patient, operator, and environment that will alter the reliability of blood pressure measurements in clinical practice (Table 47–3).

Equipment Choice

Blood pressure may be measured by either direct or indirect methods, but only the indirect techniques are applicable to most clinical settings because they require less restraint and are technically easier to perform. Indirect methods of blood pressure measurement in cats include the ultrasonic Doppler, oscillometric, and photoplethysmographic methods.[4, 11–13, 20, 21] All of these indirect techniques employ an inflatable cuff wrapped around an extremity, and cuff pressure is measured with the aid of a

Table 47–3. Blood Pressure Measurement Protocol

Factor	Considerations
Environment	Utilize a quiet room, away from other animals
	Generally, owner should be present
Timing	Allow cat to acclimate to room for at least 10 min
	Entire procedure will require 30–45 min
Device	Same device should be employed in all evaluations of a single patient
Cuff	Median or coccygeal artery placement preferred
	Same site should be employed in all evaluations of a single patient
	Cuff width should be 30–40% of limb circumference
Personnel	Same individual should conduct all studies in a patient
	Preferably, utilize a well-trained, patient technician
Patient's "state of mind"	Calm and motionless during measurements
Number of measurements	Obtain 5–7 consistent measurements from first cuff placement
	Repeat with cuff placement site 2
	Record all results, including those that "do not make sense" or are physiologically unreasonable; these can be deleted but should be recorded to avoid operator bias
Calculations	From each cuff site, delete the highest and lowest values for each parameter and average all remaining values (at least 3) to obtain blood pressure parameter estimates
	Repeat measurements if average values differ by > 20 mm Hg.
	Otherwise, use these averages to obtain an average overall estimate for each parameter being assessed
	Repeat entire measurement session ≥ 2 hr later (different day preferred)
Record keeping	Note date and time of session, cuff width, cuff site, measurement device, identity of personnel involved, "state of mind" of animal, and *all* blood pressure values (individual and average values) on a standard form

manometer or pressure transducer. Doppler flow-meters detect blood flow as a change in the frequency of reflected sound (Doppler shift) due to the motion of underlying red blood cells. Blood pressure is read by the operator from an aneroid manometer connected to the occluding cuff placed proximal to the Doppler transducer. This device generally has been used to provide an estimate of systolic arterial blood pressure. Devices utilizing the oscillometric technique detect pressure fluctuations produced in the occluding cuff resulting from the pressure pulse. Machines using the oscillometric technique generally determine systolic, diastolic, and mean arterial pressures as well as pulse rate. Photoplethysmographic devices[1] measure arterial volume by attenuation of infrared radiation, and can be employed in cats and small dogs weighing less than 10 kg.[20]

The Association for Advancement of Medical Instrumentation has established minimum criteria for accuracy and precision of instruments that measure blood pressure. Machines that do not meet these criteria generally are not accepted for clinical use in human beings. Unfortunately, the currently available machines for detection of blood pressure in cats generally have not been shown to meet these criteria for accuracy or precision. Consequently, caution must be employed in interpreting results of measurement of blood pressure by these devices.

We have evaluated the ultrasonic Doppler and oscillometric methods in conscious cats.[21] In cats, the ultrasonic Doppler method is more accurate. Although the oscillometric device has the advantage of being able to provide an estimate of diastolic and mean blood pressure, these devices tend to underestimate blood pressure by increasing amounts as the blood pressure increases, and initially require excessive time to obtain readings in cats. When evaluated in anesthetized cats, the photoplethysmograph had less of a tendency than the Doppler and oscillometric devices to underestimate blood pressure at high pressures and overestimate blood pressure at low pressures.[21] Disadvantages of the photoplethysmographic device include its cost, the need to reposition the cuff frequently for optimum traces, and the fact that its use is limited to cats and dogs weighing less than 10 kg. To the best of my knowledge, the reliability of this device has not been evaluated in conscious animals. At the present time, based on our studies in conscious animals, devices using the Doppler principle are recommended for use in cats.

Cuff Factors

There are several important considerations related to cuff selection and placement. First, indirect blood pressure measurement studies should employ a cuff width that measures 30 to 40 per cent of the circumference of the limb. An oversized cuff may give erroneously low recordings; an undersized cuff

falsely high readings.[22] If the ideal cuff width is midway between 2 available sizes, the larger cuff should be used. The cuff may be placed around the brachial, median, cranial tibial, or medial coccygeal arteries. Generally, for the Doppler technique, the cuff is placed over the median artery, and the transducer is placed between the carpal and the metacarpal pad. The cuff should be placed at the level of the aortic valve. If not, a compensation may be made for gravitational effect, with a 1.0 mm Hg change in blood pressure expected for each 1.3 cm of vertical distance between the level of the cuff and the level of the aortic valve. Clipping of hair and application of acoustic gel at the site of transducer placement may enhance the signal. For the oscillometric technique, the median artery in cats provided more reliable values than other sites in our studies, and clipping is recommended only if signal strength is inadequate to provide consistent measurements.

Errors in cuff placement can alter the values obtained, and the cuff should be removed and replaced at least once during a blood pressure measurement session. If markedly different values are obtained with the new cuff placement, a third or fourth cuff positioning will be required.

Operator Factors

There are several important considerations related to the operator of the device. These units require operator practice to master. Generally, it is not possible for a novice to apply the cuff and cycle the machine through a standard procedure and obtain reliable values. Because of available time or patience, an experienced, trained technician is preferred to a veterinarian as the individual responsible for blood pressure measurements. Consistency in personnel is critical. Written standard procedures should be maintained and followed rigorously.

Animal Factors

The visit to the veterinary clinic, hospitalization, restraint in the examination room, clipper noise and vibration, cuff placement, cuff inflation, and other stimuli in the setting of a veterinary hospital may induce anxiety in a cat during blood pressure measurement. As a consequence, a falsely increased value for blood pressure may be obtained secondary to catecholamine release associated with this anxiety, commonly referred to as the *white-coat effect*.[23] The extent of this effect may be minimized by obtaining blood pressure measurements before physical examination, performing all measurements in a quiet room utilizing a calm and reassuring manner, and allowing the animal to acclimate to its surroundings for at least 10 minutes before obtaining blood pressure measurements. Ideally, blood pressure will be obtained in a calm, motionless animal.

Environmental Factors

The variability of anxiety-induced hypertension, and the difficulty in obtaining reliable values in moving animals, dictate that blood pressure be measured in a quiet room, away from other animals, people, and background noise. The owner should be present if possible to gently restrain and console the cat, if appropriate. If a forelimb is used for cuff placement, the animal may be allowed to rest calmly in its own carrying crate or on the owner's lap, but the cuff must be observed carefully throughout the measurement sequence.

Consistency

Unless there is strongly convincing evidence (e.g., retinal detachment) of an emergency need to accept a diagnosis of systemic hypertension on the basis of a single session of blood pressure measurement, several blood pressure measurement sessions (2 or more) should be utilized, on multiple days if possible. A minimum of 2 hours should be sought between measurement sessions.

◆ MANAGEMENT

At this time, the routine measurement of blood pressure to identify systemic hypertension in all feline patients is not warranted, except as a screening exercise. Rather, blood pressure should be assessed in those patients with identifiable risk factors (see Table 47–1). Blood pressure measurement is difficult in this species, and a minimum database (see Table 47–2) should be collected to facilitate interpretation of the results of blood pressure measurement (Fig. 47–1).

There is a clear association between ocular injury and marked systemic hypertension in dogs and cats. In light of the uncertainty and difficulties associated with blood pressure measurement in cats, only those animals with marked increases of indirectly measured blood pressure or clinical abnormalities directly attributable to hypertensive injury should be considered candidates for treatment (see Fig. 47–1). Marked systemic hypertension is associated with ocular injury, and antihypertensive treatment is indicated in any cat with a sustained systolic blood pressure greater than 200 mm Hg or diastolic blood pressure greater than 120 mm Hg, regardless of other clinical findings (see Fig. 47–1). A cat with a systolic/diastolic blood pressure that consistently exceeds 170/100 mm Hg should be considered for treatment if clinical evaluation has identified abnormalities (e.g., retinal lesions or chronic renal disease) that could be caused or exacerbated by systemic hypertension. This recommendation remains speculative in cats, but it is supported by a recent report of dogs with renal failure in which a systolic blood pressure exceeding 180 mm Hg was associ-

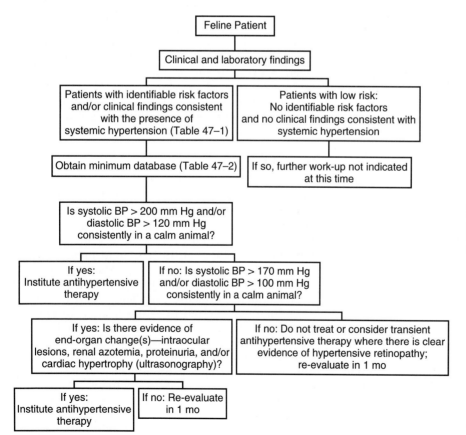

Figure 47–1. An approach to the diagnosis of systemic hypertension in cats. See text for further explanation. BP, systemic arterial blood pressure.

ated with a higher risk for complications (hypertensive retinopathy and progression of renal failure) and shorter survival time.[24] Unfortunately, a similar study has not been reported in cats, and interspecies extrapolations are necessary. In animals in which blood pressure is moderately increased (systolic/diastolic blood pressure that consistently exceeds 170/100 mm Hg) and no clinical abnormalities or risk factors related to systemic hypertension are identified, the rationale for therapy is less clear and re-evaluation is recommended (see Fig. 47–1).

◆ ANTIHYPERTENSIVE THERAPY
General

Systemic arterial blood pressure is the product of the cardiac output and total peripheral resistance, and consequently antihypertensive therapy is directed at reducing cardiac output, total peripheral resistance, or both. Therapy may be classified loosely as dietary and pharmacologic.

Treatment generally proceeds by sequential trials (Fig. 47–2). Dosage adjustments or changes in treatment should be instituted no more frequently than every 2 weeks, unless extreme hypertension necessitating emergency treatment is present. When using pharmacologic agents, a wide range of dosages should be considered, with initial dosages at the low end of the range. If an agent or combination of agents is incompletely effective, the dosage may be increased or additional agents added. Often, multiple agents will be used concurrently.

Although the duration of therapy may vary, the diagnosis of hypertension associated with chronic

Figure 47–2. An approach to the management of systemic hypertension in cats. Two to 4 weeks should be allowed after each change in therapy before assessing efficacy by repeat blood pressure (BP) measurements. All adjustments in dosage should be based on BP measurements obtained by following a standard protocol (Table 47–3). See text for further explanation.

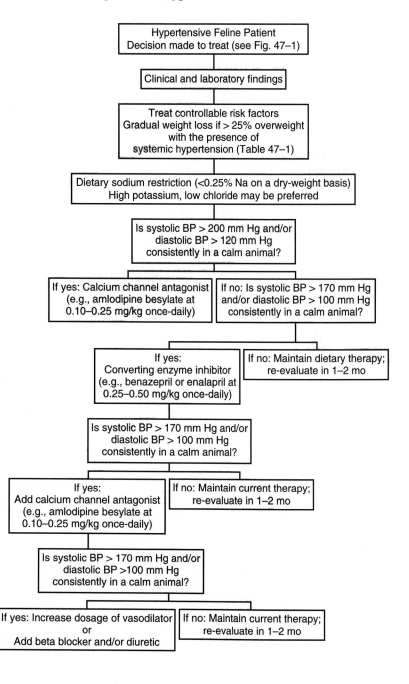

renal disease may necessitate life-long antihypertensive treatment, with periodic dosage adjustments based on blood pressure measurements. Hypertension associated with hyperthyroidism, in contrast, usually will resolve within 1 to 3 months after effective treatment of the hyperthyroidism, unless chronic renal failure also is present. In other patients, the duration of treatment cannot be predicted, but it may be required for the life of the animal. Nonetheless, periodic dosage adjustments based on blood pressure measurements are indicated in all animals.

It usually is not possible to restore blood pressure to normal when treating a hypertensive animal. The goal should be to lower blood pressure to within 25 to 50 mm Hg of the normal range, thus lowering pressure (systolic/diastolic) to less than 170/100 mm Hg. If an oscillometric unit is employed, the systolic, mean, or diastolic blood pressure may be used to judge effectiveness of therapy. If a Doppler ultrasonic device is used, the systolic blood pressure alone may be used to monitor the effectiveness of treatment.

Although it is little studied, the usual recommendation initially is to institute a low-sodium diet that provides less than 0.25 per cent sodium on a dry-weight basis (see Fig. 47–2). A diet with a low chloride and a moderately increased potassium content may provide further blood pressure–lowering benefit in cats, but this assertion is speculative. This dietary approach often is ineffective, but dietary sodium restriction may enhance the efficacy of pharmacologic agents.

Obesity can increase systemic arterial pressure[25] in human beings and dogs, and perhaps in cats. Consequently, weight loss is desirable in markedly obese, hypertensive animals. Hypertensive cats more than 25 per cent overweight should be considered candidates for gradual weight loss. However, most hypertensive cats are normal to low in body weight, and the effect of obesity on blood pressure is relatively modest, and by itself, difficult to appreciate with devices that estimate blood pressure indirectly.

Pharmacologic Agents

Medical treatment of hypertension in cats has, until recently, been extrapolated from human protocols. Recommendations for medical therapy have included vasodilators, beta blockers, and diuretics. These agents generally are given in concert with dietary sodium restriction. In human beings with systemic hypertension and renal disease, vasodilator therapy is the preferred initial choice because of the renoprotective effects of certain classes of these agents (angiotensin-converting enzyme inhibitors and calcium channel blockers).

Vasodilator therapy with either an inhibitor of angiotensin-converting enzyme (e.g., benazepril or enalapril 0.25 to 0.5 mg/kg orally [PO] every [q] 24 hr) or a calcium channel antagonist (e.g., amlodipine besylate 0.1 to 0.25 mg/kg PO q 24 hr) is an appropriate consideration for animals not responding to dietary salt restriction alone (Fig. 47–2). In cats, the role of the renin-angiotensin system in the maintenance of systemic hypertension has been questioned, and although less effective in cats,[8] a higher dosage (benazepril or enalapril 1 to 2 mg/kg orally q 24 hr) may prove efficacious. Angiotensin-converting enzyme inhibitors, specifically benazepril, lowered intraglomerular pressure in an experimental study of cats with reduced renal function, providing a theoretical advantage in that they may offer protection to the kidney from hypertensive damage.[26] Drugs classified as calcium channel antagonists seem to reduce total peripheral resistance more effectively, and are highly efficacious in decreasing systemic blood pressure in hypertensive cats. Amlodipine besylate, a long-acting dihydropyridine calcium antagonist, has been used successfully as a single agent in cats, and is recommended as first-line therapy for cats with markedly increased systemic blood pressure or with evidence of systemic hypertension associated with hypertensive retinopathy (see Fig. 47–2).[6, 7, 9] Blood pressure decreases during amlodipine treatment, and significant adverse effects (e.g., azotemia, hypokalemia, weight loss) are not identified frequently. Amlodipine has a slow onset of action, and adverse effects such as hypotension and loss of appetite usually are avoided. Alpha blockers, such as prazosin (1 to 4 mg PO q 12 to 24 hr) or phenoxybenzamine, may lower systemic arterial blood pressure by decreasing peripheral vascular resistance.

Beta blockers exert an antihypertensive effect by reducing cardiac output and decreasing renin release. A cardiospecific (beta$_1$) antagonist, such as atenolol, is preferred, with a starting dosage of 0.5 mg/kg PO q 12 to 24 hr. These agents may be combined with vasodilators or diuretics.

Diuretics such as the thiazides (e.g., hydrochlorothiazide 1 mg/kg PO q 12 to 24 hr) may be used in hypertensive cats. These agents reduce extracellular fluid volume and cardiac output, and overuse can lead to dehydration, volume depletion, and aggravation of azotemia. Hypokalemia may occur with loop diuretics as well as thiazides, and serum potassium concentrations should be monitored carefully in all animals with chronic renal disease that are receiving diuretics. The addition of spironolactone (1 to 2 mg/kg PO q 12 hr), a potassium-sparing diuretic, may be helpful in limiting potassium loss.

Each change in the therapeutic approach should be followed by assessment of the minimum database and blood pressure measurement 2 to 4 weeks later. Once blood pressure is controlled adequately, the patient should be evaluated at 2- to 3-month intervals. A complete blood count, biochemical panel, and urinalysis should be evaluated at least once every 6 months.

REFERENCES

1. Morgan RV: Systemic hypertension in four cats: Ocular and medical findings. J Am Anim Hosp Assoc 22:615–621, 1986.
2. Kobayashi DL, Peterson ME, Graves TK, et al: Hypertension in cats with chronic renal failure or hyperthyroidism. J Vet Intern Med 4:58–62, 1990.
3. Turner JL, Brogdon JD, Lees GE, et al: Idiopathic hypertension in a cat with secondary retinopathy associated with a high salt diet. J Am Anim Hosp Assoc 26:647–651, 1990.
4. Littman MP: Spontaneous systemic hypertension in 24 cats. J Vet Intern Med 8:79–86, 1994.
5. Stiles J, Polzin DJ, Bistner SI: The prevalence of retinopathy in cats with systemic hypertension and chronic renal failure or hyperthyroidism. J Am Anim Hosp Assoc 30:564–572, 1994.
6. Henik RA, Snyder PS, Volk LM: Treatment of systemic hypertension in cats with amlodipine besylate. J Am Anim Hosp Assoc 33:226–234, 1997.
7. Snyder PS: Amlodipine: A randomized, blinded clinical trial in 9 cats with systemic hypertension. J Vet Intern Med 12:157–162, 1998.
8. Jensen J, Henik RA, Brownfield M, et al: Plasma renin activity, angiotensin I and aldosterone in feline hypertension associated with chronic renal disease. Am J Vet Res 58:535–540, 1997.
9. Henik RA: Systemic hypertension and its management. Vet Clin North Am Small Anim Pract 27:1355–1372, 1997.
10. Brown SA, Henik RA: Diagnosis and management of systemic hypertension. Vet Clin North Am Small Anim Pract 28:1481–1494, 1998.
11. Labato MA, Ross LA: Diagnosis and management of hypertension. In August JR (ed): Consultations in Feline Internal Medicine, vol. 1. Philadelphia, WB Saunders, 1991, pp. 301–308.
12. Ross L: Hypertension and chronic renal failure. Semin Vet Med Surg Small Anim Pract 7:221–226, 1992.
13. Littman MP, Drobatz KJ: Hypertensive and hypotensive disorders. In Ettinger SJ (ed): Textbook of Veterinary Internal Medicine. Philadelphia, WB Saunders, 1995, pp. 93–100.
14. Lesser M, Fox PR, Bond BR: Assessment of hypertension in 40 cats with left ventricular hypertrophy by Doppler-shift sphygmomanometry. J Small Anim Pract 33:55–58, 1992.
15. Chen Q, Okeda R, Matsuo T: Selective distribution of medial thickening in the renal vessels in experimental hypertension. Pathol Int 44:569–577, 1994.
16. Mishina M, Watanabe T, Fujii K, et al: Non-invasive blood pressure measurements in cats: Clinical significance of hypertension associated with chronic renal failure. J Vet Med Sci 60:805–808, 1998.
17. Brown SA, Finco DR, Crowell WA, et al: Single-nephron adaptations to partial renal ablation in the dog. Am J Physiol 258:F495–F503, 1990.
18. Brown SA, Brown CA: Single-nephron adaptations to partial renal ablation in cats. Am J Physiol 269:R1002–R1008, 1996.
19. Brown S, Finco D, Navar L: Impaired renal autoregulatory ability in dogs with reduced renal mass. J Am Soc Nephrol 5:1768–1774, 1995.
20. Binns SH, Sisson DD, Buoscio DA, et al: Doppler ultrasonographic, oscillometric sphygmomanometric, and photoplethysmographic techniques for noninvasive blood pressure measurement in anesthetized cats. J Vet Intern Med 9:405–415, 1995.
21. Haberman C, Brown S: Unpublished observations, 1997.
22. Valtonen MH, Eriksson LM: The effect of cuff width and accuracy of indirect measurement of blood pressure in dogs. Res Vet Sci 11:258–358, 1970.
23. Belew A, Barlett T, Brown SA: Evaluation of the white-coat effect in cats. J Vet Intern Med 13:134–142, 1999.
24. Jacob F, Polzin DJ, Osborne CA, et al: Systemic hypertension in dogs with spontaneous chronic renal failure: Prevalence, target-organ damage and survival. Proceedings American College of Veterinary Internal Medicine, Annual Forum, Chicago, June 10–13, 1999, p. 719A.
25. Rocchini A, Moorhead C, Wentz E, et al: Obesity-induced hypertension in the dog. Hypertension 9:III64–III68, 1987.
26. Brown SA, Brown CA, Jacobs GJ, et al: Hemodynamic effects of angiotensin converting enzyme inhibition (benazepril) in cats with chronic renal insufficiency. Proceedings American College of Veterinary Internal Medicine, Annual Forum, Chicago, June 10–13, 1999, p. 716A.

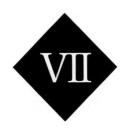

VII

Neurology

Joan R. Coates, Editor

◆ Acquired Myasthenia Gravis and Other Disorders
   of the Neuromuscular Junction 374
◆ Dysautonomia Revisited 381
◆ Cerebral Meningiomas: Diagnosis and Therapeutic
   Considerations 385
◆ Neuronal Storage Disorders 393
◆ Vascular Disorders 405
◆ Congenital Intracranial Malformations 413
◆ Inflammatory Disorders of the Central
   Nervous System 425

**Still-Current Information Found in *Consultations in
Feline Internal Medicine 2:***
Cerebrospinal Fluid Collection and Analysis (Chapter 49),
   p. 385
Diagnostic Capabilities of Computed Tomography and Mag-
   netic Resonance Imaging (Chapter 50), p. 393
Neuromuscular Disorders (Chapter 51), p. 405
Epilepsy (Chapter 55), p. 437
Circling (Chapter 56), p. 449

**Still-Current Information Found in *Consultations in
Feline Internal Medicine 3:***
Constipation, Obstipation, and Megacolon (Chapter 15), p.
   104
Diagnostic Approach and Medical Treatment of Seizure
   Disorders (Chapter 51), p. 389
Nervous System Neoplasia (Chapter 54), p. 418
Interpreting Gross Necropsy Observations in Neonatal and
   Pediatric Kittens (Chapter 74), p. 587

Elsewhere in *Consultations in Feline Internal Medicine 4:*
Cryptococcosis: New Perspectives on Etiology, Pathogenesis,
   Diagnosis, and Clinical Management (Chapter 6), p. 39
Feline Spongiform Encephalopathy and Borna Disease
   (Chapter 8), p. 62
Diseases of the Esophagus (Chapter 12), p. 99
Chylothorax (Chapter 35), p. 267
Aortic Thromboembolism (Chapter 39), p. 299
Mucopolysaccharidosis (Chapter 57), p. 450
Evaluation and Treatment of Cranial Mediastinal Masses
   (Chapter 68), p. 533
Diagnostic Imaging of Neoplasia (Chapter 70), p. 548
Molecular Diagnosis of Gangliosidoses: A Model for Elimi-
   nation of Inherited Diseases in Pure Breeds (Chapter 77),
   p. 615

48

◆ Acquired Myasthenia Gravis and Other Disorders of the Neuromuscular Junction

Julie M. Ducoté
Curtis W. Dewey

Acquired myasthenia gravis (MG) is an uncommon disorder in cats. However, it is an important differential diagnosis in a cat exhibiting focal or generalized muscle weakness. Acquired MG is an autoimmune disease in which antibodies are directed against the acetylcholine (ACh) receptors within the postsynaptic membrane of the neuromuscular junction (NMJ). MG is one of several disorders that disrupt the normal physiology of the NMJ. This chapter reviews the normal anatomy and function of the NMJ, describes the pathophysiology, clinical signs, diagnosis, and treatment of acquired MG in cats, and briefly addresses other disorders of the NMJ described in cats.

◆ ANATOMY AND PHYSIOLOGY OF THE NEUROMUSCULAR JUNCTION

The NMJ has 3 basic components: the presynaptic membrane, synaptic cleft, and postsynaptic membrane. The myelinated motor neuron branches into many nerve terminals. Each nerve terminal forms a synapse with the motor endplate of the skeletal muscle that it innervates. Many secretory vesicles containing ACh are located close to the presynaptic membrane of the nerve terminal. The postsynaptic membrane is composed of a specialized basal lamina and an associated muscle surface. ACh receptors are located within the postsynaptic membrane. This postsynaptic membrane is arranged in junctional folds, which increase the surface area for neuromuscular transmission (Fig. 48–1A). ACh receptors are concentrated near the peaks of the folds, whereas skeletal muscle voltage-gated sodium channels tend to lie in the troughs of the folds. The clustering of these ion channels has functional importance for development of the endplate potential. Acetylcholinesterase is synthesized primarily by the skeletal muscle, and is located in the basal lamina portion of the postsynaptic membrane.[1]

The ACh receptors at the NMJ of skeletal muscle are nicotinic receptors, and are anatomically and antigenically distinct from the muscarinic ACh receptors of the parasympathetic nervous system. The transmembrane portion of the ACh receptor is composed of 5 subunits: 2 α subunits, and 1 each of β, δ, and ϵ subunits (Fig. 48–2). These subunits are arranged in a circular pattern to form an ion channel (primarily an Na^+ channel).[2] The α subunits contain the ACh-binding sites. Binding of ACh to the α subunits causes a conformational change in the ACh receptor, to allow flow of ions through the channel.

Normal neuromuscular transmission begins with the propagation of an action potential in the motor neuron. This action potential reaches the nerve terminal via saltatory conduction down the myelinated axon. As the action potential reaches the nerve terminal, influx of calcium through voltage-gated calcium channels stimulates fusion of the secretory vesicles with the presynaptic membrane. ACh is released into the synaptic cleft through the process of exocytosis, and travels across the synaptic cleft where it binds to the α subunits of the ACh receptors within the postsynaptic membrane. A conformational change in the ACh receptor allows passage of cations through the receptor into the muscle cell. The influx of ions causes a small change in membrane potential called a *miniature endplate potential* (MEPP). As the endplate potential rises, more voltage-gated sodium channels open, and cause a release of calcium from the sarcoplasmic reticulum. Summation of MEPPs at the postsynaptic membrane results in an action potential and muscle contraction.

After the ACh receptor is stimulated, there is a *refractory period* in which the receptor cannot be restimulated, regardless of the amount of ACh available. In a normal animal, this refractory period is insignificant clinically. Normally, much more ACh is released into the synaptic cleft than can bind to ACh receptors. Also, more ACh receptors are located in the postsynaptic membrane than are necessary for effective neuromuscular transmission. This is referred to as the *safety factor* for neuromuscular transmission. Excess ACh is neutralized by acetylcholinesterase in the postsynaptic membrane, or diffuses into the extracellular space.

◆ ACQUIRED MYASTHENIA GRAVIS

Pathophysiology

Acquired MG is an autoimmune disorder in which antibodies (primarily immunoglobulin G) are formed against nicotinic ACh receptors (see Fig. 48–

1B). These antibodies interfere with normal neuromuscular transmission to cause skeletal muscle weakness. In dogs and human beings, autoantibodies have been shown to recognize the same epitopes on the ACh receptor in many cases.[3] These epitopes are concentrated in the *main immunogenic region* on the extracellular surface of the 2 α subunits. The main immunogenic region is in close proximity to, but distinct from, the ACh-binding site. Antibodies alter the ACh receptor by 3 mechanisms.[4] First, antibodies may bind directly to the ACh receptor and cause a blockade of the ion channel opening. This mechanism probably is the least important.[1] Second, antibodies may increase the degradation rate of ACh receptors by cross-linking, thereby lowering ACh receptor concentration at the postsynaptic membrane. The last mechanism is complement-mediated lysis of the muscle endplate.

Clinical Signs

A bimodal age distribution has been identified in cats, dogs, and human beings with acquired MG.[4, 5] Cats typically are affected at 2 to 3 years of age, or later in life, at about 9 to 10 years of age. Purebred

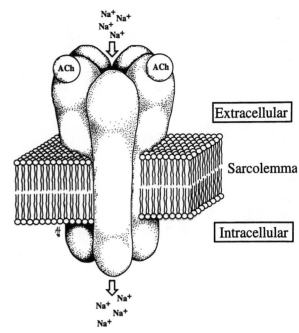

Figure 48–2. The acetylcholine (ACh) receptor is made up of 5 subunits: 2 α, and 1 each of β, δ, and ε. ACh binds at 2 sites: 1 on each of the α subunits. (Courtesy of Anton G. Hoffman, D.V.M., Ph.D., College of Veterinary Medicine, Texas A&M University.)

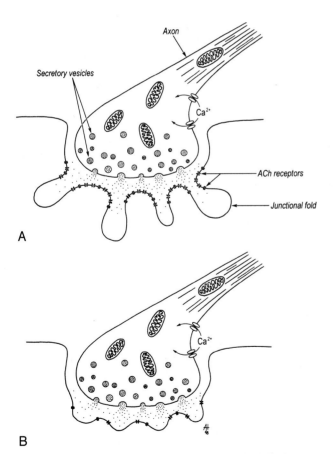

Figure 48–1. Schematic of the normal neuromuscular junction *(A)* compared with the neuromuscular junction of a patient affected with myasthenia gravis *(B)*. ACh, acetylcholine. (*A* and *B,* Courtesy of Anton G. Hoffman, D.V.M., Ph.D., College of Veterinary Medicine, Texas A&M University.)

cats have a tendency to develop acquired MG more often than mixed-breed cats. The Abyssinian and Somali breeds appear to be overrepresented, although these numbers have not been statistically significant.[5] No gender predilection has been identified.

Three different clinical forms of acquired MG have been defined in dogs[4] and cats:[5] *focal, generalized,* and *acute fulminating* MG. Cats with focal MG present with weakness of isolated skeletal muscle groups, such as esophageal, pharyngeal, laryngeal, or facial muscles. These cats do not exhibit appendicular muscle weakness. Common clinical signs include regurgitation, dysphonia, dropped jaw, diminished or absent palpebral reflexes, and dysphagia (Fig. 48–3). In a recent retrospective study,[5] 15 per cent of the cats with acquired MG had only focal disease, as opposed to 36 per cent of dogs with acquired MG.[4] This difference may be explained by the larger portion of smooth muscle in the feline esophagus, as compared with the canine esophagus (which is composed predominantly of striated muscle).[6]

Appendicular muscle weakness is the predominant clinical finding in cats with generalized MG. In dogs, this weakness may be more profound in the muscles of the pelvic limbs; however, this has not been reported in cats. The weakness in cats with MG typically is exacerbated by exercise, and improves with rest. Paresis, and ventroflexion of the neck, often are noted (Fig. 48–4). Other clinical signs of generalized MG include regurgitation, dysphagia, and dysphonia. Polymyositis has been associated with generalized MG in 1 cat.[5]

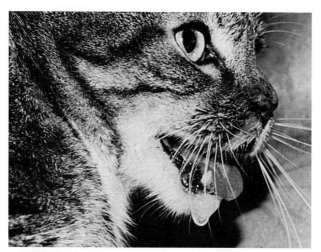

Figure 48–3. A dropped jaw and ptyalism are clinical signs of weakness in cats with acquired myasthenia gravis. (From Ducoté JM, Dewey CW, Coates JR: Clinical forms of acquired myasthenia gravis in cats. Compend Contin Educ Pract Vet 21:440–448, 1999.)

Acute fulminating MG is a severe form of generalized MG. Cats with acute fulminating MG show sudden onset and rapid progression of severe generalized muscle weakness. Skeletal muscle weakness eventually involves the intercostal muscles and/or diaphragm, causing severe respiratory distress. These cats also may develop aspiration pneumonia because of regurgitation secondary to esophageal and pharyngeal muscle weakness. In the previously mentioned study, 15 per cent of cats with acquired MG had the acute fulminating form.[5]

Common historical complaints and clinical findings in cats with acquired MG are summarized in Tables 48–1 and 48–2.

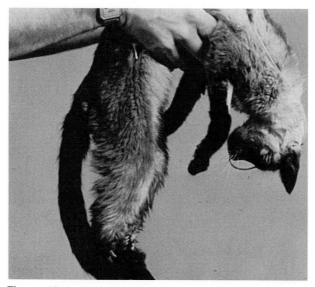

Figure 48–4. Cervical ventroflexion is a common clinical sign in cats with generalized myasthenia gravis. (From Ducoté JM, Dewey CW, Coates JR: Clinical forms of acquired myasthenia gravis in cats. Compend Contin Educ Pract Vet 21:440–448, 1999.)

Table 48–1. Owner Observations (Historical Signs) of Cats With Acquired Myasthenia Gravis

Sign	Cats	
	%	n (n = 20)
Weakness	70	14
Vomiting/regurgitation	60	12
Exercise intolerance	40	8
Difficulty swallowing	35	7
Coughing	30	6
Ventroflexion of neck	20	4
Change in voice	20	4
Nasal discharge	20	4
Acute collapse	15	3
Dropped jaw	15	3
Acute collapse	15	3
Hypersalivation	10	2
Labored breathing	5	1

From Ducoté JM, Dewey CW, Coates JR: Clinical forms of acquired myasthenia gravis in cats. Compend Contin Educ Pract Vet 21:440–448, 1999.

Diagnosis

Diagnosis of acquired MG in cats is based on demonstration of circulating antibodies to the ACh receptors. An immunoprecipitation radioimmunoassay that quantifies ACh receptor antibodies in serum has been adapted for use in cats from similar methods described in human beings and dogs. ACh receptor antibody concentrations of greater than 0.30 nM/liter are compatible with a diagnosis of acquired MG. The assay is available at the Comparative Neuromuscular Laboratory, University of California, San Diego (Basic Science Building, Room 1057, La Jolla, CA 92093–0612).

Immune complexes of the NMJ also may be detected by immunocytochemical techniques in muscle biopsy specimens. The immunoreagent staphylococcal protein A conjugated to horseradish peroxidase binds to the Fc portion of the immunoglobulins. This procedure has been used to support

Table 48–2. Clinical Findings of Cats With Acquired Myasthenia Gravis

Finding	Cats	
	%	n (n = 20)
Generalized weakness	70	14
Decreased palpebral reflex	60	12
Decreased menace response	50	10
Megaesophagus	40	8
Aspiration pneumonia	20	4
Cranial mediastinal mass	15	3
Muscle fasciculations	15	3
Decreased flexor reflexes	10	2
Polymyositis	5	1
Cardiomegaly	5	1
Muscle atrophy	5	1

From Ducoté JM, Dewey CW, Coates JR: Clinical forms of acquired myasthenia gravis in cats. Compend Contin Educ Pract Vet 21:440–448, 1999.

a diagnosis of acquired MG in cats.[7] However, the test is not specific for this disease.

Provocative testing with intravenous edrophonium chloride (Tensilon, Roche Laboratories) may aid in establishing a presumptive diagnosis of acquired MG in cats with appendicular muscle weakness. A dose of 0.25 to 0.50 mg per cat is administered intravenously through a previously placed peripheral catheter. Observation of increased muscle strength is considered a positive response. Atropine administration may be necessary, because edrophonium chloride may induce a cholinergic crisis in some patients. There are disadvantages to the edrophonium response test. Patients with neuromuscular disorders other than acquired MG may have a partial response to edrophonium chloride; therefore, a positive response is not definitive proof of acquired MG.[2] Also, the test is very subjective because it is based on observation and interpretation of muscle strength by the examiner. Results may show a small increase in strength, making interpretation difficult. The edrophonium challenge test often is not useful in cats with focal MG because they may not have detectable neurologic improvement.

Electrodiagnostic evaluation may be very helpful in the diagnosis of acquired MG. Unfortunately, general anesthesia is required, and may be contraindicated in cats with respiratory impairment. A decremental response to repetitive nerve stimulation suggests the diagnosis of MG. Stimulation at rates of 5/sec or less are used, and a decrease in the compound muscle action potential of 10 per cent or greater is considered abnormal.[8] Rarely, other NMJ disorders may produce a decremental response. Stimulation rates at 10/sec or higher usually will result in a decrement even in normal patients.[8] Single-fiber electromyography is used increasingly in human beings and dogs to aid in the diagnosis of MG.[9] Use of repetitive nerve stimulation and single-fiber EMG is limited by their lack of availability to the general practitioner, and the performance and interpretation of these tests is somewhat operator-dependent.

Thoracic radiography is indicated in cats suspected to have acquired MG. Megaesophagus with acquired MG is less common in cats than in dogs; however, its presence may imply a more guarded prognosis. Also, thymoma has been associated with acquired MG in cats, as in dogs and human beings[10, 11] (see Chapter 68, Evaluation and Treatment of Cranial Mediastinal Masses). In 2 case series of acquired MG in cats, a cranial mediastinal mass was detected on radiographs of 3 of 20 cats, and in 2 of 12 cats.[10] It has been speculated that thymectomy (for thymic hyperplasia) may result in remission of clinical signs of MG in human beings; however, this has not been demonstrated in cats. Careful consideration is recommended before a thymectomy is performed because of the stress of anesthesia and thoracotomy.

Treatment

Therapy for acquired MG in cats includes treatment with anticholinesterase and immunosuppressive agents, nutritional support, antibiotics for pneumonia, and possibly respiratory support.

Anticholinesterase drugs prevent the degradation of ACh, and prolong its availability for binding to remaining functional ACh receptors. Administration of pyridostigmine bromide (Mestinon, ICN), a long-acting cholinesterase inhibitor, may result in improved muscle strength. The recommended dose for cats is 0.25 mg/kg orally (PO) every (q) 8 to 12 hr; this dose should be titrated as needed to obtain the best clinical response.[12] Hypersalivation, vomiting, and muscle fasciculations are cholinergic side-effects of treatment, and the dose should be reduced if these signs are noticed. If the cat has megaesophagus and is at risk for aspiration, or is unable to tolerate oral intake owing to dysphagia, parenteral neostigmine (Prostigmin, ICN) may be preferred. Neostigmine has a faster onset of action and is administered intramuscularly every 6 hours. The pharmacokinetics of neostigmine in cats have not been reported. Care should be taken when choosing a dose, because cats are more sensitive than dogs to anticholinesterase drugs.[12] Placement of a gastrostomy tube may provide another method for administering pyridostigmine.

The use of immunosuppressive therapy for acquired MG in human beings and veterinary medicine has been controversial. There are 2 reasons for this controversy. First, immunosuppression may be considered to be contraindicated in patients at risk for developing, or already affected by, aspiration pneumonia. Second, glucocorticoids have been associated with muscular weakness in several species, including cats.[13] Thus, concerns exist about further weakening an already severely weak patient. The incidence of this glucocorticoid-associated weakness is unclear. Increased muscle weakness occurs in about 50 per cent of human beings treated with corticosteroids, and has been observed in dogs. In one study of cats treated with corticosteroids, an appreciable worsening of muscle weakness was not observed.[5] Prospective controlled clinical trials in human beings with acquired MG have shown an increased number of patients in clinical remission and a prolonged survival in patients treated with pyridostigmine and prednisone, or with pyridostigmine and azathioprine (Imuran, Glaxo Wellcome).[14] A recent report documents clinical remission in 4 dogs treated with azathioprine.[15] Cats are susceptible to bone marrow suppression from azathioprine, and the drug generally is not recommended for use in this species. Corticosteroids were used in conjunction with pyridostigmine to treat 14 of 20 cats with acquired MG.[5]

The pathophysiology of acquired MG, an autoimmune reduction in the number of functional ACh receptors, implies that immunosuppressive agents may be necessary to resolve the underlying disease. Doses of prednisone that have been used in cats range from 1 to 4 mg/kg/day.[5] Dexamethasone, 0.25 to 2.0 mg/kg/day, may be used in place of prednisone, but is associated with more gastrointestinal side-effects.[5]

Nutritional support is essential in cats with dysphagia or esophageal weakness causing regurgitation. Elevated feeding may be helpful, but is sometimes difficult to achieve in cats. Nutritional support, using a nasogastric tube or a percutaneously placed gastrostomy tube is an effective way of bypassing the esophagus and oropharynx, decreasing the risk of aspiration pneumonia.

Antibiotics are indicated for aspiration pneumonia. The appropriate antibiotic may be chosen based on results of culture and susceptibility tests from fluid collected by transtracheal wash. Nebulization and coupage are helpful for promoting expectoration of bronchial secretions. A recumbent patient requires frequent turning and repositioning (every 2 to 4 hours) to prevent exacerbation of the pneumonia.

Treatment of acute fulminating MG deserves special attention because the mortality rate is highest with this uncommon form of the disease. Clinical signs of skeletal muscle weakness are acute and rapidly progressive, making early diagnosis and treatment essential. Respiratory failure usually is the cause of death because of intercostal and diaphragmatic muscle weakness, which may be complicated by aspiration pneumonia. Patients need early ventilatory support and anticholinesterase treatment.[16] Immunosuppressive therapy is indicated, but should be used cautiously, because even a small decrease in muscle strength in these patients can accentuate the clinical signs. Plasmapharesis and intravenous immunoglobulin have been used successfully in human beings with acute fulminating MG. Lack of availability and expense limit their use in veterinary medicine. Use of plasmapharesis and intravenous immunoglobulin therapies for acquired MG in cats has not been reported.

Prognosis

One report of acquired MG in cats has evaluated outcome.[5] Two months after diagnosis, 11 of 20 cats (55 per cent) had improvement of clinical signs, and 6 cats (30 per cent) remained unchanged. Only 3 of 20 cats (15 per cent) had died; these were the 3 cats with acute fulminating MG, and all 3 died of respiratory failure. Two of the 5 cats (40 per cent) with follow-up at 1 year were still alive. Three cats had died or were euthanized at least 1 year after presentation for unrelated causes.[5] Two of the cats in previous reports were asymptomatic 1.5 years after diagnosis.[7, 17] These findings may suggest a better prognosis for focal or generalized MG of cats than that which has been reported in dogs. A possible explanation may relate to the lower incidence of megaesophagus and aspiration pneumonia in cats.

◆ TICK PARALYSIS

Tick paralysis in cats has been reported rarely in the veterinary literature.[18] The ticks that cause paralysis most commonly in North America are *Dermacentor andersoni* and *Dermacentor variabilis*, although other tick species have been incriminated.[19] Cats are resistant to the salivary neurotoxin produced by these ticks.[19] The toxin most likely inhibits neuromuscular transmission by its effects on the presynaptic membrane. Release of ACh is impaired, but it is not known whether this is due to inhibition of calcium influx into the motor nerve terminal or to prevention of binding of the synaptic vesicles to the presynaptic membrane.[19]

Clinical signs usually begin 5 to 9 days after attachment of the tick. Initially, pelvic limb ataxia is exhibited, which progresses rapidly to flaccid tetraplegia with absent spinal reflexes. Cranial nerve paralysis and respiratory failure secondary to intercostal and diaphragmatic muscle paralysis may occur. A diagnosis is suspected by finding an engorged tick attached to the skin. If even one tick is found (or if ticks are suspected), the patient's hair should be clipped, and the cat should be bathed and dipped in a pyrethrin solution. Removal of the tick(s) usually will result in dramatic improvement of clinical signs within 24 to 48 hours. Complete recovery from clinical signs is expected with appropriate insecticidal treatment.

◆ CORAL SNAKE ENVENOMATION

Coral snake envenomation has been reported in 3 cats that experienced acute flaccid tetraplegia.[20] Envenomation by the coral snake (*Micrurus fulvius* species) blocks post-synaptic neuromuscular transmission.[20, 21] Onset of clinical signs begins within the first 24 hours. Clinical signs include progressive flaccid tetraparesis, which affects the craniobulbar muscles preferentially. Spinal reflexes are decreased to absent. Death from respiratory muscle paralysis may occur without ventilatory support. Hemolysis and cardiac arrythmias have occurred in dogs with coral snake envenomation,[21, 22] but these abnormalities were not reported in envenomated cats.[20] Prognosis in cats is considered good with supportive care, and recovery occurs within 10 to 14 days.

Coral snake antivenin (equine origin) is available commercially, but should be used cautiously because of the risk of anaphylaxis. The dose is determined by the amount of venom injected into the cat, which is difficult to assess. Antivenin is most effective when administered within 3 to 4 hours of envenomation. Two of 3 cats in the aforementioned report were given coral snake antivenin, and showed no signs of anaphylaxis.

◆ BOTULISM

Ingestion of *Clostridium botulinum* toxin from carrion may lead to a flaccid tetraparesis. Botulinum toxin prevents ACh release at the presynaptic membrane causing neuromuscular blockade.[23] Although any species may ingest the toxin and show clinical signs of botulism, botulism in cats has not been reported in the veterinary literature. Because clinical signs are similar to other disorders causing flaccid tetraparesis, these differential diagnoses should be considered before making a presumptive diagnosis of botulism.

◆ ORGANOPHOSPHATE AND CARBAMATE TOXICITY

Organophosphate (OP) and carbamate compounds form the basis of many household pesticides and flea-control products. Although the clinical manifestations of toxicity with either of these compounds are similar, there are differences in the mechanisms of action. OP and carbamate insecticides inhibit acetylcholinesterase action at the NMJ, resulting in excess ACh and prolonged depolarization of the postsynaptic membrane. Binding of acetylcholinesterase occurs reversibly with carbamates, and irreversibly with OPs. OPs tend to "age" after several hours, making therapies ineffective.

OP causes excessive stimulation of the postsynaptic membranes,[23, 24] resulting in signs associated with the somatic and parasympathetic nervous systems. Onset of clinical signs occurs within minutes to a few hours after exposure. Common clinical signs of OP and carbamate toxicity in cats are muscle tremors (especially around the face and ears), weakness, ptyalism, vomiting, diarrhea, miosis, bradycardia, and respiratory distress.[24, 25] Restlessness, hyperactivity, and seizures occur with prolonged cholinergic stimulation of the central nervous system.

Diagnosis of OP or carbamate toxicity is based on a history of exposure and compatible clinical signs. Measurement of serum acetylcholinesterase levels in cats is not accurate, because of the presence of pseudocholinesterase in red blood cells. In other species, an acetylcholinesterase level of 50 per cent of normal or less is consistent with OP exposure.

Therapy for OP or carbamate toxicity should begin with cardiovascular stabilization, establishing a patent airway, oxygen supplementation, anticonvulsant therapy, and administration of intravenous fluids. If OP toxicity is known or suspected because of topical administration of an insecticide, the cat is bathed thoroughly to remove any residual OP after exposure. Atropine therapy counteracts the muscarinic effects of OP or carbamate toxicity. Early ad-

ministration treats the bradycardia and respiratory distress secondary to bronchoconstriction or central respiratory depression. The recommended dose is 0.1 to 0.2 mg/kg; 25 per cent of this dose is given intravenously, and the remainder intramuscularly.[24] Overadministration of atropine may result in life-threatening tachyarrythmias, delirium, and hyperthermia. Atropine is not effective for the nicotinic signs of OP toxicity; therefore, it is of little benefit in patients with muscle tremors or weakness.[24, 26]

Pralidoxime chloride (2-PAM, Protopam Chloride, Wyeth-Ayerst) should be administered as soon as possible after exposure. 2-PAM may break down the bond between OP/carbamate and acetylcholinesterase, and form a complex with OP compounds that is eliminated in the urine.[24] Because some OP insecticides "age" with time, 2-PAM is most effective when administered within the first several hours after exposure. 2-PAM is administered intramuscularly or slowly intravenously, at a dose of 20 mg/kg every (q) 8 hr until the patient is asymptomatic, or no improvement has been seen in 24 to 36 hours.[24, 26] Slow intravenous administration is recommended because rapid administration may be associated with tachycardia, muscle rigidity, transient neuromuscular blockade, and laryngospasm.[12] 2-PAM probably is not necessary for carbamate toxicity because binding between the carbamate compound and acetylcholinesterase is reversible. 2-PAM generally is free of adverse effects.

Diphenhydramine has been recommended for alleviation of the nicotinic effects of OP toxicity, but its efficacy has been controversial.[27] The dose in dogs is 1 to 4 mg/kg q 6 to 8 hours, but the appropriate dose for cats has not been investigated. If diphenhydramine is administered, the patient should be monitored carefully for worsening signs of central nervous system depression.

◆ SUMMARY

Differential diagnosis of weakness in cats should include NMJ disorders. An acquired MG is recognized more commonly in cats, and occurs in focal, generalized, and acute fulminating forms. The prognosis is favorable owing to the lower incidence of megaesophagus and aspiration pneumonia in cats compared with dogs.

Coral snake envenomation, tick paralysis, and botulism are rare disorders of the NMJ in cats. OP and carbamate toxicity is common in cats. Knowledge of the clinical signs and treatment regimens of each of these diseases is important for the feline practitioner.

REFERENCES

1. Boonyapsit K, Kaminski HJ, Ruff RL: Disorders of neuromuscular junction ion channels. Am J Med 106:97–113, 1999.
2. Drachman DB: Myasthenia gravis. N Engl J Med 330:1797–1808, 1994.

3. Shelton GD, Cardinet GH, Lindstrom JM: Canine and human myasthenia gravis autoantibodies recognize similar regions on the acetylcholine receptor. Neurology 38:1417–1423, 1988.
4. Dewey CW, Bailey CS, Shelton GD, et al: Clinical forms of acquired myasthenia gravis in dogs: 25 cases (1988–1995). J Vet Intern Med 11:50–57, 1997.
5. Ducoté JM, Dewey CW, Coates JR: Clinical forms of acquired myasthenia gravis in cats. Compend Contin Educ Pract Vet 21:440–448, 1999.
6. Banks WJ: Applied Veterinary Histology, 3rd ed. St. Louis, Mosby–Year Book, 1993, p. 337.
7. Cuddon PA: Acquired immune-mediated myasthenia gravis in a cat. J Small Anim Pract 30:511–516, 1989.
8. Sims MH, McLean RA: Use of repetitive nerve stimulation to assess neuromuscular function in dogs: A test protocol for suspected myasthenia gravis. Prog Vet Neurol 1:311–319, 1990.
9. Hopkins AL, Howard JF, Wheeler SJ, et al: Stimulated single fibre electromyography in normal dogs. J Small Anim Pract 34:271–276, 1993.
10. Joseph RJ, Carrillo JM, Lennon VA: Myasthenia gravis in the cat. J Vet Intern Med 2:75–79, 1988.
11. Malik R, Gabor L, Church DB, et al: Benign cranial mediastinal lesions in three cats. Aust Vet J 75:183–187, 1997.
12. Plumb DC: Veterinary Drug Handbook, 3rd ed. Ames, Iowa State University Press, 1998.
13. Robinson AJ, Clamann P: Effects of glucocorticoids on motor units in cat hindlimb muscles. Muscle Nerve 11:703–713, 1988.
14. Palace J, Newsom-Davis J, Lecky B, et al: A randomized double-blind trial of prednisolone alone or with azathioprine in myasthenia gravis. Neurology 50:1778–1783, 1998.
15. Dewey CW, Coates JR, Ducoté JM, et al: Azathioprine therapy for acquired myasthenia gravis in five dogs. J Am Anim Hosp Assoc 35:396–402, 1999.
16. King LG, Vite CH: Acute fulminating myasthenia gravis in five dogs. J Am Vet Med Assoc 212:830–834, 1998.
17. Mason KV: A case of myasthenia gravis in a cat. J Small Anim Pract 17:467–472, 1976.
18. Mason RW, Kemp DH, King SJ: Ixodes cornuatus and tick paralysis. Aust Vet J 50:580, 1974.
19. Malik R, Farrow BRH: Tick paralysis in North America and Australia. Vet Clin North Am Small Anim Pract 21:157–171, 1991.
20. Chrisman CL, Hopkins AL, Ford SL, et al: Acute, flaccid quadriplegia in three cats with suspected coral snake envenomation. J Am Anim Hosp Assoc 32:343–349, 1996.
21. Marks SL, Mannella C, Schaer M: Coral snake envenomation in the dog: Report of four cases and review of the literature. J Am Anim Hosp Assoc 26:629–634, 1990.
22. Kremer KA, Schaer M: Coral snake (Micrurus fulvius fulvius) envenomation in five dogs: Present and earlier findings. J Vet Emer Crit Care Soc 5:9–15, 1995.
23. Nafe LA: Selected neurotoxins. Vet Clin North Am Small Anim Pract 18:593–604, 1988.
24. Fikes JD: Organophosphorus and carbamate insecticides. Vet Clin North Am Small Anim Pract 20:353–367, 1990.
25. Jaggy A, Oliver JE: Chlorpyrifos toxicosis in two cats. J Vet Intern Med 4:135–139, 1990.
26. Hansen SR: Management of organophosphate and carbamate insecticide toxicoses, In Bonagura JD (ed): Kirk's Current Veterinary Therapy XII. Philadelphia, WB Saunders, 1995, pp. 245–248.
27. Clemmons RM, Meyer DJ, Sundlof SF, et al: Correction of organophosphate-induced neuromuscular blockade by diphenhydramine. Am J Vet Res 45:2167–2169, 1984.

49
◆ Dysautonomia Revisited

Todd W. Axlund
Donald C. Sorjonen
Dennis O'Brien

Feline dysautonomia, also known as the Key-Gaskell or dilated pupil syndrome, is a disease predominantly of the autonomic nervous system resulting in high patient morbidity and mortality. It has been diagnosed in cats from Scandinavia, Europe, the United Kingdom, New Zealand, and the United States.[1] The first reported cases in the United States involved cats imported from the United Kingdom, but it has been diagnosed in native animals.[2–5] The incidence of this disease in the United Kingdom and Scandinavia from 1982 through 1986 reached near-epidemic proportions. Subsequently, the disease has decreased spontaneously in frequency and severity.[1, 6] In the United States, feline dysautonomia is rare. However, familiarity with the clinical signs of dysautonomia is imperative both in making a diagnosis and in monitoring the spread of this disease.

◆ PATHOLOGIC FINDINGS

To date, the etiology of feline dysautonomia is unknown despite intensive efforts by several researchers; however, the associated pathologic changes provide some insight into the possible cause of this disease. The most prominent changes involve the sympathetic and parasympathetic ganglia. Initially, affected neurons in the ganglia become swollen and develop a homogeneous eosinophilic cytoplasm with slight vacuolation and pyknotic nuclei.[7–9] In the latter stages of the disease, affected neurons may become shrunken and irregular, or may disappear altogether. In the affected ganglia, these changes coincide with an increase in nonneuronal cell types.[10] The pathologic changes are not confined to the autonomic ganglia. Similar but less severe changes have been documented in dorsal root ganglia, spinal ventral horn gray matter, and motor nuclei of the oculomotor, trigeminal, facial, vagus, and hypoglossal nerves.[9, 11]

Electron microscopic analysis of acutely affected hypoglossal neurons has been performed. Within the first 2 weeks of the disease, the Nissl substance undergoes dramatic changes. Dispersion of the rough endoplasmic reticulum within the first 3 days is followed by loss of the ribosomal attachments and accumulation of electron-dense floccular material within distended cisternae.[10] Severely affected neurons show no evidence of the rough endoplasmic

reticulum or the Golgi apparatus, and become packed with proliferative smooth endoplasmic reticulum. Additionally, the number of mitochondria and lysosomes is increased.[10] Similar changes have been noted in the autonomic ganglia. These ultrastructural findings offer strong evidence that the lesion primarily involves the protein biosynthetic pathway in specific neurons.

Similarities exist between the feline disease and the dysautonomias that occur in dogs, horses, rabbits, and human beings. Whereas the clinical presentation may differ slightly among these other species, the histopathologic changes are strikingly similar. Such similarity suggests a common, albeit unknown, cause.

◆ CLINICAL SIGNS

There has been no breed, gender, or age predisposition noted. Exclusively outdoor, indoor, and free-access cats have been afflicted with this disease. Single cats in multicat households have been affected, and rarely, multiple cats from a single dwelling may develop the disease.[12, 13] No specific activities have been identified that increase the risk for development of this disease.

Clinical signs may develop acutely or insidiously. The most consistent clinical findings in cats with dysautonomia are anorexia, weight loss, and depression. Other presenting problems are related to parasympathetic dysfunction, and for the most part, are due to widespread gastrointestinal stasis and decreased secretions. Signs include dry mucous membranes and external nares, constipation, keratoconjunctivitis sicca, fixed midrange or dilated pupils, regurgitation or vomiting, dysuria, and megaesophagus. Diarrhea occurs infrequently. Signs of sympathetic dysfunction include prolapse of the nictitating membrane, bradycardia, and syncope. Signs that are seen less frequently include mild paraparesis and anal sphincteric areflexia (Table 49–1). These latter somatic signs probably result from dorsal root ganglia and ventral horn cell lesions noted in this disease. Secondary infections such as aspiration pneumonia, upper respiratory tract infections, and urinary tract infections are common.

◆ DIAGNOSIS

In cats with fulminant disease, diagnosis may be based on the combination of unusual clinical signs.

Table 49–1. Common Clinical Signs of Feline Dysautonomia

Parasympathetic Signs	Sympathetic Signs	Somatic Signs
Fixed dilated pupils	Persistent bradycardia	Paraparesis
Megaesophagus	Elevated nictitating membranes	Anal areflexia
Dry mucous membranes	Syncope	
Constipation		
Dysuria		
Regurgitation/vomiting		

However, milder cases of dysautonomia can be a diagnostic challenge. A grading scheme has been developed that assigns a numerical value to the common clinical features of this disease. A presumptive diagnosis of feline dysautonomia may be based on the overall score.[14] An accurate diagnosis may be obtained using radiography, ocular examination, and pharmacologic testing.

Contrast radiography can help confirm the presence of gastrointestinal stasis. Overt signs of megaesophagus occasionally may be seen on noncontrasted thoracic radiographs. Evidence of aspiration pneumonia with or without a grossly dilated esophagus is a valuable indicator of an esophageal motility disorder. In cats without a dilated esophagus, a motility disorder may be observed during the passage of a food bolus mixed with a radiographic contrast agent. The cervical and intrathoracic sections of the esophagus should be examined carefully for retention of the food bolus. Delayed gastric emptying and increased intestinal transit times also have been documented; however, the high degree of individual variability makes interpretation of these findings difficult.

Ocular abnormalities are prominent in this disease. Fixed, midrange-to-dilated pupils, anisocoria, mucopurulent ocular discharge, and prolapsed nictitating membranes are commonly noted problems in cats with dysautonomia (Fig. 49–1). A thorough ophthalmologic examination should be performed to help rule out primary ocular disease. A Schirmer tear test provides objective assessment of lacrimation, which often is markedly reduced in cats with dysautonomia.

Evaluation of pupillary responses to pharmacologic tests is perhaps the most valuable way to make an antemortem diagnosis of dysautonomia. Results of these tests are based on denervation supersensitivity. This concept assumes that denervation of tissue by the postganglionic nerve results in either an increased number or increased sensitivity of the postsynaptic receptors. The net result is an exuberant response to any substance that is agonistic to the postsynaptic receptor.

One to 2 drops of pilocarpine (0.1 per cent), a direct-acting cholinergic agonist, is applied topically to 1 eye of an affected cat with fixed dilated pupils, and to 1 eye of at least 1 control (normal) cat.[15] The pilocarpine concentration is too dilute to produce a response (miosis) in the control animal(s), but a denervated pupil of an affected animal will respond usually within 20 minutes. Mydriasis also may result from the administration of anticholinergic drugs. Therefore, it is essential to question the owners carefully about prior medications. If uncertainty remains, 1 to 2 drops of 1.0 per cent pilocarpine may be applied to the affected eye 1 or more hours after giving the more dilute dose. Lack of miosis after administration of the concentrated pilocarpine indicates primary iridial disease or pharmacologic blockade, not dysautonomia, as the cause of pupillary dilatation.

Testing for sympathetic (adrenergic) supersensitivity of the iris may be performed in a similar manner using dilute sympathomimetics. However, systemic absorption of the sympathetic agonist may have life-threatening consequences in a dysautonomic animal. For this reason, the authors do not recommend provocative sympathetic testing. Instead, sympathetic evaluation may be performed by assaying for catecholamines and catecholamine metabolites in urine collected over a 24-hour period.[5] Cats with dysautonomia have markedly reduced urine catecholamine levels. However, the special handling and processing required for urine samples, and the limited availability of assays, currently preclude the widespread use of this test.

Whereas ocular parasympathetic denervation is not pathognomonic for dysautonomia, mydriasis combined with signs of generalized parasympathetic or sympathetic failure (e.g., megaesophagus, dry mucous membranes, delayed gastric emptying, persistent bradycardia) are highly suggestive of feline dysautonomia. A definitive diagnosis is obtained only by histopathologic analysis of autonomic ganglia. Typically, the celiac, mesenteric, and

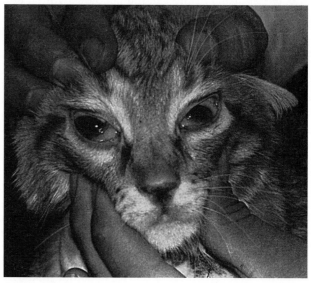

Figure 49–1. A cat with typical clinical signs of dysautonomia.

cervicothoracic ganglia are collected and submitted to an experienced pathologist for examination.

◆ TREATMENT

Management of animals with this disease is limited to supportive therapy because no underlying cause has been identified. Adequate nutrition is a major concern. Most affected cats are unable to maintain daily caloric requirements because of anorexia, vomiting, or severe regurgitation. Alimentary or parenteral nutritional support has been used with some success. Nasoesophageal, nasogastric, pharyngostomy, percutaneous gastric, and jejunostomy tubes may be used to administer caloric requirements. However, severely affected animals may continue to vomit or regurgitate food placed into the alimentary system, making this route of caloric support unacceptable. Additionally, food may be retained in the esophagus or stomach, necessitating regular radiographic evaluation of the thorax and abdomen to ensure the movement of food. Cats that respond to alimentation should be maintained exclusively with a feeding tube. Oral supplementation should begin slowly as the cat regains strength.

Cats that are unable to tolerate alimentation will benefit from parenteral nutritional support. A solution containing lipids, amino acids, vitamins, and dextrose has been used.[4] The solution should be given in a large-gauge catheter placed in the jugular vein or caudal vena cava, and the rate of administration should be increased slowly to full caloric requirements over 3 to 4 days. As with parenteral nutrition in other species, strict aseptic technique should be utilized when manipulating the catheter or changing fluids to prevent the introduction of bacteria. Oral feeding should begin after a recovery period and when it is well tolerated by the animal.

Other supportive measures are necessary. Artificial tears should be applied 2 to 3 times daily, and intermittent nebulization performed to reduce the irritation from dry mucous membranes. Animals that are unable to urinate require frequent bladder evacuations. Regular examination of the health of the urinary tract with urinalysis and urine culture is necessary. Parasympathomimetic agents may aid in urination. Pilocarpine is administered in the conjunctival sac to promote urination and defecation, and to ameliorate the ocular abnormalities. However, individual variations in response to this drug make standard dosing schedules hazardous. A dosage of 1 to 2 drops of 0.25 per cent pilocarpine given in the conjunctival sac every 6 to 8 hours may offer some relief, but close monitoring of response and tailoring of the dose often is necessary. Bethanechol also has proved helpful in a number of cases at a dosage of 2.5 to 7.5 mg orally divided 2 or 3 times daily. As with pilocarpine, careful tailoring of the dose of bethanechol is necessary. It is wise to start treatment with a low dose of the drug, and increase until the proper response is elicited. The most common side-effects of parasympathetic stimulation include vomiting, regurgitation, defecation, lacrimation, and excessive salivation.

Antiemetics may offer some relief in animals with severe vomiting. Metoclopramide (0.3 mg/kg, every [q] 8 hr subcutaneously), a gastric prokinetic and centrally acting antiemetic, may be of some benefit. Prochlorperazine (0.12 mg/kg, q 8 hr intramuscularly) may be given if no response is noted with metoclopramide. However, the response to either of these drugs is variable.

It is important to inform the owners about the goals of therapy. Treatment is exclusively supportive; it offers some palliation of the clinical signs and time for the cat to recover neurologic function. As such, careful consultation about the length of convalescence and degree of commitment on the part of the owner is essential. Recovery usually begins several months after the onset of clinical signs, and may take a year or longer for more advanced recovery. Some animals never regain full function, and will require some degree of support for the rest of their lives. Cats that are more severely affected tend to have longer and less complete recoveries. Complications of this disease, such as persistent vomiting and urinary incontinence, may necessitate euthanasia of some affected cats during the prolonged recovery phase.

Feline dysautonomia was an important disease in Britain and some European countries during the 1980s. Although it has not become a widespread disease in the United States at this time, it is important to be able to recognize the signs associated with this condition in order to monitor its propagation and to help formulate a rational treatment plan.

REFERENCES

1. Edney AT, Gaskell CJ: Feline dysautonomia around the world (Letter). Vet Rec 123:451–452, 1988.
2. Bromberg NM: Feline dysautonomia: A case report. J Am Anim Hosp Assoc 24:106–108, 1986.
3. Canton DD, Sharp NJ, Aguirre GD: Dysautonomia in a cat. J Am Vet Med Assoc 192:1293–1296, 1988.
4. Guilford WG, O'Brien DP, Allert A, Ermeling HM: Diagnosis of dysautonomia in a cat by autonomic nervous system function testing. J Am Vet Med Assoc 193:823–828, 1988.
5. Levy JK, James KM, Cowgill LD, et al: Decreased urinary catecholamines in a cat with dysautonomia. J Am Vet Med Assoc 205:842–844, 1994.
6. Blaxter A, Gruffydd-Jones T: Feline dysautonomia. In Practice 9:58–61, 1987.
7. Griffiths IR, Nash AS, Sharp NJ: The Key-Gaskell syndrome: The current situation. Vet Rec 111:532–533, 1982.
8. Pollin M, Griffiths IR: A review of the primary dysautonomias of domestic animals. J Comp Pathol 106:99–119, 1992.
9. Sharp NJ, Nash A, Griffiths IR: Feline dysautonomia (the Key-Gaskell syndrome): A clinical and pathological study of forty cases. J Small Anim Pract 25:599–615, 1984.
10. Pollin M, Griffiths IR: Feline dysautonomia: An ultrastructural study of neurones in the XII nucleus. Acta Neuropathol 73:275–280, 1987.

11. Griffiths IR, Sharp NJ, McCulloch MC: Feline dysautonomia (the Key-Gaskell syndrome): An ultrastructural study of autonomic ganglia and nerves. Neuropathol Appl Neurobiol 11:17–29, 1985.

12. Symonds HW, McWilliams P, Thompson H, et al: A cluster of cases of feline dysautonomia (Key-Gaskell syndrome) in a closed colony of cats. Vet Rec 136:353–355, 1995.

13. Nash AS, Thompson H, Rosengurt N, et al: Feline dysautonomia in group-housed cats (letter; comment). Vet Rec 134:175–176, 1994.

14. Sharp NJ: Visceral dysfunction. *In* Wheeler SJ (ed): Manual of Small Animal Neurology. London, BSAVA, 1989, pp. 215–222.

15. Collins KB, O'Brien DP: Autonomic dysfunction of the eye. Semin Vet Med Surg Small Anim 5:24–36, 1990.

50

◆ Cerebral Meningiomas: Diagnostic and Therapeutic Considerations

Richard A. LeCouteur

> It is fair to say that few procedures in surgery may be more immediately formidable than an attack upon a large tumor of the type herein to be discussed, and that the ultimate prognosis hinges more on the surgeon's wide experience with the problem in all its many aspects than is true of almost any other operation that can be named.
>
> *Harvey Cushing and Louise Eisenhardt, 1938*[1]

The term *meningioma* was first used by Harvey Cushing over 75 years ago to classify variously named tumors of the meninges of human beings.[2] Since that time, meningiomas have been identified as the most common primary central nervous system (CNS) tumor of both cats and dogs, and have been identified in many other species of domestic animals including sheep, horses, and cattle.[3–6]

Intracranial neoplasms may be classified as either primary or secondary.[7, 8] Primary neoplasms arise from brain or meningeal stem cells, whereas secondary tumors are either metastases from a primary tumor located outside the nervous system, or tumors that affect the brain by local invasion from adjacent nonneural structures such as bone, middle ear, or nasal cavity. Primary brain tumors in cats rarely metastasize outside the nervous system, although in some cases, local spread along cerebrospinal fluid (CSF) pathways may occur,[9] and a case report exists of metastasis to lung of a solitary parietal lobe meningioma in a cat.[10]

The terms *benign* and *malignant* may be used to classify tumors according to their tendency to become progressively worse, metastasize, and result in death.[7] In assessing the malignant potential of a brain tumor, the difference between cytologic and biologic malignancy should be considered.[7] Cytologic malignancy is a morphologic assessment of a tumor based on histologic characteristics. Biologic malignancy is the likelihood that a tumor will kill an animal. Although feline meningiomas usually are cytologically benign, they may be biologically malignant as a result of their location, and the secondary effects they produce, such as increased intracranial pressure (ICP), cerebral edema, or brain herniation.

◆ INCIDENCE

Cerebral meningioma is the most frequently occurring intracranial neoplasm of cats, accounting for almost 10 per cent of feline nonhematopoietic neoplasms,[3, 11, 12] and over 50 per cent of CNS neoplasms found at necropsy.[6] Of 48 cats with intracranial neoplasms in one study, 42 (88 per cent) had meningiomas.[6] In another series of 30 primary CNS neoplasms, 80 per cent were meningiomas.[12]

Primary brain tumors appear to be less common in cats than in dogs or human beings.[7] Primary brain tumors other than meningioma reported to occur in the brain of cats include ependymoma, choroid plexus papilloma, medulloblastoma, lymphoma, olfactory neuroblastoma, and gangliocytoma.[9, 12, 13]

◆ LOCATION

Meningiomas are thought to arise from mesodermal elements of the cranial or spinal meninges, most likely from arachnoid cells or arachnoid cap cells, or both.[14, 15] These are specialized cells found in arachnoid granulations. It is not surprising that the majority of rostral fossa meningiomas are clustered around venous sinuses and dural folds, where arachnoid granulations are located in large numbers.[15] The occurrence of meningiomas in the choroid plexuses of cats is believed to result from neoplastic transformation of clusters of arachnoid cells normally found within the connective tissue stroma.[3] These clusters are derived from the tela choroidea as it invaginates to form the choroid plexuses.[3]

In cats, solitary meningiomas occur most frequently over the cerebral hemispheres, with frontal, parietal, and occipital lobe sites about equally represented.[3, 16] Meningiomas also may develop along the falx cerebri, at the base of the brain, within the third ventricle or a lateral ventricle, and within the caudal fossa of the calvarium.[3, 13, 16] Cerebral meningiomas occur more frequently that spinal meningiomas.[16] In one study of meningiomas in 24 cats, 96 per cent were intracranial and 4 per cent affected the spinal cord.[12]

Although meningiomas in cats most often develop as solitary tumors, multiple primary meningiomas occur relatively commonly.[6, 17] McGrath[12] reported that multiple intracranial meningiomas were found in 11 of 23 cats.

◆ ETIOLOGY

The exact cause of meningiomas in cats remains undetermined.[14, 15] The occurrence of meningiomas in 4 of 7 young cats with mucopolysaccharidosis I may suggest that this metabolic disorder in some way predisposed to the development of this neoplasm, or that the 2 entities share a common etiologic mechanism such as a specific chromosomal deletion.[18] Chemotherapy for thymic lymphoma was postulated as a possible cause for the development of multiple meningiomas in a 2-year-old cat 5 months after initiation of the chemotherapy.[19]

Meningiomas have been induced experimentally in dogs using chemical carcinogens, Rous sarcoma virus, or perinatal x-irradiation.[3, 20] Genetic, chemical, viral, traumatic, and immunologic factors may predispose human beings to meningioma formation.[14] Radiation has been confirmed as a definite causative factor of meningiomas in children receiving scalp irradiation.[14] Several clinical features suggest that growth of meningiomas may be influenced by sex hormones (progesterone or estrogen).[14] The relationship between meningioma development in human beings, and viruses, brain trauma, sex hormones, or other factors, remains unclear.[14]

◆ PATHOLOGIC FINDINGS

Typically, feline meningiomas are well-defined, lobulated masses with a broad meningeal base of attachment.[3] They may vary in size from small nodules up to masses several centimeters in diameter, and tend to be firm to hard in consistency with a granular irregular surface. These tumors may be enucleated easily from their intraparenchymal indentation, as they derive a thin investing capsule from the leptomeninges.[3] Growth of the tumor usually occurs by local expansion and rarely by parenchymal invasion.[21] Meningiomas tend to grow slowly under the dura mater and expand toward the brain producing pressure atrophy and parenchymal displacement. They may adhere to the dura mater, or lie within the leptomeningeal tissue. The growth rate of meningiomas in cats appears to be slower than that in dogs.

Meningiomas are histologically diverse, with most tumors demonstrating more than 1 cellular subtype. Pure histologic forms are exceptional.[3] Immunohistochemistry is essential for the accurate identification and classification of feline brain tumors.[22] The meningioma subtypes identified include meningothelial, fibroblastic, transitional (mixed), psammomatous, papillary, microcystic, myxoid, angiomatous (angioblastic), and atypical.[23] Transitional and fibroblastic appear to be the most common subtypes seen in cats. Feline meningiomas commonly have multiple areas of cholesterol cleft formation. The histologic diversity of meningiomas may reflect the mixed mesodermal and neural crest origins of the brain and spinal cord leptomeninges.

The classification of meningiomas into these histologic subtypes may have little bearing on their clinical behavior.[16] An exception may be the angioblastic subtype, which is associated with a poor prognosis in human beings.[14, 15]

When confirmation of a diagnosis of meningioma is difficult with light microscopy alone, other techniques may be used. Confirmation of a meningioma is accomplished most reliably using ultrastructural criteria.[14, 15] Irrespective of their histologic subtyping, most meningiomas have very characteristic long, interdigitating, parallel-layered cytoplasmic processes with endocytotic evaginations of their cytoplasmic membrane. Their most consistent features are the various morphologic types of cell-to-cell connections between these processes. There are variable numbers of normal and abnormal desmosomal and gap junctions.[24] Tight junctions and hemidesmosomes are seen almost invariably, although their numbers may vary widely among histologic subtypes.

◆ CLINICAL FINDINGS

Meningiomas have been reported in cats from 1 to 24 years of age.[3] Approximately 70 to 75 per cent of meningiomas occur in cats over 9 years of age.[3] The occurrence of meningiomas in older cats may be related to development of senile arachnoid cell clusters with subsequent hyperplasia and calcification.[3] Although there does not appear to be a breed predisposition for the development of meningiomas, male cats are affected more frequently than females.[17]

Meningiomas in cats may occur in the absence of neurologic signs.[16] In one series of cases, 11 of 36 cats (31 per cent) with meningiomas did not have apparent neurologic signs.[17] Most of these tumors were located over the cerebral convexities. In another study of 155 cats that were neurologically normal, 8 (5.2 per cent) had an incidental finding of meningioma.[4] The meningiomas in 7 of these cats arose from the tela choroidea and were located in the third ventricle.

Clinical signs that may be associated with a meningioma affecting the brain are summarized in Table 50–1. Location within the brain and rate of growth determine the clinical signs associated with a meningioma. Localized (focal) abnormalities are seen most frequently, and result from direct compression, invasion, or irritation of a region of the brain. Generalized (nonlocalizing) signs result from secondary effects such as elevated ICP, cerebral edema, or herniation. In a study of meningiomas in 36 cats, tentorial herniation was reported in 6 (16.7 per cent) cats.[17]

The extent of peritumoral brain edema associated with cerebral meningiomas of cats is extremely variable. In human beings, development of accompanying peritumoral edema occurs in 40 to 60 per cent of meningiomas.[25] Edema also is a prominent finding associated with many canine meningio-

Table 50–1. Clinical Signs Associated With Meningiomas of Cats

*Generalized Signs**

Altered state of consciousness
Behavioral change
Head pressing
Pacing
Papilledema

Localized (Focal) Signs

Paresis (tetraparesis, hemiparesis)
Ataxia
Circling
Hemisensory abnormalities
Impaired vision (bilateral or unilateral deficits)
Cranial nerve deficits

Seizures

Focal or secondary generalized

Specific Neurologic Syndromes

Cerebellomedullary angle
Vestibular
Hypothalamohypophyseal
Cerebellar

*Often associated with increased intracranial pressure.

mas.[26] Several causative factors have been proposed for the development of peritumoral brain edema, including tumor size, location, histologic subtype, and vascularity.[25] Recently, it has been demonstrated in human beings that the expression of vascular endothelial growth factors may induce meningioma-associated peritumoral brain edema.[25]

It should be remembered that intracranial neoplasia must be considered as a possible cause for all neurologic syndromes that may be localized to the brain. Frequently, cats with a brain tumor present with a history of gradual onset of progressive signs of CNS dysfunction. Behavioral changes such as lethargy, dullness, disorientation, hiding, abnormal vocalization, and staring are described commonly.[17, 27, 28] In a number of cats with meningiomas examined by the author, decreased frequency of purring was a subtle alteration in behavior noted by the owners for up to 1 year before the onset of focal neurologic signs. These vague signs may precede more dramatic signs such as seizures. Seizure disorders in cats are nearly always the result of structural brain diseases, including brain tumors. Idiopathic and hereditary epilepsy do not appear to be common in cats.[29] Other clinical signs reported in cats with cerebral meningiomas include circling, visual deficits, hemiparesis, partial trigeminal and facial nerve palsies, and positional nystagmus.[17]

Because the brain is contained within the confines of the calvaria, even a slow-growing tumor may have devastating effects. In slow-growing lesions of the brain, surrounding structures adapt to increasing pressure. During this period of compensation, there may be a prolonged history of vague signs (e.g., subtle behavior alterations). However, even with a very slow-growing tumor, clinical signs

may progress rapidly when compensatory mechanisms have been exhausted. Rapidly growing tumors may not permit the process of compensation to occur, and in such cases a sudden onset of severe neurologic dysfunction may occur in the absence of premonitory signs. An acute onset of neurologic deficits may ensue if a neoplasm erodes or obstructs a major blood vessel, causing hemorrhage or infarction.

The precise location of a brain tumor may be masked by the more generalized secondary effects caused by the tumor, including elevated ICP, brain herniation, or hydrocephalus. Increased ICP often is associated with cerebral edema, and less commonly with hemorrhage or infarction. Increased ICP also may develop in association with either a small, rapidly growing tumor or a slowly growing tumor that has reached a significant size. Tumors that obstruct CSF flow or result in brain herniation also may result in a rapid and severe rise in ICP.

◆ DIAGNOSIS

On the basis of signalment, history, and the results of a physical and neurologic examination, it may be possible to localize a lesion to the brain, and occasionally to determine an approximate location. It should always be kept in mind that a similar neurologic syndrome will result from any one of a number of different diseases occurring at a given location. Many degenerative, metabolic, infectious, inflammatory, toxic, and vascular diseases may result in clinical signs similar to those seen with a brain tumor. These other causes must be eliminated before the diagnosis of a brain tumor is made. The diagnosis of an intracranial neoplasm is based primarily on elimination of causes outside the nervous system, and results of specialized radiographic and imaging techniques.

A minimum database for a cat suspected to have a brain lesion should include a complete blood count, serum biochemistry analysis, urinalysis, thoracic radiographs, and abdominal ultrasound examination. Results of these tests are especially important when a metastatic brain tumor is suspected, or when clinical signs of metabolic or endocrine disturbances are present.

Skull Radiographs

Before the availability of advanced imaging tools such as computed tomography (CT) and magnetic resonance imaging (MRI), an antemortem diagnosis of a brain tumor, and its exact location and extent, were difficult to determine. Plain skull radiographs were used for this purpose. General anesthesia is necessary for precise positioning of the head for plain radiographs. Radiographs of the skull appear normal in most cats with meningiomas; however, there may be evidence of mineralization within a meningioma, and hyperostosis,[3] or osteolysis[30] of the overlying calvarium may be induced by a meningioma.[6, 12] Hyperostosis was recognized radiographically in 9 of 10 (90 per cent) cats with meningiomas in one study.[31] A modified occipital projection may aid in the recognition of hyperostosis.[32] Hyperostosis may be related to direct bone invasion by tumor cells, or occur as a purely reactive change without detectable tumor cells in bone.[33] Enlarged vascular channels may be suggestive of a tumor of the dura mater or calvaria in human beings, and have been reported to occur in association with meningiomas in cats.[31]

Whereas survey radiographic abnormalities may provide indirect evidence of the presence of a meningioma, such alterations seldom provide precise information regarding location and extent of a meningioma, and its relationship to normal intracranial structures. Furthermore, deep-seated meningiomas (e.g., third ventricle meningiomas) may not induce survey radiographic changes.

Cerebrospinal Fluid

Analysis of CSF serves to help rule out inflammatory diseases and may support the diagnosis of an intracranial tumor.[7, 8] Results of CSF analysis most often seen in cats with a brain tumor include an increase in protein content in the presence of a normal cell count.[34] This is a variable finding, however, and it is possible to have normal results for these tests. Exfoliated tumor cells are seen rarely in CSF.[7–9]

CSF collection may be contraindicated in cats in which a brain tumor is suspected. It is recommended that collection of CSF be delayed until advanced imaging procedures have been completed. Care always must be taken in the collection of CSF because increased ICP may be present in association with an intracranial mass, and the ICP changes associated with the removal of CSF may lead to brain herniation. Administration of mannitol and hyperventilation may help to decrease ICP before CSF collection.

Advanced Imaging

CT and MRI provide the information required for accurate recognition of the presence and location of a mass lesion within the brain.[7, 8] Information from advanced imaging studies also provides a means to plan further diagnostic and therapeutic interventions for meningiomas of cats.

Although alterations seen with CT are not specific for any particular lesion, certain generalizations may be made regarding the CT appearance of meningiomas.[15, 35, 36] On noncontrast CT images, meningiomas appear isodense to slightly hyperdense with respect to normal gray matter. Meningiomas usually are of homogeneous density, have well-defined margins, and may be globoid, lobulated, or en plaque. Areas of mineralization may be present, and are seen more clearly on CT than on MRI. After administration of contrast medium, intense homogeneous enhancement is expected to occur. Hyperostosis, osteolysis, and apparent tumoral mineralization are readily detectable by CT. Peritumoral edema often is evident. A nonspecific sign of a meningioma is evidence of accommodation of the brain to the presence of a longstanding, slow-growing, space-occupying lesion. The falx cerebri may become bowed, and the brain may exhibit less shift than might be anticipated for the size of the tumor.

On MRI, meningiomas may be difficult to detect without contrast enhancement (Fig. 50–1).[15] On T1-weighted images, a typical meningioma is isointense or hypointense with respect to gray matter; on proton-density and T2-weighted images, a typical meningioma is isointense or hyperintense; in either sequence, a meningioma may have a "mottled" appearance (see Fig. 50–1). An interface is seen frequently between the tumor and the surrounding brain on T1- and T2-weighted images. This hypointense signal may represent a compressed arachnoid plane between tumor and brain, as well as a compressed draining venous plexus.[15] Hypointense areas within the meningioma may reflect the amount of intratumoral mineralization.[15] The so-called dural tail sign, although not specific for meningioma, is often associated with either neoplastic infiltration of meninges beyond the margin of the meningioma or hypervascularity of the dura mater.[15, 37]

CT and MRI should be viewed as complementary diagnostic imaging modalities, each with its own advantages and disadvantages.[26, 38] Whereas CT excels in the detection of osseous changes, such as skull fractures or sclerotic changes in the tympanic bullae, MRI provides superior soft-tissue detail and allows visualization of subtle changes accompanying nonenhancing or diffuse brain lesions not seen easily using CT. A percentage of intracranial mass lesions may not be visible by means of CT, probably due to diffuse distribution, similar attenuation to surrounding normal tissue, and minimum or absent contrast enhancement. The high resolution and soft-tissue contrast achieved with MRI is especially useful in the identification of these brain tumors. MRI also allows the secondary effects of a tumor to be assessed, and is generally accepted to be superior to CT in the detection of many of the features associated with brain tumors (e.g., edema, cyst formation, changes in vascularity, hemorrhage, and necrosis). Other subtle effects such as displacement of the ventricular system and gyral folds, and displacement of the external capsule or herniation of the temporal lobe, also may be visible by means of MRI. The multiplanar imaging capability of MRI also permits better definition of the anatomic relationships of a tumor and surrounding normal structures. Unlike CT scanning, beam-hardening artifact caused by thick compact bone does not occur with MRI.

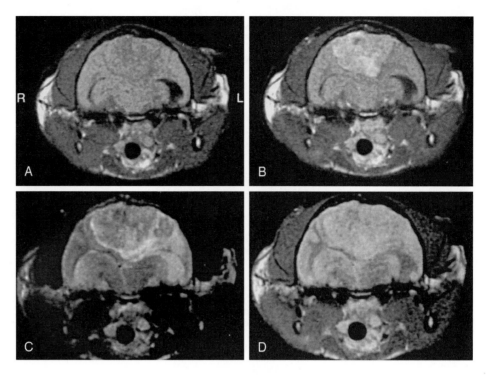

Figure 50–1. Transverse magnetic resonance images of the head of a 14-year-old castrated male domestic shorthair cat at the level of the pituitary. This cat had a 1-week history of circling to the right. A large psammomatous meningioma, characterized by whorls of spindle cells with mineralized centers, is present within the parietal lobe of the cerebrum on T1-weighted precontrast *(A)*, T2-weighted postcontrast *(B)*, T2-weighted *(C)*, and proton-density *(D)* images.

CT-Guided Brain Biopsy

Although feline meningiomas have characteristic CT and MRI features, occasionally nonneoplastic space-occupying lesions or a metastasis may mimic the CT or MRI appearance of a meningioma. Biopsy of an intracranial lesion may be an important step before initiation of any type of therapy.[7]

The most recent advance in the biopsy of brain tumors has been the modification of a CT-guided stereotactic brain biopsy system designed for use in human beings (Pelorus Mark III Stereotactic System, Ohio Medical Instruments Company, Cincinnati, OH), for use in cats and dogs.[39, 40] This CT-guided stereotactic biopsy system provides a relatively rapid and extremely accurate means of tumor biopsy, with a low rate of complications.

Cytologic evaluation of brain tumor biopsy samples may be done within minutes of biopsy collection by means of crush preparations.[8] The tissue sample is fixed rapidly in 95 per cent alcohol, and stained with hematoxylin and eosin. Diagnostically accurate information from this rapid technique generally is available from both primary and metastatic nervous system tumors, and from nonneoplastic lesions. In the author's experience, air-dried slides of crush preparations also may be stained with Wright stain and counter-stained with Giemsa to provide additional information regarding cell types present in a mass.

◆ TREATMENT AND PROGNOSIS

The major goals of brain tumor therapy are (1) to control secondary effects of a tumor (e.g., increased ICP, cerebral edema, or seizures), and (2) to eliminate a tumor, or at least reduce its size.[7, 8] Before the availability of CT or MRI, the treatment of cats with meningiomas was directed primarily toward control of the secondary effects. Palliative therapy for a cat with a meningioma consists of glucocorticoid administration for edema reduction, and phenobarbital for seizure control. Median survival times reported in cats in which only supportive therapies were used ranged from 25 to 73 days.[41]

After the development of advanced techniques for imaging of feline brain, surgical management of feline meningiomas has become accepted as the most effective method of treatment. Adjunctive therapies such as radiation therapy[42–44] or chemotherapy also may have a role in the management of feline meningiomas, particularly those that are surgically inaccessible.[14, 15] New therapies, such as gene therapy, may play a future role in the management of feline meningiomas.[8]

Neurosurgical intervention is an essential consideration in the management of a cat with an intracranial meningioma, whether for complete excision, partial removal, or biopsy of the mass.[7] Median survival times of 26 and 27 months have been reported for cats that were followed closely after undergoing surgical removal of a meningioma (Table 50–2). The precise location, size, and subtype of a neoplasm, and the physical or neurologic status of the patient will determine the extent of removal. Meningiomas, particularly those located over the frontal lobes of the cerebrum, often may be removed completely. In contrast, there may be a significant morbidity associated with the surgical removal of caudal fossa, brain stem, or third ventricular neoplasms. The treatment of multiple meningiomas is the same as for solitary tumors.

Table 50–2. Survival Data for Cats After Surgical Removal of Meningiomas

Cats (n)	Age/Gender	Postoperative Complications	Survival Infomation	Tumor Recurrence	First Author, Date
42	Median, 11.7 yr (range, 5–17 yr) 57% male 43% female	13/42 postoperative anemia 8/42 died/ euthanized immediately postoperatively [7/8 cerebral edema/ herniation; 6/8 anemic]	71% alive at 6 mo 66% at 1 yr 50% at 2 yr (not followed further) Median survival at time of writing of 18 surviving cats—26 mo	6 cats (17.6%)	Gordon, 1994[28]
17	Median, 12 yr (range, 6–21 yr) 53% male 47% female	3/17 died/ euthanized immediately postoperatively [2/3 died of brain herniation; 1/3 renal failure]	14 survived immediate postoperative period 11 were followed for 18 to 47 mo (median, 27 mo) without recurrence	3 cats (21.4%) 2 died of tumor recurrence within 1 yr 1 cat euthanized at 72 mo after surgery had a brain carcinoma causing clinical signs and an incidental finding of recurrence of meningioma	Gallagher, 1993[27]
4	Not available	1 died immediately postoperatively of brain herniation and intracranial hemorrhage	Mean survival 485 days 2-yr survival 50%	2 cats died/euthanized due to tumor recurrence	Niebauer, 1991[21]
10	Mean, 9 yr (range, 6–13 yr) 80% male 20% female	1 died immediately postoperatively due to brain herniation	2 died within 3.5 mo of surgery due to cardiomyopathy 6 alive at the time article written	1 recurrence reported 2.5 yr after surgery; this cat died of cardiomyopathy 1 mo after second surgery	Lawson, 1984[31]

Partial removal of a brain neoplasm may relieve signs of cerebral dysfunction, provide tissue for a histologic diagnosis, and may make a patient a better candidate for other therapy, such as irradiation. Surgical biopsy of a tumor must be approached with care to avoid seeding of tumor cells to normal tissue.

Although meningioma removal in cats is relatively commonplace today, the surgery is not always benign and curative. Several reviews evaluating the results of surgical removal have reported mortality rates in cats of from 10 to 25 per cent in the immediate postoperative period.[28] It is expected that recent improvements in neurosurgical techniques, neuroanesthesia, and postoperative care will result in improved morbidity and mortality statistics for cats undergoing surgical removal of a meningioma.

Hemorrhage and blood loss may be a significant problem intraoperatively, and transfusion may be necessary.[28] In human beings, meningiomas are known to produce a hypercoagulable state with pulmonary thromboembolism as a potential postoperative complication.[45]

Brain herniation would appear to be the most common cause of death during the immediate postoperative period (see Table 50–2). Life-threatening increases in ICP may occur at any time before, during, or after intracranial surgery, and if not recognized, or left untreated, may proceed rapidly to decompensation of cerebral tissues, herniation, and patient death. Preexisting intracranial hypertension may be exacerbated by various drugs, including the inhalational anesthetics, and hypoventilation. The recent development of small, easy to use ICP monitors suitable for use in cats should make monitoring of ICP more routine during the intraoperative and postoperative periods.

Recurrence of meningioma is a complication after surgical meningioma removal in cats. In several studies with long-term follow-up of cats after surgical removal of a meningioma, 17.6 to 21 per cent of cats that survived the immediate postoperative period later developed tumor recurrence, 1 as early as 1.5 months after surgery (see Table 50–2). In one study in which 6 cats experienced tumor regrowth, 3 had recurrence at the original site, 1 had recurrence at the original site and a new site, and 2 had tumor growth in a new location.[28] One cat with tumor regrowth underwent a second surgery, and was still alive at 46.2 months after the first surgery (11.8 months after the second surgery).[28] Important surgical considerations that influence tumor recurrence include removal of hyperostotic bone and removal of dura mater in the region of the tumor.

Recurrence of meningiomas occurs in 10 to 32 per cent of human patients after apparent "complete" surgical excision.[15] Recurrence of a meningioma is seen more frequently in human beings when the location of a meningioma, invasion of bone, or involvement of major vascular structures precludes total surgical excision of the mass. Although the degree of resection appears to be most important in determining meningioma recurrence, histopathologic features also are important.[14] The high rate of recurrence of meningiomas in human patients after surgical excision has resulted in the widespread use of radiation therapy after tumor resection.[44]

The use of radiation therapy for the treatment of primary brain tumors is well established, and it may be used either alone or in combination with other treatments.[7, 8] The objective of radiation therapy is to destroy a neoplasm, while at the same time minimizing damage to any normal tissue that is included in the irradiated volume. External beam, megavoltage irradiation currently is recommended for the therapy of meningiomas in cats. Although orthovoltage radiation has been used for the treatment of some brain tumors, its use is not optimum because of poor beam penetration, profile, and limited field configuration. Careful treatment planning by a qualified radiation therapist is essential for a successful outcome from radiation therapy. The selection of a radiation dose is based partly on considerations such as tumor type and location, and partly on tolerance of the surrounding normal tissues. Computerized treatment planning using images generated by CT or MRI is in use at many veterinary facilities. Effective radiation therapy generally involves fractionating the total dose into smaller fractions that are given over a 3- to 5-week period. In veterinary medicine, a wide variety of fractionating schemes have been used. It is recommended that daily fractions (Monday to Friday) of less than or equal to 3 Gy be given for up to 4 weeks, with the total normal tissue dose below 50 Gy.[46]

Although much has been published about the in vivo and in vitro effects of a variety of drugs on the growth of meningioma cells in culture and in nude mouse models,[15] there is little clinical experience with drug therapy for cats with meningiomas. Treatment using cytotoxic agents or hormone receptor-blocking agents has been recommended[15, 47]; however, more research in this area clearly is needed. Likewise, although the development of gene therapy strategies for treatment of intracranial tumors shows much promise, research in this area is still at an early stage.[7]

Since the first recorded surgical removal of a feline meningioma was reported in 1959,[48] the management of meningiomas of cats has remained a major challenge to veterinary neurosurgeons. With the advent of better imaging techniques, tumors are being identified earlier, and may be found in cats with only a seizure as the presenting problem. Improved surgical techniques and instrumentation, enhanced anesthetic management, and advanced postoperative care techniques (such as ICP monitoring), have contributed to better survival statistics. Radiation therapy may have a substantial effect in limiting tumor growth in some meningiomas. Future developments in adjunctive treatments such as chemotherapy or gene therapy are likely to contribute further to the long-term survival of cats with cerebral meningiomas. However, it appears that the key factors in the successful management of meningiomas in cats are (1) the use of good judgment in decisions relating to diagnosis and therapy, and (2) the surgical skills of the neurosurgeon involved.

REFERENCES

1. Cushing H, Eisenhardt L: Meningiomas: Their Classification, Regional Behavior, Life History and Surgical End Results. Springfield, IL, Charles C Thomas, 1938.
2. Cushing H: The meningiomas (dural endotheliomas): Their source, and favored seats of origin. Brain 45:282–306, 1922.
3. Braund KG, Ribas JL: Central nervous system meningiomas. Compend Contin Educ Pract Vet 8:241–247, 1986.
4. Luginbuhl H: Studies on meningiomas in cats. Am J Vet Res 22:1030–1040, 1961.
5. Luginbuhl H, Fankhauser R, McGrath JT: Spontaneous neoplasms of the nervous system in animals. Prog Neurol Surg 2:85–64, 1968.
6. Zaki FA, Hurvitz AI: Spontaneous neoplasms of the central nervous system of the cat. J Small Anim Pract 17:773–782, 1976.
7. LeCouteur RA: Tumors of the nervous system. In Withrow SJ, MacEwen EG (eds): Small Animal Clinical Oncology, 2nd ed. Philadelphia, WB Saunders, 1996, pp. 393–419.
8. LeCouteur RA: Current concepts in the diagnosis and treatment of brain tumours in dogs and cats. J Small Anim Pract 40:411–416, 1999.
9. Dickinson PJ, Keel MK, Higgins RJ, et al: Clinical and pathological features of oligodendrogliomas in two cats. Vet Pathol 37:160–167, 2000.
10. Dahme VE: Meningome bei Fleischfressern. Berl Münch Tierärztl Wochenschr 70:32–34, 1957.
11. Patnaik AK, Liu SK, Hurvitz AI, et al: Nonhematopoietic neoplasms in cats. J Natl Cancer Inst 54:855–860, 1975.
12. McGrath JT: Meningiomas in animals. J Neuropathol Exp Neurol 21:327–328, 1962.
13. Kornegay JN: Central nervous system neoplasia. In Kornegay JN (ed): Neurologic Disorders. New York, Churchill Livingstone, 1986, pp. 79–108.
14. Black PM: Meningiomas. Neurosurgery 32:643–657, 1993.
15. McDermott MW, Wilson CB: Meningiomas. In Youmans JR (ed): Neurological Surgery, 4th ed. Philadelphia, WB Saunders, 1996, pp. 2782–2825.
16. Holzworth J: Diseases of the Cat. Philadelphia, WB Saunders, 1987, pp. 554–556.
17. Nafe LA: Meningiomas in cats: A retrospective clinical study of 36 cases. J Am Vet Med Assoc 74:1224–1227, 1979.
18. Haskins ME, McGrath JT: Meningiomas in young cats with mucopolysaccharidosis I. J Neuropathol Exp Neurol 42:664–670, 1983.
19. Lobetti RG, Nesbit JW, Miller DB: Multiple malignant meningiomas in a young cat. J S Afr Vet Assoc 68:62–65, 1997.
20. Benjamin SA, Lee AC, Angleton GM, et al: Neoplasms in young dogs after perinatal irradiation. J Natl Cancer Inst 77:563–571, 1986.
21. Niebauer GW, Dayrell-Hart B, Speciale J: Evaluation of craniotomy in dogs and cats. J Am Vet Med Assoc 198:89–95, 1991.
22. Schwecheimer K, Kartenbeck J, Moll R, et al: Vimentin filament-desmosome cytoskeleton of diverse types of human meningiomas. Lab Invest 51:584–591, 1984.
23. Kliehues P, Burger PC, Scheithauer BW: Histological typing of tumors of the central nervous system. In World Health Organization: International Histological Classification of Tumours. Berlin, Springer-Verlag, 1993, pp. 33–42.
24. Higgins RJ, LeCouteur RA, Koblik PD, et al: Canine meningiomas: Cell to cell communication (Abstract #114). Vet Pathol 33:598, 1996.
25. Yoshioka H, Hama S, Taniguchi E, et al: Peritumoral brain edema associated with meningioma. Cancer 85:936–994, 1999.

26. Kraft SL, Gavin PR, DeHaan C, et al: Retrospective review of 50 canine intracranial tumors evaluated by magnetic resonance imaging. J Vet Intern Med 11:218–225, 1997.
27. Gallagher JG, Berg J, Knowles KE, et al: Prognosis after surgical excision of cerebral meningiomas in cats: 17 cases (1986–1992). J Am Vet Med Assoc 203:1437–1440, 1993.
28. Gordon LE, Thacher C, Mattiesen DT, et al: Results of craniotomy for the treatment of cerebral meningioma in 42 cats. Vet Surg 23:94–100, 1994.
29. Quesnel AD, Parent JM, McDonell W, et al: Diagnostic evaluation of cats with seizure disorders: 30 cases (1991–1993). J Am Vet Med Assoc 210:65–71, 1997.
30. Hague PH, Burridge, MJ: A meningioma in a cat associated with erosion of the skull. Vet Rec 84:217–219, 1969.
31. Lawson DC, Burk RL, Prata RG: Cerebral meningioma in the cat: Diagnosis and surgical treatment of ten cases. J Am Anim Hosp Assoc 20:333–342, 1984.
32. Burk RL, Corwin LA, Zimmerman D: Use of a modified occipital view for radiographic examination of the skull. Vet Med Small Anim Clin 73:460–463, 1978.
33. Pieper DR, Al-Mefty O, Hanada Y, et al: Hyperostosis associated with meningioma of the cranial skull base: Secondary changes or tumor invasion. Neurosurgery 44:742–746, 1999.
34. Rand JS, Parent J, Percy D, et al: Clinical, cerebrospinal fluid, and histological data from thirty-four cats with primary noninflammatory disease of the central nervous system. Can Vet J 35:174–181, 1994.
35. LeCouteur RA, Fike JR, Cann CE, et al: X-ray computed tomography of brain tumors in cats. J Am Vet Med Assoc 183:301–305, 1983.
36. Turrel JM, Fike JR, LeCouteur RA, et al: Computed tomographic characteristics of primary brain tumors in 50 dogs. J Am Vet Med Assoc 188:851–856, 1986.
37. Graham JP, Newell SM, Voges AK, et al: The dural tail sign in the diagnosis of meningiomas. Vet Radiol Ultrasound 39:297–302, 1998.
38. Thomson CE, Kornegay JN, Burn RA, et al: Magnetic resonance imaging—A general overview of principles and examples in veterinary neurodiagnosis. Vet Radiol Ultrasound 34:2–17, 1993.
39. Koblik PD, LeCouteur RA, Higgins RJ, et al: Modification and application of a Pelorus Mark III stereotactic system for CT-guided brain biopsy in 50 dogs. Vet Radiol Ultrasound 40:424–433, 1999.
40. Koblik PD, LeCouteur RA, Higgins RJ, et al: CT-guided brain biopsy using a modified Pelorus Mark III stereotactic system: Experience with 50 dogs. Vet Radiol Ultrasound 40:434–440, 1999.
41. Hohenhaus AE: Feline intracranial masses: Computed tomography and outcome in 50 sequential cases. Proceedings 14th American College of Veterinary Internal Medicine Forum, San Antonio, May 23–26, 1996, p. 757.
42. Barbaro NM, Gutin PH, Wilson CB, et al: Radiation therapy in the treatment of partially resected meningiomas. Neurosurgery 20:525–528, 1987.
43. Mesic JB, Hanks GE, Scotte Doggett RL: The value of radiation therapy as an adjuvant to surgery in intracranial meningiomas. Am J Clin Oncol 9:337–340, 1986.
44. Taylor BW, Marcus RB, Friedman WA: The meningioma controversy: Postoperative radiation therapy. Int J Radiat Oncol Biol Phys 15:299–304, 1988.
45. Brosnan C, Razis P: Complications of treatment: Pulmonary embolism following craniotomy for meningioma. J Neurosurg Anesth 11:119–123, 1999.
46. Gavin PR, Fike JR, Hoopes PJ: Central nervous system tumors. Semin Vet Med Surg Small Anim 10:180–189, 1995.
47. Speciale JS, Koffman BM, Bashirelahi N, et al: Identification of gonadal steroid receptors in meningiomas from dogs and cats. Am J Vet Res 51:833–835, 1990.
48. Monteagudo OG, Purpura DP: Epileptogenic effects of an auditory cortex meningioma in a cat. Cornell Vet 49:375–379, 1959.

51

◆ Neuronal Storage Disorders

Philip A. March

Neuronal storage disorders (NSDs) are lysosomal storage diseases that affect nervous system structure and function. Storage disorders occur secondary to a defect in either a lysosomal enzyme, an activator protein that promotes enzyme activity, or a transport protein that moves macromolecules into and out of the lysosome. The result is accumulation of undegraded metabolites within the cell and subsequent cellular swelling. Storage in viscera, especially liver and spleen, is observed frequently and gross organomegaly may be evident on abdominal palpation. Intracellular storage in central nervous system (CNS) tissues is the most striking feature of many NSDs, but often does not correlate with the appearance of clinical signs. Similarly, the onset and degree of storage may not coincide with the onset and severity of neurodegenerative changes that occur in the CNS. This incongruity between lysosomal storage, morphologic alterations, and clinical dysfunction underscores our inadequate understanding of disease pathogenesis. Although some pathologic changes (axonal abnormalities, demyelination, neuronal loss) have been identified as probable contributors to nervous system deficits, changes at the molecular level and their relationship to neural dysfunction require more study.

A tentative diagnosis of an NSD may be made based on a history of chronic, progressive neurologic signs in a 7- to 16-week-old kitten. A majority of NSDs are inherited as autosomal recessive traits, and affected cats are homozygous for the gene defect. Familial inbreeding leads to phenotypic expression of the recessive trait in selected offspring (usually 1 or 2 affected individuals in a litter). Cerebellar signs typically are observed early in the disease course, but progression to multifocal signs helps to rule out cerebellar hypoplasia or abiotrophy as a diagnosis.[1] Cerebrocortical signs include behavior change, dementia, blindness, seizures, circling, and conscious proprioceptive deficits. Signs of brain stem involvement include spastic upper motor neuron tetraparesis, central vestibular signs, conscious and unconscious proprioception loss, megaesophagus, and dysphagia.[2] Concurrent spinal cord involvement is common. The neurologic signs eventually observed in many NSDs resemble those manifested by cats with experimental lesions of the basal ganglia.[3] These include slow, tentative movements (bradykinesia, akinesia), "frozen" movements in the middle of an activity, feeding difficulties characterized by increased chewing, licking, and repetitive swallowing attempts, and decreased visual tracking. Additional clinical signs of many NSDs are reduced growth, skeletal deformities, hepatomegaly (see earlier), and ocular changes.

Specific diagnostic tests will aid in making a diagnosis of an NSD and in ruling out other potential causes of multifocal nervous system disease. Cerebrospinal fluid (CSF) analyses usually are normal in the NSDs. CSF pleocytosis and elevated protein values are more indicative of an infectious disease process. Appropriate titers (e.g., for cryptococcosis, toxoplasmosis) on serum and/or CSF also are helpful in ruling in or out an infectious disease. A number of NSDs are characterized by microscopically visible inclusions in circulating white blood cells. A Wright-Giemsa stain usually is the best method to demonstrate these inclusions. A definitive antemortem diagnosis usually may be made based on lysosomal enzyme assays of serum, peripheral leukocytes, cultured skin fibroblasts, or other tissues. Laboratories also are available that can screen urine samples for undegraded metabolites that are excreted in some of the NSDs.

NSDs usually are diagnosed after significant neurologic deterioration has occurred. In these circumstances, neuronal injury and dysfunction are irreversible, and treatment options are limited. Supportive therapies are necessary because affected patients are recumbent and have an increased susceptibility to infection. Although not accessible to most practitioners and not feasible for most pet owners, bone marrow transplantation (BMT) has been shown to prolong survival and either prevent or slow the progression of neurologic signs if performed early in the disease course. The underlying hypothesis in BMT is that circulating leukocytes and tissue macrophages derived from hematopoietic precursor cells of the donor can deliver lysosomal enzymes to deficient cells in all tissues of the host, through either secretion or direct cell-to-cell interaction. A limiting factor involved in the success or failure of this therapy appears to be the ability of the donor-derived cells to deliver the deficient enzyme to neurons of the CNS.

This chapter reviews the genetic defects, pathogenesis, clinical signs, and utility of BMT in those NSDs recognized in cats. Although these disorders are diagnosed rarely in clinical practice, our clinical and clinicopathologic knowledge of the NSDs is expanding owing to detailed studies in laboratory colonies of affected cats. Various feline NSDs have served as highly useful animal models of identical human conditions, and so are the focus of a great deal of interest from the standpoint of understanding pathogenesis and correction of the underlying metabolic defect.

◆ GM1 GANGLIOSIDOSIS

Genetic Defect

GM1 gangliosidosis is characterized by a deficiency of lysosomal beta-galactosidase. Type I or generalized GM1 gangliosidosis has been reported in domestic shorthair cats. This subtype is unique among the gangliosidoses in being characterized by CNS, visceral, and skeletal involvement.[4–8] Type II or juvenile GM1 gangliosidosis in Siamese, Korat, and domestic shorthair cats is characterized by CNS involvement with no skeletal lesions and mild-to-variable visceral abnormalities.[7, 8] The mutated enzyme in the juvenile form of feline GM1 gangliosidosis may have some activity toward those glycosaminoglycans required for normal bone growth.[7]

Pathogenesis

A deficiency of beta-galactosidase results in secondary accumulation of GM1 ganglioside and other complex oligosaccharides in neurons and glial cells. GM1 ganglioside is an important constituent of the plasma membrane, and is concentrated in nerve endings. Among the various putative functions of GM1 ganglioside, its neuroprotective and growth factor properties, neurotransmitter effects, and calcium-binding characteristics are described most thoroughly.[5, 7, 9, 10] In most forms of GM1 gangliosidosis, hepatocytes, endothelial cells, and cells of the macrophage/monocyte system also exhibit intralysosomal storage. Pathogenesis of brain dysfunction has been studied most extensively in GM1 gangliosidosis of Siamese cats.[4, 5, 8, 10] Ganglioside and glycolipid storage is pronounced in most areas of the CNS well before clinical signs of neurologic illness are evident. Intraneuronal periodic acid–Schiff (PAS)–positive inclusions and ballooned cell bodies are seen in frozen brain sections. Ultrastructurally, inclusions are composed of multilamellated membrane-like structures in a whorling pattern (membranous cytoplasmic bodies) or in stacked parallel arrays (zebra bodies) (Fig. 51–1).[4, 8]

As cell death is not a feature of the gangliosidoses, other biochemical and morphologic alterations have been investigated in an attempt to explain the neurologic findings. Neurochemical imbalances such as increased acetylcholine synthesis and activity, and decreased glutamate, gamma-aminobutyric acid (GABA), and norepinephrine reuptake have been found in GM1 synaptosomes.[5, 10] Focal expansions at the base of axons (swollen axon hillocks and "meganeurites") and proliferation of dendrite-like structures (ectopic spines and neurites) from these sites have been demonstrated in cerebrocortical pyramidal neurons. Excitatory synaptic inputs have been identified on these ectopic structures, but the source of these excitatory afferents is not known.[10] Neuroaxonal dystrophy characterized by more distal axonal swellings (spheroids, "torpedoes") in GABAergic (inhibitory) neurons is another important morphologic change. The severity and localization of neurologic signs in these feline patients appear to parallel the degree and regional distribution of spheroids in GABAergic axons. Neuroaxonal dystrophy is pronounced in cerebrocortical, brain stem, and cerebellar locations.[11] Dystrophic changes in inhibitory circuits suggest that an inhibitory defect is present in GM1 gangliosidosis. This may explain the signs of increased excitability in affected cats (see later).

Clinical Signs

Clinical signs of brain dysfunction and extraneural involvement vary slightly among the different cat breeds in which GM1 gangliosidosis has been identified. Typical signs in domestic shorthair and Siamese cats with type II GM1 gangliosidosis are a fine head and/or body tremor accompanied by mild ataxia at 8 to 10 weeks of age.[4, 7] More severe ataxia with dysmetria, a truncal sway, balance loss, and nystagmus occurs subsequently. Over time, an upper motor neuron spastic tetraparesis is seen that progresses to complete tetraplegia by 7 to 8 months of age. Dysphagia and abnormal swallowing movements are common findings. Cerebral signs of behavior change, dementia, vision loss, and grand mal seizures are evident by 1 year of age.[4–7] Skeletal and visceral changes are rare in this juvenile form of GM1 gangliosidosis. The generalized (type I) form, on the other hand, is typified by a domed calvarium, other craniofacial distortions, and hepatomegaly.[8, 12] Ocular abnormalities are common in both types of feline GM1 gangliosidosis. Changes include diffuse corneal opacities due to oligosaccharide storage in corneal epithelium and endothelium, and dark and pale spots in the nontapetal fundus due to accumulation of inclusions in the ganglion cell and inner nuclear layers.[13] There is no "cherry red spot" in the retina as is seen in human GM1 gangliosidosis. The cherry red spot in human beings is due to normal macular areas surrounded by a zone of grayish white, glycolipid-laden retina.[13]

Differential Diagnosis

Cerebellar hypoplasia and infectious causes of cerebellovestibular signs can mimic early signs of GM1 gangliosidosis. The progression of CNS signs and the unique ocular abnormalities in an otherwise healthy cat should help rule out these other diseases and rule in GM1 gangliosidosis.

Diagnosis

Circulating lymphocytes often are vacuolated on Wright-Giemsa blood smears.[14] Elevated urinary oli-

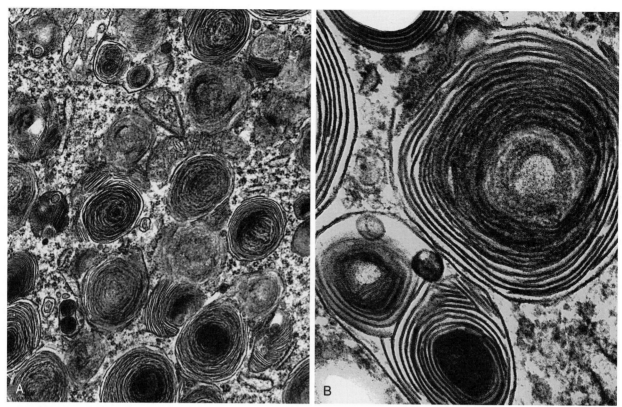

Figure 51–1. Multilamellar membranous cytoplasmic bodies with or without more dense osmiophilic inclusions and vacuolar profiles are found commonly in central nervous system neurons from cats with either gangliosidoses or Niemann-Pick disease. Low- (*A*) and high- (*B*) magnification electron micrographs depict membranous cytoplasmic bodies in a spinal cord neuron from a cat with Niemann-Pick disease type A. Original magnification, ×1800 (*A*) and ×5300 (*B*).

gosaccharides may or may not be present.[6, 8] Homozygous affected patients usually have less than 5 per cent of normal beta-galactosidase activity in tissues, whereas heterozygous individuals have approximately 50 per cent normal activity.[4, 5] Some research laboratories associated with human medical facilities will perform a battery of requested enzyme assays on peripheral white blood cells, cultured skin fibroblasts or conjunctival cells, or other tissues. Molecular techniques for diagnosis of the gangliosidoses are being developed (see Chapter 77, Molecular Diagnosis of Gangliosidoses: A Model for Elimination of Inherited Diseases in Pure Breeds).

Treatment

Treatment strategies for GM1 gangliosidosis are limited. BMT has been attempted in affected cats, and partial responses have been demonstrated.[15] Slower disease progression or prolonged survival times were observed in cats of various ages after BMT. Maximum benefit is difficult to assess because a majority of cats already were exhibiting clinical signs at the time of treatment. CNS lesions did not appear to be significantly improved after BMT.[15, 16]

◆ GM2 GANGLIOSIDOSIS

Genetic Defect

The lysosomal enzyme beta-hexosaminidase is involved in degradation of GM2 ganglioside. Beta-

hexosaminidase is made of 2 subunits, alpha and beta. The B-variant form of GM2 gangliosidosis or Tay-Sachs disease is characterized by deficient activity of hexosaminidase alpha subunit only. The 0-variant or Sandhoff's disease is characterized by deficient activity of both hexosaminidase subunits. The AB-variant denotes the absence of an activator protein that stimulates the hexosaminidase alpha subunit.[6, 8] As for the majority of NSDs, the genetic defect is autosomal recessive in character.

Pathogenesis

Neural and extraneural storage in affected cats with GM2 gangliosidosis is similar to GM1 gangliosidosis. PAS-positive, intracytoplasmic inclusions of the membranous cytoplasmic body type are present in most CNS neurons and glia. GM2 ganglioside is the predominant unmetabolized glycolipid found in lysosomes.[8, 10] As in GM1 gangliosidosis, neuronal loss is not a feature of this disorder. Instead, GABAergic neuroaxonal dystrophy and ectopic dendritogenesis are the primary morphologic abnormalities.[10, 11] In domestic shorthair cats with the 0-variant form of GM2 gangliosidosis, swollen axon hillocks with ectopic neurite growth are very common on layers II, III, and V pyramidal neurons.[10, 17]

Clinical Signs

Cats with GM2 gangliosidosis tend to exhibit a more rapid clinical course than cats with GM1 gangliosidosis. Affected cats usually are nonambulatory by 6 months of age. Domestic shorthair cats with the 0-variant form of this disease develop an intention tremor, hypermetria, and ataxia by 4 to 10 weeks of age. An upper motor neuron type of para- or tetraparesis occurs by 5 months of age and often is accompanied by dysphagia and difficulty prehending food owing to "paroxysmal episodes" during feeding.[5, 6, 8, 18] Extraneural involvement of ocular tissues (bilateral corneal opacities) and facial structures (rounded forehead, strained facial expression) may be evident.[5, 6, 13, 18] Hepatomegaly is not observed. Korat cats with the 0-variant form of GM2 gangliosidosis have a similar progression of neurologic signs. Mobility is lost by 10 to 12 weeks of age. Additional signs of tetraplegia, seizures, generalized myoclonus, vision loss, and hepatomegaly are seen in affected Korat cats at 6 months of age (see Chapter 77, Molecular Diagnosis of Gangliosidoses: A Model for Elimination of Inherited Diseases in Pure Breeds).[6, 19]

◆ DIFFERENTIAL DIAGNOSIS

See GM1 Gangliosidosis.

Diagnosis

Assays for the various beta-hexosaminidase enzyme subunits and activator protein are available, and can be performed on white blood cells or other tissues.

Treatment

BMT at 7 to 9 weeks of age does not appear to alter the disease progression (Dr. Steve Walkley, personal communication, 1999). This finding contrasts with results obtained in kittens with alpha-mannosidosis (see later). Although the reasons for this lack of efficacy are unclear, mechanics of enzyme and/or substrate transfer, relative blood-brain barrier permeability, and degree of neuronal injury at the time of transplantation all are factors that may have influenced correction of the metabolic defect.

◆ SPHINGOMYELINOSIS (NIEMANN-PICK DISEASE)

Genetic Defect

The underlying defects in various types of Niemann-Pick disease (NPD) are dissimilar. In the human classification system, types A, B, and F exhibit a sphingomyelinase deficiency. Types C, D, and E have normal sphingomyelinase activity.[6, 8] Some investigations have uncovered a cholesterol transport defect in NPD type C.[20] In cultured skin fibroblasts, there also is an inability of the cells to esterify exogenous cholesterol, leading to accumulation of unesterified cholesterol intracellularly.[20] Genetic studies reveal an autosomal recessive pattern of inheritance for all types of NPD.

Pathogenesis

The NPDs are characterized by sphingomyelin and cholesterol accumulation in tissues. Neuropathologic findings are similar to those found in the gangliosidoses. Intraneuronal inclusions are very similar to those found in the gangliosidoses (membranous cytoplasmic bodies and zebra bodies), and elevated levels of both GM2 and GM3 ganglioside are found in brain. Extraneural tissues exhibit more widespread storage than that found in the gangliosidoses. Foamy macrophages are found in the liver, spleen, bone marrow, lung, lymph nodes, adrenal glands, and intestines. In cats with NPD type C, mild-to-moderate cerebellar atrophy, moderate-to-severe Purkinje cell loss, some granule cell loss, and pronounced neuroaxonal dystrophy within cerebral cortex, basal ganglia, brain stem, and cerebellum are described.[8, 20–22] Purkinje cell axons develop multiple spherical and torpedo-like swellings before cell death (Fig. 51–2). As in GM1 gangliosidosis, neuroaxonal dystrophy in cerebrocortical gray matter affects primarily GABAergic neurons (Fig. 51–3), and an inhibitory defect in cortical processing has been hypothesized.[21] Histologic findings in NPD type A reflect both a CNS and a peripheral nervous system component of the disease. In the CNS, vacuolated neurons and neurons containing metachromatic granules are most numerous in cerebellar gray matter (Fig. 51–4), cerebellar deep nuclei, hippocampus, dorsal root ganglia, and peripheral ganglia, including the myenteric plexus. White matter changes characterized by varying degrees of myelin loss also are evident. In the peripheral nervous system, the demyelinating process is more severe. Vacuolated macrophages and/or Schwann cells containing myelin-like debris are found in peripheral nerve endoneurium. Myelin sheaths are variable in thickness, and generally much thinner than normal.[6, 8, 23, 24]

Clinical Signs

NPD type C has been described in domestic shorthair cats.[6, 20–22, 25] Affected domestic shorthair cats with NPD type C exhibit intention tremors at 8 to 12 weeks that quickly progress to ataxia, hypermetria, an absent menace response with intact vision, and an occasional positional nystagmus. By 19 to 23 weeks of age, cats have a crouched posture and a truncal sway, and fall over frequently. By 25

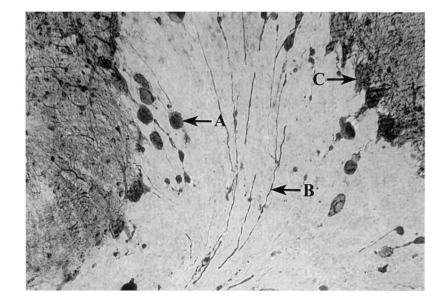

Figure 51–2. Neuroaxonal dystrophy in cerebellum is characterized by swellings or spheroids (*arrow* at A) in axons of Purkinje cells. *Arrows* at B and C depict a normal Purkinje cell axon and a Purkinje cell body, respectively. This abnormality is common in cats with either Niemann-Pick disease type C, GM1 and GM2 gangliosidosis, or alpha-mannosidosis. Calbindin immunohistochemistry, ×350.

to 33 weeks, the righting response is lost, spastic tetraparesis is seen, and cats remain in lateral recumbency. Hepatosplenomegaly and increases in serum alkaline phosphatase and alanine aminotransferase are common findings. Death usually occurs by 8 to 10 months of age.[6, 20–22, 25]

NPD type A has been described in Siamese and Balinese cats.[6, 23, 24, 26–28] Signs of head tremor, head bobbing, and dysmetria start at 3 to 4 months of age. Pelvic limbs often are more severely affected than thoracic limbs. Initial ataxia and proprioceptive loss cause pelvic limbs to splay. Paresis is seen in later stages of the disease. Cuddon and colleagues[23] found signs of a demyelinating polyneuropathy in 1 family of affected cats that develop a flaccid tetraparesis by 4 to 7 months of age. Mild-to-moderate hepatomegaly is a feature of NPD type A.[6, 23, 24, 26–28]

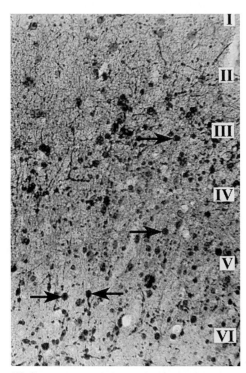

Figure 51–3. Neuroaxonal dystrophy in cerebrocortical inhibitory neurons is a feature of the same neuronal storage diseases mentioned in the legend for Figure 51–2. Numerous spheroids in GABAergic axons label with an antibody to parvalbumin (*arrows*). Parvalbumin also labels cell bodies scattered throughout the cortical gray matter. Roman numerals at right denote cerebrocortical laminae. Parvalbumin immunohistochemistry, ×350.

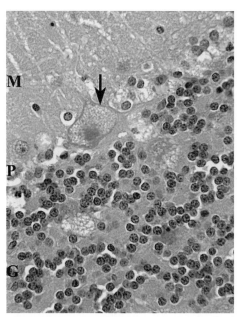

Figure 51–4. Purkinje cells often exhibit massive amounts of storage material in the form of vacuolar inclusions in many neuronal storage disorders. A single Purkinje cell (*arrow*) has a large amount of foamy cytoplasm indicative of multiple lysosomes engorged with storage material. Cerebellar cell layers are indicated by M (molecular layer), P (Purkinje cell layer), and G (granule cell layer). Toluidine blue, ×756.

Differential Diagnosis

Clinical signs of NPD type C are very similar to those in the feline gangliosidoses. Extraneural involvement (e.g., hepatosplenomgaly) tends to be more severe in NPD type C, and ocular signs are less severe. NPD type A is distinguished more easily owing to the presence of lower motor neuron signs (e.g., hyporeflexia, hypotonia). Nerve conduction studies are helpful in characterizing the peripheral nerve involvement in NPD type A.

Diagnosis

NPD type C is characterized by an inability of cultured fibroblasts to esterify exogenous cholesterol. Homozygous recessive individuals and heterozygous carriers may be screened using this fibroblast culture assay system. Fibroblasts from heterozygous cats recently have been demonstrated to possess intermediate rates of cholesterol esterification.[20, 29] Unesterified cholesterol within cultured fibroblasts or within tissue hepatocytes from both homozygous recessive individuals and heterozygous carriers also may be stained with filipin, a fluorescent polyene antibiotic.[20, 29] NPD type A may be diagnosed by routine sphingomyelinase assays of white blood cells, cultured fibroblasts, and other tissues. A peripheral nerve biopsy will reveal the characteristic inclusions in macrophages/Schwann cells, and demonstrate myelin loss.[6, 8, 23]

Treatment

BMT has not been evaluated in cats affected with NPD type A. A partial response (delay in onset of ataxia, extended survival) was observed after BMT in sphingomyelinase knock-out mice, but CNS pathology was still evident.[30] Both BMT and dietary manipulation are being evaluated as potential treatment strategies for feline NPD type C.[31, 32] Cats that underwent BMT had slowed onset and progression of CNS signs, but progressed clinically to end-stage disease.[31] A cholesterol-restricted diet resulted in a lowering of elevated hepatic enzymes and cholesterol in serum, but did not alter clinical progression of neurologic deficits.[32]

◆ MUCOLIPIDOSIS II (I-CELL DISEASE)

Genetic Defect

Feline mucolipidosis (I-cell disease in human beings) is caused by a deficiency of N-acetylglucosamine-1-phosphotransferase. This disease has been identified in domestic shorthair cats, and is inherited as an autosomal recessive trait.[33, 34]

Pathogenesis

N-Acetylglucosamine-1-phosphotransferase attaches phosphates to lysosomal enzymes, thus enabling these enzymes to be trafficked to the lysosome. If this enzyme is absent or dysfunctional, lysosomal enzymes are excreted into the extracellular compartment. Individuals with mucolipidosis often have elevated levels of lysosomal enzymes in serum, but low levels intracellularly in certain tissues. Visceral tissues such as liver and spleen are not affected as severely as skeletal tissues. The retina also is predisposed to dysfunction in this disorder. Cortical neurons exhibit some degree of storage, but histologic lesions in the CNS and peripheral nervous system apparently are rare.[33, 34] The origin of the neurologic deficits seen in this disorder (pelvic limb paresis) is uncertain.

Clinical Signs

Signs relate primarily to abnormalities of bone growth in the axial and appendicular skeleton. As early as 4 weeks of age, affected cats show retarded growth and abnormal facial features including a domed frontal area. By 7 months of age, ankylosis and fusion of the spinal column, bilateral coxofemoral luxations, and reduced bone density are seen. Other signs are a progressive upper motor neuron pelvic limb paresis, dilated pupils that are poorly responsive to light, and blindness.[33, 34]

Differential Diagnosis

The clinical signs resemble those found in mucopolysaccharidosis I and VI in cats. Both disorders can cause multiple bony deformities, and mucopolysaccharidosis VI can produce a caudal paresis secondary to proliferative thoracolumbar spinal lesions that compress the spinal cord (see later).

Diagnosis

The toluidine spot test for urinary glycosaminoglycans is negative. This helps distinguish this disease from the mucopolysaccharidoses (see later). The enzyme defect can be determined by white blood cell or cultured fibroblast assays. Serum levels of other lysosomal enzymes are elevated.[33, 34]

Treatment

No treatment protocols have been described for feline mucolipidosis II.

◆ MUCOPOLYSACCHARIDOSIS

Genetic Defect

The 3 major types of mucopolysaccharidosis (MPS) seen in cats are types I, VI, and VII (see Chapter 57,

Mucopolysaccharidosis). MPS-I is due to a deficiency of lysosomal alpha-L-iduronidase, and has been described in domestic shorthair cats.[6, 35] MPS-VI in Siamese cats is caused by a deficiency of arylsulfatase-B.[6, 8, 36, 37] MPS-VII, a deficiency of beta-glucuronidase, has been described in a domestic shorthair cat.[38]

Pathogenesis

The mucopolysaccharidoses rarely are associated with neurologic disease, even though glycosaminoglycan and glycolipid storage often can be demonstrated in CNS neurons. Glycosaminoglycans and other proteoglycans (e.g., dermatan sulfate, heparan sulfate) normally are important constituents of connective tissue, including bone. Defects in the degradation of these compounds result in their accumulation in many cell types, but the axial and the appendicular skeleton are affected most severely. Undegraded dermatan sulfate, heparan sulfate, and other glycoproteins and glycolipids accumulate within chondrocytes, bone marrow myeloid cells, keratinocytes, pericytes, skin fibroblasts, smooth muscle, hepatocytes, and neurons, and these sulfated glycosaminoglycans can be found in the urine.[6, 8, 35, 36] Ultrastructurally, neuronal inclusions are either clear vacuoles (where glycosaminoglycans have been leached out during tissue fixation) or zebra bodies, which are indicative of ganglioside (sphingolipid) accumulation.[6, 8, 35, 36, 38] An increased incidence of meningiomas has been observed in cats with MPS-I, but a causative factor for this neoplastic transformation has not been defined. Meningiomas were diagnosed at less than 3 years of age in 4 cats, and all tumors involved the tela choroidea of the third ventricle.[6, 39] Otherwise, neurohistopathologic changes are rare in the mucopolysaccharidoses. Bony proliferative lesions of the thoracolumbar spine may compress the spinal cord secondarily to produce a focal cord lesion in MPS-VI (see later). Studies in cats have failed to demonstrate GABAergic neuroaxonal dystrophy, but ectopic neuritogenesis of cerebrocortical pyramidal neurons has been reported in MPS-I.[10, 11]

Clinical Signs

The most common clinical signs observed in cats with MPS-I are lameness and an awkward gait owing to skeletal and joint changes (bony dysplasia, vertebral fusion, widened cervical vertebrae, polyarthropathies and joint immobility, coxofemoral luxations, and stunted growth).[6, 35] Corneal clouding is another consistent feature. Facial deformities include a shortened maxilla with a broad face, a depressed nasal bridge, and small ears. Thickened cardiac valves and coronary vessels are due to deposition of storage material within fibroelastic connective tissue cells. Affected cats may live to

adulthood and reproduce.[6, 8, 35] Typically, the neurologic examination is normal.[35] Hydrocephalus is an incidental finding at necropsy, and may be due to decreased CSF resorption by thickened arachnoid villi.[35]

Clinical signs in cats affected by MPS-VI are very similar to those in cats with MPS-I, but also include epiphyseal dysplasia and exostoses of long bones, severe spondylosis and kyphosis, osteoarthrosis of articular facets, odontoid process abnormalities, widened intervertebral disc spaces, and severe facial dysmorphism.[8, 36, 37, 40] Neurologic deficits are rare, and if present, are characterized by a progressive upper motor neuron paraparesis due to focal bony proliferative lesions causing extradural spinal cord compression in the thoracolumbar area.[41]

A single cat with MPS-VII has been described.[38] Clinical signs of MPS-VII included abnormal facial features, multiple axial and appendicular skeletal deformities causing an awkward gait, reduced growth, corneal clouding, and an upper motor neuron caudal paresis. An unusual clinical sign was the presence of generalized seizures, which could be induced by stimulation of the skin over the back. The authors of this case report attributed the neurologic signs to the effects of the sphingolipid found in CNS neurons, even though this storage was, in their own description, "discrete."[38]

Differential Diagnosis

All forms of MPS in cats have very similar clinical and clinicopathologic features. Feline mucolipidosis, metabolic bone diseases, and hypervitaminosis A may mimic MPS. The most reliable way to distinguish these disorders is by enzyme assays (see later).

Diagnosis

Circulating neutrophils in MPS-VI and MPS-VII contain metachromatic granules when stained with toluidine blue.[8, 14, 37, 38] Lymphocytes contain clear, vacuolar inclusions. The toluidine blue spot test for urinary sulfated glycosaminoglycans is positive in all types of feline mucopolysaccharidoses.[35, 36, 38] A definitive diagnosis may be made by enzyme assays of white blood cells or cultured skin fibroblasts.

Treatment

Partial correction of the enzyme defect and alleviation of clinical signs have been observed after allogeneic BMT in feline MPS-VI (see Chapter 57, Mucopolysaccharidosis). Improved gait, increased movement of the head, neck, and mandible, partial resolution of facial dysmorphism, and clearing of corneal opacities have been described.[42] BMT has not been attempted in feline MPS-VII, but has been performed in the canine and murine models with some success.[43, 44] Direct and vector-mediated gene transfer also has been performed in beta-glucuronidase–deficient mice.[15, 45, 46]

◆ ALPHA-MANNOSIDOSIS

Genetic Defect

Normal feline alpha-mannosidase has been purified, and the cDNA sequence is known.[47] Feline alpha-mannosidosis is an autosomal recessive trait characterized by a deficiency of alpha-mannosidase, but there is molecular heterogeneity with respect to the type of genetic defect. A 4-base-pair deletion has been reported in a group of affected Persian cats that results in completely absent enzyme activity.[47] A group of affected domestic longhair cats with 2 per cent enzyme activity did not possess these base-pair deletions, but the genomic mutation has not been identified.[47] Another line of Persian cats has been reported to have a missense mutation in the alpha-mannosidase coding region. These cats had between 3 and 5 per cent enzyme activity. The degree of residual enzyme activity may have an influence on phenotype as discussed later.

Pathogenesis

Acidic alpha-mannosidase is a lysosomal enzyme that cleaves mannose residues from complex oligosaccharides and glycoproteins. Absence of this enzyme leads to accumulation of mannose-rich materials in brain, liver, kidney, and other organs. Intraneuronal storage can be intensive early in the course of the disease without causing cell dysfunction.[48–51] Oligosaccharides spill into the urine. Cat breeds reported to have this disorder include domestic shorthair and longhair cats and Persians.[8, 48–51] Neuropathologic changes in Persian cats include severe neuroaxonal dystrophy of cerebellar gray matter (Purkinje cell axons), and mild-to-moderate neuroaxonal dystrophy of cerebrocortical GABAergic neurons.[11] Dystrophic axons and myelin loss also have been described in cerebral and cerebellar white matter of affected Persian cats.[6, 49, 50] Pronounced Purkinje cell loss is the most characteristic feature of alpha-mannosidosis in domestic longhair cats,[6, 12, 51] but neuronal loss is not a feature of other types of alpha-mannosidosis.[6, 48, 50] Ectopic neuritogenesis of pyramidal neurons in cerebral cortex occurs, but a majority of neurons do not exhibit this abnormality.[10]

Clinical Signs

Clinical heterogeneity appears to be a common feature of alpha-mannosidosis. Phenotypic differences are, in some instances, related to the genotype and the relative amount of residual enzyme activity present. For example, extraneural signs of skeletal abnormalities, hepatomegaly, and cataracts in domestic shorthair and Persian cats likely are related to the severe enzyme deficiency in these breeds.[6, 48, 49] Skeletal deformities include carpal dysplasia, luxating patellas, open suture lines in the calvarium, moth-eaten vertebrae, and other bony malformations.[48, 49] Ocular lesions are characterized by stippling of the cornea and lens, and mottled areas of the tapetal fundus.[13] Stillbirths and neonatal deaths are common in affected Persian cats,[50] but the relative contribution of other inbred potentially lethal traits to this phenomenon is unknown. Domestic longhair cats with some residual enzyme activity lack skeletal, hepatic, and ocular lesions.[51] Interestingly, even within 1 family of affected domestic longhair cats, onset, progression, and severity of clinical signs varied.[51] Despite variations in the clinical presentations of these 3 feline groups, certain clinical features are shared. Onset of clinical signs usually is between 2 and 5 months of age. Affected cats exhibit progressive cerebellar signs (tremors, ataxia, absent menace, nystagmus, incoordinated swallowing movements, opisthotonus, hypermetria, lurching, and falling).[48–51] Persian and domestic shorthair cats also may show behavior changes and dementia.[6, 49, 50]

Differential Diagnosis

Signs of cerebellar disease may be seen with cerebellar hypoplasia, infectious CNS disease, and other NSDs, especially the gangliosidoses and NPDs. Limb deformities are uncommon in the gangliosidoses or in NPD type C. Limb deformities are common features of the mucopolysaccharidoses, but usually occur in the absence of neurologic deficits.

Diagnosis

Circulating lymphocytes in Wright-Giemsa–stained peripheral blood smears often contain clear vacuoles.[14] Typical patterns of neutral oligosaccharides in urine and deficient alpha-mannosidase activity in either white blood cells or tissues (liver, kidney, placenta, or tail-tip biopsy) support a diagnosis of alpha-mannosidosis. Individuals heterozygous for the defect usually have approximately 50 per cent of normal enzyme activity.[6, 48–51]

Treatment

BMT has been attempted in a group of related cats from a laboratory colony.[52] Marrow donors were siblings. Results of this study demonstrated a clear benefit after early transplantation. Affected kittens were identified by enzyme assay within 2 to 3 days of birth, and subsequently underwent BMT between

2 and 3 months of age when clinical signs were either extremely mild or absent. The procedure effectively prevented progression of neurologic signs. Small amounts of storage were found in brain, and other neuropathologic alterations were identified rarely in treated cats sacrificed at 11 and 21 months after BMT. Important conclusions from this study were that enzyme/substrate translocation can take place after BMT of this glycoproteinosis, and that timing of the transplant may be critical.[52] Issues of blood-brain barrier integrity and progression/reversibility of neuronal dysfunction at early ages need further investigation in this and other related NSDs.

◆ GLYCOGEN STORAGE DISEASE
Genetic Defect

A variety of glycogen storage diseases (GSDs) are recognized in domestic animals, but few cause neuromuscular signs. A notable exception to this observation is GSD type IV in Norwegian forest cats. This autosomal recessive disorder is caused by a deficiency of a glycogen branching enzyme (alpha-1,4-D-glucan:alpha-1,4-glucan-6 glucosyltransferase).[53, 54]

Pathogenesis

Feline GSD type IV results in accumulation of abnormal glycogen in neurons of the CNS and peripheral nervous system and in muscle. CNS storage is most pronounced in the vestibular and deep cerebellar nuclei and in Purkinje cells of the cerebellum. Intracellular inclusions are PAS-positive, finely granular, and non–membrane-bound. Although the precise pathogenesis is not understood, this defect leads to severe degeneration of axons and myelin (both centrally and peripherally), and neuronal loss in brain stem nuclei and spinal cord. Pathologic changes are most severe in the peripheral nervous system. Neurogenic atrophy of myofibers is severe and multifocal.[8, 53, 54]

Clinical Signs

Affected cats in one case series exhibited generalized muscle tremors, weakness, and a bunny-hopping gait at about 5 months of age. This progressed to a flaccid tetraparesis with muscle atrophy, dysphagia, and femorotibial and tibiotarsal joint contractures by 8 months of age.[53] In another report, muscle tremors, mild ataxia, dysphagia, and reduced postural responses in the pelvic limbs at 4 months of age progressed to tetraparesis, muscle atrophy, joint contracture, loss of menace response, and diminished vestibuloocular and limb reflexes at 5 to 6 months of age. Seizures also were observed

at 6 months of age, and were believed to be secondary to hypoglycemia.[54]

Differential Diagnosis

Other congenital neuromuscular disorders should be ruled out. With the possible exception of NPD type A, other lysosomal storage diseases rarely produce such severe lower motor neuron signs in conjunction with joint and limb deformities.

Diagnosis

Affected cats have less than 10 per cent of normal enzyme activity in white blood cells, muscle, and liver. Ultrastructural examination of muscle and nerve biopsies reveals the finely granular inclusions typical of this disorder. Electromyography demonstrates spontaneous activity, but nerve conduction velocity is normal.[53, 54]

Treatment

Therapy for feline GSD type IV has not been described.

◆ NEURONAL CEROID LIPOFUSCINOSIS
Genetic Defect

There is no known lysosomal hydrolase defect in neuronal ceroid lipofuscinosis (NCL), and questions exist as to whether this disease is a true lysosomal storage disorder. In some affected human beings and dogs, the primary component of the storage material is subunit-c of mitochondrial adenosine triphosphate (ATP)–synthase.[6, 55, 56] This is now leading investigators to study potential defects in the proteolytic pathway and/or intracellular transport of this essential protein.[55] To this author's knowledge, there is only 1 case report of probable NCL in 2 Siamese cats. No enzyme or other protein assays were performed in these 2 cats to confirm the metabolic defect, nor were breeding or pedigree studies performed to determine mode of inheritance.[57]

Pathogenesis

Neuronal ceroid lipofuscinosis originally was named for the lipopigments, ceroid and lipofuscin, that accumulate within CNS neurons of affected patients. These autofluorescent pigments resemble, but are not the same as, those lipopigments associated with aging (lipofuscin) or peroxidation of unsaturated lipids (ceroid).[6, 8] Intraneuronal inclusions usually are membrane-bound, and may be either finely granular with globules of lipid-like material or tri- to pentilaminar membrane stacks arranged in a "fingerprint" or "curvilinear" pattern.[8, 57, 58] The latter inclusion types occasionally resemble degenerating mitochondria.[58, 59] Extraneural storage occurs in retinal pigment epithelium of some affected dogs, but was not described in cats.[58, 60] Severe neuronal loss in all cerebrocortical areas and in cerebellum is a hallmark feature of NCL in human beings and dogs. Cerebral gray matter atrophy may be so severe that sulci are expanded and ventricles are dilated. Remaining neurons have Luxol fast blue, Sudan black, and PAS-positive inclusions. An intense gliotic response is seen characteristically in these brain areas.[6, 8, 58, 61] Neither neuronal loss nor gliosis was reported in feline NCL.[57]

Clinical Signs

NCL usually causes chronic, progressive cerebral, cerebellar, and/or visual deficits in dogs and human beings. Onset of clinical signs in dogs is as early as 6 months of age and as late as 3 years of age.[6, 58, 61] Signs in both reported Siamese cats occurred at 2 years of age, and were rapidly progressive. These signs included behavior change, increased irritability, hyperesthesia, visual difficulties, and seizures.[57] These signs resemble those seen in dogs.[6, 58]

Differential Diagnosis

Feline NCL is unique among the NSDs in that signs apparently develop rapidly, and initial signs are not cerebellar in origin. Rapidly progressive cerebrocortical signs in a 2-year-old cat are commonly caused by infectious and/or toxic agents.

Diagnosis

Because a definitive enzyme or protein defect has not been identified, antemortem diagnosis in dogs and human beings is possible only by brain biopsy and identification of typical NCL inclusions by electron microscopy.[60, 61] This technique also may be possible in affected cats, but has not been reported. The feline cases described had curvilinear inclusions in neural tissue obtained at necropsy.[57]

Treatment

Treatment protocols have not been described for feline NCL. BMT in the English setter model of canine NCL did not alter the progression of the disease.[62]

◆ GLOBOID CELL LEUKODYSTROPHY (KRABBE'S DISEASE)

Genetic Defect

Globoid cell leukodystrophy (GCL) or Krabbe's disease is a lysosomal storage disease that is classified as a leukodystrophy instead of an NSD owing to its primary pathologic effects on white matter rather than gray matter. GCL is caused by a deficiency of beta-galactocerebrosidase (galactosylceramidase I), and has been reported in 2 domestic shorthair cats.[63]

Pathogenesis

The lysosomal enzyme defect results in storage of galactocerebroside in many cells of the body. Accumulation of galactocerebroside in neural cells, however, may not be related to the subsequent demyelination that occurs. Another substance that accumulates, psychosine, is toxic to oligodendrocytes and Schwann cells—the myelinating cells of the CNS and peripheral nervous system, respectively.[8] GCL is named for the globoid, foamy, PAS-positive macrophages that form in perivascular and meningeal locations in the brain and cord and in endoneurium of peripheral nerves.[6, 8] Ultrastructurally, inclusions consist of both myelin-like membranes (myelin breakdown products) and aggregates of straight, arched, or twisted tubules (galactocerebroside). The characteristic lesion in the CNS of affected dogs is one of demyelination of cerebral white matter, centrum semiovale, corona radiata, corpus callosum, optic tracts, cerebellar white matter and peduncles, and subpial white matter throughout all spinal cord funiculi. Cord lesions generally are worse cranially than caudally. In the peripheral nervous system, there usually is severe segmental demyelination and secondary axonal degeneration of both peripheral nerve fibers and nerve roots. Globoid cells are present throughout the neuraxis.[8, 64–66] Although less well-described in feline GCL, PAS-positive globoid macrophages are found in all areas of the CNS, especially the cerebellar folia and corpus callosum.[63] The peripheral nervous system was not examined in the 2 reported cases of feline GCL.[63] Visceral storage is not reported in GCL in animals.

Clinical Signs

Affected cats exhibit an ascending ataxia starting at 5 to 6 weeks of age. Both cats described in the literature were euthanized shortly after onset of clinical signs (6.5 to 8.5 weeks of age), so progression of signs was not followed over time.[63] In dogs, ascending ataxia progresses to thoracic limb ataxia and hypermetria followed by eventual tetraparesis/plegia, muscle atrophy, head tremor, and visual and cognitive dysfunction. In late stages of the disease, multifocal signs indicate widespread involvement of many areas of the nervous system.[6, 64–66]

Differential Diagnosis

Feline GCL resembles NPD type A in many respects. Both disorders are sphingolipidoses that affect both the CNS and the peripheral nervous system. Both cause a myelin defect in these areas to produce very similar clinical signs. Visceral involvement in NPD type A may aid in distinguishing between these 2 disorders. Other differential diagnoses that should be considered include a chronic ascending idiopathic or toxic neuropathy, such as chronic organophosphate toxicity. Lysosomal enzyme assays provide a definitive answer.

Diagnosis

Diagnosis may be made by standard enzyme assays or by peripheral nerve biopsy.[6, 8]

Treatment

No treatment exists for feline GCL. BMT of affected mice ("Krabbe or Twitcher mouse" model) demonstrated a beneficial effect in some mice, but not in others transplanted at the same age and under the same conditions. In those mice in which neurologic signs were less severe, morphologic changes were observed less frequently in the CNS.[67]

◆ SUMMARY AND CONCLUSIONS

The NSDs that affect cats are also found in the human population. These inborn errors of metabolism often are just as devastating in human beings as they are in animals. For this reason, there is considerable interest in developing animal models of these diseases so that different approaches to treatment may be attempted. Important lessons learned from attempted therapeutic trials in animals are that different diseases respond differently depending on the enzymatic defect, and that the timing of BMT is critical. Treatment as close as possible to the perinatal period appears to be most effective. Blood-brain barrier issues aside, neuronal dysfunction may be reversible only if BMT is performed before irreversible cellular damage has occurred. This most likely means that "rescue" therapies need to be attempted before clinical signs of neuronal dysfunction are evident. In other words, diagnostic screening in the pediatric patient should be done as early as possible in life to determine the need for BMT/gene therapy.

Although this approach might be feasible in es-

tablished NSD research colonies and private breeding facilities, it is unrealistic in small-animal practice. Most patients with these disorders have moderate-to-advanced clinical signs by the time they are brought to the veterinarian. Such patients would not be suitable candidates for therapy. In these circumstances, it is still highly advisable to recommend diagnostic screening of siblings, parents, and other relatives to determine carrier status. Spaying and/or neutering carriers from a breeding program should be the primary goal of practitioner follow-up, and will effectively prevent genetic transmission of these fatal neurodegenerative diseases.

REFERENCES

1. Kornegay JN: Ataxia of the head and limbs: Cerebellar diseases in dogs and cats. Prog Vet Neurol 1:255–274, 1990.
2. de Lahunta A: Veterinary Neuroanatomy and Clinical Neurology, 2nd ed. Philadelphia, WB Saunders, 1983.
3. Schneider JS, Yuwiler A, Markham CH: Production of a Parkinson-like syndrome in the cat with N-methyl-4-phenyl-1,2,3,6-tetrahydropyridine (MPTP): Behavior, histology, and biochemistry. Exp Neurol 91:293–307, 1986.
4. Baker HJ, Lindsey JR, McKhann GM, et al: Neuronal GM1 gangliosidosis in a Siamese cat with beta-galactosidase deficiency. Science 174:838–839, 1971.
5. Baker HJ, Reynolds GD, Walkley SU, et al: The gangliosidoses: Comparative features and research applications. Vet Pathol 16:635–649, 1979.
6. Braund KG: Clinical Syndromes in Veterinary Neurology, 2nd ed. St. Louis, CV Mosby, 1994.
7. Dial SM, Mitchell TW, LeCouteur RA, et al: GM1 gangliosidosis (type II) in three cats. J Am Anim Hosp Assoc 30:355–359, 1994.
8. Summers BA, Cummings JF, de Lahunta A: Veterinary Neuropathology. St. Louis, CV Mosby, 1995.
9. Koenig ML, Jope RS, Baker HJ, et al: Reduced calcium flux in synaptosomes from cats with GM1 gangliosidosis. Brain Res 424:169–176, 1987.
10. Walkley SU: Pathobiology of neuronal storage disease. Int Rev Neurobiol 29:191–244, 1988.
11. Walkley SU, Baker HJ, Rattazzi MC, et al: Neuroaxonal dystrophy in neuronal storage disorders: Evidence for major GABAergic neuron involvement. J Neurol Sci 104:1–8, 1991.
12. Blakemore WF: GM1 gangliosidosis in a cat. J Comp Pathol 82:179–185, 1972.
13. Nasisse M: Feline ophthalmology. In Gelatt KN (ed): Veterinary Ophthalmology, 2nd ed. Philadelphia, Lea & Febiger, 1991, pp. 529–575.
14. Alroy J, Freden GO, Goyal V, et al: Morphology of leukocytes from cats affected with alpha-mannosidosis and mucopolysaccharidosis VI (MPS VI). Vet Pathol 26:294–302, 1989.
15. Haskins M, Baker HJ, Birkenmeier E, et al: Transplantation in animal model systems. In Desnick RJ (ed): Therapy of Genetic Diseases. New York, Churchill Livingstone, 1991, pp. 183–202.
16. Baker HJ, Walkley SU, Rattazzi MC, et al: Feline gangliosidoses as models of human lysosomal storage diseases. In Desnick RJ, Patterson DF, Scarpelli DG (eds): Animal Models of Inherited Metabolic Diseases. New York, Alan R. Liss, 1982, pp. 203–212.
17. Siegel DA, Walkley SU: Growth of ectopic dendrites on cortical pyramidal neurons in neuronal storage diseases correlates with abnormal accumulation of GM2 ganglioside. J Neurochem 62:1852–1862, 1994.
18. March PA: Degenerative brain disease. In Bagley R (ed). Intracranial Disease. Vet Clin North Am Small Anim Pract 26:945–971, 1996.
19. Neuwelt EA, Johnson WG, Blank NK, et al: Characterization

of a new model of GM2-gangliosidosis (Sandhoff's disease) in Korat cats. J Clin Invest 76:482–490, 1985.

20. Brown DE, Thrall MA, Walkley SU, et al: Feline Niemann-Pick disease type C. Am J Pathol 144:1412–1415, 1994.

21. March PA, Thrall MA, Brown DE, et al: GABAergic neuroaxonal dystrophy and other cytopathological alterations in feline Niemann-Pick disease type C. Acta Neuropathol 94:164–172, 1997.

22. Lowenthal AC, Cummings JF, Wenger DA, et al: Feline sphingolipidosis resembling Niemann-Pick disease type C. Acta Neuropathol (Berl) 81:189–197, 1990.

23. Cuddon PA, Higgins RJ, Duncan ID, et al: Polyneuropathy in feline Niemann-Pick disease. Brain 112:1429–1443, 1989.

24. Snyder SP, Kingston RS, Wenger DA: Niemann-Pick disease. Sphingomyelinosis of Siamese cats. Am J Pathol 108:252–254, 1982.

25. Munana KR, Luttgen PJ, Thrall MA: Neurological manifestations of Niemann-Pick disease type C in cats. J Vet Intern Med 8:117–121, 1994.

26. Wenger DA, Sattler M, Kudoh T, et al: Niemann-Pick disease: A genetic model in Siamese cats. Science 208:1471–1473, 1980.

27. Baker HJ, Wood PA, Wenger DA, et al: Sphingomyelin lipidosis in a cat. Vet Pathol 24:386–391, 1987.

28. Chrisp CE, Ringler DH, Abrams GD, et al: Lipid storage disease in a Siamese cat. J Am Vet Med Assoc 156:616–622, 1970.

29. Brown DE, Thrall MA, Walkley SU, et al: Metabolic abnormalities in feline Niemann-Pick type C heterozygotes. J Inherit Metab Dis 19:319–330, 1996.

30. Miranda SR, Erlich S, Friedrich VL, et al: Biochemical, pathological, and clinical response to transplantation of normal bone marrow cells into acid sphingomyelinase-deficient mice. Transplantation 65:884–892, 1998.

31. Brown DE, Thrall MA, Wenger D, et al: Bone marrow transplantation for feline Niemann-Pick Type C. Vet Pathol 30:428, 1993.

32. Royals KL, Brown DE, Fulton R, et al: Effect of cholesterol restricted diet in feline Niemann-Pick Type C. Vet Pathol 33:578, 1996.

33. Hubler M, Haskins ME, Arnold S, et al: Mucolipidosis type II in a domestic shorthair cat. J Small Anim Pract 37:435–441, 1996.

34. Bosshard NU, Hubler M, Arnold S, et al: Spontaneous mucolipidosis in a cat: An animal model of human I-cell disease. Vet Pathol 33:1–15, 1996.

35. Haskins ME, Aguirre GD, Jezyk PF, et al: The pathology of the feline model of mucopolysaccharidosis I. Am J Pathol 112:27–36, 1983.

36. Haskins ME, Aguirre GD, Jezyk P, et al: The pathology of feline arylsulfatase B-deficient mucopolysaccharidosis. Am J Pathol 101:657–674, 1980.

37. Cowell KR, Jezyk PF, Haskins ME, et al: Mucopolysaccharidosis in a cat. J Am Vet Med Assoc 169:334–339, 1976.

38. Gitzelmann R, Bosshard NU, Superti-Furga A, et al: Feline mucopolysaccharidosis VII due to beta-glucuronidase deficiency. Vet Pathol 31:435–443, 1994.

39. Haskins ME, McGrath JT: Meningiomas in young cats with mucopolysaccharidosis I. J Neuropathol Exp Neurol 42:664–670, 1983.

40. Konde LJ, Thrall MA, Gasper P, et al: Radiographically visualized skeletal changes associated with mucopolysaccharidosis VI in cats. Vet Radiol 28:223–228, 1987.

41. Haskins ME, Bingel SA, Northington JW, et al: Spinal cord compression and hindlimb paresis in cats with mucopolysaccharidosis VI. J Am Vet Med Assoc 182:983–985, 1983.

42. Gasper PW, Thrall MA, Wenger DA, et al: Correction of feline arylsulfatase B deficiency (mucopolysaccharidosis VI) by bone marrow transplantation. Nature 312:467–469, 1984.

43. Haskins M, Chieffo C, Wang P, et al: Bone marrow transplantation in canine mucopolysaccharidosis VII (beta-glucuronidase deficiency). Am J Hum Genet 49:435, 1991.

44. Bou-Gharios G, Adams G, Pace P, et al: Long-term effects of bone marrow transplantation on lysosomal enzyme replacement in beta-glucuronidase-deficient mice. J Inherit Metab Dis 15:899–910, 1992.

45. Wolfe JH, Deshmane SL, Fraser NW: Herpesvirus vector gene transfer and expression of beta-glucuronidase in the central nervous system of MPS VII mice. Nat Genet 1:379–384, 1992.

46. Kyle JW, Birkenmeier EH, Gwynn B, et al: Correction of murine mucopolysaccharidosis VII by a human beta-glucuronidase transgene. Proc Natl Acad Sci U S A 87:3914–3918, 1990.

47. Berg T, Tollersrud OK, Walkley SU, et al: Purification of feline alpha-mannosidase, determination of its cDNA sequence and identification of a mutation causing alpha-mannosidosis in Persian cats. Biochem J 328:863–870, 1997.

48. Blakemore WF: A case of mannosidosis in the cat: Clinical and histopathological findings. J Small Anim Pract 27:447–455, 1986.

49. Jezyk PF, Haskins ME, Newman LR: Alpha-mannosidosis in a Persian cat. J Am Vet Med Assoc 189:1483–1485, 1986.

50. Vandevelde M, Fankhauser R, Bichsel P, et al: Hereditary neurovisceral mannosidosis associated with α-mannosidase deficiency in a family of Persian cats. Acta Neuropathol (Berl) 58:64–68, 1982.

51. Cummings JF, Wood PA, de Lahunta A, et al: The clinical and pathologic heterogeneity of feline alpha-mannosidosis. J Vet Intern Med 2:163–170, 1988.

52. Walkley SU, Thrall MA, Dobrenis K, et al: Bone marrow transplantation corrects the enzyme defect in neurons of the central nervous system in a lysosomal storage disease. Proc Natl Acad Sci U S A 91:2970–2974, 1994.

53. Fyfe JC, Giger U, Van Winkle TJ, et al: Glycogen storage disease type IV: Inherited deficiency of branching enzyme activity in cats. Pediatr Res 32:719–725, 1992.

54. Coates JR, Paxton R, Cox NR, et al: A case presentation and discussion of type IV glycogen storage disease in a Norwegian forest cat. Prog Vet Neurol 7:5–11, 1996.

55. Palmer DN, Fearnley IM, Walker JE, et al: Mitochondrial ATP synthase subunit C storage in the ceroid lipofuscinosis (Batten disease). Am J Med Genet 42:561–567, 1992.

56. Hall NA, Lake BD, Dewji NN, et al: Lysosomal storage of subunit C of mitochondrial ATP synthase in Batten's disease (ceroid lipofuscinosis). Biochem J 275:269, 1991.

57. Green PD, Little PB: Neuronal ceroid-lipofuscinosis in Siamese cats. Can J Comp Med 38:207–212, 1974.

58. Koppang N: Canine ceroid lipofuscinosis—A model for human ceroid lipofuscinosis and aging. Mech Ageing Dev 2:421–445, 1973/74.

59. March PA, Wurzelmann S, Walkley SU: Morphological alterations in neocortical and cerebellar GABAergic neurons in a canine model of juvenile Batten disease. Am J Med Genet 57:204–212, 1995.

60. Taylor RM, Farrow BRH: Ceroid lipofuscinosis in the border collie dog: Retinal lesions in an animal model of juvenile Batten disease. Am J Med Genet 42:622–627, 1992.

61. Sisk DB, Levesque DC, Wood PA, et al: Clinical and pathological features of ceroid lipofuscinosis in two Australian cattle dogs. J Am Vet Med Assoc 197:361–364, 1990.

62. Deeg HJ, Shulman HM, Albrechtsen D, et al: Batten's disease: Failure of allogeneic bone marrow transplantation to arrest disease progression in a canine model. Clin Genet 37:264–270, 1990.

63. Johnson KH: Globoid leukodystrophy in the cat. J Am Vet Med Assoc 157:2057–2064, 1970.

64. Hirth RS, Nielsen SW: A familial canine globoid cell leukodystrophy ("Krabbe type"). J Small Anim Pract 8:569–575, 1967.

65. Zaki FA, Kay WJ: Globoid cell leukodystrophy in a miniature poodle. J Am Vet Med Assoc 163:248–250, 1973.

66. Boysen BG, Tryphonas L, Harries NW: Globoid cell leukodystrophy in the bluetick hound dog. I. Clinical manifestations. Can Vet J 15:303–308, 1974.

67. Suzuki K, Hoogerbrugge PM, Poorthuis BJ, et al: The twitcher mouse. Central nervous system pathology after bone marrow transplantation. Lab Invest 58:302–309, 1988.

52

◆ Vascular Disorders

William B. Thomas

Vascular disorders may affect the brain, spinal cord, or peripheral nerves. The hallmark of a vascular disorder of the nervous system is a sudden onset of focal, often asymmetric neurologic deficits. After the acute onset, there generally is a static phase followed by improvement, if the patient survives. This chapter discusses the diagnosis and treatment of the more common vascular disorders of the brain, spinal cord, and peripheral nerves.

◆ PATHOPHYSIOLOGY OF NEURAL ISCHEMIA AND INFARCTION

Owing to its high metabolic demands, the central nervous system depends on a constant supply of oxygen and glucose from the circulation. Homeostatic mechanisms normally maintain adequate blood flow over a wide range of blood pressure. If there is a decrease in blood flow that exceeds the ability of autoregulatory mechanisms, the nervous system is deprived of the necessary oxygen and glucose, resulting in ischemia (reduction of blood flow to a level incompatible with normal function) or infarction (reduction of blood flow so severe and prolonged that an area of necrosis ensues).

The primary mechanism of damage in infarction is deranged energy metabolism caused by failure of synthesis of adenosine triphosphate (ATP) and other nucleoside triphosphates.[1] Maintaining ion homeostasis by pumping ions across the cell membrane requires ATP, and is the largest energy requirement of neurons. With inadequate ATP, there is a loss of ion pumping, resulting in an influx of Na^+, Cl^-, and osmotically obligated water (edema). Depletion of ATP also results in anaerobic glycolysis, increased H^+ production, lactic acidosis, uncontrolled rise in intracellular Ca^{2+}, and activation of proteases and phospholipases. These processes, coupled with the inability to synthesize proteins and lipids because of inadequate ATP, lead to disruption of cellular integrity and necrosis.[1]

Both the degree and the duration of reduced blood flow are important in determining whether or not infarction develops. If blood flow does not meet metabolic demand, the neurons first become unexcitable. For example, in cats, when cerebral blood flow is reduced to approximately one-half of normal levels, normal neuronal electrical activity ceases but the neurons remain viable.[2] Cellular ion homeostasis is lost when cerebral blood flow drops to about one-third of normal level.[2] Up to this point, how-

ever, neuronal changes are potentially reversible if blood flow is restored quickly enough. If not, the neurons become irreversibly damaged.[1] Complete occlusion of the middle cerebral artery for less than 3 hours causes transient neurologic deficits and minimum infarction.[3] Occlusion for longer than 5 hours causes permanent neurologic deficits associated with infarction.[3]

Reduced blood flow may be caused by arterial thrombosis or embolism. A *thrombus* is a blood clot developing within a vessel that causes vascular obstruction at the site of formation. *Embolism* is occlusion of a vessel by a fragment of blood clot or other substance that has flowed to the site of obstruction from a distant location. Vasospasm of arteries also can interrupt normal blood flow. Occlusion of veins or venous channels by a thrombus also can affect blood flow; because arterial flow is preserved initially, hemorrhage and edema tend to be more severe in venous infarction, compared with arterial infarction.

◆ CEREBROVASCULAR DISEASE

Cerebrovascular disease is an abnormality of the brain attributable to a disturbance in its blood supply. The most common cerebrovascular diseases in cats are feline ischemic encephalopathy and intracranial hemorrhage.

Feline Ischemic Encephalopathy

Feline ischemic encephalopathy (idiopathic feline cerebral infarction) causes 1 or more infarcts in the brain.[4-7] Pathologic lesions most commonly are unilateral and located along the distribution of the middle cerebral artery, but bilateral cerebral lesions and brain stem lesions also may occur.[4, 7] Primary vascular lesions, such as thromboembolism or vasculitis, are uncommon, so the pathophysiology of this syndrome was previously uncertain. Recent studies, however, suggest that the cause of feline ischemic encephalopathy is aberrant migration of *Cuterebra* larvae. Careful pathologic inspection usually reveals a *Cuterebra* larva within the brain or cribriform plate.[8, 9] *Cuterebra* migration also explains the fact that this syndrome usually occurs in summer, coinciding with the migration phase of the parasite's life cycle. Feline ischemic encephalopathy is not known to occur in regions of the world without *Cuterebra*.[9]

The life cycle of *Cuterebra* is complex. The adult

fly, which resembles a bumblebee, lays eggs near the burrows of their natural hosts, lagomorphs and rodents. Cats may become infected with the first stage larva, which are 1 to 2 mm in length. The larva penetrates the mucous membranes or skin, develops for several weeks in subcutaneous tissue, and eventually emerges through a hole it produces in the skin.[10] In some cases, the larva migrates into the brain, usually through the nares and cribriform plate.[9] The migrating parasite probably induces vasospasm of brain arteries, resulting in ischemia or infarction. The pathophysiology of the vasospasm is incompletely understood, but may be related to a toxin produced by the larva.[9]

Clinical Features

Cats of any age and both genders are affected, most commonly in summer months. Affected cats typically have access to outdoors. There is a sudden onset of focal, often asymmetric neurologic deficits. Signs referable to the cerebrum are most common, and include seizures, abnormal behavior, depression, ipsilateral circling, contralateral hemiparesis, and blindness in the contralateral visual field with normal pupillary light reflexes. Brain stem lesions (e.g., vestibular dysfunction) and involvement of the optic nerve/chiasm (blindness with dilated, unresponsive pupils) are less common. Neurologic deficits often are preceded by upper respiratory signs (such as sneezing or epistaxis), and occasionally facial swelling suggestive of an allergic reaction.[8, 10]

Diagnosis

Diagnosis is based largely on clinical features. Cerebrospinal fluid (CSF) analysis may be normal or show a mild increase in protein and mononuclear cells or eosinophils.[7, 8] Computed tomography (CT) reveals multifocal regions of decreased attenuation and abnormal enhancement. Some lesions are hyperattenuating, indicating acute hemorrhage. On magnetic resonance imaging (MRI), these lesions usually are hypointense on T1-weighted images and hyperintense on T2-weighted images. A tractlike lesion may be visualized extending from the cribriform plate through the cerebral hemisphere (Fig. 52–1).

Treatment

Antiseizure medication (diazepam at 0.5 to 1.0 mg/kg, intravenously [IV]; phenobarbital at 2 mg/kg IV, intramuscularly [IM], or by mouth [PO], every [q] q 12 hr) is indicated in patients with seizures. Antibiotic therapy (enrofloxacin at 5 mg/kg PO q 12 hr for 14 days) is indicated to prevent secondary bacterial infection. Supportive care to maintain normal hydration and nutrition are important. A treatment protocol for *Cuterebra* infection has been proposed, consisting of diphenhydramine (4 mg/kg IM) followed in 1 to 2 hours with ivermectin (400 μg/kg, subcutaneously [SQ]) and dexamethasone (0.1 mg/kg IV).[8] Neurologic deficits often improve spontaneously within several weeks. Seizures, abnormal behavior, or visual deficits may persist.

Intracranial Hemorrhage

Intracranial hemorrhage may be epidural (between the dura mater and the skull), subdural (between the dura and the arachnoid), subarachnoid (between the arachnoid and the pia mater), or intraparenchymal.[11] Causes of intracranial hemorrhage include trauma, vascular malformations, brain tumors, coagulopathies, and vasculitis.[11–13] Systemic hypertension is a common cause of intracranial hemorrhage in human beings.[14, 15] Although intracranial hemorrhage owing to hypertension is poorly documented in cats, hypertension caused by disorders such as hyperthyroidism and renal disease is well recognized[16] (see Chapters 36, Systemic Hypertension, and 47, Diagnosis and Treatment of Systemic Hypertension). Intracranial

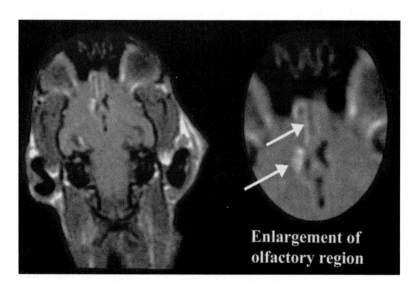

Enlargement of olfactory region

Figure 52–1. Magnetic resonance imaging of *Cuterebra* migration. Three weeks previously, this 1-year-old cat suffered an acute onset of nonprogressive depression, circling to the left, right hemiparesis, and blindness in the right visual field. The neurologic deficits were preceded by sneezing, gagging, and facial swelling. Three *Cuterebra* larvae were removed from the subcutaneous tissue of the face and neck. On the dorsal plane T1-weighted image with contrast, there is a contrast-enhancing tract (*arrows*) in the left olfactory region, extending from the cribriform plate to the area of the left caudate nucleus.

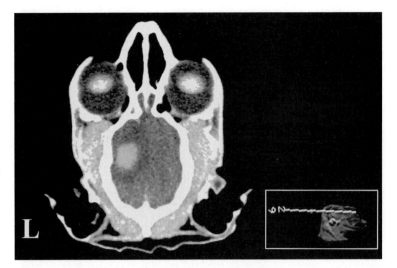

Figure 52–2. Acute intraparenchymal hematoma in a 12-year-old cat with hyperthyroidism and hypertension. The cat suffered an acute onset of depression and right hemiparesis 2 days previously. The dorsal-plane computed tomography scan shows a hyperattenuating mass within the left cerebral hemisphere. The hematoma is surrounded by hypoattenuating edema.

hemorrhage usually causes neurologic deficits referable to a focal brain lesion. Edema begins to develop in the brain tissue surrounding the hematoma within the first several hours after bleeding. The edema, combined with enlargement of the hematoma, causes progressive worsening of neurologic function.[12] In severe cases, this culminates in transtentorial or tonsillar herniation, the most life-threatening consequences of intracranial hemorrhage.[15]

Diagnosis

Diagnosis is based on CT or MRI. On CT, acute hemorrhage in a patient with a normal hematocrit is evident as increased attenuation with associated mass effect.[17, 18] Hemorrhage in patients with severe anemia may be less obvious. An acute hematoma usually is surrounded by a hypoattenuating region corresponding to edema (Fig. 52–2).[17–19] The attenuation of extravasated blood increases for the first 72 hours with clot formation and extrusion of low-density serum.[20] After that, the attenuation gradually decreases as the result of lysis and phagocytosis of erythrocytes, which starts at the periphery and progresses centrally.[19, 20] The hematoma eventually becomes isoattenuating at about 1 month after onset.[19, 20] Use of contrast agent is unnecessary in most acute hematomas, and may obscure the inherent

hyperattenuation, thus confusing the diagnosis. The use of a contrast agent may be helpful, however, if there is a small hemorrhage with mass-effect out of proportion to the size of the hematoma. In this instance, the differential diagnosis includes bleeding into a tumor, and contrast may be necessary to visualize the tumor.[20]

The MRI features of intracranial hematomas depend in part on the age of the hemorrhage, and are summarized in Table 52–1. In general, CT is the diagnostic study of choice for the initial evaluation of acute intracranial hemorrhage because it can be completed quickly, and is sensitive to acute hemorrhage. A disadvantage of MRI is the longer examination time and the difficulty in monitoring unstable patients in the MRI environment. In patients with subacute hemorrhage, MRI is more sensitive and specific, and is the procedure of choice once the patient is stabilized (Fig. 52–3).[21]

In cats with intracranial hemorrhage not caused by obvious trauma, further diagnostic evaluation is aimed at identifying any underlying cause. The owner is asked about potential exposure to anticoagulant rodenticides. The clinician should perform a careful physical examination, including fundic examination, to detect any other regions of hemorrhage. A complete blood count, coagulation profile, serum chemistry profile, urinalysis, serum thyrox-

Table 52–1. Magnetic Resonance Appearance of Intracranial Hemorrhage at Medium Field Strength (e.g., 0.5 Tesla)

Approximate Time	Stage	T1-Weighted Intensity*	T2-Weighted Intensity*
First few hours	Oxyhemoglobin	Slightly hypointense	Hyperintense
Several hours to several days	Deoxyhemoglobin	Slightly hypointense	Very hypointense
First several days	Intracellular methemoglobin	Very hyperintense	Very hypointense
Several days to several months	Hemolysis	Very hyperintense	Very hyperintense
Several days to indefinitely	Ferritin and hemosiderin		
	Center	Hypointense	Hyperintense
	Rim	Hypointense	Very hypointense

*Signal intensities are relative to normal gray matter.
Data from Spetzler RF, Hargraves RW, McCormick PW, et al: Relationship of perfusion pressure and size of hemorrhage from arteriovenous malformations. J Neurosurg 76:918–923, 1992, and Bradley WG: Hemorrhage and brain iron. In Stark DD, Bradley WG (eds): Magnetic Resonance Imaging, 2nd ed. St. Louis, Mosby–Year Book, 1992, pp. 721–769.

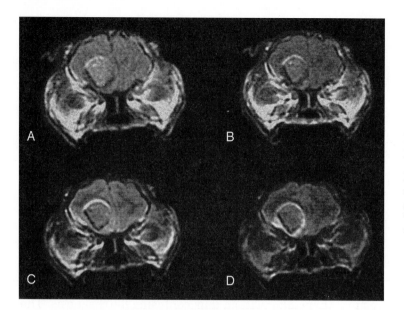

Figure 52–3. Subacute intraparenchymal hematoma in a 9-year-old cat with an acute onset of dementia and ataxia 10 days previously. There is a mass in the left cerebral hemisphere with deviation of the longitudinal fissure to the right. The mass is hyperintense on T1-weighted images without contrast (*A*) and slightly hyperintense on proton-density (*C*) and T2-weighted (*D*) images, consistent with methemoglobin. The ventral rim of the mass is hypointense on all images, consistent with hemosiderin and ferritin. There is minimum enhancement on the contrast-enhanced T1-weighted image (*B*).

ine (T₄), measurement of blood pressure, and chest radiographs also are helpful.

Treatment

The primary goals of treatment are to maintain adequate tissue oxygenation; manage any progressive neurologic sequelae, such as seizures and increased intracranial pressure; and treat any underlying disease. Supplemental oxygen should be provided. Unconscious animals require endotracheal intubation. Hypovolemia should be treated with volume expansion to prevent compromised cerebral blood flow, but overhydration and hyponatremia must be avoided because they worsen brain edema.[15] Blood glucose is maintained at normal concentration. In ischemic brain tissue, high glucose levels cause increased lactic acid production and acidosis, which exacerbate brain damage.

Hypertension may be a cause of intracranial hemorrhage, or may be secondary to sympathetic stimulation associated with brain injury. Although increased blood pressure may exacerbate edema or hemorrhage, acute normalization of blood pressure is dangerous because it may reduce cerebral perfusion to ischemic levels. For this reason, hypertension should not be treated unless there is acute systemic damage, such as renal or cardiac failure, or evidence of progressive intracranial bleeding.[22] In such cases, amlodipine (¼ of a 2.5-mg tablet, PO, q 24 hr) may be useful (see Chapters 36, Systemic Hypertension, and 47, Diagnosis and Treatment of Systemic Hypertension).

Mannitol decreases brain edema and intracranial pressure due to brain hemorrhage.[15] By increasing plasma osmolality, mannitol creates an osmotic gradient between the intravascular and the extravascular compartments, and results in movement of water out of the brain.[23] Probably more importantly, mannitol decreases blood viscosity, which enhances cerebral blood flow.[24] In the face of improved cerebral blood flow, autoregulatory mechanisms cause vasoconstriction in normal brain, reducing the volume of blood within the cranium, thereby decreasing intracranial pressure.[24]

The standard dose of mannitol is 1.0 g/kg, intravenously. This dose usually is repeated every 6 hours. Lower, more frequent doses (0.25 g/kg q 3 hr) are equally effective.[22] A fairly arbitrary goal is to increase serum osmolality to 310 to 320 mOsm/kg.[22] As with all treatments for elevated intracranial pressure, however, treatment should be guided primarily by clinical response.[22] Mannitol is contraindicated in dehydration, hypovolemia, or pulmonary edema.[25] Because mannitol can cause abnormalities in blood electrolytes, daily monitoring of electrolyte levels is recommended. Although some veterinary texts cite intracranial hemorrhage as a contraindication for mannitol administration, there is little evidence that mannitol exacerbates intracranial hemorrhage, and osmotic diuretics are used routinely in the control of intracranial pressure in human patients with known intracranial hemorrhage.[22]

Glucocorticoids do not alter the size of hemorrhage, do not decrease edema caused by brain hemorrhage, and may predispose to complications, such as infection.[14, 15] Uncontrolled seizures can cause severe increases in cerebral metabolism and intracranial pressure, resulting in further brain ischemia. Seizures are treated with diazepam (0.5–1.0 mg/kg, IV). If frequent seizures occur, phenobarbital (2 mg/kg IV, IM, or PO, q 12 hr) should be started.

Surgical removal of the hematoma should be considered in cats with head injury, deteriorating neurologic status, and CT or MRI evidence of a large hematoma.[11] The role of surgery for intracranial hemorrhage not caused by trauma is less clear. In human patients with spontaneous intracranial hemorrhage, surgery is considered for patients with deteriorating neurologic status and cerebral or cerebellar hemorrhage. Surgery rarely is beneficial in patients that are comatose at the onset of hemorrhage.[26]

Outcome is determined primarily by the size and location of the hematoma. Recovery is possible with appropriate treatment and supportive care. Deteriorating levels of consciousness, uncontrollable seizures, uncontrollable rises in intracranial pressure, and signs of brain herniation warrant a poor prognosis.

◆ FIBROCARTILAGINOUS EMBOLISM

Fibrocartilaginous embolism (FCE) is a common cause of acute spinal cord dysfunction in dogs.[27] It occurs when blood vessels of the spinal cord are occluded with fibrocartilage, originating presumably from the intervertebral disc. The mechanism by which the embolic material travels from the disc into the vessels of the spinal cord is not known.[27] Pathologically confirmed FCE has been reported infrequently in cats.[7, 28–31] However, the number of published cases may underestimate the incidence, because recognition of FCE at necropsy is dependent partly on clinical suspicion. Also, many dogs with FCE recover, precluding histologic examination, and the same may be true for cats.

Cats between 9 and 12 years old are reported to be affected most commonly. There is a sudden onset of nonpainful paraparesis or tetraparesis, which may be asymmetric. The course usually is nonprogressive, although there may be deterioration in neurologic status during the first few days. Diagnosis is based on clinical features and by excluding other causes by radiography, myelography, and analysis of CSF. In patients with FCE, myelography is normal, or shows focal spinal cord swelling.[31] Analysis of CSF may show increased protein.[31] The primary diagnostic considerations for an acute focal lesion of the spinal cord is trauma and intervertebral disc extrusion, which can be detected by radiography and myelography. Aortic thromboembolism causes ischemia to pelvic limb nerves and muscles, rather than spinal cord ischemia, but the resulting paraparesis may appear similar to spinal cord disease (see later). Myelitis and neoplasia also may appear similar, but typically have a slower, more progressive course and usually can be identified by CSF analysis and myelography.

There is no specific treatment. Based on experience in dogs with FCE, many patients recover spontaneously within several weeks.[27] Nursing care, in particular manual bladder expression in incontinent patients, is important. The prognosis is poor for patients with absent deep pain perception or no improvement within 2 to 4 weeks.

◆ PERIPHERAL NERVE ISCHEMIA

Compared with the central nervous system, peripheral nerve is relatively resistant to ischemia. The metabolic demands of nerve are relatively low—only about one-third the amount of oxygen normally supplied.[32] Furthermore, peripheral nerve, unlike most tissue, has 2 separate, functionally independent vascular systems: an intrinsic system composed of longitudinal vessels within the endoneurium, and an extrinsic system consisting of regional and epineural vessels.[33] Thus, peripheral nerve suffers ischemic damage only with widespread vascular alteration.

In cats, complete ischemia of the sciatic nerve produces conduction failure within 30 minutes. Correction of ischemia within 1 hour results in prompt recovery of nerve function. After 3 hours of ischemia, abnormally low conduction persists for up to 1 week. If the ischemia is not corrected, there is demyelination and axonal necrosis within 24 to 48 hours.[32]

Aortic Embolism

The most common cause of peripheral nerve ischemia is aortic embolism. All forms of feline cardiomyopathy predispose to thrombosis due to poor atrial emptying, endocardial injury, and hypercoagulability (see Chapter 39, Aortic Thromboembolism).[34] Thrombi form most commonly in the left atrium. All or part of the thrombus may break off and be carried through the blood stream to lodge distally at a point of narrowing of the vessel. In about 90 per cent of cases, the embolus lodges in the distal aorta ("saddle" embolism). The embolus causes release of vasoactive substances that constrict collateral circulation, resulting in ischemia of the peroneal and tibial nerves and muscles distal to the midthigh region.[34] The right brachial artery is occluded occasionally, and the left brachial artery is affected rarely.[34] The incidence of embolism in cats with cardiomyopathy ranges from 13 to 19 per cent.[34] Aortic embolism also may be caused by a foreign body, especially BB shot.[35–37] In most cases, the projectile enters the heart and subsequently moves to the abdominal aorta.[35, 36]

Clinical Features

Middle-aged cats are affected most commonly.[38] With distal aortic embolism, there is an acute onset of painful paraparesis. Sometimes there is a history of previous transient episodes of paraparesis preceding a severe attack. Although many affected cats do not have a history of preexisting heart disease, most have signs of heart disease at presentation, including a murmur, gallop rhythm, arrhythmia, or pulmonary crackles.[38] The pelvic limbs are weak, with decreased postural reactions. One leg often is more severely affected. Initially, the gastrocnemius and cranial tibial muscles are firm, painful, and contracted. Tail and sphincter function, flexion and extension of the hips, and patellar reflexes usually are preserved.[36] Deep pain perception may be absent in the distal limb.[36] Femoral pulses are weak or absent, and the distal aspect of the limbs may be cool with cyanotic nail beds. Femoral pulses may be difficult to palpate in obese or fractious cats, in which case measuring blood pressure in the pelvic limbs compared with the thoracic limbs is helpful.

Diagnosis

Laboratory evaluation often shows increased serum creatine kinase and lactic dehydrogenase. Azotemia is common, and may be severe if the embolus occludes the renal arteries. Chest radiographs usually reveal evidence of cardiac disease, such as cardiomegaly. Electrocardiography may show tachycardia, arrhythmias, or evidence of ventricular or atrial enlargement. Echocardiography usually confirms cardiomyopathy, and may identify an intracardiac thrombus.[38] Angiography or Doppler ultrasonography of the distal aorta may be used to confirm the diagnosis when results of physical examination are inconclusive (Fig. 52–4).

Treatment

Therapy includes management of concurrent heart disease, patient monitoring, and supportive care, including nutritional support, and anticoagulant treatment to prevent further thrombosis (see Chapter 39, Aortic Thromboembolism). Surgical removal of the embolus usually is not recommended because of the high rate of perioperative mortality in cats with cardiomyopathy.[34, 39] Widespread use of thrombolytic drugs, such as streptokinase and tissue plasminogen activator (t-PA), to dissolve the clot has been limited by expense and adverse effects.[34] In an uncontrolled trial evaluating t-PA, 43 per cent of cats survived and were walking within 48 hours, but 50 per cent of the patients died, usually from complications associated with reperfusion of ischemic muscles, such as severe hyperkalemia.[39]

Anticoagulation

Anticoagulants, such as heparin and warfarin, have no effect on established clots but inhibit further thrombus formation, thereby allowing the patient's natural thrombolytic mechanisms to decrease the size of the clot. Although controlled clinical trials are lacking, anticoagulant therapy is recommended for patients that can be monitored closely. After determining the baseline partial thromboplastin time (PTT), 220 IU/kg of heparin is administered intravenously. Three hours later, maintenance therapy with 66 IU/kg subcutaneously every 6 hours is started. The dose is adjusted to maintain a PTT of 2.0 to 2.5 times the baseline value.[39, 40] Heparin usually is continued until the patient is dismissed from the hospital, or until warfarin therapy has been initiated for at least 48 hours.[41]

Sodium warfarin (Coumadin) acts to block the vitamin K–dependent clotting factors. The initial dose is 0.25 to 0.5 mg PO every 24 hours.[32, 42] One-stage prothrombin time (PT) is measured before therapy and daily after starting therapy, by obtaining a blood sample at least 2 hours after warfarin administration. The dose is adjusted to prolong the PT to twice-normal values or to obtain an international normalization ratio of 2.0 to 3.0 (INR = patient's PT/control PT).[42] PT is monitored every 3 to 4 days for the first 2 weeks, weekly for a month, and monthly thereafter.[41]

The major complication of anticoagulant therapy is hemorrhage. In most patients, this is manifested as internal bleeding causing weakness, lethargy, and pale mucous membranes.[41] Adjusting the dose, temporarily stopping therapy, and/or the administration of fresh blood or plasma may be necessary. Protamine reverses the action of heparin. If given within a few minutes of heparin, the dose is 1 mg of protamine sulfate intravenously, slowly, per 100 IU of heparin. If given 1 hour after heparin, the dose is 0.5 mg per 100 IU of heparin, and if 2 hours

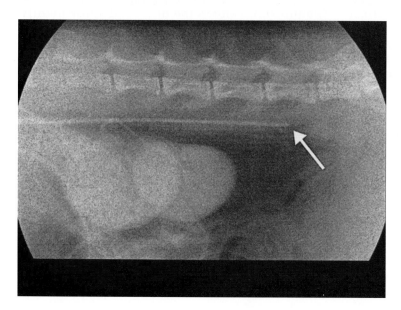

Figure 52–4. Nonselective angiogram of aortic thromboembolism. There is blockage of contrast flow (*arrow*) in the distal aorta.

have elapsed, the dose is 0.25 mg per 100 IU of heparin.[39] Vitamin K_1 (1 to 2 mg/kg PO or SQ q 24 hr for 3 days) reverses the anticoagulant effects of warfarin.[42]

Supportive Care and Patient Monitoring

Hydration and body temperature are monitored and maintained within normal ranges. Analgesics (butorphanol at 0.1 to 0.2 mg/kg IM q 8 hr) usually are necessary. Nutritional support, such as nasogastric tube feeding, is indicated in cats that do not eat. Serum chemistries and electrolytes are monitored closely. Sudden life-threatening hyperkalemia can occur owing to reperfusion. Continuous electrocardiographic monitoring is helpful to detect signs of hyperkalemia, such as P-R interval prolongation, disappearance of P waves, widening of QRS complexes, increasing T-wave amplitude, and bradycardia. Hyperkalemia may be treated with intravenous sodium bicarbonate and titrated doses of regular insulin and glucose, although severe hyperkalemia often is refractory to treatment.[34]

Prophylactic Therapy

For cats that survive an embolic episode, prophylactic therapy has been recommended by some authors in an attempt to prevent further attacks. Aspirin, at 25 mg/kg PO every 3 days, has been advocated, but results have been disappointing.[39, 40, 42] Long-term use of heparin, as discussed above previously, also has been described.[40] Some authors recommend warfarin therapy for all cats with embolic episodes or echocardiographic evidence of cardiomyopathy,[42] whereas others reserve anticoagulant therapy for patients with an embolic episode, if the cat lives indoors and is monitored closely.[34]

Prognosis

In one study, 34 of 92 patients (37 per cent) survived the initial episode with a long-term survival of 11.5 months.[33] Poor prognostic indicators include refractory heart failure, decreasing limb viability evident as progressive hardening of the gastrocnemius and cranial tibial muscles, clinical signs indicating multiple sites of embolism (acute renal failure, bloody diarrhea, central nervous system deficits), disseminated intravascular coagulation, arrhythmias, and unresponsive hypothermia.[34] For cats that survive the initial attack, motor function often improves within 2 to 3 weeks, although permanent deficits are possible. Unfortunately, most affected cats suffer additional embolic episodes within days to months.

REFERENCES

1. Siesjo BK: Pathophysiology and treatment of focal cerebral ischemia. Part 1: Pathophysiology. J Neurosurg 77:169–184, 1992.
2. Strong AJ, Venables GS, Gibson G: The cortical ischemic penumbra associated with occlusion of the middle cerebral artery in the cat: 1. Topography of changes in blood flow, potassium ion activity, and EEG. J Cereb Blood Flow Metab 3:86–96, 1983.
3. Weinstein PR, Anderson GC, Telles DA: Neurological deficit and cerebral infarction after temporary middle cerebral artery occlusion in unanesthetized cats. Stroke 17:318–324, 1986.
4. deLahunta A: Feline ischemic encephalopathy—A cerebral infarction syndrome. In Kirk RW (ed): Current Veterinary Therapy VI. Philadelphia, WB Saunders, 1977, pp. 906–908.
5. Zaki FA, Nafe LA: Ischaemic encephalopathy and focal granulomatous meningoencephalitis in the cat. J Small Anim Pract 21:429–438, 1980.
6. Bernstein NM, Fiske RA: Feline ischemic encephalopathy in a cat. J Am Anim Hosp Assoc 22:205–206, 1986.
7. Shepherd DE, deLahunta A: Central nervous system disease in the cat. Compend Contin Educ Pract Vet 2:306–311, 1980.
8. Glass EN, Cornetta AM, deLahunta A, et al: Clinical and clinicopathologic features in 11 cats with Cuterebra larvae myiasis of the central nervous system. J Vet Intern Med 12:365–368, 1998.
9. Williams KJ, Summers BA, deLahunta A: Cerebrospinal cuterebriasis in cats and its association with feline ischemic encephalopathy. Vet Pathol 35:330–343, 1998.
10. Hendrix CM, Cox NR, Clemons-Chervis C, et al: Aberrant intracranial myiasis caused by larval Cuterebra infection. Compend Contin Educ Pract Vet 11:550–559, 1989.
11. Dewey CW, Downs MO, Aron DN, et al: Acute traumatic intracranial haemorrhage in dogs and cats. Vet Comp Orthop Traumatol 6:153–159, 1993.
12. Shores A, Cooper TG, Gartrell CL, et al: Clinical characteristics of cerebrovascular disease in small animals. Proceedings 9th ACVIM Forum, 1991, pp. 777–778.
13. Fankhauser R, Luginbuhl H, McGrath JT: Cerebrovascular disease in various animal species. Ann N Y Acad Sci 127:817–859, 1965.
14. Castel JP, Kissel P: Spontaneous intracerebral and infratentorial hemorrhage. In Youmans JR (ed): Neurological Surgery, 3rd ed. Philadelphia, WB Saunders, 1990, pp. 1890–1917.
15. Minematsu K, Yamaguchi T: Management of intracerebral hemorrhage. In Fisher M (ed): Stroke Therapy. Boston, Butterworth-Heinemann, 1995, pp. 351–372.
16. Dukes J: Hypertension: A review of the mechanisms, manifestations, and management. J Small Anim Pract 33:119–129, 1992.
17. Tidwell AS, Mahony OM, Moore RP, et al: Computed tomography of an acute hemorrhagic cerebral infarct in a dog. Vet Radiol Ultrasound 35:290–296, 1994.
18. Thomas WB, Scheuler RO, Kornegay JN: Surgical excision of a cerebral arteriovenous malformation in a dog. Prog Vet Neurol 6:20–23, 1995.
19. Enzman DR, Britt RH, Lyons BE, et al: Natural history of experimental intracerebral hemorrhage: Sonography, computed tomography and neuropathology. AJNR 2:517–526, 1981.
20. Grossman RI: Intracranial hemorrhage. In Latchaw RE (ed): MR and CT Imaging of the Head, Neck, and Spine, 2nd ed. St. Louis, Mosby–Year Book, 1991, pp. 171–202.
21. Thomas WB: Nonneoplastic disorders of the brain. Clin Tech Small Anim Pract 14:125–147, 1999.
22. Diringer MN: Intracerebral hemorrhage: pathophysiology and management. Crit Care Med 21:1591–1603, 1993.
23. Donato T, Shapira Y, Artru A, et al: Effect of mannitol on cerebrospinal fluid dynamics and brain tissue edema. Anesth Analg 78:58–66, 1994.
24. Muizelaar JP, Wei EP, Kontos HA, et al: Mannitol causes compensatory cerebral vasoconstriction and vasodilation in response to blood viscosity changes. J Neurosurg 592:822–828, 1983.
25. Dewey CW, Budsberg SC, Oliver JE: Principles of head trauma management in dogs and cats—Part II. Compend Contin Educ Pract Vet 15:177–193, 1993.
26. Crowell RM, Ojemann RG, Ogilvy CS: Spontaneous brain hemorrhage: Surgical considerations. In Barnett HJM, Mohr

JP, Stein BM, Yatsu FM (eds): Stroke: Pathophysiology, Diagnosis, and Management, 2nd ed. New York, Churchill Livingstone, 1992, pp. 1169–1187.

27. Neer TM: Fibrocartilaginous emboli. Vet Clin North Am Small Anim Pract 22:1017–1026, 1992.
28. Zaki FA, Prata RG, Werner LL: Necrotizing myelopathy in a cat. J Am Vet Med Assoc 169:228–229, 1976.
29. deLahunta A, Alexander JW: Ischemic myelopathy secondary to presumed fibrocartilaginous embolism in nine dogs. J Am Anim Hosp Assoc 12:37–48, 1976.
30. Turner PV, Percy DH, Allyson K: Fibrocartilaginous embolic myelopathy in a cat. Can Vet J 36:712–713, 1995.
31. Scott HW, O'Leary MT: Fibro-cartilaginous embolism in a cat. J Small Anim Pract 37:228–231, 1996.
32. Chalk CH, Dyck PJ: Ischemic neuropathy. *In* Dyck PJ, Thomas PK (eds): Peripheral Neuropathy, 3rd ed. Philadelphia, WB Saunders, 1993, pp. 980–989.
33. McManis PG, Low PA, Lagerlund TD: Microenvironment of nerve: Blood flow and ischemia. *In* Dyck PJ, Thomas PK (eds): Peripheral Neuropathy, 3rd ed. Philadelphia, WB Saunders, 1993, pp. 453–473.
34. Fox PR: Feline cardiomyopathies. *In* Fox PR, Sisson A, Moise NS (eds): Textbook of Canine and Feline Cardiology, 2nd ed. Philadelphia, WB Saunders, 1999, pp. 621–678.
35. Horton CR, Renfroe BJ: Surgical removal of a BB shot from the abdominal aorta of a cat. Vet Med Small Anim Clin 73:321–323, 1978.
36. Langelier KM: Ischemic neuromyopathy associated with steel pellet BB shot aortic obstruction in a cat. Can Vet J 23:187–189, 1982.
37. Whigham HM, Ellison GW, Graham J: Aortic foreign body resulting in ischemic neuromyopathy and development of collateral circulation in a cat. J Am Vet Med Assoc 213:829–832, 1998.
38. Laste NJ, Harpster NK: A retrospective study of 100 cases of feline distal aortic thromboembolism. J Am Anim Hosp Assoc 31:492–500, 1995.
39. Pion PD, Kittleson MD: Therapy for feline aortic thromboembolism. *In* Kirk RW (ed): Current Veterinary Therapy X. Philadelphia, WB Saunders, 1989, pp. 295–302.
40. Harpster NK: Feline myocardial diseases. *In* Kirk RW (ed): Current Veterinary Therapy IX. Philadelphia, WB Saunders, 1986, pp. 380–398.
41. Rush JE: Therapy of feline hypertrophic cardiomyopathy. Vet Clin North Am Small Anim Pract 28:1459–1479, 1998.
42. Harpster NK, Baty CJ: Warfarin therapy of the cat at risk of thromboembolism. *In* Bonagura JD (ed): Current Veterinary Therapy XII. Philadelphia, WB Saunders, 1995, pp. 868–873.
43. Spetzler RF, Hargraves RW, McCormick PW, et al: Relationship of perfusion pressure and size of hemorrhage from arteriovenous malformations. J Neurosurg 76:918–923, 1992.
44. Bradley WG: Hemorrhage and brain iron. *In* Stark DD, Bradley WG (eds): Magnetic Resonance Imaging, 2nd ed. St. Louis, Mosby–Year Book, 1992, pp. 721–769.

53

◆ Congenital Cranial and Intracranial Malformations

Joan R. Coates
Stacey A. Sullivan

Congenital defects are developmental abnormalities that are present at or near the time of birth, and account for approximately 10 to 20 per cent of all neonatal deaths in cats.[1-3] Congenital defects may or may not be manifested during the pediatric stages of kitten growth and development. The frequency of congenital defects may be underestimated because the cause of death remains undiagnosed or unnoticed. Environmental factors such as diet, viruses, drugs, and heat (temperature extremes) have their greatest effects by induction of abortion or embryonic death and resorption.[4] Kitten death that occurs during the period immediately after birth often is referred to as *fading kitten syndrome.* Congenital malformations have been associated as a cause of fading kitten syndrome.[5] Except for a few well-described syndromes, most malformations occur sporadically and have an unknown cause.[2, 4, 6]

The nervous system has been reported as the organ system most frequently affected by congenital defects in cats.[6] Cerebellar malformation accounts for the most common congenital malformation in cats. Other intracranial and cranial malformations often are lethal or associated with high neonatal mortality.[2] This chapter reviews the embryology and congenital disorders associated with neural tube and cranial development in cats. The classification scheme for these defects is outlined in Table 53–1. Congenital malformations of the spinal cord and vertebrae have been described, and are beyond the scope of this chapter.[7]

◆ ETIOLOGY OF CONGENITAL INTRACRANIAL/CRANIAL MALFORMATIONS

Malformations of the central nervous system (CNS) often are caused by abnormalities of morphogenesis; however, other emerging causes include abnormalities in regional pattern development of the CNS, and programmed cell death (apoptosis). Morphogenic alterations associated with embryonic development include neural tube and neuronal migration defects. Pattern-specific disruption occurs very early in embryonic development, and probably results from an altered inductive influence controlled by specific genes (homeobox) of regionally specified mesoderm on the overlying ectoderm.[8, 9] *Pro-grammed cell death* refers to a process by which cells die during normal development, is an expression of terminal differentiation, and involves new gene expression.[10] This process is critical for achieving correct population size and proper morphogenesis of brain structures.

Two differential categories for causes of congenital malformations are genetic and teratogenic. Not all congenital defects are inherited; conversely, not all inherited defects are congenital. Genetic defects may arise spontaneously or inadvertently by genetic selection. Selection processes used by breeders include inbreeding, line-breeding, and out-crossing. Inbreeding and line-breeding practices result in a reduction of genetic variability and an increase in homozygous and recessive traits. Inbreeding tends to select for a particular trait. Line-breeding is a less intense form of inbreeding that augments ancestral traits. Simple inherited (mendelian) patterns have served as the basis for determining modes of inheritance of many genetic disorders. Determining inheritance pattern is more difficult for polygenic and

Table 53–1. Classification Scheme for Intracranial Defects in Cats

Forebrain Malformations

Hydrocephalus

Hydranencephaly/Porencephaly

Neural Tube Defects
Primary neural tube closure defects
   Exencephaly/anencephaly
   Craniorachischisis
Primary axial mesodermal defects
   Encephalocele/meningocele
   Craniofacial mesodermal defects in Burmese cats
   Cleft palate

Disorders of Forebrain Induction
Holoprosencephaly
Agenesis of corpus callosum

Disorders of Neuronal Migration
Lissencephaly

Malformations of the Hindbrain
Dandy Walker syndrome
Chiari malformation
Parvoviral (feline panleukopenia virus)-induced cerebellar
   degeneration (hypoplasia)
Hereditary cerebellar cortical atrophy

Table 53–2. Teratogenic Agents Causing Congenital Cranial Malformations in Cats

Teratogen	Malformation
Parvovirus (feline panleukopenia)	Hydranencephaly, porencephaly, hydrocephalus, cerebellar hypoplasia
Methylmercury	Exencephaly, ↓ cellular density in external granule cell layer, cerebellar hypoplasia
Griseofulvin	Exencephaly, hydrocephalus, holoprosencephaly, corpus callosal agenesis, cranium bifidum, spina bifida, cleft palate, absence of maxillae, cyclopia, anophthalmia
Hydroxyurea	Cyclopia, cleft palate, exencephaly, microcephaly, cyclopia
Diphenylhydantoin	Cleft palate

multifactorial traits. Polygenic inheritance refers to situations in which proper development relies on sequential activation of genes or for traits of variable penetrance that result in a variety of phenotypes for a given genotype. Multifactorial traits are determined by the interaction between environment and polygenic predisposition. No single gene or environmental factor is a major determinant of a multifactorial disease.

Teratogens are external factors that adversely affect embryonic development during the critical period for an organ system.[11] Commonly recognized teratogens include toxins, drugs, viral infections, over- and undersupplementation of nutrients, and environmental factors (e.g., radiation exposure and maternal hyperthermia). The CNS is sensitive to teratogenic insult throughout prenatal and early postnatal development.[12] Specific teratogens and their effects are reviewed as specific malformations are discussed (Table 53–2).

◆ EMBRYOLOGY

Early in development, embryos are composed of 3 germ layers: ectoderm, mesoderm, and endoderm. The ectoderm is the outermost layer, which becomes the epidermal, neural, and skeletal and connective tissues of the head. The mesoderm becomes muscle and skeletal tissue and is divided serially into somites. Each somite separates into dermatomal, myotomal, and sclerotomal regions. The endoderm forms into structures and lining of the respiratory and alimentary tracts.

Critical morphogenesis of the brain in cats occurs between 11 and 22 days of gestation.[12] The neural tube is the progenitor of the CNS, and is surrounded by the axial skeleton. Embryogenesis of the neural tube is a complex phenomenon of cellular and subcellular processes. Precise timing of these events must occur for successful neural tube development.[13] Primary neurulation begins with thickening of the midline ectoderm (cervical/occipital junction)

toward the rostral portion of the embryo; this thickening is referred to as the *neural plate.* The lateral edges of the neural plate fold dorsally to form a longitudinal neural groove and folds. The neural folds converge toward the midline to form the neural tube. Prior to neural tube closure, neuroblasts migrate without glial guidance to form the outer marginal, intermediate, and inner ventricular zone. Glial guidance allows for further neuronal migration to occur first tangentially and then radially. It was thought previously that closure of the neural tube proceeded cranially and caudally to form the future brain and spinal cord, respectively. More recently, it has been described that closure sites along the neural tube occur at multiple locations and may vary.[14, 15] The neural tube separates from the surface ectoderm after closure is complete.

The cephalic portion of the neural tube is delineated into 3 primary vesicles: forebrain (prosencephalon), midbrain (mesencephalon), and hindbrain (rhombencephalon).[16] The forebrain expands to form the prosencephalon that develops into paired telencephalic and optic structures, the diencephalon, and the third ventricle. The telencephalon subsequently becomes the cerebrum and lateral ventricles. The midbrain remains a small undifferentiated structure, which encompasses the mesencephalic aqueduct. The hindbrain subdivides rostrally into the metencephalon and caudally into the myelencephalon. The metencephalon and myelencephalon develop further to become the pons/cerebellum and medulla oblongata, respectively. The myelencephalon forms into the medulla oblongata. After primary neurulation, the neuroblasts proliferate, differentiate into neurons, and migrate. Most of the reported developmental anomalies usually occur during this process of development.

The cerebral cortical neurons and the cerebellum in cats undergo maximal development late in the third trimester and during the first 2 weeks of postnatal growth.[12] The change in cerebellar morphology is most pronounced by a transition that occurs in the external granule cell layer. The external granule cell layer increases in thickness during the first week and is followed by a decline beginning at 2 weeks, and rapid thinning by 9 weeks.[17] Postnatal development of cerebellar granule cells in kittens appears to follow a pattern and time course of development similar to that of other species.[18]

Development of head and facial structures is induced by brain development and peaks between days 12 and 32 of gestation.[12] Axial skeletal development begins when sclerotomal components of the mesodermal somites migrate around the neural tube soon after closure has been completed. In the cranial region, only the vault of the skull is formed by axial mesoderm. It is important from a pathogenesis perspective to distinguish between malformations that are a result of abnormal neural tube closure and those that are a result of bony defects associated with abnormal axial mesodermal development. Neural tube defects often are accompanied by secondary bony defects. Abnormalities of mesodermal development may result in herniation of the neural tube through the bony defect.

Neural crest cells are a condensation of neuroepithelium that form dorsal to the neural tube and give rise to the peripheral and autonomic nervous systems, the adrenal medulla, and pigmentary cells. In the cranial region, the population of neural crest cells is quite large. Cranial neural crest cells migrate from the neural folds early in embryogenesis and appear to be a prerequisite for folding of the neural tube.[13] These neural crest cells become the mesenchyme of the face and skull base, and contribute to the spiral septum in the outflow tract of the heart. Agents affecting this tissue migration process are likely to cause defects of the face and heart.

◆ DIFFERENTIAL DIAGNOSIS

Disease differentials for congenital cranial and intracranial malformations in cats include prenatal or perinatal infectious diseases (feline panleukopenia, [FPL], feline infectious peritonitis) and toxin exposure. Other causes include lysosomal storage diseases such as gangliosidosis and mannosidosis, glycogen storage disease, and hereditary neuroaxonal dystrophy. Causes for these disorders should be readdressed regularly, considering the expanding knowledge base of genetic disorders and increasing usage of molecular diagnostic techniques.

◆ MALFORMATIONS OF THE FOREBRAIN

Hydrocephalus

Hydrocephalus is discussed first because of its clinical importance and frequency of occurrence in many of the malformation disorders addressed in this chapter. Evaluation and diagnosis of hydrocephalus play a crucial role in management of these disorders. Multiple classification schemes exist with regard to cause and pathogenesis.

Cause. Hydrocephalus is one of the most common manifestations of developmental disorders. Hydrocephalus has been reported as an autosomal recessive trait in Siamese cats.[19] Hydrocephalus often represents a secondary manifestation of a developmental (e.g., Chiari malformations) or an acquired (e.g., neoplasia) disorder. Acquired causes in kittens may be due to toxin exposure or infectious inflammatory disease such as perinatal or prenatal infectious peritonitis coronaviral[20] and in utero FPL parvoviral[21, 22] infections. Kittens of queens treated with griseofulvin during pregnancy developed hydrocephalus with other brain malformations.[23] Congenital hydrocephalus of unknown cause has been described in other reports.[24–26]

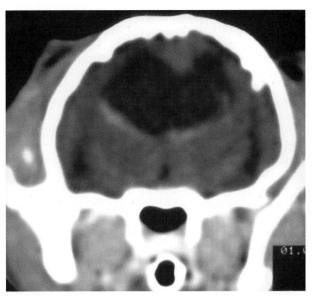

Figure 53–1. Computed tomography (CT) appearance of a feline brain with internal hydrocephalus. On this transverse image, both lateral ventricles are enlarged.

Pathogenesis. Hydrocephalus denotes an increase in volume of cerebrospinal fluid (CSF) within the intracranial compartment. Internal (Fig. 53–1) and external (Fig. 53–2) hydrocephalus refer to increased fluid accumulation within the ventricular and subarachnoid spaces, respectively. Noncommunicating (obstructive) hydrocephalus refers to increased CSF only within the ventricular system, and

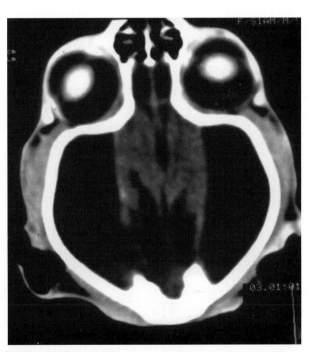

Figure 53–2. CT appearance of a feline brain with external hydrocephalus. On this dorsal image, both cerebral hemispheres are externally compressed. A defect in the right occipital cortex is apparent.

communicating refers to increased CSF within the ventricular system and subarachnoid space. Communicating hydrocephalus results from an outflow obstruction of the venous system or from an increase of CSF production. Obstructive hydrocephalus occurs rostral to the obstructive lesion. CSF flow can be obstructed along its path through the ventricles, cerebral aqueduct, subarachnoid space, or arachnoid villi. Congenital hydrocephalus can be associated with fusion of the rostral colliculi causing secondary mesencephalic aqueductal stenosis. Aqueductal stenosis has occurred in kittens exposed in utero from a queen treated with griseofulvin,[23] and with exposure to FPL virus.[22] Pre- or postnatal inflammations alter the ependymal surface of the aqueduct and can cause secondary stenosis.[27] Hydrocephalus ex vacuo refers to an increase in size of the lateral ventricles secondary to absence or loss of cerebral tissue. This form of hydrocephalus occurs when there is lack of development or destruction of cerebral tissue (e.g., hydranencephaly) and porencephaly.

Neuropathologic changes associated with hydrocephalus include focal destruction of the ependymal lining, compromise of the cerebral vasculature, damage to the periventricular white matter, and injury to the neurons.[28] The character and distribution of pathologic changes are dependent on the age at which hydrocephalus develops, the rate and magnitude of ventricular enlargement, and the duration of hydrocephalus.[28] Secondary calvarial abnormalities associated with hydrocephalus are thought to result from increased intracranial volume, and include an increased head circumference, incomplete calvarial ossification, and failure of suture closure. The degree of calvarial distortion also depends on the rate at which fluid accumulates, the severity of ventricular enlargement, and the stage of ossification of the cranial sutures at the onset of fluid accumulation.[29]

Clinical Signs. Clinical signs of hydrocephalus manifest typically as forebrain dysfunction, and can vary in severity and onset. Affected kittens may have dome-shaped heads and open fontanelles (Fig. 53–3B). Eye position often manifests as a ventrolateral deviation (see Fig. 53–3A). Typical abnormal mental states include disorientation, obtundation, and stupor. Behavioral abnormalities may include inability to learn (e.g., litter box training). Gait abnormalities may manifest as dysmetria, ataxia, and compulsive circling. Seizure activity also can be a clinical sign associated with hydrocephalus. Clinical signs of transient hypopituitarism causing a hypodipsic hypernatremia and associated myopathy have been reported in a hydrocephalic cat.[26]

Diagnostic Assessment. On physical examination, an enlarged cranium and open fontanelle often are apparent. Radiographic evidence suggestive of hydrocephalus includes doming of the calvarium with cortical thinning, decreased prominence of normal calvarial convolutions, and persistent fontanelles.[29] Diagnosis can be better confirmed by ultrasonography through persistent fontanelles,[30] and by advanced imaging (computed tomography and magnetic resonance imaging).[31, 32]

Treatment. Medical therapy can reduce the severity of clinical signs presumably by altering CSF production. Corticosteroids are believed to act by decreasing CSF production. Prednisone (0.25 to 0.5 mg/kg every [q] 12 to 24 hr) is used initially and then tapered to the lowest tolerable dose. Furosemide (0.5 to 2.0 mg/kg q 12 to 24 hr), a diuretic, decreases CSF production by inhibition of the sodium-potassium cotransport system. Acetazolamide (0.1 mg/kg orally [PO] q 8 hr), also a diuretic, decreases CSF production by inhibition of carbonic

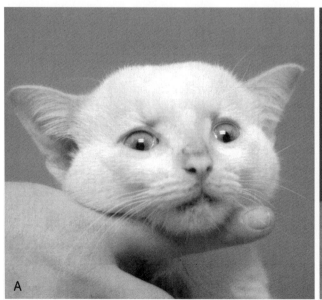
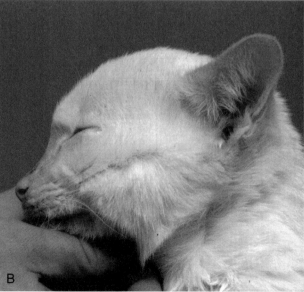

Figure 53–3. An example of ventral strabismus *(A)* and a dome-shaped calvarium *(B)* in a cat with hydrocephalus.

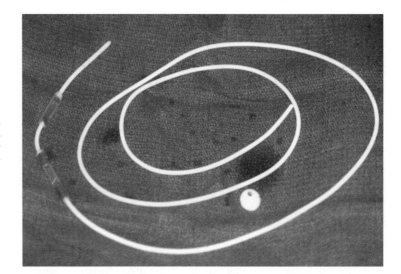

Figure 53–4. The Accura Standard Shunt system (Phoenix Biomedical Corp., Valley Forge, PA), which we use for ventriculoperitoneal shunting of cerebrospinal fluid. The shunt contains a pump and a fluid withdrawal port.

anhydrase. Anticonvulsant therapy is indicated for control of seizure activity.

The goal of surgical management is shunting of CSF from the ventricles to another space (e.g., atrium, abdominal cavity).[33, 34] This procedure traditionally has been reserved for patients refractory to medical therapy in veterinary medicine; however, shunting procedures are the mainstay of therapy for hydrocephalus in human medicine.[35] The most common location for shunting of the CSF is into the abdominal peritoneal cavity or the right atrium. Small vessel size and vasospasm in cats often preclude shunting into the jugular vein/right atrium. Shunt systems currently in use are ventriculoperitoneal or venous shunting devices with nonpressure or pressure-controlled valves placed under the skin. We currently use the Accura Standard Shunt system (Phoenix Biomedical Corp., Valley Forge, PA) (Fig. 53–4). The shunt is placed through a burr hole of the caudal parietal bone into the occipital region of the brain, and the distal tip is tunneled by undermining through the dermis of the lateral body wall into the peritoneal cavity (Figs. 53–5 and 53–6). Major complications of shunts defined in human medicine include mechanical problems, shunt-related infections, and functional problems (shunt blockage, overdrainage).[36–38]

Prognosis. Prognosis for cats with congenital hydrocephalus is influenced by coexistence of other major neural abnormalities. Medical management in cats with severe neurologic dysfunction is guarded to poor. Long-term prognosis following ventriculoperitoneal shunt placement in dogs and cats remains to be determined because of limited experience; however, we advocate early shunt placement to reduce residual neurologic and behavioral deficits.

Hydranencephaly/Porencephaly

Hydranencephaly and porencephaly are congenital cavitary anomalies of the brain. In hydranencephaly, the cerebral hemispheres are reduced to fluid-filled sacs. The defect is contiguous with the lateral ventricles but not lined completely by ependyma.[39] An anatomic distinction from hydrocephalus is that the head is of normal size with hydranencephaly. Porencephaly is characterized by multiple discrete cystic defects in the cerebrum, which may or may not communicate with the ventricles or subarachnoid space.

Hydranencephaly and porencephaly usually are associated with secondary destructive processes that represent hypoplasia and secondary atrophy in early and later stages of brain development, respectively.[27] In human beings, there is an association between hydranencephaly and twinning, possibly due to embolization or infarction after intrauterine death of a donor twin.[7] Another association is with fetal infection. Many viruses have been implicated as a cause of hydranencephaly in other domestic animal species.[27]

Hydranencephaly in kittens has been reported as

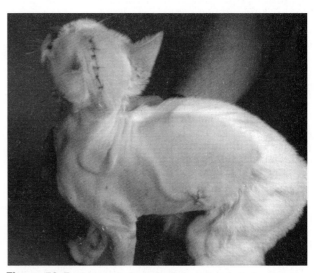

Figure 53–5. Postsurgical view of a cat demonstrates the presence of the shunt beneath the dermis.

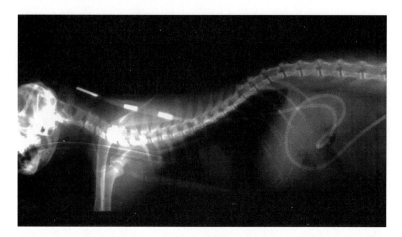

Figure 53–6. Lateral radiograph of a cat demonstrates placement of the shunt into the cranial and abdominal peritoneal cavities.

a distinct disease entity secondary to in utero feline parvovirus infection.[39, 40] Porencephaly also has been attributed to feline parvovirus infection.[41] Cerebellar hypoplasia is the more common anomaly associated with parvoviral infection, and concurrent anomalies have been reported.[41, 42] A lesion of focal or multifocal distribution depends on the stage of gestation at which the parvoviral infection occurs. Kittens with hydranencephaly are unable to ambulate and have abnormal behavior. Magnetic resonance imaging has been used to establish an antemortem diagnosis of hydranencephaly.[41, 42]

Neural Tube Defects

The neural tube is the progenitor of the CNS. Neural tube defects result in brain or spinal cord malformations, and occur early in gestation as a direct result of defective closure or reopening of the neural tube. Terminology of neural tube closure defects provides a description of the type and location of the defect. Neural tube defects are classified as open if neural tissue is exposed or covered only by membrane, or as closed if the defect is covered by normal skin. Neural tube defects also are divided into cranial (brain) and caudal (terminal spinal cord) types. Caudal defects represent anomalies associated with the secondary neurulation process that produce the neural tube in the lower sacral and coccygeal regions.[7]

Spina bifida and anencephaly, the 2 most common forms of neural tube defects, occur in 1 in 1000 pregnancies in the United States.[43] Epidemiologic studies in human beings suggest that environmental and genetic factors have a joint role in the causation of neural tube defects.[44] Recognized environmental causes include maternal diabetes, maternal use of valproic acid, and fever and hyperthermia in early pregnancy. The increased risk of neural tube defects among people of lower socioeconomic status has led to hypotheses related to poor nutrition. Together with other enzymes and cofactors, folate is involved in methylation reactions that ultimately are involved with nervous system development.[45] Certain genotypes also may be predisposing factors of neural tube defects, and the risks may vary depending on maternal factors, for example, vitamin supplementation.[46]

Primary Neural Tube Closure Defects

These defects are associated with failure of the neural tube closure, in which secondary bony defects occur owing to faulty skeletal modeling around the malformed neural tube.[8]

Exencephaly/Anencephaly

Exencephaly and anencephaly are the same anomaly that occur at different stages of development. Direct contact of the neuroepithelium and the amniotic fluid results in degeneration of the neuroepithelium and exencephaly.[47] Anencephaly occurs later in gestation, and the absence of brain and calvaria can be total or partial. Exencephaly has been reported in a Manx cat,[48] Burmese kittens,[11, 12, 49] stillborn kitten,[50] and in kittens of a teratogenicity study.[51] Exencephaly has been associated with treatment of the pregnant queen with griseofulvin,[23] methylmercury,[52] and hydroxyurea.[53]

Craniorachischisis

Craniorachischisis is characterized by anencephaly and a contiguous bony defect of the spine and exposure of neural tissue. This defect has been reported in a kitten with exencephaly.[50]

Primary Axial Mesodermal Defects

Primary axial mesodermal defects are a result of abnormal bony mesodermal development without a persistently open neural tube.[8]

Encephalocele/Meningocele

Encephaloceles and cranial meningoceles consist of a protrusion of brain or meninges through a cranial defect. These defects have been reported in kittens with other cranial and brain malformations.[11, 53] The defect is inherited as an autosomal dominant trait with incomplete expression in the Burmese cat.[11] Affected kittens have a telencephalic meningoencephalocele and hydrocephalus of varying severity. Pregnant queens treated with griseofulvin in early pregnancy will produce kittens with cranium bifidum and meningoencephalocele of varying severity.[23]

Craniofacial Malformation in Burmese Cats

The malformation in Burmese cats is linked to continuous selection since the 1970s for a rounded, brachycephalic facial appearance. The line is called the Eastern, "new look," or contemporary strain of Burmese. These selection processes have produced kittens with lethal neonatal facial deformities. Zook and colleagues[49] first characterized the presence of encephalocele with other craniofacial anomalies in Burmese cats. The anatomy, embryology, and pattern of inheritance of the abnormality were documented by Noden and Evans.[11] The anatomic abnormality is characterized by agenesis of the medial nasal prominence; duplication of derivatives of the maxillary processes, including the canine teeth and whiskers; telencephalic meningoencephalocele; and secondary ocular degeneration.

Cause. The lethal phenotype is inherited as an autosomal dominant trait with incomplete expression. Heterozygotes express a range of facial dimensions. The lethal genetic load exceeds 25 per cent. All contemporary phenotype Burmese cats are carriers of this defect.

Pathogenesis. Noden and Evans[11] have established the trait as a neural crest defect.[8] The data suggest that neural crest cells that disperse over the rostral surface of the prosencephalon become spatially programmed incorrectly. It also was observed that the width of the prosencephalon on day 21 is abnormal, by which time the crest cells have circumscribed the future forebrain. This suggests that the primary genetic lesion may originate on the rostral plate, which subsequently transmits incorrect spatial information to the overlying neural crest population.

Cleft Palate

Cleft palate is one of the most common gross anatomic defects in neonatal kittens.[2] Cleft palate has been an associated cranial anomaly in kittens with exencephaly.[48, 50, 51, 53] Cleft palate alone also has been reported as a fetal anomaly when queens were dosed with diphenylhydantoin (2 mg/kg) on days 10 to 22 of gestation[53] or with griseofulvin.[23]

Disorders of Forebrain Induction

Holoprosencephaly

Disorders associated with abnormal development of the prosencephalon are termed *holoencephaly, arhinencephaly,* and *cyclopia.* Holoencephaly refers to a single, nondivided cerebrum over the diencephalon. Arhinencephaly refers to lack of development of the olfactory region. Cyclopian malformation and anophthalmia with absence of optic nerves have been observed in kittens born from a queen exposed to griseofulvin.[23] A craniothoracopagus conjoined pair of twins in a Siamese breed had bilateral cyclopia.[27]

Agenesis of the Corpus Callosum

Agenesis of the corpus callosum has been documented in a kitten with multiple CNS anomalies, including agenesis of the septum pellucidum and hippocampal commissure and a cranial meningocele.[54] Kittens exposed to griseofulvin while in utero had agenesis of the corpus callosum along with other holoprosencephalic features.[23] Seizure activity has been associated with corpus callosal agenesis in a cat.[55]

Disorders of Neuronal Migration

Brain malformations are related commonly to defects associated with neuronal migration. Neuronal migration commences near the periventricular zone. Neuroblasts multiply and attach to radial glial cells, migrating subsequently in tangential and radial directions (radial-glial hypothesis). During migration, neuroblasts establish synaptic contacts and organize into layers from the ventricle to the pial surface of the cortex. Simultaneously, apoptosis and glial cell proliferation and differentiation occur. Cerebral cortical migrational abnormalities may be grouped into 3 categories: lissencephaly/pachygyria (lack or partial lack of gyri and sulci), polymicrogyria (extensive folds of cerebral cortex), and heterotopia (disorganized gray matter in inappropriate places).[8] Only lissencephaly has been described in cats.

Lissencephaly (Agyria/Pachygyria)

Agyria and pachygyria are reflected by gross abnormalities of the cerebral cortical surface and by microscopic thickening of the cortical laminae/layers. Agyria implies absence of gyri, and pachygyria is reduced numbers of broadened gyri. In human beings, agyria is termed Miller-Dieker syndrome. Other clinical features in human beings consist of microcephaly, small jaw, profound mental and motor retardation, hypo/hypertonia, and seizures. Lissencephaly with microencephaly has been reported in a Korat cat that manifested abnormal behavior and self-mutilation.[27]

Pathogenesis. The lesion most likely is the result of arrested neuroblast migration. Gross and microscopic anomalies vary in degree of severity.

Diagnostic Assessment. Lissencephaly can be identified by brain imaging techniques (computed tomography and magnetic resonance imaging).

Treatment. Seizure activity needs to be controlled with appropriate anticonvulsant therapy. Because lissencephaly may be a cause for the seizures, adequate control may be more difficult in these patients.

◆ MALFORMATIONS OF THE HINDBRAIN

Dandy-Walker Syndrome

Dandy-Walker syndrome (DWS) was reported first in infants by Dandy and Blackfan,[56] and by Taggart and Walker.[57] Pathologic features classic of DWS include presence or absence of the cerebellar vermis, a large cystic dilatation of the fourth ventricle, and enlargement of the caudal fossa.[8] Hydrocephalus usually is present, but may not be a consistent feature. DWS has been described in a number of domestic animal species, but there is only 1 report confirmed by necropsy in a 4-month-old domestic shorthair kitten.[58] A caudal fossa arachnoidal cyst was documented using magnetic resonance imaging in a cat with clinical signs of seizures; however, a necropsy was not performed to confirm DWS.[59]

Pathogenesis. The primary cause of DWS is undetermined. An early theory relates to foraminal atresia causing obstructive hydrocephalus. In human beings, this theory is less likely because the fourth ventricle foramina usually are patent. A more accepted theory relates to a developmental arrest of the hindbrain.[8] This concept also supports the finding of multiple brain developmental anomalies in human beings with DWS.

Clinical Signs. Clinical signs in the affected cat were associated with cerebrocortical and vestibular dysfunction. The kitten developed anorexia and lethargy. Cranial nerve examination revealed nystagmus, miosis, and an absent menace response.

Diagnostic Assessment. Diagnosis usually is determined by computed tomography or magnetic resonance imaging of the brain.

Treatment. Treatment options include medical or surgical management of the hydrocephalus.

Chiari Malformations

Chiari described 4 types of cerebellar deformities characterized by displacement of the cerebellum and hydrocephalus.[8] Chiari malformation is characterized by caudal/ventral herniation of the caudal part of the cerebellum and/or medulla oblongata into the vertebral canal. Anatomic features include a small caudal fossa and various neural abnormalities such as brain stem deformities and hydrocephalus.[8] Type I describes herniation of the cerebellar vermis. Type II (Arnold-Chiari malformation) refers to herniation of the fourth ventricle, medulla oblongata and cerebellar vermis, and myeloschisis. Type III is characterized by occipital and cranial cervical malformations with herniation of the cerebellum. A fourth type is described as cerebellar hypoplasia that is usually categorized as a separate entity. Chiari malformation most likely is due to underdevelopment of the occipital bone, possibly related to underdevelopment of the occipital somite originating from the paraxial mesoderm.[60]

Herniation of the cerebellar vermis, elongation of the fourth ventricle, and reduction in size of the caudal fossa in captive lions had similarities to Arnold-Chiari malformation; however, affected cubs lacked spinal deformities.[61] Other studies of captive lions with suspected vitamin A deficiency report thickened bones of the cranial vault with cerebellar herniation.[62–64]

Parvoviral (Feline Panleukopenia Virus)-Induced Cerebellar Degeneration (Hypoplasia)

Congenital cerebellar degeneration is the most commonly reported intracranial malformation in cats. Congenital cerebellar ataxia has been recognized in kittens since 1888,[65] and referred to as spontaneous feline ataxia.[66, 67] The disorder also is known in general terms as cerebellar hypoplasia; however, the term *hypoplasia* should be reserved for those disorders that lack tissue development with no indication of a cause.[68]

Cause. The cause is infection with FPL virus (feline parvovirus) before birth or very early in life. Carpenter and Harter[69] studied spontaneous feline ataxia extensively and implied that feline ataxia was not inherited. Kilham and Margolis[66] established involvement of a transmissible agent, feline ataxia virus, to be responsible for inducing ataxia and cerebellar hypoplasia in kittens. Further collaborations with Johnson and associates[21] confirmed that the feline ataxia virus was that of FPL virus or feline parvovirus. Csiza and coworkers also studied the pathogenesis of natural[22, 67] and experimental[70, 71] viral transmission by intracerebral, oral, and intranasal routes in neonatal kittens. In utero infection of queens has been associated with hydrocephalus[22, 66] and hydranencephaly[39, 41] either alone or in conjunction with cerebellar hypoplasia.

Pathogenesis. Cerebella from affected cats show large variations grossly and microscopically in degree of cerebellar degeneration. Gross abnormalities of the cerebellum include reduction in size of cerebellar folia, especially the hemispheres, and cerebellar cysts[67] (Fig. 53–7). In 31 of 32 kittens with cerebellar hypoplasia, the cerebellum was reduced in size by 50 to 75 per cent of normal, and consisted of only a remnant in 1 kitten.[68] Both granule and Purkinje cells are decreased in number or entirely lacking. The loss of cellularity is due to cytopathic effects on the external granule cell layer.[66, 71–73] Cellular destruction predominates in cells of the external germinal layer that is proliferating actively and differentiating into granule neurons at the time of birth and for the first few weeks of life. Destruction of this layer produces hypoplasia of the granule cell layer. Postmitotic Purkinje cells also may degenerate because of a separate cytopathic effect of the virus.[22, 68]

Other neuropathologic findings associated with FPL virus infection include hydrocephalus,[67, 72] hydranencephaly,[39–42] focal cerebral neuronal and axonal degeneration, and spinal cord demyelination.[67] Cerebral involvement is presumed to be associated with viral infection during the time of differentiation of progenitor cells, which occurs early in the second trimester. The pathogenesis of focal neuronal and axonal degenerations from FPL virus infection may relate to ischemic damage to capillaries or to direct action by the virus on the neurons.[67]

FPL virus induces cytopathic effects on other rapidly dividing cells, especially the thymus, spleen, intestinal epithelium, and mesenteric lymph nodes.[71] Systemic dissemination occurs through viral replication in all layers of blood vessels.[71]

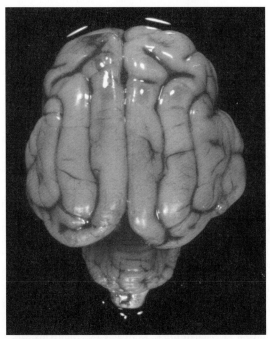

Figure 53–7. Gross appearance of a feline brain with cerebellar hypoplasia. (Courtesy of Dr. K. P. Carmichael and the University of Georgia.)

Clinical Signs. Cerebellar dysfunction is the most common neurologic sign associated with FPL virus infection. Clinical signs become observable when affected kittens become ambulatory. A wide-based stance, whole body tremor, and titubation (rocking back and forth) may be observed. Cerebellar tremor is exaggerated by goal-oriented movements (intention tremor). Gait evaluation shows symmetric ataxia with preservation of strength. Dysmetria is evident by hyper-/hypometria during limb placement. Axial and limb muscle tone are increased. An absent menace response with normal vision often is apparent on cranial nerve examination.

Diagnostic Assessment. A diagnosis of cerebellar hypoplasia due to parvoviral infection should be considered in any kitten with cerebellar dysfunction at the time of ambulation that does not progress. Magnetic resonance imaging is the procedure of choice for ante-mortem evaluation of reduction in size of the cerebellum and other associated abnormalities of FPL virus infection. Cysts within the cerebellum have been described infrequently in affected kittens.[41, 42]

In vivo tests for viral antigen and antibody assays are available. Antibodies in kittens less than 3 months of age may be maternally derived. Serum virus neutralization is the most common method.[74] Serum samples are collected 2 weeks apart. Serial dilutions of antisera are performed against predetermined amounts of FPL virus. Viral cultures are examined for specific cytopathic changes and inclusion bodies produced by the virus. A 4-fold rise in titer is indicative of acute infection. Direct fluorescent antibody testing detects viral antigens within 2 days postinfection which can persist in various tissues until 22 days postinfection and at least until 43 days postinfection in Purkinje cells.[71] Hemagglutination inhibition and hemagglutination antibody tests[75] for some strains of FPL virus are performed by use of a standard microtitration system with formalin-fixed porcine erythrocytes. These tests are considered less sensitive methods because of pH differences.[74] Enzyme-linked immunosorbent assay (ELISA) can detect virus in feces or intestinal contents, and is a more sensitive indicator.[76] Polymerase chain reaction (PCR) assay can detect parvoviral DNA in feces[77] and paraffin-embedded tissues.[41]

Definitive diagnosis is by isolation of the FPL virus from cerebellum or other organs. Virus isolation may be difficult from kittens older than 4 weeks of age.[22, 78] Viral isolation from urine and feces can be performed by indirect methods in kidney cell cultures up to 22 and 43 days after in utero inoculation, respectively.[78] Monolayer culturing techniques were able to recover the virus from trypsinized kidneys and lungs for as long as 70 days after inoculation and up to 3 years of age from the small intestines in 1 of 5 cats.[78]

Treatment. No treatment exists. Affected kittens may learn to compensate for their deficits over time.

Hereditary Cerebellar Cortical Atrophy

Hereditary ataxia in cats is a distinct clinical entity from cerebellar disorders caused by FPL virus infection and storage diseases.

Genetic Defect. Genetic studies reveal an autosomal recessive pattern of inheritance.[79] These cats may serve as an animal model for cerebellar cortical degeneration, the most common type of spinocerebellar degenerative disorders in human beings.

Pathogenesis. Neuropathologic findings include almost total loss of Purkinje cells with an increase in Bergmann's glia in the cerebellar hemisphere, preservation of some Purkinje cells in the vermis, and moderate neuronal depletion of the olivary nucleus.[80] Ultrastructural examination of the cerebellum revealed swelling of the distal dendrites of Purkinje cells without severe loss, and increase in density and mean size of presynapses in the molecular layer of the severely affected folia.[80] Prolonged existence of presynapses in the molecular and Purkinje cell layers was confirmed by positive immunoreactivity to antisynaptophysin.[80]

Clinical Signs. Affected cats develop a cerebellar ataxia at 7 to 8 weeks of age that progresses until 2.5 to 4 months of age.[79] Dysmetria and intention tremors were observed early in the disease course. Strabismus and nystagmus were not observed.

Diagnosis. Diagnosis of hereditary cerebellar ataxia was based on eliminating other acquired cerebellar disorders. Decreases in lysosomal enzyme activities were not found in affected cats, feline leukemia virus and feline immunodeficiency virus antibodies were not detected, FPL virus or other viral agents were not isolated, and amplification of FPL virus–specific capsid gene by PCR could not be achieved.[79] Magnetic resonance imaging results reveal a small cerebellum and reduced cerebellum-to-brain ratios. Neuropathologic findings are similar in affected cats.

Treatment. No treatment exists. This disorder is not considered fatal.

REFERENCES

1. Young C: Preweaning mortality in specific pathogen free kittens. J Small Anim Pract 14:391–397, 1973.
2. Lawler DF, Monti KL: Morbidity and mortality in neonatal kittens. Am J Vet Res 45:1455–1459, 1984.
3. Murtaugh RJ: Pediatrics: The kitten from birth to eight weeks. In Sherding RG (ed): The Cat: Diseases and Clinical Management. New York, Churchill Livingstone, 1994, pp. 1877–1891.
4. Saperstein G, Harris S, Leipold HW: Congenital defects in domestic cats. A special practitioner reference. Feline Pract 6:18–27, 1976.
5. Bucheler J: Fading kitten syndrome and neonatal isoerythrolysis. Vet Clin North Am Small Anim Pract 29:853–870, 1999.
6. Priester WA, Glass AG, Waggoner NS: Congenital defects in domesticated animals: General considerations. Am J Vet Res. 31:1871–1879, 1970.
7. Kroll RA, Constantinescu GM: Congenital abnormalities of the spinal cord and vertebrae. In August JR (ed): Consultations in Feline Internal Medicine, vol. 2. Philadelphia, WB Saunders, 1994, pp. 413–420.
8. Harding B, Copp AJ: Malformations. In Graham DI, Lantos PL (eds): Greenfield's Neuropathology. London, Arnold, 1997, pp. 397–533.
9. McLone DG: The biological resolution of malformations of the central nervous system. Neurosurg 43:1375–1380, 1998.
10. Honig LS, Rosenberg RN: Apoptosis and neurologic disease. Am J Med 108:317–330, 2000.
11. Noden DM, Evans HE: Inherited homeotic midfacial malformations in Burmese cats. J Craniofac Genet Dev Biol Suppl 2:249–266, 1986.
12. Noden DM, de Lahunta A: Causes of congenital malformations. In Noden DM, de Lahunta A (eds): The Embryology of Domestic Animals: Developmental Mechanisms and Malformations. Baltimore, Williams & Wilkins, 1985, pp. 81–91.
13. DeSesso JM, Scialli AR, Holson JF: Apparent lability of neural tube closure in laboratory animals and humans. Am J Med Genet 87:143–162, 1999.
14. Sakai Y: Neurulation in the mouse: Manner and timing of neural tube closure. Anat Rec 223:194–203, 1989.
15. Juriloff DM: Normal mouse strains differ in the site of initiation of closure of the cranial neural tube. Teratology 44:225–233, 1991.
16. Noden DM, de Lahunta A: Central nervous system and eye. In Noden DM, de Lahunta A (eds): The Embryology of Domestic Animals: Developmental Mechanisms and Malformations. Baltimore, Williams & Wilkins, 1985, pp. 92–119.
17. Altman J: Postnatal development of the cerebellar cortex in the rat. I: External germinal layer and the transitional molecular layer. J Comp Neurol 145:353–398, 1972.
18. Smith DE, Downs I: Postnatal development of the granule cell in the kitten cerebellum. Am J Anat 151:527–537, 1978.
19. Silson M, Robinson R: Hereditary hydrocephalus in the cat. Vet Rec 84:477, 1969.
20. Kline KL, Joseph RJ, Averill DR: Feline infectious peritonitis with neurologic involvement: Clinical and pathological findings in 24 cats. J Am Anim Hosp Assoc 30:111–118, 1994.
21. Johnson RH, Margolis G, Kilham L: Identity of feline ataxia virus with feline panleucopenia virus. Nature 214:175–177, 1967.
22. Csiza CK, Scott FW, de Lahunta A, Gillespie JH: Feline viruses. XIV: Transplacental infections in spontaneous panleukopenia of cats. Cornell Vet 61:423–439, 1971.
23. Scott FW, de Lahunta A, Schultz RD, et al: Teratogenesis in cats associated with griseofulvin therapy. Teratology 11:79–86, 1975.
24. Jackson OF: Congenital abnormalities in kittens. Vet Rec 84:76, 1969.
25. Shell LG: Congenital hydrocephalus. Feline Pract 24:10–11, 1996.
26. Dow SW, Fettman MJ, LeCouteur RA, Allen TA: Hypodipsic hypernatremia and associated myopathy in a hydrocephalic cat with transient hypopituitarism. J Am Vet Med Assoc 191:217–221, 1987.
27. Summers BA, Cummings JF, de Lahunta A: Malformations of the central nervous system. In Summers BA, Cummings JF, de Lahunta A (eds): Veterinary Neuropathology. St. Louis, Mosby, 1995, pp. 68–94.
28. Del Bigio MR: Neuropathological changes caused by hydrocephalus. Acta Neuropathol (Berl) 85:573–585, 1993.
29. Becker SV, Selby LA: Canine hydrocephalus. Compend Contin Educ Pract Vet 2:647–652, 1980.
30. Hudson JA, Simpson ST, Buxton DF, et al: Ultrasonographic diagnosis of canine hydrocephalus. Vet Radiol 31:50–58, 1990.
31. Hudson LC, Cauzinille L, Kornegay IN, Tompkins MB: Magnetic resonance imaging of the normal feline brain. Vet Radiol Ultrasound 36:267–275, 1995.
32. LeCouteur RA, Fike JR, Cann CE, et al: X-ray computed

tomography of brain tumors in cats. J Am Vet Med Assoc 183:301–305, 1983.

33. Levesque DC, Plummer SB: Ventriculoperitoneal shunting as a treatment for hydrocephalus. Proceedings 12th ACVIM Forum 1994, pp. 891–893.

34. Gage ED, Hoerlein BF: Surgical treatment of canine hydrocephalus by ventriculoatrial shunting. J Am Vet Med Assoc 153:1418–1431, 1968.

35. Kanev PM, Park TS: The treatment of hydrocephalus. Neurosurg Clin North Am 4:611–619, 1993.

36. Keucher TR, Mealey JJ: Long-term results after ventriculoatrial and ventriculoperitoneal shunting for infantile hydrocephalus. J Neurosurg 50:179–186, 1979.

37. Turner MS: The treatment of hydrocephalus: A brief guide to shunt selection. Surg Neurol 43:314–319, 1995.

38. Smely C, Van Velthoven V: Comparative study of two customary cerebrospinal fluid shunting systems in early childhood hydrocephalus. Acta Neurochir (Wien) 139:875–881, 1997.

39. Greene CE, Gorgasz EJ, Martin CL: Hydranencephaly associated with feline panleukopenia. J Am Vet Med Assoc 180:767–768, 1982.

40. Carlson ME: Hydranencephaly and cerebrocortical hypoplasia in a four-month-old kitten. Feline Pract 22:10–12, 1994.

41. Sharp NJH, Davis BJ, Guy JS, et al: Hydranencephaly and cerebellar hypoplasia in two kittens attributed to intrauterine parvovirus infection. J Comp Pathol 121:39–53, 1999.

42. Kornegay JN: Ataxia, dysmetria, tremor. Cerebellar diseases. Probl Vet Med 3:409–416, 1991.

43. Cragan JD, Roberts HE, Edmonds LD: Surveillance for anencephaly and spina bifida and the impact of prenatal diagnosis—United States, 1985–1994. MMWR CDC Surveill Summ 44(SS-4):1–13, 1995.

44. Botto LD, Moore CA, Khoury MJ, Erickson JD: Neural-tube defects. N Engl J Med 341:1509–1519, 1999.

45. Berry RJ, Li Z, Erickson JD, et al: Prevention of neural-tube defects with folic acid in China. China–U.S. Collaborative Project for Neural Tube Defect Prevention. N Engl J Med 341:1485–1490, 1999.

46. Harris MJ, Juriloff DM: Genetic landmarks for defects in mouse neural tube closure. Teratology 56:177–187, 1997.

47. Drewek MJ, Bruner JP, Whesell WO, Tulipan N: Quantitative analysis of the toxicity of human amniotic fluid to cultured rat spinal cord. Pediatr Neurosurg 27:190–193, 1998.

48. Field B: Cerebral malformation in a Manx cat. Vet Rec 96:42–43, 1975.

49. Zook BC, Sostaric BR, Draper DJ, Graf Webster E: Encephalocele and other congenital craniofacial anomalies in Burmese cats. Vet Med Small Anim Clin 78:695–701, 1983.

50. Sekeles E: Craniofacial and skeletal malformations in a cat. Feline Pract 11:28–31, 1981.

51. Khera KS, Roberts G, Trivett G, et al: A teratogenicity study with amaranth in cats. Toxicol Appl Pharmacol 38:389–398, 1976.

52. Khera KS: Teratogenic effects of methylmercury in the cat: Note on the use of this species as a model for teratogenicity studies. Teratology 8:293–303, 1973.

53. Khera KS: A teratogenicity study on hydroxyurea and diphenylhydantoin in cats. Teratology 20:447–452, 1979.

54. Griffiths IR: Abnormalities in the central nervous system of a kitten. Vet Rec 89:123–124, 1971.

55. Hiyoshi T, Wada JA: Feline agenesis of the corpus callosum. Epilepsia 28:395–398, 1987.

56. Dandy WE, Blackfan KD: Internal hydrocephalus: An experimental, clinical and pathological study. Am J Dis Child 8:406–482, 1914.

57. Taggart JK, Walker AE: Congenital atresia of the foramen of Luschka and Magendie. Arch Neurol Psychiatr 48:583–612, 1942.

58. Regnier AM, Ducos de Lahitte MJ, Delisle MB, Dubois GG:

59. Milner RJ, Engela J, Kirberger RM: Arachnoid cyst in cerebellar pontine area of a cat—Diagnosis by magnetic resonance imaging. Vet Radiol Ultrasound 37:34–36, 1996.

60. Nishikawa M, Sakamoto H, Hakuba A, et al: Pathogenesis of Chiari malformation: A morphometric study of the posterior cranial fossa. J Neurosurg 86:40–47, 1997.

61. Chandra AMS, Papendick RE, Schumacher J, et al: Cerebellar herniation in captive lions (*Panthera leo*). J Vet Diagn Invest 11:465–468, 1999.

62. Baker JR, Lyon DG: Skull malformation and cerebellar herniation in captive African lions. Vet Rec 19:154–156, 1977.

63. Bartsch RC, Imes GD, Smit JPJ: Vitamin A deficiency in the captive African lion cub *Panthera leo* (Linnaeus, 1758). Onderstepoort J Vet Res 42:43–54, 1975.

64. O'Sullivan BM, Mayo FD, Hartley WJ: Neurologic lesions in young captive lions associated with vitamin A deficiency. Austr Vet J 53:187–189, 1977.

65. Herringham WP, Andrewes FW: Two cases of cerebellar disease in cats with staggering. St Bath's Hosp Rep (Lond) 24:241–248, 1888.

66. Kilham L, Margolis G: Viral etiology of spontaneous ataxia of cats. Am J Pathol 48:991–1011, 1967.

67. Csiza CK, de Lahunta A, Scott FW, Gillespie JH: Spontaneous feline ataxia. Cornell Vet 62:300–322, 1972.

68. de Lahunta A: Comments on cerebellar ataxia and its congenital transmission in cats by feline panleukopenia virus. J Am Vet Med Assoc 158:901–906, 1971.

69. Carpenter MR, Harter DH: A study of congenital feline cerebellar malformations: An anatomic and physiologic evaluation of agenetic defects. J Comp Neurol 105:51–93, 1956.

70. Csiza CK, Scott FW, de Lahunta A, Gillespie JH: Pathogenesis of feline panleukopenia virus in susceptible newborn kittens. I. Clinical signs, hematology, serology, virology. Infect Immun 3:833–837, 1971.

71. Csiza CK, de Lahunta A, Scott FW, Gillespie JH: Pathogenesis of feline panleukopenia virus in susceptible newborn kittens. II. Pathology and immunofluorescence. Infect Immun 3:838–846, 1971.

72. Kilham L, Margolis G, Colby ED: Cerebellar ataxia and its congenital transmission in cats by feline panleukopenia virus. J Am Vet Med Assoc 158:888–901, 1971.

73. Kilham L, Margolis G: Hydrocephalus in hamsters, ferrets, rats, and mice following inoculations with reovirus type I. I. Virologic studies. Lab Invest 21:183–188, 1969.

74. Greene CE: Feline panleukopenia. *In* Greene CE (ed): Infectious Diseases of the Dog and Cat, 2nd ed. Philadelphia, WB Saunders, 1998, pp. 52–57.

75. Mochizuki H, Konishi S, Ajiki M: Comparisons of feline parvovirus subspecific strains using monoclonal antibodies against a feline panleukopenia virus. Jpn J Vet Sci 51:264–272, 1989.

76. Addie DD, Toth S, Thompson H, et al: Detection of feline parvovirus in dying pedigree kittens. Vet Rec 142:353–356, 1998.

77. Schunck B, Kraft W, Truyen U: A simple touch-down polymerase chain reaction for the detection of canine parvovirus and feline panleukopenia virus in feces. J Virol Methods 55:427–433, 1995.

78. Csiza CK, Scott FW, de Lahunta A, Gillespie JH: Immune carrier state of feline panleukopenia virus–infected cats. Am J Vet Res 32:419–426, 1971.

79. Inada S, Mochizuki M, Izumo S, et al: Study of hereditary cerebellar degeneration in cats. Am J Vet Res 57:296–301, 1996.

80. Aye MM, Izumo S, Inada S, et al: Histopathological and ultrastructural features of feline hereditary cerebellar cortical atrophy: A novel animal model of human spinocerebellar degeneration. Acta Neuropathol (Berl) 96:379–387, 1998.

Dandy-Walker syndrome in a kitten. J Am Anim Hosp Assoc 29:514–518, 1993.

54

◆ Inflammatory Disorders of the Central Nervous System

Karen R. Muñana

Etiology

Inflammation is defined as a local reaction to injury. The inflammatory response in the central nervous system (CNS) consists of the exudation of blood constituents into the neural parenchyma, the elaboration and activation of local inflammatory mediators, and the proliferation of vessels, connective tissues, and cells.[1] The initial insult and the ensuing inflammatory process both can contribute to nervous tissue damage.

Inflammation of the CNS may involve the neural parenchyma (encephalitis or myelitis), the membranous covering of the brain or spinal cord (meningitis), or a combination of both. The latter is recognized most commonly. Infectious causes of CNS inflammation in cats include viruses, protozoa, fungi, parasites, and bacterial organisms. Noninfectious causes include immune-mediated and idiopathic disorders.

Epidemiology

Inflammatory CNS disorders are a common cause of neurologic dysfunction in cats, and should be considered in the differential diagnosis of any cat presenting with signs referable to the nervous system. As a general rule, cats that have access to the outdoors or exposure to other cats are more likely to develop infections with CNS sequelae; however, this is not an exclusionary criterion, and inflammatory disease should be explored as a possible cause for neurologic dysfunction regardless of an animal's environmental history.

Pathogenesis

Most infectious agents establish a primary infection in peripheral tissues before infecting the CNS. The host's general defense mechanisms, including the reticuloendothelial system and the humoral and cellular immune responses, often are successful in clearing infections before CNS invasion occurs. Some microbial agents have evolved means of escaping these defenses, and consequently are more likely to establish an infection within the CNS. Additionally, immunocompromised cats are more likely to develop CNS infections than cats with normal immune function.

The CNS itself has a rather basic immune system, with limited local mechanisms by which to respond to infections. The main defense of the CNS is a physical one consisting of the skull, bony spinal column, meninges, and blood-brain barrier. The blood-brain barrier is the primary protection against hematogenously spread organisms. The blood-brain barrier essentially is a modified tight epithelium, consisting of specialized endothelial cells that have a dense basement membrane and connected by tight junctions and lacking fenestrations. Astrocytic foot processes surround these specialized capillaries and induce formation of tight junctions by the local endothelial cells.

Organisms that gain entrance into the CNS from the blood stream do so by several means. An organism may directly infect and replicate within the brain endothelial cells, or may infect peripheral leukocytes that enter the nervous system. In addition, organisms present in an infected embolus may occlude a vessel in the neural parenchyma, replicate, and form a local abscess. Infection of the fenestrated choroid plexus endothelial cells may introduce an organism into the cerebrospinal fluid (CSF), with extension into the neural parenchyma. For many of the infectious agents, however, the exact mechanism of entry into the CNS has not been elucidated.

The immune system of the CNS is relatively ineffective at clearing infections that become established. The CNS lacks a lymphatic system, and the concentration of lymphocytes normally present within the CSF is small. Additionally, in the normal CNS, the expression of major histocompatibility complex (MHC) molecules is low, and consequently, the cells have limited ability to function as antigen-presenting cells. During active CNS infection, the permeability of the blood-brain barrier increases, which gives rise to an influx of lymphocytes and macrophages into the neural tissue and the meninges. Cytokines are elaborated that, in turn, activate intrinsic neural cellular elements. Astrocytes and endothelial cells can be induced to express MHC class II molecules and secrete inflammatory mediators, thereby intensifying the local immune response.

An infectious agent can damage the nervous system by direct and indirect mechanisms. Some organisms are directly cytopathic to neurons or glial cells. In addition, local inflammation resulting from an infection is damaging to the neural parenchyma. Many of the inflammatory mediators are directly toxic to neural elements. Breakdown of the blood-brain barrier causes local edema, and loss of normal vascular integrity leads to local ischemia. The edema and accumulation of inflammatory cells may result in a mass effect, with compression of adjacent normal tissue. The inflammation also may occlude the ventricular system, leading to an obstructive hydrocephalus. These changes contribute to an elevation in intracranial pressure that, if great enough, predisposes the brain to herniation. Brain herniation often is the cause of a sudden, profound worsening of neurologic status in animals with CNS inflammatory disease, and is associated with a grave prognosis.

Transmission

Infectious agents can enter the nervous system through several different means. Hematogenous spread is most common, but organisms also can gain entrance by local extension through the cribriform plate, middle ear, or sinuses. Some of the most neurotropic organisms reach the CNS by retrograde transport via motor and sensory nerves. In cats, this is the case with the rabies and pseudorabies viruses.

Clinical Signs

Because many CNS infections are spread hematogenously, affected animals often display systemic signs of disease. Nonspecific clinical signs such as fever, anorexia, and lethargy may be present. In addition, evidence of ocular inflammation is identified frequently. Involvement of other organ systems also may be seen, depending on the specific tissue tropism of a particular infectious agent.

The absence of systemic signs in an animal with neurologic disease does not exclude the possibility of an infectious cause. The systemic manifestations of disease that often precede the neurologic signs may be relatively mild and go unnoticed. Some infectious agents persist latently in the CNS and become reactivated later on, usually in association with host immunosuppression. In these cases, systemic signs may be present at the time of initial infection, but not at the time of organism recrudescence. Additionally, the extremely neurotropic organisms characteristically cause nervous system disease with no systemic involvement.

Neurologic signs reflect the location and extent of the disease process. Although most inflammatory disorders cause diffuse or multifocal CNS involvement, it is not unusual for animals to present with signs referable to a focal area of the nervous system. Forebrain (cerebrum and diencephalon) disease causes signs of depression, behavioral abnormalities, seizures, circling, blindness, and contralateral postural reaction deficits with minimum gait disturbances. Cerebellar disease causes ataxia, hypermetria, intention tremor, vestibular signs, and loss of the menace response. Disease of the brain stem can cause altered consciousness, hemi- or tetraparesis, and cranial nerve deficits. Spinal cord involvement manifests as ataxia, paresis, or paralysis. Animals with meningeal involvement typically present with neck pain and fever.

Differential Diagnosis

The differential diagnosis for a cat presenting with signs of brain disease include degenerative, metabolic, toxic, neoplastic, inflammatory, traumatic, and vascular causes.

Lysosomal storage diseases probably are the most common degenerative condition to affect the CNS of cats (see Chapters 51, Neuronal Storage Disorders; 57, Mucopolysaccharidosis; and 77, Molecular Diagnosis of Gangliosidoses: A Model for Elimination of Inherited Diseases in Pure Breeds). These disorders, due to inborn errors in metabolism, are identified most commonly in young animals, and manifest with slowly progressive signs of neurologic dysfunction. Characteristic neurologic signs have been reported for the specific storage disorders, reflecting the sensitivity of different neural elements to the metabolic disturbance present.

Metabolic conditions such as hypoxia, hypoglycemia, hepatic dysfunction, and electrolyte disturbances usually cause signs of diffuse, symmetric forebrain dysfunction. Signs may be acute or chronic, and systemic evidence of disease may be identified. Toxic disorders present in a similar manner.

Primary and metastatic neoplasia can affect the CNS of cats. The most common primary CNS tumor of cats is the meningioma (see Chapter 50, Cerebral Meningiomas: Diagnostic and Therapeutic Considerations). Although tumors often are slow-growing, it is not uncommon for clinical signs to be acute in onset. Signs frequently are asymmetric and progressive.

Vascular conditions that affect the CNS of cats include hypertensive encephalopathy and feline ischemic encephalopathy (see Chapter 52, Vascular Disorders). With vascular disease, signs are acute in onset and nonprogressive. Asymmetric neurologic deficits often are present.

A list of inflammatory disorders known to affect the nervous system of cats is shown in Table 54–1.

Diagnosis

Animals with CNS inflammatory disease often have normal or nonspecific changes on their hemogram and biochemical profile. The blood-brain barrier, which effectively protects the nervous system from hematogenously spread organisms, also prevents local CNS inflammation from inciting changes in peripheral blood. Consequently, the most useful test in confirming the presence of CNS inflammatory

Table 54–1. Inflammatory Central Nervous System Disorders of Cats

Viral

Feline infectious peritonitis*
Feline immunodeficiency virus
Rabies
Pseudorabies
Borna disease virus
Feline leukemia virus

Protozoal

Toxoplasmosis*
Sarcocystis-like organism
Encephalitozoonosis

Bacterial

Aerobes
Anaerobes

Fungal

Cryptococcosis*
Blastomycosis
Histoplasmosis
Coccidioidomycosis
Aspergillosis
Candidiasis
Hyalohyphomycosis
Phaeohyphomycosis

Parasitic

Cuterebra larval myiasis*
Dirofilaria immitis

Idiopathic

Nonsuppurative meningoencephalomyelitis (presumed viral)*
Eosinophilic meningoencephalitis

*These diseases are discussed in detail in the chapter.

disease is analysis of CSF. CSF is evaluated routinely for red blood cell (RBC) count, white blood cell (WBC) count, and protein concentration. In addition, cytology is performed on a concentrated sample of fluid to determine the leukocyte differential count and to observe for the presence of any organisms. Normal CSF collected from the cerebellomedullary cistern of cats has 0 to 30 RBC/μl, 0 to 2 WBC/μl with mononuclear cells predominating, and a protein concentration of 6 to 36 mg/dl.[2]

Animals with CNS inflammation characteristically have increased numbers of leukocytes in the CSF. However, a normal CSF leukocyte count may be seen in an animal with inflammatory CNS disease. Either meningeal or ventricular inflammation must be present for inflammatory cells to be shed into the CSF. Because most inflammatory disorders are diffuse, this usually occurs. However, if a focus of inflammation is present at a distance from the ventricular system or subarachnoid space, analysis of CSF may not reflect the inflammatory process. Additionally, the location from which the sample is collected may influence the results. CSF flows from rostral to caudal in the neuraxis, and as a general rule, CSF should be collected from the closest site caudal to the suspected lesion. Therefore, CSF collected from the cerebellomedullary cistern in an animal with a focus of inflammation in the lumbar spinal cord may not accurately reflect the disease process present. Finally, animals that are immunocompromised or that have been treated with corticosteroids may have normal CSF leukocyte counts in the presence of CNS inflammatory disease.

The type of leukocytes present in the CSF provides further information about the cause of the disease. Suppurative inflammation is seen most commonly with bacterial infections and with feline infectious peritonitis (FIP). This pattern also can be seen with fungal and parasitic disease. Bacterial infections of the CNS are rare; the presence of degenerate neutrophils and the identification of intracellular bacteria support a diagnosis. The diagnosis may be confirmed by CSF culture; however, false-negative results are common because large volumes of CSF often are necessary to get a positive culture.

A predominant mononuclear inflammatory response may be seen with viral, rickettsial, protozoal, and some noninfectious causes of disease. A diagnosis of CNS lymphoma also should be considered in a cat with an increase in mononuclear cells, especially if the cells appear immature or atypical. Flow cytometry may be useful in these cases to identify the cell population definitively.

Mixed inflammation, consisting of neutrophils and mononuclear cells, typically is seen with protozoal and some fungal infections. A predominance of eosinophils should alert the clinician to the possibility of parasitic disease. Eosinophilic pleocytosis also can be seen with rickettsial disease, fungal infections, and CNS lymphoma.

The CSF is an ultrafiltrate of plasma, and normally contains protein at approximately 1/200 of the concentration found in blood.[3] Increase in the protein concentration of CSF is a nonspecific indicator of disease, and may be due to local production of antibodies or extravasation of proteins across a disrupted blood-brain barrier. The relative significance of each of these mechanisms in any individual case may be determined by further evaluation of the CSF. Protein electrophoresis may be performed to determine the relative concentrations of the different protein fractions present in a sample. In addition, albumin levels may be measured as an indication of the integrity of the blood-brain barrier. Synthesis of albumin within the CNS is negligible, and the size of the molecule limits its passage across an intact blood-brain barrier. Consequently, normal CSF albumin concentrations are low (reference range for the cat, 1 to 20 mg/dl).[4] An increase of this value usually is associated with blood-brain barrier disruption, although blood contamination of the CSF or intrathecal hemorrhage can cause similar results.

Elevated globulins in a CSF sample may be due either to serum globulins entering the CSF across a damaged blood-brain barrier or to local synthesis of globulins within the nervous system secondary to immune stimulation. Formulas have been devised to correct the CSF immunoglobulin (Ig) level for the contribution of Ig derived from the blood. These include the IgG quotient (CSF IgG/serum IgG) and the IgG index (CSF IgG/serum IgG × serum total protein/CSF total protein). Normal values reported for cats are 0.28 to 2.1 and 0.086 to 1.297, respectively.[4]

Serum may be assayed for titers to many of the infectious agents that cause CNS inflammation in cats, including FIP virus, feline immunodeficiency virus, *Toxoplasma gondii*, and *Cryptococcus neoformans*. For many of these diseases, a serum titer will establish only exposure to the organism, and does not confirm the presence of active CNS infection. Titers performed on the CSF may provide information on local infection, but blood-brain barrier compromise can lead to false-positive titers owing to leakage of serum. Specific Ig ratios (C-values), which correct for serum leakage, may be calculated utilizing the following formula: C-value = organism-specific IgG CSF/serum × total IgG serum/CSF. A C-value greater than 1 is suggestive of intrathecal antibody production, and a ratio greater than 8 is considered diagnostic for local synthesis.[5]

The increased availability of computed tomography (CT) and magnetic resonance imaging (MRI) in veterinary medicine has provided the means to evaluate the nervous system more fully. Imaging the brain of a cat with suspected encephalitis may help to confirm the diagnosis, and may provide additional clues as to the cause of the disease. Encephalitis from any cause tends to result in a heterogeneous appearance to the neural parenchyma, with focal areas of edema and contrast enhancement. Hydrocephalus is a common finding in cats with FIP, and can be diagnosed easily with brain imaging.

Despite extensive testing, an underlying cause for the CNS inflammation is not found in many patients. This reflects our limited understanding of the CNS inflammatory disorders in animals. As new diagnostic methods continue to be developed in veterinary medicine, it is likely that they will provide us with further information on this class of disease. Molecular techniques, such as the polymerase chain reaction (PCR), provide a sensitive means of examining samples for infectious agents. A commercially available PCR test has been developed for FIP, and it is likely that others will be available in the future. In addition, the ability to perform CT- or MRI-assisted stereotactic brain biopsy recently has become available in veterinary medicine, and provides a relatively noninvasive means of obtaining a tissue sample for histologic evaluation (see Chapter 50, Cerebral Meningiomas: Diagnostic and Therapeutic Considerations).

Treatment

Treatment for CNS infections entails definitive therapy for the causative agent if possible, nonspecific treatment directed at the CNS inflammation and its sequelae, and general supportive care. Because CNS disease can progress rapidly, it is important to initiate definitive treatment as soon as possible. Frequently, treatment is initiated based on preliminary CSF results because characteristic changes in leukocyte numbers and cell differential counts have been associated with the different classes of infectious agents. Treatment then can be altered if needed when final serology and culture results become available.

When considering antimicrobial treatment for CNS infections, it is important to choose an agent that is able to penetrate the blood-brain barrier. In general, antibiotics that are not highly protein-bound, have low degrees of ionization, and are lipid-soluble tend to reach higher concentrations in the CNS. In addition, because the local immune response is limited in the nervous system, microbicidal antibiotics are preferred over microbistatic drugs.

Seizures may occur in any animal with inflammation involving the forebrain. Uncontrolled seizures can exacerbate brain injury, and should be treated aggressively. Seizures are treated initially with intravenous diazepam and phenobarbital; once seizures are controlled, maintenance anticonvulsant therapy is initiated.

Brain edema is present to some extent in all cases of encephalitis. The brain is encased by the rigid bony skull and has limited room to expand. Brain edema causes an increase in intracranial pressure, which can progress to brain herniation. A cat with CNS inflammation should be observed closely for signs of increasing intracranial pressure, including depression of consciousness, change in pupil size and responsiveness, and abnormalities of cardiac rate or rhythm. Serial neurologic examinations should be performed to assess for deteriorating neurologic status. If evidence of increased intracranial pressure exists, the cats should be given mannitol (0.5 g/kg intravenously [IV], slowly over 20 to 30 minutes). Furosemide (2 mg/kg, IV) also may be administered in severe cases.

The use of corticosteroids in the treatment of CNS inflammatory disorders remains controversial. Corticosteroids may have a beneficial effect by decreasing the cerebral edema, vasculitis, and intensity of inflammation in the meninges and neural parenchyma. However, they may suppress the local immune response allowing further proliferation of the causative organism, mask or alter clinical signs and laboratory findings making definitive diagnosis more difficult, and cause systemic side-effects such as gastrointestinal bleeding. The author advocates the use of corticosteroids in 2 situations. The first is in patients with evidence of increased intracranial pressure, when it is believed that the cat is predisposed to brain herniation. In this case, corticosteroids are utilized to help reduce vasogenic edema and to decrease CSF production. Diuretics are administered concurrently. The second indication for corticosteroid administration is as a form of treatment for inflammatory disorders that have an immune-mediated component. A thorough work-up of each case is warranted to search for a treatable etiology. If no cause is identified and the disease is not self-limiting, a trial of corticosteroids is justified.

General supportive care consists of the management of any secondary complications; maintenance of adequate fluid, electrolyte, caloric, and temperature balance; and the provision of good nursing care. Recumbent cats should be turned frequently to prevent decubital ulcers and consolidation of dependent lung lobes. A cat that is unable to urinate voluntarily should have its bladder expressed 3 to 4 times daily, and should be kept clean and dry to prevent the development of urine scald.

Pathology

The hallmark of CNS inflammation is perivascular cuffing, or the accumulation of leukocytes of 1 or multiple types in the perivascular compartment around blood vessels of the CNS parenchyma and meninges.[1] Other histologic findings include evidence of edema, hypertrophy or proliferation of glial cell elements (known as gliosis), and neural cell degeneration and death. These latter changes reflect a nonspecific response to a change in the local environment, and are not seen exclusively with inflammatory disorders.

◆ FELINE INFECTIOUS PERITONITIS

Etiology

FIP is a common and serious viral disease of cats. The causative agent is a mutated form of the ubiquitous feline enteric coronavirus.

Epidemiology

FIP is the most common cause of inflammatory brain disease in cats. Approximately one-quarter to one-third of cats with the dry form of FIP will develop neurologic manifestations of disease.[6]

Pathogenesis

Neurologic involvement with FIP is seen primarily with the noneffusive or dry form of the disease. After infection, the virus disseminates hematogenously in circulating mononuclear cells, and localizes in organs such as lymph nodes, kidney, uvea, and the CNS. The pathologic changes that develop with the dry form of the disease results from a partial cell-mediated response combined with a strong humoral response to the virus. Granulomatous lesions occur around small foci of virus-laden macrophages in target organs.

Transmission

The FIP virus can be transmitted both in utero and by ingestion or inhalation postnatally. Neurologic signs are most common in those cats exposed postnatally. Most cats with FIP-associated neurologic disease arise from multiple-cat households or catteries.

Clinical Signs

The neurologic signs seen with FIP tend to have an insidious onset with no specific clinical course. Cats may present with diffuse or multifocal CNS signs, which is the most common presentation for inflammatory conditions affecting the nervous system. Alternatively, affected cats may present with signs suggestive of a focal nervous system lesion. Neurologic signs that have been described include altered consciousness, seizures, intention tremor, hypermetria, vestibular dysfunction, cranial nerve deficits, anisocoria, ataxia, paraparesis, and tetraparesis. Affected cats may have systemic manifestations of disease, including fluctuating fever, anorexia, and weight loss. Ocular lesions are identified frequently, and include anterior uveitis, keratic precipitates, hyphema, retinitis, and retinal hemorrhages. Some affected cats have evidence of disease localized only to the nervous system.

Diagnosis

The presence of hyperglobulinemia helps support a diagnosis of FIP-associated disease, but is not seen in all cases. Serum coronavirus titers are of limited value. Cats with confirmed FIP-associated neurologic disease may have negative titers because the soluble antibodies form immune complexes and escape detection by standard tests.[7] In addition, a positive coronavirus titer does not confirm infection because cross-reactivity exists between the FIP virus and the nonpathogenic enteric coronavirus.

Analysis of CSF is the most useful antemortem diagnostic test. The most characteristic finding in a cat with FIP is a neutrophilic pleocytosis with a marked increase in protein concentration greater than 200 mg/dl.[8] However, mild mononuclear inflammation or even normal CSF has been seen in cats with confirmed neurologic FIP. Titers to the FIP virus may be performed on a CSF sample; positive CSF titers were shown to be the most useful antemortem indicator of neurologic disease.[6] However, positive CSF titers must be interpreted with caution in animals with positive serum titers and high protein concentrations in the CSF because extravasation of serum proteins across a disrupted blood-brain barrier can lead to false elevations in CSF titers. Calculation of an albumin quotient and IgG index may be useful in cases in which the significance of a positive CSF titer is in question.

PCR testing recently has been developed as a diagnostic assay for FIP. In one study of cats with neurologic FIP, only a third of CSF samples were positive for FIP by PCR, and PCR analysis of brain tissue was positive in only two-thirds of the cases.[6] These results suggest that PCR testing may aid in the diagnosis, but is not a reliable test for confirming the presence of disease.

Brain imaging with CT or MRI reveals the presence of hydrocephalus in the majority of affected cats. The virus causes inflammation of the ependymal cells that line the ventricular system, which prevents the normal flow of CSF, and results in a secondary obstructive hydrocephalus.

Treatment

The prognosis for cats with neurologic FIP is poor. No effective treatment is known. The use of immunosuppressive drugs may slow the progression of disease.

Pathologic Findings

Pathologic findings may be confined to the nervous system in some affected cats. Hydrocephalus usually is apparent on gross examination of the brain. Histopathologic findings include granulomatous inflammation of the meninges, ependymal cells, and choroid plexus. Lymphocytes and macrophages are the predominant cell types, but some areas of inflammation may consist primarily of plasma cells, and others areas may appear pyogranulomatous. In the meninges, inflammation tends to be perivascular in location.

◆ NONSUPPURATIVE MENINGOENCEPHALOMYELITIS

Etiology

This disease also is known as feline polioencephalomyelitis. The etiology of this condition has not been proved, but a virus is suspected.[8, 9] The disease is characterized histopathologically by the presence of mild mononuclear inflammation within the CNS and the absence of lesions elsewhere. A variety of viruses can infect the CNS of cats, including parvovirus, calicivirus, herpesvirus, Newcastle disease virus, Near Eastern equine encephalomyelitis virus, and Powassan virus.[8] The relative significance of each of these viruses as a potential cause of clinical CNS disease in naturally infected cats has not been determined.

Epidemiology

In one study, 37 per cent of cats presenting with CNS inflammatory disease had a diagnosis of non-suppurative meningoencephalomyelitis.[8] The majority of cats diagnosed with this disorder are less than 2 years old, but cats of any age may be affected. Most patients have an acute onset of clinical signs that progress over several weeks. Environmental history does not seem to have a role because the disease has been diagnosed in exclusively indoor cats and those exposed to the outdoors.

Clinical Signs

Affected cats may have systemic signs such as fever, lethargy, anorexia, vomiting, or diarrhea. A history of respiratory signs may precede the development of neurologic signs. Evidence of chorioretinitis may be seen on fundic evaluation.

The disease may affect any area of the CNS, and neurologic signs reflect the location of the lesion within the neuraxis. Forebrain involvement is seen most frequently and seizures are a common presenting complaint.

Diagnosis

A presumptive diagnosis of nonsuppurative meningoencephalitis is based on characteristic findings of CSF analysis. Evaluation of CSF usually reveals a mild-to-moderate increase in leukocytes, with the predominant cell type being lymphocytes. Protein concentration may be normal or mildly increased. Neuroimaging of the brain may reveal multifocal areas of contrast enhancement, suggestive of inflammatory disease. Other causes of CNS inflammation must be excluded, based on negative testing for feline leukemia virus, feline immunodeficiency virus, FIP, toxoplasmosis, and cryptococcosis.

Treatment

There is no effective treatment. Supportive care should be administered, including anticonvulsant medication to control seizures as needed. The disease usually is self-limiting, and the prognosis is good for cats in which neurologic signs are not severely debilitating.

Pathology

Histologic lesions are nonspecific, and consist of mononuclear perivascular cuffing, lymphocytic-histiocytic meningeal inflammation, and gliosis.

◆ *CUTEREBRA* LARVAL MYIASIS

Etiology

Aberrant intracranial migration of *Cuterebra* larvae has been reported in cats. This *Cuterebra* larval migration has been proposed to be the cause of feline ischemic encephalopathy,[10] a disease characterized by cerebral infarction and secondary necrosis (see Chapter 52, Vascular Disorders).

Epidemiology

Aberrant migration of *Cuterebra* larvae is seen in young to middle-aged cats with access to the outdoors. Cases typically present in the summer months of July to September, with a peak in August. The adult fly lays its eggs at the entrance to burrows of its normal rodent or lagomorph hosts. The larvae enter the body through a mucous membrane–lined site, such as the eye, nose, or mouth. It is believed that the larvae enter cats through the nares and nasal cavity, and gain entrance to the brain through the cribiform plate.

Pathogenesis

Clinical signs result in part from physical disruption of the brain parenchyma and associated hemorrhage as the parasite migrates through the tissues. In addition, it has been postulated that the larvae elaborate a toxin that gains entry into the CSF.[10] This toxin is believed to be responsible for the laminar necrosis and cerebral infarcts seen on histopathologic evaluation. Cerebral infarction is the characteristic finding in feline ischemic encephalopathy, and is believed to be caused by toxin-induced local vasospasm.

Clinical Signs

Cats may have a recent history of clinical signs consistent with upper respiratory disease. Neurologic signs are peracute to acute in onset. Most cats have focal signs referable to a forebrain lesion, such as seizures, depression, blindness, and behavior change. Multifocal neurologic involvement, with signs of disease in other areas of the brain or spinal cord, also have been reported.

Diagnosis

The disease should be suspected in any cat with access to the outdoors that presents during the summer months with acute onset of forebrain signs. However, confirming a diagnosis is difficult. Clinical pathologic findings that may be seen include peripheral eosinophilia and hyperglobulinemia. Advanced imaging techniques may reveal a mottled appearance to the brain, similar to that seen with encephalitis. Results of CSF analysis also are variable. Eosinophilic inflammation helps support a diagnosis, but a normal CSF analysis does not rule out the disease.

Treatment

Experience treating intracranial *Cuterebra* myiasis is limited. The following protocol has been recommended, but has not yet been proved effective.[11] The cat is pretreated with diphenhydramine (4 mg/kg intramuscularly [IM]) 1 to 2 hours before the administration of ivermectin (400 µg/kg subcutaneously [SC]) and dexamethasone (0.1 mg/kg IV). The diphenhydramine and dexamethasone are administered to prevent any allergic or anaphylactic reactions associated with larval death. This regimen is repeated 24 and 48 hours later. Additionally, a 2-week course of antibiotics is recommended to prevent bacterial infection introduced by presumed larval migration.

Pathologic Findings

Careful inspection of the regions of the olfactory bulbs and peduncles, the cribriform plate, and the olfactory nerves and nasal cavity may reveal the larva.[10] The larva may be identified on microscopic evaluation if it is not found on gross examination. Parasitic tract lesions manifest as areas of parenchymal necrosis with small-to-moderate amounts of hemorrhage and an associated mild eosinophilic and lymphocytic inflammatory infiltrate. In addition, laminar cerebrocortical necrosis is identified commonly, as is a focal area of cerebral necrosis consistent with an infarct.

◆ CRYPTOCOCCOSIS
Etiology

Cryptococcus neoformans is a saprophytic yeast with worldwide distribution. The organism can be isolated from several sources, although it is associated most frequently with pigeon droppings. Cryptococcosis is the most common systemic mycosis of cats (see Chapter 6, Cryptococcosis: New Perspectives on Etiology, Pathogenesis, Diagnosis, and Clinical Management).

Epidemiology

Clinical cryptococcosis is seen in cats of all ages. There is no gender or breed predisposition. Cats with access to the outdoors are affected most commonly.

Transmission

The route of entry into the body usually is the nasal cavity because *Cryptococcus* spores are inhaled. Neurologic involvement may result from hematogenous spread or local extension of an infection through the cribriform plate.

Clinical Signs

Many affected cats will have a chronic nasal discharge and evidence of submandibular lymphadenopathy. These may be accompanied by cutaneous lesions on the head or nose. Ocular manifestations of disease are seen frequently with neurologic involvement, including anterior uveitis and chorioretinitis. Evidence of systemic infection is not always apparent.

Neurologic signs that have been reported include seizures, behavior change, altered mentation, circling, head pressing, blindness, apparent loss of smell, cranial nerve deficits, ataxia, and paresis. Neurologic signs typically are acute in onset and rapidly progressive.

Diagnosis

If a cat has extraneural signs of disease, a definitive diagnosis often can be made with cytology and/or culture of lesions. Enlarged lymph nodes or cutaneous masses should be aspirated. If a cat has a nasal discharge, it should be examined directly. Cytologic evaluation of these samples often reveals the presence of the encapsulated organism.

CSF analysis is the most helpful diagnostic test in those cats with neurologic signs alone. An increase in neutrophils or eosinophils may be present. Definitive diagnosis is made by visualizing the organism on cytologic preparations made with Gram stain, new methylene blue, or India ink. In cases in which the organism is not identified readily, diagnosis can be obtained by either detecting cryptococcal polysaccharide capsular antigen or culturing the organism from the CSF.

Treatment

Itraconazole and fluconazole are considered the drugs of choice for treating CNS cryptococcosis. Fluconazole at a dosage of 50 mg orally (PO) every (q) 12 hours has been used effectively to treat cats with nasal and cutaneous cryptococcosis.[12] The drug is water-soluble, and reaches therapeutic levels in the CSF.[13] Itraconazole is lipophilic, and reaches negligible levels in the CSF. However, the drug's lipid solubility enables penetration into the brain tissue, and it has proved efficacious in the treatment of CNS cryptococcosis.[14] A dose of 50 mg/day in cats weighing less than 3.2 kg and 100 mg/day in cats weighing 3.2 kg or greater has been recommended.[15] Long-term treatment is required with both of these drugs, ranging from several months to a year or more. It is difficult to rid the body completely of the organism, and relapses are common. To decrease the chance of a relapse, therapy should be continued for a minimum of 2 months beyond resolution of clinical signs.

Pathology

The organism usually is abundant in tissue and easily identified on histologic evaluation. A diffuse meningoencephalitis is seen commonly, but it is characteristic for the inflammatory response to be relatively mild compared with the numbers of organisms present. Inflammatory cells consist of macrophages, lymphocytes, and plasma cells.

◆ TOXOPLASMOSIS

Etiology

Toxoplasma gondii is an intracellular protozoan parasite of human beings and animals. Cats serve as the definitive host for the organism, and most infections in cats are clinically silent. However, infected cats occasionally will develop signs of disease, including neurologic manifestations.

Epidemiology

It has been reported that up to 54 per cent of cats in the United States are infected with *T. gondii*.[16] Cats with access to the outdoors are more likely to be exposed to the organism. There is no breed, gender, or age predisposition for clinical toxoplasmosis. Immunosuppression, either due to concurrent illness or drug-induced, can predispose to the development of clinical disease.

Transmission

Cats typically become infected with toxoplasmosis at a young age, and acquire the infection either by ingesting sporulated oocysts found in the environment or more commonly by ingesting tissue cysts found in intermediate hosts. The organism undergoes an enteroepithelial life cycle, and unsporulated oocysts are shed 10 to 14 days after initial infection. The oocysts sporulate in the environment, and subsequently are infective to other cats or intermediate hosts.

Pathogenesis

After the organism undergoes the enteroepithelial life cycle, tachyzoites are disseminated through the blood and lymph. Activation of the cat's immune system suppresses the proliferation of tachyzoites, and favors the development of tissue cysts in multiple organ systems. The brain is one site of predilection for tissue cyst formation. The tissue cysts can remain dormant for extended periods of time. Disease associated with toxoplasmosis often is due to recrudescence of local infection, with the tissue cyst being the source of the organism.

Clinical Signs

Systemic signs are seen frequently, reflecting involvement of the lungs, liver, and gastrointestinal tract. Fever is a common presenting complaint; weight loss, muscle hyperpathia, and chorioretinitis also may be seen.

Neurologic abnormalities that have been reported include seizures, behavior change, circling, blindness, ataxia, and paresis. The clinical course is variable, and signs may either be acute or have a more insidious onset.

Diagnosis

Analysis of CSF typically reveals increases in leukocyte and protein concentrations. The inflammation usually is a mix of mononuclear and polymorphonuclear cells. On rare occasions, the organism may be seen in the CSF.

Serologic testing may help to confirm a diagnosis. *T. gondii*–specific IgG and IgM can be assayed in both serum and CSF. A specific immunoglobulin ratio (C-value) may be calculated, and a C-value greater than 1 is indicative of intrathecal antibody production. However, C-values greater than 1 have been seen in clinically normal cats, and it has been postulated that nonspecific immune stimulation may lead to local production of antibodies and elevations in C-values in the absence of clinically significant infection.[17] Direct demonstration of the organism in biopsied tissue is the only definitive means of diagnosis.

Treatment

Clindamycin is utilized for the treatment of systemic and neurologic toxoplasmosis. The drug penetrates into nervous tissue effectively, and has been used successfully to treat cats with suspected CNS toxoplasmosis. A dose of 12.5 mg/kg PO q 12 hr for 4 to 6 weeks has been advocated.[18] Neurologic signs typically improve with treatment, but damage caused by the organism may be permanent and relapses can occur.

Pathology

Characteristic histopathologic findings include mononuclear perivascular cuffing, and necrotizing inflammation and granuloma formation within the brain parenchyma. Tissue cysts may be identified in the brain, and free organisms may be demonstrated frequently in macrophages, glial cells, and neurons.

REFERENCES

1. Summers BA, Cummings JF, deLahunta A: Veterinary Neuropathology. St. Louis, Mosby–Year Book, 1995, pp. 39–47.
2. Rand JS, Parent J, Jacobs R, et al: Reference intervals for cerebrospinal fluid: Cell counts and cytologic features. Am J Vet Res 51:1044–1048, 1990.
3. Fishman RA: Cerebrospinal Fluid in Diseases of the Nervous System, 2nd ed. Philadelphia, WB Saunders, 1992, p. 46.
4. Chrisman CL: Cerebrospinal fluid analysis. Vet Clin North Am Small Anim Pract 22:781–810, 1992.
5. Kennedy CR, Chrzanowska K, Robinson RO, et al: A major role for viruses in acute childhood encephalopathy. Lancet 1:989–991, 1986.
6. Foley JE, LaPointe JM, Koblik P, et al: Diagnostic features of clinical neurologic feline infectious peritonitis. J Vet Intern Med 12:415–423, 1998.
7. Kline KL, Joseph RJ, Averill DR: Feline infectious peritonitis with neurologic involvement: Clinical and pathological findings in 24 cats. J Am Anim Hosp Assoc 30:111–118, 1994.
8. Rand JS, Parent J, Percy D, et al: Clinical, cerebrospinal fluid and histological data from twenty-seven cats with primary inflammatory disease of the central nervous system. Can Vet J 35:103–110, 1994.
9. Hoff EJ, Vandevelde M: Non-suppurative encephalomyelitis in cats suggestive of a viral origin. Vet Pathol 18:170–180, 1981.
10. Williams KJ, Summers BA, deLahunta A: Cerebrospinal cuterebriasis in cats and its association with feline ischemic encephalopathy. Vet Pathol 35:330–343, 1998.
11. Glass EN, Cornetta AM, deLahunta A, et al: Clinical and clinicopathologic features in 11 cats with *Cuterebra* larvae myiasis of the central nervous system. J Vet Intern Med 12:365–368, 1998.
12. Malik R, Wigney DI, Muir DB, et al: Cryptococcosis in cats: Clinical and mycological assessment of 29 cases and evaluation of treatment using orally administered fluconazole. J Med Vet Mycol 30:133–144, 1992.
13. Vaden SL, Heit MC, Hawkins EC, et al: Fluconazole in cats: Pharmacokinetics following intravenous and oral administration and penetration into cerebrospinal fluid, aqueous humour and pulmonary epithelial lining fluid. J Vet Pharmacol Ther 20:181–186, 1997.
14. Medleau L, Greene CE, Rakich PM: Evaluation of ketoconazole and itraconazole for treatment of disseminated cryptococcosis in cats. Am J Vet Res 51:1454–1458, 1990.
15. Medleau L, Jacobs GJ, Marks MA: Itraconazole for the treatment of cryptococcosis in cats. J Vet Intern Med 9:39–42, 1995.
16. Lappin MR, Greene CE, Prestwood AK, et al: Prevalence of *Toxoplasma gondii* infection in cats in Georgia using enzyme-linked immunosorbent assays for IgM, IgG, and antigens. Vet Parasitol 33:225–230, 1989.
17. Muñana KR, Lappin MR, Powell CC, et al: Sequential measurement of *Toxoplasma gondii*–specific antibodies in the cerebrospinal fluid of cats with experimentally induced toxoplasmosis. Prog Vet Neurol 6:27–31, 1995.
18. Lappin MR, Greene CE, Winston S, et al: Clinical feline toxoplasmosis. Serologic diagnosis and therapeutic management of 15 cases. J Vet Intern Med 3:139–143, 1989.

Hematopoietic and Lymphatic Systems

Rick L. Cowell, Editor

◆ Update on Cytauxzoonosis 436
◆ Splenomegaly and Lymphadenopathy 439
◆ Mucopolysaccharidosis 450
◆ Transfusion Medicine 461
◆ Thrombocytopenia 468
◆ Use of the Polymerase Chain Reaction to Detect
  Hemoparasites 479
◆ Hereditary Erythrocyte Disorders 484
◆ Myeloid and Mast Cell Leukemias 490

Still-Current Information Found in *Consultations in Feline Internal Medicine 2*:
Arthopod-Borne Diseases (Chapter 7), p. 47
Inherited Disorders (Chapter 24), p. 183
Pancytopenia (Chapter 60), p. 495
Lymphoid Leukemias (Chapter 62), p. 509
Bone Marrow Evaluation (Chapter 63), p. 515
Transfusion Medicine (Chapter 64), p. 525
Solitary Extranodal Lymphomas: Presentation and Management (Chapter 67), p. 547
Variables in Behavior and Management of Mast Cell Tumors (Chapter 70), p. 567

Still-Current Information Found in *Consultations in Feline Internal Medicine 3*:
Cytauxzoonosis (Chapter 58), p. 474
Hemobartonellosis (Chapter 59), p. 479
Inherited Coagulopathies (Chapter 61), p. 488
Classification of Myeloproliferative Diseases (Chapter 62), p. 499
Myeloid Leukemias (Chapter 63), p. 509
Metastatic Patterns of Feline Neoplasia (Chapter 71), p. 566
Interpreting Gross Necropsy Observations in Neonatal and Pediatric Kittens (Chapter 74), p. 587

Elsewhere in Consultations in *Feline Internal Medicine 4*:
Hemobartonellosis (Chapter 2), p. 12
Rickettsial Diseases (Chapter 4), p. 28
Approach to the Icteric Cat (Chapter 10), p. 87
Clinical Approach to Chronic Diarrhea (Chapter 16), p. 127
Complications of Therapy for Hyperthyroidism (Chapter 19), p. 151
Nontuberculous Mycobacterial Diseases (Chapter 30), p. 221
Neuronal Storage Disorders (Chapter 51), p. 393
Gastrointestinal Lymphoma and Inflammatory Bowel Disease (Chapter 63), p. 499
Management of the Lymphoma Patient With Concurrent Disease (Chapter 64), p. 506
Chemotherapeutic Challenges: Special Considerations and New Agents (Chapter 65), p. 521
Evluation and Treatment of Cranial Mediastinal Masses (Chapter 68), p. 533
Diagnostic Imaging of Neoplasia (Chapter 70), p. 548
Understanding and Controlling of Feral Cat Populations (Chapter 71), p. 561
Molecular Diagnosis of Gangliosidoses: A Model for Elimination of Inherited Diseases in Pure Breeds (Chapter 77), p. 615

55

◆ Update on Cytauxzoonosis

James H. Meinkoth

Since its first description in 1976,[1] cytauxzoonosis has become recognized as a common disease of cats in areas of many southern states, and has been reported from Oklahoma, Texas, Missouri, Arkansas, Georgia, Mississippi, Louisiana, and Florida.[2] Until recently, the natural course of infection has been an acute, uniformly fatal disease that was refractory to therapy. Since 1997, we have encountered a number of cats surviving natural infection with this parasite.[3] These cats seemed to recover irrespective of treatment, and possibly represent infection with a less virulent strain of *Cytauxzoon*. Additionally, other investigators have reported apparent responses to therapy using specific antiprotozoal agents.[4]

This chapter provides a review of the salient features of the disease, and updates the practitioner to the clinical significance of recent findings regarding cats surviving cytauxzoonosis. A more detailed review of cytauxzoonosis is available in a previous edition of this text.[5]

◆ ETIOLOGY

Cytauxzoon felis, the causative agent of cytauxzoonosis, is a tick-borne protozoon classified in the family Theileriidae. The organism has 2 phases, an intraerythrocytic piroplasm (Fig. 55–1) and a tissue phase occurring in macrophages within and surrounding blood vessels in most organs of the body.[6] Within these macrophages, large schizonts are formed that greatly enlarge and distort the host cell (Fig. 55–2). The tissue phase of the organism is responsible for the production of clinical disease

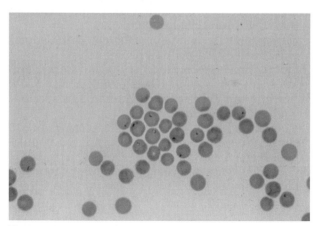

Figure 55–1. Blood smears from a cat. Numerous *Cytauxzoon felis* schizonts are present in erythrocytes. (Diff-Quik, original magnification, 330×.)

and death, probably by obstruction of vessels and release of cytokines from infected cells.[4] Infection with only the piroplasm may result in phagocytosis of infected erythrocytes, but generally is asymptomatic.

◆ EPIDEMIOLOGY

C. felis infects wild and domestic cats. In domestic cats, infection is characterized by both parasitemia and widespread development of tissue schizonts, and almost always is associated with fatal clinical disease. In studies detailing experimental infection of several hundred domestic cats, only 3 cats have been reported to survive.[7-9] In 1995, Walker and Cowell[10] reported a single cat surviving natural infection.

In bobcats, infection usually is characterized by a persistent, asymptomatic parasitemia.[11, 12] A limited, subclinical schizogenous phase can be identified immediately after infection; however, several weeks later, schizonts are absent or below limits of detection.[13] Rarely, bobcats have developed fatal disease similar to that seen in domestic cats. Other wild felids also may be infected; a 36 per cent prevalence of piroplasms in blood samples collected from free-ranging panthers and cougars was reported recently.[14] Infection of these animals generally is similar to that in bobcats, producing an asymptomatic parasitemia.

After infection of a domestic cat, developing schizonts are found in macrophages throughout the body. Schizonts produce numerous merozoites, which fill the infected macrophage and, after release, invade erythrocytes. Merozoites are detectable in macrophages a few days before organisms are seen within circulating erythrocytes.

Ticks (*Dermacentor variabilis*) are able to transmit the infection from animal to animal, and appear to be necessary for the organism to complete a portion of its life cycle.[11] Direct transfer of piroplasms to domestic cats via blood inoculation produces only an asymptomatic erythroparasitemia, without development of the tissue (schizont) phase. However, tick transfer of piroplasms to domestic cats results in development of both tissue schizonts and erythroparasitemia, as well as production of clinical disease. In contrast to the piroplasm, direct inoculation of the tissue schizonts to domestic cats results in infection with both phases and clinical disease.[15]

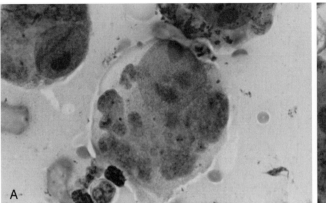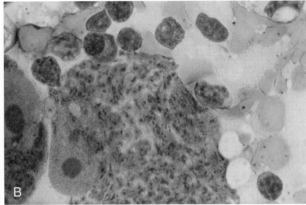

Figure 55–2. Impression smears from the spleen of a cat show *C. felis* schizonts within host macrophages. Note the large nucleoli present in the host cells. *A*, An early schizont appears as a poorly demarcated, lobulated, basophilic structure within the cytoplasm of a macrophage. *B*, A mature schizont completely fills the cytoplasm of the host macrophage. Nuclear material of the developing parasite merozoites can be seen. (*A* and *B*, Diff-Quik, original magnification, 330×.)

◆ CLINICAL FINDINGS

The prevalence of cytauxzoonosis generally is proportional to exposure of cats to the tick vector; most cases occur in the summer months in outdoor cats, especially those with access to wooded areas. Most infected cats manifest a rapidly progressive, systemic illness with nonspecific clinical signs. Initially, cats become depressed and anorexic and develop a high fever, often 41.1°C or greater.[2] Many cats are icteric, and some cry out as if in pain, particularly when handled. Hematologic changes may include any combination of nonregenerative anemia, leukopenia, or thrombocytopenia.[16] Many cats are hyperbilirubinemic.

Diagnosis generally is made by finding typical signet-ring–shaped piroplasms on peripheral blood smears (see Fig. 55–1). Parasitemia is a late event in the course of disease, and some cats do not have detectable parasites at initial presentation. In such cases, diagnosis may be confirmed by finding schizont-containing macrophages in fine-needle aspirates of lung, spleen, liver, lymph node, or bone marrow (see Fig. 55–2).

Cats generally die within a week of presentation. Historically, therapy has not been of value in clearing infection or altering the fatal course of the disease. Recently, the antiprotozoal drug imidocarb dipropionate (Imizole) has been approved for use in the United States for the treatment of canine babesiosis. Although there have been no clinical studies showing this drug to be efficacious against cytauxzoonosis, there are scattered reports of this drug being used with success, either alone or in combination with diminazine aceturate.[4] We have attempted therapy in several cats presented in the late stages of disease using imidocarb, but without success. Greene and colleagues[17] reported the successful treatment of 6 of 7 cats with cytauxzoonosis with 2 intramuscular injections of diminazene aceturate (2 mg/kg) or imidocarb dipropionate. Atropine was administered before treatments with imidocarb to prevent adverse reactions. Supportive care (fluid therapy, blood transfusions, heparin) also was important for a positive treatment outcome in these patients.

◆ RECENT EXPERIENCE WITH CATS SURVIVING *C. FELIS* INFECTION

Since the summer of 1997, we have identified more than 25 cats surviving naturally occurring *C. felis* infection. A description of many of these cases has been submitted for publication.[3] These cases all have come from a limited geographic area in northwestern Arkansas and eastern Oklahoma.

Most cats presented with clinical signs common in cytauxzoonosis: anorexia, depression, and high fever. Some cats were icteric and/or anemic. Generally, cytauxzoonosis was suspected because of clinical presentation, time of year, and a high regional rate of occurrence of this disease. In all cases, the diagnosis was confirmed by finding piroplasms in erythrocytes on peripheral blood smears. Duration of clinical illness was up to 12 days. Four cats identified were totally asymptomatic. These were housemates of one of the other survivors, whose owner had recently moved into the area. They were tested only after the diagnosis was made in their housemate. These cats presumably were all exposed to the same source of infected ticks.

Treatment of these cases was generally supportive, and was unlikely to have been responsible for the clinical outcome. The 4 asymptomatic cats received no treatment. Most clinically ill cats received intravenous fluids and a variety of antibiotics, all of which have been used without success in the past. Only 1 cat was treated twice with imidocarb dipropionate (6.6 mg/kg, IM, intramuscularly, every 14 days). Although it is possible that this drug may have had an effect in that 1 case, we have treated other cats with this drug without success.

Blood smears were checked for persistence of organisms after clinical recovery in 12 of the cats (range, 3 to 158 days from initial diagnosis). The magnitude of the parasitemia varied, but organisms could be found in all cases. Also, additional samples from the case of a naturally occurring survivor originally reported by Walker and Cowell[10] became available, and that cat was found be parasitemic more than 6 years after original diagnosis. This suggests these cats will be chronic carriers, which is consistent with what is known about the biology of cytauxzoonosis. Despite persistent parasitemia, most cats have been recovered for more than a year, with none showing ill effects related to infection.

It is possible that these cases represent infection with a less virulent strain of *C. felis*. Partial DNA sequences obtained from the organism in 2 of the cases were identical and showed greater than 99 per cent homology with the reported sequence of *C. felis*, making it unlikely that this is a novel, previously unrecognized parasite. Also, we have been able to create carriers of this organism by inoculating research cats with blood from clinical survivors. Like the clinical cases, these cats remain persistently parasitemic. Recently, we have been able to transmit the organism to a susceptible cat using *D. variabilis* ticks (Meinkoth JH, Kocan AA, unpublished observations, 1999). The recipient cat became parasitemic, but did not show clinical illness. That the organism could be transmitted via ticks without producing clinical illness also supports the notion of a less virulent strain of organism rather than innate resistance of the original cat from which the organism was isolated; however, further studies are needed.

◆ IMPLICATIONS FOR THE PRACTITIONER

It is important for the clinician to recognize that, although uncommon, some cats may survive infection with *C. felis*. Although our current cases have come from a localized area, if this represents the development of a less virulent strain, similar strains may occur elsewhere. Some of the cats identified were markedly ill at the time of presentation. High fever, icterus, and anemia all were present in at least some cases, so these factors do not preclude survival. None of the survivors became hypothermic, which is a common terminal event in cytauxzoonosis. The possibility of "naturally occurring" survival also must be considered when evaluating the efficacy of newer therapeutic regimens.

It is also important to recognize that these cats are likely to remain persistently infected and parasitemic. Possibly, organisms could be identified on blood smears from these animals even if testing is being done for an unrelated reason. Although we have not yet seen recrudescence of clinical disease in any of these cats, this possibility cannot be ruled out. Furthermore, these cats can serve as a reservoir for this organism to be spread to other animals via ticks. The clinical significance of such a transferred infection remains to be determined. Our one such experimental transfer resulted in an asymptomatic parasitemia, but it should be kept in mind that most of the cats in this study initially were clinically ill, and a range of clinical outcomes is possible. We do not yet know whether survivors will be resistant to subsequent challenge with a potentially more virulent strain of *C. felis*. Additional studies are needed to resolve this question.

REFERENCES

1. Wagner JE: A fatal cytauxzoonosis-like disease in cats. J Am Vet Med Assoc 168:585–588, 1976.
2. Cowell RL, Panciera RJ, Fox JC, et al: Feline cytauxzoonosis. Compend Contin Educ Pract Vet 10:731–736, 1988.
3. Meinkoth JH, Kocan AA, Murphy G, et al: Cats surviving natural infection with *Cytauxzoon felis*: 18 cases (1997–1999). J Vet Intern Med (In press).
4. Kier AB, Greene CE: Cytauxzoonosis. *In* Greene CE (ed): Infectious Diseases of the Dog and Cat, 2nd ed. Philadelphia, WB Saunders, 1998, pp. 470–473.
5. Meinkoth JH, Clinkenbeard KC, Theissen AE: Cytauxzoonosis. *In* August JR (ed): Consultations in Feline Internal Medicine, vol. 3. Philadelphia, WB Saunders, 1997, pp. 474–478.
6. Kier AB, Wagner JE, Kinden DA: The pathology of experimental cytauxzoonosis. J Comp Pathol 97:415–432, 1987.
7. Ferris DH: A progress report on the status of a new disease of American cats: Cytauxzoonosis. Comp Immun Microbiol Infect Dis 1:269–276, 1979.
8. Motzel SL, Wagner JE: Treatment of experimentally induced cytauxzoonosis in cats with parvaquone and buparvaquone. Vet Parasitol 35:131–138, 1990.
9. Uilenberg G, Freanssen FFJ, Perié NM: Relationships between *Cytauxzoon felis* and African piroplasmids. Vet Parasitol 26:21–28, 1987.
10. Walker DB, Cowell RL: Survival of a domestic cat with naturally acquired cytauxzoonosis. J Am Vet Med Assoc 206:1363–1365, 1995.
11. Blouin EF, Kocan AA, Glenn BL, et al: Transmission of *Cytauxzoon felis* Kier, 1979 from bobcats, *Felis rufus* (Schureber), to domestic cats by *Dermacentor variabilis* (Say). J Wildl Dis 20:241–242, 1984.
12. Glenn BL, Kocan AA, Blouin EF. Cytauxzoonosis in bobcats. J Am Vet Med Assoc 183:1155–1158, 1983.
13. Blouin EF, Kocan AA, Kocan KM, et al: Evidence of a limited schizogonous cycle for *Cytauxzoon felis* in bobcats following exposure to infected ticks. J Wildl Dis 23:499–501, 1987.
14. Rotstein DS, Taylor SK, Harvey JW, et al: Hematologic effects of cytauxzoonosis in Florida panthers and Texas cougars in Florida. J Wildl Dis 35:613–617, 1999.
15. Wagner JE, Ferris DH, Kier AB, et al: Experimentally induced cytauxzoonosis-like disease in domestic cats. Vet Parasitol 6:305–311, 1980.
16. Hoover JP, Walker BD, Hedges JD: Cytauxzoonosis in cats: Eight cases (1985–1992). J Am Vet Med Assoc 205:455–460, 1994.
17. Greene CE, Latimer K, Hopper E, et al: Administration of diminazene aceturate or imidocarb dipropionate for treatment of cytauxzoonosis in cats. J Am Vet Med Assoc 215:497–500, 1999.

56

◆ Splenomegaly and Lymphadenopathy

T. Mark Neer

In this chapter, disorders of the spleen and lymph nodes are discussed separately, but the reader is cautioned to pay close attention to disorders/diseases that may affect both systems simultaneously. In these disorders, examination/evaluation of one organ system may enable the clinician to obtain a definitive diagnosis, whereas it could not be obtained by evaluation of the other. This is due in part to the role that both of these systems play in immunity and host defense functions.

The 2 main functions of the lymph nodes are to filter material and to participate in the immunologic process. The filtering process is more active in areas rich in mononuclear-phagocytic cells, while this material transits from afferent to efferent lymphatics. During this transit, material is "taken up" and processed by the mononuclear-phagocytic cells and then presented to the lymphoid cells to generate a humoral or cell-mediated immune response.

The functions of the spleen include: hematopoiesis, filtration and phagocytosis, remodeling of red blood cells, acting as a blood reservoir in the metabolism of iron, removal of intraerythrocytic inclusions, and affecting the immunologic process.

◆ DISEASES OF THE SPLEEN
Gross and Microscopic Anatomy

The spleen is positioned in the left cranial quadrant of the abdomen. It is mobile and frequently can be palpated in the midventral region of the abdomen. It is seen most easily on abdominal radiographs between the left kidney and the fundus of the stomach, where it is folded on itself (Fig. 56–1). It is a flat organ with its length usually exceeding its width.

Microscopically, the spleen comprises red pulp, white pulp, and a fibromuscular capsule with trabeculae, which provides structure and support. The red pulp consists of venous spaces into which blood is discharged, and a loose reticular structure populated with macrophages. The white pulp consists of lymphoid nodules and follicles dispersed throughout the splenic parenchyma. The feline spleen differs from that of dogs in that it is nonsinusoidal, and has no endothelial continuity between the arterioles and the venules; rather, blood is discharged directly into the red pulp.[1] Therefore, in the feline spleen, erythrocytes are able to pass with relative ease from the arterioles to the venules and are not well scrutinized. This lack of a sinusoidal spleen may account partially for the high number of Heinz bodies observed in normal cat blood.

Diagnostic Approach to Splenomegaly

The spleen may be affected with primary disease and be the reason the patient is ill, or it may be affected secondarily by systemic disease and in this situation may act as a "sentinel organ" for an underlying disease process. Therefore, the clinician can utilize the spleen to obtain diagnostic information that might aid in defining a diagnosis or, help categorize a patient's disease (e.g., inflammatory, neoplastic, infectious). Determining, at the outset, whether the splenic enlargement is focal or diffuse (generalized) may decrease the number of possible differential diagnoses and direct the clinician's diagnostic approach (Table 56–1). In cats, causes of generalized splenomegaly are more common than diseases that result in focal splenomegaly, with mast cell tumor (mastocytosis), malignant histiocytosis,[2, 3] and lymphoproliferative neoplasia resulting in the most marked enlargement.

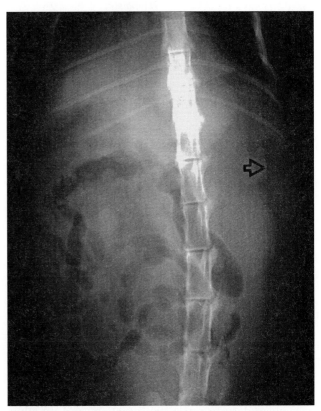

Figure 56–1. Ventrodorsal radiograph shows the normal position and size of the feline spleen (*arrowhead*).

Table 56–1. Diseases Resulting in Splenomegaly

Focal Enlargement	Diffuse Enlargement
Bacterial	**Infectious Causes**
Abscess	**Bacterial**
	Mycobacterium species
Neoplastic	Streptococcus species
Lymphoma	Staphylococcus species
Hemangiosarcoma	Salmonella species
Other sarcomas arising from spleen	Francisella tularensis
Metastatic lesions	**Mycotic**
	Sporothrix schenckii
Nonneoplastic	Histoplasma capsulatum
Extramedullary hematopoiesis	**Protozoal**
Hematoma	Toxoplasma gondii
Myelolipoma	Hemobartonella felis
Lymphoid hyperplastic nodules	**Viral**
	Feline infectious peritonitis
	Retroviral infection (FeLV and FIV)
	Congestive
	Drug-induced
	Portal hypertension
	Congestive heart failure (right-sided)
	Inflammatory/Noninfectious
	Lymphocytic-plasmacytic enteritis
	Hypereosinophilic syndrome
	Hemolytic disorders
	Neoplastic
	Mast cell tumor/mastocytosis
	Lymphosarcoma
	Multiple myeloma
	Myelo-lymphoproliferative disorders
	Malignant histiocytosis
	Nonneoplastic
	Amyloidosis
	Extramedullary hematopoiesis

Abbreviations: FeLV, feline leukemia virus; FIV, feline immunodeficiency virus.

History

The clinical signs and history of cats with splenomegaly often are vague and nonspecific, and may result from the underlying disease rather than the splenic enlargement. The history may identify anorexia, weight loss, weakness, abdominal enlargement, diarrhea, vomiting, and/or polyuria/polydipsia. Specific questions should address whether the cat lives strictly indoors, is allowed outdoors at times, and/or lives in a multicat household. This may determine the likelihood that the splenomegaly is caused by lymphoma or a myeloproliferative disease secondary to retroviral infection, and whether another infectious etiology should or should not be

considered. The signs of vomiting, diarrhea, and anorexia previously discussed could signal that the splenomegaly may be associated with gastrointestinal lymphoma, visceral mastocytosis/mast cell tumors (MCTs), feline infectious peritonitis, or lymphocytic-plasmacytic enteritis.

Physical Examination

Careful palpation of the abdomen to determine whether focal or generalized splenomegaly exists may narrow the list of differential diagnoses, and also could dictate which diagnostic tests are chosen initially. Attention to the size of the liver, abdominal lymph nodes, and the thickness of the intestinal wall may give additional information regarding the etiopathogenesis of the splenomegaly. Because abnormalities of, or size of, the spleen may be a "sentinel" for other systemic diseases, the clinician should pay close attention to the presence of other physical examination abnormalities such as edema, muffled heart sounds (pleural effusion), multiple dermal or subcutaneous nodules (Fig. 56–2), peripheral lymphadenopathy, heart murmurs, jaundice, and pallor of mucous membranes, because of their possible connection with the splenomegaly. Owing to the nature of the diseases that result in generalized splenomegaly, the cat may appear to be "systemically ill" and/or have an elevated temperature with these diseases more often than a patient with only focal splenic disease.

Diagnostic Tests

Figures 56–3 and 56–4 are algorithms for the selection and timing of appropriate tests for the feline patient with localized or generalized splenomegaly, respectively. Because generalized splenomegaly is more common, discussion focuses on this area, and the benefits/usage of the tests listed in both algorithms is discussed.

Routine laboratory testing in the patient with

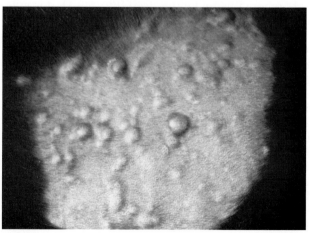

Figure 56–2. A 2 × 2 photomicrograph of the lateral thorax of a cat shows multiple, well-circumscribed dermal nodules typical of mast cell neoplasia.

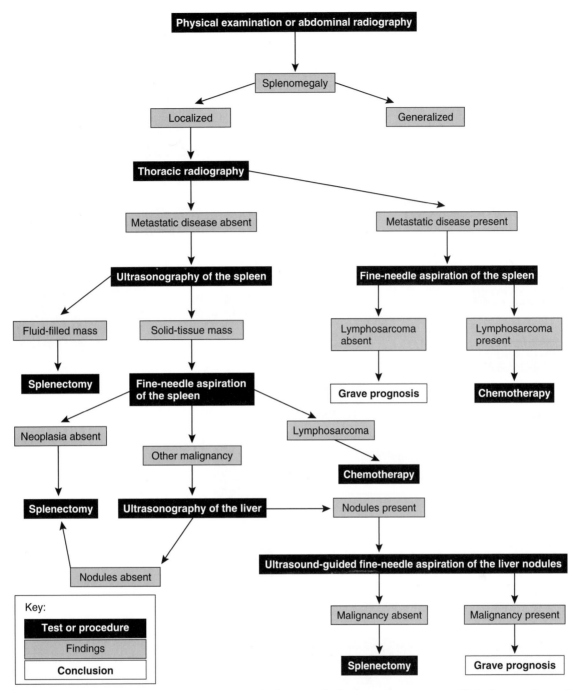

Figure 56–3. Algorithm of the clinical approach to localized splenomegaly. (Redrawn from Neer TM: Clinical approach to splenomegaly in dogs and cats. Compend Contin Educ Pract Vet 18:35–49, 1996.)

splenomegaly should include a hemogram and serum biochemical profile. These tests may not always result in a definitive diagnosis, but may direct further test selection. The erythrogram should be evaluated for anemia and for the presence of *Hemobartonella* organisms (see Chapter 2, Hemobartonellosis). If anemia is present, characterization as regenerative or non-regenerative is important so that the list of differential diagnoses may be narrowed. Splenomegaly and a regenerative anemia would be expected in a cat with hemoparasites (*Hemobartonella, Cytauxzoon*), immune-mediated

anemia, Heinz body anemias, methemoglobinemias, and possibly blood loss (splenomegaly would be unlikely in the latter situation). The presence of a non-regenerative anemia, with or without a corresponding macrocytosis, should lead one to investigate the feline leukemia virus (FeLV) and feline immunodeficiency virus status of the cat. The presence of bi- or pancytopenia or circulating blast cells warrants examination of a bone marrow aspirate. These findings would suggest diseases that result in infiltrative or myelophthisic disease such as bone marrow neoplasia (lymphoproliferative, myeloid,

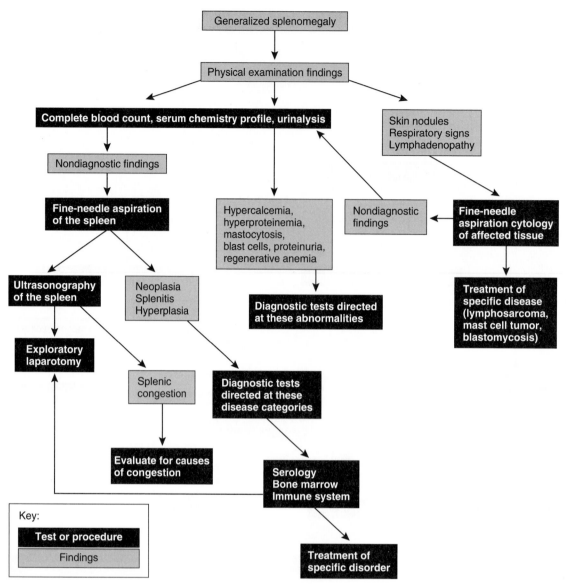

Generalized splenomegaly

↓

Physical examination findings

Complete blood count, serum chemistry profile, urinalysis

Skin nodules
Respiratory signs
Lymphadenopathy

Nondiagnostic findings

Fine-needle aspiration of the spleen

Hypercalcemia, hyperproteinemia, mastocytosis, blast cells, proteinuria, regenerative anemia

Nondiagnostic findings

Fine-needle aspiration cytology of affected tissue

Ultrasonography of the spleen

Neoplasia
Splenitis
Hyperplasia

Diagnostic tests directed at these abnormalities

Treatment of specific disease (lymphosarcoma, mast cell tumor, blastomycosis)

Exploratory laparotomy

Splenic congestion

Diagnostic tests directed at these disease categories

Evaluate for causes of congestion

**Serology
Bone marrow
Immune system**

Key:
Test or procedure
Findings

Treatment of specific disorder

Figure 56–4. Algorithm of the clinical approach to generalized splenomegaly. (Redrawn from Neer TM: Clinical approach to splenomegaly in dogs and cats. Compend Contin Educ Pract Vet 18:35–49, 1996.)

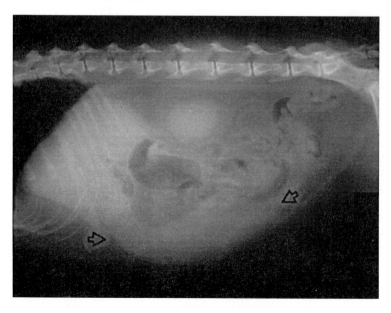

Figure 56–5. Lateral abdominal radiograph of a cat with splenic mastocytosis reveals massive splenic enlargement (*arrowheads* define the extent of the spleen).

erythremic myelosis), systemic mycoses (histoplasmosis), rickettsioses (cytauxzoonosis), or myelofibrosis. Pure red cell aplasia should be considered when only the red cell series is affected. The leukogram may reveal eosinophilia (suggestive of hypereosinophilic syndrome) or neutrophilic leukocytosis (suggestive of an inflammatory/infectious disease process). A buffy coat smear may be indicated to assess for peripheral mastocythemia.

The serum protein concentration, if elevated, may reflect possible underlying disease. Chronic inflammatory diseases, feline infectious peritonitis, and myeloma may cause hyperglobulinemia; serum protein electrophoresis subsequently is indicated to determine whether the increase is polyclonal or monoclonal in origin. Other findings on the chemistry panel should be pursued as they relate to the splenomegaly. For example, elevations in liver enzymes or azotemia in a cat with splenomegaly may indicate concurrent hepatic or renal lymphoma or feline infectious peritonitis.

Imaging of the spleen may include radiography and/or ultrasonography to determine whether there is focal or generalized enlargement (Fig. 56–5). These findings then will direct further diagnostic evaluation. Abdominal radiography often is not necessary in cats with splenomegaly, because abdominal palpation provides the same information in most cats. Ultrasonography allows for further assessment of the echogenicity of focal mass lesions and the spleen itself (Fig. 56–6). Nevertheless, palpation or radiography may identify associated abnormalities such as renomegaly, hepatomegaly, or mesenteric lymphadenopathy, which may reflect the same disease that is causing splenomegaly.

Based on the results of the laboratory evaluation and ultrasonography, a cytologic evaluation of the spleen often is indicated. Fine-needle aspiration (FNA) of an enlarged spleen is a safe, reliable method of evaluating patients with splenomegaly. The method apparently is safe even in patients with thrombocytopenia and other forms of coagulopathy.[4]

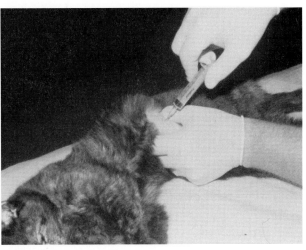

Figure 56–7. Positioning of a cat in right lateral recumbency for fine-needle aspiration of the spleen.

Diffusely enlarged spleens are aspirated readily by manual palpation, whereas focal masses are best aspirated with ultrasound guidance to ensure sampling the region of interest. A 25- or 23-gauge, ¾- to 1-inch needle and a 12-ml syringe is adequate equipment for use in cats. The cat should be positioned in right lateral recumbency (Fig. 56–7). The needle is introduced into the spleen, suction is applied 2 to 3 times without moving the needle, and then both needle and syringe are removed. Light sedation may be necessary to perform this technique.

Normal splenic cytology consists of small lymphocytes with an occasional neutrophil and large lymphocyte (Fig. 56–8). FNA may lead to a definitive diagnosis such as hematopoietic neoplasia (Figs. 56–9 and 56–10) or infectious disease (with identification of organisms) (Fig. 56–11). FNA is less effective in establishing a diagnosis in cases of focal splenomegaly than in patients with generalized splenomegaly. Also the clinician should not forget

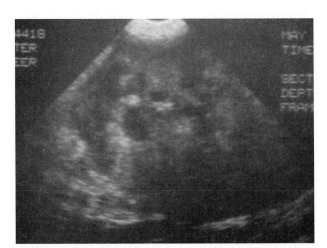

Figure 56–6. Transverse splenic ultrasonogram from a cat with splenic hemangiosarcoma. The multiple anechoic areas are consistent with hemangiosarcoma.

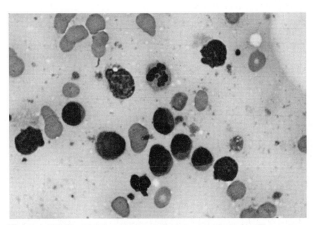

Figure 56–8. Cytologic appearance of a fine-needle aspirate from a normal spleen. Small lymphocytes predominate with an occasional neutrophil or large lymphocyte seen.

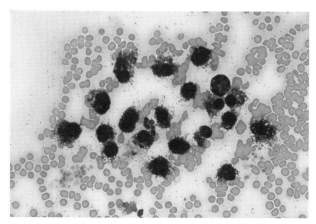

Figure 56–9. Cytologic evaluation of a fine-needle aspiration of the spleen reveals multiple large mast cells indicative of systemic mastocytosis.

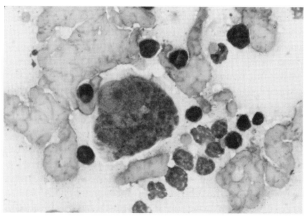

Figure 56–11. Fine-needle aspirate of a spleen reveals a macrophage containing schizonts of *Cytauxzoon felis*. (Courtesy of R. L. Cowell, Oklahoma State University.)

the potential diagnostic benefit of concurrent cytologic evaluation of other tissues such as dermal nodules (see Fig. 56–2), kidneys, liver, and/or lymph nodes (see Chapter 15, Cytologic Evaluation of Fine-Needle Liver Biopsies).

Finally, exploratory laparotomy may be indicated if a diagnosis has not been obtained with the tests discussed previously. Surgery should be preceded by thoracic radiographs to assess for metastatic disease. Surgery is indicated most commonly in situations in which focal splenic masses cannot be identified by FNA. If a focal splenic mass is identified, the entire spleen should be removed. At the time of removal, impression smears of the spleen and/or splenic mass should be performed before placing the spleen in formalin. Splenectomy may be therapeutic as well as diagnostic for cats with focal masses and MCTs (splenic mastocytosis).

Treatment

Because most of the diseases that cause generalized splenomegaly are systemic in nature (see Table 56–1), treatment should be directed at those specific diseases and not simply at the enlarged spleen. Conversely, the treatment of these diseases usually does

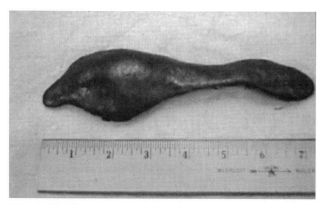

Figure 56–10. The spleen from which the aspirate was taken in Figure 56–9. Histopathologic diagnosis was splenic mastocytosis.

not require or include splenectomy. The 2 instances in which splenectomy might be beneficial in the feline patient is for lymphoreticular MCTs[5, 6] and possibly lymphoproliferative disease.[7]

Cats with lymphoreticular MCTs commonly have marked splenomegaly. Splenectomy is the treatment of choice for feline MCTs affecting the spleen; cats often survive for long periods even in the absence of other therapy.[5, 6] Median survival of cats after splenectomy is between 11 and 12 months; some survive more than 3 years from the time of splenectomy.[6] Response to splenectomy seems greater than would be explained by simple tumor-mass reduction alone, because hematologic and other organ involvements apparently resolve. It is possible that splenic suppressor-cell activity may be reduced after splenectomy, promoting some control of the tumor by the immune system. For this reason, the use of postoperative corticosteroids in these cats is controversial.[5]

Most cats with MCTs of the viscera vomit frequently from duodenal and gastric ulceration owing to chronic hyperhistaminemia. Intraoperative deaths have been reported after manipulation of the spleen during splenectomy, probably from release of vasoactive amines. For this reason, cats with MCTs should be treated before splenectomy with H_2 blockers (e.g., cimetidine 25 mg/kg orally every [q] 6 hr and diphenhydramine hydrochloride (2 mg/kg q 8 hr orally or intravenously [IV]) to reduce possible adverse effects of mast cell degranulation.

Combination chemotherapy using such agents as vincristine, cyclophosphamide, and methotrexate has not been shown to improve survival time in cats with lymphoreticular MCTs, and the indications for chemotherapy in the palliation of this disease are not well substantiated.[5, 8]

In cats with focal splenomegaly, the treatment usually consists of removal of the entire spleen. As mentioned, focal splenomegaly is less common than diffuse splenomegaly, and most often is due to neoplastic disease; however, abscess, hematoma, and infarction also may be seen.[9] Splenectomy often will be curative in cases of focal splenomegaly. The outcome of splenectomy would be determined by the tumor type in the spleen; for example, hemangiosarcoma would carry a more guarded prognosis than that of leiomyosarcoma.

◆ LYMPHADENOPATHY

Lymphadenopathy usually refers to enlargement in lymph node size. It may be due to lymphoid hyperplasia, lymphadenitis, or neoplasia (lymphoid or metastatic). In one study, neoplasia, hyperplasia, and inflammation made up 38.6, 24.8, and 15 per cent, respectively, of the histologic changes in 150 lymph node samples.[1] The remaining 21.6 per cent were lymphoid depletion (13.7 per cent), no lesions (5.2 per cent), congestion/edema (2 per cent), and amyloidosis (0.7 per cent). In addition, this study revealed that in the cases of neoplasia, lymphoma, carcinoma, MCT, and myelogenous leukemia accounted for 57.6, 23.7, 6.8, and 5.1 per cent, respectively, of the neoplasms found in excised feline lymph nodes. Because these numbers were generated from a referral institution, they may underrepresent cases of lymphadenitis in the general practice setting, given the propensity for cats to develop bite abscesses and resultant suppurative lymphadenitis.

The lymph node has 2 primary functions: (1) to filter and retain particulate matter brought to it by the afferent lymphatics and (2) to participate in the immune response. The lymph node brings all of the cell types (macrophages, B cells, T cells) necessary for immune response and antibody production together in close proximity. Therefore, a lymph node may enlarge (1) as a result of its response to antigens with proliferation of the normal immune cells, (2) owing to neoplastic proliferation of these normal immune cells, (3) because of infiltration with neoplastic cells resulting from drainage of a local malignant process such as squamous cell carcinoma, and/or (4) from miscellaneous causes.

Clinical Approach

With this basic understanding of the etiologies of lymphadenopathies in cats, how should the clinician approach and solve this problem? An algorithmic approach may be useful when evaluating the feline patient with lymphadenopathy (Fig. 56–12) (specific comments for each of the categories are addressed in the text).

The owner may present a cat for evaluation because she or he finds a "lump" (an enlarged lymph node) while petting the cat, but more frequently, the cat is presented for other complaints and the lymphadenopathy is found by the veterinarian on physical examination. Lymphadenopathy must be assessed in light of the presenting complaint, history, and other physical examination and laboratory findings.

History

Geographic location may determine the likelihood of infectious diseases peculiar to various regions of the United States and other countries; for example, fungal diseases such as histoplasmosis and blastomycosis are endemic in the Ohio and Mississippi river valleys, and sylvatic plague is found in Arizona, New Mexico, and California. Whether the cat is strictly indoors or not also may increase or decrease the likelihood of an infectious disease. The author cautions the reader in excluding infectious disease solely on the basis that the cat is strictly indoors. He has diagnosed cryptococcosis in several "strictly" indoor cats either because they sat in windows or because they went out onto screened-in patios that were close to bird-feeders and were exposed to pigeon droppings (see Chapter 6, Cryptococcosis: New Perspectives on Etiology, Pathogenesis, Diagnosis, and Clinical Management). One should always keep in mind the manner in which infectious diseases are acquired, and ask historical questions that assess this possible acquisition. The owner should be questioned regarding the cat's vaccination history, and especially whether vaccines have been administered recently.

Physical Examination

The lymph nodes superficially palpable in normal cats include the mandibular, superficial cervical, popliteal, and possibly inguinal; in addition, the ileocecocolic node often can be palpated in normal cats. All of these nodes, but especially the superficial cervical, inguinal, and ileocecocolic nodes, are more difficult to palpate than in dogs. If they are "readily" palpable, the clinician should be concerned that they are truly enlarged. In the obese cat, excessive fat surrounding the lymph node may give the clinician the impression that the node is enlarged; however, the examiner usually can palpate the firmer lymph node in the center of the softer fat.

The clinician should determine whether the lymph node enlargement is local, regional, or generalized. Local and regional lymphadenopathy suggests inflammation in the area drained by the node(s) or local/regional tumor metastasis, and a thorough evaluation of that specific anatomic region should be performed. In most cases, a visible or palpable lesion is obvious. Generalized lymphadenopathy suggests systemic lymphadenitis (i.e., systemic infectious disease), immune response, or lymphosarcoma. Even though peripheral lymphadenopathy is uncommon in cats with lymphoma, local, regional, or generalized enlargement may be seen. Also, in cats with mediastinal lymphoma, the neoplastic lymph node may protrude through the thoracic inlet, making it readily palpable (see Chapter 68, Evaluation and Treatment of Cranial Mediastinal Masses). An additional clue on physical examination that mediastinal lymphoma may exist is the

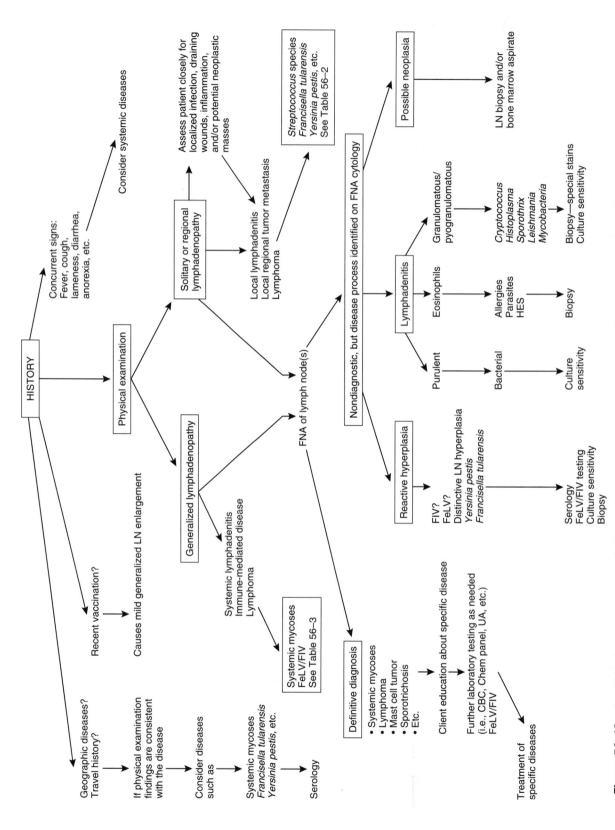

Figure 56–12. Algorithm for approach to lymphadenopathy. CBC, complete blood count; FeLV, feline leukemia virus; FIV, feline immunodeficiency virus; FNA, fine-needle aspiration; HES, hypereosinophilic syndrome; LN, lymph node; UA, urinalysis.

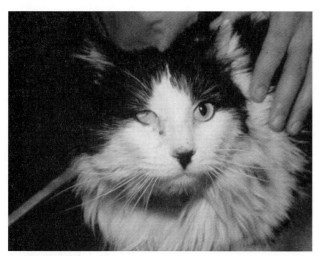

Figure 56–13. Domestic longhair cat with right-sided Horner's syndrome (sympathetic denervation to the eye) secondary to mediastinal lymphoma.

presence of Horner's syndrome (unilateral or bilateral) (Fig. 56–13). Any cat with Horner's syndrome (sympathetic denervation to the eye), and especially one with coexisting respiratory distress, should undergo thoracic radiography (Fig. 56–14). Finally, if

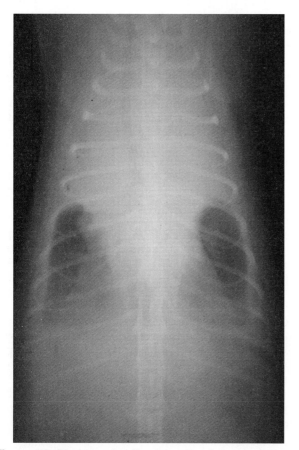

Figure 56–14. Ventrodorsal radiograph of the cat in Figure 56–13 reveals a large anterior mediastinal mass and mild pleural effusion. Fine-needle aspiration of the mass was diagnostic of lymphoma.

the lymph node is painful or warm, an acute inflammatory process (i.e., an infectious disease) should be considered most likely, and marked lymph node enlargement unaccompanied by pain usually reflects lymphoid neoplasia.

Diagnostic Approach

After the history and physical examination, the most direct and noninvasive method for lymph node evaluation is FNA. It is quick, easy, effective, inexpensive, and a virtually risk-free way to gain valuable diagnostic information.[10] In some cases, the findings establish a definitive diagnosis such as lymphosarcoma, cryptococcosis, or histoplasmosis. In other cases, the findings may aid in determining the underlying disease process, and may prompt the selection of other diagnostic procedures that may be effective in establishing a diagnosis. The reader is referred to an excellent discussion on lymph node cytology by Tyler and Cowell.[10] Based on the FNA results, further testing may include some of the following: hemogram with platelet count, biochemistry profile, urinalysis, urine culture and sensitivity, bone marrow aspiration, FeLV/feline immunodeficiency virus testing, radiology/ultrasonography, protein electrophoresis, infectious disease serology, and/or excisional lymph node biopsy.

Selected Diseases of the Lymph Nodes

This section discusses some selected diseases of the lymph nodes with a focus on diseases that probably are considered less frequently by the veterinarian. This section is certainly not all-inclusive, and the reader is referred to other texts for the remainder of the diseases listed in Tables 56–2 and 56–3.

Distinctive Peripheral Lymph Node Hyperplasia of Young Cats

Fourteen young cats (age range, 5 months to 2 years) have been reported with peripheral lymphadenopathy secondary to a distinctive hyperplasia that may be associated with FeLV infection.[11] There was no gender predisposition, and all peripheral lymph nodes were enlarged in 12 of the 14 cats. In the other 2, 1 had mandibular and popliteal enlargement and the other only had mandibular node enlargement. Nodes were judged to be 2 to 3 times normal size, with the largest measuring 6 cm in diameter. Eight of the cats were clinically normal on initial examination except for lymphadenopathy, and the remaining 6 had a combination of clinical signs that included fever, lethargy, anorexia, pale mucous membranes, hematuria, eczema, vomiting, and mastitis. Vaccination did not appear to play a role because vaccines had not been given within 4 months of the onset of signs.

Clinicopathologic abnormalities included ane-

Table 56–2. Causes of Single or Regional Lymphadenopathy

Infectious Etiology	Noninfectious Etiology
Bacterial	***Idiopathic***
Yersinia pestis	Distinctive lymph node
Corynebacterium species	hyperplasia
Streptococcus species	Plexiform vascularization of
Staphylococcus species	lymph nodes
Mycobacterium species	
Nocardia species	***Localized Inflammation***
Actinomyces species	
Francisella tularensis	***Neoplastic***
	Hemolymphatic neoplasms
Mycotic	Metastatic neoplasms
Histoplasma capsulatum	
Blastomyces dermatitidis	***Nonneoplastic***
Cryptococcus neoformans	Eosinophilic granuloma
Sporothrix schenckii	complex
Phycomycosis	
Viral	
Feline immunodeficiency	
virus	
Feline infectious peritonitis	
Feline leukemia virus	
Rickettsial/Parasitic	
Ehrlichiosis	
Hemobartonellosis	
Cytauxzoonosis	
Toxoplasmosis	

mia, neutrophilic leukocytosis, lymphocytosis, and hypergammaglobulinemia in some of the cats. Nine of 14 cats were tested for FeLV, and 6 were positive. The histologic changes in the lymph nodes were similar to those seen in some cats after experimental infection with FeLV. This suggests that the inciting cause may be viral. Lymph node excisional biopsy is needed to separate this disease from other causes of lymphadenopathy, such as lymphoma in the FeLV-positive cat.

The outcome in 10 of the 14 cats was known. Two cats were euthanized owing to their positive

Table 56–3. Causes of Generalized Lymphadenopathy

Infectious	Noninfectious
Bacterial	***Immune-Mediated***
Yersinia pestis	Chronic progressive
Francisella tularensis	polyarthritis
Streptococcus species	
	Neoplastic
Viral	Lymphoma
Feline infectious peritonitis	Myelo-lymphoproliferative
virus	disease
Feline leukemia virus	Myeloma
Feline immunodeficiency	Mast cell tumor
virus	
Postvaccinal response	***Nonneoplastic***
	Hypereosinophilic syndrome
	Distinctive lymph node
	hyperplasia

FeLV status, and the remaining 8 were followed for up to 5 years. Of these 8, 6 had resolution of the initial lymphadenopathy over a 2-week to 7-month period. One of these 8 cats developed mediastinal lymphoma, and 1 had recurrence of the distinctive lymphadenopathy periodically over 5 years.

Generalized Lymphadenopathy Resembling Lymphoma

Six cats have been described with prominent generalized lymphadenopathy that, on excisional lymph node biopsy, had histologic features similar to those of lymphoma.[12] The interesting clinical feature was that 5 of 6 cats had regression of the lymphadenopathy within 1 to 17 weeks (1 cat was euthanized after an initial diagnosis of lymphoma).

The age of these cats ranged from 1 to 4 years; 3 cats were Maine coons and the other 3 were domestic shorthair cats. Four cats were evaluated initially for signs of upper respiratory disease or urinary tract infection. The other 2 cats were from households with known FeLV-positive cats, and were evaluated because of lymphadenopathy that had developed 10 to 12 months after exposure. The lymph nodes were firm and 2 to 3 cm in diameter.

Clinicopathologic findings revealed that 4 cats had elevated white blood cell counts, and 1 had a low count (range, 4800 to 26,000/mm³). Follow-up complete blood counts over a 2-month period showed that 4 cats retained an elevated count, and that 2 of this group had atypical lymphocytes and/or lymphocytosis. Bone marrow cytology was normal in the 2 cats in which it was performed. Results of FeLV tests in 5 cats were negative (no FeLV antigen detected). The two cats from the FeLV-positive households had neutralizing antibody titers greater than 1:10 for FeLV and 1:32 for feline oncornavirus cell membrane antigen, consistent with previous transient infection with FeLV.

The lymph nodes of these cats had some histopathologic features consistent with lymphoma, but there also were features that did not indicate malignancy, including: (1) abundant nodal vascularity, (2) primary and secondary follicles with active germinal centers, (3) mixed cells, especially lymphoid cells including plasma cells, histiocytes, and granulocytes, (4) lack of capsular invasion, and (5) lack of high-grade anaplastic changes, or high rate of mitotic activity in the lymphoid cells.

Owing to the questionable nature of the clinical and histologic features, none of the 5 cats was treated, and reduction of peripheral lymphadenopathy was observed over a period of 5 to 120 days. The 5 cats were alive and had no clinical signs 12 to 84 months after diagnosis of lymphadenopathy, thus supporting a diagnosis of nonmalignant lymphadenopathy.

Plexiform Vascularization of Lymph Nodes

An unusual cause of solitary lymphadenopathy reported in cats is plexiform vascularization of the lymph nodes.[13, 14] Affected cats ranged from 3 to 14 years of age, and were clinically normal other than the problem of unilateral solitary lymphadenopathy. The lymph nodes affected most commonly were in the cervical and inguinal regions. The 2 cats with inguinal lymphadenopathy had bilateral involvement.

Histologically, the disease is characterized by replacement of the interfollicular pulp by a plexiform proliferation of small capillary-sized vessels. Decreased numbers of lymphoid cells accompany the vascular changes. The etiology of this vascular change is unknown; however, affected cats remain healthy after surgical removal of the diseased nodes.

Plague and Tularemia

Plague (*Yersinia pestis*) and tularemia (*Francisella tularenesis*) are 2 infectious diseases that may result in regional or generalized lymphadenopathy and appear very similar clinically. Whereas plague has a more geographic distribution to the western United States,[15] tularemia may be seen throughout the United States; however, an endemic area in Fairbanks, Alaska, has been reported.[16] Both of the diseases are more common in the warmer months. Owing to the significant zoonotic potential of these 2 diseases, the clinician always should be on the alert when a cat is presented with lymphadenopathy. Both of these diseases should be considered when the triad of lethargy, anorexia, and fever are found in conjunction with enlarged lymph nodes. The reader is referred to a detailed discussion of plague by Gasper.[15] With plague, the mandibular lymph nodes are affected more commonly, whereas with tularemia, the retropharyngeal, superior cervical, and mesenteric nodes (revealed as multiple firm masses on abdominal palpation) are affected most often.[17, 18] In addition, abscess formation is more likely to occur with plague than with tularemia.

A definitive diagnosis of plague or tularemia may require 1 or all of the following tests: (1) fluorescent antibody testing of lymph node or abscess aspirates, (2) culture and sensitivity (blood, lymph node, abscess, bone marrow), which is the most definitive test, and/or (3) serology. For plague, a single titer of 1:32 or greater is very suspicious for active disease. A 4-fold increase in 10 to 14 days is needed to confirm *Y. pestis* infection because cats from endemic areas frequently have high titers to *Y. pestis* that persist for a year or longer after exposure.[19] In tularemia, a negative titer is considered to be less than 1:20 (microagglutination), but again a 4-fold increase is needed to truly confirm a diagnosis.

The decision to treat for plague is seldom based on a definitive diagnosis, owing to the delay in receiving laboratory test results. Therefore, when plague is suspected based on clinical and/or epidemiologic history, specific antibiotic therapy should be instituted immediately because initiation of antibiotic therapy 24 hours after the onset of the pneumonic or septicemic forms of the disease appears to be of little benefit.[15] Antibiotics that are effective include tetracyclines, chloramphenicol, aminoglycosides, and trimethoprim-sulfamethoxazole. A more detailed discussion on treatment and management of cats with plague can be found in the paper by Gasper.[15]

The drugs of choice for treating tularemia include streptomycin, gentamicin, and tetracycline, and possibly amoxicillin-clavulanic acid or enrofloxacin.[18]

REFERENCES

1. Hammer AS, Couto CG: Disorders of the lymph nodes and spleen. *In* Sherding RG (ed): The Cat: Diseases and Clinical Management, 2nd ed. vol. 1. New York, Churchill Livingstone, 1994, p. 671.
2. Court EA, Earnest-Koons KA, Barr SC, et al: Malignant histiocytosis in a cat. J Am Vet Med Assoc 203:1300–1302, 1993.
3. Freeman L, Stevens J, Loughman C, et al: Malignant histiocytosis in a cat. J Vet Intern Med 9:171–173, 1995.
4. O'Keefe DA, Couto CG: Fine-needle aspiration of the spleen as an aid in the diagnosis of splenomegaly. J Vet Intern Med 1:102–109, 1987.
5. Ogilvie GK, Moore AS: Mast cell tumors. *In* Ogilvie GK, Moore AS (eds): Managing the Veterinary Cancer Patient, 1st ed. Trenton, Veterinary Learning Systems, 1995, p. 512.
6. Liska WD, MacEwen EG, Zaki FA, et al: Feline systemic mastocytosis: A review and results of splenectomy in seven cases. J Am Anim Hosp Assoc 15:589–597, 1979.
7. Brooks MB, Matus RE, Leifer CE, et al: Use of splenectomy in the management of lymphoma in dogs: 16 cases (1976–1985). J Am Vet Med Assoc 191:1008–1010, 1987.
8. Elmslie RE, Ogilvie GK: Variables in behavior and management of mast cell tumors. *In* August JR (ed): Consultations in Feline Internal Medicine, vol. 2. Philadelphia, WB Saunders, 1994, p. 567.
9. Spangler WL, Gilbertson MR: Prevalence and type of splenic diseases in cats: 455 cases (1985–1991). J Am Vet Med Assoc 201:773–776, 1992.
10. Tyler RD, Cowell RL: Diagnostic approach to lymph node disorders. *In* August JR (ed): Consultations in Feline Internal Medicine, vol. 1. Philadelphia, WB Saunders, 1991, p. 367.
11. Moore FM, Emerson WE, Cotter SM, et al: Distinctive peripheral lymph node hyperplasia of young cats. Vet Pathol 23:386–391, 1986.
12. Mooney SC, Patnaik AK, Hayes AA, et al: Generalized lymphadenopathy resembling lymphoma in cats: Six cases (1972–1976). J Am Vet Med Assoc 190:897–900, 1977.
13. Lucke VM, Davies JD, Wood CM, et al: Plexiform vascularization of lymph nodes: An unusual but distinctive lymphadenopathy in cats. J Comp Pathol 97:109–119, 1987.
14. Welsh EM, Griffon D, Whitbread TJ: Plexiform vascularization of a retropharyngeal lymph node in a cat. J Small Anim Pract 40:291–293, 1999.
15. Gasper PW: Plague. *In* August JR (ed): Consultations in Feline Internal Medicine, vol. 3. Philadelphia, WB Saunders, 1997, p. 12.
16. Liles WC, Burger RJ: Tularemia from domestic cats. West J Med 158:619–622, 1993.
17. Baldwin CJ, Panciera RJ, Morton RJ, et al: Acute tularemia in three domestic cats. J Am Vet Med Assoc 199:1602–1605, 1991.
18. Woods JP, Crystal MA, Morton RJ, et al: Tularemia in two cats. J Am Vet Med Assoc 212:81–83, 1998.
19. Macy DW: Plague. *In* Greene CE (ed): Infectious Diseases of the Dog and Cat, 2nd ed. Philadelphia, WB Saunders, 1998, p. 295.

57

◆ Mucopolysaccharidosis

Mary Anna Thrall

Lysosomal storage diseases are inherited disorders in which substances accumulate in lysosomes, leading to cellular dysfunction. Lysosomal enzymes are responsible for degrading many substrates found in cells, and almost all lysosomal storage disorders are due to a functional deficiency of a specific enzyme required for the catabolism of lipids, mucopolysaccharides (glycosaminoglycans [GAGs]), glycogen, or glycoprotein. However, a few storage disorders are due to the production of dysfunctional proteins other than enzymes.[1, 2] Most storage disorders are inherited as autosomal recessive traits, and result from mutations in the coding sequence of a protein. Lysosomal storage disorders and other "inborn errors of metabolism" have been of utmost importance in the understanding of the genetic, biochemical, and molecular bases of disease, as well as normal physiology, because the role of enzymes and other proteins often becomes apparent only through the consequences of their absence.

Cats that have lysosomal storage disorders serve as "animal models of human disease" and are used extensively to study the pathophysiologic and molecular basis of disease, as well as to evaluate various modes of therapy.[1] These studies, while providing useful information for human beings, also have contributed knowledge pertaining to feline medicine. To date, at least 12 different lysosomal storage diseases have been described in cats, including globoid-cell leukodystrophy (Krabbe's disease),[3] GM_1 gangliosidosis,[4-10] GM_2 gangliosidosis,[11-15] alpha mannosidosis,[16-21] Niemann-Pick disease type A,[22-27] Niemann-Pick disease type C,[28-30] a putative case of glycogen storage disease II (acid maltase deficiency or "Pompe's disease"),[31] acid lipase deficiency (cholesterol ester storage disease),[32] mucolipidosis II,[33, 34] and mucopolysaccharidoses (MPSs) I,[35-37] VI,[38-47] and VII.[48, 49] The reader is referred to Chapter 77, Molecular Diagnosis of Gangliosidoses: A Model for Elimination of Inherited Diseases in Pure Breeds, for a detailed discussion of the molecular diagnosis of the gangliosidoses affecting Korat cats.

The MPSs are a group of heritable lysosomal storage disorders caused by deficiency of lysosomal enzymes needed for the stepwise degradation of GAGs, also referred to as mucopolysaccharides. Depending on the type of enzyme deficiency, the catabolism of dermatan sulfate, heparan sulfate, keratan sulfate, chondroitin sulfate, or hyaluronan may be blocked, singly, or in combination.[50-52] In human beings and animals with MPS, undegraded GAGs accumulate in lysosomes, resulting in progressive cell, tissue, and organ dysfunction,[51, 53, 54] and phenotypic abnormalities, including facial dysmorphia (Fig. 57–1).

◆ HISTORICAL BACKGROUND

MPS was first described in children in 1917.[55] In 1952, the term *mucopolysaccharidoses* was coined for these disorders after excessive mucopolysaccharide was found in the liver and meninges of a patient.[56] In 1957, increased urinary excretion of mucopolysaccharides was reported,[57] which is now the basis of a commonly used screening test. In 1968, abnormal metabolism of mucopolysaccharides in cultured fibroblasts from affected patients was corrected by coculture with normal cells due to a "corrective factor" released in the culture medium.[58] These corrective factors were soon found to be lysosomal enzymes.[59, 60] At least 11 different enzyme deficiencies that cause MPS have now been reported in human beings.[51, 61] Clinical and biochemical characteristics of the different types of MPS depend on the specific lysosomal enzyme deficiency, the type of GAG stored, and the tissues in which storage occurs. Currently, most of the research in this area is aimed at isolation of genes and cDNAs encoding lysosomal enzymes, mutation analysis underlying the various types of MPS (see Chapter 77, Molecular Diagnosis of Gangliosidoses: A Model for Elimination of Inherited Diseases in Pure Breeds), and therapy.

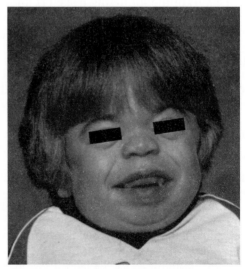

Figure 57–1. A 7-year-old child with mucopolysaccharidosis (MPS) I. The typical facial dysmorphia is present.

Table 57–1. Classification of the Feline Mucopolysaccharidoses

Number	Eponym in Human Beings	Enzyme Deficiency	GAG(s) Stored
MPS I	Hurler's syndrome	Alpha-L-iduronidase	Dermatan sulfate Heparan sulfate
MPS VI	Maroteaux-Lamy syndrome	Arylsulfatase B (N-acetylgalactosamine 4-sulfatase)	Dermatan sulfate Chondroitin sulfates
MPS VII	Sly's syndrome	Beta-glucuronidase	Dermatan sulfate Heparan sulfate Chondroitin sulfates

Abbreviations: GAG, glycosaminoglycan; MPS, mucopolysaccharidosis.

◆ FELINE MUCOPOLYSACCHARIDOSIS

Feline MPS was first described in 1976, in a Siamese cat born of a mother-son mating.[38] Three types of MPS (I, VI, and VII) have been described in cats to date.[35–50, 53, 54, 62, 63] Enzyme deficiencies and types of GAG stored in feline MPS are summarized in Table 57–1. Storage of GAG results in features common to most types of MPS, including dwarfism (except feline MPS I), severe bone disease, degenerative joint disease, facial dysmorphia, hepatomegaly (except feline MPS VI), corneal clouding, excess urinary excretion of GAG, and metachromatic granules in blood leukocytes (subtle in MPS I). Disease is progressive, with clinical signs usually apparent at 2 to 4 months of age. Affected animals may live several years, but locomotor difficulty is progressive. Central nervous system disease is not clinically apparent in any of the types of MPS reported in cats, although neuronal storage is evident microscopically. All of the types of MPS described in cats are inherited as autosomal recessive traits. The characteristic clinical and pathologic features of each type of feline MPS are described later, and important clinical and laboratory findings are summarized in Table 57–2.

◆ MUCOPOLYSACCHARIDOSIS VI (ARYLSULFATASE B DEFICIENCY)

Since the first description of mucopolysaccharidosis VI in a Siamese cat in 1976,[38, 39] numerous unrelated affected cats, including Siamese, domestic longhair,

and longhaired Siamese, have been identified.[40–44, 64, 65] Several breeding colonies have been developed for research, and the disease has been well characterized.[41, 42, 50, 54, 62, 63] Clinical features include small body size (Fig. 57–2), corneal clouding, which is usually detectable by 8 weeks of age (Figs. 57–3 and 57–4), flattened broad face, broad maxilla, slightly thickened eyelids, short ears and nose, large paws, and a progressively abnormal gait. The facial dysmorphia is particularly evident in Siamese cats, which normally have an elongated face (Fig. 57–5). Some MPS VI cats develop posterior paresis, usually between 6 and 8 months of age, owing to spinal cord compression.[66] Occasionally, affected cats have an atypical-sounding meow. A less severe type of feline MPS VI has been described recently, in which affected cats have normal growth and appearance, but have biochemical and microscopic characteristics of MPS VI.[67, 68]

Radiographic Findings

Radiographic abnormalities increase in severity with age, and include osteoporosis, shortened vertebral bodies with bony proliferation on their caudoventral border, lengthening of the intervertebral spaces, and broadening of the ribs at the costochondral junction with the costal cartilage being convex at the caudal sternebral section. Metaphyseal and epiphyseal areas of long bones have bony proliferation with irregular articular surfaces. Coxofemoral joints usually are bilaterally subluxated with shallow irregular acetabula. Femoral heads usually are flattened (Fig. 57–6). The skulls show evidence of increased width between the zygomatic arches, and

Table 57–2. Clinical and Laboratory Features of Feline Mucopolysaccharidosis I, VI, and VII and Mucolipidosis II

Feature	MPS I	MPS VI	MPS VII	Mucolipidosis II
Skeletal abnormalities	+	+	+	+
Dwarfism	−	+	+	+
Corneal clouding	+	+	+	−
Hepatomegaly	+	−	+	−
Neutrophil granulation	±	+	+	−
Urine GAG	+	+	+	−

Abbreviations: GAG, glycosaminoglycan; MPS, mucopolysaccharidosis; +, present; −, not present.

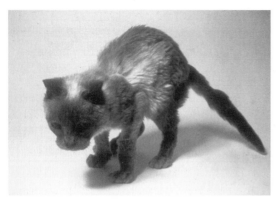

Figure 57–2. A 3-year-old cat with MPS VI. The typical crouched gait is present.

shortening from the nose to the posterior of the skull.[69] Decreased bone density also is evident when measured by dual-energy x-ray absorptiometry.[70]

Pathologic Findings

The gross pathology includes bony proliferations at the epiphyses, and in cats with posterior paresis, bony proliferations into the spinal canal that impinge on the spinal cord. Heart valves usually are thickened. Hepatosplenomegaly is not observed. The microscopic feature common to all MPSs is vacuolation or granulation of connective tissue cells, hepatocytes, and leukocytes. Neutrophils contain metachromatic granules, referred to as Alder-Reilly bodies, which are GAG-filled lysosomes (Fig. 57–7). Lymphocytes and macrophages sometimes are vacuolated, and a small metachromatic inclusion often is present within the vacuole. GAG inclusions in liver, bone marrow aspirates, and joint fluid are very apparent (Figs. 57–8 to 57–10). Ultrastructural studies have shown vacuoles and granules to be lysosomes containing GAG and lipid (Fig. 57–11). Many of the described light microscopic and ultrastructural pathologic findings in MPS VI–affected cats have been related to eye[71–76] and bone.[77–80] Corneal clouding is due to storage of GAG

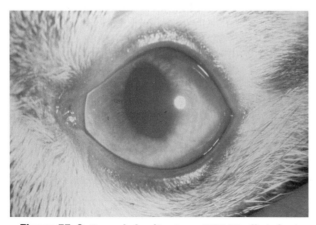

Figure 57–3. Corneal clouding in an MPS VI–affected cat.

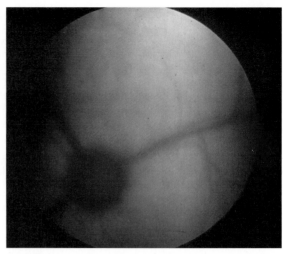

Figure 57–4. Appearance of the optic disc and vessels of an MPS VI–affected cat, as viewed through the cloudy cornea.

in stromal keratocytes, resulting in structural alterations that include abnormal spacing, size, and arrangement of collagen fibrils.[76] Histopathologic lesions in bone consist of severe osteopenia, with fewer, finer trabeculae than normal.[77–80] The GAG stored in feline MPS VI is predominantly dermatan sulfate, although chondroitin sulfate is stored excessively in some tissues, including bone and kidney.[52] Feline arylsulfatase B enzyme has been characterized, as have the abnormal properties of the enzyme from MPS VI–affected cats.[81–83] The genetic mutations resulting in feline MPS VI have been identified.[45–47, 62]

◆ MUCOPOLYSACCHARIDOSIS I (ALPHA-L-IDURONIDASE DEFICIENCY)

MPS I was first described in a domestic shorthair cat in 1979,[35] and has been well-characterized.[36, 50, 53, 62, 63, 76] Clinical features are similar to those seen in MPS VI–affected cats, and include an abnormally shaped face, comprising a broad short maxilla, frontal bossing, wide-spaced eyes, depressed nasal bridge, and small ears. Dwarfing is not seen. Corneal clouding is diffuse and bilateral. Radiographic features include bilateral hip subluxation, fusions of cervical vertebrae, and pectus excavatum. Skeletal abnormalities are less severe in cats with MPS I than in those with MPS VI. No neurologic abnormalities are apparent, although inclusions are present in neurons. A high incidence of meningiomas has been reported in young affected cats in a research breeding colony.[36, 84] These tumors were incidental findings at necropsy, and were not associated with clinical signs. MPS I–affected cats can live for several years and reproduce. Gross pathologic features include mild hepatosplenomegaly and thickening of mitral valve leaflets in chordae tendineae. Cytoplasmic vacuolation of chondrocytes, fibroblasts,

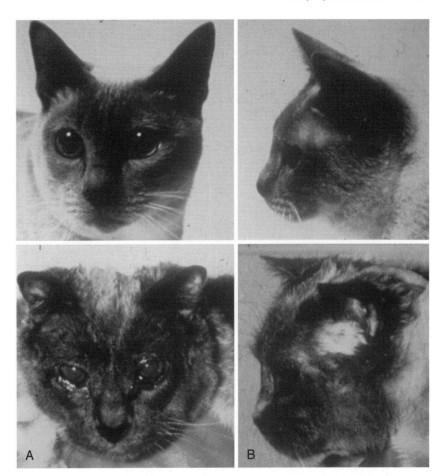

Figure 57–5. *A* and *B*, An MPS VI–affected Siamese cat with facial dysmorphia (*bottom*). Note the short ears and flat, broad face. The normal sibling of this cat (*top*).

hepatocytes, keratocytes, smooth-muscle cells, and neurons are apparent by light microscopy, and granular and lamellar inclusions can be seen by electron microscopy.[36] The GAGs stored are dermatan and heparan sulfate. The mutation causing MPS I in cats has been described and characterized recently.[37]

◆ MUCOPOLYSACCHARIDOSIS VII (BETA-GLUCURONIDASE DEFICIENCY)

MPS VII was first described in 1994 in a domestic shorthair cat from Switzerland,[48] and more recently in a domestic shorthair cat from California.[49] Clinical and radiologic features are similar to those seen in cats with MPS VI, including dwarfism, flat broad face, corneal clouding, large paws, difficulty walking, epiphyseal dysplasia, easily luxated patellas, and subluxation of coxofemoral joints. However, the 2 cats with MPS VII had hepatomegaly, and their clinical abnormalities were more severe than those that are seen typically with MPS VI. The cat from Switzerland developed grand mal seizures, was unable to walk by 6 months of age, and was euthanized at that time. The cat from California had difficulty walking by the age of 16 weeks, was paraparetic at 6 months of age, and died at 21 months of age.

Light and electron microscopic features also are

similar to those found in MPS VI cats, and include granulated neutrophils and vacuolated lymphocytes and macrophages on blood films (Fig. 57–12), and vacuolation of cells, which on electron microscopic examination appears as flocculent material (GAG) within lysosomes of most tissues examined.

◆ DIFFERENTIAL DIAGNOSIS

Mucolipidosis II

Cats with another lysosomal storage disease, mucolipidosis II (I-cell disease), may appear very similar to cats with MPS. Mucolipidosis II was reported in a 7-month-old domestic shorthair cat from Switzerland in 1996.[33, 34] This cat exhibited dwarfism, abnormal gait, large paws, flat broad face with frontal bossing, a depressed nasal bridge, short ears, and thickened eyelids, features that are very suggestive of MPS. Radiographic findings included subluxated patellas and elbows, dorsal fusion of the cervical spine, and bilateral luxation of the femoral heads. Unlike in MPS, the skin was extremely stiff, the corneas were clear, no granules were present in neutrophils, and no GAG was present in the urine.

Mucolipidosis II results from the abnormal transport of lysosomal enzymes, due to a deficiency of a Golgi enzyme (GlcNAc-phosphotransferase) that is

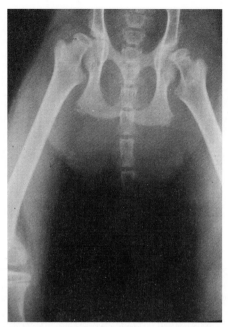

Figure 57–6. Radiograph of the pelvis of an MPS VI–affected cat demonstrates subluxated coxofemoral joints with shallow irregular acetabuli and flattened femoral heads.

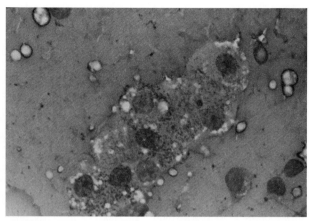

Figure 57–8. Liver aspirate from an MPS VI–affected cat. Note the numerous granules, which represent glycosaminoglycan (GAG)-filled lysosomes. Wright stain.

responsible for the mannose-6-phosphate recognition site that directs most lysosomal enzymes to lysosomes. Affected cells are thus deficient in numerous lysosomal enzymes, and various kinds of macromolecules are stored in lysosomes, resulting in inclusions in cells, thus the name inclusion (I)-cell disease.[34] GlcNAc-phosphotransferase activity was markedly decreased in the cat's leukocytes and cultured fibroblasts. The cultured fibroblast activity of several lysosomal enzymes, including alpha-L-iduronidase and arylsulfatase B, was decreased, although serum activity of several lysosomal enzymes, including alpha-L-iduronidase, arylsulfatase B, and beta-glucuronidase, was markedly increased, findings that help differentiate mucolipidosis from

the MPSs. Storage was evident on light and electron microscopy in mesenchymal tissues, and unlike in the MPSs, parenchymal cells were free of storage. Ultrastructurally, inclusions were varied in morphology, suggesting that lysosomes held not only GAG, but also oligosaccharides and lipids. Clinical and laboratory features are summarized in Table 57–2.

Other Differential Diagnoses

Whereas the radiographic appearance of MPS is quite characteristic, other disorders with similarities include congenital hypothyroidism, epiphyseal dysplasia, multiple cartilaginous exostoses, and hypervitaminosis A.[85, 86] Interestingly, the first case of MPS was misdiagnosed initially as hypervitaminosis A.[38]

Corneal clouding may be present in numerous other lysosomal storage diseases including acid lipase deficiency, GM$_1$ and GM$_2$ gangliosidosis, and alpha-mannosidosis. Corneal edema and corneal

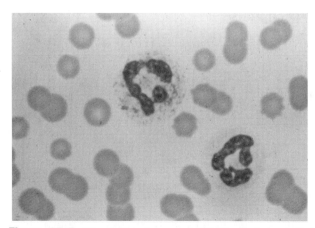

Figure 57–7. Blood film from an MPS VI–affected cat that has been treated with bone marrow transplantation. The upper neutrophil contains granules (Alder-Reilly bodies); the lower neutrophil is a donor-derived normal neutrophil with no granules. Wright stain.

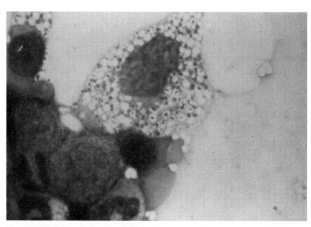

Figure 57–9. Bone marrow aspirate from an MPS VI–affected cat. Note the large macrophage filled with vacuoles containing small metachromatic granules. Wright stain.

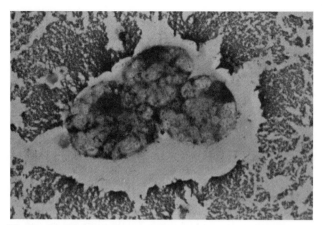

Figure 57–10. Joint fluid from an MPS VI–affected cat. Note the 3 large mononuclear cells filled with GAG. Wright stain.

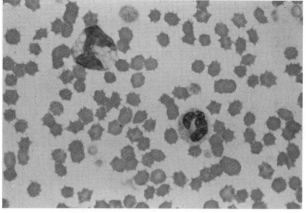

Figure 57–12. Blood film from an MPS VII–affected cat. Note the vacuolated monocyte and neutrophil that contains granules. Wright stain.

dystrophy may appear somewhat similar to storage-induced corneal clouding.

Metachromatic granules within neutrophils and occasionally within lymphocytes are quite suggestive of MPS,[87] but can be observed in GM_2 gangliosidosis, which, unlike MPS, is characterized by progressive neurologic disease and early death. Similar, but finer, granules also can be observed in neutrophils of some Birman cats.[88] Lymphocytes are normal in Birman cats, and no clinical abnormalities are exhibited. Very rarely, toxic granulation of neutrophils can have a similar appearance. Many of the other feline lysosomal storage diseases are characterized by vacuolated lymphocytes and normal-appearing neutrophils; most of these diseases present with progressive central nervous system disease.[1, 89]

◆ DIAGNOSIS

Evaluation of Wright-stained blood films is the most simple diagnostic tool; neutrophils and monocytes

from individuals with MPS contain numerous distinctive metachromatic granules. Granules usually are not apparent when stained with Diff-Quik, and granules are quite indistinct in neutrophils of cats with MPS I. Occasional lymphocytes contain vacuoles, within which may be metachromatic granules, particularly in MPS VII.

Radiographic evaluation of the skeletal system is useful diagnostically. Bone density is decreased, and cortices are thin. Epiphyseal abnormalities vary from slight irregularities to large scalloped defects in subchondral bone. Joint disease is progressive, and includes acetabular flattening and periarticular osteophyte formation. Proliferative bone is present around all articular facets of vertebrae, resulting in fusion of cervical vertebrae in some cats.

Presence of excess GAG in urine usually is indicative of MPS. Commercially available strips that detect GAG semiquantitatively are available (Figs. 57–13 and 57–14 but false-positive results may be observed when testing urine from young kittens. For more precise qualitative and quantitative measure-

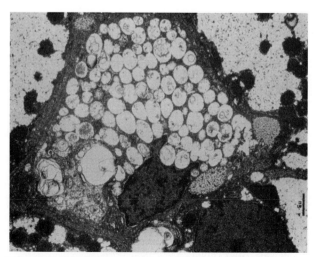

Figure 57–11. Electron micrograph of a Kupffer cell within the liver of an MPS VI–affected cat. Note the marked vacuolation, which represents distended GAG-filled lysosomes.

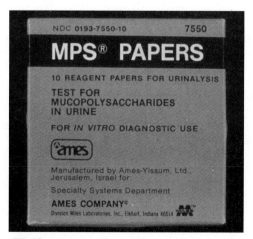

Figure 57–13. Commercially available MPS papers for detecting GAGs in urine.

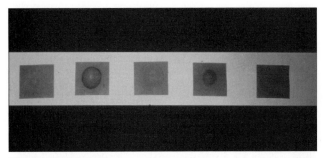

Figure 57–14. MPS papers that have been used to screen a litter of kittens for MPS VI. The second and fourth papers show spots that are positive for GAGs in the urine.

ments, frozen urine can be sent to one of the veterinary or human laboratories that routinely test for the presence of GAG in urine. Definitive diagnosis usually is made by measuring lysosomal enzyme activity in serum, leukocyte pellets, or frozen liver. For the leukocyte pellet lysosomal enzyme activity assay, approximately 4 ml of whole blood is collected in heparin (green-top tube), and nonrefrigerated blood is sent to a laboratory that routinely assays for lysosomal enzymes (Lysosomal Disease Testing Laboratory, Dr. David A. Wenger, Jefferson Medical College, Jefferson Alumni Hall, Room 394, 1020 Locust Street, Philadelphia, PA 19107, telephone: [215] 955–4923, fax: [215] 955–9554; Metabolic Screening Laboratory, Section of Medical Genetics, Veterinary Hospital of the University of Pennsylvania, 3900 Delancey Street, Philadelphia, PA 19104–6010). Blood should arrive within 24 hours of collection, and telephone consultation is recommended before sample collection. Because feline models of human disease have been so useful, any cat suspected of having a lysosomal storage disease should be tested. It is likely that previously unreported types of MPS and other lysosomal storage diseases will continue to be discovered.

◆ THERAPY

The discovery that cultured MPS–affected cells could be restored to normal by corrective factors stimulated hope that enzyme replacement therapy could be used to treat these disorders in human beings. Early unsuccessful attempts at therapy included the administration of plasma, leukocytes, fibroblasts, and amnion.[51] The feline model has been of particular value for testing new therapies, such as bone marrow transplantation (BMT), enzyme replacement, and gene transfer. BMT was first performed in a cat with MPS VI in 1982.[44, 90, 91] Dramatic improvement is seen after BMT, particularly if the BMT is performed when affected kittens are less than 12 weeks of age. BMT also has been effective in children with MPS.[92] Normal bone marrow–derived enzyme-replete cells assist in the removal of GAG from various tissues of the host. However, allogeneic BMT is a high-risk, expensive procedure. Pet cats

with MPS can be treated with BMT,[93] but by the time the disease is diagnosed, cats usually have attained skeletal maturity, after which time BMT is of little value.

The feline model of MPS VI also has been used to evaluate recombinant enzyme replacement therapy, with encouraging results.[94–96] Currently, feline models of MPS are being utilized in the development and testing of gene replacement therapy, in which a viral vector is used to introduce cDNA encoding the missing lysosomal enzyme into the affected cat's cells.[97–101]

Cats with MPS are more susceptible to viral and bacterial respiratory infections, and use of antibiotics may be indicated. Affected cats also are prone to dehydration, and subcutaneous fluids may be given as indicated. With increasing age, immobility and difficulty in eating progress; a diet of soft food may be helpful. Prognosis is reasonably good in animals treated with BMT. Untreated cats usually develop severe skeletal and joint disease, and may become nonambulatory at approximately 3 to 5 years of age.

◆ PREVENTION

Because the feline MPSs are inherited by the recessive mode, their control is simple, provided the parentage of affected animals is known. Parents of affected animals are carriers, and there is a 1 in 4 risk that the offspring will be affected. Carriers usually can be detected by leukocyte pellet lysosomal enzyme activity analysis, as they typically have approximately half-normal activity.[102] However, there often is overlap between the ranges for enzyme activity from normal and carrier cats. Accurate carrier detection can be achieved by a molecular test for the specific mutation in those diseases for which the genetic abnormality is known (see Chapter 77, Molecular Diagnosis of Gangliosidoses: A Model for Elimination of Inherited Diseases in Pure Breeds).

REFERENCES

1. Haskins M, Giger U: Lysosomal storage diseases. *In* Kaneko JJ, Harvey JW, Bruss ML (eds): Clinical Biochemistry of Domestic Animals, 5th ed. Orlando, FL, Academic, 1997, pp. 741–760.
2. Neufeld EB, Wastney M, Patel S, et al: The Niemann-Pick C1 protein resides in a vesicular compartment linked to retrograde transport of multiple lysosomal cargo. J Biol Chem 274:9627–9635, 1999.
3. Johnson KH: Globoid leukodystrophy in the cat. J Am Vet Med Assoc 157:2057–2064, 1970.
4. Blakemore WF: GM-1 gangliosidosis in a cat. J Comp Pathol 82:179–185, 1972.
5. Baker HJ Jr, Lindsey JR, McKhann GM, et al: Neuronal GM_1 gangliosidosis in a Siamese cat with beta-galactosidase deficiency. Science 174:838–839, 1971.
6. Baker HJ, Lindsey JR: Animal model: Feline GM_1 gangliosidosis. Am J Pathol 74:649–652, 1974.
7. Murray JA, Blakemore WF, Barnett KC: Ocular lesions in cats with GM_1-gangliosidosis with visceral involvement. J Small Anim Pract 18:1–10, 1977.

8. Baker HJ, Reynolds GD, Walkley SU, et al: The gangliosidoses: Comparative features and research applications. Vet Pathol 16:635–649, 1979.
9. Dial SM, Mitchell TW, LeCouteur RA, et al: GM₁ gangliosidosis (type II) in three cats. J Am Anim Hosp Assoc 30:355–359, 1994.
10. De Maria R, Divari S, Bo S, et al: Beta-galactosidase deficiency in a Korat cat: A new form of feline GM₁-gangliosidosis. Acta Neuropathol 96:307–314, 1998.
11. Cork LC, Munnell JF, Lorenz MD: GM₂ ganglioside lysosomal storage disease in cats with beta-hexosaminidase deficiency. Science 196:1014–1017, 1977.
12. Cork LC, Nummell JF, Lorenz MD: The pathology of feline GM₂ gangliosidosis. Am J Pathol 90:724–730, 1978.
13. Neuwelt EA, Johnson WG, Blank NK, et al: Characterization of a new model of GM₂ gangliosidosis (Sandhoff's disease) in Korat cats. J Clin Invest 76:482–490, 1985.
14. Muldoon LL, Neuwelt EA, Pagel MA, et al: Characterization of the molecular defect in a feline model for type II GM₂ gangliosidosis (Sandhoff disease). Am J Pathol 44:1109–1118, 1994.
15. Baker HJ, Mole JA, Lindsey JR, et al: Animal models of human ganglioside storage diseases. Fed Proc 35:1193–1201, 1976.
16. Burditt LJ, Chotai K, Hirani S, et al: Biochemical studies on a case of feline mannosidosis. Biochem J 189:467–473, 1980.
17. Walkley SU, Blakemore WF, Purpura DP: Alterations in neuron morphology in feline mannosidosis. A Golgi study. Acta Neuropathol 53:75–79, 1981.
18. Vandevelde M, Fankhauser R, Bichsel P, et al: Hereditary neurovisceral mannosidosis associated with alpha-mannosidase deficiency in a family of Persian cats. Acta Neuropathol 58:64–68, 1982.
19. Jezyk PF, Haskins ME, Newman LR: Alpha-mannosidosis in a Persian cat. J Am Vet Med Assoc 18:1483–1485, 1986.
20. Cummings JF, Wood PA, deLahunta A, et al: The clinical and pathologic heterogeneity of feline alpha-mannosidosis. J Vet Intern Med 2:163–170, 1988.
21. Berg T, Tollersrud OK, Walkley SU, et al: Purification of feline lysosomal alpha-mannosidase, determination of its cDNA sequence and identification of a mutation causing alpha-mannosidosis in Persian cats. Biochem J 328:863–870, 1997.
22. Percy DH, Jortner BS: Feline lipidosis. Light and electron microscopic studies. Arch Pathol Lab Med 92:136–144, 1971.
23. Wenger DA, Sattler M, Kudoh T, et al: Niemann-Pick disease: A genetic model in Siamese cats. Science 208:1471–1473, 1980.
24. Snyder SP, Kingston RS, Wenger DA: Niemann-Pick disease. Sphingomyelinosis of Siamese cats. Am J Pathol 108:252–254, 1982.
25. Baker HJ, Wood PA, Wenger DA, et al: Sphingomyelin lipidosis in a cat. Vet Pathol 24:386–391, 1987.
26. Yamagami T, Umeda M, Kamiya S, et al: Neurovisceral sphingomyelinosis in a Siamese cat. Acta Neuropathol 79:330–332, 1989.
27. Cuddon PA, Higgins RJ, Duncan ID, et al: Polyneuropathy in feline Niemann-Pick disease. Brain 112:1429–1443, 1989.
28. Lowenthal AC, Cummings JF, Wenger DA, et al: Feline sphingolipidosis resembling Niemann-Pick disease type C. Acta Neuropathol 81:189–197, 1990.
29. Brown DE, Thrall MA, Walkley SU, et al: Feline Niemann-Pick disease type C. Am J Pathol 144:1412–1415, 1994.
30. Muñana KR, Luttgen PJ, Thrall MA, et al: Neurological manifestations of Niemann-Pick disease type C in cats. J Vet Intern Med 8:117–121, 1994.
31. Sandstrom B, Westman J, Ockerman PA: Glycogenosis of the central nervous system in the cat. Acta Neuropathol 14:194–200, 1969.
32. Thrall MA, Mitchell T, Lappin M, et al: Cholesteryl ester storage disease in two cats. Vet Clin Pathol 21:34, 1992.
33. Hubler M, Haskins ME, Arnold S, et al: Mucolipidosis type II in a domestic shorthair cat. J Small Anim Pract 37:435–441, 1996.
34. Bosshard NU, Hubler M, Arnold S, et al: Spontaneous mucolipidosis in a cat: An animal model of human I-cell disease. Vet Pathol, 33:1–13, 1996.
35. Haskins ME, Jezyk PF, Desnick RJ, et al: Mucopolysaccharidosis in a domestic short-haired cat—A disease distinct from that seen in the Siamese cat. J Am Vet Med Assoc 175:384–387, 1979.
36. Haskins ME, Aguirre GD, Jezyk PF, et al: The pathology of the feline model of mucopolysaccharidosis I. Am J Pathol 112:27–36, 1983.
37. He X, Li CM, Simonaro CM, et al: Identification and characterization of the molecular lesion causing mucopolysaccharidosis type I in cats. Mol Genet Metab 67:106–112, 1999.
38. Cowell KR, Jezyk PF, Haskins ME, et al: Mucopolysaccharidosis in a cat. J Am Vet Med Assoc 169:334–339, 1976.
39. Jezyk PF, Haskins ME, Patterson DF, et al: Mucopolysaccharidosis in a cat with arylsulfatase B deficiency: A model of Maroteaux-Lamy syndrome. Science 198:834–836, 1977.
40. Langweiler M, Haskins ME, Jezyk PF: Mucopolysaccharidosis in a litter of cats. J Am Anim Hosp Assoc 14:748–751, 1978.
41. Haskins ME, Jezyk PF, Patterson DF: Mucopolysaccharide storage disease in three families of cats with arylsulfatase B deficiency: Leukocyte studies and carrier identification. Pediatr Res 13:1203–1210, 1979.
42. Haskins ME, Jezyk PF, Desnick RJ, et al: Animal model of human disease: Mucopolysaccharidosis VI, Maroteaux-Lamy syndrome, arylsulfatase B–deficient mucopolysaccharidosis in the Siamese cat. Am J Pathol 105:191–193, 1981.
43. Breton L, Guerin P, Morin M: A case of mucopolysaccharidosis VI in a cat. J Am Anim Hosp Assoc 19:891–896, 1983.
44. Gasper PW, Thrall MA, Wenger DA, et al: Correction of arylsulfatase B deficiency (mucopolysaccharidosis VI) by bone marrow transplantation. Nature 312:467–469, 1984.
45. Jackson CE, Yuhki N, Desnick RJ, et al: Feline arylsulfatase B (ASB): Isolation and expression of the cDNA, comparison with human ARSB, and gene localization to feline chromosome A1. Genomics 14:403–411, 1992.
46. De Luca T, Minichiello L, Leone A, et al: Preliminary molecular analysis of a case of feline mucopolysaccharidosis VI. Biochem Biophys Res Commun 196:1177–1182, 1993.
47. Yogalingam G, Litjens T, Bielicki J, et al: Feline mucopolysaccharidosis type VI. Characterization of recombinant N-acetylgalactosamine 4-sulfatase and identification of a mutation causing the disease. J Biol Chem 271:27259–27265, 1996.
48. Gitzelmann R, Bosshard NU, Superti-Furga A, et al: Feline mucopolysaccharidosis VII due to beta-glucuronidase deficiency. Vet Pathol 31:435–443, 1994.
49. Schultheis PC, Gardner SA, Owens JM, et al: Mucopolysaccharidosis VII in a cat. Vet Pathol 37:502–505, 2000.
50. Haskins ME, Otis EJ, Hayden JE, et al: Hepatic storage of glycosaminoglycans in feline and canine models of mucopolysaccharidoses I, VI, and VII. Vet Pathol 29:112–119, 1992.
51. Neufeld EF, Muenzer J: The mucopolysaccharidoses. In Scriver CR, Beaudet AL, Sly WS, Valle D (eds): The Metabolic and Molecular Bases of Inherited Disease, 7th ed. New York, McGraw-Hill, 1995, pp. 2465–2494.
52. Byers S, Rozaklis T, Brumfield LK, et al: Glycosaminoglycan accumulation and excretion in the mucopolysaccharidoses: Characterization and basis of a diagnostic test for MPS. Mol Genet Metab 65:282–290, 1998.
53. Haskins ME, Jezyk PF, Desnick RJ, et al: Animal models of mucopolysaccharidosis. Prog Clin Biol Res 94:177–201, 1982.
54. Haskins ME, Jezyk PF, Desnick RJ, et al: Feline models of mucopolysaccharidosis. Birth Defects 16:219–224, 1980.
55. Hunter C: A rare disease in two brothers. Proc R Soc Med 10:104–116, 1917.
56. Brante G: Gargoylism: A mucopolysaccharidosis. Scand J Clin Lab Invest 4:43–46, 1952.
57. Dorfman A, Lorincz AE: Occurrence of urinary acid mucopolysaccharides in the Hurler syndrome. Proc Natl Acad Sci U S A 43:443–446, 1957.

58. Fratatoni JC, Hall CW, Neufeld EF: The defect in Hurler and Hunter syndromes: II. Deficiency of specific factors involved in mucopolysaccharide degradation. Proc Natl Acad Sci U S A 64:360–366, 1968.

59. Cantz M, Chrambach A, Neufeld EF: Characterization of the factor deficient in the Hunter syndrome by polyacrylamide gel electrophoresis. Biochem Biophys Res Commun 39:936–942, 1970.

60. Neufeld EF: The biochemical basis for mucopolysaccharidoses and mucolipidoses. Prog Med Genet 10:81–101, 1974.

61. Triggs-Raine B, Salo TJ, Zhang H, et al: Mutations in HYAL1, a member of a tandemly distributed multigene family encoding disparate hyaluronidase activities, cause a newly described lysosomal disorder, mucopolysaccharidosis IX. Proc Natl Acad Sci U S A 96:6296–6300, 1999.

62. Haskins ME, Aguirre GD, Jezyk PF, et al: The pathology of the feline model of mucopolysaccharidosis VI. Am J Pathol 101:657–674, 1980.

63. Sheridan O, Wortman J, Harvey C, et al: Craniofacial abnormalities in animal models of mucopolysaccharidoses I, VI, and VII. J Craniofac Genet Dev Biol 14:7–15, 1994.

64. Di Natale P, Annella T, Daniele A, et al: Animal models for lysosomal storage diseases: A new case of feline mucopolysaccharidosis VI. J Inherit Metab Dis 15:17–24, 1992.

65. Beekman GK: Mucopolysaccharidosis VI in a kitten: A case report and discussion of feline Maroteaux-Lamy syndrome. Fel Pract 21:7–11, 1993.

66. Haskins ME, Bingel S, Northington JW, et al: Spinal cord compression and hindlimb paresis in cats with mucopolysaccharidosis VI. J Am Vet Med Assoc 182:983–985, 1983.

67. Yogalingam G, Hopwood JJ, Crawley A, et al: Mild feline mucopolysaccharidosis type VI. Identification of an N-acetylgalactosamine-4-sulfatase mutation causing instability and increased specific activity. J Biol Chem 273:13421–13429, 1998.

68. Crawley AC, Yogalingam G, Muller VJ, et al: Two mutations within a feline mucopolysaccharidosis type VI colony cause three different clinical phenotypes. J Clin Invest 101:109–119, 1998.

69. Konde LJ, Thrall MA, Gasper PW, et al: Radiographically visualized skeletal changes associated with mucopolysaccharidosis VI in cats. J Vet Radiol 28:223–228, 1987.

70. Turner AS, Norrdin RW, Gaarde S, et al: Bone mineral density in feline mucopolysaccharidosis VI measured using dual-energy x-ray absorptiometry. Calcif Tissue Int 57:191–195, 1995.

71. Aguirre G, Stramm L, Haskins M: Feline mucopolysaccharidosis VI: General ocular and pigment epithelial pathology. Invest Ophthalmol Vis Sci 24:991–1007, 1983.

72. Stramm L, Haskins M, Desnick RJ, et al: Disease expression in cultured pigment epithelium. Feline mucopolysaccharidosis VI. Invest Ophthalmol Vis Sci 26:182–192, 1985.

73. Stramm LE, Desnick RJ, Haskins ME, et al: Arylsulfatase B activity in cultured retinal pigment epithelium: Regional studies in feline mucopolysaccharidosis VI. Invest Ophthalmol Vis Sci 27:1050–1057, 1986.

74. Aguirre G, Raber I, Yanoff M, et al: Reciprocal corneal transplantation fails to correct mucopolysaccharidosis VI corneal storage. Invest Ophthalmol Vis Sci 33:2702–2713, 1992.

75. Mollard RJ, Telegan P, Haskins M, et al: Corneal endothelium in mucopolysaccharide storage disorders. Morphologic studies in animal models. Cornea 15:25–34, 1996.

76. Alroy J, Haskins M, Birk DE: Altered corneal stromal matrix organization is associated with mucopolysaccharidosis I, III and VI. Exp Eye Res 68:523–530, 1999.

77. Norrdin RW, Moffat KS, Thrall MA, et al: Characterization of osteopenia in feline mucopolysaccharidosis VI and evaluation of bone marrow transplantation therapy. Bone 14:361–367, 1993.

78. Norrdin RW, Simske SJ, Gaarde S, et al: Bone changes in mucopolysaccharidosis VI in cats and the effects of bone marrow transplantation: Mechanical testing of long bones. Bone 17:485–489, 1995.

79. Abreu S, Hayden J, Berthold P, et al: Growth plate pathology in feline mucopolysaccharidosis VI. Calcif Tissue Int 57:185–190, 1995.

80. Nuttall JD, Brumfield LK, Fazzalari NL, et al: Histomorphometric analysis of the tibial growth plate in a feline model of mucopolysaccharidosis type VI. Calcif Tissue Int 65:47–52, 1999.

81. McGovern MM, Vine DT, Haskins ME, et al: Purification and properties of feline and human arylsulfatase B isozymes. J Biol Chem 257:12605–12610, 1982.

82. Vine DT, McGovern MM, Haskins ME, et al: Feline mucopolysaccharidosis VI: Purification and characterization of the resident arylsulfatase B activity. Am J Hum Genet 33:916–927, 1981.

83. Vine DT, McGovern MM, Schuchman EH, et al: Enhancement of residual arylsulfatase B activity in feline mucopolysaccharidosis VI by thiol-induced subunit association. J Clin Invest 69:294–302, 1982.

84. Haskins ME, McGrath JT: Meningiomas in young cats with mucopolysaccharidosis I. J Neuropathol Exp Neurol 42:664–670, 1983.

85. Sande RD, Bingel SA: Animal models of dwarfism. Vet Clin North Am Small Anim Pract 13:71–89, 1983.

86. Schrader SC, Sherding RG: Disorders of the skeletal system. In Sherding RG (ed): The Cat. Diseases and Clinical Management, vol. 2. New York, Churchill Livingstone, 1989, pp. 1247–1292.

87. Alroy J, Freden GO, Goyal V, et al: Morphology of leukocytes from cats affected with alpha-mannosidosis and mucopolysaccharidosis VI (MPS VI). Vet Pathol 26:294–302, 1989.

88. Hirsch VM, Cunningham TA: Hereditary anomaly of neutrophil granulation in Birman cats. Am J Vet Res 45:2170–2174, 1984.

89. Blakemore WF: Neurolipidoses: Examples of lysosomal storage diseases. Vet Clin North Am Small Anim Pract 10:81–90, 1980.

90. Wenger DA, Gasper PW, Thrall MA, et al: Bone marrow transplantation in the feline model of arylsulfatase B deficiency. Birth Defects 22:177–186, 1986.

91. Dial SM, Byrne T, Haskins M, et al: Urine glycosaminoglycan concentrations in mucopolysaccharidosis VI–affected cats following bone marrow transplantation or leukocyte infusion. Clin Chim Acta 263:1–14, 1997.

92. Krivit W, Pierpont ME, Ayaz K, et al: Bone-marrow transplantation in the Maroteaux-Lamy syndrome (mucopolysaccharidosis type VI). Biochemical and clinical status 24 months after transplantation. N Engl J Med 311:1606–1612, 1984.

93. Thrall MA, Haskins ME: Bone marrow transplantation. In August JR (ed): Consultations in Feline Internal Medicine, vol. 3. Philadelphia, WB Saunders, 1997, pp. 514–524.

94. Crawley AC, Niedzielski KH, Isaac EL, et al: Enzyme replacement therapy from birth in a feline model of mucopolysaccharidosis type VI. J Clin Invest 99:651–662, 1997.

95. Brooks DA, King BM, Crawley AC, et al: Enzyme replacement therapy in mucopolysaccharidosis VI: Evidence for immune responses and altered efficacy of treatment in animal models. Biochim Biophys Acta 1361:203–216, 1997.

96. Byers S, Nuttall JD, Crawley AC, et al: Effect of enzyme replacement therapy on bone formation in a feline model of mucopolysaccharidosis type VI. Bone 21:425–431, 1997.

97. Yogalingam G, Bielicki J, Hopwood JJ, et al: Feline mucopolysaccharidosis type VI: Correction of glycosaminoglycan storage in myoblasts by retrovirus-mediated transfer of the feline N-acetylgalactosamine 4-sulfatase gene. DNA Cell Biol 16:1189–1194, 1997.

98. Ray J, Wolfe JH, Aguirre GD, et al: Retroviral cDNA transfer to the RPE: Stable expression and modification of metabolism. Invest Ophthalmol Vis Sci 39:1658–1666, 1998.

99. Simonaro CM, Haskins ME, Abkowitz JL, et al: Autologous transplantation of retrovirally transduced bone marrow or neonatal blood cells into cats can lead to long-term engraftment in the absence of myeloablation. Gene Ther 6:107–113, 1999.

100. Yogalingam G, Crawley A, Hopwood JJ, et al: Evaluation of fibroblast-mediated gene therapy in a feline model of mucopolysaccharidosis type VI. Biochim Biophys Acta 1453:284–296, 1999.

101. Yogalingam G, Muller V, Hopwood JJ, et al: Regulation of N-acetylgalactosamine 4-sulfatase expression in retrovirus-transduced feline mucopolysaccharidosis type VI muscle cells. DNA Cell Biol 18:187–195, 1999.

102. McGovern MM, Vine DT, Haskins ME, et al: An improved method for heterozygote identification in feline and human mucopolysaccharidosis VI, arylsulfatase-B deficiency. Enzyme 26:206–210, 1981.

58

◆ Transfusion Medicine

K. Jane Wardrop

The administration of blood or blood components can be a lifesaving form of therapy for the feline patient. Appropriate use of blood requires knowledge of (1) feline blood types, (2) how or where to obtain blood products, (3) indications for the use of these products, (4) proper administration techniques, and (5) potential adverse reactions associated with transfusions. Knowledge of blood alternatives, such as synthetic colloids and the new hemoglobin-based oxygen-carrying solutions, also is important. The purpose of this chapter is to provide information on these topics, so that safe and efficacious feline blood transfusions can be performed.

◆ FELINE BLOOD TYPES

One blood group system, the AB system, is recognized in cats. The system consists of 3 blood types—type A, type B, and type AB. These blood type antigens are determined by a form of neuraminic acid present on erythrocyte glycolipids or glycoproteins. N-glycolyneuraminic acid is the determinant of the A antigen, whereas N-acetylneuraminic acid is contained in the major erythrocyte membrane glycolipid of type B cats. A combination of both neuraminic acids is found in type AB cats.[1]

Blood type A is inherited in a dominant fashion over type B. Type B cats are homozygous for the B allele, whereas type A cats can be homozygous or heterozygous.[2] Blood type AB is not the result of codominant inheritance of type A and type B. Although the exact mode of inheritance is unknown, breeding results suggest that a third allele AB codes for an enzyme capable of producing type A and type B substances.[3]

The frequency of these antigens varies with breed and geographic location. Type A is the most common blood type. Table 58–1 summarizes the frequency of blood type B in various feline breeds in the United States. Breeds such as Exotic and British shorthair and Cornish and Devon rex have the highest frequency of type B blood, with up to 50 per cent of these cats being type B.[4] Siamese, Burmese, Tonkinese, and Russian blue cats have the lowest frequency, with no type B cats found in one study.[2] The highest frequency of type B cats in the United States is seen on the West Coast, with a frequency as high as 6 per cent.[4] Blood type AB is quite rare, and has been described in domestic shorthair and domestic longhair cats and in the Abyssinian, Birman, British shorthair, Norwegian forest, Persian, Scottish fold, and Somali breeds.[3]

The primary clinical significance of the feline blood types lies in the naturally occurring alloantibodies produced against them. Kittens develop these naturally occurring antibodies at 6 to 8 weeks of age, and have adult serum titer levels at about 3 months of age.[5] Type A cats contain a low titer of naturally occurring anti-B hemagglutinins of the immunoglobulin (Ig)M class and hemolysins consisting of both IgG and IgM.[5] Approximately one-third of type A cats have macroscopic agglutinins and hemolysins, and microscopic examination or an antiglobulin test is required to detect antibody in the remaining two-thirds of type A cats. Type B cats have a high titer of naturally occurring anti-A hemagglutinins and hemolysins, consisting primarily of IgM with a lesser amount of IgG.[5, 6] Type AB cats do not possess antibody against either type A or type B.

These alloantibodies are responsible for 2 main types of reactions—hemolytic transfusion reactions and neonatal isoerythrolysis (NI). Hemolytic transfusion reactions are discussed later in this chapter. NI, also termed hemolytic disease of the newborn, occurs when maternal antibody against neonatal red blood cells gains access to the neonatal circulation. In cats, NI has been associated with type B queens who give birth to type A kittens.[7] Because of the nature of the naturally occurring antibody in cats, NI can occur with first-time queens. The feline placenta does not allow significant passage of antibody during gestation; rather the anti-A alloantibody is

Table 58–1. Blood Type B Frequencies in Various Feline Breeds in the United States

Type B Frequency (%)	Breeds
0	Siamese, Burmese, Tonkinese, Russian blue, Ocicat, Oriental shorthair
<5	Maine coon, Norwegian forest, DSH/DLH
5–25	Abyssinian, Himalayan, Birman, Persian, Somali, Sphinx, Scottish fold, Japanese bobtail
25–50	Exotic and British shorthair, Cornish rex, Devon rex

Abbreviations: DLH, domestic longhair; DSH, domestic shorthair.
Data from Giger U, Bucheler J, Patterson DF: Frequency and inheritance of A and B blood types in feline breeds of the United States. J Hered 82:15–20, 1991; Giger U, Griot-Wenk M, Bucheler J, et al: Geographical variation of the feline blood type frequencies in the United States. Fel Pract 19:21–27, 1991; and Griot-Wenk ME, Giger U: Feline transfusion medicine: Blood types and their clinical importance. Vet Clin North Am Small Anim Pract 25:1305–1322, 1995.

contained in high titers in colostrum and is obtained during nursing. Kittens develop clinical signs within hours to days of colostrum ingestion. Kittens may die peracutely or have clinical signs of hemoglobinemia, hemoglobinuria, anemia, and icterus. Affected kittens should be removed from the queen and foster-nursed. Severely anemic kittens may need washed type B red blood cells during the first 3 days of life, and type A blood thereafter, when anti-A alloantibodies are diminished in circulation.

◆ DONOR SELECTION

Feline blood or blood products may be purchased from a commercial veterinary blood bank (Table 58–2) or collected from a clinic blood donor. The commercial veterinary blood banks provide a safe and effective product; however, it must be remembered that shipment of these products requires time. This could be a disadvantage when dealing with the anemic emergency patient, necessitating the use of in-house donors.

Cats selected as blood donors should be large (>5 kg), nonobese animals in good physical condition and with a calm disposition. Preferably, they should be 1 to 6 years of age. All cats should be blood-typed and screened for blood-borne infectious disease before becoming blood donors. Blood-typing cards are available for cats (see Crossmatching and Blood-Typing), and these cards can identify blood types A, B, and AB. Most cats are blood type A, and diligent searching or planning may be necessary to locate a type B donor.

Initial screening should include a complete blood count, serum chemistry profile, urinalysis, and fecal examination. Donor cats should be heartworm-negative, and should be tested for feline leukemia virus, feline immunodeficiency virus, the feline coronaviruses, and *Hemobartonella felis*. Testing for *Bartonella* species and *Toxoplasma gondii* also should be considered. Screening for other blood-borne infectious disease agents may be necessary, depending on specific location and environment. Maintenance

Table 58–2. Commercial Veterinary Blood Banks With Feline Blood Products*

Blood Bank	Products Available
Midwest Animal Blood Services, Inc. P.O. Box 626 120 E. Main St. Stockbridge, MI 49285 (517) 851–8244	Whole blood, packed red blood cells Fresh frozen plasma, plasma
Animal Blood Bank P.O. Box 1118 Dixon, CA 95620–1118 (800) 243–5759	Whole blood, packed red blood cells Plasma

*Regional veterinary emergency clinics or colleges of veterinary medicine also may offer these products and may be contacted.

of blood donors should include routine vaccinations for feline herpesvirus-1, calicivirus, chlamydia, panleukopenia, and rabies. Iron supplementation (10 mg/kg orally twice-weekly[8]) is required for cats donating blood frequently (at least at monthly intervals).

◆ CROSSMATCHING AND BLOOD-TYPING

All cats should be blood-typed or crossmatched before transfusion. Blood-typing is performed to identify which blood-type antigens are present on the red blood cells of the cat—A, B, or AB. Crossmatching is used to detect antibodies against those antigens. Because of the naturally occurring alloantibodies of cats, even first-time transfusions performed with untyped or uncrossmatched blood can be fatal in cats, as seen in the case of type B cats receiving type A blood.[9, 10] Transfusions also may result in accelerated destruction of the transfused cells, as seen when type B blood is given to type A cats.[11]

Feline blood-typing is performed by many veterinary laboratories. These laboratories usually require the submission of either ethylenediaminetetraacetic acid (EDTA) or anticoagulant citrate dextrose (ACD) whole blood. Blood-typing also can be performed in a clinical setting with the aid of blood-typing cards (DMS Laboratories, Inc., Flemington, NJ). The cards have wells containing lyophilized antisera or reagent, which reacts with feline red blood cell antigens. Type A blood is detected using antisera from type B cats. Type B blood is detected using a *Tritium vulgaris* lectin, previously shown to interact with feline type B red blood cells.[12] The lyophilized material is reconstituted with a diluent (phosphate-buffered saline), a drop (40 μl) of EDTA whole blood from the feline patient is added, and the card is rocked for approximately 2 minutes. Agglutination indicates a positive response (Fig. 58–1). Controls are included to aid in reading the reactions. Cats with type A, B, or AB can be identified. The advantage of these cards lies in their speed and simplicity; however, care should be taken to ensure correct interpretation. The controls included in these kits can become outdated, and may give less than satisfactory results. Weak reactions can be a source of confusion. In the case of a cat that tests as a type B blood cat on the cards, it is a good idea to back-type this cat using its plasma—that is, plasma from a type B cat contains a high titer of anti-A antibody and will strongly agglutinate red blood cells from a type A cat.

Crossmatching can be performed when typing is not available or in addition to blood-typing. It should be noted that although only the AB blood group system has been described in cats, other blood groups or antigens may exist. This is evidenced by crossmatch incompatibilities seen between frequently transfused cats and a donor of similar type. Crossmatching allows the detection of antibodies

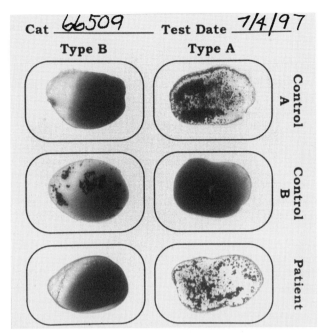

Cat ___66509___ Test Date __7/4/97__

Type B   Type A

Control A

Control B

Patient

Figure 58–1. Feline blood-typing using a typing card. Agglutination indicates a positive response. The patient in this case was a type A cat, and blood from the patient applied to the card matches the agglutination pattern seen with the type A control sample.

against red blood cells, occurring between a patient and a potential blood donor. A crossmatching procedure is included in Table 58–3. A simplified crossmatch procedure, using 2 drops of recipient plasma and 1 drop of donor EDTA red blood cells in place of washed and diluted red blood cells, has been described for use in emergency situations.[8] The plasma and cells are mixed together on a glass slide,

and the slide is examined for hemagglutination after 1 to 5 minutes. As in any crossmatch, a control sample (patient plasma and patient red blood cells) also should be processed and interpreted.

◆ BLOOD COLLECTION

Collection of blood from cats generally requires some form of sedation. A combination of ketamine (2 mg/kg), diazepam (0.1 mg/kg), and atropine (0.01 mg/kg) may be administered intravenously. Sedation using oxymorphone and diazepam, ketamine and midazolam, or chamber induction with isoflurane also may be used.[13] Maximum donation volumes range from 11 ml/kg to 15 ml/kg. With the cat in sternal or lateral recumbency, blood is collected from the jugular vein into a syringe containing ACD, citrate phosphate dextrose (CPD), or citrate phosphate dextrose adenine (CPDA-1) solutions (1 ml/7 to 9 ml blood). Either a 19- to 20-gauge needle or a butterfly infusion set may be used for collection. The author routinely uses a 60-ml syringe with 6 ml of ACD, filling with 54 ml of blood. Blood should be agitated gently during collection to ensure adequate mixing with the anticoagulant preservative solution. The blood can be transferred to a collection bag if storage is desired (see later). Crystalloid solutions at 2 to 3 times the volume of blood removed can be administered immediately after collection, either as a routine prophylactic measure or only if signs of hypotension occur.

Previously, it has been difficult to store or process feline blood owing to the lack of available storage collection systems for cats. Systems to remedy this situation are under development. In one study, a

Table 58–3. Crossmatching Procedure

1. Obtain an anticoagulated (EDTA) specimen of blood (1 to 2 ml) from both patient and donor. Centrifuge and separate plasma from RBCs.
2. Wash RBCs by adding 2–3 ml of saline solution or PBS to 0.25 ml of packed RBCs, mixing, and centrifuging for 1 min at 3400 rpm. Decant the saline solution and repeat 3 times, filling the tubes with saline solution, mixing, centrifuging, and decanting.
3. After last wash, decant supernatant and resuspend cells with saline solution to give a 2–4% ("weak" tomato juice) suspension of RBCs. The suspension also may be calculated; e.g., 0.1 ml blood in 2.4 ml saline solution gives a 4% suspension.
4. Make the following mixtures by adding the indicated amount of the well-mixed RBC suspension and plasma to small (12 × 75 mm) tubes:
   Major crossmatch: 2 drops patient plasma, 1 drop donor 2–4% RBCs
   Minor crossmatch: 2 drops donor plasma, 1 drop patient 2–4% RBCs
   Include controls: 2 drops patient plasma, 1 drop patient 2–4% RBCs
                          2 drops donor plasma, 1 drop donor 2–4% RBCs
5. Incubate tubes for 15 min at 37°C.
6. Centrifuge for 15 sec (3400 rpm).
7. Read tubes:
   Macroscopic: Rotate tubes gently and observe cells coming off the RBC "button" in the bottom of the tube. In a compatible reaction, i.e., where there is no antigen-antibody reaction, the cells should float off freely, with no clumping/hemagglutination (compare with the control tubes). Rouleaux formation can be falsely interpreted as a reaction. If rouleaux formation is suspected, a saline replacement technique can be used in which the tubes are recentrifuged, the plasma is removed and replaced with an equal volume of saline solution. The tubes again are centrifuged for 15 sec and interpreted. Rouleaux will appear as a "stacked-coin" appearance on microscopic examination. Proceed to the microscopic examination in those tubes with weak or no obvious reactions.
   Microscopic: After tubes have been viewed macroscopically, place a drop of the cells/plasma mixture on a slide, coverslip, and examine microscopically. The RBCs normally should appear as individual cells, with no clumping or rouleaux formation.

Abbreviations: EDTA, ethylenediaminetetraacetic acid; PBS, phosphate-buffered saline; RBC, red blood cell.

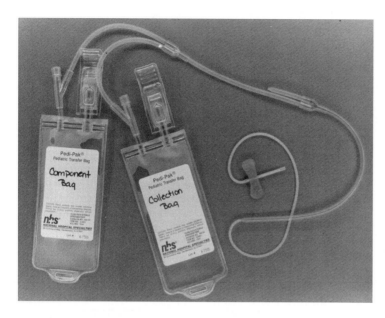

Figure 58–2. Closed-system feline blood collection set created by welding a winged infusion set to a pair of pediatric blood bags. Blood is collected using a vacuum chamber. This system allows for the sterile processing and storage of feline whole blood or blood components. (Courtesy of Dr. Urs Giger.)

tube welding instrument (Terumo Sterile Tubing Welder 312, Terumo Medical Corporation, Somerset, NJ) was used to weld a 19-gauge winged infusion set to a pair of pediatric blood packs (Fig. 58–2).[14] CPDA-1 anticoagulant was used in one of the packs. The closed system was placed within a vacuum chamber, and negative pressure was applied. After venipuncture and collection, the whole-blood unit could be used immediately, stored as whole blood, or processed into components by using the attached empty pack.[14] Another system (available from Animal Blood Bank, Dixon, CA) consists of a 60-ml syringe, donor tubing with needle adapter, small blood bag, and 3-way stopcock (Fig. 58–3). After anticoagulant is drawn into the syringe, venipuncture is performed, and blood is collected into the

syringe. At the conclusion of collection, the blood is transferred to the blood bag. The transfer tubing can be sealed, and blood in the bag can be stored at 1 to 4°C. This latter system also is available with a connected bag for component processing. If components are made, the small bags used for feline collection can be centrifuged in a standard blood centrifuge by using special plastic inserts for the centrifuge cups (Sorvall, DuPont Medical Products, Newtown, CT). The reader is referred elsewhere for a more thorough discussion of how to prepare blood components.[13]

Feline whole blood can be stored in a refrigerator for approximately 4 weeks, depending on the anticoagulant used.[15, 16] Additive solutions have been used to prepare packed red blood cells in cats and

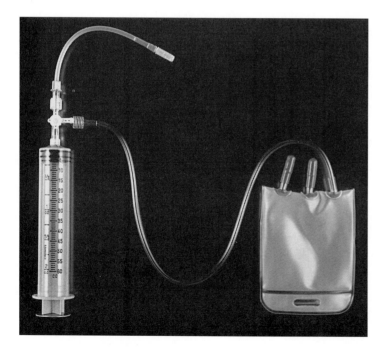

Figure 58–3. Feline blood collection set. Blood is collected into anticoagulant in the syringe and transferred to the blood bag for refrigerated storage.

may provide longer storage, but studies on the resulting storage time have not been performed.

Anemia is the most common indication for transfusion in cats. Whole blood often is administered to anemic feline patients, owing to the relative ease with which it can be obtained and prepared. However, packed red blood cells, if available, are the treatment of choice for normovolemic anemia. Packed red blood cells are obtained by removing the majority of plasma after centrifugation or settling of whole blood. The resultant product contains a higher yield of red blood cells per unit volume. The volume of whole blood or packed red blood cells to be administered can be calculated by the following formula. This formula assumes a normal blood volume of a cat to be approximately 67 ml/kg.[17]

$$Volume = Body\ weight\ (kg) \times 67 \times \frac{desired\ PCV - recipient\ PCV}{PCV\ of\ transfused\ blood}$$

Plasma transfusions also may be performed in cats, although they are administered infrequently compared with dogs. Fresh frozen plasma is plasma frozen within 6 hours of collection. Fresh frozen plasma contains both labile and stable coagulation factors, as well as albumin and globulins. Cats with coagulopathies, such as those seen with liver disease, may receive 10 ml/kg of fresh frozen plasma.

◆ ADMINISTRATION

Blood or blood products always must be administered through a blood filter. Administration sets used in cats generally are shorter than those used in dogs because the volume of blood to be infused is less. Syringe filters (Hemo-Nate filter, Utah Medical Products, Inc., Midvale, UT) or short-length component administration sets may be used, and are available through commercial veterinary blood banks. Blood is administered into the jugular, cephalic, or medial femoral vein. If access to these veins cannot be obtained, the blood may be given intraosseously, using an 18- to 20-gauge hypodermic, spinal, or bone marrow needle inserted into the intramedullary cavity of the femur, ilium, or humerus.

The initial rate of blood administration should be slow, 5 ml/kg/hr or less over the first 5 to 15 minutes. This rate also should be observed in cases of cardiac failure, to avoid circulatory overload. If no adverse reactions are seen in the first few minutes, normovolemic patients can proceed to 10 to 22 ml/kg/hr, whereas hypovolemic patients can receive as much as 66 ml/kg/hr.[18] Concurrent administration of drugs or solutions other than physiologic saline through the same intravenous catheter should be avoided.

◆ TRANSFUSION REACTIONS

The administration of blood or blood products that have been appropriately typed or crossmatched is generally a safe procedure; however, transfusion reactions may occur occasionally. In a study on feline blood component therapy, transfusion reactions were associated with 6.3 per cent of the whole-blood or packed red blood cell transfusions.[19] All cats should be monitored carefully during transfusions. Vital signs, general attitude, packed cell volume and total solids, and evaluation of plasma and urine for presence of hemoglobin should be assessed before, during, and for 2 to 4 hours after transfusion.

Transfusion reactions may be subdivided into acute or delayed reactions, and immunologic or nonimmunologic reactions. The most feared reaction is the acute hemolytic reaction, which is an immunologic reaction commonly due to anti–red blood cell antibodies present in the recipient plasma. The most severe form of this reaction is seen when a cat with type B blood is given type A blood. Clinical signs are dramatic and life-threatening.[9–11] Initial signs occur within seconds to minutes, and may be seen after infusion of as little as 1 to 2 ml of blood. Signs include transient apnea or hypopnea, bradycardia, cardiac arrhythmias, hypotension, seizures, vocalization, urination, defecation, salivation, and depression. Hemoglobinemia and hemoglobinuria also may occur. Treatment involves immediate cessation of the transfusion, followed by supportive or shock therapy. Administration of type B blood to a cat with type A blood causes much milder signs, and the reaction seen is a form of a delayed hemolytic reaction. Here the weak titer of anti-B antibodies present in type A cats will result in extravascular hemolysis of the transfused cells over a few days. Although not usually life-threatening, the transfusion is ineffective clinically.

Other immunologic reactions include febrile nonhemolytic reactions and anaphylactic (IgE-mediated) or anaphylactoid (non–IgE-mediated) reactions. Febrile nonhemolytic reactions cause a rise in temperature of 1°C or more, and occur during or shortly after transfusion. Many of these reactions are due to recipient antibody against donor white blood cells or platelets. The fever may be self-limiting, or may be treated with antipyretics. Fever also may be a sign of acute hemolysis or sepsis, and these disorders must be excluded. Anaphylactic reactions, usually due to recipient antibody to foreign proteins, may be mild (urticaria) or severe (hypotension, dyspnea). Cessation of the transfusion, along with administration of antihistamines, prednisone, and epinephrine in severe cases, is advised.

Nonimmunologic reactions include some hemolytic reactions, sepsis, circulatory overload, citrate toxicity, and infectious disease transmission. Nonimmunologic hemolytic transfusion reactions are caused by prior mechanical or chemical disruption of the transfused red blood cells during storage or handling. Causes can include inadvertent freezing of stored red blood cells, overheating of blood during administration, exposure to hypotonic solutions, and mechanical damage from fluid administration pumps. Sepsis also may produce nonimmunologic hemolysis. Sepsis is produced by infusion of blood products contaminated by bacteria or their toxins. In a well-described outbreak of bacterial contamination of feline whole blood, cats infused with blood contaminated with *Serratia marcescens* exhibited vomiting, diarrhea, collapse, icterus, and panting. Interestingly, fever was seen in only 1 of 14 cats that received the contaminated product.[20]

Circulatory overload is a reaction that results from rapid blood administration, especially in cats with cardiac disease, cats with oliguria or anuria, or cats receiving other fluids simultaneously. Signs include dyspnea and tachypnea, and can progress quickly to pulmonary edema and congestive heart failure. Management includes cessation of transfusion, treatment with diuretics, and oxygen support if required. Vomiting may be observed with rapid administration of blood, or may occur as a nonspecific reaction or in association with hemolysis. Rapid blood infusion also may potentially cause citrate toxicity, a rare reaction due to chelation of calcium by blood products containing the anticoagulant citrate. The resulting hypocalcemia causes muscle tremors and cardiac abnormalities.[21] Ionized calcium concentrations should be determined if this reaction is suspected.

Infectious disease transmission may occur as a delayed, nonimmunologic effect of transfusion. Screening of blood donors for infectious disease, as described earlier in this chapter, should be performed.

◆ SYNTHETIC COLLOIDS AND BLOOD SUBSTITUTES

Although feline blood or blood products are a lifesaving form of therapy, their supply may be limited owing to a lack of availability of donor cats or an inability to access commercial blood products. Synthetic products, such as colloid plasma expanders or the new hemoglobin-based oxygen-carrying solutions, can provide support for the patient when blood is not available.

Synthetic colloids are used in situations of hypovolemia or hypoproteinemia. They are high-molecular-weight molecules that remain in the vascular space and increase oncotic pressure. Colloids replace intravascular deficits only, and crystalloids must be administered simultaneously (reduce volume by 40 to 60 per cent) to replace interstitital deficits. Albumin contributes most of the normal plasma colloid oncotic pressure, and transfusion with 5 per cent human serum albumin solutions commonly is used in hypooncotic human patients. Use of such human albumin solutions is not recommended for cats, owing to the potential for allergic reactions.

Hetastarch, a type of hydroxyethyl starch, is a colloid composed of a heterogeneous population of starch molecules made from amylopectin.[22] The commercially available product (Hespan, B. Braun Medical Inc., Irvine, CA) contains molecules ranging in size from 10,000 to over 1 million daltons, with a number average weight of 69,000. Hespan comes as a 6 per cent solution in 0.9 per cent sodium chloride, and has a stable shelf life of approximately 1 year.[23] Pentastarch, a lower-molecular-weight hydroxyethyl starch, also is available as a synthetic colloid, but its use has not been described in cats.

Hetastarch has been shown to be equal or superior to albumin in its ability to increase colloid oncotic pressure in hypooncotic people and dogs.[24, 25] It has low toxicity after acute or long-term administration. The median lethal dose (LD_{50}) of a single acute dose in cats is greater than 4.5 g/kg (>75 ml/kg).[26] Some caution should be exercised when using hetastarch in patients with hemostatic disorders. Colloids can affect coagulation adversely, either through a dilutional effect or through interference of function of coagulation factors and platelets.[23, 26]

The dose of hetastarch recommended for cats for peracute resuscitation in hypovolemic shock is 10 to 15 ml/kg, given as a bolus over 5 to 10 minutes.[27] A lower dose of 5 to 10 ml/kg given over 4 to 6 hours is used for supporting colloid oncotic pressure in nonemergency situations.[28]

Other synthetic colloids may have more toxic side-effects and are used less commonly. Dextrans are high-molecular-weight glucose polymers synthesized from glucose. Dextran-40 has an average molecular weight of 40 kilodaltons and is used infrequently in clinical veterinary medicine. Dextran-70 has an average molecular weight of 70 kilodaltons. The deleterious effects of both dextrans are thought to be greater than those seen with hetastarch. Anaphylaxis and adverse renal and coagulation effects have been described.[26, 29, 30] For acute volume resuscitation, a slow bolus of 10 to 15 ml/kg is given in cats.[27] Chemically modified gelatins (Vetaplasma, DMS Laboratories, Flemington, NJ) are used as plasma substitutes for emergency use. They are relatively short-acting (4-hour duration of effect), and may be associated with anaphylaxis or antibody production.[28] Dosing recommendation is 3 to 5 ml/kg as a bolus over 15 minutes.[28] Vetaplasma currently is not available in the United States.

Hemoglobin-based oxygen-carrying solutions also have colloidal properties, and exert an oncotic effect. In addition, they serve as "blood substitutes," carrying oxygen and delivering oxygen to tissues. Several types of hemoglobin solutions currently are under development, and are prepared from naturally occurring hemoglobin (human, bovine) or from recombinant hemoglobin. One hemoglobin-based oxygen carrier, Oxyglobin (Biopure Corp., Cambridge, MA) has been approved by the U.S. Food and Drug Administration for use in dogs with anemia.

Oxyglobin is an ultrapure hemoglobin solution of bovine origin. The purified hemoglobin is crosslinked chemically to form stabilized tetramers and large hemoglobin polymers that are well retained in the vascular system. Oxyglobin has a hemoglobin concentration of 13 g/dl, and is prepared in a modified lactated Ringer solution. The product is stable at 2 to 30°C for up to 2 years.[31] Although approved only for use in dogs at this time, studies on the use of Oxyglobin in other species, including cats, are ongoing. In one study of experimentally induced feline hemorrhagic shock, Oxyglobin administered at 20 ml/kg was as effective as autotransfusion and superior to hetastarch in restoring oxygen transport.[32] In a clinical setting, the product has been administered to feline patients at 10 ml/kg, at a rate not to exceed 5 ml/kg/hr.[28]

Advantages of these new oxygen-carrying solutions include availability, stability, lack of disease transmission, ease of administration (no cross-matching or special blood administration sets required), and excellent oxygen delivery. Primary disadvantages include their short half-life (plasma half-life of 30 to 40 hours in dogs), discoloration of plasma and serum that may interfere with laboratory tests, inability to monitor patients by determining the packed cell volume (assess effect via clinical signs or through measurement of hemoglobin) and potential for overexpansion of the vascular volume (increased central venous pressure).[28, 31]

◆ CONCLUSION

The field of veterinary transfusion medicine, including feline transfusion medicine, has increased its knowledge base significantly in recent years. New developments and discoveries have provided a wealth of information for the practicing veterinarian. It is hoped that the information provided by this chapter, along with information from other publications or presentations, will result in improved care for those feline patients requiring blood or blood products.

REFERENCES

1. Andrews GA, Chavey PS, Smith JE, Rich L: N-glycolylneuraminic acid and N-acetylneuraminic acid define feline blood group A and B antigens. Blood 79:2485–2491, 1992.
2. Giger U, Bucheler J, Patterson DF: Frequency and inheritance of A and B blood types in feline breeds of the United States. J Hered 82:15–20, 1991.
3. Griot-Wenk ME, Callan MB, Casal ML, et al: Blood type AB in the feline AB blood group system. Am J Vet Res 57:1438–1442, 1996.
4. Giger U, Griot-Wenk M, Bucheler J, et al: Geographical variation of the feline blood type frequencies in the United States. Fel Pract 19:21–27, 1991.
5. Bucheler J, Giger U: Alloantibodies against A and B blood types in cats. Vet Immunol Immunopathol 38:283–295, 1993.
6. Wilkerson MJ, Meyers KM, Wardrop KJ: Anti-A isoagglutinins in two blood type B cats are IgG and IgM. Vet Clin Pathol 20:10–14, 1991.
7. Giger U: The feline AB blood group system and incompatibility reactions. In Kirk RW (ed): Current Veterinary Therapy XI. Philadelphia, WB Saunders, 1992, pp. 470–474.
8. Griot-Wenk ME, Giger U: Feline transfusion medicine: Blood types and their clinical importance. Vet Clin North Am Small Anim Pract 25:1305–1322, 1995.
9. Giger U, Akol KG: Acute hemolytic transfusion reaction in an Abyssinian cat with blood type B. J Vet Intern Med 4:315–316, 1990.
10. Wilkerson MJ, Wardrop KJ, Giger U, et al: Two cat colonies with A and B blood types and a clinical transfusion reaction. Fel Pract 19:22–26, 1991.
11. Giger U, Bucheler J: Transfusion of type A and type B blood to cats. J Am Vet Med Assoc 198:411–418, 1991.
12. Butler M, Andrews GA, Smith JE: Reactivity of lectins with feline erythrocytes. Comp Haematol Int 1:217–219, 1991.
13. Schneider A. Blood components. Collection, processing, and storage. Vet Clin North Am Small Anim Pract 25:1305–1322, 1995.
14. Springer T, Hatchett WL, Oakley DA, et al: Feline blood storage and component therapy using a closed collection system. Proceedings 16th ACVIM Forum, May 22–25, 1998, p. 738.
15. Marion RS, Smith JE: Posttransfusion viability of feline erythrocytes stored in acid-citrate-dextrose solution. J Am Vet Med Assoc 183:1459–1460, 1983.
16. Bucheler J, Cotter SM: Storage of feline and canine whole blood in CPDA-1 and determination of the post-transfusion viability. J Vet Intern Med 8:172, 1994.
17. Spink RR, Malvin RL, Cohen BJ: Determination of erythrocyte half-life and blood volume in cats. Am J Vet Res 27:1041–1043, 1966.
18. Giger U: Feline transfusion medicine. Prob Vet Med 4:600–611, 1992.
19. Henson MS, Kristensen AT, Armstrong PJ, et al: Feline blood component therapy: Retrospective study of 246 transfusions. J Vet Intern Med 8:169, 1994.
20. Hohenhaus AE, Drusin LM, Garvey MS: Serratia marcescens contamination of feline whole blood in a hospital blood bank. J Am Vet Med Assoc 210:794–798, 1997.
21. Cooper N, Brazier JR, Huttenrott C, et al: Myocardial depression following citrated blood transfusion. Arch Surg 107:756–763, 1973.
22. Hulse JD, Yacobi A: Hetastarch: An overview of the colloid and its metabolism. Drug Intell Clin Pharmacol 17:334–341, 1983.
23. Smiley LE, Garvey MS: The use of hetastarch as adjunct therapy in 26 dogs with hypoalbuminemia: A phase two clinical trial. J Vet Intern Med 8:195–202, 1994.
24. Rackow EC, Weil MH, Macneil AR: Effects of crystalloid and colloid fluids on extravascular lung water in hypoproteinemic dogs. J Appl Physiol 62:2421–2425, 1987.
25. Kirklin JK, Lell WA, Kouchoukos NT: Hydroxyethyl starch versus albumin for colloid infusion following cardiopulmonary bypass in patients undergoing myocardial revascularization. Ann Thorac Surg 37:40–46, 1984.
26. Smiley LE: The use of hetastarch for plasma expansion. Prob Vet Med 4:652–667, 1992.
27. Rudloff E, Kirby R: Hypovolemic shock and resuscitation. Vet Clin North Am Small Anim Pract 24:1015–1039, 1994.
28. Wall RE: Synthetic colloids and blood substitutes. Compend Contin Educ Prac Vet Suppl 20:4–9, 1998.
29. Matheson NA, Diomi P: Renal failure after the administration of dextran 40. Surg Gynecol Obstet 131:661–668, 1970.
30. Ring J, Messmer K: Incidence and severity of anaphylactoid reactions to colloid volume substitutes. Lancet 1:466–469, 1977.
31. Giger U, Rentko VT: Alternatives to blood transfusions. Proceedings 16th ACVIM Forum, May 22–25, 1998, pp. 430–431.
32. Walton RS. Polymerized hemoglobin versus hydroxyethyl starch in an experimental model of feline hemorrhagic shock. Proceedings of 5th International Veterinary Emergency and Critical Care Symposium, San Antonio, September 15–18, 1996.

59

◆ Thrombocytopenia

Claudia J. Baldwin
Rick L. Cowell

Thrombocytopenia is a common laboratory finding in small animals. The presence of this abnormality in domestic cats however, appears to be less frequent than in dogs. In a review of laboratory submissions to a veterinary teaching hospital, prevalence of thrombocytopenia in feline patients over a 5-year period was 1.2 per cent.[1] In a report of hemostatic profiles, thrombocytopenia was present in 53 per cent of cats tested.[2] In another study of hemostatic disorders, 23 per cent of cats tested were thrombocytopenic.[3] The presence of thrombocytopenia alone, in these 2 studies, was found in fewer cases, 19 and 12 per cent, respectively.[2, 3] In the study in which the incidence of thrombocytopenia alone was 12 per cent, the incidence in dogs under similar circumstances was indeed higher (23 per cent).[3]

Thrombocytopenia often is associated with an underlying disease process in which the platelets either are not produced; are sequestered; are destroyed; or are utilized or consumed too rapidly to meet demand. The presence of thrombocytopenia allows the clinician to formulate a list of differential diagnoses. Bleeding disorders associated with thrombocytopenia in cats have been reported to occur in approximately 14 to 30 per cent of patients,[1, 3] and would be expected when the thrombocytopenia is severe or the patient is challenged (e.g., surgery). Presented here is a brief review of hemostasis, followed by the initial diagnostic approach, laboratory evaluation, and clinical approach to diagnosis and management of the thrombocytopenic cat.

◆ HEMOSTASIS

Hemostasis depends on an interaction between the primary system (vessel walls and platelets) and the secondary system (soluble coagulation factors). When a vessel is injured, it undergoes local reflex vasoconstriction. This reflex vasoconstriction is short-lived, and must be maintained by release of vasoactive compounds from platelets and surrounding tissue. Maintenance of vasoconstriction decreases blood flow at the site of the injury, allowing activated platelets and soluble coagulation factors to accumulate locally and function in clot formation. When vessels become injured and epithelium is denuded, subepithelial collagen is exposed. The exposed collagen activates platelets and soluble coagulation factors. Circulating platelets accumulate, aggregate, and form a loose primary platelet plug. The simultaneous activation of the soluble coagulation factors results in the activation of thrombin, which cleaves fibrinogen into fibrin. A fibrin network is laid down on the primary platelet plug, crosslinked by Factor XIII, forming a secondary or stable plug. Descriptions of the secondary system contribution to hemostasis may be found in other reviews.[2–4]

Circulating blood platelets live for approximately 10 days. They are derived from bone marrow megakaryocyte progenitor cells. The progenitor cell progresses from the megakaryoblast to promegakaryocyte to mature platelet-producing megakaryocyte to releasable blood platelet. Maturation time from megakaryoblast to platelet is approximately 4 to 5 days. Regulation of thrombopoiesis occurs via the hormone thrombopoietin (TPO). TPO concentration is controlled by circulating platelet mass (greater mass, more platelet surface adsorption of TPO, less free TPO to stimulate bone marrow production), and not by platelet number. The liver and spleen in normal cats can house 20 to 30 per cent of the circulating platelet mass. An increased pool of platelets within these organs (sequestration) could decrease the "countable" platelets in the laboratory, but because the mass is not changed, platelet production is unchanged.[5] Recently, feline TPO was molecularly cloned from feline liver, and appears to have stimulatory activity in vitro.[6]

To summarize coagulation, vessel injury results in local vasoconstriction that decreases blood flow, allowing platelets to adhere and recruit more platelets that bind and activate soluble coagulation factors. The end result is a stable platelet plug.

◆ INITIAL DIAGNOSTIC APPROACH

When managing a patient with a suspected or potential bleeding disorder, signalment, history, physical examination findings, and coexistent disease are invaluable in clinical assessment and selection of initial diagnostic tests to allow efficient diagnosis and timely clinical management.

Signalment

In general, breed, age, and gender are important considerations when considering potential inherited

468

bleeding disorders. These parameters, however, may not be as important a consideration in the thrombocytopenic cat, because no inherited causes of thrombocytopenia have been documented in that species. Predilection for certain diseases, however, that may produce decreased numbers of platelets in *breed* (i.e., feline infectious peritonitis in Birman or Persian lines),[7] *age*, or *gender* (i.e., feline immunodeficiency virus [FIV] seropositivity in older male cats)[8] groups does exist, and thus, signalment always should be noted.

History

Past history should be obtained on all patients, inclusive of related cats and feline housemates. Episodes of historical weakness, lameness, or illness should be recorded, because these may be related to the patient's current bleeding disorder. Also, the clinician should inquire about prior bleeding episodes, inclusive of severity, age of occurrence, number of episodes, and association with disease, challenge, or drug therapy. Previous drug therapy in particular should be addressed because drugs may suppress megakaryopoeisis, inhibit platelet function, or increase platelet destruction. Dates of vaccination should be determined because transient mild-to-moderate thrombocytopenia associated with platelet and/or endothelial dysfunction (between days 1 and 10 after modified-live-virus vaccination) has been shown to occur in other species,[4, 9, 10] as has mild spontaneous clinical bleeding associated with severe thrombocytopenia and concurrent underlying disease.[11]

History of the current bleeding episode, such as environmental factors, whether bleeding was spontaneous or associated with some event (e.g., trauma), site and severity of bleeding, and treatment should be recorded, because these may aid in assessment of the disorder and interpretation of the laboratory findings.

Physical Examination

Physical examination should be complete, including a fundic examination. Note should be taken of the type of bleeding present, along with the site and severity of bleeding. Primary system abnormalities (platelet and vascular disorders) manifest more typically as superficial bleeding into the skin or mucous membranes or from body orifices. *Purpura*, defined as hemorrhage into the skin or mucous membranes, may be small (petechia) or large (ecchymosis) areas of extravasation. Petechiation is most typical of primary system abnormalities, and signifies prolonged bleeding time resulting from thrombocytopenia, thrombopathia, or vascular disease. Blood loss from primary system abnormalities generally is not as severe as blood loss associated with the secondary system (soluble coagulation factor deficiency/defect).

With a pure secondary system disorder, ecchymoses may be seen, but hematomas, hemarthrosis, and bleeding into body cavities are more typical. Severe bleeding does not support a diagnosis of primary system hemorrhage, but rather the secondary system's inability to stabilize the platelet plug. Combined disorders of the primary and secondary systems (e.g., disseminated intravascular coagulation [DIC]) may occur and result in both petechiation (primary system) and deep hemorrhage (secondary system). A careful examination for a concurrent, and possibly causal, disease should be done. Other disorders associated with bleeding also should be considered in some patients, along with differential diagnoses of disorders of hemostasis. Although epistaxis is characteristic of primary system abnormalities, it may be unilateral and therefore also characteristic of nasal disease, such as foreign body or neoplasia.

Clinical signs reported in a review of thrombocytopenia in cats included epistaxis, bruising, retinal hemorrhage, hyphema, hemothorax, hematemesis, hemorrhagic enteritis, petechiation, and thrombosis.[1] Physical examination, the type and severity of hemorrhage, knowledge of signalment, and history usually suggest possible etiologies and/or helpful diagnostic procedures.

Laboratory Evaluation

Initial laboratory evaluation in the feline patient with a suspected bleeding disorder should include not only tests to differentiate between primary and secondary system abnormalities but also tests to assess the overall condition of the patient. A complete blood count should be performed to detect the presence and severity of anemia and whether there is evidence of appropriate bone marrow response (regenerative) to an anemia by means of a reticulocyte count. Evaluation of a blood film should be conducted to detect presence of hemoparasites (e.g., *Cytauxzoon*; see Chapter 55, Update on Cytauxzoonosis). Alterations in white blood cell numbers or morphology, or white blood cell inclusions (e.g., *Ehrlichia* morulae) may suggest a certain causative disease for the hemorrhage. At the same time, platelet numbers should be evaluated on the stained blood smear to determine whether they are adequate (see later). Serum biochemistries are useful in detection of underlying or concurrent disease and evaluation of the cat's overall health. A urinalysis should be performed to detect hemorrhage or other abnormalities. Seropositivity for feline leukemia virus (FeLV) and FIV should be assessed to determine whether there is a relationship between these infections and the disease process.

Most domestic animals have platelet counts ranging from 200,000 to 500,000/µl. Platelet counts must drop below 50,000/µl before the patient has increased bleeding secondary to trauma, and below 25,000/μl before spontaneous hemorrhage occurs owing to thrombocytopenia alone. Automated platelet counts are readily available with current in-house instrumentation. Unfortunately, most instrumentation cannot count feline platelets accurately because platelet size is too similar to that of the red blood cell, and because of the tendency for clumping. Because of this, other methods for assessing platelet number should be used. Automated counts using platelet-rich plasma, rather than whole blood, have been described, although the authors report a lowered reference range with this methodology.[12] In a recent publication of evaluation of methods of platelet counting in cats, the authors compared hemacytometer manual counts (their "gold standard") to other methods (e.g., automated, estimates, special stains). They reported the highest correlation (0.776) and diagnostic accuracy (88 per cent) to exist between the hemacytometer method and blood film estimates.[13]

Manual hemacytometer platelet counts can be performed readily in-hospital by the Unopette method, which is very similar to doing a Unopette white blood cell count. Platelet counts typically are performed on ethylenediaminetetraacetic acid (EDTA)–anticoagulated blood, but may be done on blood collected in sodium citrate. The platelet count should be done within 5 hours of blood collection, otherwise erroneously low platelet counts may be reported. Also, platelet clumping (common in feline samples) may occur in any sample, causing erroneously low platelet counts.

When estimating platelet numbers from a blood smear, platelet numbers should be evaluated within the monolayer of the blood film. Platelet numbers are assessed subjectively as increased, decreased, or adequate. An average of 6 to 35 platelets/oil power field (OPF) in the monolayer of the slide merits classification as *adequate*. If platelet numbers are greater than 35 platelets/OPF, they are reported as *increased*, and if less than 6 platelets/OPF, they are reported as *decreased*. If platelet numbers appear decreased, the blood slide, especially the feathered edge, should be scanned to ensure that the decrease is not due to clumping. If there are platelet clumps, the platelets should be reported as clumped instead of decreased; however, the clinician should realize that if there are sufficient platelets to cause platelet clumps, platelet numbers are sufficient to prevent spontaneous hemorrhage due to thrombocytopenia alone.

Mild thrombocytopenias are not recognized on subjective evaluations of peripheral blood smears. Each platelet seen in the monolayer of the blood film represents about 15,000 platelets/μl. Therefore, if an average of 6 to 7 platelets/OPF are seen, and platelets are reported as adequate, the patient still may be thrombocytopenic, because 6 to 7 platelets/OPF is equivalent to about 100,000 platelets/μl. Hence, only moderate and marked thrombocytopenias are detected by subjective evaluation of platelet

numbers using the procedure and ranges described previously. When spontaneous hemorrhage occurs due to thrombocytopenia alone, the platelet count must be 25,000/μl or less. Platelet counts this low are readily discernible on well-made blood smears (≤2 platelets/OPF).

Another cause of laboratory-reported thrombocytopenia that must be kept in mind is *artifactual*. As mentioned previously, platelet estimates and/or counts may be decreased falsely secondary to platelet clumping in vitro. Feline blood is prone to platelet clumping, especially if difficulty is encountered during the venipuncture. Time delay in making blood smears or performing a platelet count also may result in an artifactual thrombocytopenia. Platelet counts and/or high-quality blood smears for platelet estimation should be made from the EDTA sample within 5 hours of collection.

The clinician should look for large (>5 μm) platelets whenever thrombocytopenia is present. These large platelets typically are referred to as either *megaplatelets*, *stress platelets*, or *shift platelets*. They account for up to 1 per cent of the platelet population in normal animals. Whenever thrombocytopenia is present owing to platelet utilization and/or destruction, these large platelets increase in number and typically account for more than 1 per cent of the platelet population. Therefore, assessing the number of large platelets can help differentiate decreased platelet production or sequestration from increased platelet utilization or destruction.

Bone marrow evaluation with special emphasis on megakaryocyte number, stage, and morphology may be extremely useful for differentiating the general mechanisms of thrombocytopenia. Bone marrow aspirates can be collected safely even in severely thrombocytopenic animals. Because the marrow cavity is solidly enclosed and marrow is high in tissue thromboplastin, intramarrow hemorrhage resulting from a bone marrow aspirate is controlled quickly by the release of tissue thromboplastin and the increase in intramarrow pressure secondary to the hemorrhage. Thrombocytopenia due to increased platelet utilization, consumption, or destruction results in normal-to-increased marrow megakaryocyte numbers; thrombocytopenia due to platelet sequestration results in normal marrow megakaryocyte numbers; and thrombocytopenia due to decreased platelet production results in decreased marrow megakaryocyte numbers. Bone marrow cytologic evaluation also facilitates the detection of abnormal cells (creating myelopthisis) or causative infectious agents (e.g., histoplasmosis).

Bleeding time is used to assess the function of the primary system. Prolonged bleeding time is caused by quantitative or qualitative platelet disorders and/or vascular disease. Bleeding times may be prolonged by thrombocytopenia alone in patients with platelet counts of less than 40 to 50 × 10³/μl; therefore, testing of bleeding time usually is not performed once severe thrombocytopenia has been demonstrated.

◆ CLINICAL APPROACH TO DIAGNOSIS AND MANAGEMENT

Traditionally, thrombocytopenic disorders have been presented in the basic categories of decreased production, sequestration, increased destruction, and excessive utilization/consumption (Table 59–1). Organization of basic mechanisms of thrombocytopenia in this manner allows the clinician to better understand the development of the thrombocytopenia, and then choose specific tests; for example, bone marrow evaluation for suspected decreased production, or thorough abdominal evaluation (radiographs and ultrasound studies) for suspected sequestration. To that end, a review of the basic mechanisms of thrombocytopenia is presented. However, disease processes are not always straightforward, and associated thrombocytopenia may be due to more than 1 mechanism (e.g., histoplasmosis may cause thrombocytopenia by means of sequestration, destruction, and possibly utilization or consump-

Table 59–2. DAMNITT Scheme for Differential Diagnosis

D	=	Degenerative
		Developmental
A	=	Allergic
		Autoimmune (Immune-mediated)
M	=	Metabolic
N	=	Neoplastic, nutritional
I	=	Iatrogenic
		Idiopathic
		Inflammatory
		Infectious
		Immune-mediated
T	=	Toxic
T	=	Traumatic

tion), or organ dysfunction. For this reason, organization of the causes of thrombocytopenia may be better considered in the clinical setting by process of disease utilizing the DAMNITT scheme (Table 59–2) or by organ system causes.

Basic Mechanisms of Thrombocytopenic Disorders (see Table 59–1)

Decreased Production of Platelets

Decreased production of platelets may be due to a variety of causes. Defects in production of bone marrow cells may be generalized or platelet-specific. Decreased production of platelets is supported by the finding of less than 1 per cent of circulating platelets being megaplatelets, and cytologic evidence of decreased megakaryopoiesis in bone marrow aspirates. This basic category includes autoimmune (immune-mediated), neoplastic, infectious, idiopathic, and iatrogenic/toxicity disorders. The key to establishing this mechanism is cytologic evaluation of the bone marrow.

Aspiration of bone marrow in cats usually requires some sort of short-acting chemical restraint. Impressions, based on initial evaluation of cellularity, can be formed quickly in well-prepared aspirates, whereas aspirates contaminated with peripheral blood may be difficult to evaluate for cellularity. Aspiration technique and details of cytologic evaluation may be found in a review.[14] Core biopsies, to evaluate cellularity, are indicated when marrow cannot be obtained. A hypocellular marrow is consistent with aplastic anemia (pancytopenia), myelofibrosis, and myelonecrosis, whereas hypercellular marrow is consistent with ineffective erythropoiesis, increased peripheral destruction or utilization/consumption, preleukemic syndrome (myelodysplasia) or myeloproliferative disease, and myelophthisis. When decreased production of platelets alone occurs, cellularity of the marrow may be normal except for the absence of adequate numbers of megakaryocytes.

As mentioned previously, harvested marrow may be used for cytologic identification of organisms, or for bacteriologic, viral, or immunologic studies.

Table 59–1. Basic Mechanisms of Thrombocytopenia in Cats

Disorders of Decreased Production

Idiopathic aplasia
Immune-mediated disease
Infectious diseases
    Bacterial *(Francisella tularensis)*
    Viral (panleukopenia virus, FeLV, FIV)
    Rickettsial (*Ehrlichia canis* and *platus*)
Neoplastic disorders
    Myeloproliferative disease
    Myelophthisis
Toxicity disorders
    Chemotherapeutic drugs
    Heavy metal (thallium)
    T2 toxin

Disorders of Sequestration

Splenic inflammatory, infiltrative, congestive disease
Hyperplastic splenomegaly
Hepatomegaly/hepatopathy
Endotoxemia

Disorders of Increased Destruction

Primary immune-mediated
Secondary immune-mediated
    Infectious disease
    Other immune-mediated disease
    Neoplasia
    Toxicity (drug-induced)
Postvaccination
Microangiopathy

Disorders of Excessive Utilization/Consumption

Disseminated intravascular coagulation
Thrombotic thrombocytopenic purpura (hemolytic/uremic syndrome)
Vascular disease (immune-mediated, parasitic, infectious)
Early viral disease response
Severe hemorrhage (e.g., vitamin K antagonism)

Abbreviations: FeLV, feline leukemia virus; FIV, feline immunodeficiency virus.

Sequestration of Platelets

Sequestration of platelets is an important category of disease. With sequestration, the body mass of platelets is unchanged; therefore, megakaryopoiesis, as determined by evaluation of a bone marrow aspirate, is not changed. However, circulating platelets may be markedly decreased, resulting in increased bleeding time, especially with surgical challenge. Table 59–1 lists some of the many causes.

Platelets circulate throughout the vascular system with 20 to 30 per cent normally pooled within the liver and spleen. With splenic enlargement from any cause, increased numbers of platelets may be sequestered, resulting in thrombocytopenia. Splenomegaly creating sequestration thrombocytopenia (hypersplenism) may be associated with a variety of inflammatory or infectious processes, neoplastic and nonneoplastic infiltrative diseases, congestion (pharmacologic, portal hypertension), and hyperplastic splenomegaly.[15] The liver, when enlarged or diseased, also serves as a site of platelet sequestration.[16] Reduced survival times of sequestered platelets may be seen.[17] Additionally, pulmonary sequestration may occur in cats. In dogs with experimentally induced endotoxemia, vasodilatation occurred as a response to prostacyclin, and platelets were sequestered within the pulmonary vasculature, resulting in thrombocytopenia.[16]

Patients with sequestration may or may not exhibit evidence of a primary bleeding disorder on physical examination. In the thrombocytopenic patient, the spleen and liver should be assessed carefully. Even if the size of these organs appears normal on physical examination, radiographic and possibly ultrasonographic studies are indicated, because disease alone, rather than enlargement, may be responsible for the thrombocytopenia. Fine-needle aspiration of these organs may lead to a cytologic diagnosis in some cases (e.g., histoplasmosis, lymphosarcoma). Additionally, thoracic radiographic studies may be indicated in some patients.

Increased Destruction of Platelets

Thrombocytopenia due to increased platelet destruction is considered a common cause of bleeding disorders (see Table 59–1) in companion animals. Platelets may be destroyed by immune- or non–immune-mediated mechanisms. Immune-mediated destruction, whether primary or secondary, is reported to be the most common cause of bleeding disorders in cats and dogs.[18] Primary immune-mediated thrombocytopenia in cats appears, however, to be the less common disorder of the 2, based on clinical experience, the few reports in the literature,[19, 20] and a review of 41 cases of thrombocytopenia in which only 1 cat met the criteria for a diagnosis of primary immune-mediated thrombocytopenia.[1] In addition, of the 6 cases of thrombocytopenia alone in a case series of hemostatic disorders, only 1 cat was diagnosed with primary immune disease.[3]

Secondary immune-mediated thrombocytopenias may be associated with viral diseases, rickettsial diseases *(Ehrlichia)*, neoplasia, other primary immune-mediated diseases, and drug administration.[17, 21–23] Many mechanisms have been proposed for immune destruction of the circulating platelets, ranging from autoantibodies, which occur in autoimmune disease, to isoantibodies, which occur in response to a foreign protein. The end result is destruction of platelets. Historically, drug exposure is very important in these patients.

Other causes of increased platelet destruction include microangiopathy, associated with neoplastic disease involving the spleen or liver, or pulmonary thromboembolic disease, and in other species, vaccination with modified live adenovirus and myxovirus products.[16]

Excessive Platelet Utilization/Consumption

Consumptive coagulopathies, such as DIC, may represent the most common causes of excessive platelet utilization, although other causes, such as vascular disease, also occur. In a report of sick cats screened for coagulation defects, 38 of 85 had 1 or more abnormalities of the coagulation profile. Twenty of the 38 affected cats exhibited thrombocytopenia as well as other hemostatic abnormalities. These findings suggested that hemostatic disorders develop more frequently than clinical signs would suggest, and that more than 50 per cent of the cats with coagulopathies had thrombocytopenia.[2] Regardless of the cause, bone marrow megakaryocytes typically are increased and megaplatelets account for more than 1 per cent of the circulating platelets when excessive utilization/consumption is occurring. Some diseases that cause increased utilization of platelets also may create thrombocytopenia by other mechanisms (e.g., destruction, decreased production).[16, 22, 24, 25]

Thrombocytopenia associated with DIC results from consumption of platelets, because of excessive formation of thrombin and intravascular fibrin thrombi. Similarly, thrombotic thrombocytopenic purpura (TTP), also known as hemolytic-uremic syndrome, has been described. This disorder usually is due to an unknown stimulus, resulting in formation of intravascular platelet thrombi, and worsening thrombocytopenia. The TTP syndrome has been described with renal transplantation/cyclosporine therapy in domestic cats.[26] In addition, diseases in which vascular damage is present (e.g., immune-mediated vasculitis, heartworm disease, infectious diseases, septicemia) may result in thrombosis, due to exposure of subendothelial components and decreased endothelial production of prostacyclin, which normally help to repel platelets. Early viral infection may induce platelet release of adenosine diphosphate, resulting in intravascular aggregation of platelets that then are removed by the mononuclear phagocytic system. Hemorrhage should not be overlooked as a cause of platelet utilization; however, blood loss would be expected to be severe. It has been reported that vitamin K antagonism (rodenticides) may be associated with significant thrombocytopenia in dogs,[27] and the same scenario might be expected in the nondiscriminant feline hunter.

Thrombocytopenia due to utilization or consumption always is secondary to an underlying disease. The only identified cause of TTP thus far is iatrogenic. History of exposure to infectious diseases (e.g., bacterial, fungal, viral, rickettsial, parasitic) may be helpful. Physical examination may reveal evidence of an underlying disease. Evaluation of the secondary (activated partial thromboplastin time, one-stage prothrombin time) and fibrinolytic (fibrin degradation products) systems, and the circulating natural anticoagulant antithrombin III, may help distinguish DIC from the other causes.[2]

DAMNITT Scheme Approach
(see Table 59–2)

Thrombocytopenia often is a laboratory diagnosis without overt evidence of primary bleeding. A complete history and physical examination, obtained before the laboratory finding of thrombocytopenia, should allow the clinician to formulate a list of differential diagnoses. Because thrombocytopenia may be due to ill-defined mechanisms, or more than 1 mechanism, it often is helpful to utilize the DAMNITT scheme. Included in this section are confirmed or highly likely causes of documented thrombocytopenia in cats.

Neoplastic Causes

Cancer is becoming a more important disease process in the lives of cats, now that we are able to identify and manage other medical problems, and prolong life. Additionally, our diagnostic skills and equipment have improved such that definitive diagnoses can be made less invasively. Treatment modalities also have improved, and cat owners have kept pace in their acceptance of alternatives to euthanasia.

Hematologic abnormalities are seen commonly with neoplastic disease. In a review of thrombocytopenia in cats, 16 of the 41 cats (39 per cent) had 1 or more neoplastic disorders.[1] Neoplasia affecting the bone marrow was involved most often, although lymphoma, hemangiosarcoma, and adenocarcinoma were present in some of the thrombocytopenic cats. Proposed mechanisms of thrombocytopenia included decreased production, increased destruction (involving vascular lesions and microangiopathies), utilization (owing to hemorrhage) and consumption (through DIC).[1] In addition, sequestration should be considered when hepatosplenic involvement occurs. In one study of cats with hemostatic disorders, neoplasia was identified both in the group affected by thrombocytopenia alone, and in the group with

hemostatic disorders. In this study of 85 cats with hemostatic disorders, neoplasia was 1 of the 3 largest categories of underlying disease identified.[2] These findings were similar to those from an earlier study of 101 cats with hemostatic disorders that reported malignant neoplasms (primarily lymphoma) to be one of the 3 largest categories of underlying disease.[3] In addition to the basic mechanisms of thrombocytopenia (e.g., decreased production, sequestration), the low platelet count also is considered to be a paraneoplastic syndrome. This diagnosis would be made by eliminating all other causes of thrombocytopenia, and documenting correction of the problem when the apparently unrelated tumor is removed.[28]

Nutritional Causes

Thrombocytopenia generally is not thought to be associated with nutrition or feeding, but was observed in 7 normal cats maintained on total parenteral nutrition (TPN). During the 2 weeks of TPN, anemia and thrombocytopenia developed to varying degrees. These abnormalities were reversible when TPN was discontinued and the cats were returned to enteral feeding.[29] In that study, the mechanism of thrombocytopenia was not determined. Finding of decreased platelets in clinical patients receiving TPN should prompt investigation of other potential causes; however, the thrombocytopenia may be self-resolving after the termination of TPN.

Iatrogenic Causes

Renal Transplantation

In recent years, renal transplantation has become available for cats with renal failure (see Chapter 43, Renal Transplantation in the Management of Chronic Renal Failure). The procedure is best suited for the stable patient in very early decompensated renal failure.[30] TTP or hemolytic uremic syndrome has been described as an uncommon sequela to transplant and cyclosporine therapy. Two of the 3 cases described in the literature probably were the result of cyclosporine immunosuppression, and the third case was thought to have been associated with allograft rejection. Mortality rate was 100 per cent. Hemolytic anemia, thrombocytopenia, and azotemia were present in all cases. Interestingly, platelet counts were mildly to moderately depressed (99,000 to 125,000/μl). Histologic lesions were compatible with utilization/consumption of platelets.[26] Clinicians caring for renal transplant patients should be aware of this syndrome, because early recognition and treatment may be critical to survival.

Bone Marrow Transplantation

Bone marrow transplantation studies have been under way since the early 1990s. In one experimental study, 1 of 7 cats developed immune-mediated hemolytic anemia and thrombocytopenia in the immediate posttransplant period, which were responsive to immunosuppressive therapy.[31] In 1996, a feline patient was reported to have received an allogeneic bone marrow transplant for treatment of acute myeloid leukemia. The most life-threatening complication after the transplant was hemorrhage secondary to severe thrombocytopenia. The patient survived, and was reported to be doing well 4 years after transplant.[32] Although bone marrow transplant still is not widely available today, it may become more feasible in the future; attending clinicians should be aware of thrombocytopenia as a possible complication.

Drug Therapy

See Toxicity

Idiopathic Causes

Idiopathic causes for any disorder always must be considered. In the thrombocytopenic patient, every effort should be made to identify known causes of the problem. However, the cause of persistent thrombocytopenia may go undiagnosed. In a retrospective study of 41 cats with thrombocytopenia, a cause could not be found for 20 per cent of the patients. Interestingly, 88 per cent of these cats were nonpurebred females.[1] Idiopathic thrombocytopenia should be a diagnosis of exclusion, and should be the final diagnosis only when all other potential causes (including DIC and immune-mediated disorders) have been excluded. This approach differs somewhat from that in dogs, in which idiopathic TTP is synonymous for immune-mediated thrombocytopenia, and a diagnosis of exclusion leads one to assume that the thrombocytopenia is immune in nature.

Inflammatory Causes (Table 59–3)

Infectious Causes

Infectious causes of thrombocytopenia have represented a large percentage of the cases appearing in reviews of thrombocytopenia and hemostatic disorders. In one study, infectious disease represented

Table 59–3. Inflammatory Causes of Feline Thrombocytopenia

Infectious	Viral
Bacterial	Feline leukemia virus
Francisella tularensis	Feline immunodeficiency
Fungal	virus
Histoplasma capsulatum	Feline coronavirus
Protozoal	Panleukopenia virus
Cytauxzoon	
Rickettsial	*Immune*
Ehrlichia canis	Primary
Ehrlichia risticii	Secondary

29 per cent (12/41) of the cases, the largest group reported.[1] When including cats from the multiple-disorder group, another 7 cats were identified with infectious disease, bringing the incidence of infection in these cases to 46 per cent. FeLV infections were identified in 27 per cent (11/41) of thrombocytopenic cats. Most of the remaining cases were attributed to other viral causes (FIV, feline infectious peritonitis virus, and panleukopenia virus).[1] In a report on hemostatic abnormalities, systemic infections were 1 of the 3 largest categories of disease identified. In cats with thrombocytopenia alone, diseases identified included FeLV, FIV, and *Histoplasma capsulatum* infections.[2] In both of these studies, infectious disease or systemic infection was ranked in the top 3 categories of disease, and viral disease predominated.

Regional differences exist in the prevalence of infectious diseases. The viral diseases, already mentioned as being associated with or causing thrombocytopenia, are less dependent on environment and vectors, and as such, are seen throughout North America. Other infectious diseases, newly emerging or seen regionally, are associated with thrombocytopenia and are covered briefly.

H. capsulatum is a fungal organism that causes a noncontagious infection in cats in the midwestern and southern United States. The disease may be localized to the pulmonary system or may disseminate. In one study of 12 cases, 4 cases displayed thrombocytopenia with normal megakaryopoiesis.[24] Another notable disease associated with thrombocytopenia is tularemia, caused by the bacterium *Francisella tularensis*. Although the disease has been reported nationwide in a variety of mammalian hosts, it is seen most commonly in the southern and western regions of the United States. An acute systemic (typhoidal) form of the disease has been described with all 3 cats succumbing.[33] A second clinical report described successful treatment and survival of 2 cats.[34] All cats in these reports developed thrombocytopenia. As this is a zoonotic disease, care should be taken in handling potential cases, and a high index of suspicion is needed to make an antemortem diagnosis.[35] Cytauxzoonosis is a highly fatal disease caused by the protozoan *Cytauxzoon felis* (see Chapter 55, Update on Cytauxzoonosis). It has been reported in domestic cats in the south-central and southeastern United States. The natural reservoir appears to be the bobcat, with transmission through ticks (*Dermacentor variabilis*). Thrombocytopenia is common, and in a recent report, all 7 cats had low platelet counts.[12] In this latest report, 6 of 7 cats survived with treatment. Another emerging disease, possibly transmitted by ticks or mice, is ehrlichiosis (see Chapter 4, Rickettsial Diseases). The seroprevalence is 33.1 per cent, based on 583 cats tested in the continental United States. Twenty-three cases have been described with clinical signs. One-third of cases with available hematologic data were found to be thrombocytopenic.[36]

Immune Causes

Immune causes of thrombocytopenia also must be considered in the inflammatory category. Immune disease may be primary, in which the immune system attacks the platelet directly, or secondary to another offending agent or disease whereby the platelet is destroyed in the immune reaction. Primary immune destruction of platelets is not common in cats (see earlier discussion in Basic Mechanisms). A recent case report describes a single case, with reference to only 2 other primary immune thrombocytopenia cases in the literature.[20] Primary immune destruction of platelets should be considered when no other predisposing disorders can be identified. Accurate (specific and sensitive) tests to evaluate immune destruction of feline platelets may not be readily available. In the most recent report, indirect immunohistochemisty using serum, and direct immunohistochemisty utilizing bone marrow, were performed.[20] A diagnosis of primary immune destruction was made with a positive result on the direct immunohistochemistry test, and with exclusion of secondary causes. Treatment should include immunosuppressants (glucocorticoids, azathioprine) and supportive care. Response to treatment is viewed by some veterinarians as confirming the diagnosis; however, the clinician must use caution with this approach. Idiopathic, artifactual, or transitory thrombocytopenia also may appear to respond to immunosuppressive treatment but may, in fact, have been self-resolving.

Toxic Causes

Most toxic causes of thrombocytopenia probably are associated with medications that are prescribed. These include anthelmintics, antibiotics, antifungals, antithyroid drugs, antivirals, and chemotherapeutics. Table 59–4 lists the drugs that are known to cause thrombocytopenia in cats.

Albendazole has been reported to have better efficacy against giardiasis in a number of species, compared with fenbendazole and metronidazole. Since the report of reversible pancytopenia associated with albendazole administration, including thrombocytopenia of a significant level (30,000/μl) in 1 cat, the authors have been hesitant to prescribe this medication.[37] Although neither benzimidazole is licensed for use in domestic cats, fenbendazole, although perhaps not as effective, is considered safer.

Chloramphenicol was once used widely in cats, but concern for human health and the availability of other antibiotics have lessened its use. A reversible form of cytopenia has been described experimentally in domestic cats.[38] Bicytopenia (leukopenia and thrombocytopenia) was detected in FeLV-negative cats treated with chloramphenicol for 2 weeks; however, the effect was reversible when the drug was discontinued. Griseofulvin is an antifungal antibiotic, with fungistatic properties. It is indicated

Table 59–4. Toxicities Associated With Feline Thrombocytopenia

Pharmacologics

Anthelmintics
  Albendazole
Antibiotics
  Chloramphenicol
Antifungals
  Griseofulvin
Antithyroids
  Methimazole
  Propylthiouracil
Antivirals
  Ribavirin
Chemotherapeutics
  Azathioprine
  Carboplatin
  Dacarbazine
  Doxorubicin
  Liposome-encapsulated *cis-bis*-neodecanoato-trans-R,R,-1,2-diaminocyclohexane platinum (II)

Toxins

Envenomation *(Vipera palaestinae)*
T-2 toxin
Vitamin K antagonists

in the treatment of dermatophyte infections in cats. Hematologic findings associated with griseofulvin toxicity include anemia, leukopenia, and occasionally pancytopenia.[39] Bone marrow evaluation may reveal severe hypoplasia of all hematopoietic cell lines. Concurrent infection with FeLV or FIV, both of which can cause thrombocytopenia or pancytopenia, should be investigated, because patients infected with either of these viruses may be at increased risk for the drug-induced hematopoietic dyscrasias. Treatment for toxicity involves discontinuation of the drug, with blood counts usually returning to normal within 2 weeks. An antiviral drug, ribavirin, was investigated in cats infected experimentally with calicivirus. The treatment failed to have any beneficial effect on clinical course of disease or to decrease viral excretion. However, treated cats developed symptomatic thrombocytopenia, presumably from the ribavirin. The adverse effects were reversed within 1 week of discontinuation of treatment.[40]

Antithyroid drugs have been associated with immune disease in cats, as demonstrated by positive immune testing (antinuclear antibody testing and direct Coombs). The incidence of thrombocytopenia with evidence of primary bleeding was 11 and 3.8 per cent, respectively, associated with propylthiouracil and methimazole.[41, 42] Administration of propylthiouracil no longer is advocated, and methimazole still is utilized, with monitoring, as a short- or long-term treatment for hyperthyroidism. Hematologic abnormalities associated with methimazole should resolve within 1 week of discontinuation of the drug.

Chemotherapeutic agents are the most common drugs causing thrombocytopenia in cats (see Table

59–4). Studies were performed in normal cats to determine hematologic and systemic toxicities that might preclude the use of these drugs.[43–46] Currently, azathioprine, carboplatin, and doxorubicin all are used in cats at dosages that usually do not cause thrombocytopenia; however, platelet counts are evaluated regularly to monitor for this side-effect.

Environmental toxins causing thrombocytopenia in cats are listed in Table 59–4. A recent report of venomous snake bites in cats in Israel indicated that thrombocytopenia was present, and varied from mild to severe.[47] Poisonous snakes exist in North America, and although cats may be more resistant than other species to snake bites, bite wounds in cats with concurrent thrombocytopenia and other hematologic or hemostatic changes should prompt the clinician to consider this differential diagnosis.

Alimentary toxic aleukia is a disorder in human beings caused by a trichothecene metabolite, T-2 toxin. This mycotoxin is produced by *Fusarium* species, and is found in moldy grains. Although not reported clinically as an intoxicant in cats, this species is a useful model to study the disease in human beings. Chronic oral administration of T-2 toxin to cats resulted in clinical illness and death in all 10 subjects. The hematologic picture included pancytopenia with hypocellular marrow. Evidence of bleeding was present, and death was attributed to hemorrhagic diathesis, as a result of severe thrombocytopenia.[48] Whether cats become infected with T-2 toxin naturally is unknown. A presumptive diagnosis might be made based on clinical and necropsy findings. A definitive diagnosis can be made by submission of feed samples to an analytical laboratory.

Vitamin K antagonists are useful to control rodent populations, and cats are known to be affected from eating either bait or rodents that are toxic. The bleeding associated with vitamin K antagonists is due to disruption of activation of the vitamin K procoagulant group of clotting factors—a secondary system disorder. Platelet numbers generally are not thought to be affected significantly. A report in dogs, however, confirmed the clinical suspicion that significant thrombocytopenia (as low as 17,000/μl) may be seen, most likely due primarily to utilization.[27] Clinicians should remember that utilization, due to hemorrhage, may produce significant thrombocytopenia.

Not included in this list of toxicities are phenobarbital and estrogens. Phenobarbital is used widely as an anticonvulsant in cats. In one large study of 30 cases of seizure disorders in cats, due to a variety of etiologies, 1 cat receiving phenobarbital developed ecchymoses and was found to be severely thrombocytopenic (20,000/μl). Platelet count returned to normal within a few days of discontinuation of the drug, and institution of diazepam and glucocorticoids. The report did not elaborate on other diagnostic evaluations that were performed to find other causes of thrombocytopenia, nor did it report on the number of cats receiving phenobarbital.[49] In these authors' opinion, a stronger association is needed between phenobarbital and thrombocytopenia before this drug can be added to the list of causes of this hematopoietic dyscrasia. Thrombocytopenia or pancytopenia resulting from the effects of endogenous or exogenous estrogen is a well-documented clinical entity in dogs.[50] Fatal bone marrow suppression is seen in ferrets, another species apparently sensitive to the effects of estrogen, if they are allowed to have repeated anovulatory estrous cycles. Administration of diethylstilbestrol to cats has resulted in death,[51] and reviews of toxicologic disorders in cats suggest that thrombocytopenia and pancytopenia develop secondary to estrogen administration. However, to the authors' knowledge, there are no investigatory or clinical reports that indicate thrombocytopenia or pancytopenia develop after administration of estrogenic compounds (e.g., diethylstilbestrol, estradiol cyclopentaneopropionate) or after repeated anovulatory estrous cycles in cats.

Organ System Dysfunction Associated With Thrombocytopenia

In an earlier report of 41 thrombocytopenic cats, 7 per cent (3/41) were identified to have only cardiac disease.[1] In a report of hemostatic studies, of the 6 cats with thrombocytopenia alone, 2 were identified to have only cardiac disease.[3] In a third review, cardiac disease again was identified in the cats with thrombocytopenia alone.[2] The causal effects of cardiac disease are unknown, but altered blood flow and microangiopathy (as evidenced by shearing effect on red blood cells) with utilization are proposed. Liver disease also was identified in both hemostatic studies as one of the 3 largest categories of diseases identified.[2, 3]

◆ MANAGEMENT OF THE THROMBOCYTOPENIC CAT

Once thrombocytopenia is suspected or identified, testing of the remainder of the hemostatic system may be necessary to appreciate fully the extent for potential bleeding. This is most important when invasive diagnostics are planned. An atraumatic environment should be afforded and care, even with clipping haircoat or collecting blood samples, should be taken to avoid prolonged bleeding. Intramuscular injections should be avoided.

Treatment should be directed toward the underlying cause of the thrombocytopenia. Although administration of fresh plasma or platelet-rich plasma sometimes is discussed in severely thrombocytopenic patients, it is not offered commonly, because the number of platelets delivered is small, and their viability is questionable. In addition, they may be destroyed, consumed, or utilized quickly by the primary disease process.[52] Administration of vincristine sulfate increases platelet numbers by stimulating megakaryocyte endomitosis, leading to the premature release of platelets from the bone marrow. Results may be seen in 4 or more days. It is unclear whether the platelets generated by this drug are functional, because they are immature and platelet aggregation may be hindered.[53] Future treatment may include administration of TPO. Recombinant human TPO has been beneficial in the management of thrombocytopenia associated with chemotherapeutics and increases platelet numbers in normal dogs.[54] With the cloning of feline TPO,[6] it may be possible to employ this cytokine in the future management of thrombocytopenia.

REFERENCES

1. Jordan HL, Grindem CB, Breitschwerdt EB: Thrombocytopenia in cats: A retrospective study of 41 cases. J Vet Intern Med 7:261–265, 1993.
2. Thomas JS, Green RA: Clotting times and antithrombin III activity in cats with naturally developing diseases: 85 cases (1984–1994). J Am Vet Med Assoc 213:1290–1295, 1998.
3. Peterson JL, Couto CG, Wellman ML: Hemostatic disorders in cats: A retrospective study and review of the literature. J Vet Intern Med 9:298–303, 1995.
4. Baldwin CJ, Cowell RL, Kostolich M, et al: Hemostasis: Physiology, diagnosis and treatment of bleeding disorders in surgical patients. *In* Slatter D (ed): Textbook of Small Animal Surgery, 2nd ed. Philadelphia, WB Saunders, 1993, pp. 29–52.
5. Duncan JR, Prasse KW, Mahaffey EA: Hemostasis. *In* Duncan JR, Prasse KW, Mahaffey EA (eds): Veterinary Laboratory Medicine: Clinical Pathology, 3rd ed. Ames, Iowa State University Press, 1994, p. 76.
6. Matsushiro H, Kato H, Tahara T, et al: Molecular cloning and functional expression of feline thrombopoietin. Vet Immunol Immunopathol 66:225–236, 1998.
7. Foley JE, Pedersen NC: The inheritance of susceptibility to feline infectious peritonitis in purebred catteries. Fel Pract 24:14–22, 1996.
8. Sellon RK: Feline immunodeficiency virus infection. *In* Greene CE (ed): Infectious Diseases of the Dog and Cat, 2nd ed. Philadelphia, WB Saunders, 1998, pp. 84–95.
9. Pineau S, Belbeck LN, Moore S: Levamisole reduces the thrombocytopenia associated with myxovirus vaccination. Can Vet J 21:82–84, 1979.
10. Straw B: Decrease in platelet count after vaccination with distemper-hepatitis (DH) vaccine. Vet Med Small Anim Clin 73:725–726, 1978.
11. McAnulty JF, Rudd RG: Thrombocytopenia associated with vaccination of a dog with a modified live paramyxovirus vaccine. J Am Vet Med Assoc 186:1217–1219, 1985.
12. Greene CE, Latimer K, Hopper E, et al: Administration of diminazene aceturate or imidocarb dipropionate for treatment of cytauxzoonosis in cats. J Am Vet Med Assoc 215:497–500, 1999.
13. Tasker S, Cripps P, Mackin A: Evaluation of methods of platelet counting in the cat (Abstract). J Vet Intern Med. 13:254, 1999.
14. Tyler RD, Cowell RL, Meinkoth JH: Bone marrow. *In* Cowell RL, Tyler RD, Meinkoth JH (eds): Diagnostic Cytology and Hematology of the Dog and Cat, 2nd ed. St. Louis, Mosby, 1995, pp. 284–304.
15. Couto CG: Diseases of the lymph nodes and the spleen. *In* Ettinger SJ (ed): Textbook of Veterinary Internal Medicine. Diseases of the Dog and Cat, 3rd ed. Philadelphia, WB Saunders, 1989, pp. 2225–2245.
16. Davenport DJ, Carakostas MC: Platelet disorders in the dog and cat. Part I. Physiology and pathogenesis. Compend Contin Educ Pract Vet 4:762–772, 1982.
17. Feldman BF: Disorders of platelets. *In* Kirk RW, Bonagura JD (eds): Current Veterinary Therapy X. Philadelphia: WB Saunders, 1989, pp. 457–464.
18. Dodds WJ, Wilkins RJ: Animal model of human disease: Canine and equine immune-mediated thrombocytopenia and idiopathic thrombocytopenia purpura. Am J Pathol 86:489–491, 1977.
19. Smith J, Schaer M, Chandra S: Chronic thrombocytopenia and epistaxis in a cat. Fel Pract 27:5–8, 1999.
20. Tasker S, Mackin AJ, Day MJ: Primary immune-mediated thrombocytopenia in a cat. J Small Anim Pract 40:127–131, 1999.
21. Axthelm MK, Krakowka S: Canine distemper virus–induced thrombocytopenia. Am J Vet Res 48:1269–1275, 1987.
22. Breitschwerdt EB: Infectious thrombocytopenia in dogs. Compend Contin Educ Pract Vet 10:1177–1186, 1988.
23. Thomason KJ, Feldman BF: Immune-mediated thrombocytopenia: diagnosis and treatment. Compend Contin Educ Pract Vet 7:569–576, 1985.
24. Clinkenbeard KD, Cowell RL, Tyler RD: Disseminated histoplasmosis in cats: 12 cases. J Am Anim Hosp Assoc 20:119–122, 1984.
25. Hibler SC, Hoskins JD, Greene CE: Rickettsial infections in dogs. Part I. Rocky mountain spotted fever and *Coxiella* infections. Compend Contin Educ Pract Vet 7:856–865, 1985.
26. Aronson LR, Gregory C: Possible hemolytic uremic syndrome in three cats after renal transplantation and cyclosporine therapy. Vet Surg 28:135–140, 1999.
27. Lewis DC, Bruyette DS, Kellerman DL, et al: Thrombocytopenia in dogs with anticoagulant rodenticide-induced hemorrhage: Eight cases (1990–1995). J Am Anim Hosp Assoc 33:417–422, 1997.
28. Ogilvie GK, Moore AS: Paraneoplastic syndromes: Thrombocytopenia. *In* Ogilvie GK, Moore AS (eds): Managing the Veterinary Cancer Patient. Trenton, Veterinary Learning Systems, 1995, pp. 211–212.
29. Lippert AC, Faulkner JE, Evans AT, et al: Total parenteral nutrition in clinically normal cats. J Am Vet Med Assoc 194:669–676, 1989.
30. Kochin EJ, Gregory CR: Renal transplantation: Patient selection and post-operative care. *In* August JR (ed): Consultations in Feline Internal Medicine, vol. 2. Philadelphia, WB Saunders, 1994, pp. 339–342.
31. Cain JL, Cain GR, Turrel JM, et al: Clinical and lymphohematologic responses after bone marrow transplantation in sibling and unrelated donor-recipient pairs of cats. Am J Vet Res 51:839–844, 1990.
32. Gasper PW, Rosen DK, Fulton R: Allogeneic marrow transplantation in a cat with acute myeloid leukemia. J Am Vet Med Assoc 208:1280–1284, 1996.
33. Baldwin CJ, Panciera RJ, Morton RJ, et al: Acute tularemia in three domestic cats. J Am Vet Med Assoc 199:1602–1605, 1991.
34. Woods JP, Crystal MA, Morton RJ, et al: Tularemia in two cats. J Am Vet Med Assoc 212:81–83, 1998.
35. Baldwin CJ, Ledet AE: Pancytopenia. *In* August JR (ed): Consultations in Feline Internal Medicine, vol. 2. Philadelphia, WB Saunders, 1994, pp. 495–502.
36. Lappin MR: Feline ehrlichiosis. *In* Greene CE (ed): Infectious Diseases of the Dog and Cat, 2nd ed. Philadelphia, WB Saunders, 1998, pp. 149–154.
37. Stokol T, Randolph JF, Nachbar S, et al: Development of bone marrow toxicosis after albendazole administration in a dog and cat. J Am Vet Med Assoc 210:1753–1756, 1997.
38. Watson DJ, Middleton DJ: Chloramphenicol toxicosis in cats. Am J Vet Res 39:1199–1203, 1978.
39. Rottman JB, English RV, Breitschwerdt EB, et al: Bone marrow hypoplasia in a cat treated with griseofulvin. J Am Vet Med Assoc 198:429–431, 1991.
40. Povey RC: Effect of orally administered ribavirin on experimental feline calicivirus infection in cats. Am J Vet Res 39:1337–1441, 1978.
41. Peterson ME, Hurvitz AI, Leib MS, et al: Propylthiouracil-associated hemolytic anemia, thrombocytopenia and antinuclear antibodies in cats with hyperthyroidism. J Am Vet Med Assoc 184:806–808, 1984.

42. Peterson ME, Kintzer PP, Hurvitz AI: Methimazole treatment of 262 cats with hyperthyroidism. J Vet Intern Med 2:150–157, 1988.
43. O'Keefe DA, Schaeffer DJ: Hematologic toxicosis associated with doxorubicin administration in cats. J Vet Intern Med 6:276–282, 1992.
44. Beale KM, Altman D, Clemmons RR, et al: Systemic toxicosis associated with azathioprine administration in domestic cats. Am J Vet Res 53:1236–1240, 1992.
45. Hahn KA, McEntee MF, Daniel GB, et al: Hematologic and systemic toxicoses associated with carboplatin administration in cats. Am J Vet Res 58:677–679, 1997.
46. Fox LE, Toshach K, Claderwood-Mays M, et al: Evaluation of toxicosis of liposome-encapsulated *cis-bis*-neodecanoato-trans-R,R-1,2-diaminocyclohexane platinum (II) in clinically normal cats. Am J Vet Res 60:257–263, 1999.
47. Michal MT, Eran L: Suspected *Vipera palaestinae* envenomation in three cats. Vet Hum Toxicol 41:145–148, 1999.
48. Lutsky II, Mor N: Alimentary toxic aleukia (septic angina, endemic panmyelotoxicosis, alimentary hemorrhagic aleukia): T-2 toxin–induced intoxication of cats. Am J Pathol 104:189–191, 1981.
49. Quesnel AD, Parent JM, McDonell W: Clinical management and outcome of cats with seizure disorders: 30 cases (1991–1993). J Am Vet Med Assoc 210:72–77, 1997.
50. Weiss DJ, Klausner JS: Drug-associated aplastic anemia in dogs: Eight cases (1984–1988). J Am Vet Med Assoc 196:472–475, 1990.
51. Wilkinson GT: A review of drug toxicity in the cat. J Small Anim Pract 9:21–32, 1968.
52. de Gopegui RR, Feldman BF: Use of blood and blood components in canine and feline patients with hemostatic disorders. Vet Clin North Am Small Anim Pract 25:1387–1402, 1995.
53. Couto CG: Disorders of hemostasis. *In* Nelson RW, Couto CG (eds): Small Animal Internal Medicine, 2nd ed. St. Louis, Mosby, 1998, pp. 1192–1206.
54. Thomas JS: Advances in the diagnosis and therapeutic management of platelet disorders. American College of Veterinary Internal Medicine, 17th Annual Forum, Chicago, 1999, pp. 567–569.

60

◆ Use of the Polymerase Chain Reaction to Detect Hemoparasites

Joanne B. Messick
Linda M. Berent

The traditional method of identifying a pathogen relies on culturing to establish the causal link between a particular disease and a specific organism. However, many infectious organisms, including mycoplasmas, rickettsiae, mycobacteria, fungi, and viruses, either are fastidious and grow very slowly or cannot be cultured at all. In such instances, serologic or histologic methods may be used to identify the infectious agent. However, these methods often yield only indirect or circumstantial evidence of infection. Molecular techniques have been developed by several investigators for direct and specific detection of small numbers of parasites in the blood. In this chapter, we review the use of a molecular test, the polymerase chain reaction (PCR), for diagnosis of hemoparasite infections in cats.

◆ POLYMERASE CHAIN REACTION

By mimicking the phenomenon of in vivo DNA replication, the PCR permits selective in vitro amplification of a particular DNA sequence. With in vivo replication, a series of enzyme-mediated reactions within the dividing cell produces a faithful copy of the entire genome. PCR, on the other hand, allows a "target" DNA sequence to be copied selectively and amplified exponentially in a test tube (Fig. 60–1).[1] During PCR, high temperature is used to separate (denature) the DNA molecules into single strands. Short synthetic sequences (primers) of DNA then can bind or anneal to specific sites at the beginning of the target region on one strand and at the end of the target region on the opposite strand. DNA polymerase, in the presence of excess amounts of nucleotides, is able to copy the target sequence starting from these primed ends (extension). By repeating the steps of denaturing, annealing, and extending, upward of a billion copies of a specific piece of DNA can be made in only a few hours. The amplified sequence then is visualized by ethidium bromide staining after gel electrophoresis. The ability of PCR to amplify minute amounts of specific microbial DNA sequences despite a background mixture of host cell DNA makes it a powerful diagnostic tool. However, PCR just now is beginning to have an impact on the diagnosis of infectious diseases in small-animal medicine.

Advantages of PCR Assays

In contrast to tests that rely on indirect evidence such as antibody response, PCR directly amplifies DNA of the infectious organism within host tissues. The sensitivity of PCR-based methods is exquisite, reportedly detecting as few as 10 to 100 copies of a particular gene in clinical samples. The sensitivity of an assay depends on many variables including the type of sample, method of DNA extraction, primer set used, and conditions of the PCR.[1] Therefore, it is essential that the sensitivity of each PCR assay be established. This can be done by limiting dilution of a known positive sample to determine the smallest number of organisms that can be detected or by using more sophisticated methods such as quantitative-competitive PCR.[2] For example, the actual limit of detection in blood using the PCR assay for *Haemobartonella felis* developed at the University of Illinois was between 50 and 704 organisms.[3] In experimentally infected cats, this level of sensitivity translated to the detection of a positive sample 2 days after infection, whereas organisms were not seen microscopically on a stained peripheral blood smear until day 6 after infection.[4]

Limitations of PCR Assays

It is essential to understand that there are limitations and inherent problems in PCR testing.[1] The extreme sensitivity of PCR may lead to one of its greatest drawbacks, the occurrence of false-positive results. The massively amplified target sequence can contaminate reagents and equipment easily, especially when a diagnostic PCR is performed repeatedly for one particular DNA sequence. Strict procedures must be followed to minimize carryover, including the use of chemical and enzymatic reagents and irradiation to degrade contaminating PCR products. It also is crucial to include negative and positive controls in every PCR assay. In a diagnostic assay, negative control samples should be subjected to the same extraction, purification, and PCR amplification as the patient sample. High and low copy number positive controls are included in each PCR run for a particular infectious agent. These controls check the overall quality of the assay, and ensure that the assay is working properly.

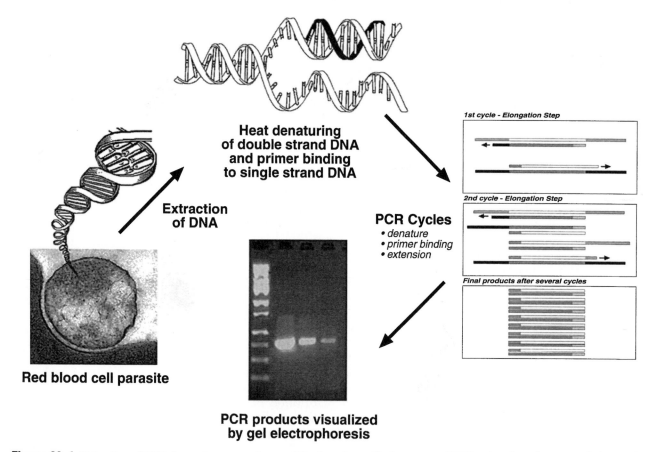

Figure 60–1. Extraction of DNA from a hemoparasite, amplification of specific fragments of DNA using the polymerase chain reaction (PCR), and visualization of PCR products by gel electrophoresis.

After DNA is extracted from the hemoparasite, a reaction mixture for PCR is prepared that contains the target DNA sequence, nucleotides (deoxyribonucleoside triphosphates [dNTPs]), 2 primers, and a heat-stable polymerase. At a high temperature, the double strands of DNA separate. The primers bind to opposite strands of the DNA at either end of the target DNA sequence. After annealing, the reaction mixture is raised to an intermediate temperature. Now the polymerase extends the primers into new strands, using the dNTPs in the reaction mix. The cycle is repeated about 30 times, creating billions of copies of the specific fragments of DNA. The amplified sequences are visualized by ethidium bromide staining after gel electrophoresis. A molecular-weight marker for determination of size is shown in the far left lane, and PCR products amplified from 3 samples containing decreasing amounts of DNA are shown in the next 3 lanes.

◆ *HAEMOBARTONELLA FELIS*

Development of PCR Assay

Perhaps the most exciting clinical application of PCR would be to detect and identify a bacterial pathogen that cannot be cultured and for which an efficient diagnostic test is not available,[5] such as *H. felis* infections in cats. A prerequisite for designing primers to be used in this or any diagnostic assay is the availability of genomic sequence information, making the lack of sequence data for *H. felis* a potential problem. However, it was reported previously that nearly the entire sequence of the 16S rRNA gene of any bacterium could be amplified using a set of universal primers. This approach was used by 2 separate groups of researchers to amplify target sequences successfully in blood specimens obtained from cats that were naturally or experimentally infected with *H. felis*.[3, 6] The sequence information obtained from the 16S rRNA gene was used to develop a species-specific PCR assay and to provide

objective information about the molecular evolution of *H. felis*.[3, 4, 6, 7] Based on morphologic characteristics alone, *H. felis* had been classified for the past 50 years as a rickettsial species. The nucleotide sequence analysis of the PCR products, however, has now firmly established that *H. felis* is a mycoplasma.

The 16S rRNA gene is the basis for all of the PCR assays developed to date for identifying the red cell parasite *H. felis* (Table 60–1).[3, 4, 7] Several different primer pairs for detection and amplification of *H. felis* have been reported. To be useful in a diagnostic assay, primers must be designed specifically to bind to unique regions of the 16S rRNA gene of *H. felis*, and not to genomic DNA of the cat or to similar gene sequences in other bacteria. Once a primer set has been designed, it must be evaluated critically to ensure that it is specific for *H. felis* and detects all strains[7] of the organism. There is, however, a paucity of information about the primers currently used and the performance of the various PCR assays. Regardless, PCR-based assays offer a vast improvement

Table 60–1. Universities and Veterinary Laboratories That Currently Perform Polymerase Chain Reaction for Detection of Hemoparasites That Infect Cats

Organism	PCR	Gene(s) Used
Haemobartonella felis	U of I; OSU; U of Calif; Heska; Antech; Symbiotics*	16S rRNA
Bartonella henselae† B. clarridgeiae B. koehlerae	Antech; Heska†; Symbiotics*	16S rRNA, citrate synthase, heat shock protein, 16S-23S intergenic spacer
Ehrlichia species‡	U of Calif§; U of G; Cornell U; OSU; Heska‡; LSU§	16S rRNA

Abbreviation: PCR, polymerase chain reaction.
Key: U of I = University of Illinois, 2001 South Lincoln Ave., College of Veterinary Medicine, Urbana, IL (217–333–1620).
U of Calif = University of California–Davis, School of Veterinary Medicine, Box 1770, Davis, CA (530–752–8709).
OSU = Ohio State University, College of Veterinary Medicine, 1925 Coffee Rd., Columbus, OH (614–292–5661).
U of G = University of Georgia, Department of Medical Microbiology, College of Veterinary Medicine, Athens, GA (706–542–5812).
Cornell U = Cornell University, New York State College of Veterinary Medicine, Ithaca, NY (607–253–3900).
Antech Diagnostics, 17672-A Cowan Ave., Suite 200, Irvine, CA (800–542–1151).
Heska Corporation, 1825 Sharp Point Dr., Fort Collins, CO (970–493–7272).
*Kit available for use.
†In development.
‡Commercial laboratories for human testing also offer PCR for *Bartonella* and granulocytic *Ehrlichia* species.
§U of Calif = University of California–Davis (*E. equi, E. risticii, E. canis*); LSU = Louisiana State University (*E. canis* and *E. platys*).

over microscopic methods for the diagnosis of *H. felis* infection.

Samples for *H. felis* PCR Assay

PCR test results may be affected by the nature of the sample that is submitted. About 75 per cent of cats that are treated with appropriate antibiotics will survive an uncomplicated episode of anemia induced by *H. felis*. However, recovered cats are chronically infected.[8] Work at the University of Illinois has shown that experimentally infected cats might have negative PCR assays during or immediately after doxycycline treatment. The numbers of organisms in the blood are greatly diminished after antibiotic treatment, falling to levels that are below the threshold for detection by PCR or disappearing completely from the peripheral blood.[4] The PCR assay will not detect infection in these carrier animals until about 6 weeks after the completion of antibiotic therapy. Therefore, it is recommended that blood samples for PCR be collected before the initiation of treatment.

Transport conditions also may affect the outcome of the PCR test. Extremes in temperature, especially heat, during shipment can lead to degraded DNA

that cannot be amplified. Before submitting specimens for PCR, it is advisable to consult the PCR laboratory for instructions regarding proper sample selection and shipping recommendations. In addition, it is still unknown whether all strains of *H. felis* are detected by the PCR assays currently available. Therefore, it is suggested that a freshly prepared, unstained peripheral blood smear be submitted concurrently for evaluation.

Future of PCR Assay for *H. felis*

The first generation of PCR-based assays for detection of *H. felis* have used primers designed to anneal to the 16S rRNA gene sequence. Several groups currently are working on the development of a multiplex PCR in which several different regions of the 16S rRNA gene are amplified to ensure that all strains of *H. felis* are detected. However, in the case of *H. felis*, the sensitivity of any assay based on the 16S rRNA is limited by there being only 1 or, at the most, 2 copies of this gene. The development of an even more sensitive test in the near future should not be difficult. For example, a PCR test could be developed around a gene that encodes some adhesion epitope, which is much more likely to be present in high copy numbers.[9]

◆ *BARTONELLA* SPECIES

Bartonella henselae is the etiologic agent of most cases of cat-scratch disease in human beings. There now is epidemiologic, microbiologic, and molecular evidence for the involvement of domestic cats in the life cycles of *Bartonella* species, including *B. henselae, B. clarridgeiae*, and *B. koehlerae*.[10, 11] Although infected cats often fail to show clinical signs of disease, PCR is an efficient means of demonstrating organisms in blood samples due to high levels of bacteremia in this host.[10] PCR followed by restriction fragment length polymorphism (RFLP) to confirm the diagnosis was used recently to show that the virulence of *B. henselae* in cats may, however, be strain-dependent.[12] *B. henselae* also has been detected by PCR in fleas infesting bacteremic cats.[13]

The development of specific PCR-based assays for the diagnosis of *Bartonella* infections has focused on the 16S rRNA, citrate synthase, and heat shock genes.[14–17] Relman and associates[14] were the first to design *Bartonella*-specific PCR primers based on unique regions of the 16S rRNA gene. The specificity of these primers was verified subsequently in several different studies by sequencing of the PCR products. The primers used for amplification of the citrate synthase gene fragment of *Bartonella* species were not specific. However, RFLP of the PCR products allowed for the discrimination of *Bartonella* species from other bacteria.[16] Anderson and colleagues[17] described an alternative approach in which amplification of the gene for heat shock protein was followed by hybridization. These PCR assays and others that have been developed recently (see Table 60–1) will be invaluable tools for more clearly defining the role that *Bartonella* species play in diseases of cats.

There are many PCR-based assays available today, both commercially and in research settings. For the most part, these assays are specific for a particular *Bartonella* species. In cats, it may be more appropriate to use a PCR assay that will detect infection at the level of the genus *Bartonella*. A more specific assay could be run thereafter, or the PCR products sequenced or subjected to RFLP, to identify the particular *Bartonella* species infecting the cat.

◆ *EHRLICHIA* SPECIES

Whereas the species of *Ehrlichia* that infect cats after natural exposure have not been determined, cats can be infected experimentally with *Ehrlichia* species that target both monocytic and granulocytic cells (see Chapter 4, Rickettsial Diseases). The granulocytic ehrlichia, including a recently characterized feline isolate, are very closely related, both antigenically and on the basis of nucleotide sequence analysis of the 16S rRNA gene.[18] Several PCR assays based on this gene have been developed recently for detecting DNA of the various granulocytic ehrlichiae.[19–21] These assays are not species-specific and also should be useful for detecting the granulocytic ehrlichia in cats. This test is available commercially (see Table 60–1). PCR tests also have been developed for detecting the monocytic *Ehrlichia* species; however, these tests are species-specific,[22, 23] and available currently only on a research basis.

◆ *CYTAUXZOON FELIS* AND OTHER PROTOZOANS

The small subunit ribosomal RNA (srRNA) of *Cytauxzoon felis* was amplified recently using PCR, cloned, and sequenced[24] (see Chapter 55, Update on Cytauxzoonosis). The sequence data clearly indicate that *C. felis* is related to other protozoans, including *Babesia* species and *Theileria* species. The srRNA is the only gene of *C. felis* for which sequence data are currently available; however, a PCR assay based on this information has not been developed. A number of PCR-based tests are available for species that cause human and bovine babesiosis; however, none has been developed specifically to detect species that have been reported to infect cats.[25–27]

Whereas infection of domestic and wild cats by protozoans belonging to the genus *Hepatozoon* has been reported in India, Africa, Israel, and the United States, no molecular test has been developed for its diagnosis.[28] In South and Central America, infection of cats by *Trypanosoma* species has been recognized. Several groups have developed PCR tests re-

cently for detection of *Trypanosoma cruzi*,[29, 30] for which cats may act as an animal reservoir in endemic areas.[31] There is little information regarding the susceptibility of cats to infection by *Trypanozoon* species found in Africa. Nevertheless, PCR-based tests have been reported for the diagnosis of infection by *T. brucei* and *T. congolense*,[32, 33] and could be used to detect infection by these species in cats. Cats are clinically infected only rarely with protozoons of the genus *Leishmania*. The PCR tests that have been developed for the different Old World and New World leishmanial species also may be useful to detect the presence of local or systemic infection in cats.[34–37] PCR has proved to be a valuable tool for the diagnosis of protozoal diseases in species other than cats and the technique is likely, in the near future, to provide us with valuable information about the susceptibility of cats to these organisms in endemic countries.

◆ CONCLUSIONS

The use of PCR for detection and identification of hemoparasites that infect cats is presently, with a few noted exceptions, still a research tool. PCR assays will continue to be used in the research setting to refine taxonomic relationships of these organisms, characterize the sequelae of infection, and determine the role that cats play in the epidemiology of infection. The PCR assays currently available for making day-to-day diagnoses are limited to *H. felis*, *Bartonella* species, and *Ehrlichia* species. In the near future, however, PCR will play a major role in the diagnosis of hemoparasitic as well as other common infectious diseases of cats.

REFERENCES

1. Rolfs A, Schuller I, Finckh U, et al: PCR principles and reaction components. *In* PCR: Clinical Diagnostics and Research. New York, Springer Laboratory, 1992, p. 1.
2. Cooper SK, Berent LM, Messick JB: Competitive, quantitative PCR analysis of *Haemobartonella felis* in the blood of experimentally infected cats. J Microbiol Methods 34:235–240, 1999.
3. Messick JB, Berent LM, Cooper SK: Development and evaluation of a PCR-based assay for detection of *Haemobartonella felis* in cats and differentiation using restriction fragment length polymorphism J Clin Microbiol 36:462–466, 1998.
4. Berent LM, Messick JB, Cooper S: Detection of *Haemobartonella felis* in cats with experimentally induced acute and chronic infections, using a polymerase chain reaction assay. Am J Vet Res 10:1215–1220, 1998.
5. Turner CMR, Bloxham PA, Cox FE, et al: Unreliable diagnosis of *Haemobartonella felis*. Vet Rec 119:534, 1986.
6. Rikihisa Y, Kawahara M, Wen B, et al: Western immunoblot analysis of *Haemobartonella muris* and comparison of 16S rRNA gene sequences of *H. muris*, *H. felis*, and *Eperythrozoon suis*. J Clin Microbiol 35:823–829, 1997.
7. Foley JE, Harrus S, Poland A, et al: Molecular, clinical, and pathologic comparison of two distinct strains of *Haemobartonella felis* in domestic cats. Am J Vet Res 12:1581–1588, 1998.
8. Harvey JW: Haemobartonellosis. *In* Greene CE (ed): Infectious

Diseases of the Dog and Cat, 2nd ed. Philadelphia, WB Saunders, 1998, p. 166.

9. Bott KF Fraser CM: *Mycoplasma genitalium. In* de Bruijn FJ, Lupski JR, Weinstock GM (eds): Bacterial Genomics: Physical Structure and Analysis. New York, Chapman & Hall, 1998, p. 508.

10. Kordick DL, Brown TT, Shin K, et al: Clinical and pathologic evaluation of chronic *Bartonella henselae* or *Bartonella clarridgeiae* infection in cats. J Clin Microbiol 37:1536–1547, 1999.

11. Droz S, Chi B, Horn E, et al: *Bartonella koehlerae* sp. nov., isolated from cats. J Clin Microbiol 37:1117–1122, 1999.

12. O'Reilly KL, Bauer RW, Freeland RL, et al: Acute clinical disease in cats following infection with a pathogenic strain of *Bartonella henselae* (LSU16). Infect Immunol 67:3066–3072, 1999.

13. Chomel BB, Carlos ET, Kasten RW, et al: *Bartonella henselae* and *Bartonella clarridgeiae* infection in domestic cats from the Philippines. Am J Trop Med Hyg 60:593–599, 1999.

14. Relman DA, Loutit JS, Schmidt TM, et al: The agent of bacillary angiomatosis. An approach to the identification of uncultured pathogens. N Engl J Med 323:1573–1580, 1990.

15. Raoult D, Drancourt M, Carta A, et al: *Bartonella (Rochalimaea) quintana* isolation in patient with chronic adenopathy, lymphopenia, and a cat. Lancet 343:977, 1994.

16. Joblet C, Roux V, Drancourt M, et al: Identification of *Bartonella (Rochalimaea)* species among fastidious gram-negative bacteria on the basis of the partial sequence of the citrate-synthase gene. J Clin Microbiol 33:1879–1883, 1995.

17. Anderson B, Sims K, Regnery R, et al: Detection of *Rochalimaea henselae* DNA in specimens from cat scratch disease patients by PCR. J Clin Microbiol 32:942–948, 1994.

18. Bjoersdorff A, Svendenius L, Owens JH, et al: Feline granulocytic ehrlichiosis—A report of a new clinical entity and characterization of the infectious agent. J Small Anim Pract 40:20–24, 1999.

19. Engvall EO, Pettersson B, Persson M, et al: A 16S rRNA–based PCR assay for detection and identification of granulocytic *Ehrlichia* species in dogs, horses, and cattle. J Clin Microbiol 34:2170–2174, 1999.

20. Massung RF, Slater K, Owens JH, et al: Nested PCR assay for detection of granulocytic ehrlichiae. J Clin Microbiol 36:1090–1095, 1998.

21. Pusterla N, Huder JB, Leutenegger CM, et al: Quantitative real-time PCR for detection of members of the *Ehrlichia phagocytophila* genogroup in host animals and *Ixodes ricinus* ticks. J Clin Microbiol 37:1329–1331, 1999.

22. McBride JW, Corstvet RE, Gaunt SD, et al: PCR detection of acute *Ehrlichia canis* infection in dogs. J Vet Diagn Invest 8:441–447, 1996.

23. Barlough JE, Rikihisa Y, Madigan JE: Nested polymerase chain reaction for detection of *Ehrlichia risticii* genomic DNA in infected horses. Vet Parasitol 68:367–373, 1997.

24. Allsopp MT, Cavalier-Smith T, De Waal DT, et al: Phylogeny and evolution of the piroplasms. Parasitology 108:147–152, 1994.

25. Salem GH, Liu X, Johnsrude JD, et al: Development and evaluation of an extra chromosomal DNA-based PCR test for diagnosing bovine babesiosis. Mol Cell Probes 13:107–113, 1999.

26. Calder JA, Reddy GR, Chieves L, et al: Monitoring *Babesia bovis* infections in cattle by using PCR-based tests. J Clin Microbiol 34:2748–2755, 1996.

27. Krause PJ, Telford S 3rd, Spielman A, et al: Comparison of PCR with blood smear and inoculation of small animals for diagnosis of *Babesia microti* parasitemia. J Clin Microbiol 34:2791–2794, 1996.

28. Baneth G, Aroch I, Tal N, et al: *Hepatozoon* species infection in domestic cats: A retrospective study. Vet Parasitol 79:123–133, 1998.

29. Dorn PL, Engelke D, Rodas A, et al: Utility of the polymerase chain reaction in detection of *Trypanosoma cruzi* in Guatemalan Chagas' disease vectors. Am J Trop Med Hyg 60:740–745, 1999.

30. Vallejo GA, Guhl F, Chiari E, et al: Species specific detection of *Trypanosoma cruzi* and *Trypanosoma rangeli* in vector and mammalian hosts by polymerase chain reaction amplification of kinetoplast minicircle DNA. Acta Trop 72:203–213, 1999.

31. Gurtler RE, Cohen JE, Cecere MC, et al: Influence of humans and domestic animals on the household prevalence of *Trypanosoma cruzi* in *Triatoma infestans* populations in northwest Argentina. Am J Trop Med Hyg 58:748–758, 1998.

32. Clausen PH, Waiswa C, Katunguka-Rwakishaya E, et al: Polymerase chain reaction and DNA probe hybridization to assess the efficacy of diminazene treatment in *Trypanosoma brucei*–infected cattle. Parasitol Res 85:206–211, 1999

33. Katakura K, Lubinga C, Chitambo H, et al: Detection of *Trypanosoma congolense* and *T. brucei* subspecies in cattle in Zambia by polymerase chain reaction from blood collected on a filter paper. Parasitol Res 83:241–245, 1997.

34. Aviles H, Belli A, Armijos R, et al: PCR detection and identification of *Leishmania* parasites in clinical specimens in Ecuador: A comparison with classical diagnostic methods. J Parasitol 85:181–187, 1999.

35. Pirmez C, da Silva Trajano V, Paes-Oliveira Neto M, et al: Use of PCR in diagnosis of human American tegumentary leishmaniasis in Rio de Janeiro, Brazil. J Clin Microbiol 37:1819–1823, 1999.

36. Minodier P, Piarroux R, Gambarelli F, et al: Rapid identification of causative species in patients with Old World leishmaniasis. J Clin Microbiol 35:2551–2555, 1997.

37. Roura X, Sanchez A, Ferrer L: Diagnosis of canine leishmaniasis by a polymerase chain reaction technique. Vet Rec 144:262–264, 1999.

61

◆ Hereditary Erythrocyte Disorders

Urs Giger

Anemia is a common presentation of cats in clinical practice. Reduced erythropoiesis due to chronic renal failure or to feline leukemia virus (FeLV) infections probably is the most frequent mechanism of anemia in cats. Blood loss anemia typically is induced by trauma/surgery, or is associated with acquired or hereditary coagulopathies, although bleeding occurs only rarely due to a primary hemostatic disorder in cats. Hemolytic anemias generally were thought to be acquired in cats. For example, acute Heinz body anemia (and methemoglobinemia) can be triggered by chemicals and food components and also by metabolic disorders. Cats with hemolytic anemia may harbor an infectious disease such as hemobartonellosis, cytauxzoonosis, and FeLV infection. Finally, immune-mediated hemolytic anemia often is assumed to be present in a cat with hemolysis—likely by extrapolation from the situation in dogs—although primary forms of immune-mediated hemolytic anemia have been documented rarely in cats.[1] However, recent studies indicate that cats with chronic or intermittent hemolytic anemia may suffer from an intrinsic erythrocyte defect, and there are other clinical presentations that could be associated with an erythrocyte defect. This chapter characterizes the clinical and pathologic features, the pathogenesis and molecular basis, and the limited therapeutic options in cats with hereditary erythrocyte disorders. A review of feline erythrocyte features and the diagnostic approach to erythrocyte defects is followed by a discussion of several specific hereditary disorders in cats, including methemoglobin (Met-Hb) reductase deficiency, porphyria, pyruvate kinase (PK) deficiency, and increased osmotic fragility of erythrocytes.

◆ ERYTHROCYTES

Before focusing on abnormal erythrocytes, the peculiar features of feline erythrocytes are reviewed.[2] With a size of 4.0 μm on a blood smear and a volume of 38 to 49 femtoliters, feline erythrocytes are much smaller than canine and human erythrocytes. In fact, owing to their small size, the central pallor of feline erythrocytic discocytes hardly is appreciated on a blood smear, and by particle count, their size can overlap with that of large feline platelets. In cases of anemia and thrombocytosis (cats generally have high platelet counts), the red blood cell count may be overestimated, making the erythrocyte indices invalid. Thus, it is imperative to use validated hematology instruments, and to review a

blood smear carefully to recognize any inconsistencies.

Evidence of active erythropoiesis may be difficult to appreciate on analysis of a blood sample; thus, a regenerative response may be missed. Polychromasia may not be readily evident on a peripheral blood smear. On a supra-vital–stained (new methylene blue) blood smear, 2 types of feline reticulocytes can be recognized. Aggregated reticulocytes with blue-staining aggregates, or at least 10 granules of reticulin, are the best indicators of a regenerative response. In a nonanemic cat, less than 0.4 per cent or 40,000/μl reticulocytes are seen normally, and they typically remain in circulation for less than a day. The reticulocyte response in anemic animals often is mild, thus any degree of reticulocytosis should be noted; however, reticulocyte numbers can reach very high levels in certain hemolytic and blood loss anemias. Furthermore, punctate reticulocytes, which have a few blue granules and should not be confused with Heinz bodies and Howell-Jolly bodies or parasites, may be present in very large numbers and indicate an earlier erythropoietic response. They remain in circulation for up to 3 weeks. Although the bone marrow from healthy cats does not contain any appreciable Prussian blue–stainable iron, the iron availability appears to be adequate for hematopoiesis. In fact, iron deficiency has been recognized only in kittens with external blood loss or in those fed an iron-deficient diet. In contrast, excessive iron stores may be recognized not only in the bone marrow but also in the spleen and liver in cats with hemolysis.

The survival time of feline erythrocytes is only 70 to 75 days, as assessed by various labeling methods. Radioactive labeling with ^{14}C-glycine and ^{59}Fe-iron or potassium ^{14}C-cyanide and ^{51}chromium has been used to determine the apparent half-life of erythrocytes in vivo. More recently, biotinylation offers an attractive nonradioactive labeling alternative. Because the spleen is very ineffective in pitting and culling erythrocytes, erythrocytes with Heinz bodies, Howell-Jolly bodies, and parasitized erythrocytes may be found readily on peripheral blood smears.

For decades, it was thought that cats have 2 adult hemoglobins, HbA and HbB, which differ only in their β-globin chain, and are present in different HbA:HbB ratios from 90:10 to 50:50. However, more recent studies indicate that the feline hemoglobin system is composed of 1 α-globin chain, but at least 6 different β-globins, 2 of them being acetylated at the N-terminal end. Each cat may have 1 to 4 different β-globin chains. The β-globin pattern of each cat is controlled genetically, and appears to remain fixed throughout life in health and disease.[3, 4]

Because feline hemoglobins have high numbers of sulfhydryl groups, they are more likely a target for oxidation and Heinz body formation. Furthermore, Heinz body production is exaggerated by the fact that oxidative agents are less likely inactivated in cats, because they lack a drug-metabolizing glucuronide transferase, and their ability for sulfation and glutathione binding also is limited. In contrast to canine hemoglobin, oxygen release from feline hemoglobin is not 2,3-diphosphoglycerate–dependent, but chloride-dependent. The partial oxygen tension at which half of hemoglobin is oxyhemoglobin and deoxyhemoglobin with 30 to 35 torr is relatively high, thereby allowing for adequate oxygen delivery (release) to tissue in the absence of 2,3-diphosphoglycerate. Cats do not contain appreciable concentrations of 2,3-diphosphoglycerate in their erythrocytes.

Similar to normal canine erythrocytes, the Na-K-ATPase of feline erythrocyte membranes is lost during reticulocyte maturation. Thus, the sodium and potassium content of feline erythrocytes is similar to plasma, and intravascular hemolysis and in vitro lysis will not affect serum/plasma electrolyte concentrations; that is, will not cause (pseudo-)hyperkalemia.

◆ ERYTHROCYTE DEFECTS

Disorders of erythrocytes are divided conveniently into (1) heme or hemoglobinopathies, (2) membrane defects, and (3) glycolytic erythroenzymopathies, although one abnormality also may affect other erythrocyte components[5] (Table 61–1). Classic hemoglobinopathies, such as thalassemia and sickle-cell anemia in human beings, have not been documented in cats, although the feline globins are now better characterized to detect these defects. Recently, we discovered a juvenile severely anemic domestic shorthair cat with Heinz bodies and unstable hemoglobin form. Whereas classic hemoglobinopathies affect the globin chains, there are others affecting the heme component such as defects of porphyrin ring synthesis, known as porphyrias, or iron oxidation called methemoglobinopathies. Many membrane protein defects are well-characterized in human beings and other species, whereas these disorders are poorly defined in cats. We found 1 anemic domestic shorthair kitten with extremely fragile erythrocytes and severe erythrocytic shape changes likely due to a membrane defect (Fig. 61–1). Recently, an increased osmotic fragility of erythrocytes causing intermittent anemia and splenomegaly was discovered in several Abyssinian and Somali cats (Fig. 61–2). The most common glycolytic erythroenzymopathy in human beings and dogs is erythrocytic PK deficiency, which now has been recognized in cats. Since about 1990, feline PK deficiency has been characterized from its clinical presentation to its underlying molecular defect.

The mode of inheritance has not been identified for all feline erythrocyte defects. At least 1 form of porphyria appears to have an autosomal dominant mode of inheritance, whereas the Met-Hb reductase

Table 61–1. Hereditary Erythrocyte Disorders

Disease	Breed	Mode of Inheritance	Defect	Signs
Heme and Hemoglobin				
Porphyria	DSH	AD	Porphobilinogen deaminase deficiency	Brown, discolored fluorescing teeth No anemia
	Siamese	U	U	Anemia Brown, discolored fluorescing teeth
	DSH	AD	U	Discolored teeth and episodic anemia
Methemoglobinemia	DSH	AR	Methemoglobin (cytochrome B_5 reductase deficiency)	Cyanosis, hypoxia Polycythemia
Unstable hemoglobin	DSH	U	U	Heinz body anemia
Membrane Defects				
Increased OF	Abyssinian Somali	U	Extremely fragile erythrocytes	Intermittent anemia, splenomegaly, increased OF test
Poikilocytosis	DSH	U	Highly abnormal erythrocyte shapes	Severe anemia
Glycolytic Erythroenzymopathies				
PK deficiency	Abyssinian Somali DSH	AR	R-PK deficiency in erythrocytes (splicing defect)	Recurrent anemia DNA test for Abyssinians and Somalis

Abbreviations: AD, autosomal dominant; AR, autosomal recessive; DSH, domestic shorthair; PK, pyruvate kinase; OF, osmotic fragility; R-PK, R-type pyruvate kinase; U, unknown.

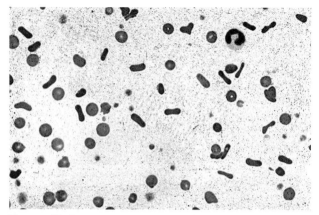

Figure 61–1. Severe poikilocytosis in a 1-year-old domestic shorthair cat with severe chronic hemolytic anemia.

and PK deficiencies are inherited in an autosomal recessive pattern, which is typical for enzyme deficiencies. For other disorders, either the molecular basis has been defined incompletely and/or relatives were not available for study to determine the inheritance pattern.

◆ DIAGNOSTIC APPROACH

Generally, hereditary disorders should be considered whenever:

1. No other underlying disease such as infection, intoxication, and cancer can be identified.
2. Some other littermates or relatives are/were similarly affected.
3. Kittens to 1-year-old cats are affected, albeit some mild or intermittent diseases may not be recognized until later in life.
4. The clinical signs are progressive, persistent, or recurrent. Some cases appear to respond to conventional therapy only to have recurrences later in life.

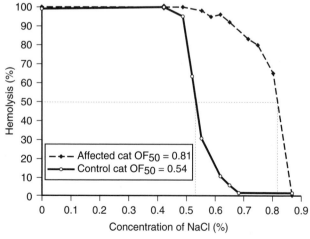

Figure 61–2. Increased osmotic fragility (OF) of erythrocytes from an Abyssinian cat.

Because any erythrocyte defect conceivably affects cell function and thereby cell deformability and integrity, hemolysis and anemia represent the key clinical manifestations. However, in some cases, the degree of hemolysis is so well-compensated by accelerated erythropoiesis and heme breakdown metabolism that clinical signs are not evident. Cats with their leisurely lifestyle usually adapt very well, and show only minimal overt signs of anemia. However, exposure to infectious agents and chemicals may exaggerate the degree of hemolysis by activating the macrophage system and/or by damaging the erythrocytes directly. Furthermore, underlying disease may hamper the regenerative response of the bone marrow. Splenomegaly may be present because of extravascular hemolysis, extravascular hemopoiesis, and hemosiderosis. In certain forms of porphyria, the dental porphyrin deposits may be all that are recognized in kittens, although the same disorder also may lead to fetal losses. Furthermore, there is a notable exception to the hemolytic anemia presentation: Met-Hb reductase deficiency presents with a mild compensatory erythrocytosis in response to tissue hypoxia, because Met-Hb is incapable of carrying oxygen.

Before focusing on an intrinsic erythrocyte defect, the following routine laboratory tests should be performed: complete blood cell count, urinalysis, serum chemistry analysis, direct Coombs' test, blood-typing, and screening for infectious diseases such as FeLV and feline immunodeficiency virus infections, *Haemobartonella felis,* and in certain parts of the world, *Babesia* and *Cytauxzoon.* The complete blood count should include red blood cell indices and a reticulocyte count. The packed cell volume may be higher than the calculated hematocrit, because fragile erythrocytes may lyse in the automated blood cell analyzer; this also will increase the mean corpuscular hemoglobin concentration (MCHC) artificially. In contrast, the counting of (large) platelets within the window of erythrocytes may falsely increase the calculated hematocrit and decrease the MCHC; thus, review of an erythrogram is indicated. The direct Coombs' test generally is negative, but false-negative immune-mediated hemolytic anemias also are suspected to occur.

Bilirubinuria and hyperbilirubinemia, the hallmark findings of hemolysis in an anemic cat, often are minimal. In fact, icteric cats are much more likely to have a hepatopathy than hemolysis, which may proceed without appreciable bilirubinuria. The presence of hemolyzed plasma or serum may indicate intravascular hemolysis or lysis of blood from time of collection until analysis. Intravascular hemolysis is further supported by hemoglobinuria and depletion of plasma haptoglobin. Because lysis of red blood cells may trigger or be associated with an inflammatory process, hyperglobulinemia commonly is observed. This has led to the suspicion of a feline infectious peritonitis infection in several anemic cats; however, this virus does not appear to cause severe anemia. Nevertheless, the most advanced techniques should be used to exclude infectious diseases.

Most cats with hemolytic anemia initially are treated with doxycycline and prednisone for presumptive hemobartonellosis and immune-mediated hemolytic anemia (see Chapter 2, Hemobartonellosis). Because intrinsic erythrocyte disorders cause severe anemia, affected cats may require transfusions during a hemolytic crisis. In contrast to the patient's defective erythrocytes, transfused cells likely will have a near-normal survival. However, only blood-typed and, after more than 1 transfusion (>4 days), cross-matched blood should be administered, and compatible blood donors or stored blood should be made readily available. Except for methemoglobinemia, there is no specific treatment available for intrinsic erythrocyte defects. However, cats with certain erythrocyte defects can adapt very well without treatment, and may reach a near-normal life expectancy.

A variety of specific erythrocyte studies are available in specialized laboratories; for example, the author's laboratory at the University of Pennsylvania (www.vet.upenn.edu/penngen). Depending on signalment, clinical signs, and routine laboratory test results, some of the following special tests may be indicated:

- Erythrocyte osmotic fragility test
- Erythrocyte membrane electrophoresis
- Erythrocyte glycolytic enzyme activities
  PK (also DNA test for Abyssinian and Somali)
  Met-Hb reductase
  Heme synthesis enzymes
- Metabolic analyses
  Met-Hb (whole blood)
  Porphyrins (urine, erythrocytes)
  Glycolytic metabolites (erythrocytes)
- Hemoglobin high-pressure liquid chromatography
- Hemoglobin-oxygen dissociation curve

◆ PORPHYRIA

Hereditary porphyrias result from enzyme deficiencies in heme biosynthesis. This leads to tissue accumulation and urinary excretion of porphyrins. The pattern of porphyrin metabolites may reveal the metabolic block. Depending on the enzyme deficiency observed in human patients, clinical signs vary from porphyrin staining of teeth and bones to cutaneous photosensitivity, hemolysis, and hepatic/neurologic attacks.

Although several cats with porphyria have been described in the literature, and a small number of feline colonies with affected cats have been established, the specific biochemical defects have been defined incompletely.[6–10] In 2 independent research colonies of domestic shorthair cats, the mode of inheritance is autosomal dominant; in 1 of them, porphyria also contributes to fetal resorption and

stillborn kittens. The most consistent finding of porphyric cats is their brown discolored teeth (from gum lines to the tips) that fluoresce pink when exposed to ultraviolet light. None of the affected cats developed ulcerative dermatitis due to cutaneous porphyrin accumulation and associated photosensitivity, a clinical sign in porphyric cattle and some human patients. Similarly, intermittent neurologic signs and abdominal pain attacks seen with acute hepatic porphyria in human patients were not observed in cats; however, the cats may not have been exposed to seizure-inducing agents.

The hematologic abnormalities of porphyric cats are considerably more variable, Some cats had either a normal hematocrit or only mild nonregenerative anemia. Nucleated red blood cells, siderocytes, or erythrocytes with nuclear remnants (Howell-Jolly bodies) indicating an erythroid maturation defect may be observed on a peripheral blood smear. These cats appear to have a normal life expectancy. Others developed intermittent moderate-to-severe macrocytic hypochromic anemia along with the morphologic changes discussed previously. These cats may die because of anemia and renal failure (Siamese). Some cats may develop episodic severe pigmenturia probably due to free hemoglobin, bilirubin, and porphyrin metabolites that are light-sensitive.

Although teeth discoloration and anemia suggest porphyria, a definitive diagnosis requires porphyrin analysis in urine and blood as well as the specific enzyme deficiency in heme-synthesizing tissue.

◆ METHEMOGLOBIN REDUCTASE DEFICIENCY

Feline hemoglobin is particularly susceptible to oxidative damage and, thereby, to the formation of Met-Hb and Heinz bodies in erythrocytes. Heinz bodies represent precipitated hemoglobin attached to the erythrocyte membrane. The heme iron of Met-Hb is in the ferric (Fe^{3+}) form, and is unable to carry oxygen. Nicotinamide adenine dinucleotide, reduced form (NADH)– Met-Hb reductase (EC 1.6.2.2; cytochrome b^5 reductase; NADH diaphorase) is important in the reduction of Met-Hb to oxyhemoglobin with iron in the ferrous (Fe^{2+}) form, and is thus capable of transporting oxygen.

$$\text{Met-Hb} + \text{NADH} \xrightarrow[\text{Reductase}]{\text{Met-Hb}} \text{Hb} + \text{NAD}^+$$
$$(Fe^{3+}) \qquad\qquad\qquad\qquad (Fe^{2+})$$

Met-Hb reductase deficiency, previously described in human beings and dogs, recently has been reported in cats.[11–13] Affected domestic shorthair cats have dark brown mucous membranes and tongues on physical examination, or cyanotic blood vessels during surgery that will not turn pink-red even when giving 100 per cent oxygen. These cats experienced no apparent exercise intolerance; however, they were kept indoors.

Affected cats have severe methemoglobinemia (up to 52 per cent; normal, <0.5 per cent). Because of their inability to transport oxygen, they develop a mild erythrocytosis (secondary absolute polycythemia; hematocrit, 45 to 55 per cent) and mild reticulocytosis. Erythrocyte Met-Hb reductase activity measured using ferricyanide as substrate was either completely deficient or severely reduced. This enzyme deficiency appears to be inherited in an autosomal recessive pattern. Heterozygote animals are asymptomatic, have a normal hematocrit and low Met-Hb level, but their Met-Hb reductase activity in erythrocytes is intermediate.[13]

Generally, affected cats may not need treatment; however, they are at an increased risk for developing life-threatening methemoglobinemia (>60 per cent). Therefore, these cats should not be exposed to oxidative agents (onions, drugs, certain food components). Reducing agents such as ascorbic acid and methylene blue appear helpful in lowering the Met-Hb concentration.

◆ INCREASED OSMOTIC FRAGILITY OF ERYTHROCYTES

Many anemic Abyssinian and Somali cats, 2 related breeds, and rare domestic shorthairs were found to have extremely fragile erythrocytes; however, the exact erythrocyte abnormality has not been identified.[14] The initial presentation of affected cats varies from a few months to several years of age, but because of the recurrent nature of the anemia, anemic episodes may be missed or mistaken for other diseases. The typical signs of anemia can be associated with severe splenomegaly (reaching 225 g) and weight loss, particularly as the animal ages; the clinical signs may wax and wane over months and years, the oldest known affected cat had reached 12 years of age. The mode of inheritance has not been defined, but domestic shorthair and other breeds of cats also may experience this disorder.

During a crisis, the hematocrit may dip below 10 per cent, but remains most commonly between 15 and 25 per cent. The anemia is characterized by macrocytosis and mild-to-moderate reticulocytosis, but the high degree of lysis often invalidates the complete blood cell count results. A few stomatocytes may be recognized. Interestingly, most cats developed recurrent hyperglobulinemia (polyclonal) and lymphocytosis (as high as 50,000/μl), as well as mild hyperbilirubinemia and increases in serum liver enzymes.

In vitro erythrocyte studies were hampered severely by the extreme cell fragility. In fact, anticoagulated blood kept cold (refrigerator) often is severely hemolyzed the next day. The osmotic fragility test, which measures the stability of erythrocytes to lyse in saline concentrations decreasing from physiologic strength to plain water is markedly increased (see Fig. 61–2). Although the increased osmotic fra-

gility of erythrocytes suggests a membrane defect, no specific membrane protein abnormality has been discovered by additional studies. The erythrocyte PK activity of these patients is normal. Because a simple PK-DNA screening test is readily available, it is recommended to screen anemic Abyssinian and Somali cats first for PK deficiency and then for increased osmotic fragility. However, it is possible that a cat may have both diseases.

Treatment with prednisone during hemolytic crises may inhibit the macrophage system and erythrocyte destruction. With transfusion support, splenectomy has been performed in several symptomatic cats with severe anemia, lethargy, and inappetence, and resulted in regaining appetite and weight, although a moderate anemia often persisted. Particularly in the postoperative period, splenectomized cats appear to be prone to sepsis.

◆ PYRUVATE KINASE DEFICIENCY

Pyruvate kinase (PK; EC 2.7.1.40) is one of the key regulatory enzymes of anaerobic glycolysis, also known as Embden-Meyerhof pathway. Erythrocytes express one of the PK isoforms R-type PK, and this enzyme reaction generates energy for stability and deformability as well as function of erythrocytes. Erythrocytic PK deficiency causes hemolytic anemia and has been described in human beings, dogs, mice, and cats.[15, 16]

$$\text{Phosphoenolpyruvate} + \text{ADP} \xrightarrow[\text{Enzyme}]{\text{PK}} \text{Pyruvate} + \text{ATP}$$

where ADP is adenosine diphosphate and ATP is adenosine triphosphate.

Feline PK deficiency has been reported in Abyssinian, Somali, and domestic shorthair cats, all of which had the same disease-causing mutation in the R/L-PK gene. A splicing defect at the 3' end of exon 6 causes a 13-base-pair deletion. Affected cats therefore have very low PK activity in erythrocytes. The mode of inheritance is autosomal recessive; therefore, carriers are asymptomatic, but have intermediate PK activity and a normal and mutant PK allele.

Clinical signs of anemia may be first noted at a few months to several years of age. The anemia and associated signs often are intermittent. Despite severe anemia with a packed cell volume of as low as 8 per cent, the clinical signs, except for pale or slightly icteric mucous membranes, often are mild. Crises of anemia may be induced by infection or toxin exposure. Based on erythrocyte parameters, the anemia is slightly macrocytic-hypochromic and usually mildly to strongly regenerative. Hyperbilirubinemia, hyperbilirubinuria, and splenomegaly are mild. Intravascular hemolysis is not observed, and the erythrocyte osmotic fragility is only slightly increased. In contrast to dogs, PK-deficient cats do not develop a progressive osteosclerosis. They die usually during an acute hemolytic crisis, but may reach advanced age; the oldest PK-deficient cat reached 13 years of age. Prednisone therapy may be helpful during hemolytic crises. Splenectomy also has been tried and may ameliorate hemolytic crises.

Because not only PK deficiency but also increased erythrocytic osmotic fragility is responsible for anemia in Abyssinian and Somali cats, it is important to differentiate these 2 disorders. A simple DNA test is available to screen anemic cats, asymptomatic Abyssinians and Somalis that have relatives with anemia, and cats that are used for breeding. General screening of Abyssinians and Somali cats could reduce the frequency of PK deficiency rapidly in these related breeds.

ACKNOWLEDGMENTS

The original studies performed at the University of Pennsylvania were supported in part by grants from the National Institutes of Health (RR02512 and HL02355). The author would like to thank Drs. Osheiza Abdulmalik, Toshio Asakura, Beth Callan, Sarah Ford, Ann Hohenhaus, Barbara Kohn, Andrea Niggemeier, Yashoda Rajpurohit, and Ping Wang, as well as the many referring veterinarians and feline breeders.

REFERENCES

1. Giger U: Regenerative anemias caused by blood loss or hemolysis. *In* Ettinger SJ, Feldman EC (eds): Textbook of Veterinary Internal Medicine, 5th ed. Philadelphia, WB Saunders, 2000, pp. 1784–1804.
2. Weiser G: Erythrocyte responses and disorders. *In* Ettinger SJ, Feldman EC (eds): Textbook of Veterinary Internal Medicine, 4th ed. Philadelphia, WB Saunders, 1995, pp. 1864–1891.
3. Kohn B, Reilly MP, Asakura T, Giger U: Polymorphism of feline β-globins studied by reversed-phase high-performance liquid chromatography. Am J Vet Res 59:830–835, 1998.
4. Kohn B, Henthorn PS, Rajpurohit Y, et al: Feline adult β-globin polymorphism in restriction fragment length patterns. J Hered 90:177–181, 1999.
5. Giger U: Hereditary erythrocyte disorders. *In* Bonagura JD (ed): Kirk's Current Veterinary Therapy XIII: Small Animal Practice. Philadelphia, WB Saunders, 2000, pp. 414–420.
6. Kaneko J: Porphyrias and porphyruria. *In* Feldman BF, Zinkle JG, Jain NC (eds): Schalm's Veterinary Hematology. Baltimore, Lippincott Williams & Wilkins, 2000, pp. 1002–1007.
7. Giddens WE Jr, Labbe RF, Swango LJ, Padgett GA: Feline congenital erythropoietic porphyria associated with severe anemia and renal disease. Clinical, morphologic, and biochemical studies. Am J Pathol 80:367–386, 1975.
8. Glenn BL, Glenn HG, Omtvedt IT: Congenital porphyria in the domestic cat (*Felis catus*): Preliminary investigations on inheritance pattern. Am J Vet Res 29:1653–1657, 1968.
9. Glenn BL: An animal model for human disease: Feline porphyria. Comp Pathol Bull 2:2–3, 1970.
10. Haskins ME, Patterson DF: Inherited metabolic disorders. *In* Holzworth J (ed): Diseases of the Cat. Philadelphia, WB Saunders, 1987, pp. 808–819.
11. Harvey JW: Hereditary methemoglobin reductase deficiency. *In* Feldman BF, Zinkle JG, Jain NC (eds): Schalm's Veterinary Hematology. Baltimore, Lippincott Williams & Wilkins, 2000, pp. 1008–1011.
12. Harvey J, Dahl M, High M: Methemoglobin reductase deficiency in a cat. J Am Vet Med Assoc 205:1290–1291, 1994.
13. Giger U, Bowden M, Wang P: Familial methemoglobin reductase deficiency. Proceedings, First International Feline Genetic Disease Conference, Philadelphia, June 25–28, 1998.
14. Kohn B, Hohenhaus A, Goldschmidt M, Giger U: Anemia, splenomegaly and increased osmotic fragility of erythrocytes in Abyssinian and Somali cats. J Am Vet Med Assoc (in press).
15. Giger U: Erythrocyte phosphofructokinase and pyruvate kinase deficiency. *In* Feldman BF, Zinkle JG, Jain NC (eds): Schalm's Veterinary Hematology. Baltimore, Lippincott Williams & Wilkins, 2000, pp. 1020–1025.
16. Giger U, Rajpurohit Y, Wang P, et al: Molecular basis of erythrocyte pyruvate kinase (R-PK) deficiency in cats. Blood 90:5b, 1997.

62

◆ Myeloid and Mast Cell Leukemias

Wayne Shapiro

Myeloid leukemias (myeloproliferative disorders [MPDs]) are a group of malignant conditions characterized by excessive proliferation of 1 or more of the nonlymphoid bone marrow elements.[1-3] Mast cell leukemia (systemic mastocytosis) is considered to arise from solid-tissue mast cells (i.e., not of true bone marrow origin); however, because it involves the hematopoietic organs primarily,[4, 5] it is included at the end of this discussion.

MPDs are more common in cats than in other domestic species, but they are still relatively rare, accounting for only 10 per cent of all hemolymphatic malignancies.[6-8] The mean age at diagnosis is 3 to 4 years.

Classification of MPDs relies on morphologic and cytochemical staining characteristics[2, 9, 10] (Tables 62–1 and 62–2). The reader's first impression usually is that these categories seem rather complicated and comprehensive. In reality, though, each case of MPD arises as a unique disorder in an individual cat. Not only can there be great variability in clinical signs and diagnostic findings from case to case, but even within an individual case, there may be progression from one form of MPD to another over the course of the illness. These classification schemes, although they may serve to describe a particular case when staging diagnostics are collected, still may be inadequate to represent fully the extent of disease or allow precise predictions of the disease course. Traditionally, the term *acute* has been used to describe the poorly differentiated leukemias with immature (*blastic*) cell types predominating. *Chronic* has been used to describe the well-differentiated leukemias with mature (erythrocytic, granulocytic, thrombocytic) cell types predominating. *Myelodysplasia* has been used to describe any of a number of bone marrow disorders manifesting as peripheral cytopenias with normal-to-hypercellular bone marrow.[11] Myelodysplasia may progress to leukemia, chronic leukemias may enter a "blast" crisis that is indistinguishable from acute leukemia, and the final stage of any MPD can be myelofibrosis with replacement of the bone marrow by scar tissue. Regardless of classification, the most important factor is the overall condition of the individual patient. Although the extremely high circulating cell counts of leukemia occasionally will cause thromboembolic complications, it is usually the cytopenias of normal blood elements that produce the life-threatening manifestations. In general, the more severe these cytopenias, the more difficult the management will be, and the poorer the long-term prognosis.

◆ CLINICAL SIGNS

The clinical signs of MPDs are vague and entirely nonspecific. Cats are presented for evaluation of anorexia, weight loss, malaise, weakness, or lethargy.[11, 12] Occasionally, abdominal distention, abdominal discomfort, vomiting, or diarrhea is described. Physical examination findings can include mucous membrane pallor, petechiation, mild lymphadenopathy, hepatosplenomegaly, and fever.

◆ DIAGNOSIS

Because the clinical signs of MPDs are so variable and nonspecific, the first clear indication of MPD usually is found on the hemogram. This is an example of the importance of a minimum database for evaluation of any sick cat. Although high numbers of a single immature (blastic) cell type is an obvious clue of MPD, in many cases, a profound nonregenerative anemia, thrombocytopenia, neutropenia, bi- or pancytopenia, or increased numbers of immature blood cells (metarubricytes or rubricytes, white blood cell precursors, or giant platelets) are found.[9] Any of these changes can occur singly or in combination. A reticulocyte count will allow characterization of an anemia as regenerative or nonregenerative. Bleeding tendencies should be evaluated by a full coagulation profile. A serum biochemistry pro-

Table 62–1. Classification of Myeloid Leukemia/Myeloproliferative Disorders

Acute Myeloid Leukemias

Undifferentiated myeloid leukemia (M0)
Acute myelogenous leukemia (M1–M2)
   Basophilic differentiation (M2-B)
Progranulocytic leukemia (M3)
Acute myelomonocytic leukemia (M4)
Acute monoblastic/monocytic leukemia (M5a/M5b)
Erythroleukemia (M6)
   Erythroid predominance/erythremic myelosis (M6-Er)
Acute megakaryoblastic leukemia (M7)
Acute undifferentiated leukemia (AUL)

Chronic Myeloid Leukemias

Chronic myelogenous leukemia
   Eosinophilic leukemia
   Basophilic leukemia
Polycythemia rubra vera
Essential thrombocythemia

Myelodysplastic Syndrome (Preleukemia)

Table 62–2. Cytochemical Staining Characteristics of Feline Leukemias

Stain	AML	AMoL	AMMoL	ALL
MPO	+	−	±	−
CAE	+	−	±	−
ANBE	−	+	±	±
LIP	−	+	±	−
LAP	+	−	±	±

ALL, acute lymphoblastic leukemia; AML, acute myeloid leukemia; AMMoL, acute myelomonocytic leukemia; AMoL, acute monocytic/monoblastic leukemia; ANBE, alpha-naphthyl butyrate esterase; CAE, chloracetate esterase; LAP, leukocyte alkaline phosphatase; LIP, lipase; MPO, myeloperoxidase.

file and urinalysis are vital for determination of overall metabolic status. Because both the MPD itself and drugs used for its management may be associated with immune compromise, aerobic culture of an aseptically collected urine sample is recommended. Feline leukemia virus (FeLV) and feline immunodeficiency virus status should be determined. By 1 report, the majority of cats with MPDs (with the exception of those with eosinophilic leukemia and polycythemia vera) tested positive for FeLV.[13] Some reports have suggested that even cats that were consistently negative for FeLV by routine screening tests may develop disease secondary to latent (nonviremic) FeLV infection.[14, 15] Use of polymerase chain reaction (PCR)–based tests identified FeLV-related DNA sequences in samples from nonviremic cats with malignant lymphoma. As PCR testing becomes routinely available, the application of the test to samples from cats with MPDs may be of value.

The single most important procedure for evaluation of MPDs is bone marrow aspiration cytology. This not only confirms the diagnosis of MPDs, but also allows assessment of normal bone marrow elements. Morphologic characteristics alone often are inconclusive; when additional slides are stained cytochemically for cell-line–specific identifying enzymes and biologic products (see Table 62–2), 17 per cent of leukemia diagnoses based on morphology were reclassified.[16] As immunophenotyping based on detection of cluster of differentiation (CD) surface markers becomes available, categorization of MPDs should become even more precise.

◆ ACUTE LEUKEMIAS

Acute Myelogenous Leukemia (M0–M3)

The hallmark of acute myelogenous leukemia (AML) is excessive numbers of myeloblasts in the peripheral blood and/or bone marrow[6–9, 17–19] (Fig. 62–1). Circulating malignant cell numbers may range from undetectable (aleukemic) to greater than 250,000/μl. Diagnosis frequently is followed by euthanasia; even with chemotherapy, reported survival times range from only 4 to 8 weeks.[18]

Myelomonocytic Leukemia (M4)

Acute myelomonocytic leukemia (AMMoL) is reported rarely in cats.[16, 20, 21] It is diagnosed by finding malignant cells in peripheral blood and/or bone marrow that have morphologic and cytochemical characteristics of both myeloid and monocytic precursors.

Monocytic/Monoblastic Leukemia (M5)

Acute monocytic leukemia (AMoL/M5b) and the more poorly differentiated monoblastic leukemia (AMoL/M5a) are rare in cats.[16, 22, 23] Owing to the immature appearance of the monocytes and short clinical course, it usually is considered an acute form of leukemia. Whereas variability occurs in total white blood cell counts, anemias, and thrombocytopenias, the anemia may not be as severe as in other manifestations of MPDs.

Erythremic Myelosis and Erythroleukemia (M6)

Both erythremic myelosis (EM) and erythroleukemia (ELE) (Fig. 62–2) manifest as severe nonregenerative anemia with large numbers of nucleated erythrocytes.[7, 12, 13, 23] In ELE, immature myeloid cells also are present. The anemias of either condition tend to be normocytic or macrocytic with anisocytosis, nucleated erythrocytes in the peripheral blood, and concurrent thrombocytopenia. One cat with ELE was reported to have responded well clinically to chemotherapy with doxorubicin, cyclophosphamide, and prednisone, but was found dead of unknown causes after 66 days.[24]

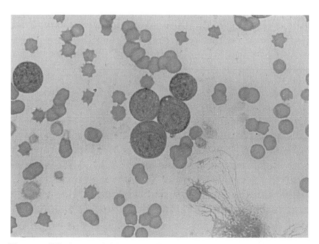

Figure 62–1. Myeloblasts with prominent nucleoli and scant agranular cytoplasm in a peripheral blood smear of a cat with acute myeloid leukemia without differentiation (M1). Wright-Giemsa, ×1000. (Courtesy of Lon J. Rich, D.V.M., Ph. D., Antech Diagnostics, Irvine, CA.)

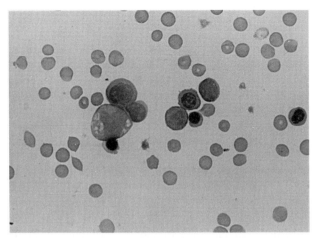

Figure 62–2. Myeloblasts, rubriblasts, and rubricytes in a peripheral blood smear from a cat with erythroleukemia (M6-Er). Wright-Giemsa, ×1000. (Courtesy of Lon J. Rich, D.V.M., Ph. D., Antech Diagnostics, Irvine, CA.)

Megakaryocytic/Megakaryoblastic Leukemia (M7)

Leukemias of the megakaryocytic cell line (ML) are extremely rare in cats.[25–28] Excessive numbers of abnormal megakaryocytes or even more primitive megakaryoblasts accumulate in the bone marrow, spleen, liver, and/or peripheral blood. Platelet counts may be high, normal, or low; severe nonregenerative anemias are observed commonly. One cat with acute megakaryocytic leukemia was managed with multiple blood transfusions and cytosine arabinoside therapy until progression of the disease prompted euthanasia at day 122.[26]

Acute Undifferentiated Leukemia

Acute undifferentiated leukemia (AUL, previously reticuloendotheliosis) is composed of blast cells so poorly differentiated that neither morphologic characteristics nor cytochemical stains allow categorization of the cell line of origin (speculation suggests either pluripotential or erythroid). Severe nonregenerative anemia is common.[12]

◆ CHRONIC LEUKEMIAS
Chronic Myelogenous Leukemia

Chronic myelogenous leukemia (CML) is extremely rare in cats. One case of CML was seen in a cat 3 years after it was diagnosed with polycythemia vera and maintained in remission with hydroxyurea.[11]

Eosinophilic Leukemia

Both eosinophilic leukemia (EL) and hypereosinophilic syndrome (HES) are characterized by persistent and markedly increased peripheral eosinophilia, bone marrow hyperplasia of eosinophilic precursors, and multiple organ infiltration by eosinophils (spleen, lymph nodes, and gastrointestinal tract).[29] EL is distinguished from HES by the relative immaturity of the eosinophilic cells. Cats with EL tend to have a higher myeloid-to-erythroid (M:E) ratio on bone marrow aspirates, higher circulating eosinophil counts, and more severe anemia than those with HES. In human beings, EL is considered a variant of CML, and the similarity of EL in cats to human CML has been described.[11, 29] Corticosteroids have been the mainstay of treatment for EL and HES, with minimal responses and poor long-term prognosis for both.

Basophilic Leukemia

Basophilic variants of CML (BL) are extremely rare. These should be distinguished from mast cell leukemia by the hypersegmented nuclei, staining characteristics of the cytoplasmic granules, and more uniform granulation of the neoplastic basophils.

Polycythemia Rubra Vera

Polycythemia rubra vera (PV) is rare in cats, and is caused by neoplastic expansion of the erythroid cell line resulting in an increased red cell mass.[11, 30, 31] Clinical signs develop as hematocrits rise to over 70 per cent, and include weakness, depression, syncope, petechiation, bright red mucous membranes, polyuria, and polydipsia. Central nervous system signs of dementia, blindness, ataxia, and seizures may be the most obvious or alarming presenting complaints. Splenomegaly is common.

Relative polycythemia may occur with dehydration or splenic contraction. Traditionally, measurement of erythropoietin (EPO) and blood gases was recommended to distinguish the secondary polycythemias of cardiopulmonary disease (increased EPO, decreased arterial oxygen saturation) and EPO-secreting tumors of the kidney or liver (increased EPO, normal arterial oxygen saturation) from PV (decreased EPO, normal arterial oxygen saturation). In 1 report, EPO levels were measured in clinical cases of canine (n = 8) and feline (n = 7) PV, canine (n = 7) and feline (n = 2) secondary polycythemias, and canine (n = 15) polycythemias of unknown origin.[32] All EPO values for cases of PV and secondary polycythemia were within the normal range, and there was no significant difference between rank sum values of EPO in PV or secondary polycythemia in either species, suggesting that EPO levels may be of limited diagnostic value for evaluation of polycythemia.

Treatment with hydroxyurea (Table 62–3) to slow the proliferation of the erythroid cells and periodic phlebotomy (removing 20 ml/kg of whole blood while concurrently infusing an equal volume of iso-

Table 62–3. Treatment of Feline Leukemia/
Myeloproliferative Disorders

Acute Myeloid Leukemias

1. Cytosine arabinoside, 100 mg/m^2, IV as 4 hr drip in saline
   solution;
   Mitoxantrone, 4–6 mg/m^2, IV drip over 4 hr, mixed with
   cytosine arabinoside;
   Repeat every 2–4 wk.
2. Cytosine arabinoside, 5–10 mg/m^2, SC, q 12 hr for 2–3 wk,
   then on alternate weeks (7 days on, 7 days off).

Chronic Myeloid Leukemias

1. Hydroxyurea, 30–50 mg/kg, orally q 24 hr for 1 wk; then q
   2–3 days.

Abbreviations: IV, intravenously; q, every; SC, subcutaneously.

tonic crystalloid solution intravenously) to maintain
the hematocrit at or below 60 per cent may provide
some cats with an acceptable quality of life for several years.

Essential Thrombocythemia

Essential thrombocythemia (ET, primary thrombosis) is an excessive proliferation of morphologically
and functionally abnormal platelets or megakaryocytes.[33] As with other forms of MPDs, the presenting
signs are nonspecific. Despite circulating platelet
counts that exceed 1,000,000/μl, the abnormal platelet function can result in petechiation, ecchymoses,
gastrointestinal, or other gross hemorrhage. One cat
with ET that was treated with fresh whole-blood
transfusion and melphalan died of sepsis before a
response to therapy could be demonstrated.[34]

◆ MYELODYSPLASTIC SYNDROME

Myelodysplastic syndrome (MDS) is considered to
be a form of MPD. Clinical signs are similar to those
of the leukemias: lethargy, inappetence, and weight
loss.[21, 35–37] Moderate-to-severe nonregenerative anemia, other single cytopenias, or bi- or pancytopenia
may be found. Dysplastic changes commonly found
in feline MDS include increased nucleated erythrocytes (metarubricytes), macrocytosis, poikilocytosis,
giant platelets, and giant, hypersegmented, or toxic
neutrophils.[9, 10, 20] Indeed, because bone marrow aspirates from cases of CML and MDS will have less
than 30 per cent blast forms, the distinction between
the 2 conditions is based on degree of dysplastic
changes.[3] If the M:E ratio is less than 1 (erythroid
predominance), the MDS can be further described
as MDS-Er. The majority of cats with MDS are reported to be positive for FeLV infection. The older
term *preleukemia* still applies; approximately one-
third of cats with MDS will progress to acute leukemia.

Treatment

Treatment of various forms of MPDs have been reported occasionally.[8, 11, 18, 22, 24, 31] The only consistent
aspect to these reports has been the poor prognosis
of AML; CML and MDS may (at least initially) be
more rewarding to treat. For all cases of MPD, supportive care (fluids, blood products, antibiotics, anabolic steroids, appetite stimulants, and nutritional
support) is an intrinsic part of therapy. Glucocorticoids seem less effective for MPDs than for lymphoproliferative malignancies. In the last volume of this
book, 3 chemotherapy protocols were presented for
management of MPDs[11] (see Table 62–3). These are
adaptations of human protocols and use established
veterinary drug dosages. As with previous chemotherapy protocols, these have had limited application in veterinary medicine; indeed, there have been
no additional reports of treatment for MPDs. The
high-dose cytosine arabinoside (Cytosar-U, Upjohn)
and mitoxantrone (Novantrone, Immunex) are appropriate for induction of an AML patient with high
peripheral leukemic cell counts (≥100,000/μl). The
low-dose cytosine arabinoside protocol is not expected to clear leukemic cells from the circulation
as rapidly, but should be less likely to suppress
normal bone marrow elements or induce "tumor
lysis syndrome," in which rapid destruction of neoplastic cells precipitates renal failure or consumptive coagulopathy. This protocol may be more appropriate for management of extremely debilitated
patients, those with peripheral cell counts less than
100,000/μl, or after induction with the high-dose
protocol. It also was suggested in the previous volume that the low-dose cytosine arabinoside protocol
(with or without nandrolone decanoate, 1 to 4 mg/
kg intramuscularly, once-weekly) may be used in an
attempt to induce differentiation of dysplastic cells
in some cases of MDS.[11] Hydroxyurea (Hydrea, Immunex) is the consensus drug of choice for chronic
leukemias, and seems to be well tolerated by cats,
although once again, there is a frustrating paucity
of published experience with treatment of this condition.

◆ MAST CELL LEUKEMIA

Mast cell leukemia (systemic mastocytosis) is a
manifestation of mast cell neoplasia, which mainly
involves the spleen, peripheral blood, and bone
marrow.[12] It is not a true leukemia because it arises
from tissue mast cells; however, as it mainly involves hematopoietic organs and is obviously distinct in most cases from cutaneous manifestations
of mast cell tumors,[4, 5] it deserves inclusion in this
chapter. Although systemic mastocytosis may occur
as frequently as the cutaneous form of mast cell
tumor in cats,[38] it is reported rarely in the veterinary
literature.[5, 39, 40] Presenting signs usually include
poor appetite, vomiting, and/or abdominal distention. Splenomegaly will be found commonly on

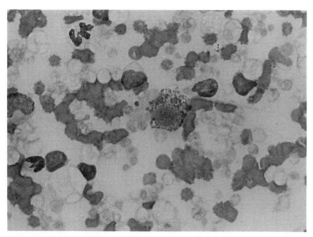

Figure 62–3. Circulating mast cell with ovoid nucleus and fine metachromatic cytoplasmic granules in the buffy coat smear of a cat. Wright-Giemsa, ×500. (Courtesy of Lon J. Rich, D.V.M., Ph. D., Antech Diagnostics, Irvine, CA.)

physical examination, radiographs, or ultrasonography. Circulating mast cells can range from none (even on a buffy coat smear) to greater than 50 per cent of the total white blood cell count. (Fig. 62–3).[12] Anemia, if present, usually is not as severe as with other (true) leukemias. Splenic aspirates for cytology demonstrate numerous mast cells. Bone marrow aspiration cytology has been recommended for staging of mast cell tumors in dogs. In the published reports of systemic mastocytosis in cats, bone marrow aspirates were not performed, and their value for such cases, especially if the hemogram shows no other cytopenias, is undetermined. Screening tests for FeLV infection have been consistently negative.

Splenectomy may result in remission of circulating mast cell leukemia and prolonged survival times (6 months to > 3 years).[5, 40] If systemic signs persist after surgery, palliative therapy with antihistamines (H₁- and H₂-receptor blockers), gastrointestinal protectants, and corticosteroids may be instituted. Treatment of systemic mastocytosis in cats with modern chemotherapeutics has not been reported.

REFERENCES

1. Young KM: Myeloproliferative disorders. Vet Clin North Am Small Anim Pract 15:769–781, 1985.
2. Evans RJ, Gorman NT: Myeloproliferative disease in the dog and cat: Definition, aetiology and classification. Vet Rec 121:437–443, 1987.
3. Raskin RE: Myelopoiesis and myeloproliferative disorders. Vet Clin North Am Small Anim Pract 26:1023–1042, 1996.
4. Lemarie RJ, Lemarie SL, Hedlund CS: Mast cell tumors: Clinical management. Compend Contin Educ Pract Vet 17:1085–1101, 1995.
5. Liska WD, MacEwen EG, Zaki FA, et al: Feline systemic mastocytosis: A review and results of splenectomy in seven cases. J Am Anim Hosp Assoc 15:589–597, 1979.
6. Holzworth J: Leukemia and related neoplasms in the cat. II: Malignancies other than lymphoid. J Am Vet Med Assoc 136:107–121, 1960.
7. Hardy WD: Hematopoietic tumors of cats. J Am Anim Hosp Assoc 17:921–940, 1981.
8. Theilen GH, Madewell BR: Leukemia-sarcoma disease complex. In Theilen GH, Madewell BR (eds): Veterinary Cancer Medicine. Philadelphia, Lea & Febiger, 1979, pp. 204–288.
9. Jain NC: Classification of myeloproliferative disorders in cats using criteria proposed by the Animal Leukaemia Study Group: A retrospective study of 181 cases (1969–1992). Comp Haematol Int 3:125–134, 1993.
10. Jain NC, Blue J, Grindem CB, et al: Proposed criteria for classification of acute myeloid leukemia in dogs and cats. Vet Clin Pathol 20:63–82, 1991.
11. Ward H, Couto CG: Myeloid leukemias. In August JR (ed): Consultations in Feline Internal Medicine, vol. 3. Philadelphia, WB Saunders, 1997, pp. 509–513.
12. Gilmore CE, Holzworth J: Naturally occurring feline leukemia: Clinical, pathologic, and differential diagnostic features. J Am Vet Med Assoc 158:1013–1025, 1971.
13. Harvey JW, Shields RP, Gaskin JM: Feline myeloproliferative disease: Changing manifestations in the peripheral blood. Vet Pathol 15:437–448, 1978.
14. Jackson ML, Haines DM, Meric SM, et al: Feline leukemia virus detection by immunohistochemistry and polymerase chain reaction in formalin-fixed, paraffin-embedded tumor tissue from cats with lymphosarcoma. Can J Vet Res 57:269–276, 1993.
15. Toby JC, Houston DM, Breur GJ, et al: Cutaneous T-cell lymphoma in a cat. J Am Vet Med Assoc 204:606–609, 1994.
16. Facklam NR, Kociba GJ: Cytochemical characterization of feline leukemia cells. Vet Pathol 23:155–161, 1986.
17. Fraser CJ, Joiner GN, Jardine JH, et al: Acute granulocytic leukemia in cats. J Am Vet Med Assoc 165:355–359, 1974.
18. Henness AM, Crow SE: Treatment of feline myelogenous leukemia: Four case reports. J Am Vet Med Assoc 171:263–266, 1977.
19. Bounous DI, Latimer KS, Campagnoli RP, et al: Acute myeloid leukemia with basophilic differentiation (AML, M-2b) in a cat. Vet Clin Pathol 23:15–18, 1994.
20. Raskin RE, Krehbiel JD: Myelodysplastic changes in a cat with myelomonocytic leukemia. J Am Vet Med Assoc 187:171–174, 1985.
21. Stann SE: Myelomonocytic leukemia in a cat. J Am Vet Med Assoc 174:722–725, 1979.
22. Henness AM, Crow SE, Anderson BC: Monocytic leukemia in three cats. J Am Vet Med Assoc 170:1325–1328, 1977.
23. Grindem CB, Perman V, Stevens JB: Morphological classification and clinical pathologic characteristics of spontaneous leukemia in 10 cats. J Am Anim Hosp Assoc 21:227–236, 1985.
24. Yates RW, Weller RE, Feldman BF: Myeloproliferative disease in a cat. Mod Vet Pract 7:753–757, 1984.
25. Michel RL, O'Handley P, Dade AW: Megakaryocytic myelosis in a cat. J Am Vet Med Assoc 168:1021–1025, 1976.
26. Hamilton TA, Morrison WB, DeNicola DB: Cytosine arabinoside chemotherapy for acute megakaryocytic leukemia in a cat. J Am Vet Med Assoc 199:359–361, 1991.
27. Colbatzky F, Hermanns W: Acute megakaryoblastic leukemia in one cat and two dogs. Vet Pathol 30:186–194, 1993.
28. Burton S, Miller L, Horney B, et al: Acute megakaryoblastic leukemia in a cat. Vet Clin Pathol 25:6–9, 1996.
29. Huibregtse BA, Turner JL: Eosinophilic leukemia: A comparison of 22 hypereosinophilic cats. J Am Anim Hosp Assoc 30:591–599, 1994.
30. Reed C, Ling GV, Gould D, et al: Polycythemia vera in a cat. J Am Vet Med Assoc 157:85–91, 1970.
31. Khanna C, Bienzle D: Polycythemia vera in a cat: Bone marrow culture in erythropoietin-deficient medium. J Am Anim Hosp Assoc 30:45–49, 1994.
32. Cook SM, Lothrop CD: Serum erythropoietin concentrations measured by radioimmunoassay in normal, polycythemic, and anemic dogs and cats. J Vet Intern Med 8:18–25, 1994.
33. Chisholm-Chait A: Essential thrombocythemia in dogs and cats. Part I. Compend Contin Educ Pract Vet 21:158–167, 1999.

34. Hammer AS, Couto CG, Getzy D, et al: Essential thrombocythemia in a cat. J Vet Intern Med 4:87–91, 1990.
35. Schalm OW: Progression of a myeloproliferative disorder in a cat. Fel Pract 8:14–17, 1978.
36. Madewell BR, Jain NC, Weller RC: Hematologic abnormalities preceeding myeloid leukemia in three cats. Vet Pathol 16:510–519, 1979.
37. Blue JT, French TW, Kranz JS: Non-lymphoid hematopoietic neoplasia in cats: A retrospective study of 60 cases. Cornell Vet 78:21–42, 1978.
38. Rogers KS: Mast cell tumors: Dilemmas of diagnosis and treatment. Vet Clin North Am Small Anim Pract 26:87–102, 1996.
39. Guerre R, Millet P, Groulade P: Systemic mastocytosis in a cat: Remission after splenectomy. J Small Anim Pract 20:769–772, 1979.
40. Jeraj KP, O'Brien TD, Yeno BL: Systemic mastocytoma associated with lymphosarcoma in an aged cat. Can Vet J 24:20–23, 1983.

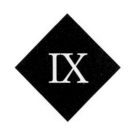

Oncology

Kenita S. Rogers, Editor

◆ Gastrointestinal Lymphoma and Inflammatory
  Bowel Disease 499
◆ Management of the Lymphoma Patient
  With Concurrent Disease 506
◆ Chemotherapeutic Challenges:
  Special Considerations and New Agents 521
◆ Approach to Oral Tumors 526
◆ Intranasal Neoplasia 529
◆ Evaluation and Treatment of Cranial Mediastinal
  Masses 533
◆ Update on Vaccine-Associated Sarcomas 541
◆ Diagnostic Imaging of Neoplasia 548

Still-Current Information Found in *Consultations in Feline Internal Medicine 2:*

Plasmacytic-Lymphocytic Stomatitis (Chapter 9), p. 59
Inflammatory Bowel Disease (Chapter 11), p. 75
Chronic Sneezing (Chapter 36), p. 273
Pleural Effusion: Physical, Biochemical, and Cytological
    Characteristics (Chapter 38), p. 287
Chylothorax: Diagnosis and Management (Chapter 39),
    p. 297
Diagnostic Capabilities of Computed Tomography and Mag-
    netic Resonance Imaging (Chapter 50), p. 393
Selective Therapy for Lymphoma (Chapter 66), p. 539
Solitary Extranodal Lymphomas: Presentation and Manage-
    ment (Chapter 67), p. 547
Postvaccination Sarcomas (Chapter 72), p. 587

Still-Current Information Found in *Consultations in Feline Internal Medicine 3:*

Evaluation and Management of Oral Disease (Chapter 9),
    p. 53
Current Concepts in Gastrointestinal Neoplasia (Chapter
    14), p. 99
Gastrointestinal Endoscopic Biopsy Techniques (Chapter
    16), p. 113
Bladder Neoplasia: Difficulties in Diagnosis and Treatment
    (Chapter 41), p. 319
Advances in Chemotherapy (Chapter 65), p. 527
Safe Handling of Chemotherapy Drugs (Chapter 66), p. 534
Clinical Perspectives on Vaccine-Associated Sarcomas
    (Chapter 67), p. 541
Metastatic Patterns of Feline Neoplasia (Chapter 71), p. 566
Recommendations for FeLV- and FIV-Positive Cats With
    Cancer (Chapter 72), p. 572

Managing Oral Health in Breeding Catteries (Chapter 80), p. 647

Elsewhere in *Consultations in Feline Internal Medicine 4*:
Update on Vaccine-Associated Sarcomas and Current Vaccine Recommendations (Chapter 1), p. 3

Contrast Radiography for Evaluation of the Gastrointestinal Tract (Chapter 9), p. 73

The Gastrointestinal Tract and Adverse Reactions to Food (Chapter 14), p. 113

Clinical Approach to Chronic Diarrhea (Chapter 16), p. 127

Acquired Myasthenia Gravis and Other Disorders of the Neuromuscular Junction (Chapter 48), p. 374

Splenomegaly and Lymphadenopathy (Chapter 56), p. 439

63

◆ Gastrointestinal Lymphoma and Inflammatory Bowel Disease

Elizabeth A. Carsten
Michael D. Willard

◆ IMPORTANCE

Inflammatory bowel disease (IBD) and alimentary lymphosarcoma (LSA) are the 2 most common feline intestinal infiltrative disorders, and are diagnosed primarily in middle-aged to older cats with anorexia, weight loss, vomiting, and/or diarrhea. Diagnosing LSA requires demonstrating neoplastic lymphocytes, whereas the diagnosis of IBD requires eliminating known causes of gastrointestinal disease in addition to demonstrating inflammatory infiltrates. However, IBD infiltrates can range from mild to so severe as to mimic neoplasia, and differentiating IBD from LSA may be difficult. To add to the confusion, IBD and LSA may coexist in intestinal tissue. The prognosis for cats with IBD can be good with appropriate dietary and medical therapy, whereas LSA may be palliated but ultimately remains fatal.

◆ ETIOPATHOGENESIS

Alimentary LSA is the most common anatomic form of feline LSA, accounting for approximately 20 per cent of all intestinal malignancies and 15 to 40 per cent of all LSA in cats.[1, 2] Alimentary LSA usually arises from gut-associated lymphoid tissue, and is of B-lymphocyte origin. This is not surprising, because feline leukemia virus (FeLV) usually affects T-lymphocytes, and cats with alimentary LSA usually are negative when tested for FeLV.

IBD is idiopathic intestinal inflammation. The pathogenesis of IBD is postulated to include 2 stages. First, an intestinal insult occurs that damages the mucosa and increases its permeability.[3] This insult may be caused by dietary antigens, bacteria, or viruses, or may result from an intrinsic defect in the mucosal barrier. Alternatively, an abnormal mucosal immune system may allow an exaggerated inflammatory response to luminal antigens by failing to down-regulate the mucosal response.[4]

Next, the initial inflammatory response is amplified inappropriately, and inflammatory cells are attracted to the injured site with subsequent production of cytokines, eicosanoids, and/or free radicals. This amplification probably is what causes the clinical signs associated with IBD.[4] Increased leukotrienes and hydroxyeicosatetraenoic acids occur in the intestinal mucosa of human beings with ulcerative colitis, in which disease severity correlates positively with leukotriene concentrations, whereas inhibition of leukotriene synthesis is associated with decreased colonic inflammation.[3] Persistent small-intestinal inflammation ultimately may produce atrophy and fibrosis of the mucosa and villi.

Feline lymphocytic-plasmacytic gastroenteritis has been suggested to be preneoplastic in some patients. In human beings, immunoproliferative small-intestinal disease predisposes to primary intestinal LSA, whereas treatment of the immunoproliferative condition decreases the risk of subsequent malignancy.[5] Concern was raised that the same predisposition toward malignancy may be true of cats with IBD, when 3 of 9 cats diagnosed as having IBD by full-thickness gastrointestinal biopsies were reported to develop alimentary LSA 9 to 18 months later.[6] However, cause and effect are not clear from this report. These cats might have developed LSA independent of the IBD, or they may have had well-differentiated LSA from the beginning that was misdiagnosed initially as IBD. If IBD is a preneoplastic lesion or does predispose some cats to LSA, this does not appear to be a common occurrence.

◆ CLINICAL SIGNS

The median age for cats presenting with IBD is 5.1 to 6.9 years (range, 6 months to 20 years).[7–9] Purebred cats have been suggested to have a higher incidence of IBD.[8, 9] Reported pure breeds affected include Siamese, Persian, Himalayan, and Abyssinian. A gender predilection for IBD has not been reported. Cats presenting with alimentary LSA tend to be older (median age, 10 years) than cats with IBD, but the age range (1 to 18 years) overlaps with that of IBD.[10] A breed or gender predisposition for alimentary LSA has not been reported. Affected pure breeds that have been reported include Abyssinian, Siamese, Persian, and Himalayan.[10]

Vomiting, anorexia, and weight loss are the most common historical findings for both IBD and alimentary LSA.[7–10] The mean duration of clinical signs in cats presenting with IBD is 7.4 to 8.5 months (range, 0.5 to 24 months),[8, 9] and probably is similar in cats with alimentary LSA. Severity of clinical signs is not necessarily associated with the histologic grade of IBD.[8, 9] A cyclical or progressive clinical course may be associated with both IBD and alimentary LSA.

Physical examination may be unremarkable, but weight loss is the most consistent physical examination finding in cats with IBD.[9] Other findings may include mildly to moderately thickened or fluid-filled intestines. In one report, an abdominal mass could be palpated in 24 of 28 cats with alimentary LSA.[10] However, this experience is not universal, and most cats with alimentary LSA seen by the authors did not have a discrete mass at physical examination, abdominal imaging, or laparotomy. It is particularly noteworthy that mesenteric lymphadenopathy may be associated with both IBD (reactive lymphadenopathy) and LSA (neoplastic or reactive lymphadenopathy). Thus, physical examination findings in cats with LSA may be identical to those with IBD.

◆ DIAGNOSIS

Complete blood count, serum biochemistries, urinalysis, FeLV and feline immunodeficiency virus tests, heartworm antigen, serum free thyroxine (T_4) concentration, fecal examinations, and diagnostic imaging typically are performed in cats with chronic vomiting, anorexia, and/or weight loss. These tests help exclude metabolic diseases (renal failure, diabetes mellitus), and provide a preanesthetic evaluation before gastrointestinal biopsy. However, these tests generally do not diagnose or exclude infiltrative bowel disease.

Hematologic abnormalities are uncommon and usually nonspecific in cats with infiltrative intestinal disease (e.g., anemia owing to chronic inflammation), although bone marrow neoplastic infiltrates may cause anemia in cats with alimentary LSA.[11] Neutrophilia, lymphopenia, and monocytosis may occur with severe IBD, and probably represent a stress response and/or chronic inflammation.[8, 9] Alternatively, absorption of endotoxins through a compromised intestinal barrier might be responsible.[11] Eosinophilia and basophilia have been described in cats with gastrointestinal tract diseases, and may reflect a type-1 hypersensitivity immune response to allergens. However, T-lymphocytes can produce substances that stimulate marrow eosinopoiesis, and 2 cats with alimentary LSA reportedly had eosinophilia.[11]

Serum biochemical abnormalities in cats with infiltrative intestinal disease usually are nonspecific, when present. Mild increases in hepatic enzyme activities (alanine transferase [ALT], alkaline phosphatase [ALP]) occur in cats with IBD.[7-9] Hepatocellular degeneration may be caused by toxins absorbed through a compromised intestinal mucosal barrier.[8] However, an association of IBD with cholangiohepatitis and pancreatitis also has been reported, and may represent ascending bacterial infection within the biliary and pancreatic ducts.[12]

Neoplastic hepatic infiltrates are a potential, although uncommon, cause of increased ALT or ALP in cats with alimentary LSA.

Altered protein metabolism sometimes occurs. Hyperproteinemia may reflect dehydration and/or chronic inflammation. Hypoalbuminemia is uncommon, but may be multifactorial when it occurs. Protein loss through damaged mucosa probably is the most important mechanism of severe hypoalbuminemia (<2.0 g/dl), with reduced protein intake and malabsorption of nutrients also contributing.[11] Hypoglobulinemia without concurrent hypoalbuminemia occurs in some cats with IBD, but its significance and cause are uncertain.[9]

Electrolyte disturbances often are secondary changes, rather than direct reflections of infiltrative intestinal disease. Hypokalemia is the most commonly reported electrolyte abnormality.[7, 8] Decreased intake (anorexia) plus loss of potassium-rich fluids owing to vomiting and/or diarrhea likely contribute to hypokalemia when present.

Survey abdominal radiographs may be normal, or may reveal fluid- and/or gas-distended loops of small intestine.[7, 9] An abdominal mass may be noted in cats with LSA; however, the absence of a mass does not eliminate neoplasia.[10] Luminal narrowing, decreased mucosal fimbriation, "thumb-printing" lesions, and bowel spasticity observed on gastrointestinal contrast studies support small bowel infiltrative disease. However, the positive and negative predictive values of such radiographic observations for LSA are unknown, and their presence or absence generally does not negate the need for intestinal biopsy.[13]

Abdominal ultrasonography is particularly valuable when alimentary LSA is suspected.[10, 14, 15] Ultrasonographic abnormalities identified in cats with alimentary LSA may include thickening of the stomach or bowel wall, loss of the normal layered appearance of the gastrointestinal wall, a hypoechoic mass associated with the gastrointestinal tract, and abdominal lymphadenopathy.[14, 15] Intestinal layer identification seemingly is more commonly preserved in inflammatory diseases than in infiltrative tumors.[14] Ultrasound-guided fine-needle aspiration and core biopsy are relatively safe, and cytologic diagnosis of certain types of alimentary LSA (especially the lymphoblastic types) seems to have good specificity, but unknown sensitivity. At this time, LSA cannot be eliminated definitively, nor can IBD be diagnosed confidently, based on aspirate cytology. Malignancies and intestinal lesions that have a bowel wall thickness greater than 2.0 cm seemingly are associated with a high percentage of correct diagnoses of neoplasia.[15] In addition, ultrasonography can aid in determining whether the lesion is within reach of the endoscope, or if laparotomy is necessary to biopsy the lesion(s).

Biopsy

Definitive diagnosis of IBD, and often LSA, requires mucosal biopsies obtained by endoscopy, laparoscopy, or laparotomy. Endoscopy is minimally invasive and usually allows procurement of diagnostic tissue samples. However, it is easy for untrained clinicians to obtain poor-quality samples with an endoscope (Fig. 63–1). Some clinicians prefer full-thickness intestinal biopsies obtained at laparotomy or laparoscopy as a means to avoid such problems. However, it is surprisingly easy to likewise obtain poor-quality, full-thickness biopsies. If endoscopy is used to obtain tissue samples, multiple samples of duodenum, ileum, colon, and (if possible) proximal jejunum (e.g., 6 to 10/site) should be obtained. If a laparotomy is performed, biopsies from duodenum, ileum, jejunum (preferably 2 samples of jejunum), and mesenteric lymph node should be obtained. Hepatic and pancreatic biopsies also should be performed if a laparotomy or laparoscopy is done.

During endoscopy, mucosal structures should be examined carefully before biopsy. The mucosa should be evaluated for erythema, granularity, friability, erosions, ulcers, and mass lesions. Be sure to biopsy such lesions as well as more normal-appearing mucosa. Sometimes, focal lesions have so much secondary inflammation that the diagnosis is best obtained from tissue away from that site, and

vice versa. One study comparing endoscopic and histologic findings in dogs and cats found that 82 per cent of tissue samples taken from animals with endoscopic evidence of increased granularity and friability were associated with increased lamina propria cellularity.[16] It was suggested that the likelihood of obtaining a diagnosis was low when the mucosa appeared normal. However, multiple mucosal biopsies should be obtained in all patients regardless of the endoscopic appearance of the mucosa.

After obtaining a mucosal sample, it should be evaluated for adequacy. Endoscopic mucosal biopsies should include the full thickness of the mucosa from the tips of the villi to the border of the muscularis mucosa (see Fig. 63–1B). Typically, when such samples are viewed grossly at the time of biopsy, they are obviously more substantive than ones composed primarily of villi. Although there is currently no documentation that tissue samples composed of villus fragments are always less diagnostic than samples that include villi and the full depth of lamina propria, it seems reasonable to assume (until proved otherwise) that such poor-quality tissue samples are much more likely to be nondiagnostic and/or lead to misdiagnosis.

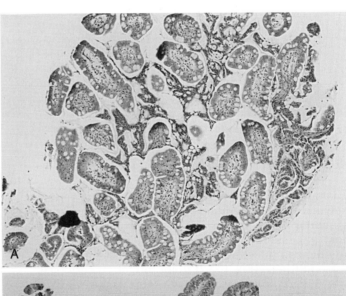
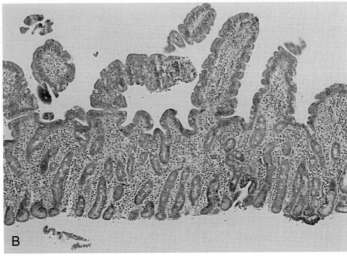

Figure 63–1. *A,* Photomicrograph of endoscopically obtained duodenal tissue that is composed primarily of fragments of villi. Although such a sample might allow diagnosis, it is probable that important changes in the lamina propria would go unsuspected. This is considered an inadequate tissue sample. *B,* Photomicrograph of endoscopically obtained duodenal mucosa from a cat without intestinal disease. This sample, in distinction to the sample in *A,* is well oriented, and includes the total depth of mucosa from the villi to the border with the muscularis mucosa. The smooth ventral border of the sample shows that this piece was "lifted" off the muscularis mucosa. Such a sample is more likely to allow the pathologist to recognize all pathologic processes present.

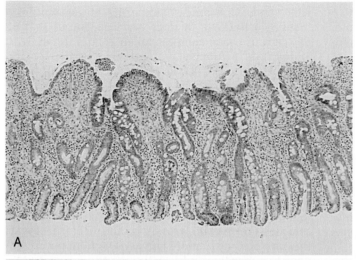

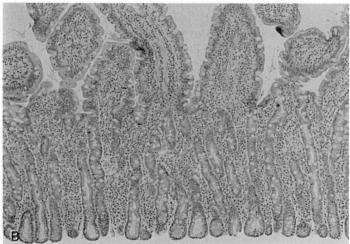

Figure 63–2. *A,* Photomicrograph of endoscopically obtained duodenal mucosa from a cat diagnosed as having mild-to-moderate lymphocytic/plasmacytic inflammatory bowel disease. The mucosal infiltrate is not particularly dense, but there is marked and consistent villus atrophy. *B,* Photomicrograph of duodenal mucosa from another cat diagnosed as having mild-to-moderate lymphocytic/plasmacytic inflammatory bowel disease. In contrast to *A,* the villi in this section are normal in length; however, there is an increase in the number of mononuclear cells in the subvillus lamina propria that is a little more obvious than the infiltrate seen in *A.*

◆ HISTOPATHOLOGY

Histopathologic assessment of good-quality, representative mucosal biopsies is necessary for distinguishing normal, inflammatory, and neoplastic intestinal lesions. However, it can be difficult to distinguish intestinal tissue with modest inflammatory infiltrates (Fig. 63–2) from normal mucosa (see Fig. 63–1*B*). Likewise, although some tissue samples obviously have LSA (Fig. 63–3), it can be difficult to distinguish well-differentiated LSA (Fig. 63–4) from severe IBD in some patients. A major problem of gastrointestinal histopathology is the lack of uniformity with which various pathologists evaluate intestinal tissue samples (i.e., different pathologists may call the same tissue sample "normal," "mild lymphoplasmacytic enteritis," or "moderate lymphoplasmacytic enteritis"). This variability in the interpretation of intestinal histopathology has caused some to raise questions regarding the value of intestinal biopsy.

Many types of inflammatory cells may infiltrate the intestinal mucosa, including eosinophils, neutrophils, lymphocytes, and plasma cells. Of these, lymphocytes and plasma cells are the ones most commonly associated with IBD.[17, 18] Part of the confusion about evaluation of intestinal tissue stems from a lack of information regarding exactly what constitutes "normal," especially for lymphocytes and plasma cells in the lamina propria and villi.

Different investigators have published varying

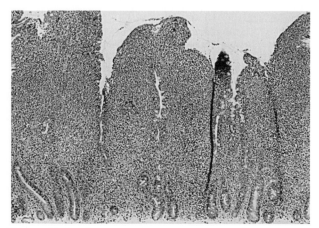

Figure 63–3. Photomicrograph of endoscopically obtained ileal mucosa that is heavily infiltrated by neoplastic lymphocytes.

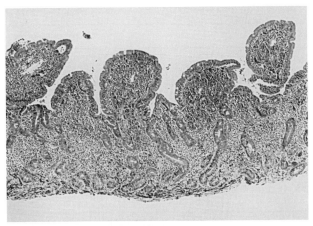

Figure 63–4. Photomicrograph of endoscopically obtained duodenal mucosa. There was disagreement as to whether this represented inflammatory bowel disease or lymphoma. The cat was treated initially with prednisolone, metronidazole, and chlorambucil. The cat improved initially but became clinically worse within 2 months. The post-mortem diagnosis was lymphoma.

criteria for histologic grading of various inflammatory bowel disorders.[7, 9, 19] Unfortunately, there are no generally agreed-on criteria for distinguishing normal and diseased intestinal mucosa, nor for grading diseased mucosa.[17] Consequently, clinicians not only should provide the best-quality tissue samples possible, but also should communicate routinely with their pathologists. Preferably, this should be the same pathologist, so that both the clinician and the pathologist become familiar with the relationship between his or her interpretation of intestinal histopathology and the cat's response to therapy.

Most clinicians are aware that IBD can be diagnosed mistakenly when the patient has alimentary LSA. Lymphocytic-plasmacytic infiltrates surrounding LSA foci may produce this misinterpretation.[20] However, LSA may be diagnosed when, in fact, the patient has a nonneoplastic infiltrate. One cat with chronic diarrhea was diagnosed as having duodenal LSA on 2 separate sets of endoscopic biopsies, but all clinical signs resolved for years after the diet was changed to a hypoallergenic one.[21] Therefore, several criteria should be considered before diagnosing LSA (especially if euthanasia will be the result of such a diagnosis). First, the cellular infiltrate should be evaluated for uniformity and evidence of neoplastic characteristics (e.g., abnormal/multiple nucleoli, multinucleation, abnormal mitotic figures); a homogeneous cellular infiltrate with strong neoplastic characteristics is more typical of LSA than IBD. Next, finding lymphocytes and especially lymphoblasts in abnormal locations may suggest LSA. Third, immunohistochemical stains for B- and T-lymphocytes allow one to distinguish a homogenous B-cell infiltrate (more suggestive of LSA) from a mixed B- and T-cell infiltrate (more suggestive of IBD). If the history, physical examination, or both do not clearly support the histologic diagnosis of alimentary LSA in a patient with a debatable histologic interpretation, then treating the

cat as though it had severe IBD may be the most reasonable option. Successful long-term response (≥2 years) to anti-inflammatory therapy suggests IBD, even if histologic evaluation suggests LSA.[21] Similarly, a cat diagnosed with severe IBD that is not responding to apparently appropriate therapy should be reevaluated for the possibility of a well-differentiated LSA.

◆ TREATMENT

Dietary manipulation, antimicrobial agents, corticosteroids, metronidazole, and cytotoxic drugs have been the mainstay of therapy for IBD. An elimination diet can resolve an underlying food allergy or intolerance. However, even if an allergy or intolerance is not present, dietary modification may allow the patient's diseased intestinal tract to better compensate. For example, an elemental diet may permit the intestines to absorb nutrients despite their disease. However, elemental diets (e.g., Vivonex) are used infrequently in veterinary patients owing to the cost and lack of patient acceptance. However, esophagostomy and gastrostomy tubes may overcome some of these problems.

Corticosteroids typically are used to treat both IBD and LSA. Most patients with either disease will show some response to prednisolone at a dosage of 2.2 mg/kg/day orally (PO). In patients with IBD, the prednisolone dose is decreased gradually by 50 per cent at 2- to 4-week intervals after clinical remission is achieved, until a maintenance dose of 0.5 to 1 mg/kg every other day is reached.[18, 22] Cats with mild inflammatory changes usually respond well to lower doses, and alternate-day or every-third-day treatment often can be employed. Occasionally, corticosteroid treatment may be discontinued by 3 to 6 months, and the cat maintained with dietary and/or metronidazole therapy. Patients with moderate-to-severe IBD may require higher doses of prednisolone (2 to 4 mg/kg/day PO) for longer periods of time to maintain clinical remission. Alternatively, dexamethasone (0.22 mg/kg/day PO) may be useful in cats with IBD that are poorly responsive to prednisolone.[17] Most feline LSA chemotherapy protocols include oral prednisolone (25 to 50 mg/m² every [q] 24 to 48 hr, or 2 mg/kg/day) as part of therapy.[2, 10, 23]

Metronidazole is used commonly to treat feline IBD. Besides its antibacterial and antiprotozoal activities, metronidazole also is purported to inhibit cell-mediated immune responses.[18] A low dose of metronidazole is used (10 to 15 mg/kg q 12 hr PO), which helps to prevent vomiting or neurologic signs. Metronidazole therapy usually is combined with corticosteroid administration; however, it may be tried as the sole drug therapy if corticosteroids are contraindicated or not tolerated by a patient.

Azathioprine, an antimetabolite, is a cytotoxic drug used in cats with IBD. Because of the potential side-effects of azathioprine (especially myelosup-

Table 63-1. Chemotherapy Protocols

Protocol	Drug	Administration Schedule
COP*	Vincristine	0.5 mg/m², IV, once a wk for 8 wk
	Cyclophosphamide	50 mg/m², PO, 4 days a wk for 8 wk; then 100 mg/m², PO, once a wk for maintenance
	Prednisone	40 mg/m², PO, once daily for 8 wk; then 20 mg/m², PO, every other day for maintenance
	Methotrexate	5 mg/m², PO, twice a wk *after* 8-wk induction therapy
		Repeat 1 wk of induction therapy every 7 wk
COAP†	Vincristine	0.5 mg/m², IV, once a wk for 6 wk; then once every 4 wk for maintenance
	Cyclophosphamide	50 mg/m², PO, every other day for 6 wk
	Cytosine arabinoside	100 mg/m², SQ, first 2 days
	Prednisone	40 mg/m², PO, once daily for 1 wk; then 20 mg/m², every other day for maintenance
	Methotrexate	2.5 mg/m², PO, three times a wk *after* 6-wk induction therapy
	Chlorambucil	20 mg/m², PO, every 2 wk *after* 6-wk induction therapy

Abbreviations: COAP, cyclophosphamide, Oncovin, ara-C, prednisone; COP, cyclophosphamide, Oncovin, prednisone; IV, intravenously; PO, by mouth; SQ, subcutaneously.
*Purdue University, West Lafayette, IN.
†Veterinary Referral Clinic, Cleveland, OH.
Modified from Hamilton TA, Morrison WB: Selective therapy for lymphoma. *In* August JR (ed): Consultations in Feline Internal Medicine, vol. 2. Philadelphia, WB Saunders, 1994, pp. 539–545.

pression), its use generally is reserved for patients with histologically proven severe IBD that is resistant to corticosteroid and metronidazole therapy.[24] Even though azathioprine is a potent immunosuppressive drug, it typically must be used for 3 to 5 weeks at the correct dosage (0.3 mg/kg q 48 hr PO) before clinical effects are seen.[24] Chlorambucil seems to be safer (less myelosuppressive) than azathioprine, but about as effective. It too requires 3 to 5 weeks to be effective. There are different methods of dosing chlorambucil PO (e.g., 2 mg/m² q 48 hr; or 0.1 mg/kg daily; or 1 mg twice-weekly for cats weighing < 7 lb and 2 mg twice-weekly for cats weighing > 7 lb). Other cytotoxic agents may be used in chemotherapeutic protocols for alimentary LSA (Table 63–1).

Occasionally, the clinician is faced with a case in which one cannot distinguish between well-differentiated LSA and severe IBD, despite excellent biopsies and competent histologic evaluation. For these patients, an aggressive medical treatment protocol should be tried, including prednisolone, metronidazole, dietary manipulation, and chlorambucil. This therapeutic combination can be effective for IBD, and is reasonable therapy for well-differentiated LSA. Chlorambucil therapy probably should be initiated concurrently with the corticosteroid therapy so as to avoid acquired chemotherapy resistance in LSA that occurs with prednisolone therapy alone. Periodic monitoring for myelosuppression is recommended whenever using azathioprine or chlorambucil for long periods.

◆ SUMMARY

It can be a challenge to differentiate IBD and LSA in the older cat with chronic vomiting, anorexia, weight loss, and/or diarrhea. If the history, physical examination, or both do not clearly support a histologic diagnosis of LSA, treating for IBD may be a

reasonable option. This is especially true if euthanasia is being considered by the client.

REFERENCES

1. Zwahlen CH, Lucroy MD, Kraegel SA, et al: Results of chemotherapy for cats with alimentary malignant lymphoma: 21 cases (1993–1997). J Am Vet Med Assoc 213:1144–1149, 1998.
2. Couto CG: Gastrointestinal neoplasia in dogs and cats. *In* Kirk RW, Bonagura JD (eds): Current Veterinary Therapy XI. Philadelphia, WB Saunders, 1992, pp. 595–601.
3. Magne ML: Pathophysiology of inflammatory bowel disease. Semin Vet Med Surg (Small Anim Pract) 7:112–116, 1992.
4. Yang VW: Eicosanoids and inflammatory bowel disease. Gastroenterol Clin North Am 25:317–332, 1996.
5. Ryan JC: Premalignant conditions of the small intestine. Semin Gastrointest Dis 7:88–93, 1996.
6. Davenport DJ, Leib MS, Roth L: Progression of lymphocytic-plasmacytic enteritis to gastrointestinal lymphosarcoma in three cats. Proceedings, Veterinary Cancer Society. Madison, WI, Veterinary Cancer Society, 1987, pp. 54–56.
7. Jergens AE, Moore FM, Haynes JS, et al: Idiopathic inflammatory bowel disease in dogs and cats: 84 cases (1987–1990). J Am Vet Med Assoc 201:1603–1608, 1992.
8. Dennis JS, Kruger JM, Mullaney TP: Lymphocytic/plasmacytic colitis in cats: 14 cases (1985–1990). J Am Vet Med Assoc 202:313–318, 1993.
9. Dennis JS, Kruger JM, Mullaney TP: Lymphocytic/plasmacytic gastroenteritis in cats: 14 cases (1985–1990). J Am Vet Med Assoc 200:1712–1718, 1992.
10. Mahony OM, Moore AS, Cotter SM, et al: Alimentary lymphoma in cats: 28 cases (1988–1993). J Am Vet Med Assoc 207:1593–1598, 1995.
11. Willard MD, Tvedten H, Turnwald GH: Small Animal Clinical Diagnosis by Laboratory Methods, 3rd ed. Philadelphia, WB Saunders, 1999.
12. Weiss DJ, Gagne JM, Armstrong PJ: Relationship between inflammatory hepatic disease and inflammatory bowel disease, pancreatitis, and nephritis in cats. J Am Vet Med Assoc 209:1114–1116, 1996.
13. Weichselbaum RC, Feeney DA, Hayden DW: Comparison of upper gastrointestinal radiographic findings to histopathologic observations: A retrospective study of 41 dogs and cats with suspected small bowel infiltrative disease (1985 to 1990). Vet Radiol Ultrasound 35:418–426, 1994.
14. Pennick DG, Moore AS, Tidwell AS, et al: Ultrasonography

of alimentary lymphosarcoma in the cat. Vet Radiol Ultrasound 35:299–304, 1994.

15. Crystal MA, Penninck DG, Matz ME, et al: Use of ultrasound-guided fine-needle aspiration biopsy and automated core biopsy for the diagnosis of gastrointestinal diseases in small animals. Vet Radiol Ultrasound 34:438–444, 1993.

16. Roth L, Leib MS, Davenport DJ, et al: Comparisons between endoscopic and histologic evaluation of the gastrointestinal tract in dogs and cats: 75 cases (1984–1987). J Am Vet Med Assoc 196:635–638, 1990.

17. Wilcock B: Endoscopic biopsy interpretation in canine or feline enterocolitis. Semin Vet Med Surg 7:162–171, 1992.

18. Tams TR: Feline inflammatory bowel disease. Vet Clin North Am Small Anim Pract 23:569–586, 1993.

19. Yamasaki K, Suematsu H, Takahashi T: Comparison of gastric and duodenal lesions in dogs and cats with and without lymphocytic-plasmacytic enteritis. J Am Vet Med Assoc 209:95–97, 1996.

20. Guilford WG, Strombeck DR: Neoplasms of the gastrointestinal tract, APUD tumors, endocrinopathies and the gastrointestinal tract. In Guilford WG, Center SA, Strombeck DR, et al (eds): Strombeck's Small Animal Gastroenterology, 3rd ed. Philadelphia, WB Saunders, 1996, pp. 519–531.

21. Wasmer ML, Willard MD, Helman RG, et al: Food intolerance mimicking alimentary lymphosarcoma. J Am Anim Hosp Assoc 31:463–466, 1995.

22. Wolf A: Feline lymphocytic-plasmacytic enterocolitis. Semin Vet Med Surg 7:128–133, 1992.

23. Hamilton TA, Morrison WB: Selective therapy for lymphoma. In August JR (ed): Consultations in Feline Internal Medicine, vol. 2. Philadelphia, WB Saunders, 1994, pp. 539–545.

24. Willard MD: Inflammatory bowel disease: Perspectives on therapy. J Am Anim Hosp Assoc 28:27–32, 1992.

64

◆ Management of the Lymphoma Patient With Concurrent Disease

Glenna E. Mauldin
Samantha C. Mooney

Lymphoma is the most common neoplasm in cats, accounting for approximately one-third of reported tumors in this species.[1] Lymphoma in cats is associated with the feline leukemia virus (FeLV), a horizontally transmitted retrovirus.[2] Signalment and primary site of disease (i.e., thymus, kidney, gastrointestinal tract) are known to vary with FeLV-test status.[3-5] In early reports of cats with disease, 70 to 80 per cent were young and FeLV-test positive, and thymic involvement was most common.[5, 6] Studies have documented that the prevalence of FeLV antigenemia among cats with lymphoma has decreased to 10 to 20 per cent. Affected cats now are more likely to be 10 years of age or older with the gastrointestinal form of disease.[7, 8] An important practical implication for the veterinarian is that the patient with lymphoma is often an older cat with a variety of concurrent diseases. The goal of this chapter is to describe the ways in which concurrent disease may alter the clinical presentation and management of disease in cats with lymphoma—specifically, to examine the staging and diagnostic testing that are necessary not only for an accurate diagnosis of lymphoma but also for the identification of overt or underlying concurrent disease; and to provide practical recommendations for the management of some of the most important concurrent disease conditions encountered in cats undergoing treatment for lymphoma.

◆ CLINICAL PRESENTATION

Clinical signs associated with lymphoma are nonspecific. Lethargy, anorexia, and weight loss are the most common clinical findings, and could be caused by numerous diseases other than lymphoma.[3] Although the diagnosis of lymphoma might be probable, the clinician also must consider the possibility that some or even all of the patient's clinical signs are secondary to nonmalignant concurrent disease. Clinical signs of vomiting and diarrhea, for example, exhibited by a cat with thymic lymphoma, might be indicative of secondary gastrointestinal involvement of lymphoma; however, common disorders such as hyperthyroidism, renal disease, and inflammatory bowel disease also might be present, and they must be ruled out.

◆ STAGING AND DIAGNOSTIC TESTS

Detailed pretreatment diagnostic testing is essential in all patients to enable the clinician to confirm the diagnosis of lymphoma and to evaluate the extent of disease. Diagnostic testing provides a baseline value against which changes or abnormalities that develop during the course of treatment may be compared and followed. Finally, a detailed clinical evaluation is necessary to definitively diagnose most paraneoplastic syndromes and concurrent but unrelated diseases in cats with lymphoma. The minimum database for any cat suspected of having lymphoma should consist of the following diagnostic tests: a complete blood count, serum biochemical profile and urinalysis; current serologic testing for FeLV and feline immunodeficiency virus (FIV) infection; thoracic and abdominal radiography, in 2 views; a bone marrow aspirate; and a tissue biopsy specimen for histopathologic examination.[3] Cytologic diagnoses are acceptable when obtained from pleural or abdominal effusions, or aspirates of the bone marrow, kidney, or liver. However, caution must be exercised when interpreting lymph node or splenic aspirates in cats. Cytologic differentiation of lymphoma from severe lymphoid hyperplasia may be very difficult or even impossible in some cases. Severe, nonmalignant peripheral lymphadenopathy has been reported in young cats secondary to viral infection (see Chapter 56, Splenomegaly and Lymphadenopathy). This condition can be differentiated from lymphoma only by careful examination of clinical findings and histopathologic lymph node biopsy specimens.[9, 10]

Clinical staging should be performed in all cats with lymphoma, according to results of baseline testing (Table 64-1).[3] Clinical staging enables the clinician to assess the extent of disease objectively, and is important because clinical stage affects both prognosis and likelihood of treatment-related toxicity. This information is very important to owners trying to decide whether to pursue therapy, especially in an elderly cat that may have concurrent disease. Cats with signs of illness associated with lymphoma (substage b)[7, 8] or advanced-stage disease (stages III, IV, and V) have been shown in some studies to have a poorer prognosis than cats with early-stage disease (stages I and II).[4] In the authors'

Table 64–1. Clinical Staging System for Feline Lymphoma

Stage I	Single tumor (nodal or extranodal)
Stage II	Single extranodal tumor with lymph node involvement; 2 or more nodal or extranodal tumors on the same side of the diaphragm; resectable primary gastrointestinal tumors
Stage III	Two or more nodal or extranodal tumors on opposite sides of the diaphragm; paraspinal or epidural tumors; primary nonresectable abdominal tumors
Stage IV	Stages I through III with initial liver or spleen involvement or both
Stage V	Stages I through IV with initial central nervous system or bone marrow involvement or both
Substage a	No systemic signs of illness
Substage b	Signs of systemic illness

Adapted from Mooney SC, Hayes AA. Lymphoma in the cat: An approach to diagnosis and management. Semin Vet Med Surg (Small Anim) 1:51–57, 1986.

experience, cats with advanced disease also are more likely to experience serious treatment-related side-effects such as myelosuppression.

Additional diagnostic testing may be indicated in many animals, particularly older ones. Hyperthyroidism is a very common disease in older cats, and a serum thyroxine concentration probably should be considered part of the minimum database in all cats older than 8 or 9 years. Coagulation profiles, necessary in cats with overt evidence of hemorrhage, also may be indicated in asymptomatic cats that are scheduled to undergo invasive diagnostic procedures, such as ultrasound-guided needle biopsy and exploratory laparotomy. Anemia, a common finding among cats with lymphoma, should be analyzed for etiology. Careful analysis of red-cell indices, together with reticulocyte counts and the results of bone marrow aspiration cytology, will allow differentiation of anemia due to blood loss, chronic disease, bone marrow infiltration by lymphoma, and paraneoplastic immune-mediated hemolysis. Evaluation of blood smears for the presence of *Haemobartonella felis* as well as a direct Coombs' test will be indicated in some patients. Anemia often is present in cats with abnormal renal function. Concurrent renal dysfunction is common in older cats with lymphoma, and lymphoma itself rarely is the primary cause. Urine of all cats with active urine sediments or renal azotemia should be cultured to rule out bacterial urinary tract infection.

The use of ultrasonography may enable the clinician to better define the extent of neoplastic disease in the thorax or abdomen and to investigate the presence of concurrent diseases. Evaluation of cardiac function is possible with thoracic ultrasonography, including a baseline analysis that can be useful for later comparisons in patients. The use of abdominal ultrasonography allows for the assessment of size, shape, position, echogenicity, and architecture of organs including the liver, spleen, kidneys, pan-

creas, and adrenal glands. Abdominal ultrasonography is helpful in differentiating the more common conditions of chronic renal failure and pyelonephritis from lymphoma, which is relatively rare.[7, 8] Sonographic evaluation of the intestinal tract may be limited by the presence of gas, but imaging in these areas often is aided by the presence of liquid contents in the stomach and proximal small intestine.[11] Masses always should be measured carefully to facilitate later ultrasonographic comparisons and assessment of response to treatment. Ultrasound also may be used to guide fine-needle aspirates or Tru-Cut biopsies of organs or mass effects. Liver aspirates are particularly useful, because alterations in size, shape, and echogenicity are typical of common feline liver diseases such as lipidosis and cholangiohepatitis, which must be differentiated from lymphoma to provide appropriate treatment (see Chapter 15, Cytologic Evaluation of Fine-Needle Liver Biopsies). Ultrasound-guided aspiration cytologies of mesenteric lymph node or spleen must be interpreted with care, as described previously.

All necessary diagnostics should be performed to define the etiology and extent of any significant abnormality detected during baseline testing. It is not appropriate to assume that all abnormalities are the direct result of organ infiltration by lymphoma, and incomplete evaluation of concurrent or paraneoplastic disease will result in less than optimum treatment.

◆ GENERAL RECOMMENDATIONS FOR MANAGEMENT OF COMPLICATIONS DURING THERAPY

Continued close monitoring is essential in all cats receiving chemotherapy for the treatment of lymphoma. A thorough physical examination, weight documentation, and complete blood count should be repeated at each chemotherapy visit. Routine biochemical profiles should be performed every 3 to 4 months. These diagnostic tests permit accurate assessment of the patient's response to chemotherapy, as well as document complications and the development of unrelated concurrent diseases. The earlier potential problems are identified, the more successful intervention is likely to be.

Lymphoma is a rapidly progressive malignant disease, with a currently reported median survival of 7 to 9 months in cats receiving aggressive therapy.[7, 8] Every effort should be made to administer all treatments on time and according to protocol: postponement of scheduled therapy can compromise disease control and make relapse more likely. Fortunately, such delay rarely is necessary. Treatment is well tolerated by the majority of cats, and quality of life improves and remains excellent in most cases. Leukopenia secondary to chemotherapy-induced myelosuppression occurs infrequently.

Gastrointestinal side-effects usually are mild and self-limiting, and cats respond quickly to simple supportive measures.[3, 4, 7]

When continued clinical signs or significant complications occur, complete re-evaluation of the patient is strongly recommended. Chemotherapy may need to be deferred during this process. The assumption that all clinical signs are due to lymphoma must be avoided, or concurrent diseases might be overlooked. Specific diagnostic testing varies in each cat (see discussion of specific disease states later), but almost without exception will include complete blood count, serum biochemical profile, and urinalysis. Imaging studies are necessary in many cases. In most patients, identification of optimum therapy requires an accurate diagnosis of concurrent or complicating disease processes as well as an objective assessment of the response of the patient's lymphoma to treatment. Specific consideration must be given to the potential immunosuppression caused by cytotoxic therapy. Although many conditions can be managed successfully in cats that are receiving concurrent chemotherapy for lymphoma, pursuit of aggressive treatment is difficult to recommend in cats with preexisting, poorly responsive malignant disease.

The potential adverse effects of chemotherapy must be considered as a cause of illness; however, the clinician should not assume that illness is related to treatment. Often patient behavior, including appetite and interaction, treatment schedule, client observation, and weight documentation are useful indications of specific problems. Alterations in protocol are beneficial for some cats that develop serious side-effects or complicating diseases. Drugs that cause consistent problems may be deleted. Significant or progressive organ dysfunction also may require alteration of protocol owing to the pharmacokinetics and unique toxicities of specific drugs. Doxorubicin is potentially cardiotoxic, and should be avoided in cats with significant cardiac disease. Decreased dosage of drugs with significant renal excretion should be considered when renal function is compromised (see Chronic Renal Failure, later). Likewise, the dosage of drugs whose half-life depends on hepatobiliary excretion might need to be decreased if liver function is not normal. The dosage of vincristine is routinely decreased by 50 per cent in human patients with serum total bilirubin concentrations in excess of 3.0 mg/dl.[12] Some authors also recommend dosage reduction for doxorubicin when hepatic compromise is present, but this is not always necessary: the primary factor limiting the rate of doxorubicin clearance is its very slow release from tissue-binding sites, and liver dysfunction must be extremely severe to affect drug elimination.[13] Drugs requiring hepatic activation, such as cyclophosphamide and chlorambucil, are reported to be less effective in patients with significant liver disease.[12]

◆ IMPORTANT CONCURRENT DISEASES

Infectious Diseases

Retroviral Infections

FeLV is a horizontally transmitted retrovirus that causes hematopoietic malignancy in cats by insertion of nuclear material into the host genome. At one time, virtually all feline lymphoid malignancies were believed to be the result of FeLV infection.[14] However, it is important to recognize that immunosuppression and myelosuppressive syndromes such as nonregenerative anemia together account for approximately 80 per cent of all FeLV-related deaths.[14–16] Immunosuppression in FeLV-infected cats is caused by suppression of both cell-mediated and humoral immunity, and affected animals are predisposed to a wide variety of bacterial, viral, fungal, rickettsial, and protozoal infections. Anemia is the most common manifestation of FeLV-related myelosuppression, and occurs owing to viral interference with erythropoiesis and erythroid differentiation at the level of the bone marrow.[16] Severe, nonregenerative, normochromic, normocytic to macrocytic anemia is the typical result. Macrocytosis often is dramatic, but is not associated with reticulocytosis or other evidence of regeneration.

Although concurrent detectable infection with FeLV is much less common among pet cats with lymphoma today than it was in the mid-1970s,[2, 6–8] determination of FeLV status remains one of the most important tests in the assessment of the feline patient with lymphoma. Enzyme-linked immunosorbent assay (ELISA) or immunofluorescent antibody (IFA) test techniques that detect the FeLV core viral antigen p27 are widely available,[14, 16] and results are very reliable when interpreted carefully.[17] Several studies have shown that immediate response to chemotherapy is not affected by FeLV status in cats with lymphoma, and FeLV-test–positive cats are just as likely to attain remission as FeLV-test–negative cats.[4, 7, 18] However, FeLV status has a significant effect on long-term prognosis.[4, 8] Remission durations and survival times are significantly shorter in FeLV-test–positive cats, with an expected median survival time approximately half that of FeLV-test–negative cats.[4] In addition, FeLV-infected cats with lymphoma are still susceptible to virally induced immunosuppression with secondary infection and the development of cytopenias, and these potential complications affect prognosis as well.

The owners of FeLV-test–positive cats should not be discouraged from treating their pets for lymphoma. The initial response to treatment is likely to be good, and individual animals may enjoy extended remission and survival times. The authors recommend the same doxorubicin-containing combination chemotherapy protocol for the treatment of FeLV-test–positive and FeLV-test–negative cats with lymphoma. However, the overall prognosis for the FeLV-test–positive cat with lymphoma is guarded. Owners should be advised to keep FeLV-infected cats indoors, and to avoid the introduction of new animals. These precautions decrease the chances of exposure to infectious agents, which may pose a significant risk in infected cats owing to the combined immunosuppressive effects of cancer therapy and FeLV. Cats with concurrent FeLV infections should be monitored closely for signs of illness, and when present, these should be pursued aggressively with further diagnostics. Appropriate specific therapy should be instituted immediately when concurrent infectious diseases are diagnosed.[19] Anemias should be investigated to determine etiology and optimum treatment. Owners also should be prepared for the likelihood that an increased level of supportive care will be necessary in the FeLV-test–positive cat: intermittent administration of subcutaneous crystalloids, antibiotics, and nursing measures such as hand-feeding or even tube-feeding might be necessary to maintain good quality of life in infected cats. Transfusion support, subcutaneous human recombinant erythropoietin with oral iron and vitamin B supplementation, as well as treatment with oral human recombinant interferon alpha,[20] also may provide benefit in some cats.

The first report describing FIV was published in 1987.[21] FIV is a lentivirus that is closely related to the human immunodeficiency virus. It is transmitted between cats largely through bite wounds. Male cats are predisposed to infection.[22] FIV causes chronic, progressive immunosuppression owing to selective destruction of CD4+ lymphocytes, and infected cats develop a wide spectrum of opportunistic and secondary infectious processes.[23] Fever, weight loss, dermatitis, stomatitis and gingivitis, upper respiratory tract infections, neurologic disease, and enteritis with chronic diarrhea are reported commonly. The course of disease often is protracted, lasting years in many cats.[23, 24]

Several studies suggest that cats infected with FIV are at increased risk for the development of lymphoma, presumably secondary to chronic immunosuppression.[25–28] As with FeLV, serologic testing for FIV is part of the staging process in any cat with lymphoma. An initial diagnosis of FIV infection is made through ELISA detection of FIV-specific antibodies. Confirmation of the presence of FIV-specific antibodies by Western blot usually is recommended, owing to the potential for false-positive ELISA results in some cats.[23] Baseline diagnostic testing in FIV-test–positive cats with lymphoma also may reveal additional nonspecific abnormalities such as anemia, neutropenia or neutrophilia, thrombocytopenia, azotemia, or hyperglobulinemia. Monoclonal gammopathy has been reported in an FIV-test–positive cat with concurrent lymphoma.[29]

The effects of FIV infection on prognosis among cats with concurrent lymphoma are not well established. A negative effect might be expected as a result of augmented immunosuppression and the varied complications of FIV infection, but this has yet to be demonstrated convincingly. No difference in remission duration or survival time was found between FIV-test–positive and FIV-test–negative cats in 1 study, but the number of FIV-test–positive cats included in the study population was very small.[7] Antiviral agents such as azidothymidine (AZT) and phosphonylmethoxyethyladenine (PMEA) may ameliorate some of the immunologic changes and clinical signs associated with FIV infection,[30–33] but have no effect on FIV-associated malignancy. These agents also are expensive, and may cause significant hematologic complications in some cats. At the present time, the most practical approach for FIV-test–positive cats with lymphoma appears to be very similar to that described previously for FeLV-test–positive cats: optimum therapy for lymphoma, thorough and consistent monitoring for evidence of FIV-related complicating disease, and immediate institution of appropriate supportive measures.

Upper Respiratory Tract Infections

Viral infection is one of the most common causes of primary upper respiratory tract disease in cats. The 2 viruses most often implicated are the feline herpesvirus-1, and the feline calicivirus. The feline strain of the obligate intracellular bacterium *Chlamydia psittaci,* as well as a small number of other etiologic agents, is believed to be the cause of a minority of feline upper respiratory tract infections. Vaccination programs against the feline herpesvirus-1 and feline calicivirus have significantly reduced the incidence of viral respiratory disease in cats, although outbreaks still are common in catteries, shelters, and hospitals.[34]

Development of upper respiratory tract infections is not uncommon among cats receiving chemotherapy for lymphoma. Vaccination against feline calicivirus is made difficult by the existence of multiple strains of virus, and vaccines cannot provide equivalent protection against all strains.[34] Other factors that may predispose these cats to viral upper respiratory tract infections include the immunosuppression caused by anticancer drugs and corticosteroids; infection with FIV, which is known to increase the severity of clinical signs in cats exposed to feline herpesvirus-1 or calicivirus[35, 36]; and the existence of long-term carrier states for both respiratory viruses. Glucocorticoid treatment has been shown to increase viral shedding and induce recrudescence of severe clinical signs in cats that are long-term carriers of feline herpesvirus-1.[34] Chemotherapeutic agents could be expected to have a similar effect.

A clinical diagnosis of feline viral upper respiratory tract infection is made routinely on the basis of characteristic clinical signs. Virus isolation techniques may provide a definitive diagnosis but are impractical in most clinical situations, and treatment will be unchanged regardless of the specific etiologic agent involved. Typical clinical signs of feline herpesvirus-1 infection initially include pyrexia, lethargy, anorexia, and sneezing, progressing to serous and finally mucopurulent oculonasal discharge. Conjunctivitis usually accompanies the nasal signs and may be severe, with pronounced scleral injection and chemosis. Corneal ulceration and keratitis may occur, and are more likely to be present in immunosuppressed animals (see Chapter 7, Update on the Diagnosis and Management of Feline Herpesvirus-1 Infections). Feline calicivirus infection also causes fever and lethargy early in its course, and may progress to sneezing and oculonasal discharge. However, severe oral ulcerations are much more common with feline calicivirus than with feline herpesvirus-1 infection, and may be the only clinical sign of infection. Feline calicivirus also may result in polyarthropathy and lameness.[34]

Effective antiviral medications for the treatment of cats with viral upper respiratory tract infections are not widely available. Cats that are undergoing concurrent chemotherapy may suffer much more pronounced clinical signs than immunocompetent animals, and successful recovery often will depend on conscientious supportive care. Cats that are less severely affected may be managed at home, but the sickest cats require hospitalization. Chemotherapeutics and glucocorticoids should be discontinued when clinical signs of upper respiratory tract infection are first detected, although physiologic doses of glucocorticoids may be considered in cats that have received long-term therapy. Basic supportive care consists of oral antibiotics, preferably in liquid form, to address secondary bacterial infection; gentle cleaning of accumulated discharge from the eyes and nose at least 3 to 4 times daily with a soft material moistened with warm water; an antibiotic ophthalmic ointment instilled in the eyes after cleaning; and a 0.025 per cent solution (pediatric strength) of oxymetazoline nasal drops to decrease nasal congestion in some animals. Probably most important, appetite should be monitored carefully, and every effort made to maintain voluntary intake, including hand-feeding of highly palatable, aromatic foods. Intermittent trips to the hospital for outpatient administration of subcutaneous crystalloids are necessary in cats that do not maintain adequate food and water intake.

Hospitalization should be encouraged in more severely affected cats and in cats that do not respond to home care. More aggressive monitoring and supportive care can be instituted in the hospital setting, in addition to the measures described previously. Intravenous administration of crystalloids is indicated in dehydrated or persistently febrile animals. Once an intravenous catheter is in place, it also may be used to administer antibiotics, avoiding uncomfortable manipulation of the face and mouth. Judicious use of acetylsalicylic acid (*never* acetaminophen) at a dosage of 15 mg/kg every (q) 72 hours orally (PO) may be helpful in controlling pyrexia. Nebulization may assist in clearing respiratory secretions. Finally, feeding tubes should be placed immediately in those cats unable to maintain an adequate food intake. (Attempts at pharmacologic appetite stimulation frequently are unsuccessful, and often delay appropriate tube placement.) In the authors' experience, nasopharyngeal tubes are very poorly tolerated in cats with upper respiratory tract signs. Pharyngostomy tubes are a better choice, and can be placed in heavily sedated cats by an experienced clinician. Esophagostomy or percutaneous endoscopic gastrostomy tubes also may be considered, but require general anesthesia for placement. Complete and balanced, nutrient-dense, paste-type commercial formulations are the optimum rations for use with pharyngostomy, esophagostomy, and percutaneous endoscopic gastrostomy tubes.

Full recovery of a severely affected cat may take several weeks, and resumption of chemotherapy and glucocorticoids should be delayed, if possible. However, evidence of progressive lymphoma may necessitate earlier treatment in some cats. Owners should be informed that repeated episodes of upper respiratory tract signs might occur over the course of chemotherapy, owing to chronic immunosuppression of carrier animals. Chronic bacterial rhinitis and sinusitis also are potential sequelae of severe viral upper respiratory tract infections in some cats, and may be frustrating to manage in immunosuppressed patients. Discontinuation of chemotherapy usually is not possible owing to the long-term nature of the condition. More detailed diagnostic testing, including thoracic and skull radiography, computerized tomography or magnetic resonance imaging, and a nasal flush or biopsy with cultures, cytology, and histopathology may be indicated to confirm the diagnosis and to eliminate the possibility of underlying fungal disease or neoplasia. Long-term antibiotic therapy may be necessary to control clinical signs, but generally does not resolve them completely. Waxing and waning anorexia, sneezing, and mucopurulent nasal discharge may significantly affect quality of life in affected cats.

The role of vaccination is unknown in the treatment and prevention of active viral upper respiratory disease in cats receiving concurrent chemotherapy. Injectable or intranasal modified-live vaccines, as well as injectable inactivated vaccines, are available and appear to provide equivalent protection against disease in normal animals, although they do not prevent infection or establishment of the carrier state.[34] However, the ability of a cat receiving concurrent chemotherapy to mount an effective immune response to any vaccine must be questioned. Furthermore, in healthy animals, modified-live vaccines may induce clinical signs of disease that easily could be intensified in an immunosuppressed patient. Finally, killed, adjuvanted multivalent vaccines against feline panleukopenia and upper respiratory tract viruses have been implicated in the induction of vaccine site–associated sarcomas.[37] At the present time, all these factors make it difficult to recommend routine vaccination for upper respiratory tract viruses in cats with lymphoma receiving concurrent chemotherapy.

Salmonellosis

The Salmonellae are motile, gram-negative bacteria belonging to the family Enterobacteriaceae. They are ubiquitous within the environment, and capable of causing disease in numerous species including reptiles, birds, mammals, and human beings. Salmonellosis usually is acquired through ingestion of food or water contaminated with infective fecal material, but contaminated objects within the hospital environment also may transmit the organism. Salmonellae are capable of long-term survival outside an animal host.[38] The serovar isolated most commonly in cases of feline salmonellosis is *Salmonella typhimurium*,[38] although *S. newport*[39] and *S. arizonae*[40] as well as other serovars have been reported.

Most *Salmonella* infections are enteric, but systemic disease with involvement of multiple organs occurs in some individuals. Based on published studies that suggest a lower prevalence of positive cultures compared with other species,[38] cats are believed to be more resistant to infection by *Salmonella* species. Regardless, certain host characteristics may predispose an animal to more severe gastrointestinal or widespread systemic infection, and several of these are relevant to cats receiving chemotherapy for the treatment of lymphoma. Compromise of the host immune response by underlying malignancy, glucocorticoid therapy, or chemotherapy has been implicated in the development of salmonellosis in dogs and cats. Clinical or fatal *Salmonella* infections have been reported in cats with underlying lymphoma[41] or retroviral infections,[39] and in both cats and dogs receiving chemotherapy for the treatment of lymphoma.[7, 41, 42] Antibiotic therapy also reduces host resistance to infection,[38] and may increase the likelihood for development of an asymptomatic carrier state.[43]

The morbidity and mortality associated with symptomatic feline salmonellosis are high,[7, 39, 41, 44] although the specific clinical signs are variable. Gastroenteritis is the most common presenting sign, with affected animals usually exhibiting signs of illness within 3 to 5 days of exposure to the organism.[38, 44] Lethargy, anorexia, and pyrexia are detected initially, followed by abdominal discomfort, vomiting, and diarrhea. Fecal material usually is malodorous and watery in consistency, with mucus and fresh blood in some cases.[38, 39, 44] Severe dehydration, weight loss, jaundice, and shock are observed terminally. Central nervous system and respiratory signs occasionally are present.[38]

A systemic syndrome more similar to so-called enteric fever in human beings also has been reported in cats,[39] and may be more likely to occur in immunosuppressed patients, such as those receiving chemotherapy.[38] *Salmonella* bacteremia appears to result in a more nonspecific clinical presentation in these animals, characterized by chronic fever, lethargy, and vague signs of illness. Gastrointestinal signs may not be present. Clinical signs compatible with cardiovascular collapse such as pallor, tachycardia, weakness, and hypothermia eventually develop as the disease progresses. Disseminated intravascular coagulation with thrombosis and multiorgan failure are reported terminally.[38, 39]

Results of clinical pathology testing in cats with salmonellosis vary depending on the severity and form of the disease. Classically, neutropenia with a left shift is present.[38] However, mature neutrophilia has been documented in some cats, particularly those with chronic infections.[38, 39, 41] Nonregenerative anemia, secondary to either blood loss (microcytic hypochromic) or chronic disease (normocytic normochromic), also may be observed.[38] Thrombocytopenia, accompanied by prolonged clotting times, has been detected in severely affected cats with disseminated intravascular coagulation.[38, 39] Biochemical abnormalities such as hypoproteinemia, azotemia, hyperbilirubinemia, increased serum liver enzyme activities, hypoglycemia, and hypokalemia also are most likely to be present in cats with overwhelming infection.[38, 39, 41]

The challenge for the veterinarian is to separate clinical signs caused by side-effects of chemotherapy or progressive lymphoma from those potentially caused by superimposed salmonellosis. Failure to accomplish this task is highly likely to result in the death of the patient. Clinical history should be evaluated first, and owners should be questioned carefully to determine the type, duration, and severity of clinical signs. It often is helpful to compare these findings with the previous course of an individual cat's response to chemotherapy. For instance, a cat with acute onset of vomiting and diarrhea within 48 hours of the administration of a chemotherapy drug that previously has caused similar gastrointestinal signs in that patient is less likely to have salmonellosis. Conversely, the chances of *Salmonella* infection are higher in a cat with the same clinical signs that has been in long-term remission and never has experienced any side-effects after chemotherapy.

A thorough physical examination is important in distinguishing the effects of lymphoma or chemotherapy and salmonellosis. Nonspecific findings such as dehydration, weight loss, and pallor are common to all 3 situations. However, the presence of fever and abdominal pain associated with acute onset of gastrointestinal signs should prompt the clinician to consider the possibility of *Salmonella* infection. On the other hand, vomiting and diarrhea with recurrence of palpable abdominal masses, especially when fever is absent, are signs more suggestive of progressive lymphoma.

Additional diagnostics are necessary to differentiate chemotherapy toxicity, progressive lymphoma, and salmonellosis definitively. Samples should be collected in all cases for complete blood count, serum biochemical profile, and urinalysis, and test results evaluated for the presence of abnormalities consistent with *Salmonella* infection. Abdominal radiography and ultrasonography are helpful in differentiating infiltrative disease (lymphoma) from *Salmonella* infection and chemotherapy toxicity in many patients, although results must be interpreted with care when cats are early in the course of treatment and not yet in complete remission. Repeat retroviral screening, coagulation profile analysis, and thoracic radiography may be considered in some animals, depending on clinical signs and the results of baseline testing. Ultimately, however, a positive culture is the strongest supporting evidence for salmonellosis. Detection of *Salmonella* organisms from sites that normally are sterile, such as blood, urine, or cerebrospinal fluid, is highly suggestive of *Salmonella* bacteremia.[38] Positive fecal cultures are more difficult to interpret because of the existence of the asymptomatic carrier state,[39] but can be dependable when they are obtained from a patient with concurrent clinical signs compatible with salmonellosis. However, negative cultures from any site do not preclude the possibility of *Salmonella* infection, as the organism often is difficult to grow. Most commercial laboratories utilize enrichment broths and specialized plating techniques to improve yield.[38]

Unfortunately, the prognosis usually is poor for cats undergoing chemotherapy for lymphoma that are diagnosed with concurrent *Salmonella* infections.[7, 41, 42] Therapy must be timely and aggressive. All immunosuppressive therapy should be discontinued initially, including both glucocorticoids and chemotherapeutics (although cats that have received long-term glucocorticoid treatment may require physiologic replacement therapy). Parenteral administration of intravenous crystalloids is the mainstay of treatment, and must replace gastrointestinal losses and prevent further volume depletion. Blood products for the treatment of anemia or coagulopathies may be required in some patients. Overall, the use of antibiotics for the treatment of salmonellosis is controversial owing to the risk of inducing a chronic carrier state.[43] However, antibiotics clearly are indicated in the management of *Salmonella* infections that occur in cats receiving chemotherapy for the treatment of lymphoma owing to host immunosuppression. Standard antibiotics such as trimethoprim-sulfa combinations or amoxicillin may be effective in animals with less severe disease, but parenterally administered high-dose quinolones currently appear to be the best choice for patients with overwhelming infection.[38] Infection should not be considered resolved nor cytotoxic therapy resumed until at least 3 negative *Salmonella* cultures have been obtained over a 2- to 3-week period.

Meticulous attention to environmental contamination in the home and hospital, and recognition of the zoonotic potential of this organism are critical components of the management of salmonellosis in cats. Animals suspected of having *Salmonella* infections should be isolated from other household pets, and maintained separately from the general hospital population. Cages, litter pans, food bowls, and utensils must be disinfected appropriately or autoclaved.[38] Owners of infected cats should be made aware of the potential symptoms associated with human salmonellosis, and urged to seek a physician's advice if illness develops.

Dermatophytosis

Feline dermatophytosis is caused most commonly by the keratinophilic fungus *Microsporum canis. Microsporum gypseum* and *Trichophyton mentagrophytes* are isolated in a minority of cases.[45] An adequate host immune response is necessary to terminate dermatophyte infections effectively, so it is not surprising that immunodeficient animals, such as those receiving chemotherapy, have been shown to be at risk for acquiring more frequent, severe, and prolonged infections.[48] Cats infected with FIV have an increased frequency of dermatophytosis,[47] and generalized, poorly responsive dermatophytosis caused by *M. canis* has been reported in a cat that received oral busulfan, total-body irradiation, and cyclosporine therapy to facilitate a bone marrow transplant for acute myeloid leukemia.[48] Glucocorticoids, included in many chemotherapy protocols for the treatment of feline lymphoma, also increase host susceptibility to dermatophytosis by decreasing the local inflammatory response.[46]

Definitive diagnosis of feline dermatophytosis by clinical signs alone is not possible in normal cats, and is even less likely in cats receiving chemotherapy for lymphoma. Feline dermatophytosis is characterized most commonly by patchy alopecia. Scale and hair-shaft breakage often are present as well. However, clinical presentation can be extremely variable: classic, circular patches of alopecia, crusted papules, pruritic dermatitis, and ulcerated dermal granulomas all are possible. Some cats are asymptomatic carriers.[48] Furthermore, chemotherapy may alter clinical signs by decreasing the local inflammatory response in cats with lymphoma. Thus, definitive diagnosis requires culture of the causative organism. Hair and scale from active lesions should be submitted in dermatophyte test medium. Procedures including examination of hair and scale mounted in potassium hydroxide, examination of the hair coat for fluorescence under a Wood's lamp, and tissue biopsy with histopathology are not as sensitive, although they may be useful in some cases.[46]

Topical and systemic therapy have both been recommended for the treatment of dermatophytosis in cats. Simultaneous use of both modalities appears to be the most logical approach in cats receiving concurrent chemotherapy. Insufficient objective data currently exist to recommend the use of commercial *Microsporum* vaccines. Lime sulfur dips, miconazole shampoos and creams, and ketoconazole shampoos are the most effective topical treatments,[46] removing infective spores from the hair shafts. Clipping of the hair at the periphery of localized lesions or shaving of the whole body in cats with generalized dermatophytosis often is recommended to facilitate topical therapy, but both are controversial. Although some studies show that clipping can worsen and spread existing lesions,[49] it also may reduce the amount of potentially infective material released into the infected cat's environment.[46]

Systemic treatment provides antifungal therapy at the hair-follicle level, and should be strongly considered in all cases of dermatophytosis in cats that are receiving concurrent chemotherapy. Infection in the immunocompromised host may be much more widespread than clinical lesions suggest, and recovery may be prolonged without systemic treatment. Griseofulvin (microsized preparation; 25 to 50 mg/ kg PO q 12 hr for 4 to 8 weeks) and itraconazole (capsules; 5 to 10 mg/kg PO for 3 to 4 weeks) are the antifungals of choice for feline dermatophytosis.[46] Both are expensive and have potentially serious side-effects, and neither should be prescribed without a definitive diagnosis of dermatophytosis through culture. Itraconazole probably is superior to griseofulvin: it has equal or even greater efficacy against *M. canis*,[50] and tends to be better tolerated in cats.[46] Potential side-effects include anorexia and hepatotoxicity, characterized by increased serum concentrations of hepatocellular leakage enzymes. Itraconazole also is an inhibitor of the cytochrome P450 3A system, and therefore, may increase the plasma concentration of the vinca alkaloids.[51]

In general, chemotherapy should be continued during systemic antifungal therapy for dermatophytosis in cats with lymphoma. Systemic antifungals should be administered until the isolated pathogen cannot be cultured from 3 separate hair samples collected 1 week apart,[45] and this may represent weeks to months of treatment in some cats. Progression of lymphoma could occur within this time frame, and remission may be difficult or impossible to re-establish. Close patient monitoring through serial physical examination, complete blood count, and serum biochemical profile is essential. Anticancer and antifungal therapy should be modified according to the results of these tests.

Chronic Renal Failure

Chronic renal failure is defined as primary renal failure that has persisted for an extended period, usually months to years. It is common in cats of all ages, although older cats are more likely to be affected. The underlying causes of chronic renal failure are extremely variable, and include numerous inherited, congenital, and acquired conditions. Renal damage is irreversible and progressive. Cats with chronic renal failure are asymptomatic early in the course of disease, but clinical signs develop with worsening azotemia.[52]

Concurrent chronic renal failure does not pre-clude treatment for lymphoma or necessarily affect prognosis for response. However, cats with both diseases must be evaluated thoroughly and monitored closely in order to diagnose causes of renal insufficiency that may respond to intervention, to predict potential complications, and to prepare for the additional supportive measures that may be required. History and physical examination findings should be scrutinized so that nonspecific abnormalities compatible with chronic renal failure or lymphoma may be identified and separated from findings specifically suggestive of one disease or the other: for example, polyuria and polydipsia, oral ulcerations with halitosis, small irregular kidneys, and retinopathy are findings most consistent with chronic renal failure, whereas palpable abdominal masses are seen more often in cats with lymphoma. Baseline staging tests, as well as blood work repeated during the course of treatment, should be examined for evidence of chronic renal failure and clues regarding its etiology. Abnormalities such as azotemia, hyperphosphatemia, anemia, acidosis, hypokalemia, and isosthenuria are common in many cats with renal failure, but findings such as severe proteinuria or an active urine sediment with bacteriuria suggest specific underlying pathology. Abdominal radiography and ultrasonography may provide further evidence of renal disease; for example, kidneys that are abnormal in size or contour, renal parenchymal mineralization, nephroliths, ureteroliths, or cystic calculi.

Concurrent bacterial urinary tract infection must be diagnosed and treated aggressively in cats receiving treatment for lymphoma. All cats that are azotemic or have active urine sediments on baseline or repeat laboratory evaluation should have urine bacterial cultures with antibiotic sensitivity testing performed. Failure to institute an effective antibiotic regimen in an immunosuppressed patient may result in irreversible renal damage. Chemotherapy should be postponed and glucocorticoids discontinued temporarily in patients with fulminant infection, but risk of progressive lymphoma may necessitate concurrent administration of antibiotics with chemotherapy in some animals. Urine cultures should be repeated periodically in cats with a history of infection, even after negative culture results suggest that the initial infection has been cleared; immunosuppression secondary to chemotherapy predisposes these animals to recurrent disease.

It also is essential to differentiate renal failure secondary to renal lymphoma from chronic renal failure due to other causes. Cats with renal lymphoma usually have dramatically enlarged kidneys with characteristic macronodular texture. Ultrasonographic examination is very helpful in distinguishing renal lymphoma from typical chronic renal failure, and characteristically reveals bilateral renomegaly with increased echogenicity when lymphoma is present. Renal architecture usually is maintained, although a subcapsular rim of hypoechoic material and multifocal hypoechoic masses with indistinct margination may be visualized in the renal cortex (B. Partington, Louisiana State University, Baton Rouge, personal communication, 1999). The degree of azotemia is highly variable, ranging from none to severe; it is neither diagnostic of neoplasia nor indicative of prognosis. Fluid diuresis should be initiated in cats with significant azotemia and continued until renal function has stabilized. Urine should be cultured, and coexisting urinary tract infections treated appropriately. Definitive diagnosis of renal lymphoma usually can be made by aspiration cytology.

Chemotherapy is the most appropriate treatment for cats with renal lymphoma. Although renal function test results may suggest the extent of renal impairment, a cat's response to treatment is a better indication of prognosis.[53] Some early reports of treatment in cats with renal lymphoma were discouraging,[54] but a later study reported some complete responses, especially among early stage, FeLV-test–negative cats.[53] Several large studies have since shown that anatomic form of disease does not affect prognosis.[4, 7, 8] Systemic illness associated with lymphoma (substage b) is more likely responsible for decreased duration of remission and survival in some cats with renal lymphoma.[7, 8]

Cats with lymphoma that have renal insufficiency of any etiology must be monitored closely throughout treatment. Blood pressure should be checked on a regular basis. Repeat serum biochemical profiles may be indicated weekly or biweekly in cats with worsening clinical signs, significant and progressive azotemia, or electrolyte abnormalities, and only quarterly in cats with mild, stable renal dysfunction. Dose reduction for chemotherapy drugs excreted by the renal route should be considered in cats with persistent azotemia, to avoid increased treatment-related toxicity caused by prolongation of drug half-life. Carboplatin and procarbazine have primarily renal excretion, and decreased doses of these agents should be considered in cats with even relatively mild azotemia.[12] The dose of drugs with partial renal excretion, for example, cyclophosphamide or methotrexate, also could be decreased once renal failure is more severe, but specific guidelines do not exist for cats. Dose modification is not necessary for drugs that are minimally excreted or not excreted through the kidney, including chlorambucil, nitrogen mustard, cytosine arabinoside, vincristine, and L-asparaginase.

Doxorubicin is one of the most effective cytotoxic agents ever developed, and studies have shown that inclusion of this drug in protocols for cats with lymphoma results in improved response to treatment, remission duration, and survival times.[7, 8] Early work suggested that a significant proportion of cats receiving doxorubicin developed serious nephrotoxicity,[55, 56] but very high total cumulative doses were administered in these studies. Many reports now document the use of this highly effective drug in cats with minimum or no evidence of significant renal toxicity.[7, 8, 57–61] The benefit of doxoru-

bicin outweighs the potential risk in the majority of cats with lymphoma, and the authors routinely recommend it for the treatment of lymphoma in cats with mild chronic renal failure, as well as renal lymphoma.

Various supportive measures assist in the amelioration of the clinical signs and complications associated with chronic renal failure in cats receiving concurrent chemotherapy for lymphoma, improving quality of life and, in some cases, extending survival time (see Chapter 44, Medical Management for Chronic Renal Failure).[62] The true role of dietary modifications such as protein or phosphorus restriction is controversial early in the course of renal failure. However, there is no doubt that therapeutic diets are beneficial once clinical signs of uremia develop, as long as an adequate food intake can be maintained, and depletion of lean body mass does not occur. Home administration of subcutaneous crystalloids is learned easily by most owners, and regular diuresis will improve quality of life significantly in symptomatic cats. Oral potassium supplementation is indicated in cats with hypokalemia, and may help to stabilize renal function. Gastrointestinal signs associated with uremic gastritis may resolve with the use of gastrointestinal protectorants or H_2 blockers. Cats with clinically significant anemia often respond to oral iron and vitamin B supplementation in addition to injections of human recombinant erythropoietin; however, cats treated with recombinant erythropoietin must be monitored for evidence of development of antierythropoietin antibodies. Finally, treatment for documented hypertension secondary to chronic renal failure should be considered. Renal function must be followed very closely in cats receiving these medications, because deterioration secondary to hypotension and decreased renal perfusion may occur in some animals.

Hyperthyroidism

Hyperthyroidism is the most commonly diagnosed endocrine disorder in cats. It occurs in middle-aged to older cats, with a median age at diagnosis of 13 years.[63] As the average age increases in cats with lymphoma,[7, 8] concurrent hyperthyroidism is encountered more frequently. The clinical signs and physical examination findings in hyperthyroid cats vary with the severity and duration of disease. The most frequent owner complaints are weight loss, vomiting, polyphagia, polyuria and polydipsia, and behavior changes (hyperactivity). Some owners may delay veterinary evaluation not only because their pets' clinical signs develop gradually but also because certain signs, such as increased appetite and hyperactivity, actually are misinterpreted as signs of good health in their elderly cats.

Physical examination most commonly reveals a palpable thyroid nodule, weight loss, and tachycardia with a heart murmur,[64] but additional laboratory testing is necessary for definitive diagnosis of hyperthyroidism. An increased total serum thyroxine concentration (T_4) is present in over 95 per cent of symptomatic hyperthyroid cats.[64] Total T_4 concentrations also should be assessed routinely in older cats that develop recurrent weight loss or new gastrointestinal signs during chemotherapy for lymphoma. Additional diagnostics should be considered when progressive lymphoma or chemotherapy side-effects have been ruled out, and hyperthyroidism seems likely but cannot be confirmed by total T_4 concentrations. Further testing may include serial serum total T_4 concentrations, determination of serum free T_4, the triiodothyronine suppression test, and the thyrotropin-releasing hormone stimulation test (see Chapter 18, Diagnosis of Occult Hyperthyroidism). Specific protocols for the performance of all of these tests have been previously published.[63, 65]

Hyperthyroid cats with clinical signs should be treated to avoid development of serious complications secondary to thyrotoxicosis. However, owners must be informed that food intake is likely to decrease with treatment, and that this is evidence of effective therapy. Appetite is one of the parameters monitored most closely by the owners of cats receiving chemotherapy for lymphoma, and owner compliance may be less than ideal if the goals of treatment for hyperthyroidism are not explained carefully beforehand. Medical treatment is the most appropriate therapy for the majority of hyperthyroid cats with lymphoma, and methimazole is the drug of choice. Methimazole is administered initially at a dose of 10 to 15 mg PO each day, and then decreased gradually to the lowest dose that will maintain serum T_4 concentrations in the low-normal range.[63] Cats should be monitored on a biweekly basis during the first 2 months of methimazole therapy for evidence of side-effects such as excoriation and pruritus, and hematologic abnormalities. Thereafter, serum T_4 concentrations should be rechecked quarterly in stable patients. The prognosis for hyperthyroidism alone is good, and if it can be managed medically, it is unlikely to affect either quality or duration of life in cats with lymphoma.

Treatment with surgery or radioactive iodine results in permanent resolution of feline hyperthyroidism, but these treatments require extended hospitalization, and in the short term, are more expensive than methimazole. The realistic long-term prognosis for a hyperthyroid cat with lymphoma must be assessed carefully and discussed frankly with the owner before choosing one of these alternative treatments. Currently reported median survival times for cats with lymphoma treated with aggressive doxorubicin-containing combination protocols are 7 to 9 months.[7, 8] Although surgery or radioactive iodine treatment is indicated occasionally in cats that are unable to tolerate methimazole or in "healthy" lymphoma patients in stable and extended remission, both are inappropriate choices for the majority of cats receiving concurrent treatment for lymphoma.

Diabetes Mellitus

Diabetes mellitus is another common endocrine disease that occurs in some cats with lymphoma. Most cats have type 2 diabetes, which is characterized early in its course by glucose intolerance and hyperinsulinemia. Post-insulin receptor defects are hypothesized to exist in peripheral and hepatic target cells, and result in concurrent peripheral insulin resistance as well as increased hepatic gluconeogenesis. Eventually, the ability of pancreatic beta cells to synthesize and secrete insulin is exhausted, and hypoinsulinemia ensues.[66, 67] Deposition of islet amyloid and production of its precursor peptide amylin seem to play central roles in the pathogenesis of feline type 2 diabetes, both peripherally and at the level of the pancreatic beta cells and ganglia.[66–68] Type 3 or secondary diabetes is more rare in cats. It results from destruction of pancreatic beta cells by an unrelated disease process, or from insulin resistance caused by conditions such as acromegaly, hyperadrenocorticism, hyperthyroidism, or chronic administration of glucocorticoids or progesterone.[66, 69–72] Most chemotherapy protocols for the treatment of lymphoma in cats incorporate glucocorticoids.[4, 7, 8, 18, 73] Consequently, the proportion of type 3 diabetics is likely to be much higher among cats being treated for lymphoma than among the general feline population. However, the insulin resistance caused by glucocorticoid therapy also complicates the management of preexisting type 2 diabetes.

The presence of clinically significant hyperglycemia and persistent glucosuria should be confirmed carefully in cats apparently developing diabetes while on chemotherapy. Several supporting blood glucose concentrations should be obtained. It also may be helpful to have owners use commercial urine dipsticks at home to document glucosuria. Insulin therapy should not be started unless clearly indicated: some cats receiving glucocorticoids have intermittent periods of mild hyperglycemia that resolve without treatment. Cats that are truly diabetic will have compatible clinical signs, particularly polyuria and polydipsia. Polyphagia with weight loss also may be observed. Baseline diagnostics should be repeated in cats with lymphoma that are suspected of developing diabetes. Detection of characteristic abnormalities including hyperglycemia, hyperbilirubinemia, increased serum liver enzyme activities, increased serum pancreatic enzyme activities, glucosuria, ketonuria, and active urine sediment will help to confirm a diagnosis of diabetes, and also guide optimum therapy. Abdominal radiography or ultrasonography is indicated in some animals to separate biochemical abnormalities secondary to diabetes from those potentially due to progressive lymphoma. Ultrasound-guided hepatic aspirates may be necessary to differentiate infiltrative hepatic disease from lipidosis, which may occur with diabetes (see Chapter 15, Cytologic Evaluation of Fine-Needle Liver Biopsies).

Glucocorticoids are extremely effective agents in the treatment of cats with lymphoma. Type 3 diabetes is an unusual complication among cats receiving treatment for lymphoma, as long as glucocorticoids are administered by mouth: in the authors' experience, substitution of injectable forms increases risk significantly. Concerted attempts should be made to control both preexisting and newly diagnosed diabetes with appropriate insulin therapy while continuing glucocorticoid treatment as prescribed by protocol. Acceptable glycemic control usually can be achieved in type 2 or type 3 diabetic cats if their diet is consistent, and if they are treated with an intermediate-acting insulin such as NPH or Lente, administered twice-daily. A cautious weight loss program usually will improve the response to insulin in very overweight cats; obesity is one of the most important predisposing factors for cats with diabetes.[74]

Significant insulin resistance occasionally is encountered in diabetic cats that receive concurrent chemotherapy for lymphoma. The response to insulin in these animals is unpredictable, and blood glucose concentrations may fluctuate widely. Detailed evaluation of the patient is strongly recommended so that specific etiology and thus optimum therapy may be determined precisely. Failure to identify underlying disease eventually may lead to life-threatening complications. A glucose curve consisting of serial blood glucose concentrations obtained over a period of 12 to 24 hours should be constructed to confirm the diagnosis. Owners should be questioned in detail regarding their insulin injection technique and feeding regimen. Consumption of large meals during periods when insulin activity is likely to be low may result in clinically significant hyperglycemia.[75] Owners should be encouraged to feed the same complete and balanced commercial ration consistently in 2 or more meals, scheduled so that predicted increases in blood glucose concentration will coincide with periods of greatest insulin activity. Free-choice feeding is a reasonable alternative for cats that consume very small amounts of food throughout the day.[69]

Patient history and physical examination should be reviewed and may provide important clues regarding the cause of insulin resistance such as obesity or the presence of a thyroid nodule. Additional diagnostics may be indicated to rule out conditions such as ketoacidosis, hyperthyroidism, and renal or hepatic insufficiency as the cause of insulin resistance, and to identify potential sources of infection. Several factors are known to predispose all diabetic patients to infection,[69] but diabetic cats receiving concurrent chemotherapy probably are at even greater risk owing to the accumulated immunosuppressive effects of cytotoxic therapy. Thus, any evidence for occult bacterial infection should be assessed carefully. Thoracic and abdominal radiography and ultrasonography may be helpful, sug-gesting further diagnostic testing such as transtracheal wash or hepatic aspiration cytology. Appropriate treatment then should be initiated based on the results of this diagnostic testing. Chronic immunosuppression secondary to antineoplastic therapy also may justify an empirical broad-spectrum antibiotic trial in some insulin-resistant cats with concurrent lymphoma, even if the existence of bacterial infection cannot be proved definitively. Addition of regular insulin to the intermediate-acting form already in use may be helpful in resolving severe hyperglycemia.[69]

Acromegaly and primary hyperadrenocorticism are 2 very rare causes of insulin-resistant diabetes in older cats. Acromegaly is suggested in cats with severe insulin-resistant diabetes and associated clinical signs including enlargement of internal organs (heart, liver, and kidneys), weight gain, and degenerative joint disease.[70] Cats with pituitary-dependent hyperadrenocorticism or cortisol-secreting adrenal tumors also may be insulin-resistant diabetics, and characteristic clinical signs in these animals usually include polyuria, polydipsia, pendulous abdomen, and thinning of the skin with alopecia.[71] Hyperadrenocorticism is an extremely uncommon disease in cats, but it still may be difficult for clinicians to distinguish between cats with true hyperadrenocortism and those with iatrogenic hyperadrenocorticism due to chronic administration of glucocorticoids. Abdominal ultrasonography, computed tomography, and magnetic resonance imaging of the pituitary fossa are helpful if adrenal or pituitary masses are visualized. Specialized tests such as adrenocorticotropic hormone (ACTH) stimulation, dexamethasone suppression, and plasma ACTH concentrations may be indicated, but are less reliable in cats with hyperadrenocorticism than in dogs,[71] and they are even more difficult to interpret in cats with nonadrenal disease that are receiving chronic glucocorticoid therapy. A diagnosis of true hyperadrenocorticism should be avoided in cats with lymphoma until their response to discontinuation of glucocorticoid therapy has been assessed. Replacement glucocorticoids may be required by some cats during this process.

Second Cancers

A relatively high proportion of cats achieve long-term survival after chemotherapy for lymphoma; 30 to 40 per cent live 1 year or longer.[7] Some cats survive long enough to develop second cancers. Second cancers are a well-described phenomenon among human cancer patients, and their occurrence may or may not be related to the patient's primary malignancy. Some second cancers develop by chance, but others are believed to be associated with continued exposure to environmental carcinogens, host risk factors such as genetic alterations or immunosuppression, or the carcinogenicity of antineoplastic treatment itself.[76] Cats with lymphoma most often are treated with chemotherapy alone, and several alkylating agents are known to cause acute nonlymphoid leukemias in human patients years after their initial therapy has been completed.[76] The alkylating agent cyclophosphamide also is capable of inducing transitional cell carcinoma of the bladder in dogs and human beings.[76, 77]

The decision to pursue treatment for a second cancer in a cat with lymphoma depends on a number of factors. Prognosis probably is the most important factor, and the clinician must carefully weigh the prognosis of the second cancer against that of the underlying lymphoma. Treatment efforts should be directed toward the neoplastic disease that is most likely to be life-limiting. Aggressive treatment of a second cancer that is unlikely to affect quality or duration of life will not benefit a cat with lymphoma.

The basic principles of tumor diagnosis and staging apply to second cancers, and the information obtained during this process is essential in determining the prognosis and most appropriate treatment. A thorough clinical re-evaluation also provides the opportunity to document the remission status of the patient's underlying lymphoma objectively. A histologic diagnosis based on tissue biopsy of the second cancer is necessary in most cases. Imaging studies should include radiography of the second tumor site, as well as likely sites of metastasis. Thoracic or abdominal ultrasonography adds valuable information in many patients, and is particularly useful in assessment of preexisting lymphoma.

Chemotherapy for lymphoma (including glucocorticoid treatment) should be discontinued temporarily if a surgical procedure is planned. The potential effects of chemotherapy on wound healing must be considered, including myelosuppression and chronic immunosuppression resulting in an increased risk of infection. Myelosuppression secondary to the chemotherapy drugs cyclophosphamide or doxorubicin peaks 7 to 10 days after administration,[78] and low white blood cell counts during this period may predispose the patient to infection of the surgical wound. Both of these drugs also may delay wound healing during the proliferative phase, which begins 3 to 5 days after injury and lasts approximately 2 weeks.[79] Ideally, surgery probably should not be attempted for 14 days after administration of either of these agents, and neither should be given until the proliferative phase of wound healing is complete, an additional 14 days. The commonly used chemotherapy drug vincristine has minimum myelosuppressive effect,[78] and has been suggested to have little impact on wound healing[79]; however, the authors still recommend a postoperative period of 14 days without chemotherapy of any kind to promote optimum wound healing. Antibiotic coverage during the perioperative period is indicated in all patients that have received chemotherapy previously.

The advisability of adjuvant treatment for second

cancers in cats with lymphoma varies from case to case. A short course of palliative radiation therapy (e.g., three 8- to 10-Gy fractions delivered on days 0, 7, and 21) could be administered to most patients without significantly increased risk of complications. Incorporation of definitive radiation therapy delivered over several weeks and with a prescription to a much higher total dose is more complex. Definitive radiation therapy carries a greater potential for complications when combined with concurrent chemotherapy, particularly in protocols that contain radiation sensitizers such as doxorubicin. Increased risk and toxicity also would be expected of intensified chemotherapy administered to address metastasis of a second cancer. The benefit of such treatments must be very clear to outweigh the possible side-effects and expense, especially in a patient with an already limited lifespan owing to preexisting lymphoma.

REFERENCES

1. Dorn CR, Taylor DON, Schneider R, et al: Survey of animal neoplasms in Alameda and Contra Costa Counties, California. II. Cancer morbidity in dogs and cats from Alameda County. J Natl Cancer Inst 40:307–318, 1968.
2. Hardy WD Jr: Hematopoietic tumors of cats. J Am Anim Hosp Assoc 17:921–941, 1981.
3. Mooney SC, Hayes AA: Lymphoma in the cat: An approach to diagnosis and management. Semin Vet Med Surg (Small Anim) 1:51–57, 1986.
4. Mooney SC, Hayes AA, MacEwen EG, et al: Treatment and prognostic factors in lymphoma in cats: 103 cases (1977–1981). J Am Vet Med Assoc 194:696–699, 1989.
5. Francis DP, Cotter SM, Hardy WD, et al: Comparison of virus-positive and virus-negative cases of feline leukemia and lymphoma. Cancer Res 39:3866–3870, 1979.
6. Cotter SM, Hardy WD, Essex M: Association of feline leukemia virus with lymphosarcoma and other disorders in the cat. J Am Vet Med Assoc 166:449–454, 1975.
7. Mauldin GE, Mooney SC, Meleo KA, et al: Chemotherapy in 132 cats with lymphoma (1988–1994). Veterinary Cancer Society, Proceedings of the 15th Annual Conference, Tucson, AZ, Oct. 21–24, 1995.
8. Vail DM, Moore AS, Ogilvie GK, et al: Feline lymphoma (145 cases): Proliferation indices, cluster of differentiation 3 immunoreactivity, and their association with prognosis in 90 cats. J Vet Intern Med 12:349–354, 1998.
9. Moore FM, Emerson WE, Cotter SM, et al: Distinctive peripheral lymph node hyperplasia of young cats. Vet Pathol 23:386–391, 1986.
10. Mooney SC, Patnaik AK, Hayes AA, et al: Generalized lymphadenopathy resembling lymphoma in cats: Six cases (1972–1976). J Am Vet Med Assoc 190:897–900, 1987.
11. Miles KG: Sonography of the liver, pancreas, and alimentary tract. In August JR (ed): Consultations in Feline Internal Medicine, vol. 3. Philadelphia, WB Saunders, 1997, pp. 79–90.
12. Haskell CM: Principles of cancer chemotherapy. In Haskell CM (ed): Cancer Treatment, 4th ed. Philadelphia, WB Saunders, 1995, pp. 31–57.
13. Doroshow JH: Anthracyclines and anthracenediones. In Chabner BA, Longo DL (eds): Cancer Chemotherapy and Biotherapy: Principles and Practice, 2nd ed. Philadelphia, Lippincott-Raven, 1996, pp. 409–434.
14. Hoover EA, Mullins JI: Feline leukemia virus infection and diseases. J Am Vet Med Assoc 199:1287–1297, 1991.
15. Reinacher M: Diseases associated with spontaneous feline leukemia virus (FeLV) infection in cats. Vet Immunol Immunopathol 21:85–95, 1989.

16. Cotter SM: Feline viral neoplasia. *In* Greene CE (ed): Infectious Diseases of the Dog and Cat, 2nd ed. Philadelphia, WB Saunders, 1998, pp. 71–84.

17. Jacobson RH: How well do serodiagnostic tests predict the infection or disease status of cats? J Am Vet Med Assoc 199:1343–1347, 1991.

18. Cotter SM: Treatment of lymphoma and leukemia with cyclophosphamide, vincristine, and prednisone: II. Treatment of cats. J Am Anim Hosp Assoc 19:166–172, 1983.

19. Bell FW: Recommendations for FeLV- and FIV-positive cats with cancer. *In* August JR (ed): Consultations in Feline Internal Medicine, vol. 3. Philadelphia, WB Saunders, 1997, pp. 572–578.

20. Weiss RC, Cummins JM, Richards AB: Low-dose orally administered alpha interferon treatment for feline leukemia virus infection. J Am Vet Med Assoc 199:1477–1481, 1991.

21. Pedersen NC, Ho E, Brown ML, et al: Isolation of a T lymphotropic virus from domestic cats with an immunodeficiency-like syndrome. Science 235:790–793, 1987.

22. Cohen ND, Carter CN, Thomas MA, et al: Epizootiologic association between feline immunodeficiency virus infection and feline leukemia virus seropositivity. J Am Vet Med Assoc 197:220–225, 1990.

23. Sellon RK: Feline immunodeficiency virus infection. *In* Greene CE (ed): Infectious Diseases of the Dog and Cat, 2nd ed. Philadelphia, WB Saunders, 1998, pp. 84–96.

24. Pedersen NC, Barlough JE: Clinical overview of feline immunodeficiency virus. J Am Vet Med Assoc 199:1298–1305, 1991.

25. Fleming EJ, McCaw DL, Smith JA, et al: Clinical, hematologic, and survival data from cats infected with feline immunodeficiency virus: 42 cases (1983–1988). J Am Vet Med Assoc 199:913–916, 1991.

26. Hutson CA, Rideout BA, Pedersen NC: Neoplasia associated with feline immunodeficiency virus infection in cats of Southern California. J Am Vet Med Assoc 199:1357–1362, 1991.

27. Callanan JJ, McCandish IAP, O'Neil B, et al: Lymphosarcoma in experimentally induced feline immunodeficiency virus experimental infection. Vet Rec 130:293–295, 1992.

28. Poli A, Abramo F, Baldinotti F, et al: Malignant lymphoma associated with experimentally induced feline immunodeficiency virus infection. J Comp Pathol 110:319–328, 1994.

29. Rosenberg MP, Hohenhaus AE, Matus RE: Monoclonal gammopathy and lymphoma in a cat infected with feline immunodeficiency virus. J Am Anim Hosp Assoc 27:335–337, 1991.

30. Egebrink HF, Hartmann K, Horzinek MC: Chemotherapy of feline immunodeficiency virus infection. J Am Vet Med Assoc 199:1485–1487, 1991.

31. Hartmann K, Donath A, Beer B, et al: Use of two virustatics (AZT, PMEA) in the treatment of FIV and FeLV seropositive cats with clinical symptoms. Vet Immunol Immunopathol 35:167–175, 1992.

32. Philpott MS, Ebner JP, Hoover EA: Evaluation of 9-(2-phosphonomethoxyethyl)adenine for feline immunodeficiency virus using a quantitative polymerase chain reaction. Vet Immunol Immunopathol 35:155–166, 1992.

33. Smyth NR, Bennett M, Gaskell RM, et al: Effect of 3′azido-2′-3′deoxythymidine (AZT) on experimental feline immunodeficiency virus infection in domestic cats. Res Vet Sci 57:220–224, 1994.

34. Gaskell R, Dawson S: Feline respiratory disease. *In* Greene CE (ed): Infectious Diseases of the Dog and Cat, 2nd ed. Philadelphia, WB Saunders, 1998, pp. 97–106.

35. Reubel GH, George JW, Barlough JE, et al: Interaction of acute feline herpesvirus-1 and chronic feline immunodeficiency virus infections in experimentally infected specific pathogen free cats. Vet Immunol Immunopathol 35:95–119, 1992.

36. Reubel GH, George JW, Higgins J, et al: Effect of chronic feline immunodeficiency virus infection on experimental feline calicivirus–induced disease. Vet Microbiol 39:335–351, 1994.

37. Lester S, Clemett T, Burt A: Vaccine site–associated sarcomas in cats: Clinical experience and a laboratory review (1982–1993). J Am Anim Hosp Assoc 32:91–95, 1996.

38. Greene CE: Salmonellosis. *In* Greene CE (ed): Infectious Diseases of the Dog and Cat, 2nd ed. Philadelphia, WB Saunders, 1998, pp. 235–240.

39. Dow SW, Jones RL, Henik RA, et al: Clinical features of salmonellosis in cats: Six cases (1981–1986). J Am Vet Med Assoc 194:1464–1466, 1989.

40. Krum SH, Stevens DR, Hirsh DC: *Salmonella arizonae* bacteremia in a cat. J Am Vet Med Assoc 170:42–44, 1977.

41. Hohenhaus AE, Rosenberg MP, Moroff SD: Concurrent lymphoma and salmonellosis in a cat. Can Vet J 31:38–40, 1990.

42. Calvert CA, Leifer CE: Salmonellosis in dogs with lymphosarcoma. J Am Vet Med Assoc 180:56–58, 1982.

43. Wall PG, Davis S, Threlfall EJ, et al: Chronic carriage of multidrug resistant *Salmonella typhimurium* in a cat. J Small Anim Pract 36:279–281, 1995.

44. Timoney JF, Neibert HC, Scott FW: Feline salmonellosis: A nosocomial outbreak and experimental studies. Cornell Vet 68:211–219, 1978.

45. Lewis DT, Foil CS, Hosgood G: Epidemiology and clinical features of dermatophytosis in dogs and cats at Louisiana State University: 1981–1990. Vet Dermatol 2:53–58, 1990.

46. Foil CS: Dermatophytosis. *In* Greene CE (ed): Infectious Diseases of the Dog and Cat, 2nd ed. Philadelphia, WB Saunders, 1998, pp. 362–370.

47. Mancianti F, Gianelli C, Bendinelli M, et al: Mycological findings in feline immunodeficiency virus–infected cats. J Med Vet Mycol 30:257–259, 1992.

48. Gasper PW, Rosen DK, Fulton R: Allogeneic marrow transplantation in a cat with acute myeloid leukemia. J Am Vet Med Assoc 208:1280–1284, 1996.

49. Moriello KA: Treatment of feline dermatophytosis: Revised recommendations. Feline Pract 24:32–36, 1996.

50. Moriello KA, DeBoer DJ: Efficacy of griseofulvin and itraconazole in the treatment of experimental dermatophytosis. J Am Vet Med Assoc 207:439–444, 1994.

51. Anonymous: Package insert, Sporanox.® Titusville, NJ, Janssen Pharmaceutica Inc., 1997.

52. Polzin DJ, Osborne CA, Bartges JW, et al: Chronic renal failure. *In* Ettinger SJ, Feldman EC (eds): Textbook of Veterinary Internal Medicine, 4th ed. Philadelphia, WB Saunders, 1995, pp. 1734–1760.

53. Mooney SC, Hayes AA, Matus RE, et al: Renal lymphoma in cats: 28 cases (1977–1984). J Am Vet Med Assoc 191:1473–1477, 1987.

54. Weller RE, Stann SE: Renal lymphosarcoma in the cat. J Am Anim Hosp Assoc 19:363–367, 1983.

55. Cotter SM, Kanki PJ, Simon M: Renal disease in five tumor-bearing cats treated with Adriamycin. J Am Anim Hosp Assoc 21:405–409, 1985.

56. O'Keefe DA, Sisson DD, Gelberg HB, et al: Systemic toxicity associated with doxorubicin administration in cats. J Vet Intern Med 7:309–317, 1993.

57. Madewell BR, Leighton RL, Theilen GH: Amputation and doxorubicin for treatment of canine and feline osteogenic sarcoma. Eur J Cancer 14:287–293, 1978.

58. Jeglum KA, deGuzman E, Young KM: Chemotherapy of advanced mammary adenocarcinoma in 14 cats. J Am Vet Med Assoc 187:157–160, 1985.

59. Mauldin GN, Matus RE, Patnaik AK, et al: Efficacy and toxicity of doxorubicin and cyclophosphamide used in the treatment of selected malignant tumors in 23 cats. J Vet Intern Med 2:60–65, 1988.

60. Hahn KA, Frazier DL, Cox SK, et al: Effect of infusion regime on doxorubicin pharmacokinetics in the cat. J Am Anim Hosp Assoc 33:427–433, 1997.

61. Zwahlen CH, Lucroy MD, Kraegel SA, et al: Results of chemotherapy for cats with alimentary malignant lymphoma: 21 cases (1993–1997). J Am Vet Med Assoc 213:1144–1149, 1998.

62. Polzin DJ, Osborne CA, James KM: Medical management of chronic renal failure in cats: Current guidelines. *In* August JR (ed): Consultations in Feline Internal Medicine, vol. 3. Philadelphia, WB Saunders, 1997, pp. 325–336.

63. Peterson ME: Hyperthyroid diseases. *In* Ettinger SJ, Feldman EC (eds): Textbook of Veterinary Internal Medicine, 4th ed. Philadelphia, WB Saunders, 1995, pp. 1466–1487.

64. Broussard JD, Peterson ME, Fox PR: Changes in clinical and laboratory findings in cats with hyperthyroidism from 1983 to 1993. J Am Vet Med Assoc 206:302–305, 1995.
65. Kemppainen RJ, Clark TP: CVT update: Sample collection and testing protocols in endocrinology. *In* Bonagura JD (ed): Kirk's Current Veterinary Therapy XII: Small Animal Practice. Philadelphia, WB Saunders, 1995, pp. 335–339.
66. Lutz TA, Rand JS: Pathogenesis of feline diabetes mellitus. Vet Clin North Am Small Anim Pract 25:527–552, 1995.
67. Lutz TA, Rand JS: A review of new developments in type 2 diabetes in human beings and cats. Br Vet J 149:527–536, 1993.
68. O'Brien TD, Johnson KH, Hayden DW: Pancreatic ganglioneuronal amyloid: Occurrence in diabetic cats with islet amyloidosis. Am J Pathol 119:430–435, 1985.
69. Peterson ME: Diagnostic and therapeutic approach to insulin resistance. *In* August JR (ed): Consultations in Feline Internal Medicine, vol. 3. Philadelphia, WB Saunders, 1997, pp. 132–141.
70. Peterson ME, Taylor RS, Greco DS, et al: Acromegaly in 14 cats. J Vet Intern Med 4:192–201, 1990.
71. Feldman EC, Nelson RW: Hyperadrenocorticism in cats. *In* Canine and Feline Endocrinology and Reproduction, 2nd ed. Philadelphia, WB Saunders, 1996, pp. 256–261.
72. Middleton DJ, Watson ADJ: Glucocorticoid intolerance in cats given short-term therapies of prednisolone and megestrol acetate. Am J Vet Res 46:2623–2625, 1985.
73. Matus RE: Chemotherapy of lymphoma and leukemia. *In* Kirk RW (ed): Current Veterinary Therapy X: Small Animal Practice. Philadelphia, WB Saunders, 1989, pp. 482–488.
74. Nelson RW, Himsel CA, Feldman EC, et al: Glucose tolerance and insulin response in normal-weight and obese cats. Am J Vet Res 51:1357–1362, 1990.
75. Ihle SL: Nutritional therapy for diabetes mellitus. Vet Clin North Am Small Anim Pract 25:585–597, 1995.
76. van Leeuwen FE: Second cancers. *In* DeVita VT, Hellman S, Rosenberg SA (eds): Cancer: Principles and Practice of Oncology, 5th ed. Philadelphia, Lippincott-Raven, 1997, pp. 2773–2796.
77. Weller RE, Wolf AM, Oyejide A: Transitional cell tumor of the bladder associated with cyclophosphamide therapy in the dog. J Am Anim Hosp Assoc 15:733–736, 1979.
78. Ogilvie GK: Chemotherapy. *In* Withrow SJ, MacEwen EG (eds): Small Animal Clinical Oncology, 2nd ed. Philadelphia, WB Saunders, 1996, pp. 70–86.
79. Laing EJ: Problems in wound healing associated with chemotherapy and radiation therapy. *In* Lindsay WA (ed): Problems in Veterinary Medicine, vol. 2. Philadelphia, JB Lippincott, 1990, pp. 433–441.

65

◆ Chemotherapeutic Challenges: Special Considerations and New Agents

Ruthanne Chun

Whereas a plethora of information exists regarding the treatment for dogs with a variety of neoplasms, traditionally there have been few data to guide the chemotherapeutic management of the feline oncology patient. In the past few years, a number of clinical trials evaluating a variety of chemotherapeutic agents for the treatment of feline malignancies have been completed and published. This chapter summarizes recent advances in the medical management of cats with cancer. Updates on the more familiar drugs as well as information on administration, toxicities, and indications for some of the newer chemotherapy agents are included.

◆ UPDATES ON COMMONLY USED DRUGS

Doxorubicin

Doxorubicin is an anthracycline antibiotic that has activity against a wide range of feline neoplasms including lymphoma, mammary gland tumors, and soft-tissue sarcomas.[1, 2] Doxorubicin is a severe vesicant; perivascular administration results in major tissue damage. Therefore, this drug always is given as an intravenous injection through a cleanly placed indwelling catheter. Doxorubicin is likely to cause anorexia in cats. Along with the general side-effects of myelosuppression and gastrointestinal upset, some of the early publications on the use of doxorubicin in cats reported the development of renal failure.[1–4] Nephrotoxicity was described originally by Cotter and coworkers in 1984.[3] Five cats with naturally occurring malignancies were treated with 30 to 40 mg/m² doxorubicin at 3-week intervals; total cumulative doses ranged from 130 to 320 mg/m². Renal failure was documented in all cats within 4 to 7 months. Four of these cats were necropsied; histologic kidney changes included cytomegaly of tubular epithelial cells and stromal fibrosis, changes that are typical of renal lesions in other species with anthracycline-induced nephrotoxicity.[3] Two subsequent publications on combination chemotherapy of doxorubicin and cyclophosphamide by Jeglum and colleagues[1] and Mauldin and associates[2] reported minimum nephrotoxicity in their patient populations. The dose of doxorubicin used was 30 and 25 mg/m², respectively, and cyclophosphamide was administered at 100 mg/m² and 50 mg/m² on days 3, 4, 5, and 6 after doxorubicin, respectively.

None of the 14 cats reported by Jeglum and colleagues,[1] and only 2 of the 17 cats reported by Mauldin and associates,[2] developed azotemia. A thorough study by O'Keefe and coworkers[4] reported the systemic toxicity associated with doxorubicin administered to 6 normal cats at 30 mg/m² to a cumulative dose of 300 mg/m². The cats were euthanized 3 weeks after the last dose, with 1 cat dying at a total cumulative dose of 225 mg/m². All 6 cats had renal lesions including thickening of the mesangial matrix and cytomegaly of tubular cells. Only 2 of these 6 cats had developed azotemia by the time of euthanasia. (See discussion of stealth liposome-encapsulated doxorubicin for further information on doxorubicin and nephrotoxicity in cats.)

Although the pathogenesis of the renal damage is unknown, it is believed to be a dose-dependent cumulative toxicity. Therefore, the currently recommended dose of doxorubicin for cats is 1 mg/kg intravenously (IV) every 3 weeks; a maximum cumulative dose remains to be determined. It is likely that the traditionally recommended dose of doxorubicin (20 to 25 mg/m²) holds no therapeutic advantage over the currently recommended dose of 1 mg/kg.[5] Most chemotherapy doses are calculated using body surface area (BSA) rather than body weight. Whereas BSA correlates with metabolic rate and glomerular filtration rate, smaller patients have a greater BSA:body weight ratio than larger patients. Therefore, dosing on a BSA basis results in a much higher milligram-per-kilogram dose in smaller patients and a greater potential for toxicity. A study by Hahn and colleagues[5] supports the use of a dose of 1 mg/kg rather than the 25 mg/m² dose traditionally recommended. Additionally, these investigators demonstrated that a slower infusion rate results in a greater area under the plasma-concentration-versus-time curve and a longer distribution phase, compared with a faster infusion rate. The recommended dosage for doxorubicin in cats is 1 mg/kg IV over 15 to 20 minutes every 3 weeks.

Vincristine

Vincristine is a plant alkaloid derived from the common ground-cover plant *Vinca rosea*. The most common indication for vincristine is as a component of combination chemotherapy for the treatment of lymphoma.[6–10] This drug also is a vesicant, causing tissue irritation and sloughing if perivascular administration occurs. Vincristine is given through a "clean" venipuncture technique as a rapid bolus. Although vincristine traditionally has been considered a relatively nontoxic chemotherapeutic agent, some reports suggest that neutropenia may occur after single-agent vincristine administration at conventional doses (0.5 to 0.75 mg/m² IV).[6, 8, 9] Whereas recommendations for use have not changed, it is prudent to monitor closely the complete blood counts in patients that are receiving vincristine chemotherapy. As with other myelosuppressive drugs, if the neutrophil count drops below 2500 cells/µl, additional chemotherapy should be delayed by 1 week. If the neutrophil count drops below 1000 cells/µl, broad-spectrum antibiotic therapy should be initiated.

Mitoxantrone

Mitoxantrone is a dihydroxyquinone derivative of anthracycline, similar in structure to doxorubicin.[11] Ogilvie and associates[11] completed a combined toxicity and efficacy study of this drug in cats. Based on their work, mitoxantrone has activity against a variety of carcinomas (17.6 per cent response) and sarcomas (37.5 per cent response), as well as lymphoma (11.8 per cent response). Mitoxantrone appears to be beneficial when combined with external-beam radiation therapy for the management of oral squamous cell carcinoma, with 8 out of 11 cats undergoing a complete remission when treated with this combination. Unfortunately, the remission duration was brief, with a median of 170 days. Overall, mitoxantrone is well-tolerated with potential side-effects being anorexia, lethargy, and gastrointestinal upset. The recommended dosage is 6.5 mg/m², diluted in 10 to 20 ml of 0.9 per cent NaCl solution, given over 5 to 10 minutes IV once every 3 weeks.

Because mitoxantrone has limited activity as a single agent, Henry and coworkers[12] undertook a study to determine the timing and severity of myelosuppression, as well as the incidence of concurrent toxicities with combined mitoxantrone and cyclophosphamide ("Cyclone") administration in normal cats. Three normal cats were used in this study. Mitoxantrone was administered as described previously, and cyclophosphamide (100 mg/m²) was given immediately afterward as a rapid intravenous bolus. This regimen was repeated every 21 days for a total of 3 cycles. The neutrophil nadir occurred between 2 and 10 days after each dose of chemotherapy. Interestingly, all 3 cats had elevated platelet counts 8 days after their last treatment. Other side-effects included inappetence, soft stool, and vomiting. No appreciable weight change was observed in the study cats. Although the therapeutic efficacy of this protocol remains to be determined, it appears to be well-tolerated by healthy cats. Investigations into the toxicity and efficacy in tumor-bearing cats are warranted.

Carboplatin

Carboplatin is a cisplatin analogue that is safe after intravenous and intralesional administration in cats.[13–17] Several phase I (toxicity) trials have attempted to determine the maximally tolerated dose in cats.[15–17] Hahn and colleagues[17] administered carboplatin to 9 healthy 6- to 7-month-old cats with the objective of determining the prevalence and severity of carboplatin-induced dose-limiting toxicoses in cats. Three cats each were treated with 1 dose of carboplatin at 150, 200, and 250 mg/m² IV, and complete blood counts were obtained every 3 to 4 days. The 250 mg/m² dose resulted in neutrophil and platelet nadirs on days 17 and 14, respectively, with values of 560 ± 303 cells/µl and 96,500 ± 11,815 cells/µl, respectively. None of the cats showed signs of illness throughout the duration of the study. Necropsies on the study cats 4 weeks after drug administration did not reveal any abnormalities to the lungs, kidneys, gastrointestinal tract, bone marrow, and other tissues.

Two separate groups, Kisseberth and associates[15] and Wood and coworkers,[16] undertook similar studies, administering progressively higher doses of carboplatin to cats with naturally occurring tumors. Kisseberth and associates[15] reported that the cats tolerated doses up to 240 mg/m² with no clinical signs of drug toxicity. The neutropenia nadir occurred at 21 days. Out of 55 cats treated, 10 had partial responses (Table 65–1). This study went on to identify a maximally tolerated dose of 260 mg/m² (DM Vail, personal communication, 1999).

Wood and coworkers[16] treated 54 cats with 105 doses of carboplatin. As in Kisseberth's group, the neutrophil nadir occurred at 21 days. Dose escalation in this study stopped at 210 mg/m². Eight patients (with a variety of adenocarcinomas, vaccine-associated fibrosarcoma, and squamous cell carcinoma) experienced a complete remission, 5 (vaccine-associated sarcoma, oral melanoma, cutaneous squamous cell carcinoma, and nasal osteosarcoma) obtained a partial remission. Because both of these were dose-escalation studies, the maximally tolerated dose was not given to all cats. Therefore, the true range of activity remains unknown.

The author routinely treats cats at 260 mg/m² IV once every 4 weeks. Whereas most cats do experi-

Table 65–1. Tumors That Showed Response to Carboplatin in a Phase I Clinical Trial

Tumor Type	Cats Treated (n)	Cats With PR (n)
Fibrosarcoma	16	6
Squamous cell carcinoma	6	2
Malignant fibrous histiocytoma	1	1
Lymphoma	1	1

Abbreviation: PR, partial remission, none of the cats underwent a complete remission.

ence myelosuppression at 3 to 4 weeks after therapy, patients rarely show clinically significant signs.

Another route by which to administer carboplatin is intratumoral. Theon and colleagues[14] described a technique whereby carboplatin is mixed with purified sesame oil and injected into the neoplasm. They evaluated this technique in cats with squamous cell carcinoma of the nasal planum, and found that therapy was well-tolerated by all cats, with 73 per cent of the cats experiencing a complete remission that was durable for greater than 12 months in over 50 per cent of the patients. Intralesional injections require general anesthesia, are technically demanding, and raise chemotherapy safety issues.

Idarubicin

Idarubicin is a synthetic anthracycline analogue that has the advantage of being effective after oral administration. Moore and associates[18] treated 34 cats with oral idarubicin at 1 to 3 mg/cat/day for 3 consecutive days every 3 weeks. The maximally tolerated dose is 2 mg/cat/day for 3 consecutive days every 3 weeks. A maximum cumulative dose has yet to be determined. In the study population of cats, observed toxicities included anorexia (7 cats), leukopenia (6 cats), and vomiting (5 cats). Lymphoma was the only tumor type that went into remission after idarubicin therapy. Although this preliminary study by Moore and associates supports further investigation of idarubicin's efficacy, unfortunately this drug is not yet available commercially.

◆ NEW AGENTS

Stealth Liposome-Encapsulated Doxorubicin and Cisplatin

Liposomes are self-assembling colloidal particles in which a lipid bilayer encapsulates a fraction of the surrounding aqueous medium. There are several different forms of liposomes, including conventional, polymorphic (cationic or fusogenic), and stealth (sterically stabilized or nonreactive). Conventional liposomes are used in veterinary oncology for the encapsulation of nonspecific immunostimulatory agents.[19] Polymorphic liposomes exhibit high reactivity to nucleic acids and cell membranes, and therefore have potential application to gene therapy by improving transfection by exogenous DNA. Stealth liposomes are constructed of lipid bilayers surrounded by glycolipids or ethylene glycol, which provide a steric barrier. When chemotherapy is encapsulated in such liposomes, the drug half-life and thus the duration of exposure of the tumor cells to the chemotherapy are increased greatly.[20]

Multiple chemotherapy drugs are undergoing evaluation in stealth liposome-encapsulated form, including doxorubicin, mitoxantrone, and cisplatin.[20–23] Stealth liposome-encapsulated doxorubi-

cin (Doxil) is undergoing evaluation in cats by Thamm and coworkers.[21] Thirty-nine cats with naturally occurring tumors have been treated with Doxil at either 0.75 (n = 3), 0.8 (n = 2), 1.0 (n = 21), 1.1 (n = 5), 1.2 (n = 18), 1.3 (n = 20), 1.4 (n = 15), or 1.5 (n = 55) mg/kg. Because this was a dose-escalation trial, if cats tolerated their initial dose of Doxil, subsequent treatments were administered at a higher dose. Inappetence was reported by 5 owners; 1 of these cats had a dose reduction because of the severity of the inappetence. Myelosuppression was not evident on blood counts obtained before each treatment. Unique skin toxicity included mild-to-moderate alopecia, hyperpigmentation, erythema, and papule formation primarily of the perioral area and the distal limbs (DM Vail, personal communication, 1999). Thirty-six per cent of the cats enjoyed a measurable response in tumor burden. Unfortunately, 15 per cent of the study cats have shown evidence of renal dysfunction (elevated blood urea nitrogen and creatinine, low urine specific gravity) on follow-up evaluation. The median time of onset of renal changes was 180 days after therapy. Significantly, 36 per cent of the cats treated with a 1.5 mg/kg dose developed the kidney changes; none of the cats treated with 1 mg/kg or less was affected. The recommended dosage of Doxil is 1 mg/kg as a 5- to 10-minute intravenous injection every 3 weeks.

Thamm and Vail[23] completed a toxicity trial of stealth liposome-encapsulated cisplatin in 2 clinically normal cats. Unlike free cisplatin, this formulation did not cause fatal pulmonary edema in the study animals.[24] Both cats received 70 mg/m² (free cisplatin equivalent) as a 10-minute intravenous bolus every 3 weeks for 4 treatments. Thorough monitoring of complete blood counts, chemistry profiles, urinalysis, and thoracic radiographs failed to identify any evidence of significant toxicity. Both cats experienced pyrexia, beginning approximately 12 hours after administration and continuing for 18 hours. The pyrexia appears to be self-limiting. Based on the fact that this drug was not fatal to cats, clinical studies to evaluate efficacy are warranted.

◆ SPECIAL CONSIDERATIONS

Nutritional Support

Anorexia is one of the most devastating side-effects that cats experience from chemotherapy. This problem, coupled with the fact that many tumor-bearing cats are presented with a history of inappetence, obliges the clinician to address the nutritional status of the feline oncology patient. Early recognition of the need for aggressive nutritional support is an important component of the management of the oncology patient. Nutritional support can be provided through pharmacologic or mechanical methods. Cyproheptadine and megestrol acetate have been used as appetite stimulants in human beings, but only megestrol acetate has been documented to enhance weight gain in cancer patients.[25, 26] There are no veterinary studies of appetite stimulants. This author has used both cyproheptadine (2 mg/cat 2 to 3 times daily) and megestrol acetate (2.5 mg/cat daily for 4 days, then every other day) with varying and limited success in feline patients.

Esophagostomy and gastrostomy tubes are easy to place and manage in cats; both tubes are excellent routes for providing calories. The techniques for placing these tubes have been described in depth.[27, 28] There are several commercially available diets for cancer patients that are formulated specifically for tube-feeding.

Marks and associates[29] compared healthy cats that were given methotrexate and fed either a commercial (i.e., containing intact proteins and fiber) or an elemental diet. Cats on the commercial diet had far fewer gastrointestinal side-effects than cats on the elemental diet. These results support the important role that intact proteins and dietary fiber play in intestinal health.

Client-Related Issues

An essential component of veterinary cancer therapy is client communication. Slater and coworkers[30] performed standardized telephone interviews of owners of cats with cancer. The goals of the study included identifying owner characteristics associated with a decision of euthanasia or intervention, identifying factors associated with an owner's satisfaction with euthanasia or intervention, and evaluating inappropriate expectations of the owners who selected an intervention. No significant factors affecting the likelihood of the owner deciding to euthanize or treat the cat were identified. Owners whose cats were able to groom, eat, and play normally were 15 times more likely to be dissatisfied with their decision to euthanize, rather than treat, their cats. Cat owners who understood the number of return visits and had a realistic expectation of life expectancy, and whose cats had a good or excellent quality of life were more likely to be satisfied with their decision. The conclusion of this study was that veterinarians must be both knowledgeable and approachable in their client interactions.

◆ SUMMARY

As access to the Internet continues to increase, cat owners will develop increasingly higher expectations of their veterinarians. Although much work remains to be completed, the amount of information regarding cancer therapy for cats is improving. Chemotherapy options are becoming clearer, and veterinary oncologists are involved in several cooperative studies in an effort to obtain a better grasp on how best to manage our feline oncology patients.

REFERENCES

1. Jeglum KA, deGuzman E, Young K: Chemotherapy of advanced mammary adenocarcinoma in 14 cats. J Am Vet Med Assoc 187:157–160, 1985.
2. Mauldin GN, Matus RE, Patnaik AK, et al: Efficacy and toxicity of doxorubicin and cyclophosphamide used in the treatment of selected malignant tumors in 23 cats. J Vet Intern Med 2:60–65, 1988.
3. Cotter SM, Kanki PJ, Simon M: Renal disease in five tumor-bearing cats treated with adriamycin. J Am Anim Hosp Assoc 21:405–409, 1984.
4. O'Keefe DA, Sisson DD, Gelberg HB, et al: Systemic toxicity associated with doxorubicin administration in cats. J Vet Intern Med 7:309–317, 1993.
5. Hahn KA, Frazier DL, Cox SK, et al: Effect of infusion regime on doxorubicin pharmacokinetics in the cat. J Am Anim Hosp Assoc 33:427–433, 1997.
6. Golden DK, Langston VC: Uses of vincristine and vinblastine in dogs and cats. J Am Vet Med Assoc 193:1114–1117, 1988.
7. Hahn KA: Vincristine sulfate as single-agent chemotherapy in a dog and a cat with malignant neoplasms. J Am Vet Med Assoc 197:504–506, 1990.
8. Mahony OM, Moore AS, Cotter SM, et al: Alimentary lymphoma in cats: 28 cases (1988–1993). J Am Vet Med Assoc 207:1593–1598, 1995.
9. Hahn KA, Fletcher CM, Legendre AM: Marked neutropenia in five tumor-bearing cats one week following single-agent vincristine sulfate chemotherapy. Vet Clin Pathol 25:121–123, 1996.
10. Zwahlen CH, Lucroy MD, Kraegel SA, et al: Results of chemotherapy for cats with alimentary malignant lymphoma: 21 cases (1993–1997). J Am Vet Med Assoc 213:1144–1149, 1998.
11. Ogilvie GK, Moore AS, Obradovich JE, et al: Toxicoses and efficacy associated with administration of mitoxantrone to cats with malignant tumors. J Am Vet Med Assoc 202:1839–1844, 1993.
12. Henry CJ, Brewer WG, Royer NS: Hematological and clinical responses to combined mitoxantrone and cyclophosphamide administration to normal cats. Can Vet J 35:706–708, 1994.
13. Page RL, McEntee MC, George SL, et al: Pharmacokinetic and phase I evaluation of carboplatin in dogs. J Vet Intern Med 7:235–240, 1993.
14. Theon AP, VanVechten MK, Madewell BR: Intratumoral administration of carboplatin for treatment of squamous cell carcinomas in the nasal plane in cats. Am J Vet Res 57:205–210, 1996.
15. Kisseberth WC, Vail DM, Jeglum JA, et al: Evaluation of carboplatin in tumor bearing cats: A phase I study from the Veterinary Cooperative Oncology Group (VCOG). Proc Vet Cancer Society Ann Conf 16:21, 1996.
16. Wood CA, Moore AS, Frimberger AE, et al: Phase I evaluation of carboplatin in tumor bearing cats. Proc Vet Cancer Society Ann Conf 16:39–40, 1996.
17. Hahn KA, McEntee MF, Daniel GB, et al: Hematologic and systemic toxicoses associated with carboplatin administration in cats. Am J Vet Res 58:677–679, 1997.
18. Moore AS, Ruslander D, Cotter SM, et al: Efficacy of, and toxicoses associated with, oral idarubicin administration in cats with neoplasia. J Am Vet Med Assoc 206:1550–1554, 1995.
19. MacEwen E, Kurzman ID, Rosenthal RC, et al: Therapy for osteosarcoma in dogs with intravenous injection of liposome-encapsulated muramyl tripeptide. J Natl Cancer Inst 81:935–938, 1989.
20. Vail DM, Kravis LD, Cooley AJ, et al: Preclinical trial of doxorubicin entrapped in sterically stabilized liposomes in dogs with spontaneously arising malignant tumors. Cancer Chemother Pharmacol 39:410–416, 1997.
21. Thamm DH, MacEwen E, Chun R, et al: Phase I clinical trial of Doxil®, a stealth liposome encapsulated doxorubicin in cats with malignant tumors. Proc Vet Cancer Society Ann Conf 17:38, 1997.
22. Ruslander D, Kaser-Hotz B, Klink B, et al: Liposome-encapsu-

lated mitoxantrone: Interim results of a phase I study in dogs. Proc Vet Cancer Society Ann Conf 17:97, 1997.

23. Thamm DH, Vail DM: Evaluation of SPI-77, a sterically stabilized (stealth) liposome encapsulated cisplatin in cats. Proc Vet Cancer Society Ann Conf 16:74, 1996.

24. Knapp DW, Richardson RC, DeNicola DB, et al: Cisplatin toxicity in cats. J Vet Intern Med 1:29–35, 1987.

25. Loprinzi CL: Management of cancer anorexia/cachexia. Support Care Cancer 3:120–122, 1995.

26. Kardinal CG, Loprinzi CL, Schaid DJ, et al: A controlled trial of cyproheptadine in cancer patients with anorexia and/or cachexia. Cancer 65:2657–2662, 1990.

27. Levine PB, Smallwood SH, Buback JL: Esophagostomy tubes as a method of nutritional management in cats: A retrospective study. J Am Anim Hosp Assoc 3:405–410, 1997.

28. Armstrong PJ, Hardie EM: Percutaneous endoscopic gastrostomy: A retrospective study of 54 clinical cases in dogs and cats. J Vet Intern Med 4:202–206, 1990.

29. Marks SL, Cook AK, Griffey S, et al: Dietary modulation of methotrexate-induced enteritis in cats. Am J Vet Res 58:989–996, 1997.

30. Slater MR, Barton CL, Rogers KS, et al: Factors affecting treatment decisions and satisfaction of owners of cats with cancer. J Am Vet Med Assoc 208:1248–1252, 1996.

66

◆ Approach to Oral Tumors

G. Neal Mauldin

Oral tumors account for roughly 3 to 10 per cent of all neoplasms reported in cats.[1, 2] The majority of these tumors occur in older cats, with median age at diagnosis reported to be 10 to 13 years. There does not appear to be any gender predilection. Approximately 90 per cent of these tumors will be malignant, because the 2 most common tumors of the feline oral cavity are squamous cell carcinoma (SCC) and fibrosarcoma (FSA). Other tumors that have been reported in the oral cavity of cats include lymphoma, rhabdomyosarcoma, osteosarcoma, salivary gland carcinoma, melanoma, granular cell tumor, and plasmacytoma.[1, 3, 4] There also are rare reports of different variants of odontogenic tumors in cats.[1, 5–7]

◆ CLINICAL PRESENTATION

The most common presenting complaint for cats with oral tumors is facial asymmetry. However, one prospective study of mandibular swellings in cats revealed that nonneoplastic dental lesions accounted for 50 per cent of these cases, demonstrating the essential role that biopsy plays in the diagnosis of oral disease in cats.[8, 9] Other clinical signs include hypersalivation, weight loss, dysphagia, anorexia, halitosis, bloody saliva, difficulty in prehending food, and facial pain. These clinical signs may mimic those associated with the feline stomatitis/pharyngitis complex.[10] A nasal discharge may be seen if there is extension of an oral tumor into the nasal cavity. Any cat presenting with clinical signs referable to the oral cavity should have an appropriate diagnostic evaluation. Conservative medical management rarely is beneficial, even for dental causes of these signs, and may delay the timely diagnosis of malignant disease.

◆ DIAGNOSIS AND STAGING

As with all diseases of geriatric cats, a minimum database should be obtained before any anesthetic procedures. This includes a complete blood count and differential, serum biochemical profile, and urinalysis. Retroviral screening should be performed when appropriate. These will offer little information specific to the nature of the oral cavity disease, but will help to identify concurrent diseases that may be present. Thoracic radiographs also should be considered part of the routine staging protocol of oral tumors, and may be performed before anesthe-

sia as well. The regional lymph nodes, primarily the mandibular and superficial scapular nodes, should be examined as part of the staging process. If there is nodal enlargement or asymmetry, or if the nodes are invasive into surrounding tissues, they should be biopsied for the presence of metastatic disease. A fine-needle aspiration of the affected node may be beneficial if it reveals obvious neoplastic disease. These regional nodes are frequently reactive and enlarged if the tumor is ulcerated or necrotic, so the presence of lymphadenopathy should not be equated automatically with metastasis. In fact, it is uncommon for oral tumors in the cat, with the exception of oral lymphoma, to metastasize to regional lymph nodes.

A good oral examination, preferably with the patient under sedation or anesthesia, should be performed in cats presenting with clinical signs suggestive of oral neoplasia. The oral examination should include a visual inspection of the caudal pharynx, pharyngeal pillars, mucosal linings of the maxilla and mandible, upper and lower dental arcade, hard and soft palates, and the sublingual region. Palpation of the soft palate may identify masses in the oropharynx that are not apparent visually. Any loose teeth, especially in the absence of significant dental disease, warrant further exploration, usually in the form of dental/skull radiographs (Fig. 66–1). Radiographically, oral tumors may have either an osteoproductive or an osteolytic appearance. It is imperative that good-quality radiographs be obtained to evaluate the oral cavity adequately. Some of the radiographic changes seen with oral neoplasia may be very subtle, and require excellent positioning and technique to be seen. For this reason, cranial/dental radiographs always should be performed with the patient under anesthesia. Complete radiographic evaluation of the maxilla and mandible requires that oblique lateral, open-mouth lateral, intraoral, dorsoventral, and ventrodorsal views be obtained.[11] Advanced imaging techniques, such as computed tomography scans or magnetic resonance imaging, may be necessary to evaluate fully the extent of the tumor and to determine whether surgery has a reasonable chance of cure (Figs. 66–2 and 66–3). These cross-sectional imaging modalities can be valuable in helping the clinician to determine the type and magnitude of surgery necessary to achieve a complete resection.

A good clinical approach is to sedate the cat for an oral examination, and to be prepared to perform radiographs or other diagnostic imaging studies if necessary after the visual examination of the oral

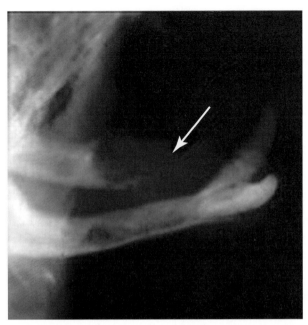

Figure 66–1. Lytic lesion of the body of the left mandible (*arrow*). Minimum soft-tissue changes were visible grossly, and the cat has had multiple "loose" teeth removed. Biopsy done subsequent to these radiographs revealed a diagnosis of lymphoma.

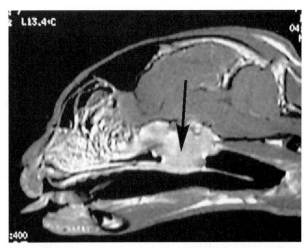

Figure 66–3. Transverse magnetic resonance imaging section of the cat in Figure 68–2. Note the large mass extending into the oropharynx and nasopharynx, and invading dorsally through the palatine and sphenoid bones into the thalamic region. Surgical cure is not possible, necessitating adjuvant therapy if local control is to be achieved. The owners declined radiation therapy. Histopathology revealed a diagnosis of rhabdomyosarcoma.

cavity. Any masses, ulcers, or suspicious gingival swellings should be evaluated. Fine-needle aspiration of an oral mass or scraping of an ulcerated lesion may provide a diagnosis before the definitive surgical procedure, and may allow for better surgical planning. However, mesenchymal tumors such as FSA exfoliate very poorly, and a diagnosis of neoplasia usually is not possible without tissue biopsy. It is imperative that any biopsies performed be in a manner that will not compromise future

surgical approaches. The amount of normal tissue around an oral tumor frequently is the limiting factor for surgical resection, so care must be taken to avoid compromising normal tissues that cannot be resected easily with the primary tumor. It also is important to choose an appropriate site within the tumor from which to obtain the biopsy material. Because oral tumors frequently are ulcerated and may have secondary bacterial contamination, a superficial biopsy may reveal only necrotic tissue and inflammation. In general, it is appropriate to take a deep biopsy sample at the margin of the tumor–normal tissue interface.[9]

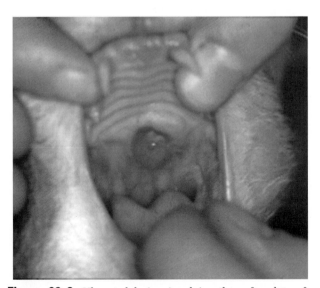

Figure 66–2. Ulcerated lesion involving the soft palate of a young cat. The cat was being evaluated for surgical resection of the mass. The decision to perform a magnetic resonance imaging study before surgery was made for staging purposes.

◆ THERAPY AND PROGNOSIS

Appropriate therapy for oral tumors follows the same principles applied to tumors arising from other anatomic sites. Cats with locally aggressive tumors—for example, SCC or FSA—should be treated with therapies designed to achieve adequate local control, such as surgery and/or radiotherapy.[12–15] Oral tumors with a high metastatic potential, such as lymphoma or anaplastic sarcomas, will need some form of systemic chemotherapy in order to increase survival times significantly. Local therapies may provide some palliation of clinical signs associated with the oral mass, but will not alter the metastatic behavior of these tumors. Other treatment modalities such as immunotherapy, photodynamic therapy, and cryosurgery have not been used extensively in the treatment of oral tumors in cats.

Squamous Cell Carcinoma

SCC is a tumor that exhibits an extremely aggressive clinical course in cats. Metastasis is unusual, owing in part to the fact that most cats die from the local effects of this tumor within a few weeks to months of initial presentation. The most common site for oral SCC in cats is sublingual, making a timely diagnosis difficult unless a good oral examination is performed. One study of 7 cats with mandibular SCC produced a median survival time of 14 months when mandibulectomy with apparently complete resection was combined with radiation therapy.[15] Unfortunately, most cats present with advanced-stage disease, and complete surgical resection is not possible. These cats warrant an extremely grave prognosis, even in the face of aggressive combined-modality therapy. A retrospective study of 52 cats with oral SCC revealed a median survival time of only 2 months in those treated with surgery alone, surgery plus radiotherapy, radiotherapy plus chemotherapy, or radiation and hyperthermia.[16] Improved supportive-care techniques, such as percutaneous endoscopic gastrostomy tube placement, may increase our ability to support these cats and improve their overall survival. However, these cats still will die from the local effects of this tumor unless more effective treatments are found.

Mesenchymal Tumors

FSA is the most common mesenchymal tumor of the feline oral cavity. These tumors usually present as soft-tissue swellings along the gingiva of the mandible or maxilla, but may be found anywhere in the oral cavity. Radiographs may not reveal any evidence of bony invasion or lysis. However, the invasive nature of these tumors makes it imperative that aggressive local resection, including removal of underlying bone, be performed if a surgical cure is to be achieved. The most common mistake made in the surgical treatment of mesenchymal tumors of the oral cavity is failure to resect an appropriate margin of normal tissue with the tumor. Normal tissue margins frequently are the limiting factor in oral cancer surgery. This means that a poorly planned or executed first surgical procedure may make the difference between a curative procedure and a purely palliative one. Performing multiple soft-tissue resections, while leaving underlying bone intact, is a strategy doomed to failure. Radiation therapy may be used if complete surgical resection is not possible. The prognosis is poor for cats with incompletely resected tumors.

Chondrosarcoma, osteosarcoma, and rhabdomyosarcoma also have been reported in the feline oral cavity. As with FSA, the first goal of therapy is to achieve local control. The metastatic potential of these tumors is not known in cats; chemotherapy may be of benefit in cats with aggressive or anaplastic tumors.

Odontogenic and Periodontal Tumors

Tumors of odontogenic origin have a bewildering array of names and classifications. However, they are relatively rare tumors in cats, and share the characteristics of local invasion without systemic spread. Odontogenic tumors may arise from epithelial or mesenchymal dental structures. Epithelial odontogenic tumors such as ameloblastoma, odontoma, and inductive fibroameloblastoma are more common than their mesenchymal counterparts.[13, 17] Odontogenic tumors warrant a good prognosis with complete surgical excision, although recurrence after incomplete excision is common. Radiation therapy may be used as an adjunct to surgery for cases in which complete excision is not possible.

Epulides are mesenchymal tumors arising from the periodontal ligament. These tumors behave in a manner similar to the odontogenic tumors, and usually are cured with appropriate local control.

REFERENCES

1. Stebbins KE, Morse CC, Goldschmidt MH: Feline oral neoplasia: A ten-year survey. Vet Pathol 26:121–128, 1989.
2. Cotter SM: Oral pharyngeal neoplasms in the cat. J Am Anim Hosp Assoc 17:917–920, 1981.
3. Patnaik AK, Mooney S: Feline melanoma: A comparative study of ocular, oral, and dermal neoplasms. Vet Pathol 25:105–112, 1988.
4. Rothwell JT, Valentine BA, Eng VM: Peripheral giant cell granuloma in a cat. J Am Vet Med Assoc 192:1105–1106, 1988.
5. Gardner DG: Ameloblastomas in cats: A critical evaluation of the literature and the addition of one example. J Oral Pathol Med 27:39–42, 1998.
6. Gardner DG, Dubielzig RR: Feline inductive odontogenic tumor (inductive fibroameloblastoma)—A tumor unique to cats. J Oral Pathol Med 24:185–190, 1995.
7. Poulet FM, Valentine BA, Summers BA: A survey of epithelial odontogenic tumors and cysts in dogs and cats. Vet Pathol 29:369–380, 1992.
8. Kapatkin AS, Marretta SM, Patnaik AK, et al: Mandibular swellings in cats, prospective study of 24 cats. J Am Anim Hosp Assoc 27:575–580, 1991.
9. Withrow SJ: The three rules of good oncology: Biopsy, biopsy, biopsy! J Am Anim Hosp Assoc 27:311–314, 1991.
10. Marretta SM: Feline dental problems: Diagnosis and treatment. Fel Pract 20:16–20, 1992.
11. Oakes MG, Lewis DD, Hedlund CS, Hosgood G: Canine oral neoplasia. Compend Contin Educ Pract Vet 15:15–30, 1993.
12. Marretta SM, Matthiessen D, Matus R, Patnaik A: Surgical management of oral neoplasia. In Bojrab MJ, Tholen MA (eds): Small Animal Oral Medicine and Surgery. Philadelphia, Lea & Febiger, 1989, pp. 96–120.
13. Birchard S, Carothers M: Aggressive surgery in the management of oral neoplasia. Vet Clin North Am Small Anim Pract 20:1117–1140, 1990.
14. Salisbury SK, Richardson DC, Lantz GC: Partial maxillectomy and premaxillectomy in the treatment of oral neoplasia in the dog and cat. Vet Surg 15:16–26, 1986.
15. Hutson CA, Willauer CC, Walder EJ, et al: Treatment of mandibular squamous cell carcinoma in cats by use of mandibulectomy and radiotherapy: Seven cases (1987–1989). J Am Vet Med Assoc 201:777–781, 1992.
16. Postorino-Reeves NC, Turrel JM, Withrow SJ: Oral squamous cell carcinoma in the cat. J Am Anim Hosp Assoc 29:438–441, 1993.
17. Poulet FM, Valentine BA, Summers BA: A survey of epithelial odontogenic tumors and cysts in dogs and cats. Vet Pathol 29:369–380, 1992.

67

◆ Intranasal Neoplasia

Annette Smith

◆ ETIOLOGY

Intranasal tumors are primarily a disease of older animals, likely due to accumulation of irreparable damage to the DNA with age. The only causative factor that has been linked consistently with any intranasal tumor is the presence of feline leukemia virus infection, which can be associated with the development of lymphoma; however, most primary intranasal lymphoma is seen in virus-negative patients.[1]

◆ EPIDEMIOLOGY

Intranasal tumors are considered rare, accounting for 1 to 5 per cent of all tumors in cats.[2, 3] The mean age is 8 to 10 years, although reports have been made in animals ranging from 3 to 15 years of age.[2, 4] There may be a gender predilection, because some reports have indicated a relative risk of greater than 2 in castrated males.[4]

◆ PATHOPHYSIOLOGY

Most intranasal tumors are malignant (>90 per cent),[3] and are classified as carcinomas or adenocarcinomas because they arise from the respiratory or olfactory epithelium that lines the nasal passages, paranasal sinuses, and the nasal turbinates.[5, 6] Cells of the supportive tissues such as bone, cartilage, fibrous connective tissue, and lymphoid tissue also can develop into tumors, and are classified as osteosarcomas, chondrosarcomas, fibrosarcomas, and lymphosarcomas, respectively.[7] Malignant neuroblastoma,[7] arising from neuroectoderm, and hemangiosarcoma,[8] arising from endothelial cells, also have been reported in cats. Benign tumors, such as adenomas and chondromas, are rare. Polyps, which probably are inflammatory in origin, also may be seen in the nasopharyngeal area, although usually they arise from the tympanic bulla.[9]

These tumors are quite locally invasive, but occasionally metastasize, usually to the regional lymph nodes and the lungs.[4, 10] Local invasion through the cribriform plate may be seen in as many as 25 per cent of cases,[4] and extension into the orbit (Fig. 67–1) and other sites external to the nasal cavity may be seen in advanced cases.[11] Lymphoma may be seen as multicentric disease, although primary intranasal lymphoma is a clinical entity recognized in cats.[1]

◆ CLINICAL SIGNS

Clinical signs associated with intranasal tumors can mimic many other upper respiratory diseases (Table 67–1). Chronic nasal discharge, ocular discharge, sneezing, epistaxis, dyspnea with inspiratory stridor, and facial deformity are typical signs of intranasal neoplasia.[3, 4, 10] Neurologic signs such as seizures, behavior change, and mental dullness may be associated with invasion of the tumor into the cranial vault, and may occur without the presence of nasal discharge.[12] Clinical signs usually are chronic, with reported durations of 1 week to as long as 4.5 years.[3, 4, 10] Most affected cats have had clinical signs for longer than 2 months, and had been treated, with transient responsiveness, with antibiotics or corticosteroids.[4]

◆ DIAGNOSIS

Survey bloodwork and urinalysis usually are unremarkable. Epistaxis may be due to coagulopathies; therefore, a coagulation profile and clotting times may be necessary to rule out platelet or clotting

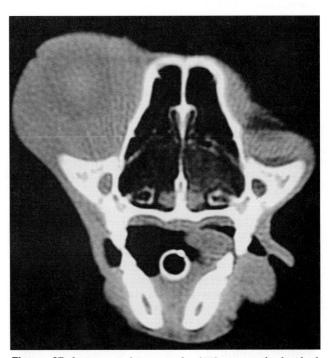

Figure 67–1. Computed tomography (CT) scan at the level of the eye demonstrates exophthalmos due to tumor invasion into the retrobulbar space. Lymphosarcoma was diagnosed.

Table 67-1. Differential Diagnosis of Chronic Nasal Discharge

Allergic disease/atopy/food allergy
Bacterial rhinitis/sinusitis
   Acinetobacter species
   Bordetella bronchiseptica
   Chlamydia psittaci
   Mycoplasma species
   Pasteurella multocida
   Pseudomonas aeruginosa
   Staphylococcus epidermidis
Dental disease
Foreign body
Fungal rhinitis/sinusitis
   Aspergillus species
   Blastomyces dermatitidis
   Cryptococcus neoformans
   Histoplasma capsulatum
   Sporothrix schenckii
Lymphocytic-plasmacytic rhinitis
Nasopharyngeal polyp
Neoplasia
Parasites
   Capillaria aerophila
   Cuterebra larvae
   Mammomanogamus ierei
Viral rhinitis/sinusitis
   Calicivirus
   Coronavirus
   Herpesvirus
   Reovirus

factor disorders. Radiographs taken with the patient under general anesthesia may be suggestive of neoplasia when unilateral aggressive lesions (lysis of lateral bones, nasal turbinate destruction, loss of teeth) are present.[13] The intraoral dorsoventral view is valuable for identifying these changes. Increased soft-tissue opacity of the nasal cavity may be indicative of a mass lesion.[4] Bilaterally symmetric lesions are more indicative of chronic rhinitis.[13] In one study, facial masses (Fig. 67–2) and deviation or lysis of the nasal septum occurred with similar frequency with rhinitis and neoplasia.[13]

Computed tomography (CT) scans are more sensitive than radiographs in determining the extent of disease and in differentiating neoplasia from infectious/inflammatory disease in dogs.[14–16] In addition, treatment planning for radiation therapy and predicting the potential for complications with this modality is best accomplished with a CT scan.[14] Studies in cats likely would yield similar findings.

Various techniques have been used for distinguishing inflammatory from neoplastic disease. Nasal washing or flushing rarely yielded a diagnosis in a study of canine intranasal tumors,[17] and the same likely is true in cats. However, this technique may be helpful in removal of foreign bodies, if present. Brush cytology may be more useful. A recent study found an 87 per cent correlation between diagnosis of inflammation and tumor, with a sensitivity of 73 per cent, a specificity of 97 per cent, a positive predictive value of 94 per cent, and a negative predictive value of 83 per cent.[18]

Definitive diagnosis of this disease is made through biopsy and histopathology. Rigid urinary catheters, bone curettes, endoscopic biopsy instruments, and alligator forceps all have been used to obtain biopsy samples. Penetration of the cribriform plate is possible if the instrument is advanced beyond the medial canthus of the eye, so the instrument should be measured and marked before inserting it into the nostril. Care must be taken to obtain large and deep tissue samples because these tumors often are associated with secondary superficial inflammation and bacterial infections. Rhinoscopy has been advocated in dogs to visualize the biopsy site,[16] but in the author's experience, blind biopsies after review of radiographs or CT scan have been adequate for a diagnosis in most cases. The small size of the feline nose, friability and bleeding of diseased tissue, and profuse nasal discharge can make rhinoscopy difficult.

If a pathologist reports only inflammation, but the index of suspicion is very high for a tumor, multiple and/or serial biopsies may be necessary to arrive at the correct diagnosis. Impression smears of the biopsy sample and cytology may help to determine whether a sample is adequate before recovering the patient from anesthesia. In some cases, surgical rhinotomy is the only means available to obtain an accurate biopsy sample.

Staging of intranasal neoplasia involves determining the extent of the local invasion, which is best accomplished with a CT scan, mandibular lymph node cytology or histopathology, and 3-view thoracic radiographs.

◆ TREATMENT

Surgery is not considered curative for most malignant tumors,[10] although rhinotomy or curettage may

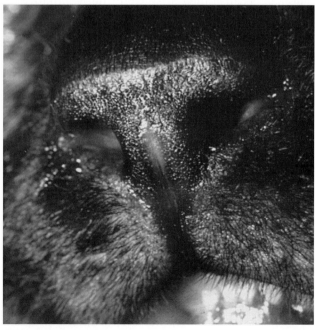

Figure 67–2. Mass protruding from the right nostril. Cryptococcosis was diagnosed.

play some role in palliation of the upper respiratory obstruction and dyspnea in selected patients. In 4 cats with adenocarcinoma, survival after surgery was only 2.5 weeks.[4] Benign tumors and chondrosarcomas may have good results with surgery alone, although local recurrence is reported.[4, 10]

Chemotherapy plays a role in the management of lymphoma, although other intranasal tumor types have not responded with increased survival times. Cisplatin has been reported to improve quality of life in dogs, however, with a decrease in clinical signs.[19] Because this drug can not be used in cats, carboplatin may be of some benefit, although clinical studies have not been performed. Cisplatin also has been proposed as a radiation sensitizer in dogs, although a treatment advantage with its use has not been apparent. No studies have been reported in cats.

Radiation therapy is the treatment of choice for intranasal neoplasia[4, 20–24] (Figs. 67–3 and 67–4). Total dosages of 40 to 60 Gy usually are given, with variable fractionation, 3 to 5 times weekly. Normal tissue effects include both early and late tissue reactions.[11] Dermatitis, oral mucositis, rhinitis, and keratitis may be seen beginning in week 2 or 3 of therapy, and may last for a few weeks after therapy has been completed. Supportive care usually resolves these effects without lasting damage. Permanent effects can include keratoconjunctivitis sicca, cataracts, alopecia, or hyper- or hypopigmentation of skin and hair. Ocular lubricants may be necessary to prevent ulceration and pigmentary changes. Normal nasal function usually does not return after therapy because the tumor typically destroys much of the turbinates. Frequently, chronic nasal discharge and secondary infection must be managed. Antihistamines, antibiotics, humidification, and periodic cleaning of the nostrils may be helpful to keep the cat comfortable.

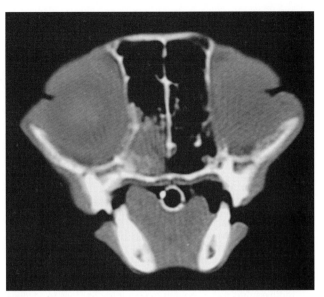

Figure 67–4. CT scan of the same cat, 3 months after radiation therapy, demonstrates significant regression of the mass in the left nasal cavity.

◆ PROGNOSIS

Cats with intranasal lymphoma appear to have an excellent prognosis with radiation therapy, which may be curative in some cases.[22, 24] The optimum dose and schedule have not been determined, as complete remissions have been achieved with doses of 8 to 40 Gy. Chemotherapy in conjunction with local irradiation must be recommended, however, owing to the incidence of systemic disease development after treatment of localized disease.[22, 24] With radiation of other intranasal tumors, the survival times appear to be prolonged, with a 1-year survival rate of 44 per cent and a 2-year survival of 17 per cent.[21] One cat was still alive after 41 months before being lost to follow-up.[23] Cats with olfactory neuroblastomas, often accompanied by brain invasion, appear to have a guarded-to-grave prognosis.[4]

REFERENCES

1. Holzworth J: Leukemia and related neoplasms in the cat. I. Lymphoid malignancies. J Am Vet Med Assoc 136:47–69, 1960.
2. Engle GC, Brodey RS: A retrospective study of 395 feline neoplasms. J Am Anim Hosp Assoc 5:21–31, 1969.
3. Madewell BR, Priester WA, Gillette EL, et al: Neoplasms of the nasal passages and paranasal sinuses in domestic animals as reported by 13 veterinary colleges. Am J Vet Res 37:851–856, 1976.
4. Cox NR, Brawner WR, Powers RD, et al: Tumors of the nose and paranasal sinuses in cats: 32 cases with comparison to a national database (1977 through 1987). J Am Anim Hosp Assoc 27:339–347, 1991.
5. Patnaik AK: Canine and feline nasal and paranasal neoplasms: Morphology and origin. In Reznik G, Stinson S (eds): Nasal Tumors in Animals and Man, vol. 2. Boca Raton, FL, CRC, 1983, pp. 199–227.
6. Elkan D: Olfactory esthesioneuroblastoma. In Reznik G, Stinson S (eds): Nasal Tumors in Animals and Man, vol. 2. Boca Raton, FL, CRC, 1983, pp. 129–147.

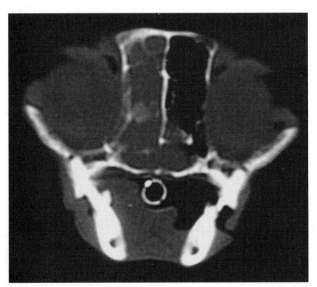

Figure 67–3. CT scan of a cat with nasal adenocarcinoma demonstrates soft-tissue opacity primarily in the left nasal passage.

7. Becker LE, Hinton D: Primitive neuroectodermal tumors of the central nervous system. Hum Pathol 14:538–550, 1983.

8. Scavelli TD, Patnaik AK, Mehlhaff CJ, Hayes AA: Hemangiosarcoma in the cat: Retrospective evaluation of 31 surgical cases. J Am Vet Med Assoc 187:817–819, 1985.

9. Kapatkin AS, Matthiesen DT, Noone KE, et al: Results of surgery and long-term follow-up in 31 cats with nasopharyngeal polyps. J Am Anim Hosp Assoc 26:387–392, 1990.

10. Legendre AM, Krahwinkel DJ, Spaulding KA: Feline nasal and paranasal sinus tumors. J Am Anim Hosp Assoc 17:1038–1039, 1981.

11. Ogilvie GK, Larue SM: Canine and feline nasal and paranasal sinus tumors. Vet Clin North Am Small Anim Pract 22:1133–1144, 1992.

12. Smith MO, Turrel JM, Bailey CS, Cain GR: Neurologic abnormalities as the predominant signs of neoplasia of the nasal cavity in dogs and cats: Seven cases (1973–1986). J Am Vet Med Assoc 195:242–245, 1989.

13. O'Brien RT, Evans SM, Wortman JA, Hendrick MJ: Radiographic findings in cats with intranasal neoplasia or chronic rhinitis: 29 cases (1982–1988). J Am Vet Med Assoc 208:385–389, 1996.

14. Thrall DE, Robertson ID, McLeod DA, et al: A comparison of radiographic and computed tomographic findings in 31 dogs with malignant nasal cavity tumors. Vet Radiol 30:59–66, 1989.

15. Park RD, Beck ER, LeCouteur RA: Comparison of computed tomography and radiography for detecting changes induced by malignant nasal neoplasia in dogs. J Am Vet Med Assoc 201:1720–1724, 1992.

16. Codner EC, Lurus AG, Miller JB, et al: Comparison of computed tomography with radiography as a noninvasive diagnostic technique for chronic nasal disease in dogs. J Am Vet Med Assoc 202:1106–1110, 1993.

17. MacEwen EG, Withrow SJ, Patnaik AK: Nasal tumors in the dog: Retrospective evaluation of diagnosis, prognosis, and treatment. J Am Vet Med Assoc 170:45–48, 1977.

18. Caniatti M, Roccabianca P, Ghisleni G, et al: Evaluation of brush cytology in the diagnosis of chronic intranasal disease in cats. J Small Anim Pract 39:73–77, 1998.

19. Hahn KA, Knapp DW, Richardson RC, Matlock CL: Clinical response of nasal adenocarcinoma to cisplatin chemotherapy in 11 dogs. J Am Vet Med Assoc 200:355–357, 1992.

20. Withrow SJ: Tumors of the respiratory system: Nasal tumors. *In* Withrow SJ, MacEwen EG (eds): Small Animal Clinical Oncology, 2nd ed. Philadelphia, WB Saunders, 1996, pp. 281–286.

21. Theon AP, Peaston AE, Madewell BR, Dungworth DL: Irradiation of nonlymphoproliferative neoplasms of the nasal cavity and paranasal sinuses in 16 cats. J Am Vet Med Assoc 204:78–83, 1994.

22. Evans SM, Hendrick M: Radiotherapy of feline nasal tumors. Vet Radiol 30:128–132, 1989.

23. Straw RC, Withrow SJ, Gillette EL, McChesney AE: Use of radiotherapy for the treatment of intranasal tumors in cats: Six cases (1980–1985). J Am Vet Med Assoc 189:927–929, 1986.

24. Elmslie RE, Ogilvie GK, Gillette EL, McChesney-Gillette S: Radiotherapy with and without chemotherapy for localized lymphoma in 10 cats. Vet Radiol 32:277–280, 1991.

68

◆ Evaluation and Treatment of Cranial Mediastinal Masses

Kenita S. Rogers

The presence of a mass within the cranial mediastinal compartment of the feline thorax frequently is associated with neoplasia. In many instances, however, this neoplasm is quite treatable, with the possibility of complete remission or long-term survival seen with lymphoma and thymoma, respectively. In addition, several nonneoplastic disorders that are very amenable to treatment may result in a cranial mediastinal mass. Discovery of a mass often is as simple as reviewing a thoracic radiograph. Making a definitive diagnosis may be more difficult because the intrathoracic location limits the number of noninvasive techniques available for routine use, and the cytologic distinction between some of the etiologies may be subtle. This chapter focuses on the clinical presentation of patients with cranial mediastinal masses, the most commonly reported differential diagnoses, the options available for diagnostic evaluation, and the most appropriate therapeutic modalities for each disease process.

◆ CLINICAL SIGNS

Masses arising within the cranial mediastinum may be incidental findings on thoracic radiographs (Fig. 68-1), but in most circumstances, the patient presents with clinical abnormalities caused by 1 of 3 primary mechanisms: local infiltration, pleural effusion, or systemic manifestations of paraneoplastic syndromes. If the mass is particularly large or invasive, clinical signs may be related to direct compression or infiltration of normal thoracic structures.[1] Manifestations may include regurgitation, dysphagia, drooling, cardiac abnormalities, and respiratory compromise with compression of the trachea or segmental bronchi. A large mass may cause the cranial thorax to be subjectively less compliant with external compression, and occasionally may even extend through the thoracic inlet and be palpable. Distended jugular veins may be noted, as well as edema of the face, neck, and forelimbs if the mass leads to vena cava syndrome.[2] Peripheral nerve entrapment may cause Horner's syndrome, stridor, changes in vocalization, and laryngeal paralysis with resultant upper-airway obstruction. On auscultation, bilateral muffled heart sounds and absent ventral lung sounds may be appreciated. Development of pleural effusion is expressed clinically as changes in respiratory effort. Effusions may occur with neoplastic or inflammatory processes, or may develop secondary

to disruption of thoracic duct dynamics, leading to chylothorax[3, 4] (see Chapter 35, Chylothorax). The underlying etiologies associated most consistently with development of pleural effusion are lymphoma and thymoma. When a chylous effusion is documented in association with a cranial mediastinal mass, it is usually due to obstruction of flow, which results in lymphatic hypertension, lymphangiectasia, and subsequent chyle transudation through dilated lymphatic walls.[3] Concurrent paraneoplastic syndromes or extrathoracic abnormalities may be recognized with diseases including lymphoma (hypercalcemia, lymphadenopathy, cytopenias, coagulopathy), thymoma (hypercalcemia, myasthenia gravis, exfoliative dermatitis), and fungal infection (organomegaly, cytopenia).

◆ DIFFERENTIAL DIAGNOSES

The cranial mediastinum is bounded by the sternum and thoracic inlet and follows the dorsal pericardial surfaces to the cardiophrenic ligament.[1] Structures encompassed within this space include the ascending segments of the great vessels, cranial vena cava, thymus, sternal and cranial mediastinal lymphatics, right and left vagosympathetic trunks, portions of the trachea and esophagus, and remnants of embryonic tissues.[5] Ectopic thyroid or parathyroid tissue also may be found within this space. Abnormalities of any of these structures may result in development of a mass lesion within the cranial mediastinum. Whereas the delicate mediastinal tissue offers little resistance to the spread of disease processes to other compartments within the mediastinum, neoplastic and inflammatory diseases tend to remain preferentially within a given compartment.[1]

Mass lesions of the mediastinum include space-occupying lesions within the mediastinal pleura and enlargement of lymph nodes.[1] Conditions that produce space-occupying lesions within the mediastinum include infectious abscesses or granulomas, lymphadenopathy, cysts, neoplasia, and a variety of miscellaneous processes, such as hemorrhage secondary to trauma or coagulopathy, edema due to heart failure or lymphatic obstruction, exudative fluid due to feline infectious peritonitis, and excessive fat associated with obesity.[1, 5, 6]

Lymphadenopathy of the sternal and mediastinal lymph nodes may be infectious or inflammatory in origin, or may result from metastatic or primary

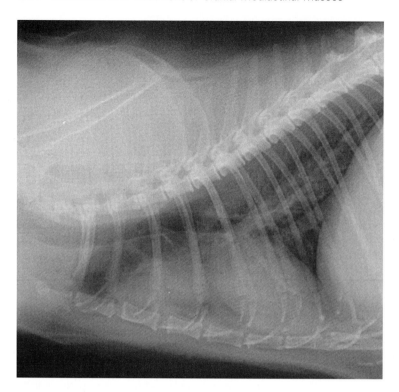

Figure 68–1. Lateral radiograph of a 16-year-old domestic shorthair cat being evaluated for nasal adenocarcinoma. Although the cat was asymptomatic for intrathoracic disease, routine thoracic radiographs revealed the presence of a discrete mass within the cranial mediastinum. Cytology of the mass was consistent with a thymoma.

lymphoid neoplasia. The infectious agents associated most commonly with marked enlargement of these lymph nodes are fungal, particularly blastomycosis, histoplasmosis, and coccidioidomycosis. Lymphadenopathy attributed to metastatic neoplasia typically is due to carcinoma (mammary, thyroid, pulmonary, or head and neck), but the site of origin may be distant (urogenital or gastrointestinal).[7] Other tumor types that may spread to these lymph nodes include mast cell tumor, malignant melanoma, and histiocytic disorders. When evaluating lymphadenopathy of unknown cause, it is helpful to recall that the regional drainage pattern to the sternal lymph nodes is the diaphragm, mediastinum, thymus, pleura, cranial portions of abdominal muscles, first 3 mammary glands, muscles of the lateral and ventral thoracic wall, superficial and deep pectoral muscles, and serratus ventralis muscle.[8] Afferent lymphatics to the cranial mediastinal nodes are from the mediastinum; pleura; heart; esophagus; trachea; thymus; muscles of the neck, shoulder, and trunk; and the bronchial lymphocenter.

Mediastinal cysts are uncommon, benign, and located most frequently in the cranial compartment. Cysts may originate from diverse cell lines including pleural, lymphatic, bronchogenic, and thymic.[9] Patients usually are asymptomatic, and the cysts frequently are inadvertent findings on thoracic radiographs obtained for other reasons. They must be differentiated from solid neoplasia by needle aspiration because some tumors may have a cystic component.[10, 11] Benign cysts should be diminished substantially in size or absent radiographically after aspiration.

Whereas neoplastic ectopic thyroid or parathyroid tissue is identified occasionally, the most common types of neoplasia involving the mediastinum arise spontaneously from a mediastinal structure such as lymphatics (lymphoma) and the thymus (thymoma, squamous cell carcinoma).[1, 12, 13] Although other neoplasms may have cranial mediastinal lymphadenopathy as a systemic part of their disease (multiple myeloma, leukemias), lymphoma and thymoma are the tumors most likely to present with a cranial mediastinal mass as their primary manifestation.

The cranial mediastinal form of lymphoma may be solitary or associated with extrathoracic organ involvement. *Mediastinal lymphoma* is a more appropriate term than thymic lymphoma for this disease process because the cranial and caudal mediastinal nodes are involved rather than the thymus.[14] This form often affects young cats, many of which are feline leukemia virus (FeLV)–test–positive.[15, 16] The mediastinal form is one of the most common anatomic forms of lymphoma in cats, but there appear to be regional differences in its prevalence.[14] Indeed, this particular form may have decreased in frequency over time. It has been suggested that vaccination and testing for FeLV may be altering the demographics of feline lymphoma, with an increase in the proportion of anatomic forms that are often FeLV-test–negative, such as the gastrointestinal form.[17] Pleural effusion secondary to mediastinal lymphoma is common, often contains neoplastic lymphocytes, and contributes to clinical signs of respiratory compromise.[18] Hypercalcemia is a rare complication in cats with lymphoma.

Thymomas are rare tumors in cats, with no age,

gender, or breed predisposition.[19] Development of thymoma does not appear to be related to retrovirus infection. Thymomas arise from thymic epithelial cells, and usually are benign in their histologic appearance; however, local invasiveness and occasional metastasis indicate the potential for malignant behavior.[20] When used to describe thymoma, the terms *benign* and *malignant* are more useful if they are used in the context of the degree of invasiveness rather than their microscopic appearance, because histologic appearance has not been shown to have prognostic importance.[20,21] Metastasis is uncommon, but has been reported in the lungs, liver, and bone. These tumors often are encapsulated, particularly in cats. However, they also may be minimally invasive, with adhesion to intrathoracic structures such as pleura and pericardium, or may be very infiltrative and encompass important structures such as the cranial vena cava.

Pleural effusion is a common sequela of thymoma, and may be chylous.[3,19] Paraneoplastic syndromes are not as common in cats with thymomas as in dogs. Those reported include myasthenia gravis (MG), polymyositis, myocarditis, hypercalcemia, and exfoliative dermatitis.[20, 22–25] MG is a rare disease in cats, and is associated only occasionally with a cranial mediastinal mass (see Chapter 48, Acquired Myasthenia Gravis and Other Disorders of the Neuromuscular Junction). In 20 cats diagnosed with MG, only 3 had a mass documented.[26] Thoracotomy in 2 of the 3 cats confirmed a diagnosis of thymoma. Compared with dogs, megaesophagus is a relatively less common sequela to MG. In the previously cited study, only 8 of 20 cats had megaesophagus. This disparity between species likely results from the smaller proportion of skeletal muscle in the feline esophagus, and probably contributes to the lower mortality rate in cats with acquired MG because aspiration pneumonia is less likely.[26] Exfoliative dermatitis developed in 3 cats with thymoma.[24] This condition began as nonpruritic scaling with mild erythema on the head and pinnae. The dermatosis progressively involved the rest of the body, scaling intensified, and alopecia developed. The digits and claw beds also were affected.

◆ DIAGNOSTIC EVALUATION
Physical Examination

Owing to the possibility of systemic manifestations, particularly with lymphoma and thymoma, patients should receive a complete physical examination. This examination should include palpation of the anterior thorax, palpation of peripheral lymph nodes, assessment of muscular weakness or other signs of MG, assessment of mucous membrane color, and an ophthalmic examination.

Minimum Database

Laboratory evaluation should include a complete blood count, biochemical profile, and urinalysis for overall assessment of the cat's health. Specific findings that may be related to causes of the cranial mediastinal mass include hypercalcemia (lymphoma, thymoma, granulomatous fungal disease) and cytopenias of bone marrow origin associated most commonly with lymphoma. Tests for FeLV and feline immunodeficiency virus are indicated to help establish a prognosis and guide decisions regarding other cats in the household.[14] A coagulation profile may be indicated in the patient with thrombocytopenia or if active hemorrhage into the mediastinum is suspected. For selected patients, thyroid and parathyroid hormone levels may be appropriate, and if MG is suspected, serum acetylcholine receptor antibody titers may be performed.

Radiography

The most commonly used and practical test for assessing the location and size of a cranial mediastinal mass is survey thoracic radiography. The radiographic appearance of most mediastinal masses is similar, and the ventrodorsal or dorsoventral projection is more helpful than the lateral projection in differentiating whether a lesion is within the mediastinum or originates from the lung.[5] In the ventrodorsal or dorsoventral position, most of the cranial mediastinum is superimposed on the spine, and the width of the mediastinum usually is less than 2 times the width of the spine (Fig. 68–2). In obese patients, the cranial mediastinum may be widened by fat accumulation, and the resultant opacity can be confused with a mediastinal mass. Masses within the cranial mediastinal compartment often elevate the trachea, but so can large volumes of pleural fluid not associated with a mediastinal mass.[5] Pleural fluid alone does not result in tracheal compression, which may be helpful if a patient has a large amount of pleural fluid that obscures the mediastinum. If tracheal compression is noted, a mass lesion should be suspected (Fig. 68–3). If pleural fluid interferes with evaluation of the cranial mediastinum, thoracocentesis may be performed and the radiographs repeated. However, before fluid removal, the diagnostic utility of ultrasound should be considered because the presence of pleural fluid can substantially facilitate visualization of a mass. It also should be remembered that fluid within the mediastinum typically resembles a mass lesion radiographically. For example, esophageal perforation and secondary bacterial mediastinitis in a cat may appear radiographically as a mass lesion that is indistinguishable from a neoplastic process. Contrast studies that may be helpful in some circumstances to locate and outline specific mediastinal masses include esophograms, angiograms, and lymphangiograms.

Ultrasonography

Ultrasound can image the cranial mediastinum, and is particularly helpful in patients in which pleural

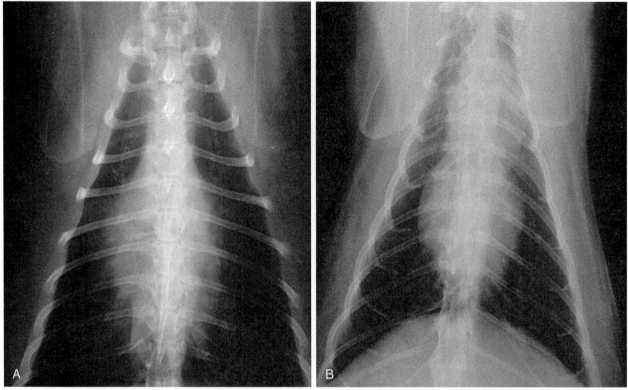

Figure 68–2. *A*, Ventrodorsal thoracic radiograph in a normal cat. The mediastinum is superimposed on the spine and is less than twice its width. *B*, Ventrodorsal thoracic radiograph of a cat with a thymoma in the cranial mediastinum. The mediastinal mass exceeds twice the width of the spine.

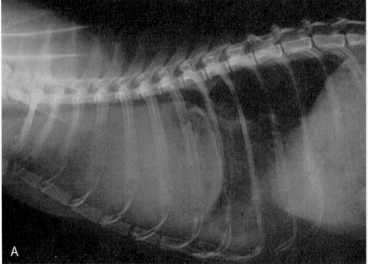

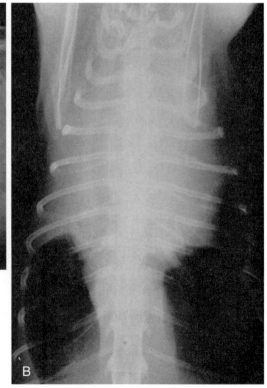

Figure 68–3. *A*, Lateral radiograph of a 9-year-old domestic shorthair cat with a large invasive thymoma. The mass effect is not likely to be due to pleural effusion because the trachea is deviated dorsally. *B*, Ventrodorsal radiograph of the same patient shows deviation of the trachea to the right.

fluid obscures structures within the thorax. Indeed, pleural fluid may facilitate visualization of mediastinal masses by serving as an acoustic window.[27] Ultrasound also can be used to guide fine-needle aspirates or needle-core biopsies of mediastinal masses, delineate the extent of cardiac and extracardiac masses, and determine whether a mass is cystic. When the mediastinal mass is small or a limited amount of fluid is present, it may be helpful to image the patient from the dependent side. This approach takes advantage of atelectasis in the dependent lungs, flow of fluid toward the dependent side, and physical displacement of the mediastinal mass toward the dependent side as a result of gravity.

Advanced Imaging

Computed tomography (CT) and magnetic resonance imaging (MRI) are used routinely to evaluate the mediastinum in human beings. Disadvantages of use in veterinary patients include limited availability, expense, and requirement of general anesthesia in a patient that already may be in respiratory compromise.[28] However, these procedures can help the veterinarian identify the specific site of origin of many diseases, distinguish fat and fluid-filled cysts from other lesions, and evaluate thoracic areas that are difficult to image on survey radiographs. In some settings, imaging a cranial mediastinal mass by CT or MRI may be helpful in the decision-making process, as these modalities are more likely to yield information about the precise extent of the mass and what structures are involved when surgical resection is contemplated (Fig. 68–4). However, CT and MRI have a poor ability to distinguish between mediastinal masses and adjacent collapsed or consolidated lung lobes, and cannot differentiate benign from malignant causes of lymphadenopathy reliably.

Cytology

Cytology may be used to assess the fluid that may be collected by thoracocentesis and direct aspirates of the mass. Collection of pleural fluid may be useful both diagnostically and therapeutically. If pleural fluid obscures the mediastinum and a mass lesion is suspected, removing the fluid and repeating thoracic radiographs may be helpful in assessing the cranial mediastinum. Fluid samples should be collected for culture as well as cytology if the patient's clinical signs and fluid analysis suggest bacterial mediastinitis.[1] When evaluating fluid from a body cavity, the inexperienced cytologist must remember that the population of reactive mesothelial cells that are exfoliated into the fluid may show a number of cytologic changes that can be confused with malignancy, regardless of the underlying cause of the effusion.

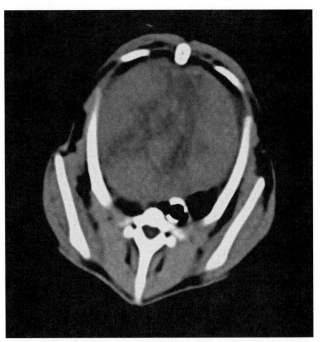

Figure 68–4. Computed tomography scan of the thorax of the patient in Figure 68–3. The patient is positioned in dorsal recumbency. The large mass fills most of the thorax, and displaces the trachea and esophagus dorsally.

Cytologic evaluation of thoracocentesis fluid collected from cats with mediastinal lymphoma frequently reveals the presence of serosanguinous fluid containing numerous vacuolated, neoplastic lymphoid cells.[14] Recall that chylothorax may be present secondary to obstruction or rupture of the thoracic duct, and may contain numerous mature, small lymphocytes that should not be confused with lymphoma. Confirmation of a chylous effusion can best be made by simultaneous comparison of the pleural fluid and serum triglyceride concentrations.[3] In all cases of chylothorax, the fluid triglyceride concentration should exceed that in serum, and in general is greater than 100 mg/dl. The actual triglyceride concentration depends on the dietary fat content and the postprandial state of the cat.

Direct aspiration of a mediastinal mass can be accomplished with ultrasonographic guidance or by triangulation based on assessment of the position of the mass on orthogonal thoracic radiographs.[1] Diseases that may be diagnosed by this technique include lymphoma, thymoma, cysts, and bacterial, fungal, or metastatic lymphadenopathy. Contraindications for this technique include severe dyspnea, coagulopathy, and difficulties in restraining the patient. Before aspiration, the skin site should be clipped and prepared for surgery. Twenty-five- to 22-gauge needles generally are adequate for aspiration and are available in various lengths. The needle is inserted between the ribs and into the mass, with no redirection once the needle has been advanced. After aspiration and needle withdrawal, material within the needle is ejected onto a clean glass slide.

If sufficient material is available, horizontal smears as well as vertical pull-apart slides are prepared because of the fragility of cells important in some disease processes, particularly lymphoma.[1]

In the normal lymph node, small lymphocytes account for 75 to 95 per cent of the total cell population.[29] A small number of medium and large lymphocytes also are found, with occasional other cell types noted, including plasma cells, macrophages, neutrophils, eosinophils, and mast cells. Most lymph nodes are reactive, and there is no clear line of cytologic separation between a normal node and a hyperplastic one because the small lymphocyte is the predominant cell type in both normal and hyperplastic nodes.[29] Reactive hyperplasia typically is characterized by increased numbers of medium and large lymphocytes; the number of other infiltrating inflammatory cells varies. Lymphadenitis is characterized cytologically by the accumulation of substantial numbers of inflammatory cells, although the cell type varies with the inciting cause. For example, most bacterial infections elicit a neutrophilic response, and macrophage numbers often are increased within a node secondary to fungal, protozoal, and higher bacterial infections, and in regional drainage from a neoplasm. Metastatic neoplasia is suggested by the presence of cells not normally found within a lymph node, or by an increase in numbers of certain cell types that normally can be found in a node (e.g., mast cells).[29] The node in question usually is within the regional drainage pattern of an identified primary tumor. Neoplasms that metastasize preferentially to a lymph node include carcinoma, malignant melanoma, and mast cell tumors. In addition, plasma cell myeloma and many leukemias may present with lymphadenopathy caused by neoplastic infiltration of nodes peripheral to the bone marrow.

Lymphoma is characterized by immature lymphocytes that eventually replace the entire normal cell population.[29] Mediastinal lymphoma most often is of a large cell type. These cells may be recovered by aspiration of the intrathoracic mass or identified within pleural fluid. Occasionally, cranial mediastinal lymphoma is manifested as a small, well-differentiated lymphocyte type. This form is difficult to differentiate cytologically from reactive hyperplasia and thymoma.

The cytologic preparation from a thymoma typically contains many small lymphocytes and a variable number of thymic epithelial cells.[30] In most circumstances, small lymphocytes predominate, but in some tumors, large lymphocytes may be present in substantial numbers.[31] Thymic epithelial cells are medium to large, and may vary in shape from round to oval to stellate. The epithelial cells appear infrequently in some cytologic preparations, making definitive diagnosis of thymoma difficult. With numerous small lymphocytes and a paucity of malignant epithelial cells, the cytology also could be consistent with reactive lymphadenopathy or small-cell lymphoma. Cytology from a cranial mediastinal

mass in an older FeLV-test–negative cat that has a preponderance of small lymphocytes rather than lymphoblasts suggests that the tumor may be thymoma rather than lymphoma. Mast cells are present in up to 50 per cent of aspirates from thymomas in cats.[19] Invasive and noninvasive thymomas cannot be differentiated on cytologic examination alone[30]; imaging or exploratory thoracotomy usually are required. Needle-core biopsies were successful in providing a definitive diagnosis of thymoma in approximately 50 per cent of the cats in one study because histopathology demonstrated the malignant epithelial component more readily.[22]

Recovery of several milliliters of a clear-to-yellow, poorly cellular fluid from a mediastinal mass is suggestive of a cyst. Aspiration of this fluid often will lead to collapse of the structure so that it is no longer visualized on thoracic radiographs.

Thyroid Scintigraphy

Performing a thyroid scan with technetium-99m, or occasionally iodine-131, may be indicated in the appropriate patient.[1] A scan may detect ectopic thyroid tissue, as well as metastatic thyroid carcinoma in mediastinal lymph nodes. Limited availability and the requirement of an overnight stay in the hospital are disadvantages of this technique.

Histopathology

Tissue may be collected from a mass in the cranial mediastinum for histologic evaluation. It is collected most commonly during an exploratory thoracotomy, but may be attained by needle biopsy or via thoracostomy. Care must be taken with these less invasive procedures to avoid excessive hemorrhage or puncture of a vital structure. Ultrasound guidance may help substantially to ensure accurate and safe placement of the biopsy needle. Percutaneous biopsy of intrathoracic lesions with CT guidance has been described in cats and dogs.[32] Although thoracotomy is an invasive procedure, it can serve as a therapeutic intervention as well as supply tissue for definitive diagnostic evaluation. A median sternotomy approach is appropriate for most mediastinal disorders. The goals of the surgical procedure are to obtain an incisional or excisional biopsy for histopathology and culture, and to assess resectability of the lesion.

◆ TREATMENT

Reactive lymphadenopathy generally is found incidentally, and treatment and prognosis will be based on the underlying etiology. For example, fungal disease will be treated with systemic antifungal therapy. A diagnosis of lymphadenopathy as a sequela of metastatic disease generally equates with a poor long-term prognosis, and limits performing surgery or radiation of the primary tumor site with curative intent.

Treatment of ectopic neoplastic or metastatic thyroid tissue generally can be accomplished with radioactive iodine. In most of these patients, the finding of radioactive nuclide uptake in the cranial mediastinum is associated with metastasis of a thyroid carcinoma, and the patients are presented for clinical signs of hyperthyroidism. Aspiration of cysts generally will diminish their size on radiographs. If they recur, surgical removal may be considered.

Treatment of the mediastinal form of lymphoma will depend to some extent on the stage of disease and availability of radiation therapy. Lymphoma is a very chemotherapy-sensitive tumor, and systemic cytotoxic drug therapy generally is the treatment of choice, particularly if extrathoracic disease has been documented. The mediastinal form of lymphoma had the highest rate of complete remission (92 per cent) in one study of feline lymphoma treated with a combination of vincristine, cyclophosphamide, and prednisone, with a median remission duration of 24 weeks.[33] In another study, only 45 per cent of 31 cats with mediastinal lymphoma attained complete remission, for a median remission of 8 weeks after a cyclical combination protocol including vincristine, cyclophosphamide, and methotrexate.[34] Regardless of the clinical form of lymphoma, cats that achieve complete remission after chemotherapy have longer survival times than cats that obtain only a partial remission.[15] Cats that are positive for FeLV have shorter survival times, but FeLV status does not influence initial response to therapy.[15, 33] There are a number of chemotherapy protocols available for use in the feline lymphoma patient. One of the most commonly used protocols has been the combination of cyclophosphamide, vincristine (Oncovin), and prednisone (COP).[14] Whereas this protocol has been used quite effectively and tolerated well by the majority of feline lymphoma patients, remission durations and survival times have not been optimum. The advantage of using doxorubicin for maintenance therapy in cats achieving complete remission after COP induction has been documented.[35] In this study, cats receiving doxorubicin maintenance therapy for up to 6 months had a median remission duration of 281 days compared with 83 days in cats receiving COP maintenance therapy.

Cranial mediastinal lymphoma also may be treated with radiation therapy. Radiation causes rapid reduction in tumor burden, and may be considered for cats that have life-threatening obstructive or space-occupying forms of lymphoma, such as those with mediastinal, nasal, pharyngeal, or retrobulbar involvement. Response rates to radiation therapy in cats with localized lymphoma are quite high.[36] Eight of 10 cats in one study achieved a complete remission after treatment with radiation.[36] Five of the 8 responding cats received radiation alone with no adjunctive chemotherapy. The primary disadvantage of radiation therapy is the need for sedation or general anesthesia in an animal that often presents in respiratory distress. However, radiation remains a useful treatment that may be administered as the sole form of therapy or as an adjunct to chemotherapy. For the critical patient with respiratory compromise, our current approach is to perform thoracocentesis and initiate chemotherapy. Dramatic clinical improvement often is noted within 24 to 48 hours. We may add radiation therapy when the patient's respiratory status is more stable and if no evidence of extrathoracic lymphoma is found. It has been our clinical impression that lymphoma patients with tumors that are poorly chemoresponsive often do not respond as well as expected to radiation therapy and vice versa.

Surgical excision is the treatment of choice for noninvasive thymomas. In a report of 12 feline thymomas treated with surgery, 5 were well-encapsulated and easily excised.[22] Seven tumors were found to be adhered to the pericardium, parietal pleura, and cranial vena cava; 3 of these tumors were poorly encapsulated and considered incompletely excised. Two of the 12 cats were euthanized in the early postoperative period, but each of the 10 remaining cats had long-term survival with no evidence of local tumor recurrence or metastasis. The most common complication of thymoma surgery in these cats was postoperative intrathoracic hemorrhage. Unlike dogs, cats with thymoma often can be offered a good prognosis, particularly if the tumor appears encapsulated. Postoperative median survival has been reported to be 16 months.[22] Because of the prominent lymphoid component of this tumor, thymomas also may have some response to chemotherapy or radiation, either alone or after incomplete surgical resection.[20, 37, 38] Chemotherapy protocols suitable for lymphoma may be used with modest success in some of these patients. Indeed, corticosteroid responsiveness of a cranial mediastinal mass is not always helpful in distinguishing thymoma from lymphoma.[10]

Symptomatic care of feline patients with a cranial mediastinal mass may include thoracocentesis with fluid removal to aid respiration, assisted nutrition, medical management of hypercalcemia, or treatment of MG. If MG is a complicating factor, treatment with anticholinesterase and immunosuppressive drugs may be indicated.[26]

REFERENCES

1. Rogers KS, Walker MA: Disorders of the mediastinum. Compend Contin Educ Pract Vet 19:69–83, 1997.
2. Sottiaux J, Franck M: Cranial vena cava thrombosis secondary to invasive mediastinal lymphosarcoma in a cat. J Small Anim Pract 39:352–355, 1998.
3. Pardo AD: Chylothorax: Diagnosis and management. In August JR (ed): Consultations in Feline Internal Medicine, vol. 2. Philadelphia, WB Saunders, 1994, pp. 297–307.
4. Forrester SD, Fossum TW, Rogers KS: Diagnosis and treatment of chylothorax associated with lymphoblastic lymphosarcoma in four cats. J Am Vet Med Assoc 198:291–294, 1991.

5. Thrall DE: The mediastinum. *In* Thrall DE (ed): Textbook of Veterinary Diagnostic Radiology, 3rd ed. Philadelphia, WB Saunders, 1998, pp. 309–321.

6. Day MJ: Review of thymic pathology in 30 cats and 36 dogs. J Small Anim Pract 38:393–403, 1997.

7. Rogers KS: Metastatic patterns of feline neoplasia. *In* August JR (ed): Consultations in Feline Internal Medicine, vol. 3. Philadelphia, WB Saunders, 1997, pp. 566–571.

8. Rogers KS, Landis M, Barton CL: Canine and feline lymph nodes. Part I. Anatomy and function. Compend Contin Educ Pract Vet 15:397–408, 1993.

9. Bauer T, Woodfield JA: Mediastinal, pleural, and extrapleural diseases. *In* Ettinger SJ, Feldman EC (eds): Textbook of Veterinary Internal Medicine, 4th ed. Philadelphia, WB Saunders, 1995, pp. 812–842.

10. Malik R, Gabor L, Hunt GB, et al: Benign cranial mediastinal lesions in three cats. Aust Vet J 75:183–187, 1997.

11. Galloway PEJ, Barr FJ, Holt PE, et al: Cystic thymoma in a cat with cholesterol-rich fluid and an unusual ultrasonographic appearance. J Small Anim Pract 38:220–224, 1997.

12. Carpenter JL, Valentine BA: Squamous cell carcinoma arising in two feline thymomas. Vet Pathol 29:541–543, 1992.

13. Anilkumar TV, Voigt RP, Quigley PJ, et al: Squamous cell carcinoma of the feline thymus with widespread apoptosis. Res Vet Sci 56:208–215, 1994.

14. Vonderhaar MA, Morrison WB: Lymphosarcoma. *In* Morrison WB (ed): Cancer in Dogs and Cats. Medical and Surgical Management. Baltimore, Williams & Wilkins, 1998, pp. 667–695.

15. Mooney SC, Hayes AA, MacEwen EG, et al: Treatment and prognostic factors in lymphoma in cats: 103 cases (1977–1981). J Am Vet Med Assoc 194:696–699, 1989.

16. Gabor LJ, Malik R, Canfield PJ: Clinical and anatomical features of lymphosarcoma in 118 cats. Aust Vet J 76:725–732, 1998.

17. Moore AS: Treatment of feline lymphoma. Fel Pract 24:17–20, 1996.

18. Davies C, Forrester SD: Pleural effusion in cats: 82 cases (1987–1995). J Small Anim Pract 37:217–224, 1996.

19. Ogilvie GK, Moore AS: Tumors of body cavities. *In* Ogilvie GK, Moore AS (eds): Managing the Veterinary Cancer Patient. Trenton, NJ, Veterinary Learning Systems, 1995, pp. 441–450.

20. Morrison WB: Nonpulmonary intrathoracic cancer. *In* Morrison WB (ed): Cancer in Dogs and Cats. Medical and Surgical Management. Baltimore, Williams & Wilkins, 1998, pp. 537–550.

21. Atwater SW, Powers BE, Park RD, et al: Thymoma in dogs: 23 cases (1980–1991). J Am Vet Med Assoc 205:1007–1013, 1994.

22. Gores BR, Berg J, Carpenter JL, et al: Surgical treatment of thymoma in cats: 12 cases (1987–1992). J Am Vet Med Assoc 204:1782–1785, 1994.

23. Scott-Moncrieff JC, Cook JR, Lantz GC: Acquired myasthenia gravis in a cat with thymoma. J Am Vet Med Assoc 196:1291–1293, 1990.

24. Scott DW, Yager JA, Johnston KM: Exfoliative dermatitis in association with thymoma in three cats. Fel Pract 23:8–13, 1995.

25. Foster–van Hijfte MA, Curtis CF, White RN: Resolution of exfoliative dermatitis and *Malassezia pachydermatis* overgrowth in a cat after surgical thymoma resection. J Small Anim Pract 38:451–454, 1997.

26. Ducote JM, Dewey CW, Coates JR: Clinical forms of acquired myasthenia gravis in cats. Compend Contin Educ Pract Vet 21:440–448, 1999.

27. Konde LJ, Spaulding K: Sonographic evaluation of the cranial mediastinum in small animals. Vet Radiol 32:178–184, 1991.

28. Burk RL: Computed tomography of thoracic diseases in dogs. J Am Vet Med Assoc 199:617–621, 1991.

29. Duncan JR: The lymph nodes. *In* Cowell RL, Tyler RD, Meinkoth JH (eds): Diagnostic Cytology and Hematology of the Dog and Cat, 2nd ed. St. Louis, Mosby, 1999, pp. 97–103.

30. Cowell RL, Tyler RD, Baldwin CJ: The lung parenchyma. *In* Cowell RL, Tyler RD, Meinkoth JH (eds): Diagnostic Cytology and Hematology of the Dog and Cat, 2nd ed. St. Louis, Mosby, 1999, pp. 174–182.

31. Rae CA, Jacobs RM, Couto CG: A comparison between the cytological and histological characteristics in thirteen canine and feline thymomas. Can Vet J 30:497–500, 1989.

32. Tidwell AS, Johnson KL: Computed tomography–guided percutaneous biopsy in the dog and cat: Description of technique and preliminary evaluation in 14 patients. Vet Radiol Ultrasound 35:445–456, 1994.

33. Cotter SM: Treatment of lymphoma and leukemia with cyclophosphamide, vincristine, and prednisone: II. Treatment of cats. J Am Anim Hosp Assoc 19:166–172, 1983.

34. Jeglum KA, Whereat A, Young K: Chemotherapy of lymphoma in 75 cats. J Am Vet Med Assoc 190:174–178, 1987.

35. Moore AS, Cotter SM, Frimberger AE, et al: A comparison of doxorubicin and COP for maintenance of remission in cats with lymphoma. J Vet Intern Med 10:372–375, 1996.

36. Elmslie RE, Ogilvie GK, Gillette EL, et al: Radiotherapy with and without chemotherapy for localized lymphoma in 10 cats. Vet Radiol 32:277–280, 1991.

37. Hitt ME, Shaw DP, Hogan PM, et al: Radiation therapy for thymoma in a dog. J Am Vet Med Assoc 190:1187–1190, 1987.

38. Smith AN: Thymomas: Future directions in therapy. Vet Cancer Soc Newsletter 23:8–9, 1999.

69

◆ Update on Vaccine-Associated Sarcomas

Carolyn J. Henry

◆ ETIOLOGY

The occurrence of sarcomas at vaccination sites in cats was first reported in a letter to the editor of the *Journal of the American Veterinary Medical Association* in 1991.[1] The recognition of a possible relationship between vaccination and sarcoma development followed the 1985 approval of a subcutaneous (SQ) killed aluminum-adjuvant rabies vaccine (replacing high egg passage modified-live vaccines, which had been administered intramuscularly), and the introduction of a killed aluminum-adjuvant feline leukemia virus (FeLV) vaccine the same year. In their letter to the editor, Drs. Hendrick and Goldschmidt noted an increase in the number of feline nonoral fibrosarcomas since 1988, and reported that these tended to occur in the interscapular and dorsal cervical regions. Whereas their biopsy population from 1987 to 1991 had an overall 61 per cent increase in fibrosarcomas, there was no increase in the proportion of fibrosarcomas occurring at non–vaccine-associated sites.[1] At that time, the tumors were believed to be related to a vaccine adjuvant. The tumors had become more common after the enactment of a mandatory rabies vaccination law and the shift from intramuscular (IM) to SQ rabies vaccine administration.

Since the recognition of this tumor, now referred to as *vaccine-associated feline sarcoma* (VAFS), researchers and practitioners have sought to determine its cause. In 1996, the Vaccine Associated Feline Sarcoma Task Force (VAFSTF) was developed through the combined efforts of the American Animal Hospital Association, the Veterinary Cancer Society, the American Association of Feline Practitioners, and the American Veterinary Medical Association. The research objectives of the group were divided into 3 categories: epidemiology/pathology, etiology, and treatment.

The efforts of the VAFSTF are enhancing our knowledge of the tumor, but in order to understand why VAFSs occur, several important questions must be answered. First, *What has changed in our vaccination or injection practices that has led to an increased incidence of sarcoma development?* The initial circumstantial evidence provided by reports of increased tumor development at vaccine sites has been supported by epidemiologic studies. In their retrospective study of 345 cats in Hawaii and California, Kass and colleagues[2] showed causal and temporal relationships between FeLV and rabies vaccinations and sarcoma development. Since that time, other vaccines, including feline viral rhinotra-

cheitis, calicivirus, and panleukopenia virus (FVRCP),[3, 4] and injectable products (lufenuron[5]) also have been incriminated in the development of sarcomas. To date, no single vaccine type (adjuvanted, nonadjuvanted, attenuated, inactivated), brand, or antigen class has been linked definitively with the sudden increase in sarcoma development at injection sites. Although aluminum adjuvant initially was suspected as a primary cause, subsequent studies have shown that these tumors also develop in the absence of an aluminum-adjuvanted product.[4, 6, 7] In 1 review of clinical cases from a private practice in Canada, an association was suggested between killed panleukopenia and respiratory virus vaccine administration in the interscapular area and subsequent sarcoma development.[4] The affected cats had not received other types of injections or vaccinations in that site, and no new cases were noted when the practice began using a modified live FVRCP vaccine.

Other factors such as vaccine temperature at the time of injection, reuse of needles and syringes, needle gauge, and injection technique (e.g., whether or not the area is massaged after vaccination) have been suggested to be important in tumor development. However, because this variability in vaccination technique existed long before an increased incidence of VAFSs was noted, it is considered unlikely to be a major factor in tumor development.

The key to understanding the etiology of VAFS during the 1990s lies in understanding what has changed during the same time frame. Have components of vaccines or other injectable products, syringes, or needles changed such that they now elicit an inflammatory response in cats that ultimately may lead to tumorigenesis? One difficulty in pursuing the answer to this question is that adjuvants are considered proprietary information. In an attempt to determine which vaccines are most likely to induce postvaccinal reactions, Macy[8] evaluated 6 inactivated feline vaccines (3 rabies and 3 FeLV) for evidence of local reactions 21 days after vaccination in 36 cats (see Chapter 1, Update on Vaccine-Associated Sarcomas and Current Vaccine Recommendations). Inactivated rabies vaccines most consistently (80 to 100 per cent) produced local reactions, and the presence or absence of aluminum in the adjuvant was not related to the size of the reaction. Conversely, an aluminum-adjuvanted FeLV vaccine was more likely to produce local postvaccinal reactions than was a non–aluminum-adjuvanted FeLV vaccine. An FeLV vaccine containing no adjuvant did not produce histologic evidence of a local reaction.

Perhaps some of the most useful information regarding VAFS etiology will come from a multicenter study currently under way. This study, led by Dr. Philip Kass, will compare adjuvanted to nonadjuvanted vaccines and attenuated organism vaccines to inactivated organism vaccines to determine whether risk factors can be identified. The study also will examine vaccine antigen classes and vaccination protocols (vaccination site, mixing vaccines, reusing syringes) in an attempt to find causal relationships. In addition, responsible reporting of vaccination and other injection reactions (see Control and Prevention) by practitioners will provide valuable information regarding risk factors.

The second question with regard to etiology is: *What is unique about cats that leads to tumor formation at these sites?* The role of feline viruses in the development of VAFS has been investigated as a species-unique cause of these tumors. Ellis and coworkers[9] examined 136 VAFSs using polymerase chain reaction and immunohistochemical staining in an attempt to identify evidence of FeLV in association with these tumors. Neither method provided evidence of such a link. As feline sarcoma virus requires FeLV as a helper virus in oncogenesis, the absence of FeLV particles in the tumors decreases the likelihood that feline sarcoma virus is involved in their pathogenesis.

Investigations of the role of the *p53* tumor-suppressor gene in feline sarcoma development are currently under way. Two of 10 fibrosarcomas were found to have mutations in *p53* in a previous study.[10] A tissue bank of sarcomas, normal-appearing tissue margins, and blood has been established and is being evaluated for *p53* gene mutations as a VAFSTF study.[11] Sites of polymorphism in the *p53* gene have been identified in tissues (including normal surrounding tissues), suggesting a link to tumor development in cats. Other factors being investigated in VAFSTF-sponsored studies include growth factors such as platelet-derived growth factor and insulin-like growth factor and the role of lymphocytes. Preliminary data suggest that T-lymphocytes, rather than B-lymphocytes, tend to infiltrate VAFSs,[11] although the relevance to tumorigenesis is uncertain.

Inflammation remains one of the most likely underlying causes in the development of VAFS. Previous work has established evidence for fibrosarcoma development at the site of wounding in cats.[12] A similar model that may provide insight regarding tumor formation and prevention in cats is the Rous sarcoma virus model in chickens. V-src–infected chickens have been shown to develop tumors at wound sites 10 to 15 days after wounding.[13] By suppressing postwounding inflammation, it is possible to suppress tumor development in this model.[14] Presuming inflammation plays an initiating role in tumorigenesis in cats, efforts to decrease inflammation at injection sites may be important in prevention of VAFS. Recently, a nonadjuvanted rabies vaccine (Pure Vax, Merial Ltd., Iselin, NJ) was developed, and other vaccine manufacturers are likely to follow suit.

The final crucial question regarding VAFS etiology is: *Are vaccinations solely responsible for the initiation of these tumors, or could other injections be linked, as well?* A recent case report described a 17-year-old female spayed cat that developed a fibrosarcoma at the site of an interscapular lufenuron injection.[5] The mass first appeared 1 month after the injection, and a biopsy was obtained from the mass 6 months later. Histopathologic examination revealed intersecting bundles of spindle-shaped neoplastic fibroblasts within the mass and aggregates of small lymphocytes at the periphery. The cat had not been vaccinated in the year prior to the development of this mass, although influence of earlier vaccines could not be ruled out as a causative factor. The package insert for lufenuron (Program, Novartis Animal Health US, Inc., Greensboro, NC) lists injection site lumps/granulomas as possible adverse effects of its use. Although this is an isolated case, it raises the possibility that injectable products other than vaccines are capable of inducing an inflammatory response that can progress to fibrosarcoma in cats.

◆ EPIDEMIOLOGY AND PATHOGENESIS

Current estimated prevalence of VAFS is approximately 5 in 10,000 vaccinated cats.[3] The median age of cats with VAFS is 8 years, compared with 11 years for cats with non–vaccination-site sarcomas.[15] The latency period for tumor development varies from 3 months to 3 years (average = 340 days).[2, 16] Although fibrosarcomas are reported most often, other sarcomas including soft-tissue osteosarcoma, chondrosarcoma, rhabdomyosarcoma, malignant fibrous histiocytoma, anaplastic sarcoma, myofibroblastic sarcoma, and liposarcoma may occur with this syndrome.[2, 17, 18]

◆ CLINICAL SIGNS

Development of an inflammatory nodule after vaccination is the earliest warning sign for VAFS. Nodules that continue to increase in size more than 1 month after vaccination, are larger than 2 cm in diameter, or persist for greater than 3 months should be suspected to be VAFSs and managed according to the guidelines in Table 69–1. VAFSs vary from solitary, firm nodules to diffuse masses that attach to underlying bone (scapulae, dorsal spinous processes) and can become cystic (Fig. 69–1). Metastatic disease occurs in 10 to 24 per cent of cases,[19–22] but is unlikely to be the cause of initial presenting signs.

Table 69–1. Vaccine-Associated Feline Sarcoma Task Force Guidelines

Diagnosis and Treatment of Suspected Sarcomas

The following recommendations are based on information available as of April 1999 and are subject to revision as new information becomes available.

1. **Diagnosis**
   Record anatomic location, shape, and size (measured by caliper and recorded in 3 dimensions) of all masses that occur at the site of an injection.
2. **Manage a mass that develops at a previous injection site as if it were malignant until proven otherwise.**
   A lesion should be fully assessed and aggressively treated if it meets any 1 of the following criteria:
   a. Persists more than 3 months postinjection.
   b. Is larger than 2 cm in diameter.
   c. Is increasing in size after 1 month postinjection.
3. **If a mass meets 1 or more of the above criteria, we recommend that you perform a diagnostic biopsy prior to surgical excision.**
   A Tru-Cut needle biopsy or incisional wedge biopsy is preferred for diagnosing lesions. Tru-Cut biopsy should be done in such a way that subsequent surgical removal can readily include the entire needle tract. Wedge biopsy should be performed so that subsequent surgery can remove all tissue affected by the biopsy. Fine-needle aspiration cytology is considered unreliable for the diagnosis of vaccine-associated feline sarcomas (VAFSs) and is not recommended.
4. **Management (masses confirmed as malignant should be handled as listed below):**
   a. Perform routine thoracic radiographs and preoperative labwork for any malignant mass.
   b. When feasible, cats with histologically confirmed VAFSs should be imaged by computed tomography (CT) or magnetic resonance imaging (MRI). Soft-tissue sarcomas often spread along fascial planes and may be undetectable visually in early stages of tumor growth. Advanced imaging data are very useful in determining the extent of surgery and/or the size of the radiation field that will be needed to maximize the chances for successful treatment.
5. **Consult with an oncologist for current treatment options prior to initiating therapy.**
6. **Never "shell out" a sarcoma. Incomplete surgical removal of a sarcoma is the most common cause of treatment failure.**
   Employ oncologic surgical techniques to avoid seeding malignant cells. Remove at least a 2-cm margin in all planes, including the deep side. In some instances, this will involve reconstruction of the body wall, removal of bone, or other advanced surgical techniques.
7. **Submit the entire excised specimen for histopathology.**
   Mark the excised mass with India ink or suture tags to provide an anatomic reference to facilitate subsequent treatment.
8. **Report all histologically confirmed VAFSs to the manufacturer and to U.S. Pharmacopoeia Veterinary Practitioners' Reporting Program.**
   To make a report or request reporting forms, call 800–4–USP–PRN (800–487–7776) or visit the USP Web site at www.usp.org.
9. **After a sarcoma has been removed:**
   a. Recheck by physical examination monthly for the first 3 months, then at least every 3 months for 1 year.
   b. Perform additional diagnostic procedures as appropriate for the abnormalities detected.

◆ DIAGNOSIS AND TREATMENT

Diagnosis of VAFS is based on historical case information, tumor site, and cytologic and histopathologic evaluation of the mass. Cytologic features do not distinguish VAFSs from other soft-tissue sarcomas, but may aid in differentiating inflammatory injection reactions from malignant mesenchymal tumors and in monitoring for recurrence after surgery.[23] Cytologic findings suggestive of injection reactions include moderate cellularity and a predominance of lymphocytes and fewer activated macrophages and nondegenerate neutrophils. Reactive fibroblasts, eosinophils, mast cells, plasma cells, and multinucleated giant cells also may be noted. Basophilic to azurophilic, amorphous or globular intracytoplasmic material within multinucleate giant cells or macrophages is considered one hallmark of an injection reaction.[23] Previous work has shown that this amorphous material is related to the adjuvant used in some vaccines.[24] Fibrosarcomas are distinguished cytologically by a high degree of cellularity and nuclear and nucleolar characteristics of malignancy.[23] There frequently is an abundance of wispy pink extracellular matrix material, and pink cytoplasmic granules (suggestive of secretory granules) may be present.[23] Histologic features of VAFS include stellate or irregular spindle-shaped fibroblastoid cells with irregular large nuclei containing euchromatin, thin cytoplasmic extensions into the collagenous interstitium, and cells showing features of myofibroblasts.[7, 25] In 1 series, unique features of some VAFSs included multinucleated giant cells, glycogen, needle-like crystalline material, intratumoral endocytosed erythrocytes, and hemoglobin crystals. No viruses were seen in these tumors. The infiltrating white blood cells included macrophages, neutrophils, and lymphocytes.[25] When attempting to distinguish VAFS from other sarcomas, younger age of the cat, subcutaneous location of the mass, and presence of inflammation suggest VAFS.[15] Those with histologic features of necrosis, increased mitotic activity, and pleomorphism are more likely to be aggressive tumors.[15]

Once a diagnosis of VAFS is established, appropriate case management requires accurate treatment planning and early aggressive therapy. A summary of the current Task Force Guidelines is provided in Table 69–1. Contrast-enhanced computed tomography or magnetic resonance imaging of the affected area appears to be a much better indicator of tumor extent than are palpation and radiographs[26] (Figs.

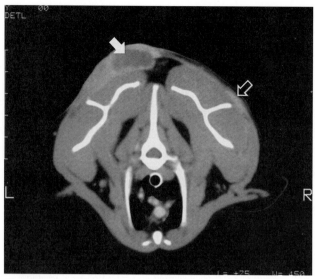

Figure 69–1. Computed tomography (CT) scan demonstrates the cystic nature *(closed arrow)* of some vaccine-associated feline sarcomas (VAFSs). Note the tendril extending over the scapular spine *(open arrow)* that can be visualized with contrast enhancement.

69–2 and 69–3). Thoracic radiographs are performed because this is the most commonly reported site of metastasis. Multimodality treatment is likely to provide the best outcome for VAFS, but controlled clinical studies are limited in the literature, owing to the recent recognition of this tumor. Until the findings of the VAFSTF treatment subgroup are reported, therapy for cats with VAFS should be based on current knowledge regarding responses to surgery, radiation therapy, chemotherapy, and immunotherapy. This information is summarized later.

Surgery

Early aggressive surgery is recommended for the treatment of VAFS. In general, excision with greater than 3-cm margins (often including bone) is recommended. The borders of excised tissue should be marked such that the pathologist can differentiate surgical margins from artifactual borders. Because complete surgical excision is difficult, it is wise to use radiodense materials (hemaclips or stainless steel sutures) to delineate borders of surgical dissection, should radiotherapy become necessary. A retrospective study of 45 cats with soft-tissue fibrosarcoma revealed an overall median survival of 11.5 months for treated cats (n = 35) versus less than 1 month for untreated cats.[27] Cats with complete tumor excision (46 per cent) survived longer (median, >16 months) than those with incomplete excisions (median survival = 9 months) and had longer disease-free intervals (>16 months versus 4 months). Ten cats survived greater than 12 months, and 3 cats were alive after 2 years. Although radiation therapy was not shown to improve survival in this study group, a selection bias was present in that the radiotherapy group comprised cats with recurrent or progressive disease.

Preliminary results of a prospective study at the University of Pennsylvania and the University of Wisconsin—Madison suggest that surgical excision alone is inadequate for control of VAFS.[22] Of 24 cats receiving surgery without adjuvant therapy, only 2 were long-term survivors. The majority of cats developed recurrence within 400 days of surgical excision. Interestingly, the investigators reported a 24 per cent metastatic rate, which is higher than that reported previously. Therefore, chemotherapy is likely to play a role in the successful treatment of VAFS.

A second preliminary report of treatment outcome in cats with VAFS treated at North Carolina State University since 1994 was presented recently.[28] Cats without metastatic disease were treated with radiation therapy (48 Gy in 16 daily fractions of 3 Gy), followed in 2 to 3 weeks by excision (including vertebral spinous process exci-

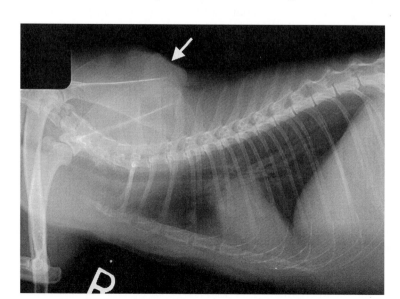

Figure 69–2. Radiographic appearance of a vaccine-associated fibrosarcoma *(arrow)* in the interscapular region of a cat.

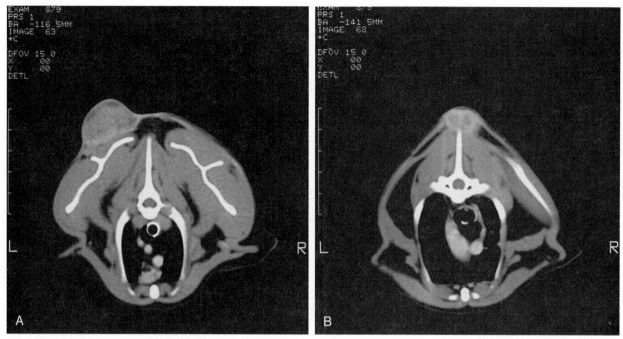

Figure 69–3. *A* and *B*, Two CT images from the same cat (Fig. 69–2) reveal 2 masses, rather than 1. The extent of some lesions may be underestimated radiographically.

sion, scapulectomy, and hemipelvectomy when indicated). Some cats also received chemotherapy (carboplatin, doxorubicin, or mitoxantrone). Of 168 cats with fibrosarcomas treated since 1994, 148 had fibrosarcomas at injection sites (7 cervical, 89 thorax/scapular, 36 lumbar/flank, and 16 proximal extremity). Forty-three cats were not treated, and 10 received surgery only. Ninety-three cats received a full course of radiation therapy, and 80 had follow-up surgery. Metastasis was observed in 13 of 148 cats, and local recurrence was noted in 22 of 148. Treatment failure was not related to tumor location. The median time to treatment failure was 204 days. The investigators concluded that VAFS could be treated effectively using radiation therapy and surgery.

Radiation Therapy

As described in the previous section, radiation therapy has been advocated in the postoperative setting for treatment of incompletely excised sarcomas and in the preoperative setting for cytoreduction. A clear benefit of one schedule over the other has not been established. Meleo and Mauldin[29] reported on 9 cats treated with postoperative radiation therapy (63 Gy over 21 fractions) for fibrosarcoma. Forty-four per cent of the cats had died at the time of the report, with a median survival of 343 days. A retrospective evaluation of 33 cats treated with preoperative radiation therapy for fibrosarcoma indicated improvement in responses over those reported with postoperative radiation.[30] The median disease-free interval was 398 days, and the median overall survival was

600 days. The only prognostic variable identified was presence of tumor cells at the excised margins after radiation therapy. The number of prior surgeries, tumor volume, and doxorubicin chemotherapy did not affect the disease-free interval. Although postoperative radiation therapy recently has been suggested as the treatment of choice for VAFS,[16] the results reported by Cronin and associates[30] and those more recently presented by Price and colleagues[28] provide support for the use of radiation before surgical intervention.

Chemotherapy

Reports of controlled studies examining the efficacy of chemotherapy against VAFS are limited. In 1 report of 10 cats treated with doxorubicin and cyclophosphamide for nonresectable fibrosarcoma, 60 per cent had an objective response (tumors made amenable to surgery and regression of metastatic lesions).[31] However, another report demonstrated no improvement in disease-free interval for cats treated with low-dose doxorubicin (10 mg/m^2 once-weekly) in conjunction with radiation.[31] More recently, a phase I clinical trial of liposome-encapsulated doxorubicin (Doxil, Sequus Pharmaceuticals Inc., Menlo Park, CA) revealed a response in 5 of 13 cats with soft-tissue sarcomas.[32] A multicenter randomized trial comparing standard doxorubicin with Doxil for the presurgical or postsurgical treatment of cats with VAFS currently is under way.[11] Owing to delayed renal toxicity noted in cats treated with Doxil, the dosage has been reduced from 1.5 mg/kg to 1.0 mg/kg. Preliminary results of case outcome are not yet available.

Carboplatin has been suggested for adjuvant therapy of VAFS.[16] In a phase I dose-escalation study, carboplatin (160 to 240 mg/m²) provided partial responses in 6 of 16 cats with fibrosarcoma.[33] However, phase II and III clinical trials are needed to determine the efficacy of carboplatin against VAFS.

In a recent report, chemotherapy agents administered in conjunction with radiation therapy and surgery included carboplatin (n = 25 cats), doxorubicin (n = 10 cats), and mitoxantrone (n = 5 cats).[28] The failure (recurrence or metastasis) rate for cats receiving chemotherapy was 22 per cent as compared with 44 per cent for cats not receiving chemotherapy. However, this was not statistically significant using a Fisher exact test. The findings presented were preliminary results, and conclusions should be based on analysis of final study data.

Immunotherapy

Acemannan, an extract of the aloe vera plant, has been touted as a valuable adjuvant therapy for fibrosarcomas in cats. The mechanism of action proposed for acemannan is the enhanced release of tumor necrosis factor, interleukin-1α, interferon, and prostaglandin E_2 after macrophage uptake of the product. In 1 report of 3 cats with VAFS treated with surgery and acemannan, a positive response was noted in 1 cat.[34] In another study, 4 of 5 cats treated with acemannan in conjunction with radiation and surgery were reported to have responded.[35] Whereas acemannan therapy appears to be safe, prospective controlled studies are needed to determine its efficacy in the treatment of VAFS.

◆ CONTROL AND PREVENTION

In an effort to reduce the prevalence of vaccine-associated sarcomas, the VAFSTF has made recommendations regarding vaccination of cats. The initial recommendations were published in the *Journal of the American Veterinary Medical Association* in 1997,[36] and are shown in Table 69–2 (see also Chapter 1, Update on Vaccine-Associated Sarcomas and Current Vaccine Recommendations).

◆ SUMMARY

Since the last edition of this textbook, new insights regarding etiology, clinical behavior, and treatment options for VAFS have been gained. Research efforts of the Vaccine Associated Feline Sarcoma Task Force have begun to elucidate molecular mechanisms of VAFS formation. Concerns regarding post-vaccination inflammation due to adjuvants have resulted in development of at least 1 nonadjuvanted vaccine to date. Public awareness of VAFS has been heightened and the profession has responded by publishing informational brochures and attempting to standardize vaccination protocols and case management recommendations. We now know that the metastatic rate for these tumors may approach 25 per cent and treatment planning should bear this in mind. Contrast-enhanced computed tomography or magnetic resonance imaging has been shown to provide a much better estimate of tumor extent than do palpation and radiographic imaging. These imaging modalities have become part of standard pretreatment evaluations and are likely to improve treat-

Table 69–2. Recommendations Regarding Feline Vaccinations

1. The manufacturer's label recommendation is the only official item a veterinarian currently has to demonstrate the basis for vaccination.
2. Alternate vaccination routes (e.g., nasal, topical) should be considered if and when available.
3. The use of vaccines packaged in single-dose vials should be encouraged.
4. Vaccination is a medical procedure and protocols should be individualized to the patient. Administration of any vaccine should proceed only after duly considering the medical significance and zoonotic potential of the infectious agent, the patient's risk of exposure, and germane legal requirements.
5. Any occurrences of vaccine-associated sarcomas or other adverse reactions should be reported directly to the vaccine manufacturer and to the United States Pharmacopoeia (USP). Information about the USP Practitioners' Reporting Programs and a sample submission form can be found in the JAVMA, Vol. 208, No. 3, Feb. 1, 1996, pp. 361–363. Additional reporting forms can be obtained by calling 1–800–4–USP–PRN. Submission of the form can be facilitated by diagnostic laboratories if the laboratories include a report form with each diagnosis of vaccine-associated sarcoma. The record should include vaccine type, lot number, and vaccination site; this information should also be incorporated into the patient's permanent medical file.
6. To further characterize the causal link and to facilitate treatment of vaccine-associated sarcomas, the following general guidelines for vaccine (and other injectable product) administration are suggested:
   a. Veterinarians should standardize vaccination (and other injection) protocols within their practice and document the location of the injection, the type of vaccine or other injectable product administered, and the manufacturer and serial number of the vaccine, in the patient's permanent medical record.
   b. It is recommended that:
      i. Vaccines containing antigens limited to panleukopenia, feline herpesvirus type-1, and feline calicivirus (± chlamydia) should be administered on the right shoulder, according to the manufacturer's recommendations.
      ii. Vaccines containing rabies antigen (+ any other antigen) should be administered on the right rear limb, as distally as possible, according to the manufacturer's recommendations.
      iii. Vaccines containing feline leukemia virus antigen (± any other antigen except rabies) should be administered on the left rear limb, as distally as possible, according to the manufacturer's recommendations.
      iv. Injection sites of other medications should be recorded.

From Romatowski J: Recommendations of the Vaccine-Associated Feline Sarcoma Task Force. J Am Vet Assoc 210:890, 1997.

ment outcome. Multimodality therapy, including surgery, radiation, and chemotherapy, is being investigated, but peer-reviewed reports of treatment outcome are sparse at this point. However, with the continued research efforts of the VAFSTF, responsible reporting of injection reactions and adherence to recommended guidelines by concerned practitioners, support and cooperation of vaccine manufacturers and public demand for answers, the likelihood of resolving this problem within the next decade is strong.

REFERENCES

1. Hendrick MJ, Goldschmidt MH: Do injection site reactions induce fibrosarcomas in cats? J Am Vet Med Assoc 199:968, 1991.
2. Kass PH, Barnes WG Jr, Spangler L, et al: Epidemiologic evidence for a causal relation between vaccination and fibrosarcoma tumorigenesis in cats. J Am Vet Med Assoc 203:396–405, 1993.
3. Hendrick MJ, Shofer FS, Goldschmidt MH, et al: Comparison of fibrosarcomas that developed at vaccination sites and at nonvaccination sites: 239 cases (1991–1992). J Am Vet Med Assoc 205:1425–1429, 1994.
4. Lester S, Clemett T, Burt A: Vaccine site–associated sarcomas in cats: Clinical experience and a laboratory review (1982–1993). J Am Anim Hosp Assoc 32:91–95, 1996.
5. Esplin DG, Bigelow M, McGill LD, et al: Fibrosarcoma at the site of a lufenuron injection in a cat. Vet Cancer Soc Newsl 23(2):8, 1999.
6. Macy DW: Current understanding of vaccination site–associated sarcomas in the cat. J Feline Med Surg 1:15–21, 1999.
7. Hendrick MJ, Brooks JJ: Postvaccinal sarcomas in the cat: Histology and immunohistochemistry. Vet Pathol 31:126–129, 1994.
8. Macy DW: The potential role and mechanism of FeLV vaccine–induced neoplasms. Semin Vet Med Surg (Small Anim) 10:234–237, 1995.
9. Ellis JA, Jackson ML, Bartsch RC, et al: Use of immunohistochemistry and polymerase chain reaction for detection of coronaviruses in formalin-fixed, parathion-embedded fibrosarcomas from cats. J Am Vet Med Assoc 209:767–771, 1996.
10. Mayr B, Schaffner G, Kurzbauer R, et al: Mutations in tumor suppressor gene p53 in two feline fibrosarcomas. Br Vet J 151:707–713, 1995.
11. Starr RM: Update: Vaccine-Associated Feline Sarcoma Task Force (VAFSTF) Veterinary Cancer Society meeting—Bodega Bay, California. Vet Cancer Soc Newsl 23(2):10, 1999.
12. Hardy WD Jr: The feline sarcoma viruses. J Am Anim Hosp Assoc 17:981–982, 1981.
13. Dolberg DS, Hollingworth R, Hertle M, et al: Wounding and its role in RSV-mediated tumor formation. Science 230:676–678, 1985.
14. Martins-Green M, Boudreau N, Bissel MJ: Inflammation is responsible for the development of wound-induced tumors in chickens infected with Rous sarcoma virus. Cancer Res 54:4334–4345, 1994.
15. Doddy FD, Glickman LT, Glickman NW, et al: Feline fibrosarcomas at vaccination sites and non-vaccination sites. J Comp Pathol 114:165–174, 1996.
16. Leveque NW: Update on vaccine-associated sarcoma. J Am Vet Med Assoc 212:1350, 1998.
17. Dubielzig RR, Hawkins KL, Miller PE: Myofibroblastic sarcoma originating at the site of rabies vaccination in a cat. J Vet Diagn Invest 5:737–738, 1993.
18. Esplin DG, McGill LD, Meininger A, et al: Postvaccination sarcomas in cats. J Am Vet Med Assoc 202:1245–1247, 1993.
19. Briscoe C, Tipscomb T, McKinney LA: Pulmonary metastasis of a feline postvaccinal fibrosarcoma. Abstr Vet Pathol 32:5, 1995.
20. Esplin DG, Campbell R: Widespread metastasis of a fibrosarcoma associated with a vaccination site in a cat. Feline Pract 23:13–16, 1995.
21. Rudmann DG, Van Alstine WG, Doddy F, et al: Pulmonary and mediastinal metastasis of a vaccination site sarcoma in a cat. Vet Pathol 33:466–469, 1996.
22. Hershey AE, Sorenmo K, Hendrick M, et al: Feline fibrosarcoma: Prognosis following surgical treatment: A preliminary report. Proc Vet Cancer Soc—Am Coll Vet Radiol Combined Conf 1997, p. 36.
23. Borjesson D: Cytology of sarcomas. Vet Cancer Soc Newsl 23(2):1–4, 1999.
24. Hendrick MJ, Goldschmidt MH, Shofer FS, et al: Postvaccinal sarcomas in the cat: Epidemiology and electron probe microanalytical identification of aluminum. Cancer Res 52:5391–5394, 1992.
25. Madewell BR: Feline vaccine-associated sarcomas: Ultrastructural features. Vet Cancer Soc Newsl 23(2):4, 1999.
26. Samii VF: Contrast-enhanced computed tomographic imaging of feline vaccine-associated sarcomas. Vet Cancer Soc Newsl 23(2):7, 1999.
27. Davidson EB, Gregory CR, Kass PH, et al: Surgical excision of soft tissue fibrosarcomas in cats. Vet Surg 26:265–269, 1997.
28. Price GS, Thrall DE Hauck LE, et al: Preliminary review of feline injection site fibrosarcoma treatment and outcome. Vet Cancer Soc Newsl 23(2):8, 1999.
29. Meleo KA, Mauldin GN: Post-operative radiotherapy for the treatment of fibrosarcoma in 9 cats. Proc 14th Annu Vet Cancer Soc 1994, pp. 127–128.
30. Cronin K, Page RL, Spodnick G, et al: Radiation therapy and surgery for fibrosarcoma in 33 cats. Vet Radiol Ultrasound 39:51–56, 1998.
31. Barber LG, Sorenmo KU, Cronin KL, et al: Effect of combined doxorubicin and cyclophosphamide therapy on non-resectable feline fibrosarcoma. Proc 16th Annu Vet Cancer Soc 1996, p. 53.
32. Thamm DH, MacEwen EG, Chun R, et al: Phase I clinical trial of Doxil®, a stealth liposome encapsulated doxorubicin, in cats with malignant tumors. Proc Vet Cancer Soc—Am Coll Vet Radiol Combined Conf 1997, p. 38.
33. Kisseberth WC, Vail DM, Ward H: Evaluation of carboplatin in tumor bearing cats: A phase I study from the Veterinary Cooperative Oncology Group (VCOG). Proc 16th Annu Vet Cancer Soc 1996, p. 21.
34. Kent EM: Use of an immunostimulant as an aid in the treatment and management of fibrosarcoma in three cats. Feline Pract 21:13–17, 1993.
35. King GK, Yates KM, Greenlee PG, et al: The effect of acemannan immunostimulant in combination with surgery and radiation therapy on spontaneous canine and feline fibrosarcomas. J Am Anim Hosp Assoc 31:439–447, 1995.
36. Romatowski J: Recommendations of the Vaccine-Associated Feline Sarcoma Task Force. J Am Vet Med Assoc 210:890, 1997.

70

◆ Diagnostic Imaging of Neoplasia

Anne Bahr

Diagnostic imaging plays a large role in the diagnosis, staging, and monitoring of cancer. Commonly used imaging modalities in veterinary medicine include conventional radiography, ultrasonography, computed tomography (CT)/magnetic resonance imaging (MRI), and nuclear medicine imaging. The first 2 now are widely available at veterinary teaching hospitals as well as at many referral and private practices. The latter 2 modalities are somewhat more limited in their availability, but are becoming commonplace in major referral centers.

With all of these methods available to image our feline patients, it is important to understand the specific strengths and weaknesses of each modality and to choose the most appropriate imaging procedure for each patient (Table 70–1). This chapter reviews only the indications and basic principles for each modality. If more detailed information is required, the reader is directed to the suggested readings at the end of the chapter. The strengths and weaknesses of each modality as it pertains particularly to imaging cancer, as well as some basic interpretation of the imaging studies, also are discussed.

◆ CONVENTIONAL RADIOGRAPHY
General Indications

Radiography often is the first step in establishing a diagnosis of cancer. It often is used to assess a palpable mass in a crude attempt to determine the origin, extent, and invasiveness of the mass. Alternatively, a mass may not be palpable, but the patient may be showing clinical signs indicating a problem with a particular organ system, and radiographs of that organ system may reveal a neoplasm. Furthermore, once a primary neoplasm is identified, radiography may be useful in evaluating likely metastatic sites that depend on the type of cancer and mode of metastasis. Basic understanding of the different behaviors of cancer and metastasis is necessary to determine which sites to radiograph.

Evaluating Thoracic Radiographs

Many types of cancer may grow within the thoracic cavity. Radiographs help primarily with determining the location and distribution of neoplasia. To

Table 70–1. Strengths and Weaknesses of Imaging Modalities

Imaging Modality	Strength	Weakness
Thoracic radiography	Commonly available Good for evaluation of primary/secondary lung neoplasia Noninvasive	Requires 3 views Hindered by pleural fluid Provides crude anatomic visualization/location of neoplasia owing to superimposition
Abdominal radiography	Commonly available Noninvasive	Often relies on displacement of normal structures to identify abnormalities Difficult to determine precise origin of mass owing to superimposition Hindered by presence of fluid
Ultrasonography	Provides information on internal architecture Enhanced in presence of fluid Can be used to guide sample acquisition Minimally invasive	Limited by operator expertise Provides narrow field of view Hindered by gas
Computed tomography	Provides information on internal architecture without superimposition Provides excellent bone detail and reasonably good soft-tissue detail Good for evaluation of the lung Provides wide field of view Can be used to plan radiation therapy	Usually requires general anesthesia Usually much more expensive and more limited in availability
Magnetic resonance imaging	Provides information on internal architecture without superimposition Excellent soft-tissue detail No radiation exposure Can be used to plan radiation therapy	Poor bone and lung detail Requires general anesthesia No metals can be in field or will cause large artifact Usually much more expensive and more limited in availability
Nuclear medicine imaging	Provides functional information	Requires special radiation safety procedures Provides poor anatomic detail

obtain the most information from thoracic radiographs, proper technique and positioning must be employed. Specifically, when evaluating the thorax for neoplasia, it generally is accepted that a minimum of 3 views are required, 2 opposite recumbent lateral views and a ventrodorsal or dorsoventral view (either is acceptable).[1] The 2 recumbent lateral views are necessary because the dependent lung may become slightly atelectatic, and may hide a small lesion that may be visualized if the lung was more air-filled. The smallest soft-tissue pulmonary nodule that can be detected is 2 mm in diameter, and must be distinguished from other normal structures such as end-on vessels.[2] The best way to determine whether a suspected nodule is an end-on vessel is to try to visualize similarly sized branching vessels entering or exiting the nodule. If a branching vessel is identified, the suspected nodule is more likely to be an end-on vessel. If questions regarding a suspicious nodule are still present, one option is to re-radiograph the animal in 2 to 4 weeks. If the nodule increases in size, it is likely to represent a neoplasm.

Once proper radiographs are obtained, evaluation for neoplasia includes determining the location and extent of the disease. It must be determined whether there is cancer involving the pulmonary parenchyma, pleural space, or mediastinum, or a combination of these. In 1 study, 50 per cent of cats with primary lung neoplasia also had pleural involvement.[3] In that same study, pulmonary adenocarcinomas tended to be either focal, solitary, well-circumscribed masses or multiple, poorly circumscribed masses. Bronchioloalveolar carcinomas tended to be more pleomorphic and often were ill-defined. Cavitation and mineralization were seen occasionally. It is important to remember that these same general radiographic findings also could be compatible with nonneoplastic disease processes such as abscesses and granulomas.

The literature is scant regarding radiographic findings of pulmonary metastatic neoplasia. In 1 cat with metastatic squamous cell carcinoma, multiple cavitary lesions were identified in the lungs.[4] In the author's experience, metastatic neoplasia may be very pleomorphic, and cavitation is more common than in dogs (Figs. 70–1 to 70–4). Early in the disease process, cavitary metastatic neoplasia sometimes mimic bronchiolar changes seen in feline asthma.

One of the most common neoplasms involving the mediastinum is lymphoma (see Chapter 68, Evaluation and Treatment of Cranial Mediastinal Masses). Often, it is accompanied by pleural effusion, which can make diagnosis difficult on survey radiographs alone owing to silhouetting of the fluid with the heart and cranial mediastinum. Furthermore, both a mediastinal mass and pleural effusion can cause tracheal elevation. However, displacement of the carina caudal to the fifth intercostal space may be 1 finding that is more suggestive of a cranial mediastinal mass (Fig. 70–5). Ultimately, ultrasound usually is employed to examine for potential masses; however, if this is not available, other techniques also may be employed (Fig. 70–6). Often, the effect of gravity may be used to promote visualization of the cranial mediastinum. If effusion is present, a ventrodorsal radiograph with the cat held vertically and using a horizontally directed x-ray beam may be helpful. This technique should allow free pleural fluid to collect in the diaphragmatic recesses and provide a clearer view of the cranial mediastinum. However, this technique will fail if the pleural fluid is compartmentalized.

Evaluating Abdominal Radiographs

As in the thorax, a definitive diagnosis of cancer usually is not possible based solely on the radio-

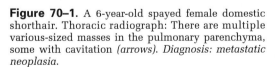

Figure 70–1. A 6-year-old spayed female domestic shorthair. Thoracic radiograph: There are multiple various-sized masses in the pulmonary parenchyma, some with cavitation *(arrows). Diagnosis: metastatic neoplasia.*

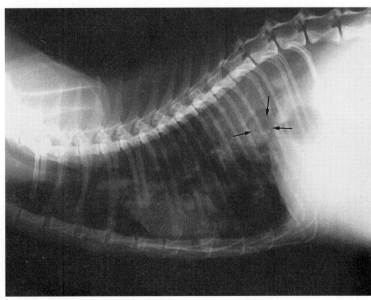

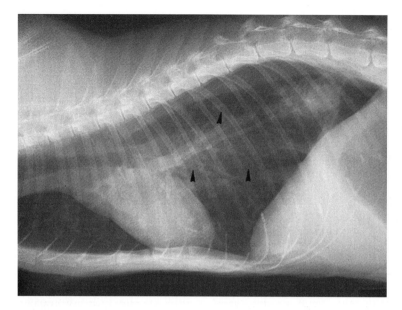

Figure 70–2. An 18-year-old spayed female domestic shorthair. Thoracic radiograph: Note the multiple cavitated nodules throughout the pulmonary parenchyma. Some of the smaller nodules look similar to thickened bronchi that may be seen in "feline asthma" *(arrowheads). Diagnosis: metastatic neoplasia.*

graphic findings. However, much information may be gained through close scrutiny, and radiographs are used to provide a general overview of the abdominal structures. In general, organ enlargement or displacement, or masses seen arising from abdominal structures, may be due to cancer. Knowledge of the normal size and anatomic position of the abdominal structures is critical to detection of these abnormalities.

Most of the liver should be contained within the rib cage, and it should have a sharp ventral margin. The stomach axis should be parallel to the ribs on the lateral view. The pylorus of the stomach should not cross the midline on the ventrodorsal view. A mass involving the liver often causes displacement

of the stomach (Fig. 70–7). The kidneys should be 2.4 to 3 times the length of L2, as measured on the ventrodorsal view.[5] They should have a smooth "bean-shaped" contour. Neoplasia of the kidneys usually causes enlargement with or without a concurrent shape change (Fig. 70–8). The spleen usually is small, and should have smooth contours. The small intestines should be looped lazily in the mid abdomen, and their serosal detail should be good in the average-size cat (Fig. 70–9). If the urinary bladder is full, it should be teardrop-shaped. Some cats have a particularly long bladder neck, which is of no clinical consequence. Lymph nodes are not visualized normally. Mesenteric lymphadenopathy often is visualized as an ill-defined mass in the mid abdo-

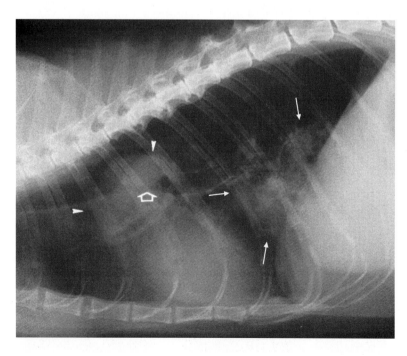

Figure 70–3. A 17-year-old castrated male exotic shorthair. Thoracic radiograph: There is an ill-defined irregular cavitated infiltrate in the caudal lung fields *(solid arrows).* Note the ill-defined opacity encircling the distal trachea and narrowing its lumen *(arrowheads). Diagnosis: metastatic carcinoma with involvement of regional lymph nodes (open arrow).*

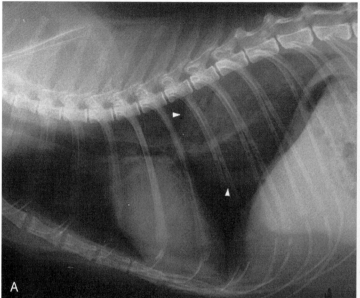

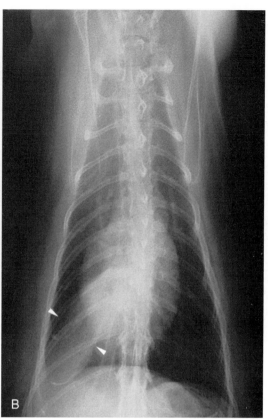

Figure 70–4. *A* and *B*, An 11-year-old castrated male domestic shorthair. Thoracic radiographs: Note the homogeneous opacity involving the right caudal lung lobe *(arrowheads)*. The infiltrate extends to the lobar borders. *Diagnosis: metastatic carcinoid.*

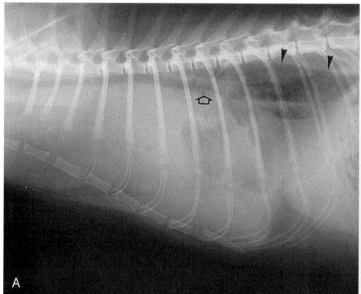

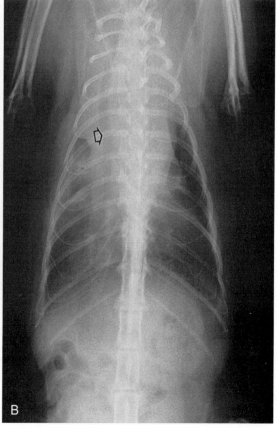

Figure 70–5. *A* and *B*, A 1-year-old castrated male domestic shorthair, feline leukemia virus (FeLV)–positive. Thoracic radiograph: There is retraction of the caudal lung lobes that indicates a small amount of pleural effusion *(arrowheads)*. There is a cranial mediastinal opacity that silhouettes with the heart. The carina is displaced caudally to the 7th intercostal space *(open arrow in A)*. *B*, the trachea is deviated to the right on the ventrodorsal view *(open arrow)*. *Diagnosis: mediastinal lymphoma.*

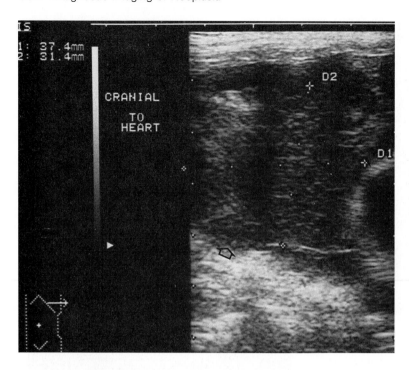

Figure 70–6. A 1 year-old castrated male domestic shorthair, FeLV-positive. Thoracic ultrasound: A large hypoechoic mass *(open arrows)* is seen cranial to the heart *(arrowheads)* consistent with a mediastinal mass. *Diagnosis: lymphoma.*

men, or it may manifest simply as a decrease in the serosal detail of the intestines (Fig. 70–10). Overall, serosal detail in the feline abdomen should be excellent, particularly ventral to the liver where cats of-

ten store a large amount of fat in the falciform fat pad. Effusion within the abdomen also will cause decreased serosal detail, and may be associated with neoplasia.

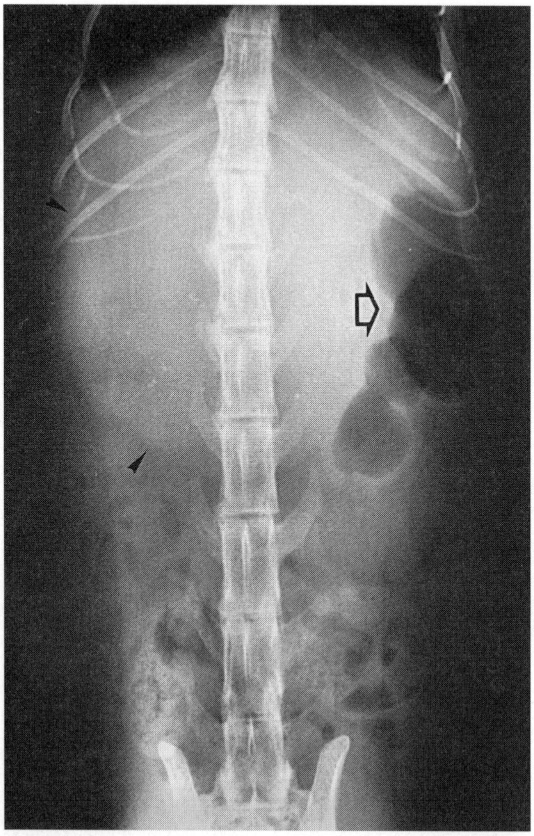

Neoplasia may involve any of the structures in the abdomen, and cause changes in the shape, position, or visibility of the involved structure. However, many other disease processes can cause similar findings, and it must be reiterated that microscopic evaluation is necessary for a definitive diagnosis.

◆ ULTRASONOGRAPHY

Ultrasonography has become widely used because it provides a real-time view of the internal anatomy of the body. It allows the clinician to examine the internal organs for diffuse or focal derangements that may not be visualized readily on radiographs. The presence of fluid, which is a hindrance in radiography, actually enhances sonographic images. Most importantly, ultrasound may be used to help guide sample acquisition to obtain a definitive diagnosis of cancer.

Ultrasonography is extremely operator-dependent. A good sonographer must be thorough in her or his examination, and must have a firm understanding of the normal anatomy to identify abnormalities accurately. In the abdomen, the spleen usually is the most echogenic (brightest), and has a uniform fine granular echotexture. The liver is slightly hypoechoic compared with the spleen, but has a slightly coarser echotexture. The kidney cortex is isoechoic to hypoechoic in echogenicity compared with the liver. It should be noted that in some obese cats, especially intact males, the kidney cortex may be more hyperechoic than the liver owing to fat deposition.[6]

Figure 70–7. A 13-year-old castrated male Himalayan. Abdominal radiograph: Note the large mass with multiple areas of mineralization *(arrowheads)* that is causing displacement of the pylorus to the left *(arrow)*. *Diagnosis: biliary cystadenoma.*

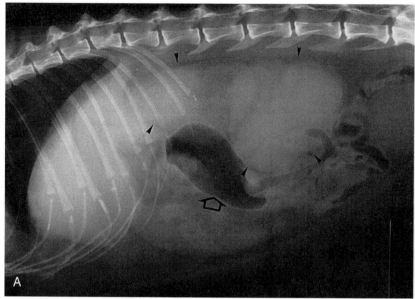

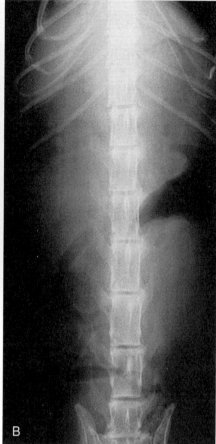

Figure 70–8. *A* and *B,* A 17-year-old castrated male domestic shorthair. Abdominal radiograph: Both kidneys are enlarged and have irregular contours *(arrowheads).* Note the ventral displacement of the colon/bowel due to the kidney mass effect *(arrow in A). Diagnosis: lymphoma.*

Ultrasonography is used to detect cancer by visualizing changes in the echogenicity or size of the organ, or by finding masses. Neoplasia does not have any specific changes on ultrasound that are pathognomonic (Figs. 70–11 to 70–13). Alteration from the normal organ echogenicity, size, and shape is a key aspect of evaluation. It often is helpful to obtain radiographs of the area of interest to help guide the ultrasound examination. Only a small area can be imaged at 1 time using ultrasound, and the images obtained are dependent on the placement of the transducer. If the operator is not consistent and thorough, a small mass or abnormality may be missed easily. Once an abnormality is identified, it is classified as diffuse, focal, or multifocal, as well as hypo-, iso-, or hyperechoic. To obtain a definitive diagnosis, a sample of the abnormal area is necessary. Ultrasound-guided aspirates and biopsies are

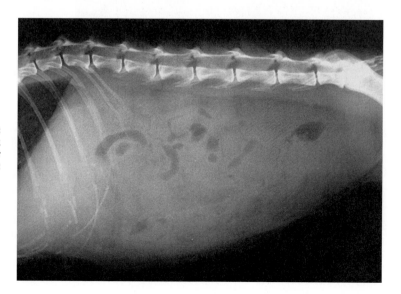

Figure 70–9. A 12-year-old spayed female domestic shorthair. Abdominal radiograph: Note the severe lack of serosal detail throughout the abdomen. *Diagnosis: decreased serosal detail due to minimum effusion and lymphadenopathy secondary to lymphoma.*

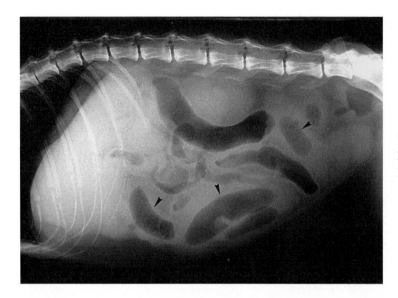

Figure 70–10. An 11-year-old castrated male Siamese. Abdominal radiograph: Note the multiple loops of distended small intestines *(arrowheads)* and the diffuse lack of serosal detail. *Diagnosis: lymphoma.*

minimally invasive, and in experienced hands often provide a definitive diagnosis (see Chapter 15, Cytologic Evaluation of Fine-Needle Liver Biopsies).[7]

Ultrasound-guided aspirates or biopsies may be obtained either free-hand under ultrasound guidance or by using a manufactured biopsy guide that attaches to the transducer. With the biopsy guides, a guide line is projected onto the ultrasound image along the needle path to aid in guiding the needle into the area of interest. A great deal of practice is necessary to develop the skill required to accurately guide a needle free-hand. However, the biopsy guides tend to be rather expensive. If the free-hand technique is employed, practice using a phantom (gelatin with fruit mixed in works well) is highly recommended before attempting this technique in a patient. Using either technique, the key is to direct the needle parallel to the ultrasound beam, allowing

visualization of the needle in the ultrasound image. A needle guide maintains this alignment for the benefit of the sonographer. If using a free-hand technique and the needle plane is not aligned, the needle will not be visualized, an accurate sample may not be obtained, or damage to adjacent structures may be caused inadvertently.

Commonly, aspirates are obtained using a 22-gauge needle attached to a syringe or extension set. Samples are obtained with active suction or by moving the needle in and out of the area of interest. The sample subsequently is sprayed onto a slide for cytologic examination. Biopsies usually are obtained using a Tru-Cut–type needle system. These systems are available in a variety of sizes; however, smaller-gauge varieties are recommended for cats. This author commonly uses 18-gauge biopsy needles with an 11-mm throw to obtain samples from cats. The smaller systems are recommended to help minimize possible complications, which include significant hemorrhage and inadvertent damage to surrounding structures.

Before attempting sample collection, proper patient preparation is necessary. Commonly, aspirates can be obtained safely in calm animals with manual restraint. It is strongly recommended that fractious animals be restrained chemically for aspirates and biopsies. Biopsies may be obtained with the use of only local anesthesia, but chemical restraint often is necessary. The demeanor of the patient, as well as the area of sample collection, should be considered when determining methods of restraint. If aspirates or biopsies are to be obtained from areas that are very vascular or near major vessels, this author recommends short-acting intravenous anesthesia.

In experienced hands, ultrasound is a useful way to examine the internal architecture of structures that may be affected by neoplasia, as well as to help obtain the definitive diagnosis by guiding sample acquisition. It is relatively fast, minimally invasive, and commonly available to most practitioners, and

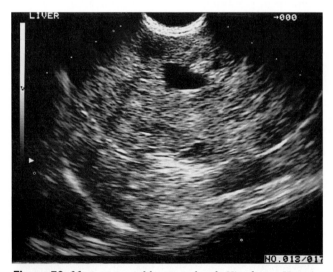

Figure 70–11. A 13-year-old castrated male Himalayan. Hepatic ultrasound: Note the patchy areas of hypo- and hyperechogenicity scattered throughout the hepatic parenchyma. *Diagnosis: biliary cystadenoma.*

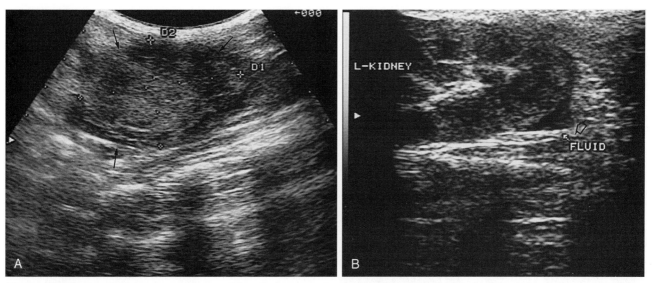

Figure 70–12. *A* and *B*, A 12-year-old spayed female domestic shorthair. Abdominal ultrasound: Multiple heterechoic masses were detected within the mid abdomen consistent with lymphadenopathy (*solid arrows in A*). A small amount of effusion is present (*open arrow in B*). *Diagnosis: lymphoma.*

has become one of the mainstays of diagnostic imaging of neoplasia.

◆ COMPUTED TOMOGRAPHY/ MAGNETIC RESONANCE IMAGING

Both CT and MRI are modalities that provide cross-sectional images of the area of interest. This is advantageous because it allows examination of specific internal structures without superimposition of superficial structures. In CT procedures, the plane from which these images are produced is dependent on patient position, whereas any plane can be obtained in MRI regardless of patient position.

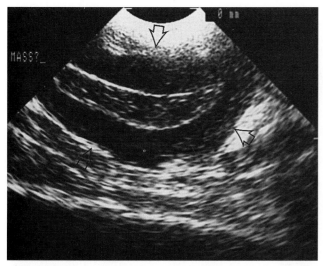

Figure 70–13. An 11-year-old castrated male Siamese. Abdominal ultrasound: Note the severely thickened loop of small intestine with loss of wall layering *(arrows). Diagnosis: lymphoma.*

CT uses the same principles as routine radiography in that x-rays are used to generate the image. Instead of radiographic film as the receiver of the transmitted x-rays, specialized detectors monitor the amount of penetrating radiation from a variety of angles around the patient. A computer takes this information and generates the resultant cross-sectional image. Not only does CT provide images unencumbered by superimposition, it also is much more sensitive in detecting a difference in densities. A 0.5 per cent difference in density is detectable on CT, whereas a 10 per cent difference is necessary to detect a change on conventional radiographs.[8] Thus, CT is especially useful for evaluating bones, but it also is satisfactory for imaging many soft-tissue structures.

MRI uses the inherent magnetic dipole of primarily hydrogen molecules in the patient's body to create images. When an animal is placed in a strong magnetic field, the inherent magnetic dipoles align themselves with the external field (much like a compass works in the Earth's magnetic field). If this alignment is disturbed using an external pulsed radiofrequency, the dipoles become unaligned. When the radiofrequency is turned off, the dipoles start to realign themselves with the external magnetic field. As they do this, they emit other radiofrequencies. Coils in the MRI unit detect these emitted radiofrequencies, and a computer uses this information to create the images. Because hydrogen is one of the primary molecules supplying the MRI signal, most tissues that contain a large amount of water are well-imaged using this technique. Structures such as bone and lung do not provide good signals for MRI. Also, metallic objects such as orthopedic implants can cause severe artifacts.

Both MRI and CT images are enhanced using contrast agents. In CT, an iodinated contrast agent usually is administered intravenously. Gadolinium

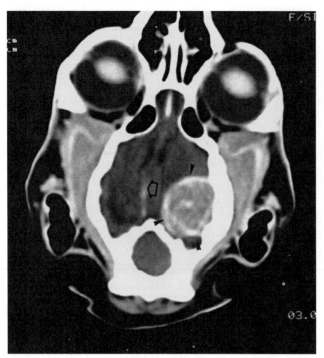

Figure 70–14. An 11-year-old castrated male mixed breed. Computed tomography (CT) scan—brain: There is a large mass with inhomogeneous contrast enhancement in the left cerebrum *(arrowheads)* that is causing a shift of the falx to the right *(arrow)*. *Diagnosis: meningioma.*

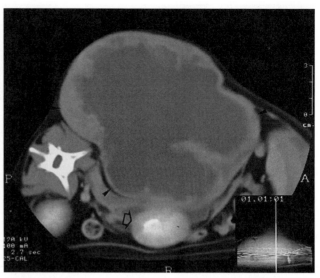

Figure 70–16. A 13-year-old castrated male domestic shorthair. CT scan—abdomen (axial image with contrast enhancement): Note the large contrast-enhancing mass arising from the left body wall *(arrowheads)*. It is causing displacement of the abdominal structures such as the left kidney *(arrow)* but not invading them. *Diagnosis: fibrosarcoma.*

diethylenetriaminetetraacetic acid (DTPA) is the contrast agent used for MRI. These agents distribute within the vascular space, and accumulate in areas of increased vascularity. This is particularly useful in delineating tumors with increased vasculature. Areas of decreased contrast enhancement also may be noted in tumors that have outgrown their blood supply and thus do not accumulate the contrast material. In the brain, these agents also accumulate in areas owing to the breakdown of the blood-brain

barrier that many neoplasms tend to destroy. Thus, contrast may help to "highlight" abnormal areas of an organ. In general, a preliminary scan is performed, followed by the identical acquisition after administration of contrast material (Figs. 70–14 to 70–18).

The cross-sectional images obtained from CT and MRI often are used in the treatment of cancer because they are critical in the planning stages of a radiation-therapy regimen. Images containing the tumor are integrated into a computer program that can utilize that information to tailor a radiation-treatment plan to each individual. Specific body contours and size of organs are integrated to allow the radiation therapist to predict accurately the

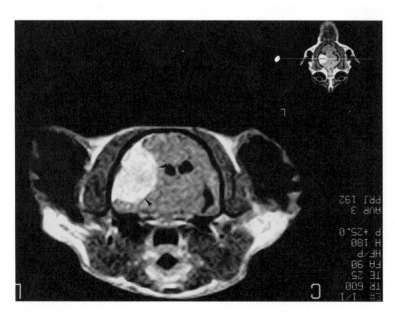

Figure 70–15. A 12-year-old spayed female domestic shorthair. Magnetic resonance imaging (MRI) study—brain (axial image with contrast enhancement): There is a large mass in the left cerebrum that shows intense uniform contrast enhancement *(arrowheads)*. *Diagnosis: meningioma.*

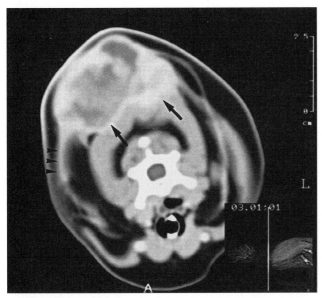

Figure 70–17. A 9-year-old spayed female Maine coon cat. CT scan of cervical region: Note the contrast-enhancing mass dorsal to the cervical vertebrae *(arrows)*. "Finger-like" projections of contrast-enhancing tissue can be seen extending into the adjacent tissues *(arrowheads)*. *Diagnosis: fibrosarcoma.*

amount of radiation that will reach the tumor, which in turn allows much more accurate delivery of the radiation with lessening of the risk to normal tissue.

Interpretation of CT and MRI requires an in-depth knowledge of normal anatomy. As cross-sectional images are obtained, identification of symmetry of bilateral structures is paramount. For example, in the brain, the lateral ventricles should be approximately the same size and position within the cerebral hemispheres. Furthermore, detection of areas of contrast agent accumulation helps in identification of abnormalities. In CT and MRI, contrast enhancement usually is displayed as whiter areas in the gray-scale representation.

◆ NUCLEAR MEDICINE IMAGING

The imaging modalities discussed thus far generally provide information regarding the anatomy of an organ or part of the body. Nuclear medicine imaging often is used to obtain functional information. It involves the use of a radionuclide, usually technetium-99m, that emits gamma rays, and usually is injected alone or linked to a pharmaceutical agent. A gamma camera is used to image the distribution and accumulation of the radioactivity in the body.

Injected technetium-99m accumulates in the salivary tissue, thyroid gland, stomach, and choroid plexus. Because of this, it often is used to evaluate the functional ability of the thyroid. Technetium-99m accumulates through the same pathway as iodine in the thyroid, but it is not organified. Thus, the amount of activity found in the thyroid after

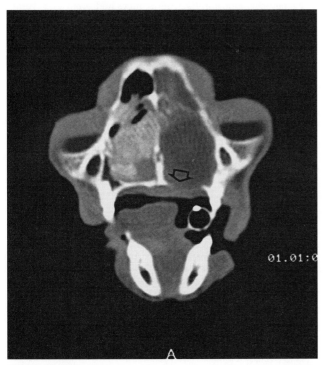

Figure 70–18. A 12-year-old castrated male domestic shorthair. CT scan of nasal cavity: Axial image just rostral to the orbits shows a soft-tissue opacity within the nasal cavities. There is bone lysis of the left side of the hard palate *(arrow)*. *Diagnosis: possible epithelial neoplasm.*

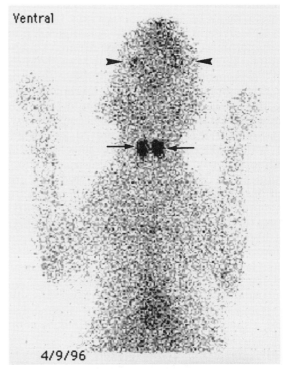

Figure 70–19. A 14-year-old spayed female domestic shorthair. Thyroid scintigraphy: There is increased uptake of the radionuclide in the thyroid *(arrows)* compared with the salivary glands *(arrowheads)* consistent with hyperthyroidism. Notice the uniform and bilateral uptake in the thyroid. *Diagnosis: bilateral adenomatous hyperplasia.*

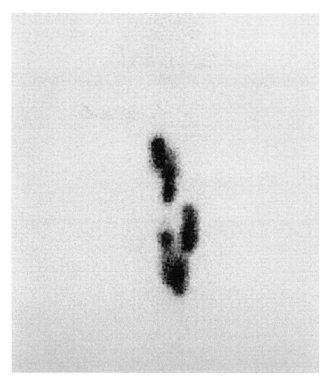

Figure 70–20. A 16-year-old spayed female domestic shorthair. Thyroid scintigraphy: There are multiple areas of increased radionuclide uptake in the cervical region. Note the inhomogeneous uptake in these regions. *Diagnosis: thyroid adenocarcinoma.*

injection is indicative of the functional state. The anatomic detail of the region, however, is poor.

In cats, hyperthyroidism due to benign adenomatous hyperplasia is a common syndrome. A technetium-99m thyroid scan is considered the "gold standard" for diagnosis of hyperthyroidism. In normal cats, the amount of activity in the thyroid compared with that of the salivary glands should be approximately 1:1.[9] Elevation in this ratio is consistent with hyperthyroidism (Figs. 70–19 and 70–20). In addition, a thyroid scan is useful for detecting ectopic functional thyroid tissue. This is critical particularly if surgical excision is being considered as a treatment option for hyperthyroidism. If there is ectopic tissue present within the thorax, surgery is unlikely to cure the patient. In most patients with adenomatous hyperplasia, the uptake of the radionuclide is uniform, and the gland has smooth borders. If the uptake is inhomogeneous, or if the gland is irregular in shape, a malignancy should be suspected. A biopsy usually is advisable in these cases if iodine-131 is considered as the definitive treatment, because a higher dosage may be required to abolish the hyperthyroid state.

Other nuclear medicine imaging procedures may be useful in evaluation of cancer. Functional studies of the kidneys, liver, and gastrointestinal tract may be performed using a variety of techniques involving technetium-99m labeled to various pharmaceuticals that alter the uptake and excretion of the radionuclide. For example, technetium-99m-DTPA often is used to evaluate the blood flow, glomerular filtration rate, and excretion rate of the kidneys. This may be important if neoplasia is infiltrated into 1 kidney. The function of the opposite kidney can be assessed before surgical removal of the affected kidney.

Nuclear medicine studies provide functional information that usually is not available from other imaging modalities. However, these studies require special imaging equipment and facilities, and the animals must be isolated for a short time as a radiation safety precaution. In spite of this, nuclear medicine imaging is becoming available in many private referral centers.

REFERENCES

1. Carlisle HC, Thrall DE: A comparison of normal feline thoracic radiographs made in dorsal versus ventral recumbency. Vet Radiol 23:3–9, 1982.
2. Suter PF: Methods of radiographic interpretation, radiographic signs and dynamic factors in the radiographic diagnosis of thoracic disease. In Suter PF, Lord PF (eds): Thoracic Radiography: A Text Atlas of Thoracic Diseases of the Dog and Cat. Wettswil, Switzerland, Peter F. Suter, 1984, pp. 79–126.
3. Koblik PD: Radiographic appearance of primary lung tumors in cats: A review of 41 cases. Vet Radiol 27:66–73, 1986.
4. Silverman S, Poulos PW, Suter PF: Cavitary pulmonary lesions in animals. J Am Vet Radiol Soc 17:134–146, 1976.
5. Feeney DA, Johnston GR: The kidneys and ureters. In Thrall DE (ed): Textbook of Veterinary Diagnostic Radiology, 3rd ed. Philadelphia, WB Saunders, 1995, pp. 466–479.
6. Yeager AE, Anderson WI: Study of association between histologic features and echogenicity of architecturally normal cat kidneys. Am J Vet Res 50:860–863, 1989.
7. Leveille R, Partington BP, Biller DS, et al: Complications after ultrasound guided biopsy of abdominal structures in dogs and cats: 246 cases (1984–1991). J Am Vet Med Assoc 203:413–415, 1993.
8. Assheuer J, Sager M: MRI and CT Atlas of the Dog. London, Blackwell Science, 1997, p. v.
9. Brawner WR: Thyroid and parathyroid imaging. In Berry CR, Daniel GB (eds): Handbook of Veterinary Nuclear Medicine. Raleigh, North Carolina State University, 1996, pp. 71–79.

SUGGESTED READING

Assheuer J, Sager M: MRI and CT Atlas of the Dog. London, Blackwell Science, 1997.
Berry CR, Daniel GB (eds): Handbook of Veterinary Nuclear Medicine. Raleigh, North Carolina State University, 1996.
Green RW (ed): Small Animal Ultrasound. Philadelphia, Lippincott-Raven, 1996.
Nyland TG, Mattoon JS (eds): Veterinary Diagnostic Ultrasound. Philadelphia, WB Saunders, 1995.
Thrall DE (ed): Textbook of Veterinary Diagnostic Radiology, 3rd ed. Philadelphia, WB Saunders, 1995.

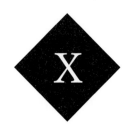

Population Medicine

Dennis F. Lawler, Editor

◆ Understanding and Controlling of Feral
  Cat Populations 561
◆ Feline Animal Shelter Medicine 571
◆ Immunocontraception to Help Control
  Feral Cat Populations 577
◆ Cognitive Dysfunction in Geriatric Cats 583
◆ Hip Dysplasia 592
◆ Understanding the Feline Genome 600
◆ Molecular Diagnosis of Gangliosidoses: A Model for
  Elimination of Inherited Diseases in Pure Breeds . . . 615
◆ Quality of Life in Long-Term Confinement 621

Still-Current Information Found in *Consultations in Feline Internal Medicine 2*:

Dermatophytosis (Chapter 29), p. 219
Congenital Abnormalities of the Spinal Cord and Vertebrae
    (Chapter 52), p. 413
Epidemiological Investigation of Disease and Health in Fe-
    line Populations (Chapter 73), p. 593
Surveillance, Prevention, and Control of Viral Diseases in
    Catteries (Chapter 75), p. 615
Surveillance and Management of Parasites in Catteries
    (Chapter 76), p. 621
Control and Prevention of Dermatophytes in Catteries
    (Chapter 77), p. 627
Nutritional Management and Nutrition-Related Diseases in
    Feline Populations (Chapter 80), p. 653

Still-Current Information Found in *Consultations in Feline Internal Medicine 3*:

The Role of *Bordetella* in Feline Respiratory Disease (Chap-
    ter 6), p. 34
Dermatophytosis: Advances in Therapy and Control (Chap-
    ter 25), p. 177
Nervous System Neoplasia (Chapter 54), p. 418
Radiographic and Myelographic Diagnosis of Spinal Dis-
    ease (Chapter 55), p. 425
Recommendations for FeLV- and FIV-Positive Cats With
    Cancer (Chapter 72), p. 572
Strategies for Controlling Viral Infections in Feline Popula-
    tions (Chapter 76), p. 603
Public Health and Important Zoonoses in Feline Popula-
    tions (Chapter 77), p. 611

Elsewhere in *Consultations in Feline Internal Medicine 4*:

Hemobartonellosis (Chapter 2), p. 12

Cat Ownership by Immunosuppressed People (Chapter 3), p. 18

Update on the Diagnosis and Management of Feline Herpesvirus-1 Infections (Chapter 7), p. 51

Diagnosis of Occult Hyperthyroidism (Chapter 18), p. 145

Complications of Therapy for Hyperthyroidism (Chapter 19), p. 151

Adrenocortical Disease (Chapter 20), p. 159

Heartworm Disease (Chapter 33), p. 253

Medical Management of Chronic Renal Failure (Chapter 44), p. 328

Cerebral Meningiomas: Diagnostic and Therapeutic Considerations (Chapter 50), p. 385

Neuronal Storage Disorders (Chapter 51), p. 393

Mucopolysaccharidosis (Chapter 57), p. 450

71

◆ Understanding and Controlling of Feral Cat Populations

Margaret R. Slater

What is a feral cat? What should be done about them? Feral cats are the offspring of owned or abandoned outdoor, intact cats. They are too poorly socialized to be handled. They can be found in cities, in suburbs, on farms, and in wilderness areas. They are seen near hospitals, schools, restaurants, barns, and abandoned buildings, or anywhere adequate food and shelter are available.[1] Although the cats themselves are at the center of the storm, feral cats really are a result of a "people problem." Some people feed them, whereas others are willing to provide more in-depth care. Some people sympathize with them, but others believe they should be killed. Even the veterinary profession is divided, as demonstrated by conflicting and often passionate letters published in the *Journal of the American Veterinary Medical Association*[2-8] (AVMA) after an article on controlling feral cats through neuter and release,[9] and a later AVMA news report on cat welfare and overpopulation.[10] Several of these letters were based on personal experiences and anecdotes, which adds to the emotion and the confusion.

Historically, feral cats were trapped and euthanized, because this was believed to be the kindest approach for a homeless, unwanted cat. This still is the approach used in many parts of the country, especially where rabies is a problem or where public interest in cats is low. This, however, rarely is an effective or humane long-term solution. In general, trap and remove/euthanize is a only a short-term solution, unless food and shelter suitable for cats are removed from the habitat.[9, 11, 12] If food sources (including feeders) are not eliminated, cats from nearby areas move into the environmental vacuum left by the cats that were trapped and euthanized. Usually, there also are 1 or 2 cats that elude trappers, and these invariably contribute to repopulating the area. During the 1990s, as the animal welfare movement has continued to evolve and to re-evaluate positions on killing healthy animals, various trap, neuter, and return programs (TNR) have been proposed and adopted. Denmark and the United Kingdom have been leaders in this approach.[13] In the past several years, the AVMA, Cat Fanciers Association, American Humane Association, and Humane Society of the United States all have suggested that a form of TNR commonly referred to as trap, test, vaccinate, alter, return, and monitor (TTVAR-M) should be considered as an option to euthanasia. This is the level of care referred to in this chapter as a *managed feral cat colony.*

Another continuing source of conflict exists between wildlife and bird enthusiasts and cat owners.[14] This conflict is not limited to feral cats, because any outdoor cat may hunt. Whereas a relatively large literature addresses some elements of the impact of cats on wildlife, most of the work has been done within island ecosystems that are not representative of most of the United States. In addition, a number of these studies have been cited out of context or extrapolated inappropriately.[14]

◆ EXTENT OF THE PROBLEM

The exact magnitude of the feral cat problem is unknown. Not all authors use the same definitions, and wide geographic variability likely exists in the numbers of feral cats and the extent of the associated problems. Two surveys of pet ownership in California provided estimates of the magnitude of the "unowned" cat problem.[15, 16] The first study (in 1993) included a question about the number of cats fed that were not owned by the household.[15] The responses indicated that 10 per cent of householders in Santa Clara County fed cats that they do not own.[15] This included 49 householders (47 per cent) who did not claim to own any cats. Respondents to the survey estimated that they fed 351 unowned cats, accounting for 40 per cent of the cats enumerated in the survey. A similar survey done in San Diego County (in 1995) was comparable: 9 per cent of householders fed cats they did not own, with these accounting for about 30 per cent of the cats reported in the survey.[16] In Massachusetts, during a 3-year period, 15 per cent of pet-owning households fed cats that were not their own.[17] Some of the "unowned" cats described in these studies probably were owned but unconfined and free-roaming. However, if these cats do not receive veterinary care and are not sterilized or vaccinated, they will contribute to pet overpopulation and the potential for zoonotic disease problems. Accurate extrapolation of these observations to other geographic areas is not possible, but these data do suggest that feral cat numbers are sizable in some parts of the country. Alley Cat Allies, one of the largest nonprofit feral cat organizations, estimates that 30 to 60 million feral cats live in the United States.[18]

Statistics on the numbers of cats acquired as strays, or that leave the household by "straying," also support the idea that the numbers of feral cats are substantial. In a study in 2 western United States cities, 20 per cent of cats left the household as strays.[19] In one of these cities, 7 of 27 cats were acquired as strays.[20] In 2 studies in Massachusetts, 17 per cent of cats were acquired as strays in 1991, and 17 per cent of cats left the household by "disappearing."[17]

Feral cats clearly are part of the pet overpopulation problem that results in millions of cats being euthanized each year. Feral cats are both a cause and an effect of overpopulation: a cause by producing more kittens, and an effect of irresponsible or uninformed cat ownership. Furthermore, cat popularity has increased to the point that cats have become the most popular pet in the United States since 1996, with some 59.1 million cats owned.[21] Although sterilization rates in some parts of the country are quite high, cats continue to have litters before sterilization. One study in Massachusetts revealed that 91.5 per cent of female cats were spayed, and 90 per cent of male cats were neutered. Yet, 15 per cent of the sterilized females had produced an average of 2 litters each before sterilization.[22] Another study in Massachusetts examined reasons for these litters.[17] These reasons in rank order were: owners could not afford sterilization of pet cats; owners thought the cat was too young to become pregnant; an intact indoor cat got out; owners did not get around to pet sterilization; and the cat was still nursing kittens. A San Diego County study reported that 84 per cent of cats were sterilized; yet 19 per cent of females had a litter before being spayed.[16] Fifty-eight per cent of these litters were the result of people not realizing that the cat could become pregnant at a young age, or that the cat was in estrus. Similar figures were reported in Santa Clara County.[15] Clearly, more cats need to be sterilized at younger ages, and owners must be educated more thoroughly about feline reproduction.

Cat owners have been exposed increasingly to the issues surrounding feral cats through the lay press[23-25] and a multitude of Internet sites. Local and national seminars have been developed by a range of agencies and organizations, including Alley Cat Allies, the San Francisco Society for the Prevention of Cruelty to Animals (SPCA), and (jointly) the American Humane and Cat Fanciers Associations. Alley Cat Allies was one of the first national organizations to provide useful information about caring for feral cats, and advice for veterinarians working with feral cats. Their website (www.alleycat.org) and that of the Feral Cat Coalition (www.feralcat.com) in California have information and links to many Internet sources.

Veterinarians also are being drawn into the feral cat arena. Sixty-three veterinarians (37 per cent of attendees) at a Texas continuing education seminar (in 1999) responded to a survey about feral cats. (Dawn Fradkin, veterinary student at Texas A&M University and founder of the Aggie Feral Cat Alliance, personal communication, May 1999). Of these respondents, 70 per cent saw feral cats in their prac-

Table 71–1. Current and Potential Participation in Individual Feral Cat Care and Potential Involvement in Trap, Neuter, and Return Programs by 63 Veterinarians Attending a Feline Continuing Education Seminar

Type of Participation*	Willingness to Treat Individual Feral Cats (%)	Willingness to Participate in a Community TNR Program (%)
Discounted services	57	54
Euthanasia	40	n/a
Like any other client	33	n/a
Volunteer services	25	29
Donated supplies	8	14
Use of facilities	n/a	14
Use of equipment	n/a	11
No participation	6	27

Abbreviations: n/a, not applicable; TNR, trap, neuter, and return.
*Respondents could choose more than 1 answer. Of these respondents, 79 per cent currently treat individual feral cats. Only 6 respondents currently were aware of TNR programs in their area.

tices, although only 9.5 per cent indicated that there was a formal TNR program in their location. Table 71–1 indicates the types of services for feral cats that veterinarians currently are providing or would be willing to provide.

For veterinary respondents not willing to participate in a formal program, personal injury was cited as the number 1 reason by 65 per cent, followed by liability and time commitment (53 per cent). Risks to pets (41 per cent), zoonotic diseases (41 per cent), and risks to local wildlife (35 per cent) were listed next. Among all respondents, most of whom do see feral cats in their practices, only 6 per cent believed that feral cats posed a serious threat to wildlife in their area. Twice this number of respondents indicated that owned cats were a threat to wildlife.

◆ DEFINITIONS

One reason for the confusion about definitions is that cats can and will change lifestyles during their lifetimes.[14] For the purposes of animal care and control, or veterinary care and follow-up, any cat that is too-poorly socialized to be handled (must be trapped or sedated for examination) and that cannot be placed into a typical pet home is *feral*. This is the definition of feral for the remainder of this chapter.

A cat's lifestyle can be defined by 4 parameters: confinement status, ownership level, sociability spectrum, and location description. The first 3 parameters are not yes/no classifications but should be considered to vary across a spectrum. They are designed to be functional descriptions in the context of the welfare and environment of the cats. For example, if all owned cats received adequate health care, there still would be a large number of unowned cats (cats that receive little or no care from people) that were never brought to a veterinary practice. If the veterinary profession could find a way to encourage people to become more responsible and committed pet owners (e.g., move people along the ownership scale toward the most committed and responsible endpoint), these owners then would provide veterinary care for their cats for the first time, and many cats also would receive a higher level of care than they currently enjoy, because improved veterinary care is one result of owner commitment.

Confinement Status

Confinement ranges from totally indoor to indoor/outdoor to always outdoors.[14] Cats may be outdoors but also confined to a pen, run, or fenced yard. Cats that are not confined to the house or an enclosure are *free-roaming*. These are the cats that usually are problematic with regard to pet overpopulation and nuisance. Feral cats usually are a subpopulation of free-roaming cats.[14]

Ownership Level

Ownership ranges from a cherished pet cat with all the health care, food, and attention necessary (committed owner) to cats that are completely unnoticed by any person.[26] Other graduated levels of ownership include: cats for which some person claims ownership but does not provide more than the most basic care; cats that are cared-for on a daily basis by a person, but are free-roaming; and "loosely-owned" cats that have been fed and cared for at some level, but are not claimed by any person. *Stray cats* are free-roaming cats that are currently or recently owned, but are lost or missing from the home. Stray cats may be returned to their owners if the owners are looking for them, or if they are found and have some kind of identification. Stray cats not reunited with their owners may be adopted, euthanized, or killed, or may remain free-roaming and eventually become feral. *Abandoned* cats are strays whose owners deliberately leave them behind when they move, or the cats may be dropped at some distant location. Stray cats usually are at least somewhat socialized after their initial separation from their owners. Veterinarians typically see cats that are owned by a relatively responsible person, but also may find themselves dealing with stray or never-owned cats.

Sociability Spectrum

Socialization level ranges from highly social pets, seeking attention from any and all people (lap-cat type) to cats that never have had contact with people and fear people (born in the wild, completely feral). Cats also may fear people but have some interactions with them, or they may be "at ease"

with people but not seek attention. These estimations of sociability also can be modified by location. For example, most veterinarians are familiar with owned, indoor cats that are difficult to handle in the veterinarian's office, but are well-socialized in the home setting.

Location Descriptions

These are phrases like *barn* or *farm cat, neighborhood cat, doorstep colony*, or *house cat*. These terms were used historically to describe cats with regard to their sociability (e.g., a farm cat was feral, or an alley cat was a feral stray). But these underlying assumptions contribute to the confusion regarding definitions. In some settings, the barn cat may be as well-socialized, provided-for, and loved as the indoor cat.

Veterinarians have patients that could be described by many different combinations of these parameters. The implications of these descriptions are important to the degree that they reflect the owner's level of commitment, the ability to provide care, and the cat's exposures to health risks. Any free-roaming cat may become feral or contribute to the feral cat population if it is unsterilized. This means that any unaltered, owned, stray, or abandoned cat can be part of the overpopulation problem. Any cat born "in the wild" unless caught and tamed, will start its life as a feral cat. Feral adult cats sometimes can be socialized to varying degrees, but the time, patience, and commitment needed rarely are practical or available. Typically, socialized previously-feral cats will be socialized only with 1 or 2 people; however, on rare occasions, they may become well-socialized to strangers.

◆ CONCEPTUAL FRAMEWORK

There are 3 main elements that affect feral cat control in the United States. The first is grass-roots efforts; the second, service providers; and the third, resource and teaching providers. These are not always clear-cut and mutually exclusive categories, but they do provide a useful framework for discussion. Veterinarians may be approached by people or may become involved with these elements in a wide variety of ways.

Grass-roots efforts include individuals with interest in feral cats, loose networks of caretakers, and established nonprofit organizations. Cat owners, shelter workers or volunteers, and veterinarians all may find themselves involved at the grass-roots level in various ways including caring for colonies, helping established grass-roots or service groups, and starting nonprofit groups. Nonprofit organizations tend to have 1 of 2 philosophical approaches: providing a broad range of programs (trapping, sterilization, fostering, and adopting), or providing a primary focus on free or very low-cost sterilization for a large number of feral cats. The choice of approaches will vary with the organizers' interests and expertise, as well as with the availability of subsidized sterilization in their geographic location.

Service providers consist of 3 main kinds of organizations: animal care and control agencies or humane societies, veterinary hospitals, and animal industry businesses. Donations by service providers to nonprofit groups of feral cat caretakers and supporters may be tax-deductible. Animal care and control organizations or humane societies may be involved at various levels, such as loaning traps; providing trapping assistance, humane euthanasia, pet placement, or subsidized spay/neuter vouchers or programs; or coordinating feral colony management. They also may offer referrals to veterinarians or caretakers with expertise in feral cat work. They may hire veterinarians to do in-house subsidized spay/neuter programs that can benefit feral cat caretakers. Animal care and control programs usually have the additional task of enforcing local ordinances.

Veterinary hospitals also provide spaying and neutering services. This may be done by individual arrangements with established clients or groups, use of vouchers or coupons for subsidized services, or a major commitment to reduced-cost surgical sterilization. Offering early-age spay/neuter is a very important service for feral cat caretakers, because kittens over age 8 weeks rarely can be tamed but should not be returned to the feral colony unsterilized. Studies on prepubertal gonadectomy demonstrate that sterilization for kittens as young as age 6 weeks is safe and practical.[27, 28] Rabies vaccinations, testing for feline leukemia virus (FeLV) and feline immunodeficiency virus (FIV), advice on control of infectious diseases (especially respiratory), and euthanasia also are key services provided by veterinarians.

Animal industry businesses include providers of food, cages, microchips, traps and other handling equipment, materials to build shelters for colonies, and other animal care equipment. Pet food companies, home and garden retailers, and pharmaceutical companies may be willing to donate, or provide at reduced cost, products for feral cat caretakers or veterinarians. Incorporation of nonprofit groups gives the whole program more legitimacy, and direct association with veterinarians also is helpful in obtaining needed equipment at prices below retail.

The third element, *resource and teaching providers*, often comes from the previously mentioned groups. These individuals and groups are critical to the discovery and dissemination of helpful, accurate, and timely information about all aspects of feral cat care and ecology. These may be people who have years of experience in trapping feral cats, or in starting grass-roots organizations, or who have access to large networks of people who have experience with feral cats. Scientists slowly are becoming involved in data collection and analysis of feral cat issues, and there is a continuing need for veterinarians with special orientation to cats to contribute their knowledge of "herd health," public health, and general health care for cats.

◆ ISSUES INVOLVING FERAL CATS

The issues involving feral cats can be divided into 5 main areas: (1) public health, particularly rabies control; (2) impact on wildlife and birds; (3) complaints about nuisance problems; (4) welfare of the cats themselves; and (5) people's perceptions of cats and their role as pets and working animals.[29] The relative importance of each of these areas depends on the specific circumstances.

Any free-roaming cat, owned or unclaimed, socialized or feral, potentially can be involved in transmission of zoonotic diseases. Lists of diseases have been published.[30] However, the diseases most likely to be issues with regard to feral cats are rabies, toxoplasmosis, plague, toxocariasis, dermatophytosis, and bartonellosis. It is important to remember that feral cats are only 1 component of the free-roaming population, and that veterinarians also must work toward getting client-owned animals that are free-roaming protected from or treated for these zoonoses. The goal is to prevent owned patients from spreading zoonotic diseases, while at the same time implementing actions to decrease the risks from zoonotic diseases in feral cats.

Rabies is by far the disease that causes the most concern in most parts of the United States. This is true particularly in light of the increasing numbers of cats diagnosed with rabies in the last several years (more than twice as many cats [300] as dogs in 1997).[31] Among the 22 large-scale human exposures to rabid or potentially rabid animals between 1990 and 1996, 3 were caused by cats.[32] Two of these cats had been vaccinated recently. Most of these large-scale exposures could have been avoided if very young animals that could be incubating rabies (having unknown medical histories), or that had been vaccinated only recently, were screened more carefully before being taken to public facilities and handled by large numbers of people. This type of large-scale exposure to feral cats is likely to occur if young kittens that are incubating the disease are fostered, adopted, or taken to schools or parties. It is important to keep rabies in perspective and remember that nearly 93 per cent of reported rabies cases in 1997 were in wild animals, and that none of the human rabies cases that occurred between 1990 and 1997 had exposure history that included cats.[31]

Several practical points should be made with regard to feral cats and rabies. Inexperienced feral cat caretakers and the general public should be cautioned against cornering or trying to handle unknown free-roaming cats. Cat bites often are due to people trying to pick up or catch by hand a cat they have been feeding or watching for some time. Cats in managed colonies all should be vaccinated for rabies at the time of sterilization, using a 3-year vaccine. Caretakers should make serious efforts to recapture cats in feral colonies to provide revaccination at 3-year intervals. Because many cats become more social with their caretakers over time, revaccination should be possible for the majority of cats. By keeping a critical mass of feral cats vaccinated against rabies in managed colonies, a herd immunity effect may be produced,[33] potentially providing a barrier between wildlife and human beings, and decreasing one of the major public health considerations regarding feral cats.

Toxoplasmosis has become of increasing concern but is a disease that is not confined to feral cats.[14] Estimated prevalence of *Toxoplasma gondii* antibodies in cats is quite variable, likely owing to the range of populations tested, and the choice of tests. Prevalence in various groups of free-ranging cats has been reported at 11, 33, 68, and 80 per cent.[34–37] In 1 study, risk factors for infection of women during pregnancy included cleaning a cat litter box, eating unwashed vegetables and fruits and undercooked or raw meat, drinking untreated surface water, and playing with children in a sandbox.[38] However, living in a neighborhood with cats was not by itself a risk factor in that study. While vaccines intended to prevent shedding of oocysts in cats are being evaluated, no real prevention is available currently.[30, 39] Because most cats shed oocysts for only a few weeks after primary infection and usually do not shed again, young cats that are hunters are most likely to be shedding oocysts.[36, 39] It is possible that keeping feral cats in well-managed colonies where food is provided and no kittens are born could help decrease shedding of oocysts into the environment by these cats.

Plague *(Yersinia pestis)* is a disease that is seen with increasing frequency, although it is much more limited geographically than toxoplasmosis. Human beings most often acquire the disease by contact with infected fleas, but contact with infected animals also may result in transmission.[40, 41] Cats can carry infected fleas and, when ill, transmit the disease directly. Feral cats, because they hunt and are likely to be in proximity to rodents and fleas, can be at risk for plague in the southwestern United States.[14] Flea control and care in handling feral cats, particularly those with signs of pneumonia, will decrease the risk of zoonotic transmission.[42]

Other zoonotic diseases that may be transmitted by feral cats include toxocariasis, dermatophytosis, and bartonellosis. However, these diseases likewise are not confined to feral cats. Owned cats also may have roundworms, and dogs can contribute to environmental contamination. Whereas it is easy to say that dogs and cats infected with roundworms should not be allowed to roam, enforcement is extremely difficult and control of this disease has not been accomplished.[43, 44] Dermatophytosis is most likely to be a problem in caretakers who are treating injured or ill feral cats, or who are fostering kittens.

Direct exposure otherwise is more limited if public contact with these cat populations is restricted by leaving only feral cats in colonies. Dermatophytosis also is a health problem in owned indoor cats, farm or barn cats, pet outlets, and in other populations that include numbers of young cats. *Bartonella* species (primarily *B. henselae* but also *B. quintana*) can produce a variety of clinical diseases in human beings.[45–47] Cat-scratch disease is the most common manifestation of *B. henselae* infection in immunocompetent human beings, and generally is self-limiting.[47] Several less common manifestations include Parinaud's oculoglandular syndrome with neurologic signs and central nervous system disease, among others.[47] In immunosuppressed or immunocompromised human beings, bacillary angiomatosis and bacillary parenchymal peliosis may occur; these diseases require appropriate antibiotic therapy and usually respond well to treatment.[46, 47] The level of risk for bartonellosis from different populations of cats still is unclear, but feral cats most likely would expose persons fostering kittens, because free-roaming kittens have been implicated in the spread of cat-scratch disease.[14, 45]

Killing birds and wildlife is a common complaint about free-roaming cats in general. Cats often are portrayed as hunting machines, and implicated in decreasing bird populations and biodiversity. Studies of cats and prey are of 3 main types: those of island ecosystems; those of pet or free-ranging owned cats; and those of mostly feral cats. These studies have been conducted in a variety of habitats, and have used various study designs. The authors of these reports have cautioned against extrapolation, and have recognized sources of bias.[14, 48, 49] Yet, their results are extrapolated[50, 51] and sensationalized ("Is there a killer in your house?").[52] Although free-roaming cats, both owned and feral, can and do hunt, no one has shown that they have a detrimental impact on prey species in mainland ecosystems. In many cases, the cats are one of many predators,[53] and may be filling the role of some other small predator that is no longer present.[48, 54] In fact, habitat destruction for birds is cited as the most serious problem.[55, 56] Pollution, competition by other bird species, and predators such as raccoons and opossums are other major problems for bird populations.[55] Window collisions, hunting of birds by native predators, and cats are much lower on the list of causes of bird deaths.[56] Conclusions about the impact of cats on wildlife and birds, therefore, depend on accurate, situation-specific data regarding a particular area or ecosystem.

Despite a lack of data supporting cats as playing a major part in decreasing numbers of prey at the species level, free-roaming cats do hunt and kill some number of individual prey animals. This leads to a philosophical view that cats, as a domestic species, should not be killing wildlife. Allowing cats to do so indicates that owners place more value on the cats' "need" to hunt than on the lives of the wildlife species. Furthermore, because cats (especially owned cats) are well-fed, their numbers and interactions with prey species are not controlled in the same way as wild predators. This means that cats do not fit into the ecosystem in an integrated fashion.

Nuisance complaints regarding cats frequently are directed to animal care and control agencies and, at times, to local government. Specific complaints include spraying; fecal contamination; yowling and fighting; presence of sick, injured, or dead cats; digging in gardens; and dirty footprints on cars. Some of these problems are minimized by sterilization, but others will occur anytime cats are found outdoors. One animal control agency in Florida found that cat complaints in a 6-square-block area were cut in half the year after a TNR program was instituted. (Linda Haller, Animal Services Department, Orange County Government, FL, personal communication, February 1999).

When the issue of the welfare of feral cats themselves is raised, 4 general approaches to control are outlined: (1) trap, remove, and euthanize; (2) trap, remove, and either relocate or place in sanctuaries; (3) TNR feral cats, adopting tame adults and kittens; and (4) do nothing. Veterinarians may be asked to euthanize feral cats in situations in which the cats are living in an unsafe environment and there is no caretaker. However, veterinarians increasingly are likely to be involved in some nonlethal management system, which would be a variation of options 2 and 3 (TNR). Relocation rarely is recommended owing to difficulty of finding a suitable site, time involved, stress on the cats, and low survival rates at new sites. Sanctuaries typically are enclosed, outdoor or indoor homes for groups of cats. Sanctuaries may include cats that are partly or very socialized; a subset of these cats often is available for adoption to appropriate homes.

In TTVAR-M, all cats in the colony should be: (1) too unsocialized to place in a typical home, (2) tested for FeLV and FIV; (3) spayed or neutered (or in the process of being trapped for that purpose); (4) vaccinated, at least for rabies; (5) provided with appropriate shelter, food, and water; and (6) monitored on a daily or alternate-day basis by a concerned caretaker. There is some debate about the need for FeLV and FIV testing, particularly if funds are scarce and testing cats will mean that fewer are able to be sterilized. These arguments sometimes are based on testing of cats in an area for a period of time to establish that the diseases are rare. Other arguments state that rates of infection are low in feral cat populations, and that spaying and neutering will decrease fighting and hence transmission of the diseases. Part of the job of the caretaker is to watch for health problems in colony cats,[57] trap and sterilize new feral cats, trap and remove tame cats, and trap and remove kittens young enough to be tamed (usually less than 8 weeks of age). Whereas placement of tame cats and kittens into good homes is the ideal, this can be surprisingly difficult, as can finding suitable foster homes in which to tame the kittens.

Doing nothing is an approach that historically has been taken as well, often by default. Many communities have no organized program for dealing with feral cats, and have few caretakers. Usually, this approach results in continued breeding and death of cats and continuing complaints and cost to animal control agencies. High kitten mortalities (greater than 50 per cent) are common.

◆ ROLES OF THE VETERINARIAN

The veterinarian's involvement in the feral cat solution is 2-fold. The first and most obvious role is to provide surgical sterilization of feral cats. This service often is a key factor in the success of a feral cat control program. Veterinarians may provide this service at an animal shelter or a subsidized or reduced-cost spay/neuter clinic, as a component of their regular practice routine, or as volunteers for grass-roots organizations. Spaying and neutering are a critical part of coping with pet overpopulation and feral cats, and are controlled solely by veterinarians.[26, 58] Prepubertal gonadectomy has been shown to be safe and to have no negative side-effects.[59–61]

The second veterinary role is education of clients, the general public, and local and state officials. For clients, education is about responsible pet ownership: (1) spaying or neutering of pets; (2) providing identification to improve the likelihood of getting the cat back if it wanders; (3) preventing public health problems like toxocariasis and rabies; (4) matching owners with pets, so that those pets remain in the household; (5) providing assistance with behavior questions and problems; and (6) finding new homes for cats that no longer can be kept by original owners, so that cats are not turned out of the house, left behind, or abandoned in the countryside. Veterinarians also can provide education to the public or city government about public health risks and options for control of feral cats. When working with feral cat caretakers, advice on infectious disease control, vaccination protocols, nutrition, parasite control, and basic hygiene and disinfection guidance also can be invaluable, as can accessible written material concerning quarantine procedures for sanctuaries.

Veterinarians may volunteer to help in established feral cat grass-roots groups. This most often takes the form of surgical services for one of the large-scale feral cat surgery programs such as that of the Feral Cat Coalition in California or Operation Catnip in North Carolina and Florida. These programs offer free subsidized sterilization once each month to anyone caring for a feral cat. Veterinary volunteers perform the surgeries, with dozens of cats being spayed or neutered, ear-tipped (removal of the top third of 1 ear), and vaccinated in 1 day. Some veterinarians feel a more personal pull toward working with the feral cat problem. Serving as an organizer for a new or developing grass-roots group or as an advocate for feral cats, representing oneself or a group, can be very effective ways to be involved. Veterinarians are highly respected and regarded in most such circles, and often their opinions carry a great deal of weight.

◆ FERAL CATS IN THE PRACTICE SETTING

When dealing with feral cat caretakers individually or with caretakers as part of organized groups, the most important thing is to determine a personal comfort level for services and health care. Table 71–2 lists some important considerations. As part of learning about feral cats, some caretakers may offer a veterinarian the opportunity to see their colonies and the level of care provided. Caretakers usually are extremely dedicated to their cats, and can be very intense when trying to obtain care for them. If one offers discounted services, keep a record of the full costs and then discount the services to keep track of what is being spent on this part of the practice. Veterinarians working with feral cat caretakers emphasize the need to be empathetic, have flexibility, and avoid judgmental attitudes. But some caretakers, like any other clients, may try to take advantage of a veterinarian's compassion and generosity. They also may "test" a veterinarian by bringing in a few cats before revealing that they care for hundreds. For these reasons, working out a personal philosophy for care of feral cats ahead of time will be very helpful. Putting these guidelines in writing when dealing with caretakers also may help preclude friction.

From a practical perspective, dealing with feral cats in private practice requires some specific considerations.[12] It is important that cats arrive in cages

Table 71–2. Questions That Will Help to Determine Comfort Level and General Philosophy of Care

1. What services will the practice offer (e.g., spay/neuter only, spay/neuter with other health care, required rabies vaccination, education and advice about cat population medicine)?
2. What is the policy for feline leukemia virus and/or feline immunodeficiency virus testing (e.g., all cats tested and positives euthanized, test a few cats from each colony to determine disease frequency, no testing)?
3. What level of follow-up care must be provided by the caretaker (very limited or only well-managed and monitored colonies)?
4. What is the fee structure (e.g., no discounts, discounts on only spaying and neutering, flat percentage discount, discounts for nonprofit feral cat organizations only)?
5. What numbers of cats can be seen (e.g., number of surgeries per week, on only specific days)?
6. What are the logistics of scheduling and delivering care (e.g., scheduling of cats to be done through routine channels like any other client or by only one representative of the group, all feral cats must be in traps, all people who deal with the feral cats must be vaccinated for rabies)?

that truly will contain them, such as a humane trap or strong carrier, with only 1 cat per trap or carrier. Providing feral cats with a 15- to 30-minute quiet period after they arrive, and before doing anything else, will decrease stress and should improve the smoothness of anesthetic induction. Some programs and veterinarians accept feral cats only in humane traps, because cats can be confined for injection more easily than in an airline-type plastic carrier. Cats may be kept in their traps for the duration of their stay in the clinic. This decreases the likelihood of escape. If cats are to be transferred to different housing, the transfer always should be done in a closed room with a solid ceiling (cats can escape through a suspended tile-type ceiling with great speed).

Most cat cages in private practices are poorly suited to hold feral cats, especially for any length of time, and the cats may be difficult to remove or restrain. A specially designed feral cat box that will fit into a regular cage is available (Animal Care Equipment & Services, Inc., Crestline, CA. For a picture of the feral cat handling system, see www.animal-care.com/cata06a). It was designed by animal shelter professionals, including veterinarians who handle large numbers of feral cats. This box has a guillotine front door for transferring cats from a humane trap, and a swivel side door that can be closed or opened to allow the cat access to the box or to contain the cat in the box so the regular cage can be cleaned. Holes on the sides allow a cat to be injected while inside the box.

Squeeze cages have been designed to fit against the end of humane traps (Tomahawk Live Trap Company, Tomahawk, WI; Animal Care Equipment & Services, Inc., Crestline, CA). These wire cages allow the handler to press the cat against the side of the cage for injection. Cats also may be restrained in the bottom of a tipped-up wire humane trap with a comb-type slide-in wall (Fig. 71–1) (available in metal version Trap Isolator from Animal Care Equipment & Services, Inc., Crestline, CA). These types of arrangements have the least risk for personnel. Some technicians and veterinarians are adept at catching and restraining feral cats with gloves, towels, and/or blankets, but these methods risk personal safety and are more stressful for the cats, and so they are not recommended.

Another housing consideration is the unknown medical histories of feral cats. In some areas, high rates of respiratory disease exist. Keeping feral patients in a separate area of the clinic may be a good practice to decrease the likelihood of diseases being spread in the clinic.

Education of the staff, any technicians who are not familiar with feral cats, and caretakers is critical for a smooth-running feral cat care program. Human rabies prophylaxis can be important for peace of mind in endemic areas. It is critical to remind staff that a truly feral cat will not allow handling; they are not just frightened or excited pets. Most will hide in a back corner of the cage, but some may

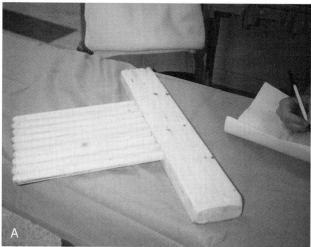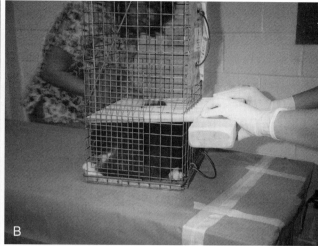

Figure 71–1. *A*, A homemade "comb"-type of device to squeeze cats into the bottom of a trap for injection. *B*, A feral cat squeezed into the bottom of the trap before injection using a comb device.

behave aggressively. Even cats that are frightened will bite and scratch if cornered or threatened. A quiet, dark location for holding feral cats can help decrease their stress.

Criteria for euthanasia should be determined in advance. Obviously, the decision will be made in consultation with the client, but because of limited ability to provide follow-up treatment, difficulties of retrapping some cats, and rigorous demands of an outdoor lifestyle, the decision to euthanize a feral cat may need to be made sooner than for a pet cat. Establishing general guidelines with caretakers before such a decision becomes necessary may be helpful in determining what is best for an individual cat.

Anesthetic protocols usually require some adjustment, the most notable being the use of an injectable combination to immobilize the cat for examination and/or surgery. A number of combinations may be used (usually including ketamine), some of which provide better analgesia and muscle relaxation than others. Combinations of ketamine and xylazine, or ketamine and tiletamine-zolazepam, with or without butorphanol, are efficacious and safe for the cats.

After the cat has been anesthetized, a physical examination can be performed and the gender of the animal established. Remember the importance of basic health care in this population of cats. Internal and external parasites and infectious diseases rarely seen in indoor cats that are well-cared for may be seen commonly in some populations of feral cats. Because many of these cats have unknown health histories and cannot be examined before anesthesia, it is important to advise caretakers that there may be increased risk of complications during anesthesia and surgery. Furthermore, a cat diagnosed with a serious health problem often should not be returned to the colony; caretakers should be reminded that euthanasia, rather than sterilization, may be the choice at this point.[62]

After examination and testing (if performed), cats usually are sterilized using absorbable skin sutures or intradermal closure for spays. There has been some debate regarding the strengths and weaknesses of the flank incision versus the ventral abdominal incision for females. In general, the argument for flank incisions is prevention of evisceration if the closure fails, and decreased risk of infection. In actual practice, both of these are extremely rare. The only situation in which the flank incision has clear benefits is in the case of recently nursing mothers, in which the mammary gland tissue makes the ventral approach and closure more difficult. Because feral cats usually must be spayed whenever they are trapped, veterinarians dealing with feral cats likely will have to handle this situation. If a ventral abdominal approach is used, intradermal sutures are recommended. Flank incisions can make it difficult to reach the contralateral ovary. The flank approach also is not appropriate for pregnant females. Thousands of feral cats have been spayed successfully using the usual ventral midline approach, so the final choice of approach is made by the surgeon.

After surgery, the cats should be vaccinated and ear-tipped. Ear-tipping involves the removal of 1 cm from the tip of 1 ear (usually the left).[63] Blunt scissors, crushing with a hemostat and then cutting with a scalpel, or laser surgery has been used to perform this procedure. Hemostasis with cautery, pressure, or a styptic powder is very important to avoid bleeding or scarring, which can distort the distinctive silhouette.[63] Ear-tipping has become the internationally recognized method for identifying that a cat has been sterilized, and is designed to be seen from a distance. Although some people are concerned by the aesthetics of this procedure, ear-tipping prevents additional risk to cats that have been trapped previously for anesthesia and surgery. The Royal College of Veterinary Surgeons in England approved this approach many years ago.[13, 63] Cats generally are held for 24 to 48 hours (females longer than males) after surgery by the veterinarian or caretaker before return to the site of trapping.

◆ CONCLUSIONS

The feral cat problem in the United States is large and complex. Quantifying the problem is difficult because different locations often have very different climates, laws, and issues. Often, individuals involved are emotional, and may speak from anecdotal experience. Definitions and terminology have been vague and inconsistent. Approaches have ranged from doing nothing to trap and euthanize, relocation, or TNR. People's perspectives range from an animal welfare view (a well-cared-for feral cat is better off in a colony than euthanized) to a practical view (trapping and euthanizing has not worked well) to a view that cats do not belong in the wild to a more pragmatic approach that it is nearly impossible to get public support (financial and volunteer help) for a program to trap and euthanize. During discussions and debates, people often present the arguments as completely opposing positions. In reality, each situation must be evaluated individually, and the solution generally turns out to be some compromise between the different positions.

It is becoming increasingly clear that feral cats are part of a larger problem related to lack of responsible pet ownership, to ignorance, and to apathy. Veterinarians are in an unique position to make a difference and help handle feral cat populations and problems. They can become involved in a wide variety of ways, according to each veterinarian's employment situation, personal philosophy, and types of local grass-roots and animal care and control programs. At present, surgical sterilization is a key component of feral cat management, and its performance is limited to veterinarians. But there are many additional ways that veterinarians can become involved. Some of these may be considered part of routine practice such as vaccination, pet selection, and advice on behavior problems. However, more emphasis is needed on health care issues that would decrease the numbers of unwanted or unexpected litters, and on general cat physiology and behavior, resulting in more cats remaining in their homes, and a stronger commitment to responsible ownership of cats.

REFERENCES

1. Mahlow JC, Slater MR: Current issues in the control of stray and feral cats. J Am Vet Med Assoc 209:2016–2020, 1996.
2. Heerens S: More on feral cats. J Am Vet Med Assoc 204:328–329, 1994.
3. Hughes JE: Feral cats. J Am Vet Med Assoc 203:1256–1257, 1993.
4. DeBrito PG, Doffermyre ML: Still more on feral cats. J Am Vet Med Assoc 204:1547, 1994.
5. McGrath M: Domestic concern about feral cats. J Am Vet Med Assoc 208:1961, 1996.
6. Gross EM, Hoida G, Sadeh T: Opposition to trap-sterilize-release programs for feral cats. J Am Vet Med Assoc 208:1380–1381, 1996.
7. Heerens S: Different viewpoints on trap-sterilize-release programs. J Am Vet Med Assoc 209:33–34, 1996.
8. Patronek GJ: Another viewpoint on trap-sterilize-release programs. J Am Vet Med Assoc 209:1061–1062, 1996.
9. Zaunbrecher KI, Smith RE: Neutering of feral cats as an alternative to eradication programs. J Am Vet Med Assoc 203:449–452, 1993.
10. Kahler SC: Welfare of cats depends on humankind. J Am Vet Med Assoc 208:169–171, 1996.
11. Neville PF, Remfry J: Effect of neutering on two groups of feral cats. Vet Rec 114:447–450, 1984.
12. Universities Federation for Animal Welfare: Feral cats: Suggestions for Control, 3rd ed. South Mims, England, Universities Federation for Animal Welfare, 1995, pp. 1–19.
13. Remfry J: Feral cats in the United Kingdom. J Am Vet Med Assoc 208:520–523, 1996.
14. Patronek GJ: Free-roaming and feral cats—Their impact on wildlife and human beings. J Am Vet Med Assoc 212:218–226, 1998.
15. Johnson K, Lewellen L, Lewellen J: Santa Clara County's Pet Population. San Jose, CA, National Pet Alliance, 1993, pp. 1–15.
16. Johnson K, Lewellen L: San Diego County: Survey and Analysis of the Pet Population. San Diego, CA, San Diego Cat Fanciers, Inc., 1995, pp. 1–29.
17. Luke C: Animal shelter issues. J Am Vet Med Assoc 208:524–527, 1996.
18. Holton L, Manzoor P: Managing and controlling feral cat populations: Killing the crisis and not the animal. Vet Forum, March 1993, pp. 100–101.
19. Nassar R, Mosier JE: Understanding the dynamics of your community's pet population. Vet Med, December 1986, pp. 1120–1125.
20. Nassar R, Mosier JE, Williams LW: Study of the feline and canine populations in the Greater Las Vegas area. Am J Vet Res 45:282–287, 1984.
21. Wise JK: U.S. Pet Ownership and Demographics Sourcebook. Schaumburg, IL, American Veterinary Medical Association, 1997, pp. 1–135.
22. Manning AM, Rowan AN: Companion animal demographics and sterilization status: Results from a survey in four Massachusetts towns. Anthrozoos 5:192–201, 1998.
23. Berkeley EP: Feral cats. Cat Fancy, July 1990, pp. 20–27.
24. Easterly S: Heeding the call of the wild. Cat Fancy, September 1998, pp. 37–42.
25. Black JC: Feral fix works wonders. SF/SPCA Our Animals, summer 1996, pp. 7–12.
26. Miller J: The domestic cat: Perspective on the nature and diversity of cats. J Am Vet Med Assoc 208:498–505, 1996.
27. Aronsohn MG, Faggella AM: Surgical techniques for neutering 6- to 14-week-old kittens. J Am Vet Med Assoc 202:53–55, 1993.
28. Faggella AM, Aronsohn MG: Anesthetic techniques for neutering 6- to 14-week-old kittens. J Am Vet Med Assoc 202:56–62, 1993.
29. Olson P: A critical evaluation of free-roaming/unowned/feral cats in the United States: Proceedings. Denver, American Humane Association, 1998, pp. 1–73.
30. Olsen CW: Vaccination of cats against emerging and reemerging zoonotic pathogens. Adv Vet Med 41:333–346, 1999.
31. Krebs JW, Smith JS, Rupprecht C, et al: Rabies surveillance in the United States during 1997. J Am Vet Med Assoc 213:1713–1728, 1998.
32. Rotz LD, Hensley JA, Rupprecht CE, et al: Large-scale human exposures to rabid or presumed rabid animals in the United States: 22 cases (1990–1996). J Am Vet Med Assoc 212:1198–1200, 1998.
33. Hugh-Jones ME, Hubbert WT, Hagstad HV: Zoonoses: Recognition, control, and prevention. Ames, IA, Iowa State University Press, 1995, p. 94.
34. Nogami S, Moritomo T, Kamata H, et al: Seroprevalence against *Toxoplasma gondii* in domiciled cats in Japan. J Vet Med Sci 60:1001–1004, 1998.

35. D'Amore E, Falcone E, Busani L, et al: A serological survey of feline immunodeficiency virus and *Toxoplasma gondii* in stray cats. Vet Res Commun 21:355–359, 1997.
36. Dubey JP, Weigel RM: Epidemiology of *Toxoplasma gondii* in farm ecosystems. J Eukaryot Microbiol 43:124S, 1996.
37. Hill RE Jr, Zimmerman JJ, Wills RW, et al: Seroprevalence of antibodies against *Toxoplasma gondii* in free-ranging mammals in Iowa. J Wildl Dis 34:811–815, 1998.
38. Kapperud G, Jenum PA, Stray-Pedersen B, et al: Risk factors for *Toxoplasma gondii* infection in pregnancy: Results of a prospective case-control study in Norway. Am J Epidemiol 144:405–412, 1996.
39. Dubey JP: Strategies to reduce transmission of *Toxoplasma gondii* to animals and humans. Vet Parasitol 64:65–70, 1996.
40. Cleri DJ, Vernaleo JR, Lombardi LJ: Plague pneumonia disease caused by *Yersinia pestis*. Semin Respir Infect 12:12–23, 1997.
41. Lopez T: Plague, finding ways to stop a killer. J Am Vet Med Assoc 211:280, 1997.
42. Eidson M, Thilsted JP, Rollag OJ: Clinical, clinicopathologic, and pathologic features of plague in cats: 119 cases (1977–1988). J Am Vet Med Assoc 199:1191–1197, 1991.
43. Hendrix CM, Bruce HS, Kellman NJ, et al: Cutaneous larva migrans and enteric hookworm infections. J Am Vet Med Assoc 209:1763–1767, 1996.
44. Schantz PM: Of worms, dogs, and human hosts: Continuing challenges for veterinarians in prevention of human disease. J Am Vet Med Assoc 204:1023–1028, 1994.
45. Breitschwerdt EB, Kordick DL: Bartonellosis. J Am Vet Med Assoc 206:1928–1931, 1995.
46. Schwartzman MD: *Bartonella (Rochalimaea)* infections: Beyond cat scratch. Annu Rev Med 47:355–364, 1996.
47. Wolf AM: *Bartonella henselae*: An important emerging zoonosis. *In* August JR (ed): Consultations in Feline Internal Medicine, vol. 3. Philadelphia, WB Saunders, 1997, pp. 7–11.
48. Mead CJ: Ringed birds killed by cats. Mamm Rev 12:183–186, 1982.
49. Dunn EH, Tessaglia DL: Predation of birds at feeders in winter. J Field Ornithol 65:8–16, 1994.
50. Coleman JS, Temple SA: Effects of free-ranging cats on wildlife: A progress report. Proc East Wildl Damage Contr Conf 4:9–12, 1989.
51. Mitchell JC, Beck RA: Free-ranging domestic cat predation on native vertebrates in rural and urban Virginia. Va J Sci 43:197–207, 1992.
52. Harrison GH: Is there a killer in your house? Natl Wildl 10–13:1089, 1992.
53. Fitzgerald BM: Diet of domestic cats and their impact on prey populations. *In* Turner DC, Bateson P (eds): The Domestic Cat. Cambridge, England, Cambridge University Press, 1988, pp. 123–147.
54. Coman BJ, Brunner H: Food habits of the feral house cat in Victoria. J Wildl Mgmt 36:848–853, 1972.
55. Terborgh J: Why American songbirds are vanishing. Sci Am, May 1992, pp. 98–104.
56. Robinson SK: The case of the missing songbirds. Consequences 3:3–15, 1998.
57. Passanisi WC, Macdonald DW: The Fate of Controlled Feral Cat Colonies. South Mims, England, Universities Federation for Animal Welfare, 1990, pp. 1–49.
58. Stubbs WP, Bloomberg MS: Implications of early neutering in the dog and cat. Semin Vet Med Surg 10:8–12, 1995.
59. Stubbs WP, Bloomberg MS, Scruggs SL, et al: Effects of prepubertal gonadectomy on physical and behavioral development in cats. J Am Vet Med Assoc 209:1864–1871, 1996.
60. Howe LM: Short-term results and complications of prepubertal gonadectomy in cats and dogs. J Am Vet Med Assoc 211:57–62, 1997.
61. Howe LM: Prepubertal gonadectomy in dogs and cats—Part I. Compend Contin Educ Pract Vet 21:103–111, 1999.
62. Universities Federation for Animal Welfare: Feral cats: Notes for veterinary surgeons. Vet Rec 108:301–303, 1981.
63. Cuffe DJC, Eachus JE, Jackson OF, et al: Ear-tipping for identification of neutered feral cats. Vet Rec 112:129, 1983.

72

◆ Feline Animal Shelter Medicine

Richard H. Evans

Feline animal shelter medicine is a form of population medicine, practiced on a very transient and heterogeneous population, in contrast to the more defined and relatively stable population seen by most practicing clinicians.[1] Cats impounded at animal shelters may be classified into several *lifestyle* categories:

- True *feral* cats are those that are not family pets. Their usual and consistent response to human beings is extreme fear, and they actively resist any human contact. In recent years, managed colonies of these cats have appeared across the United States (see Chapter 71, Understanding and Controlling Feral Cat Populations).
- *Semiferal* cats may or may not be owned, but are allowed to roam at will. Usually, they are fed by an owner or other persons in the neighborhood, resulting in a degree of cautious socialization with human beings.
- *Day-trippers* are owned cats that are allowed to roam free during specific times of the day (usually at night), returning to an owner's home for food and rest. They generally are moderately well-socialized to human beings, but still may resist handling.
- *Family house pets* are those that occasionally escape or become lost.

These lifestyle categories obviously have features in common, but also are decidedly different in terms of previous disease exposure, nutritional status, and behavior.[1, 2] When there is no source control on impounded cats, extremely heterogeneous populations are encountered, especially in terms of health management.[1] The nature of impounded cat populations is influenced by wide variability in policies and management practices among animal shelters, especially regarding the numbers and types of cats that they will accept and subsequently adopt (see Chapter 78, Quality of Life in Long-Term Confinement). Small, private shelters managed by humane groups may restrict impounds to healthy, well-socialized individuals that have a good chance of adoption, whereas large, municipal shelters often must take all subjects.

The key factor in this lifestyle categorization is the degree to which cats are kept as family house pets. A significant proportion of impounded cats are not suitable, behaviorally or medically, as family house pets, and therefore it is not difficult to understand why so many are euthanized in animal shelters across the United States every year. Whereas programs may be developed and funded to overcome this problem, solutions generally involve a very considerable financial burden to taxpayers, as well as high rates of behavioral reversion (e.g., failure of cats to maintain desirable socialization behaviors). As a result, many governing municipal bodies hesitate to spend precious financial resources "rehabilitating" adult cats that were not properly socialized to human beings at critical stages of kittenhood. Herein lies a basic dilemma of the pet overpopulation problem. Debate regarding appropriate management and disposition of cats that are impounded to shelters can create significant community, financial, and social issues, and often becomes surrounded by considerable emotion.

◆ RESTRAINT

One of the most important differences between private veterinary practice and shelter medicine is the need for shelter veterinary staff to be well-trained in the use of various methods for manual and chemical restraint of cats that are not accustomed to handling by human beings. The author has experienced many episodes in which restraint methods commonly used in private practice resulted in catastrophe and injury to the handler and the patient when used with impounded shelter cats.

Regardless of the type of restraint selected for individual cats, the safety of the shelter staff must be held paramount. The appropriate restraint device also should be one that causes the least discomfort or trauma to the patient. A contingency plan must be developed, and must be available immediately in cases in which the selected restraint method fails. Official policies and procedures should be prepared, and continuing training programs maintained for shelter veterinary staff. To neglect this issue may leave the supervising veterinarian liable when a staff member becomes injured because adequate tools and sufficient training were not provided.

The choice of manual or chemical restraint may be very difficult because feral cats usually will not permit an examination that is adequate to allow accurate assessment of the associated potential risks of one restraint method relative to another. In addition, behavior exhibited while in a cage may change dramatically when attempts are made to remove the cat from the cage. A caged cat that appears to be relatively docile may become highly agitated and aggressive when attempts are made to handle it. Thus, reliance on behavioral observations, training, and experience becomes very important for veterinarians and technicians who work in shelter environments.

For manual restraint, the shelter staff must understand feline behavior well enough to be able to decide which device or procedure to use. Several excellent texts are available; they should be part of the official restraint training program, and should be available at the shelter for reference.[3-5] Manual restraint may involve direct handling (e.g., stretch grip, neck grip), or may be assisted (e.g., cat bags, nets, snare poles). The disadvantage of many device-assisted handling methods is that they still require some degree of manual restraint to place the cat in the device. In the author's experience, gentle manual restraint and judicious use of the snare pole (e.g., Ketch-all) are sufficient in the vast majority of cases. One major disadvantage of the snare pole is that proper use requires significant training and experience. However, in the hands of a skilled and experienced animal health technician or animal control officer, even the most fractious cat can be restrained without injury to the handler or the cat.

Chemical restraint, although it is a valuable tool, also requires some degree of manual restraint to accomplish the injection. Intravenous injections are very difficult or impossible when managing feral cats, and therefore intramuscular injections usually are employed. A variety of agents are available for chemical immobilization of cats in shelter situations; however, in the author's experience, the cycloheximine tiletamine, combined with the tranquilizer zolazepam (Telazol), gives very reproducible effects at a dose of 6.6 to 11 mg/kg, despite a wide variety of temperaments encountered.

◆ IMPOUNDMENT PROCEDURES

All incoming cats should receive a standardized physical examination, including auscultation of the heart and lungs, and examination of the coat for evidence of arthropod parasites. A problem-oriented medical records system using an initial SOAP (subjective data, objective data, assessment, and plan) is recommended, and now is mandated in some states (e.g., Senate Bill 1785, State of California, July 1999).

When all attempts at manual restraint for examination are resisted, the cat should be allowed to acclimate quietly in its cage for an hour or more, unless there is obvious need for urgent care. After this time, if examination still is not possible with manual restraint, chemical restraint should be used. In any event, allowing a recently impounded cat to remain caged for an extended time, without diagnosis and treatment, is not appropriate medical care and must be avoided.

Treatments given at the time of impoundment should include responses to particular problems noted on physical examination, as well as vaccinations and preventive treatments for intestinal para-

sites and cutaneous arthropods. All of these should be administered before release from restraint. In shelters, products that are used for intestinal parasites should include those with spectra for common helminths and cestodes (e.g., Drontal Plus). Cutaneous arthropods, such as fleas and ticks, can be controlled by various means, but the clinical condition of the patient, along with specific knowledge of target organisms and the product, is very important. For example, a new "spot-on"–type topical product carries a claim for parasite control lasting 30 to 90 days, but is less satisfactory for tick control than for flea control. In another case, the manufacturer applies a claim for tick control, but fails to indicate that tick control requires over 15 times the amount of product needed to kill fleas.

Standard vaccinations should include those for feline herpesvirus, calicivirus, panleukopenia, *Bordetella*, and rabies, at appropriate ages. *Bordetella bronchiseptica* often is overlooked as a major primary or secondary cause of upper and lower respiratory disease in cats. In the author's experience, intranasal respiratory vaccines are very useful in animal shelter settings, provided that a proper disease management program is used concurrently. One minor disadvantage of intranasal vaccines is a higher post-vaccination incidence of short-term nasal discharge, sneezing, and even pyrexia. If adoption follows soon after vaccination with an intranasal product, new owners may become concerned when these signs appear, if proper explanation has not been provided. A problem-oriented medical records system should be used to track treatments and monitor responses. Ideally, records also should be computerized to allow veterinary staff to analyze demographics and disease trends within the shelter, but computer software that is available at present generally does not allow this degree of analytic flexibility.

◆ HOUSING, FEEDING, AND FOLLOW-UP CARE

One of the most commonly overlooked components of shelter medicine is development of a comprehensive nutrition program. In many cases, shelter personnel who are not educated in the intricacies of feline nutrition are allowed to develop such programs. The end result usually is a polyglot of types and manufactures of feeds, used in disorderly fashion, resulting in a high incidence of gastrointestinal disorders, poor weight gain for young and malnourished individuals, and increased susceptibility to other diseases.

The veterinarian should bear the responsibility for establishing a nutrition program that addresses the needs of the various life stages likely to be present in the shelter, and encompassing daily nutritional maintenance requirements and special dietary needs for ill, injured, malnourished, and older cats. This plan should include at the very least the following points:

- Standardized selection of nutritionally balanced feeds
- Discussion of shelf life of commercial feeds, and their proper storage, with shelter staff
- Requirements for daily food amounts and feeding intervals for all life stages in the shelter[6, 7]
- Standardized plan for kennel attendants and veterinary personnel to evaluate food consumption and nutritional status
- Discussion with shelter staff of the problems that may result from indiscriminate feeding and/or overfeeding
- Appropriate (and inappropriate) use of specialty diets
- Education to evaluate fecal consistency, and presence of blood or mucus, during daily litterpan cleaning procedures

◆ DISEASE CONTROL AND PREVENTION

For practicing clinicians, managing infectious diseases in animal shelters can be a new and formidable challenge. Many problems seen rarely or not at all in private practice may be commonplace in shelters. The veterinarian who has become accustomed to seeing 1 patient and 1 problem at a time must learn to use concepts of population medicine. He or she must understand the pathogenesis of common feline infectious diseases, especially those that are caused by viruses, in order to design effective management and primary prevention programs.[1]

A healthy population of cats must be housed in a way that will reduce the effects of psychological and environmental stress, because unmanaged stress may result in recrudescence from infectious carrier states.[7] It is a grave error to assume that vaccination programs alone, even with new "point-of-infection" (intranasal, conjunctival) vaccines, will resolve infectious problems in feline populations. In feline population medicine, management practices are of much more importance in reducing risk factors for infectious diseases. For example, a shelter had experienced repeated outbreaks of upper respiratory disease in impounded cats that did not have clinical evidence of respiratory infection at entry. In this facility, cats of all life stages were housed in a large 400-square-foot room, in banks of individual cages spaced 3 feet apart, with a commercial home air-purifier placed on each bank of cages. Multiple vaccinations failed to control the outbreaks. The problem was managed by placing cages in rows 5 feet apart. Cats in the facility also were grouped by life stages, and an inexpensive ventilation system was installed to maintain a thermoneutral environment. After these environmental changes were instituted, the incidence of clinical upper respiratory disease dropped 90 per cent in 2 weeks. A comprehensive vaccination program then further reduced the incidence of clinical disease, and significantly reduced as well the incidence of clinical respiratory disease during the first week after adoption.

In almost any shelter, some proportion of impounded cats will be showing clinical signs of common infectious diseases. These individuals should be separated and housed in a manner that prevents both direct and indirect contact with the healthy population.[7] Unfortunately, significant capital expense is required to be able to use "disease rooms" or "dirty rooms" to prevent disease dissemination to other parts of the shelter. Beyond the need to hold cats (especially those that probably are pets) for some time so that redemption is possible, shelter veterinarians must develop cost-effective programs for dealing with cats that have problematic diseases. The cost of treating cats with serious infectious diseases for periods sufficient to ensure recovery before adoption must be balanced against revenues obtained from adoption. If large amounts of money are spent recovering very ill cats, funds for maintaining impounded healthy cats may be depleted. Further, maintaining and treating cats that have terminal diseases (feline leukemia virus infection, feline immunodeficiency virus infection, neoplasia), and are not candidates for adoption, also drain funds that usually are limited already. California recently has enacted legislation to prevent adoption of animals with genetic or other medical problems that may affect their long-term health adversely.

◆ ADOPTION OF UNCLAIMED CATS

Unfortunately, many cats that are impounded into animal shelters are never redeemed. Some authorities believe that they are not family pets, but rather feral cats. However, in the author's experience, a very significant number of these cats are behaviorally well-adjusted, and are socialized to human beings. It is more likely that many of these cats are pets that have been allowed to roam free. When they are lost, their owners are not responsible enough to attempt to find them through searches of local shelters, leaving shelters with a tremendous surplus of cats. What can be done? Adoption of this surplus certainly is a potential answer, but by no means is one that will solve the problem. Because significant numbers of owners of these cats do not accept appropriate ownership responsibility, the pool of qualified potential adopters usually is reduced locally. Just as obviously, adopting cats to owners who are likely to take them home and allow them to roam at will serves only to perpetuate the impoundment-adoption cycle.

Criteria for adoption of unredeemed cats should include both medical and behavioral parameters. The medical evaluation should detect any condition (congenital, hereditary, age-based, or infectious) that might cause significant deterioration of health after adoption. This is an important consideration, because prospective owners of affected cats may not understand fully the issues, or may not agree to be morally and financially responsible for obtaining needed veterinary treatment after adoption. Shelter veterinarians are encouraged to consult recent legislation in California (Senate Bill 1785) that has addressed this problem by establishing guidelines for age and medical condition of potential pets, before adoption.

◆ EUTHANASIA OF UNREDEEMED CATS

One of the most emotionally charged and controversial aspects of feline shelter medicine involves disposition of unredeemed and unadopted cats. Redemption and adoption do not deal adequately with the large numbers of cats impounded into animal shelters throughout the United States. What is to be done with the surplus? On one side of this issue are those who feel that euthanasia is the appropriate answer. They are opposed by others who do not accept euthanasia of medically healthy cats as a solution for any problem. In addition, the emotional nature of this subject usually prevents even exploratory discussion of "mixed" solutions. Advocates of euthanasia frequently are fearful of raising the issue, lest they become labeled as uncaring sadists, whereas antieuthanasia groups seldom offer effective and fiscally responsible solutions.

The truly unfortunate reality of this debate is that euthanasia frequently is the only available avenue, in the absence of intervention proposals to curb the mammoth overpopulation problem that shelters are left to address with minimum assistance and little financial support. Further, allowing animals to sit confined for extended periods in cages, or even in small rooms, waiting for adoption that becomes progressively more unlikely, is considered by many authorities to be a form of cruelty. In fact, the author is aware of several animal shelters in California that have policies and procedures requiring that all cats be assessed for "cage neuroses" after 30 to 45 days of confinement.

A responsible euthanasia program should include the following:

- Precisely defined criteria for choosing specific cats for euthanasia
- Policies and procedures for appropriate restraint to prevent injury to handlers, and to reduce as much as possible the stress of cats being euthanized
- Methods and techniques for the procedure of euthanasia, including the pharmacology of the pharmaceutical agent selected[7]

Whereas the first program component, criteria for selection, should be developed through a combined effort of all shelter personnel, the latter 2 are the responsibility of the attending or consulting veterinarian. The veterinarian should review the most current body of accepted veterinary knowledge, and develop a written euthanasia procedure.[8] The veterinarian also should be aware that many lay humane advocacy groups do not feel that veterinarians give enough emphasis to the humane aspects of euthanasia (e.g., selection of the most painless procedure), but rather select the most expedient or cost-effective method. A good case in point is the present heated debate that is raging in California over nonspecific intraperitoneal injection versus site-specific intraperitoneal (intrahepatic) injection. The veterinarian is left with the unenviable task of countering these arguments by responding that veterinary medical technology has developed, not only as an avenue to maintain animal health but also to relieve suffering and pain. It is especially distressing that many lay persons feel that veterinarians, especially those employed in animal shelters, practice medicine with little regard to pain and suffering of patients.

Viewed in societal context, neither euthanasia nor caging cats in close confinement for extended periods of time represents a viable long-term solutions to the shelter cat problem. Ultimately, solutions will require sophisticated programs that change cultural concepts of responsible pet ownership, including reproduction control. However, as a society, we seldom seem willing to invest the effort needed for such innovative solutions. When we do, the effort usually takes the form of attempting to legislate normal responsibility, an act doomed to failure.

◆ EMPLOYEE RELATIONS

The potential for employment in shelter medicine to compromise the psychological health of veterinary and lay employees has been recognized for some time. In addition to the problem of performing euthanasia on a frequent basis, inconsiderate comments by citizens (and unfortunately by "colleagues" in other areas of veterinary medicine) can influence emotional well-being very negatively.

Maintaining the mental health and positive outlook of shelter workers is extremely important, and the veterinarian must require development of a mental health support program. Regular visits to animal shelters should be made by mental health workers who are trained to work with the problems that such employment engenders. In-house group sessions for employees also should be instituted, and recommendations that accrue from these discussions should be considered seriously by management staff. Further, local education programs should be instituted, so that communities learn to understand the formidable problems of animal shelter medicine, and the difficulties encountered by veterinary workers and caretakers. Myths about animal shelters staffed by incompetent veterinarians and deranged, ghoulish caretakers who delight in euthanasia must be dispelled. Society in general must realize that all citizens are responsible for the current state of affairs in many animal shelters, and for the pet overpopulation problem. Communities cannot continue to criticize animal shelters on the one hand, demanding more staff and facilities, while voting down sufficient funds to run and improve these facilities on the other hand. The shelter veterinarian therefore must anticipate that considerable effort may need to be directed to interface with local government and influential community groups, in order to ensure that adequate funding is maintained.

The shelter veterinarian should establish a comprehensive injury and illness program that includes recognition and prevention of zoonotic diseases.[9] In addition to being a part of good veterinary medical practice, state and federal occupational safety laws require such programs. These programs should include but not be limited to:

- Periodic educational seminars on common zoonotic diseases, their biology and symptoms, means of transmission, and their course in human beings[9]
- Veterinary staff programs to develop means to recognize and report suspected zoonotic diseases
- Comprehensive programs for shelter staff on diagnosis, treatment, and reporting of zoonotic diseases to veterinarians and Workmen's Compensation physicians
- Maintaining and posting U.S. Department of Labor accident, injury, and illness statistics
- Physical trauma (including animal bites) treatment and reporting programs

◆ FELINE POPULATION CONTROL AND THE VETERINARIAN

The present societal trend to allow pets to roam and to remain active reproductively has resulted in a tremendous pet overpopulation problem. Keeping cats as house pets but allowing them to roam at will has been a long-standing custom in the United States. Many cat owners feel that their pets still retain a vestige of "wildness," and that they must be allowed to roam in order to maintain positive mental balance. In fact, examination of many community ordinances dealing with animal control reveals that the proclivity of domestic cats to roam is recognized in law.

Many solutions to this problem have been proposed. However, none is effective without adjunct programs, such as owner responsibility awareness education. Most animal control agencies use the "traditional" control program that involves impoundment and removal of stray cats from urban areas. This method is rooted in the original legislated mandates of animal control agencies to control rabies. This, of course, requires that stray, biting, and deceased animals be removed from the environment, and requires massive antirabies vaccination and licensing programs to be implemented. Unfortunately, these ordinances generally have not kept pace with trends in domestic animal rabies. There are few legislated feline rabies control programs, despite increased incidence of feline rabies. Most agencies will pick up cats that have been confined by citizens, and some maintain active "sweep and destroy" programs that involve capturing and destroying stray cats. Obviously, these are at best short-term solutions that accomplish little, if anything at all, to manage the tide of uncontrolled reproduction in stray cats.

Recently, many lay and professional advocacy groups, including the American Veterinary Medical Association, have given support to "trap, sterilize, vaccinate, and release" programs as long-term solutions to feline overpopulation (see Chapter 71, Understanding and Controlling Feral Cat Populations). These programs have much to recommend them, and when conducted along with other programs such as community education and new legislative initiatives, they may in fact produce a comprehensive long-term solution to the overpopulation problem. However, managed alone, they are not likely to be truly effective, contrary to many published statements. Whereas proponents advocate long-term control of feral cat populations through management of reproductively active cohorts within the population, they usually fail to evaluate and incorporate applicable principles of population dynamics (e.g., recruitment from other areas, morbidity and mortality patterns adjusted to gender and age distributions). Even if we accept without data the claimed reductions in population expansion because of these programs, it does not necessarily follow that impact is made on the current epidemic of animal bites in the United States, on feline disease patterns, and on transmission of zoonotic diseases.

◆ SUMMARY

Feline overpopulation is a serious national problem, contributing very significantly to the epidemic of animal bites, and to transmission of zoonotic diseases to human beings. What is needed is a national consortium to study in-depth the population dynamics of free-roaming cats. From these studies should come models that facilitate development of legislative mandates for a series of mutually dependent programs with the ultimate goal of requiring responsible pet ownership, including generalized spay/neuter programs. It is inconceivable that we have allowed this problem to exist for so long without bringing the fruits of our intelligence to bear in the form of a solution. It is unfortunate indeed that, as with many of our social problems, we appear unwilling to attack the "root" of the problematic tree (irresponsible pet ownership), but rather have chosen to develop all manner of plans to "prune" the tree.

REFERENCES

1. Lawler DF, Evans RH: Strategies for controlling viral infections in feline populations. *In* August JR (ed): Consultations in Feline Internal Medicine, vol. 3. Philadelphia, WB Saunders, 1997, pp. 603–610.
2. Leyenhausen P: Cat Behaviour: The Predatory and Social Behaviour of Domestic and Wild Cats. New York, Garland STPM, 1979.
3. Turner DC, Bateson P: The Domestic Cat: The Biology of Its Behaviour. Cambridge, England, Cambridge University Press, 1988.
4. Fogel B: The Cat's Mind: Understanding Your Cat's Behavior. New York, Macmillan, 1992.
5. Fowler ME: Restraint and Handling of Wild and Domestic Animals. Ames, IA, Iowa State University Press, 1978.
6. Lawler DF: Designing health programs for breeding catteries. *In* August JR (ed): Consultations in Feline Internal Medicine, vol. 3. Philadelphia, WB Saunders, 1997, pp. 595–602.
7. Lawler DF, Bebiak DM: Nutrition and management of reproduction in the cat. Vet Clin North Am Small Anim Pract 16:495–519, 1986.
8. Greyhavens T: Handbook of Pentobarbital Euthanasia. Salem, OR, Humane Society of Willamette Valley, Inc., 1999.
9. Evans RH: Public health and important zoonoses in feline populations. *In* August JR (ed): Consultations in Feline Internal Medicine, vol. 3. Philadelphia, WB Saunders, 1997, pp. 611–629.

73

◆ Immunocontraception to Help Control Feral Cat Populations

Stephen M. Boyle
Amin Ahmadzadeh

The estimated number of feral cats in the United States and the number euthanized each year are subject to debate. Nonetheless, there is little argument that too many unwanted and unsupervised cats exist in this country. It is estimated that 8.5 million unwanted cats are euthanized in shelters each year in the United States. In addition to their population size, stray cats present several problems to the communities in which they live (see Chapter 71, Understanding and Controlling of Feral Cat Populations). They can act as predators of songbirds, introduce zoonotic diseases, and spread garbage while foraging, thus attracting other nuisance feral and wild animals. Some citizens are disturbed by the noise that is generated from courting and territorial behaviors, and are concerned by fecal and urinary wastes.

Spay and neuter programs are a permanent individual solution, but these programs are labor-intensive, require significant resources, and are limited by economic considerations. In addition, these catch-release programs can produce anxiety in refractory feral cats, which places the animals and their handlers at risk of injury. Removing cats for placement does not reduce population numbers, but only opens a niche for other stray or feral cats to migrate into the area. In addition, relocating cats draws additional resources, resulting in an increased kitten survival rate. The development of reliable, convenient, safe, and affordable oral contraceptives for cats would be a humane alternative to other population control programs. Oral contraceptives delivered via baited food deposited in feral cat colonies would reduce the stray cat population by controlling reproductive capacity, and at the very least, would augment other forms of population control.

During the latter half of the 20th century, a variety of oral contraceptives were developed successfully in animal models, and used in the human population. The success of human oral contraceptives appears to be limited only by economic and educational standards. In the case of feral cats, success of an oral contraceptive placed in food would necessitate overcoming a number of hurdles, the most problematic of which is developing a product that is relatively long-lasting and affects only cats. In this article, we review the concept of immunocontraception, some associated aspects of the feline immune system, the choice and delivery of antigens, and the progress of our research effort in developing a vaccine for oral delivery to cats.

◆ IMMUNOCONTRACEPTION

The notion that a vertebrate's own immune system could be used to control fertility has received increasing attention since about 1980. For such regulation to occur, the immune system must recognize a protein or carbohydrate component (an antigen) involved in the process of fertilization, and produce antibodies that interfere with the production of a fertilized egg. In the case of vertebrates, the most frequently used antigens are the protein (e.g., structural and enzymatic) components making up the sperm or the egg, or alternatively, the peptides or steroid hormones involved in oogenesis and spermatogenesis.

Immune Responses

The feline immune system is capable of generating both humoral and cell-mediated immune responses to foreign antigens. The classes of antibodies[3] include immunoglobulins IgG, IgA, IgM, and IgE, found in a variety of fluids, including serum, colostrum, milk, saliva, nasal secretions, tracheal secretions, tears, bile, and intestinal fluids.[4, 5] The fluids with the highest concentrations of immunoglobulins are serum and colostrum, with levels ranging from 1 to 35 mg/ml. IgG is predominant. It is safe to assume that, as with other vertebrates, both IgG and IgA are found in the feline reproductive tract, and that their respective quantities differ between vagina and uterus. In a number of nonfeline species, evidence exists that there is some local production of immunoglobulins in the reproductive tract.[6] However, the majority of immunoglobulins present result from transudation from serum. Therefore, measuring serum immunoglobulins should correspond directly to the types of antibodies in the reproductive tract.

In the case of cell-mediated responses, cats have T-cells consisting of the 2 major lymphocyte subpopulations, CD4 and CD8.[7] In healthy cats, approximately 25 per cent of peripheral blood lymphocytes are CD4 and 15 per cent are CD8 cells. Additionally, monocytes and macrophages produce a variety of cytokines,[8] and delayed-type hypersensitivity can be developed in response to foreign antigens.[9] Once sensitized to a specific antigen, the T-cells are responsible for destroying cell types containing the antigen. Thus, if a T-cell epitope is derived from gonadal tissue as part of a contraceptive vaccine, one would expect to see tissue damage resulting in either oocyte or sperm destruction.

In developing an immunocontraceptive vaccine, the chosen antigen could induce a humoral and/or a cellular immune response. The antigen could consist of B-cell epitopes and induce only a humoral response. In this case, the possible contraceptive effect is likely to be reversible and to not lead to autoimmune disease. Alternatively, the antigen could contain a T-cell epitope and induce a cell-mediated response that could lead to an autoimmune complication. The contraceptive effect by T-cell epitopes is likely to lead to loss of intraovarian oocytes and ovarian dysfunction, and therefore would be essentially irreversible. This latter effect actually may be desirable if indeed destruction of the gonads is the equivalent of elective surgical spay or neuter procedures.

Hormones

Effector hormones associated with the hypothalamic-pituitary-gonadal axis are obvious targets for a vaccine because specific antibodies would interfere with the ability to produce a mature, competent egg, or would prevent implantation. Studies in a variety of species include production of antibodies against follicle-stimulating hormone (FSH), gonadotropin-releasing hormone (GnRH), luteinizing hormone (LH), and choriogonadotropin (CG). Although some significant contraceptive effects have been observed by modulation of these hormones,[10] a number of side-effects make them unsuitable for market development. Some of these negative side-effects are the result of the hormones having identical protein components (the alpha subunit of LH, CG, FSH, and thyroid-stimulating hormone [TSH]). For example, antibodies raised against CG will cross-react and inactivate LH, FSH, and TSH. Although steroid hormones are necessary for maintaining specific reproductive functions, they also have important functions in other specific tissues. Therefore, antibodies that alter steroid and peptide hormone levels (e.g., LH, GnRH) could lead to serious endocrine dysfunction. Despite some of these drawbacks, vaccines that alter reproductive efficiency are being developed using antigens directed toward steroid and protein hormones.

Sperm Antigens

A variety of structural and enzymatic proteins have been isolated from sperm and used as antigens to induce infertility. One of the most characterized sperm proteins is the enzyme lactate dehydrogenase (LDH). Antibodies to LDH reduced fertility in mice, rabbits, rats, and baboons.[11] Other sperm antigens include fertilization antigen (FA-1),[12] rabbit sperm antigen (RSA),[13] PH20, fertilin, PH30,[14, 15] SP-10,[16] and zonadhesin.[17] Most of these proteins exhibit considerable homology across species, and thus are good candidates for a vaccine that affects more than 1 species. Zonadhesin appears to be a species-specific sperm antigen[17] that may provide a good opportunity to produce a vaccine that will not induce cross-reactive antibodies among species. More knowledge about the efficacy and safety of these proteins as antigens needs to be acquired before a vaccine can be considered seriously.

Oocyte Antigens

The ovum and its associated proteins also are attractive targets for a contraceptive vaccine. Most of the surface proteins associated with ova are found in the zona pellucida (ZP) layer or the oolemma membrane surrounding the cytoplasm. The ZP is a glycoprotein extracellular matrix surrounding mammalian oocytes. The functions of the ZP include roles in gamete recognition, sperm activation, and prevention of polyspermy. A number of studies in the 1970s and 1980s showed that the ZP from one animal species, when injected into another species, stimulated an immune response and, in many cases, inhibited fertilization. These observations led to further studies to test the feasibility of using ZP antigens for development of contraceptive vaccines.[18] Although initial studies revealed that immunization with ZP inhibited fertilization, this effect was accompanied by ovarian dysfunction, follicle deletion, and premature menopause.[19] Further studies have shown that antibodies to the amino-terminal region of porcine ZP1 glycoprotein are effective in blocking fertilization, without resulting in ovarian dysfunction.[20] Moreover, because this ZP epitope is present in many mammalian species, these antibodies could serve as a general model for production of a contraceptive vaccine.

The oolemma is the membrane layer surrounding the egg cytoplasm and underlying the ZP. Several types of oolemma proteins have been implicated in sperm binding. One type is an integrin proposed to be the receptor for the sperm surface ligand termed fertilin. Antibodies specific for integrin reduce binding of sperm in the mouse oocyte.[21] A 94-kDa protein is released from trypsin-treated oocytes, and its presence is required for sperm penetration.[22] Two recently discovered proteins associated with the oolemma membrane are the 75-kDa and 40-kDa proteins released by phosphatidylinositol-specific phospholipase C from mouse oocytes.[23] These 2 glycosyl-phosphophatidylinositol–anchored proteins have been shown to be absolutely necessary for mouse sperm binding. Whether antibodies specific for the 75-kDa and 40-kDa proteins will result in a decreased rate of fertilization in vitro or in vivo remains to be determined.

Delivery of Immunocontraceptive Antigens

Most of the immunocontraceptive studies conducted in animals have used purified or partially purified antigens administered intramuscularly or subcutaneously with careful control of the dose. This is a particularly important feature of vaccines that use some portion of the oocyte ZP. It has been shown that high doses of ZP result in an irreversible contraceptive effect. Moreover, high doses of ZP can induce autoimmunity, in which T-cells mediate a cell-mediated immune response against the ovaries, and cause ovarian dysfunction that is irreversible.[24]

We chose to evaluate an oral delivery system for a vaccine intended for feral cats, in which the vaccine had the opportunity to pass from the intestinal tract to the gut-associated lymphoid tissue to initiate an immune response. The capacity for this type of transit has evolved naturally in certain bacteria and viruses, thus providing vehicles for immunization studies. Specifically, genetically engineered vaccinia poxvirus has been shown to be a very effective means of oral delivery of the rabies virus glycoprotein to stimulate a protective immune response in foxes.[25] Alternatively, the enteric bacterium *Salmonella typhimurium* has been attenuated by deleting several genes required for virulence (i.e., spreading from infected macrophages within the lymphatics).[26] After oral delivery, this genetically engineered *Salmonella* vaccine strain induces its own uptake from the lumen of the intestinal tract via the M cells.[27] After phagocytosis and subsequent killing of the vaccine strain, the antigen is released and triggers an immune response. This vaccine strain of *Salmonella* has been approved for use in poultry to protect against *Salmonella* as well as other pathogens.[26]

◆ CHOICE OF *SALMONELLA* STRAIN AND TYPE OF ZONA PELLUCIDA

Salmonella was chosen over vaccinia as a delivery system because it is easy and inexpensive to engineer genetically. Once the *Salmonella* is in the gut-associated lymphoid tissue, both humoral and cell-mediated arms of the immune system can be induced. Thus, if the effectiveness of a contraceptive antigen depended on either arm of the immune system, *Salmonella* would be able to stimulate an immune response if the appropriate antigen was engineered into the vaccine strain. Using these techniques, *Salmonella* expressing a mouse ZP3 epitope has been used orally to immunize mice and reduce fertility by 50 per cent.[28]

The aforementioned attenuated *Salmonella* strain requires a gene for cell-wall synthesis. This gene has been removed from its chromosome and placed on a plasmid (an extrachromosomal, autonomously replicating piece of DNA) to create a balanced-lethal system.[29] Thus, the bacterium will not grow without the plasmid. If the plasmid is lost, the bacterium will die as its cell-wall synthesis fails. This same plasmid also can serve as a minichromosome that can be used to express additional genes (e.g., one encoding ZP).

In our studies, the plasmid was engineered into the attenuated *Salmonella* to express the gene encoding a region of swine ZP termed ZP4. In swine, ZP1 protein is responsible for secondary binding of the sperm to the egg, and ZP4 is 1 of 2 proteins making up the ZP1 protein.[30] Studies have shown that ZP4 contains a highly conserved region of amino acids, to which specific antibodies block sperm-binding or fertilization in vitro.[31] The critical epitope from ZP4 has been identified as the amino acid sequence CTYVLDPENL.[32] When this synthetic peptide was used to immunize mice, the resulting antibodies interacted with the purified peptide and swine ZP. The antibodies inhibited porcine fertilization in vitro. More importantly, this peptide induced antibody production without causing ovarian dysfunction. The studies also showed that this ZP epitope is present in human beings, dogs, cats, cows, and rabbits, and that mouse ZP antibodies interacted with the ova of these species.[32] The commonality of the ZP epitopes among vertebrate ova makes swine ZP a common immunocontraceptive antigen. In fact, injected swine ZP has been shown to be an effective contraceptive in over 25 different animal species.[33]

Genetic Engineering of *Salmonella* and Expression of ZP4

Figure 73–1 is an outline of the genetic engineering technology used in our studies to place a gene encoding a 14-kDa portion of the approximately

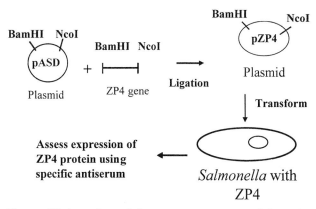

Figure 73–1. Outline of the genetic engineering of the swine zona pellucida (ZP) ZP4 gene into the plasmid aspartate semialdehyde dehydrogenase (pASD) plasmid[26] and transformation into *Salmonella* vaccine strain.

25-kDa swine ZP4 on a plasmid, which then was introduced into *Salmonella* by transformation. The proteins from *Salmonella* were separated based on molecular mass and then visualized with antiserum specific for ZP4. It is clear from the immunoblotting results in Figure 73–2 that the vaccine strain of *Salmonella* (pZP4 in lane 3) is expressing an approximately 14-kDa portion of purified ZP4 (lane 2). The ZP4 protein in *Salmonella* is smaller than purified swine ZP4, because only a portion of the ZP4 gene was cloned. This portion has the conserved epitope that induces antibodies capable of blocking fertilization in other nonfeline species.

Immune Response to *Salmonella*/ZP

To test the ability of a *Salmonella*/ZP strain to induce an immune response, 1-year-old, group-housed, female mixed-breed cats were fed the vaccine strain by oral gavage. They were assigned randomly (3 cats per group) to receive either (1) saline solution, (2) 1×10^{10} *Salmonella*, or (3) 5×10^9 *Salmonella*/ZP. Cats were immunized orally by gavage at week 0 and boosted at weeks 5 and 10. Jugular blood samples were taken before immunization and at 2-week intervals thereafter, and assayed for IgG antibodies by an enzyme-linked immunosorbant assay (ELISA). Fecal swabs were collected up to 7 days after the immunizations and analyzed for excretion of *Salmonella*. The results of fecal analyses (data not shown) revealed *Salmonella* in 6 of 9 cats on day 1 and in 3 of 9 cats on day 2. No fecal

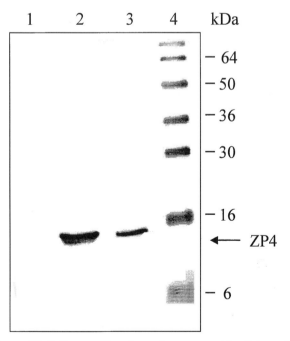

Figure 73–2. Immunoblot of proteins expressed by *Salmonella* using antiserum specific for swine *ZP4*. Lanes (1) extract from *Salmonella*/pASD; (2) extract from *Salmonella*/ZP4; (3) ½ of extract in lane 2 from *Salmonella*/ZP4; and (4) molecular weight markers—prestained.

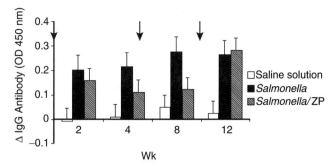

Figure 73–3. Change in serum anti–lipopolysaccharide (LPS) immunoglobulin G (IgG) levels in cats after oral immunization with *Salmonella*/ZP4 (10^9 cfu), *Salmonella* (10^{10} cfu), or saline solution given at weeks 1, 5, and 10. Serum was diluted 1:50 in phosphate-buffered saline solution–0.1 per cent gelatin, and IgG level measured by enzyme-linked immunosorbent assay (ELISA). *Arrows* indicate time of immunizations.

Salmonella was found beyond day 2 in vaccine-treated cats, or at any time in any of the saline solution–treated cats. The data in Figure 73–3 illustrate the serum levels of IgG against *Salmonella*. All cats immunized with *Salmonella* showed an increase in serum IgG levels, compared with saline solution–treated controls. This also indicates indirectly that the *Salmonella* migrated into the gut-associated lymphoid tissue. The data in Figure 73–4 illustrate the levels of IgG against ZP in sera. The ZP4 serum IgG level increased by 2-fold after the second immunization and remained elevated during weeks 8 and 12. Breeding trials are under way to assess measurable contraceptive effect in the *Salmonella*/ZP–immunized cats, relative to the saline solution– or *Salmonella*-immunized cats.

◆ SUMMARY

The usefulness of immunocontraception to help control feral cat populations has yet to be shown, in light of the results with a *Salmonella*/ZP vaccine discussed previously. However, the research results

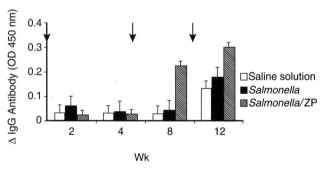

Figure 73–4. Change in serum anti-ZP4 IgG levels in cats following oral immunization with *Salmonella*/ZP4 (10^9 cfu), *Salmonella* (10^{10} cfu), or saline solution given at weeks 1, 5, and 10. Serum was diluted 1:50 in phosphate-buffered saline solution–0.1 per cent gelatin and IgG level measured by ELISA. *Arrows* indicate time of immunizations. One cat did not show an increase in ZP4 IgG; however, data from this cat were included.

obtained in our laboratories suggest that *Salmonella* expressing ZP is capable of inducing serum IgG antibodies specific for ZP. Given that this ZP4 antigen has been shown to induce contraceptive effects in other animal species, and that serum antibodies will be transported to the reproductive tract of cats, there is the distinct possibility that a contraceptive effect will be observed with further studies.

◆ FUTURE DEVELOPMENTS

As with any vaccine development, there remain several hurdles to be cleared before production of a practical oral *Salmonella*/ZP vaccine for feral cats. Our initial studies, in which *Salmonella* was mixed with moist food, revealed that cats did not mount a noticeable immune response to *Salmonella* or ZP. We therefore administered (by gavage) a 10 per cent sodium bicarbonate solution to neutralize stomach acidity just before immunization. The implications of these observations are that it will be necessary to incorporate some type of polymeric enteric coating for the *Salmonella* or to use another treatment in order for the vaccine strain to survive stomach acidity and reach the intestine. Another aspect that we currently are investigating is the specificity of the ZP vaccine. Because of the relatively high degree of homology among the vertebrate ZP proteins, most ZP vaccines would be expected to be effective in a range of animals. As there is no guarantee that animals other than cats would not eat a *Salmonella*/ZP vaccine placed in food, it will be necessary to define regions of the ZP protein that are unique to cats. This should be possible, because the ZPs from many vertebrates have been sequenced at either the DNA or the protein level. In turn, this information will allow selection and testing of unique vaccine determinants that should produce a contraceptive effect only in cats.

ACKNOWLEDGMENTS

The authors thank the Cassidy Foundation and the Scott Charitable Trust for their financial support, and Dr. Koji Koyama of the Hyogo College of Medicine (Japan) for providing the gene and antiserum for swine ZP4. Veterinary students Michelle Weissbarth and Virginia Clarke were supported by the Gerald R. Dodge Foundation and have provided the enthusiasm and effort for much of the genetic engineering and ELISA assay development. The help of Dr. Beverly Purswell (Department of Large Animal Clinical Sciences) in designing immunization protocols and bleeding the cats is greatly appreciated. In addition, we thank the staff of the Non-client Animal Holding Facilities at Virginia Tech for the care provided to the cats.

REFERENCES

1. Olson PN, Johnston SD: Animal welfare forum: Overpopulation of unwanted dogs and cats. New developments in small animal population control. J Am Vet Med Assoc 202:904–909, 1993.

2. Stevens VC, Jones WR: Vaccines to prevent pregnancy. *In* Levine MM, Walker GC, Kaper JB, Cobon GS (eds): New Generation Vaccines. New York, Marcel Dekker, 1997, pp. 1131–1143.

3. Tizard IR: Veterinary Immunology, An Introduction, 5th ed. Philadelphia, WB Saunders, 1996, p. 163.

4. Schultz RD, Scott FW, Duncan JE, et al: Feline immunoglobulins. Infect Immunol 9:391–393, 1974.

5. Barlough JE, Jacobson RH, Scott FW: The immunoglobulins of the cat. Cornell Vet 71:397–407, 1981.

6. Stokes C, Bourne JF: Mucosal immunity. *In* Halliwell REW, Gorman NT (eds): Veterinary Clinical Immunology. Philadelphia, WB Saunders, 1988, p. 164.

7. Willet BJ, Callanan JJ: The expression of leucocyte differentiation antigens in the feline immune system. *In* Willet BJ, Jarret O (eds): Feline Immunology and Immunodeficiency. New York, Oxford University Press, 1995, p. 3.

8. Lin DS: Feline immune system. Comp Immunol Microbiol Infect Dis 15:301–304, 1992.

9. Kern MR, Nelson PD: Development of the feline immune system. Proceedings 17th Annual Meeting American College of Veterinary Internal Medicine, Chicago, June 10–13, 1999, p. 14.

10. Reeves JJ, Chang CF, deAvila DM, et al: Vaccines against endogenous hormones: A possible future tool in animal production. J Dairy Sci 72:3363–3371, 1989.

11. Goldberg E, Wheat TE, Powell JE, et al: Reduction in female baboons immunized with lactate dehydrogenase C4. Fertil Steril 35:214–217, 1981.

12. Naz R, Menge A: Development of antisperm contraceptive vaccines for humans: Why and how? Hum Reprod 5:511–518, 1990.

13. O'Rand MG, Widgren EE, Nikolajezk BS, et al: Receptors for zona pellucida on sperm. *In* Alexander NJ, Griffin D, Speiler JM, Waites GMH (eds): Gamete Interaction: Prospects for Immunocontraception. New York, Wiley-Liss, 1990, p. 213.

14. Primakoff P, Lathrop W, Wollman L, et al: Fully effective contraception in male and female guinea pigs immunized with the sperm protein PH.20. Nature 335:543–546, 1988.

15. Primakoff P, Myles DG: Progress towards a birth control vaccine that blocks sperm function. *In* Alexander NJ, Griffin D, Speiler JM, Waites GMH (eds): Gamete Interaction: Prospects for Immunocontraception. New York, Wiley-Liss, 1990, p. 89.

16. Herr JC, Wright RM, John E, et al: Identification of human acrosomal antigen SP-10 in primate and pigs. Biol Reprod 42:377–382, 1990.

17. Hardy DM, Garbers DL: Species-specific binding of sperm proteins to the extracellular matrix (zona pellucida) of the egg. J Biol Chem 269:19000–19004, 1994.

18. Naz RK, Sacco A, Singh O, et al: Development of contraceptive vaccines for humans using antigens derived from gametes (spermatozoa and zona pellucida) and hormones (human chorionic gonadotrophin): Current status. Hum Reprod Update 1:1–18, 1995.

19. Mahi-Brown CA, Yanigimachi R, Nelson ML, et al: Ovarian histopathology of bitches immunized with porcine zonae pellucidae. Am J Reprod Immunol 18:94–103, 1988.

20. Hedrick JL: The pig zona pellucida: Sperm binding ligands, antigens and sequence homologies. *In* Dondero F, Johnson PM (eds): Reproductive Immunology, New York, Raven, 1993, p. 59.

21. Almeida EA, Huovila AP, Sutherland AE, et al: Mouse egg integrin alpha 6 beta 1 functions as a sperm receptor. Cell 81:1095–1104, 1995.

22. Kellon T, Vick A, Boldt J: Recovery of penetration ability in protease-treated zona-free mouse eggs occurs coincident with recovery of a cell surface 94 kD protein. Mol Reprod Dev 33:46–52, 1992.

23. Coonrod SA, Naaby-Hansen S, Shetty J, et al: Treatment of mouse oocytes with PI-PLC releases 70-kDa (pI 5) and 35- to 45-kDa (pI 5.5) protein clusters from the egg surface and inhibits sperm-oolemma binding and fusion. Dev Biol 207:334–349, 1999.

24. Henderson CJ, Hullme MJ, Aitken RJ: Contraceptive potential

of antibodies to zona pellucida. J Reprod Fertil 83:325–343, 1988.

25. Winker WG, Bogel K: Use of vaccinia virus to prevent rabies. Sci Am 266:86, 1992.

26. Curtiss R, Kelly SM, Gulig CR, et al: Avirulent Salmonellae expressing virulence antigens from other pathogens for use as orally administered vaccines. *In* Roth J (ed): Virulence Mechanisms of Bacterial Pathogens, Washington, DC, American Society for Microbiology, 1988, p. 311.

27. Madara JL: The chameleon within: Improving antigen delivery. Science 277:910–911, 1997.

28. Zhang X, Lou Y-H, Koopman T, et al: Antibody responses and infertility in mice following oral immunization with attenuated *Salmonella typhimurium* expressing recombinant murine ZP3. Biol Reprod 56:33–41, 1997.

29. Nakayama K, Kelly SM, Curtiss R: Construction of an asd+ expression-cloning vector: Stable maintenance and high level

30. Hasegawa A, Koyama K, Inoue M, et al: Amino acid sequence of a porcine zona pellucida glycoprotein ZP4 determined by peptide mapping and cDNA cloning. J Reprod Fertil 100:245–255, 1994.

31. Koyama K, Hasegawa A, Inoue M, et al: Studies on the epitope of pig zona pellucida recognized by a fertilization-blocking monoclonal antibody. J Reprod Fertil Suppl 50:135–142, 1996.

32. Hasegawa A, Yamasaki N, Inoue M, et al: Analysis of an epitope sequence recognized by a monoclonal antibody MAb-5H4 against a porcine zona pellucida glycoprotein (pZP4) that blocks fertilization. J Reprod Fertil 105:295–302, 1995.

33. Kirkpatrick JF, Turner JW, Liu IK, et al: Applications of pig zona pellucida immunocontraception to wildlife fertility control. J Reprod Fertil Suppl 50:183–189, 1996.

expression of cloned genes in a *Salmonella* vaccine strain. Biotechnology 6:693–695, 1986.

74

◆ Cognitive Dysfunction in Geriatric Cats

Katherine A. Houpt

Forty-seven per cent of American pet cats are over age 6 years, with old age in cats defined as greater than 12 years.[1] Cats may begin to show signs of aging between 7 and 10 years, and most show signs by age 12. Landsberg[2] surveyed clients who owned older cats, and found that 36 per cent of owners of cats aged 7 to 11 years reported behavior problems, compared with 60 per cent of owners of cats 12 to 15 years old, and 88 per cent of owners of 16- to 19-year-old cats.

Behavioral changes are the reason many cats are euthanized. In 1 case history, a 20-year-old cat was much loved by its owners, but within 48 hours of the onset of house soiling, the cat was euthanized. A diabetic cat was euthanized in another case, not because its blood glucose could not be controlled, but because it was urinating outside the litter pan.

◆ SIGNS

House Soiling

Improper hygiene probably is the most frequent cause of house soiling by cats of any age. This also can be a cause in geriatric cats, particularly geriatric cats that are diabetic and polyuric, those with chronic renal disease, or those treated with diuretics. Typically, the cat is producing much more urine, but the owners still clean the litter boxes as they have for the past dozen or so years. Either the cleaning frequency or the number of boxes should be increased in cats that are diabetic or polyuric for other reasons.

Cats may urinate or defecate outside the litter box. In our experience, the most common geriatric cat house-soiling problem is defecation outside the box. Younger cats exhibit this behavior infrequently. The geriatric cat usually defecates in close proximity to the box. Whether an older cat is more uncomfortable jumping into the box, or more uncomfortable assuming the defecation posture, is unknown. In these cases of inappropriate fecal placement, we recommend either placing papers under and around the litter box so that feces can be removed easily, or using a low-sided tray, such as a cafeteria tray, for a litter box.

Constipation often is exhibited by old cats. The primary causes may be inflammatory bowel disease or megacolon. These cats crouch in the litter box and strain repeatedly and unsuccessfully to defecate, and then defecate when they are inches or yards from the litter box. One owner reported that his cat was lying in lateral recumbency on his bed, and was purring when it defecated without arising. That is truly abnormal elimination. When stool softeners and cisapride were not effective in resolving the problem, this cat was referred to our facility, where a biopsy revealed lack of smooth muscle in the colon. Once the owner was aware of the problem, he was willing to accept the cat's involuntary behavior.

The final type of geriatric house soiling is the cat that is somnolent most of the day, but does have periods of activity during which it may run from one end of the house to the other, and yet may urinate and defecate close to where it sleeps. This may occur because the cat is not motivated to travel far, especially not down a flight of stairs to the basement litter box, or because its period of activity does not correspond to its elimination periods. The solution is to relocate the litter box within a few yards of the cat's resting place, but not closer than 2 feet. The owners should be aware that cats often change their preferred resting area. This probably is an innate behavior that functions to avoid ectoparasites (e.g., the cat moves before the next batch of flea eggs hatch). The litter box should move with the cat.

Vocalization

Some breeds of cats, particularly Oriental breeds, are more vocal than others. Owners may teach their cat to meow knowingly, by talking to it when it meows and encouraging it to meow again, or unknowingly, by feeding the cat so it will stop meowing. A cat can learn to meow for food quickly. In a laboratory setting, a cat would meow 15 times for each small food reward.[3] The longer the owner waits before feeding the cat, the higher the ratio of responses (meows) to reward (food), and the more difficult it will be to stop the behavior. The behavior will extinguish only after hundreds of meows.

All of the meowing behavior problems described previously can occur in any age cat. Cats that begin to vocalize too much only in old age probably are disoriented and/or fearful. They may meow at all times of day, but the behavior is most likely to be a problem at night because the owner cannot sleep. Confinement of the cat may not be possible, either because the cat still can be heard or because it attempts to escape so vigorously that it injures itself or damages property. The lack of rest resulting from the cat's hypervocalization may cause the owner to request euthanasia of an otherwise healthy pet. Not only will the cat's life be lost, but the owner will feel very guilty about the decision.

Over- and Underresponsiveness

Fear and Anxiety. Old age can be associated with increased fear. For example, cats that may have been nervous about visitors now disappear under the bed.

Overattachment. Some cats demand attention from kittenhood. These cats are always on the owners' laps, meowing for attention, rubbing against their legs, jumping on their papers. If this type of cat withdraws, a medical or behavioral consequence of aging should be considered. Even more startling to the owner is a cat that once was aloof, friendly enough but not demanding, usually near, but not on the owner. In old age, the cat now follows the owner and must be in physical contact, especially at night when it purrs, treads, and sleeps on top of the owner. If isolated from the owner, it cries inconsolably for hours. Disturbing the owner's sleep is one of the primary reasons for euthanasia of old, but otherwise healthy cats. Night-time misbehavior is second only to house soiling as a behavioral cause of euthanasia of geriatric cats.

Increased Aggression

Aggression Toward People. Aggression is a common problem in cats of any age, but may be exaggerated in older cats. The exaggeration may be caused by irritability, pain, hyperthyroidism, or any of the central neural problems. A cat that used to nip when petted once too often now may bite the owners unprovoked while they are sleeping. This can be complicated if the cat must be given painful injections to treat diabetes or chronic renal disease. Even giving oral medication can be a dangerous task, and may aggravate an aggression problem. Medications that can be used to reduce aggression in younger cats must be used with caution in older cats, but should be tried for the sake of the owner who is being bitten and the cat that may be euthanized. Amitriptyline (5 mg/cat [2 mg/kg] orally [PO] every [q] 24 hr) or paroxetine (2.5 mg/cat [1 mg/kg] PO q 24 hr or 5 mg PO q 48 hr) has been most efficacious in reducing aggression. See Pharmacologic Treatment for drugs used specifically to treat cognitive dysfunction.

Aggression Toward Other Cats. All too often, owners try to avoid grieving for a pet by replacing it before it dies. Rarely, the older animal is rejuvenated. In some cases, replacing a cat before it dies results in introduction of a kitten that claims all the attention, while the old cat is neglected. In an even worse situation, the old cat is tormented by a playful kitten. Introduction of another adult cat may result in aggression between them. This can be treated as in younger cats. Separate the cats completely. Rub each cat daily with the same towel, concentrating on the cheek area. The cats then can be introduced at meals. Either both cats or the aggressor cat (if identified) can be put in cat carriers to eat. At each meal, the cages are moved closer if the cats do not growl, hiss, or otherwise aggress against one another. If they can eat next to one another without incident, the process can be repeated with dishes far apart and the cats in the same room only for meals. If necessary, the more aggressive cat can be restrained on a harness and leash. The dishes are moved closer with each meal if there is no aggression. Finally, the cats are allowed to remain together for longer and longer periods after meals. This process can be hastened by use of the synthetic cheek gland pheromone (Feliway, Abbott Laboratories), which tends to calm cats.[4] Amitriptyline (5 to 10 mg/cat PO q 24 hr) or paroxetine (2.5 mg/cat PO q 24 hr) can be used for the aggressor, and buspirone (2.5 to 5 mg/cat PO q 8 to 12 hr) can be given to the victim. A cat that is fearful may trigger aggression in an otherwise nonaggressive cat.

◆ DIFFERENTIAL DIAGNOSIS

A change in the cat's behavior with time is the key to diagnosis of a geriatric behavior problem. In order to diagnose and treat a feline behavioral problem, a clinical history (see Behavior History), a physical examination, and diagnostic testing should be performed. The minimum diagnostic database for a geriatric cat would be a serum chemistry panel, complete blood count, urinalysis, evaluation of thyroid function, and a cardiac examination.

Any of the major classes of etiologies (anomalous, degenerative, metabolic, neoplastic, nutritional, idiopathic, inflammatory, traumatic or toxic) can cause behavior problems in older cats. Anomalous causes should not arise often in advanced life because most anomalies would be recognized at an earlier age, but acquired hydrocephalus can occur secondary to an intracranial mass. Degenerative diseases such as arthritis and sensory loss are not as obvious in cats, because owners do not expect them to be athletic, and seldom train them to perform to verbal commands. Cats may experience pain when jumping into the litter box or traveling up and down stairs, and old cats, like old dogs, may lose their sight or hearing. Owners seldom are aware of these losses because most impaired cats can navigate well in familiar surroundings. If owners complain that their cat is not responsive, does not come when called even at meal times, or does not greet them when they return, hearing loss should be ruled out before diagnosing cognitive dysfunction. Similarly, the cat may be afraid because it cannot see, or it may not want to go to the basement to eliminate for the same reason.

Metabolic diseases, such as liver dysfunction in obese cats, can affect behavior if hepatic encephalopathy develops. The most common endocrinologic problem is hyperthyroidism. The classic behavioral signs are hyperactivity, weight loss despite ravenous appetite, and aggression. The feces usually are voluminous.

Nutritional problems also can contribute to geriatric problems in cats. Overnutrition in the form of obesity is more common, but cats also may refuse food or refuse a balanced diet, leading to anorexia. Inflammatory disease can be secondary to a compromised immune system in the old cat. Interstitial cystitis, as well as the more common problems caused by calculi and renal disease, can lead to changes in elimination[5] (see Chapter 42, New Treatments in the Medical Management of Feline Interstitial Cystitis).

Traumatic injuries can occur in an old cat that can no longer see well. For example, a cat struggling to escape from confinement fell down basement stairs, sustaining traumatic injury to its skull, followed by behavioral changes. Older cats are less likely to ingest poisonous plants or antifreeze because they are less exploratory. They are, however, at greater risk of iatrogenic toxins if administering too many medications leads to drug interactions. Another iatrogenic toxicosis occurs when some medications are given at levels too high for a geriatric kidney or liver to metabolize or excrete effectively.

Brain tumors should be suspected when an older cat exhibits seizures, circling, marked increase in aggression, or other behavior changes. Meningiomas are the most common brain tumors of cats. Diagnosis is confirmed by using computed tomography or magnetic resonance imaging. Treatment may be attempted at referral centers[6] (see Chapter 50, Cerebral Meningiomas: Diagnostic and Therapeutic Considerations).

Cardiomyopathies are the most common geriatric feline cardiac problem.[7] Heart disease should not cause behavior changes directly unless blood flow to the brain is compromised. The cat may be inactive, less playful, or less willing to jump in a lap or on a bed. Most chronic heart failure is treated with a diuretic such as furosemide, among other drugs. The owner should be aware that the cat's urine production will increase if a diuretic is given, and that the litter box should be cleaned more often or another box added.

Feline Cognitive Dysfunction

Cats can develop pathology and behavioral abnormalities similar to those seen in human senility. Senile neural plaques are the hallmark of human Alzheimer's disease. The major constituent of these plaques is beta-amyloid. In 3 cats aged 15, 16, and 20 years, there were behavior changes, including wandering, confusion, and night-time howling.

Neuropathologically, the cats had extensive amyloid plaque deposition, in some areas spanning the entire cortical depth. There were no neuritic plaques or neurofibrillary tangles, features that are seen in human Alzheimer's disease.[8, 9] The signs of true cognitive dysfunction are disorientation, nonresponsiveness, disruption of sleep patterns, and hypervocalization.[10] Owners complain of disorientation in the cat that does not remember how to go outside, or forgets the location of its cat door or litter box. Many cats that "crawl away to die" may be disoriented with cognitive dysfunction, and cannot find their way home. More common is nonresponsiveness. The cat no longer greets the owner at the door with raised tail and evident interest. The cat may no longer seek out or appear to recognize its favorite person. Recognition may be based not on visual cue, but on smell. Cats appear to use olfactory cues to recognize individuals, and olfaction is one of the first senses to be compromised in human beings with cognitive dysfunction. Circadian rhythms are disrupted in human beings and dogs with dementia, and this may account for unusual night-time wakefulness of some geriatric cats.[11] Stress may hasten cognitive decline. An increase in endogenous corticosteroid, especially a chronic increase, hastens hippocampal dysfunction.[12] The hippocampus is the area of the brain that is essential for some types of memory.

◆ PHARMACOLOGIC TREATMENT

Drug treatments for dementias of elderly human beings have changed as theories of their causation have changed. When lack of blood flow to the brain was considered to be the cause, drugs that improved blood flow were prescribed. With the discovery that most senile changes result from multiple infarcts or from Alzheimer's disease, different therapies have been recommended. Alzheimer's disease is associated with lack of cholinergic function, and acetylcholine is a necessary neurotransmitter for memory.[13] Acetylcholinesterase and monoamine oxidase type B (MAOB) increase in older animals.[14] Inhibitors of cholinesterase such as tacrine (Cognex), or cholinergic agonists, are used to treat human cognitive dysfunction. There are 2 main receptor types for acetylcholine, nicotinic and muscarinic. Because smoking seems to have a protective effect against Alzheimer's disease, targeting nicotinic rather than muscarinic receptors may be more important therapeutically, but the concept awaits clinical testing.

Other related therapies have included dopamine-enhancing drugs such as deprenyl, a monoamine oxidase inhibitor (see later). Neuroprotective agents block the effect of the excitatory amino acid glutamate or its receptors; there are several types of glutamate receptors, including N-methyl-D-aspartate (NMDA), kainate and alpha-amino-3-hydroxy-5-methyl-4-isoxazole-propionic acid (AMPA). Some studies indicate a positive effect of antagonists of the NMDA–calcium channel complex on cognitive function.

Accumulation of free radicals is another theory of aging of all tissues, including neural tissue. Antioxidants such as vitamin E and more powerful compounds such as the lazarads, so named because of their putative Lazarus-like effects on restoring neurons, have been suggested for treatment of age-related problems.[15]

Three drugs have been used for treatment of cognitive dysfunction in cats, L-deprenyl, nicergoline, and propentofylline.

Selegeline or L-deprenyl (Anipryl) selectively and irreversibly inhibits the activity of MAOB, the enzyme that metabolizes dopamine, hydrogen peroxide, and possibly other cytotoxic free radicals. Free radicals are believed to be involved in cognitive dysfunction because they react with polyunsaturated fatty acids within cellular membranes. L-deprenyl increases the synthesis and release of dopamine and inhibits dopamine re-uptake. L-deprenyl has been used in the United States to treat canine cognitive dysfunction.[16] Landsberg[2] treated cats 14 years or older with L-deprenyl at 0.5 mg/kg q 24 hr when they exhibited behavior changes including decreased appetite, increased irritability, increased vocalization, disorientation, wandering, decreased affection, and overgrooming. Ten of 13 improved.

Propentofylline (Karsivan, Vivitonin) is a xanthine derivative. It improves blood flow, especially in small blood vessels, dilates bronchioles, and is neuroprotective.[17, 18] It also has been used with some success to treat canine cognitive dysfunction in Europe.

Nicergoline is a drug with alpha-adrenergic effects that increases cerebral blood flow and metabolic activity of cerebral neurons. It has been reported to increase activity in aging dogs by 75 per cent.[16]

◆ ENVIRONMENTAL MANAGEMENT

Life can be made easier for old cats by some simple environmental modifications. Ramps can be purchased or constructed that allow the cat to reach beds, window sills, or other elevated structures to which they no longer can jump. A cafeteria tray or cardboard box lid can replace a high-sided litter box. Alternatively, newspaper can be spread in the area around the litter box, so that if the cat does defecate there, cleaning will be easier. Lights can be left on in the basement or other areas to help the cat find the litter box at night. One common sign of illness in cats is failure to groom. It is very distressing to the cat and owner if mats must be combed from the coat. It may be kinder to shave the cat, as long as it can be kept warm.

Perhaps the most important behavior modifier is to change the social and physical environment as little as possible. As mentioned previously, stress aggravates cognitive decline, so moving, addition of a new cat, or other significant household changes may trigger geriatric behavioral dysfunction.

◆ CASE STUDIES

Case 1. A neutered male, domestic longhair cat named Carl was presented at age 13 years for house soiling. As a young cat, he was struck by a car and his right hind limb was amputated as a result. The cat was diagnosed with diabetes mellitus 6 months previously and received twice-daily insulin injections. He was 1 of 3 cats; the other 2 were 5-year-old litter-mate females. There were 3 litter boxes in the basement, but Carl had urinated and sprayed in several places on the first floor of the house. A few months before, the owner had taken in a kitten that urinated indiscriminantly all over the house before it was euthanized for neurologic problems. The rugs had been replaced, and the floor scrubbed and refinished. A few weeks previously, the owner had kept a friend's cat for several days. Carl exhibited aggression to the cat, and would quickly climb the stairs to the second floor in pursuit of the strange cat. The owner had been carrying Carl to the basement to use the litter box, but decided that if he could run that quickly, he did not need help.

There are several medical and behavioral aspects to this case. The cat was producing more urine, but the number of boxes had not changed. Even for healthy cats, there should be 1 more box than there are cats in the household.[19] Furthermore, the cat was having increasing difficulty walking. The owner was advised that Carl's behavior when agitated was not an indication of his normal ability to move, but rather, pain would have been forgotten in the excitement. The owner was encouraged to take the cat to the litter boxes in the basement, and to provide a box or boxes on the first floor. Cat diapers also were suggested because the owner felt that her husband would tolerate no more urination in the house. An alternative plan was to provide an exercise pen or large cage where the cat could be with the family, but not able to reach the rugs or furniture. Paroxetine (2.5 mg q 24 hr) was prescribed to reduce the cat's anxiety in response to the odors of the visiting cat and house-soiling kitten. The medication was to be administered in tuna fish because the cat was difficult to medicate orally.

Case 2. A cat had been treated by the behavior clinic for house soiling 10 years ago. The behavior had resolved, but the owner called again when the cat became aggressive to her and to her other cat. One thyroid gland had been removed, but on examination, another nodule was palpated and, later, removed surgically. Next, the owner reported that the cat was ravenously hungry. Diabetes mellitus was diagnosed after laboratory evaluation. Finally, the cat began to lose its vision. Although not as common in cats as in dogs, a pituitary tumor producing adrenocorticotropic hormone (ACTH) and thyroid-stimulating hormone (TSH) was suspected, with diabetes secondary to hyperadrenocorticism. The hyperthyroid condition may have been due to TSH stimulation. On post-mortem examination, the tumor was found to be pressing on the optic chiasma, which accounted for the visual deficit, and on the base of the hypothalamus, which explained the aggression. The owner was grateful to know why her cat's personality had changed, and to know that all of the cat's signs could be explained by an inoperable tumor.

Case 3. Fluffy was owned by 2 veterinarians. She always had been a friendly cat, but now would not leave her owners alone. She tried to sleep on their heads, and generally disturbed them at night. If she was kept out of the bedroom, she meowed loudly and could be heard all over their apartment and by neighbors. When treated with L-deprenyl, her behavior became much more like her original non-demanding behavior. Discontinuation of medication resulted in a recurrence of the problem behavior

within 2 days. Anipryl therapy again relieved the signs.

Case 4. Magoo always had been an obstreperous cat, demanding and aggressive. With age, these characteristics intensified, and he developed chronic renal disease. The owners had been administering prescribed fluid subcutaneously. Although a difficult patient, he learned that injections were followed by a treat of imported German ham, and he accepted the owners' interventions. He was constipated, and was treated with cisapride. At night, he occasionally would begin to yowl as if he wanted to jump on the bed but could not. If the owner tried to pick him up he would bite her. Sometimes, he would bite both husband and wife if they stepped out of bed. The wife began to sleep on the couch, and petted the cat whenever he yowled. Behavior modification was recommended—that is, do not reward the meowing by petting him. To allow the cat to reach the bed without being picked up, a ramp was to be built. It was suggested that he might be in pain when the cisapride stimulated intestinal motility; therefore, he did not want to be touched. L-Deprenyl (0.5 to 1 mg/kg q 24 hr) was recommended.

◆ BEHAVIOR HISTORY

◆ **General Information**

Client's name: _____ Name of pet: _____

Address: _____ Breed: _____

_____ Date of birth: _____

_____ Age: _____

Home phone: _____ Sex: _____ Neutered/spayed: _____

Work/day phone: _____ Age at acquisition: _____

Color: _____

◆ **Behavior Problem**

What is the main behavior problem or complaint?

Describe the chronology of the behavior problem, i.e., how it developed over time.

When did it first become a *serious* concern?

In what general circumstances does the cat misbehave?

How frequently does the problem (or problems) occur (how many times daily, weekly or monthly)?

a. Problem: _____ Frequency: _____
b. Problem: _____ Frequency: _____
c. Problem: _____ Frequency: _____

◆ **Litter Box and Usage**

Does your cat ever eliminate in the house but outside the litter pan? _____ yes _____ no

If yes, does your cat urinate _____ or defecate _____ or both _____?

How many litter pans do you have? _____

Where are they (please be specific: which room, which floor)?

What kind of pans are they (indicate number)?

_____ commercial litter pan (size: _____)

_____ commercial litter pan with removable "lip"

_____ covered box, "cave"-type front door

_____ covered box, "Booda"-type (cat crawls into hole)

_____ dishpan

_____ cardboard box

_____ other (please describe)

How old is each pan? _____

Do you use a liner? _____ yes _____ no   If yes, what type (plastic, newspaper, etc.)? _____

What kind of litter is used (please be specific)?

Have you changed brands recently?

How often is litter scooped? How often is litter replaced?

How do you clean the box(es), and how often (please be specific)?

Where and how do you dispose of used litter (please be specific)?

Does the cat cover urine and feces in the box?

◆ **Cat's Environment**

Please list all animals in the household:

Name	Species	Breed	Sex	Age Obtained	Age Now

In what sequence were the above animals obtained? (Please number animals in the table above.)

What is your cat's relationship to the other animals (e.g., friendly, hostile, fearful)? Please describe.

What type of area do you live in? (Circle one)

CITY   SUBURBS   RURAL

What type of house do you live in? (Circle one)

APARTMENT—STUDIO OR 1 BEDROOM
APARTMENT—2 + BEDROOMS
DUPLEX/ATTACHED HOUSE
HOUSE—SINGLE FAMILY
TRAILER
FARM
OTHER: _____

◆ Behavior Changes With Age

1. In comparison to the cat's behavior at 3 to 5 years old, does the cat purr

more often	no difference	less often

2. In comparison to the cat's behavior at 3 to 5 years old, does the cat meow

more often	no difference	less often

3. In comparison to the cat's behavior at 3 to 5 years old, does the cat hiss

more often	no difference	less often

4. In comparison to the cat's behavior at 3 to 5 years old, does the cat scratch people

more often	no difference	less often

5. In comparison to the cat's behavior at 3 to 5 years old, does the cat scratch furniture, rugs, etc.

more often	no difference	less often

6. In comparison to the cat's behavior at 3 to 5 years old, does the cat bite people

more often	no difference	less often

7. *In comparison to the cat's behavior at 3 to 5 years old, does the cat fight with other cats

more often	no difference	less often

8. *In comparison to the cat's behavior at 3 to 5 years old, does the cat associate with other cats

more often	no difference	less often

9. In comparison to the cat's behavior at 3 to 5 years old, the cat sits on the laps of the family or familiar people

more often	no difference	less often

10. In comparison to the cat's behavior at 3 to 5 years old, does the cat solicit attention by rubbing

more often	no difference	less often

---

*Only for cats in multicat households.

11. In comparison to the cat's behavior at 3 to 5 years old, is the cat's appetite

greater	no difference	less often

12. In comparison to the cat's behavior at 3 to 5 years old, does the cat urinate

more often	no difference	less often

13. In comparison to the cat's behavior at 3 to 5 years old, does the cat defecate

more often	no difference	less often

14. In comparison to the cat's behavior at 3 to 5 years old, does the cat spray (back up to objects and twitch tail and deposit urine on vertical objects)

more often	no difference	less often

15. In comparison to the cat's behavior at 3 to 5 years old, does the cat hide

more often	no difference	less often

16. In comparison to the cat's behavior at 3 to 5 years old, is the cat found alone

more often	no difference	less often

17. In comparison to the cat's behavior at 3 to 5 years old, does the cat play

more often	no difference	less often

18. †In comparison to the cat's behavior at 3 to 5 years old, does the cat go outside

more often	no difference	less often

19. In comparison to the cat's behavior at 3 to 5 years old, the cat responds to people

more often	no difference	less often

20. In comparison to the cat's behavior at 3 to 5 years old, the cat walks or paces

more often	no difference	less often

21. In comparison to the cat's behavior at 3 to 5 years old, the cat becomes lost or disoriented

more often	no difference	less often

---

†Only for cats who are allowed outdoors.

REFERENCES

1. Richards JR, Rodan I, Beekman GK, et al: Panel Report on Feline Senior Care. Albuquerque, NM, American Association of Feline Practitioners/Academy of Feline Medicine, 1998.
2. Landsberg GM: Behavior problems of older cats. *In* Proceedings of the 135th Annual Meeting of the American Veterinary Medical Association, Schaumburg, IL, 1998, pp. 317–320.
3. Molliver ME: Operant control of vocal behavior in the cat. J Exp Anal Behav 6:197–202, 1963.
4. Frank DF, Erb HN, Houpt KA: Urine spraying in cats: Presence of concurrent disease and effects of a pheromone treatment. Appl Anim Behav Sci 61:263–272, 1999.
5. Bagley RS: Common neurologic diseases of older animals. Vet Clin North Am Small Anim Pract 27:1451–1486, 1997.
6. Buffington CA, Chew DJ, Woodworth BE: Feline interstitial cystitis. J Am Vet Med Assoc 215:682–685, 1999.
7. Bright JM, Mears E: Chronic heart disease and its management. Vet Clin North Am Small Anim Pract 27:1305–1329, 1997.
8. Cummings BJ, Satou T, Head E, et al: Diffuse plaques contain C-terminal $A\beta_{42}$ and not $A\beta_{40}$: Evidence from cats and dogs. Neurobiol Aging 17:653–659, 1996.
9. Geula C, Wu C-K, Saroff D, et al: Aging renders the brain

vulnerable to amyloid β-protein neurotoxicity. Nat Med 4:827–831, 1998.

10. Houpt KA, Beaver B: Behavioral problems of geriatric dogs and cats. Vet Clin North Am Small Anim Pract 11:643–652, 1981.

11. Hineno T, Mizobuchi M, Hiratani K, et al: Disappearance of circadian rhythms in Parkinson's disease model induced by 1-methyl-4-phenyl-1,2,3,6-tetrahydropyridine in dogs. Brain Res 580:92–99, 1992.

12. Lupien S, Lecours AR, Lussier I, et al: Basal cortisol levels and cognitive deficits in human aging. J Neurosci 14:2893–2903, 1994.

13. Houpt KA: Domestic Animal Behavior for Veterinarians and Animal Scientists, 2nd ed. Ames, Iowa State University Press, 1998.

14. Landsberg G, Ruehl W: Geriatric behavior problems. Vet Clin North Am Small Anim Pract 27:1537–1559, 1997.

15. Stahl SM: Essential Psychopharmacology: Neuroscientific Basis And Practical Applications. Cambridge, UK, University of Cambridge Press, 1996.

16. Ruehl WW, Hart BL: Canine cognitive dysfunction. In Dodman NH, Shuster L (eds): Psychopharmacology of Animal Behavior Disorders. Oxford, Blackwell Science, 1998, pp. 283–304.

17. Hudlicka O, Komarek J, Wright AJA: The effect of a xanthine derivative, 1-(5′oxohexyl)-3-methyl-7-propylxanthine (HWA 285), on heart performance and regional blood flow in dogs and rabbits. Br J Pharmacol 72:723–730, 1981.

18. Wright AJA, Hudlicka O, Tyler KR, et al: The effect of vasoactive drugs on capillary density and performance in skeletal muscles. Bibl Anat 20:362–365, 1981.

19. Overall KL: Clinical Behavioral Medicine For Small Animals. St. Louis, Mosby–Year Book, 1997, p. 170.

75

◆ Hip Dysplasia

Anke Langenbach
Todd P. Murphy
Gail K. Smith

Historically, feline hip dysplasia (FHD) has not been recognized as a clinically important orthopedic condition. Accordingly, there is little published information regarding the mode of inheritance, clinical incidence, and radiographic evaluation of the feline coxofemoral joint. Recent reports suggest that FHD is more prevalent than once thought, particularly in some breeds.[1, 2] Like canine hip dysplasia (CHD), FHD is a developmental malformation of the coxofemoral joint that is characterized by hip-joint laxity early, and by remodeling of the femoral head and acetabulum later in the disease process.

The disease in cats is believed to be similar in origin and pathogenesis to CHD. It is not a congenital disorder, meaning that it is not apparent clinically or radiographically at birth. It generally is agreed that pedigreed cats are affected more often, and males and females appear to be affected with similar frequency. The majority of cats with hip dysplasia (HD) are asymptomatic, and the disease often is diagnosed incidentally by abdominal radiography for unrelated health conditions.

Nonsteroidal anti-inflammatory drugs (NSAIDs) are the mainstays of conservative treatment for CHD. Differences in metabolism of NSAIDs raise concern over the safety and efficacy of their use for treatment of degenerative joint disease (DJD) in cats, but conservative treatment of DJD frequently is unrewarding nonetheless. The surgical treatment most commonly chosen for management of pain associated with the feline hip joint is femoral head and neck ostectomy. Long-term results are favorable regarding control of pain and return to function. The focus of this chapter is on the pathogenesis, clinical presentation, treatment, and control of FHD.

◆ ETIOLOGY

The exact etiology and pathogenesis of HD in dogs and human beings is understood poorly.[3, 4] HD is very common in dogs, and much has been published regarding the pathogenesis, clinical incidence and presentation, and treatment options. In contrast to the high awareness of CHD, FHD is not diagnosed frequently, and very little has been written in veterinary literature. FHD is assumed, however, to be similar to the canine and human forms. In 1966, Henricson and associates[5] proposed empirically that hip-joint laxity in dogs was the primary condition leading to development of DJD. Specifically, hip-joint laxity is thought to lead to subluxation during weight-bearing (incongruency of femoral head and acetabulum), causing microfractures, cartilage erosion, and subchondral bone exposure and sclerosis, resulting in functional impairment and pain.[6, 7] As a result, years of research have gone into studying hip-joint laxity, its cause, and its association with development of DJD.*

Studies of the genetics of CHD have demonstrated the condition to be multifactorial and developmental.[8] It is not congenital; therefore, the hip joint at birth is congruent. Genetic and nongenetic (environmental) factors affect expression of CHD. Genetically, CHD is a polygenic trait, meaning that multiple gene pairs are involved. The genetics of HD in cats is believed to be similar to that in dogs, but definitive published studies are not available at present. Pedigreed cats appear to have a higher incidence of radiographic disease than domestic shorthair cats, but the incidence of clinical disease still is low among all cats. In the case of pedigreed cats, the narrower gene pool increases the chance of pairing alleles for HD, which may explain the perceived increased incidence of disease.

Environmental factors are those that modify the expression of the genotype and therefore influence the observed phenotype. In dogs, environmental factors include breed, size, rapid growth rate, restricted versus ad libitum feeding, dietary electrolyte balance, weight, association between pelvic muscle mass and incidence of CHD, intramuscular glycosaminoglycan injections, and endocrine factors.[9–17] Similar studies in cats have not been done.

Heritability describes the relationship of phenotype to genotype. It is the proportion of a phenotypic trait that is attributable to the average effects of the genes. That portion of the phenotype that is not attributable to the genotype is attributable to environmental factors, including diagnostic error. Reports of CHD heritability ranging from 0.2 to 0.6 have been published.[3, 4, 18] A heritability of 0.6 is considered very high, but it means also that 40 per cent of the variation in disease expression is due to environmental factors. To the authors' knowledge, there are no published estimates of the heritability of FHD. Therefore, it is not possible at present to

---

*See references 5, 9–11, 28, 30–33, and 35.

determine with certainty whether the disease can be controlled through selective breeding of phenotypically normal cats.

◆ EPIDEMIOLOGY

Epidemiologic data on FHD in veterinary literature also are scant. Riser[19] first described FHD in 1964. He considered the main deformity to be bilaterally shallow, poorly formed acetabula. He suggested that the Siamese breed is affected most commonly, but included no substantiating data regarding breed prevalence.[19] In 1974, Holt[20] described a 3½-year-old Siamese cat with HD, and Kolde[21] reported an 8-year-old Siamese cat showing signs consistent with HD. Kolde[21] also noted 5 cats diagnosed radiographically at the University of Minnesota, 3 of which were Siamese. Hayes and coworkers[22] reported the largest epidemiologic study in 1979. In a retrospective study of records of patients seen by veterinary teaching hospitals collaborating with the National Cancer Institute between March 1964 and June 1977, 16 cats were diagnosed with HD, among approximately 270,000 visits. Fourteen of the 16 cats had radiographic or surgical documentation. Of those 14 cats, 8 were purebred, and 9 were females. The hospital incidence of HD in cats was 1/180 of that in dogs at the same facilities, over the same time period. In another retrospective study at a European veterinary teaching hospital from 1975 to 1986, examining all ventrodorsal pelvic radiographs, the radiographic incidence of FHD was 18 per cent (53 of 293).[23] There was no mention of clinical incidence in this group. In the early 1990s, there were 2 case reports describing 4 cats with HD, 1 male and 1 female domestic short hair, and 2 female Siamese.[24, 25]

In more recent studies, Langenbach and colleagues[1] evaluated a group of 78 purebred cats selected nonrandomly, with a radiographic FHD prevalence of 32 per cent (25 of 78). Ten per cent (8 of 78) of these cats had history of clinical signs related to FHD. Two of these 8 cats also had concurrent medial patellar luxation. There was no gender bias in this group, in contrast to the report by Hayes and coworkers.[22] Murphy and colleagues[2] examined a select group of 82 Maine coon cats, in which the radiographic prevalence of FHD was 51 per cent (42 of 82). Of this group, only 2 showed clinical signs referable to FHD. The same study included a group of 23 domestic shorthair cats presented for elective castration. In this set, 17 per cent (4 of 23) had radiographic evidence of HD, with 1 cat exhibiting clinical signs of hindlimb muscle atrophy and lameness. Although HD in cats has been considered previously to be an uncommon condition, the radiographic prevalence appears to be quite high. Studies incorporating large randomized populations of pedigreed and domestic shorthair cats are necessary to gain a more thorough understanding of actual FHD prevalence.

◆ PATHOGENESIS

Hip-joint laxity has been thought to be a major pathophysiologic factor in CHD,[6, 26–28] and evidence suggests that it plays a similar role in the pathogenesis of FHD.[1] Hip-joint laxity allows for damage to the femoral and acetabular cartilage and microfractures of the subchondral bone, which in turn can lead to DJD.[29] Laxity of the coxofemoral joint can be evaluated subjectively by Orthopedic Foundation for Animals (OFA)–like scoring, or measured using the Norberg angle (NA) or the distraction index (DI).[30, 31] The NA measures laxity of the femoral head from the acetabulum, evaluated on the ventrodorsal hip-extended radiograph. An NA of greater than 105 degrees is considered normal in dogs by some investigators.[32] The mean NA for cats that were free of HD was 98 degrees in 2 studies,[1, 23] and 90.7 degrees in a third.[2] Normal cats appear to have a lower NA than that deemed normal in dogs.

The DI was developed to measure maximum hip-joint laxity in dogs.[30] The mean DI in cats in 1 study was 0.51,[1] and 0.63 in another.[2] A relationship between laxity and DJD in the coxofemoral joint was demonstrated clearly in a recent study measuring laxity using NA and DI in a group of cats.[1] Cats that developed DJD had significantly lower mean NAs and higher DIs than cats without DJD. The mean NA for cats with DJD was 84 degrees ± 10, compared with 95 degrees ± 5 for cats without DJD. The mean DI for cats with DJD was 0.6 ± 0.11, compared with 0.49 ± 0.14 for cats without DJD. The mean DI of disease-free cats was greater than that of several dog breeds, including the Rhodesian ridgeback (0.34), Doberman pinscher (0.39), and borzoi (0.25). It was similar to the DI of the Labrador retriever (0.5) and the Gordon setter (0.48). Like these 2 dog breeds, cats in this study had substantial hip-joint laxity that could lead to development of DJD. Not all cats or dogs with hip-joint laxity develop DJD. Some cats with low hip-joint laxity (NA > 100 degrees) on the hip-extended radiograph developed DJD, and some cats with high hip-joint laxity (NA < 80 degrees) did not develop DJD.

A threshold was found in dogs (DI ≤ 0.3), below which DJD did not develop.[31] In the study by Langenbach and associates,[1] no cat below a DI of 0.4 had DJD, and only 1 cat with an NA greater than 93 degrees developed DJD. Cats were tested only once. A longitudinal study radiographing cats at several times during their lives would be necessary to verify the existence of a threshold. Although hip-joint laxity was the only factor that could be associated statistically with development of DJD (as in dogs), laxity alone could not explain all the variation in hip-joint phenotype, including DJD.

A weak association between HD and medial patellar luxation (MPL) was detected in a group of cats.[33] Cats with MPL were 3 times more likely to have HD than to have either condition alone. A trend also was identified to indicate that cats with more severe HD were more likely to have more severe stifle laxity, as measured by the Putnam grading system.[33] It is unknown whether cat joints, in general, have more laxity than corresponding joints in dogs. Greater laxity may be typical for cats, and may allow their inherent facile and agile movements. Greater hip-joint laxity, however, could be pathologic, and could predispose to DJD in joints other than the hip. This relationship has been studied in dogs, where it was found that about 30 per cent of young dogs predisposed to HD had pathologic changes in shoulder and stifle joints.[34] An associated factor that has been evaluated in CHD is increased synovial-fluid volume.[35] Similar studies in feline medicine are lacking.

◆ CLINICAL SIGNS

Clinical signs of FHD often are subtle and certainly are variable. Although recent reports have documented high radiographic prevalence of FHD (32 to 51 per cent),[1, 2, 23] the clinical incidence (and awareness) of disease is low. The owner may note slowly progressive changes in behavior and gait, or intermittent lameness. Young kittens may be less vigorous at play when compared with their littermates, or the older cat may seem more sessile in nature. Signs reported most commonly include unwillingness to jump or play, difficulty climbing stairs, intermittent lameness, crouched gait, pain on posturing to urinate or defecate, constipation secondary to pain and reluctance to defecate, pain on touching the hindquarters, howling for unknown reasons, or decreased appetite.[20–22, 24, 25] Again, however, the majority of affected cats are asymptomatic. The lack of clinical expression of disease may be explained by the cat's small size, greater tolerance to DJD of the hips, or anatomic differences in the feline pelvis that result in a less harsh biomechanical environment compared with the dog. The low clinical incidence of FHD also may be related to the owner's lack of performance expectations of the cat as a pet. The old adage "he's just a fat and lazy cat" may cloud an owner's recognition of decreased function, discomfort, or lameness. This is in contrast to the typical dog owner, who expects her or his pet to run, play, and be active, even at an older age.

◆ DIFFERENTIAL DIAGNOSIS

A number of orthopedic and neurologic conditions may share similar clinical signs, and result in physical findings similar to those of FHD. The most common causes of lameness in cats are trauma and animal-bite wounds.[36] Recently, the authors (unpublished data) have seen a number of young cats presented for evaluation of hindlimb lameness and suspected to have FHD. These cats, however, were found to have capital physeal fractures of unknown origin. Langenbach and coworkers[33] reported on a group of 78 purebred cats in which a weak correlation was found between MPL and hip dysplasia. Several cats in that group, as well as several other cats presented to the clinic for evaluation of FHD, were found to have pain on manipulation of the luxating patellae. Surgical repair of the luxating patellae resulted in resolution of clinical signs of pain and lameness. Although not common, cruciate ligament injuries also have been reported.[37, 38] Neurologic conditions including spinal cord neoplasia[39–43] and neuromuscular conditions such as myasthenia gravis[44] or primary myopathy may mimic the pelvic limb weakness seen in cats with HD. Other metabolic conditions, such as diabetic neuropathies (see Chapter 17, Diabetic Neuropathy) and lysosomal storage diseases,[45, 46] also may present with signs of hindlimb weakness or lameness. A group of lysosomal storage diseases has been shown to cause, among other problems, severe degenerative disease in several joints, including the coxofemoral joint. A urine spot test should be performed in cats with compatible clinical signs to rule out mucopolysaccharidoses (see Chapter 57, Mucopolysaccharidosis). Owing to the high radiographic incidence and low clinical incidence of FHD, whenever a cat is presented with signs referable to FHD, other orthopedic conditions must be ruled out before treatment for FHD is prescribed.

◆ DIAGNOSIS

Diagnosis of FHD is based on clinical signs, physical examination findings, and radiographic evaluation of the coxofemoral joints. Owing to the cat's independent nature and reluctance to be gaited on a leash, physical examination often is difficult and unrewarding for the veterinarian. Physical examination findings are similar to those in dogs, and include lameness, atrophy of hindlimb muscles, pain on extension and abduction of the hip joint, and palpable hip-joint laxity by means of the Bardens method or Ortolani technique.[20–22, 24] As in the canine patient, physical examination findings and radiographic findings do not necessarily correlate. Often, cats with severe DJD are not in pain on palpation, nor clinically lame.

By convention, definitive diagnosis of FHD is by radiographic findings of a poorly conforming femoral head and acetabulum. A ventrodorsal pelvic radiograph is made with the cat's hindlimbs fully extended, femurs parallel to each other, and patellae superimposed over the femoral condyles, as described by the American Veterinary Medical Association council on veterinary services for evaluation of the canine hip.[47] Subluxation of the femoral head from the acetabulum, DJD, or both is a hallmark finding of CHD.[48] Radiographic description of the dysplastic feline coxofemoral joint has been reported[19–21]; however, there are no standard scoring systems established for cats as there are for dogs. Radiographic findings reported in cats include subluxation of the femoral head from the acetabulum (Fig. 75–1), shallow acetabulum, and DJD of the acetabular rim and femoral head and neck (Fig. 75–2).

The NA can be measured from the ventrodorsal hip-extended radiographic view. The NA indicates displacement of the femoral head relative to the acetabulum, and implies HD. The NA is the included angle between a line joining the centers of the femoral heads and a line from the center of the femoral head with the effective craniolateral acetabular rim on the ipsilateral side. As mentioned in a previous section (see Pathogenesis), an NA of 105 degrees or greater is considered "normal" for dogs by some authors. An NA less than 105 degrees indicates displacement of the canine femoral head relative to the acetabulum and implies HD. There is no readily definable "normal" NA for cats; it is yet to be defined. The NA has been used primarily for research purposes, evaluating hip laxity from the hip-extended view. Heritability studies on the NA as a selection criterion for breeding or diagnostic purposes have not been published to date.

Recently, stress radiography has been used to

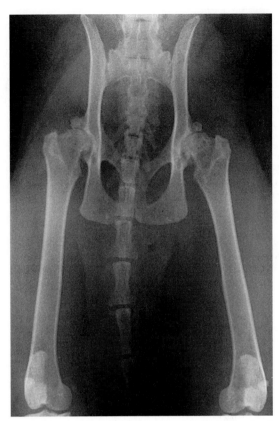

Figure 75–2. Standard hip-extended pelvic radiograph of a cat with severe hip dysplasia. Note bilateral subluxation, severe degenerative joint disease including remodeling of the femoral head and neck, and changes in the acetabular rim and edge.

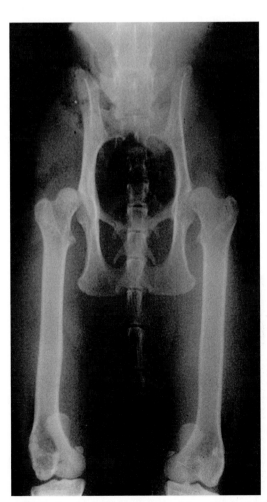

Figure 75–1. Standard hip-extended pelvic radiograph of a cat with bilateral hip dysplasia. Note bilateral subluxation, shallow acetabulum, and medial patellar luxation.

evaluate the hip joints of cats.[1, 2] In 1990, a stress-radiographic means of evaluating hip joints for passive laxity was introduced for dogs.[30] It is well-documented by the work of Smith and colleagues[30] that joint laxity is the most important predisposing factor for development of coxofemoral DJD in dogs. Radiographic evaluation of the hips is done using 3 views. First, the hip-extended view is taken for subjective evaluation of the hip joint for congruency and presence or absence of DJD (see Fig. 75–1). Next, compression (Fig. 75–3) and distraction (Fig. 75–4) radiographs are made, from which passive hip-joint laxity is measured. With the dog in a neutral, stance-phase position, a custom-designed distracter is used as a fulcrum to produce measurable lateral displacement of the femoral head from the acetabulum. The geometric centers of the acetabulum and femoral head are determined. The lateral displacement of the center of the femoral head from the acetabulum (in millimeters), divided by the radius of the femoral head (in millimeters), gives a unitless measure known as the distraction index (see Fig. 75–4). The DI ranges from 0 to 1. A DI of zero is a highly congruent joint, whereas a DI of 1 is a loose hip joint with minimal acetabular coverage. The DI has been shown to correlate highly with development of DJD in dogs.[30, 31] As the DI increases, so too does the risk of development of DJD. The

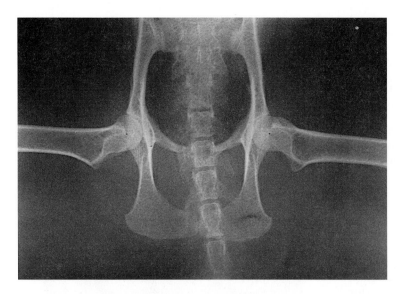

Figure 75–3. Compression view of a feline pelvis demonstrates highly congruent joint surfaces and good dorsal acetabular coverage.

major benefit of the DI is the ability to determine those dogs that are not at risk for development of DJD. A biologic threshold of 0.3 has been shown to be protective against DJD in dogs.[31] Recently, the DI has been shown to correlate with development of DJD in a group of cats.[1] Research is in progress to determine the biologic threshold for protection against DJD in cats, as well as the heritability of the DI and its usefulness as a selection criterion for breeding purposes.

◆ TREATMENT
Conservative Management

Conservative management of CHD is prescribed frequently, with good long-term clinical results.[49, 50] Conservative treatment includes weight reduction, NSAIDs for treatment of inflammation, and avoidance of those activities that exacerbate clinical pain and lameness. Owing to the low clinical incidence of FHD, little is published regarding conservative

treatment of coxofemoral DJD. Aspirin is not licensed for use in companion animals; however, it is the most commonly used NSAID in dogs and cats.[51] Aspirin has been recommended as the only NSAID for the treatment of osteoarthritis in cats.[51] Owing to the cat's lack of phase II conjugating abilities with glucuronic acid, drug dosage, frequency, and risk of toxicity limit some clinicians' use of aspirin. In the authors' experience, aspirin doses of 20 mg/kg every (q) 72 hr orally can be used safely with few side-effects. Although use of corticosteroids for treatment of DJD is controversial, these drugs have been used for the treatment of pain associated with DJD in cats. The anti-inflammatory properties of corticosteroids are quite good, and cats are more tolerant of the metabolic side-effects than dogs. However, at high dosages, corticosteroids have a negative effect on cartilage metabolism, are destructive to collagen, suppress proteoglycan synthesis, and contribute to chondrocyte death.[52, 53] As a result, many clinicians consider use of corticosteroids for treatment of DJD only after exhausting other treatment options.[54] Re-

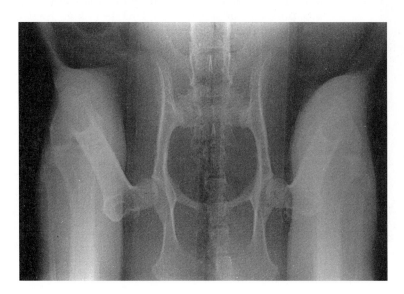

Figure 75–4. Distraction view of a feline pelvis demonstrates obvious passive hip joint laxity. The distraction index is 0.50 for both hips.

cently, neutraceuticals have become more popular among pet owners and veterinarians for treatment of the pain of DJD in dogs. Neutraceuticals currently on the market are labeled for use in cats. Clinical improvement has been noted empirically; however, there are no controlled, double-blind studies currently available to support these clinical impressions. Until such time, the perceived benefits gained from the use of neutraceuticals should not be over-interpreted.

Surgical Management

Surgical control of DJD of the feline hip joint is aimed at relieving pain associated with the synovitis of cartilage erosion and with the bone-on-bone contact of osteoarthritis. Surgical correction is recommended when the cat does not respond to conservative management, or when the quality of life or function is not acceptable to the owner. Early reports of pectineus resection for the control of FHD are limited and have mixed outcomes.[20, 21] In dogs, use of pectineus resection for treatment of pain associated with CHD has been abandoned because the procedure does not alter the course of disease, and recurrence of hip-joint pain is common. The most frequently reported technique of surgical management for FHD is femoral head and neck ostectomy. Postoperatively, cats no longer experience pain associated with DJD, and usually return to normal function. In severely affected cats with bilateral disease, the procedure can be performed from a ventral approach with low morbidity. It is the authors' impression that cats do very well clinically after femoral head and neck ostectomy. Currently, there is no commercially available total-hip replacement for use in cats.

◆ CONTROL/PREVENTION

There are no reports addressing the prevention of HD in cats. We suspect the mode of inheritance of FHD is similar to that of dogs. As mentioned previously, the heritability of HD in cats is unknown, and reports of the heritability of CHD range from 0.2 to 0.6. The heritability is the proportion of a phenotypic trait that is attributable to the average effects of the genes.[55] The most important use of heritability is its predictive role in expressing the reliability of the phenotypic value as a guide to the breeding value. Traits that are highly heritable, greater than 20 per cent, can be reduced through selective breeding programs when that trait is used as a selection criterion.[55] Without knowledge of the heritability of a measurable trait, one cannot tell how closely the phenotype represents the genotype, or whether that trait can be reduced through selective breeding programs.

Currently, there are several options open to the dog breeder wishing to prevent CHD. The most com-monly followed method for controlling HD is breeding "normal-to-normal" dogs based on an assessment of hip-joint conformation by the OFA.[26] Owing to the polygenic mode of inheritance of hip dysplasia, radiographically "normal" dogs and cats carry genes for HD. As a result, these breedings often result in dysplastic offspring, and the incidence of CHD has remained high despite well-meaning efforts to reduce its frequency. A major disadvantage has been the subjective nature by which the hips are scored traditionally. Hip-joint laxity, which in dogs is the major contributing factor leading to development of CHD, is masked in the hip-extended view.[56] Evaluation of hip joints in the hip-extended view is not physiologic, and the resulting forces on the hip-joint capsule lead to a tightening effect. Recently, the OFA has recommended the screening of breeding cats using the same subjective criteria as those used in dogs. However, to the authors' knowledge, the OFA has published no data on cats (or dogs) proving the efficacy of the method when used as a criterion for selecting breeding animals. We encourage the OFA to perform such studies and to estimate the heritability of its diagnostic phenotype.

In 1990, a stress-radiographic means of evaluating the hip joints for passive laxity was introduced for dogs.[30] It is well-documented that hip-joint laxity in dogs is the most important predisposing factor leading to development of DJD of the hip joint.[31] The DI from distraction stress radiography has been shown to correlate with development of DJD in dogs.[30-32] Risk for development of DJD increases with increasing DI in dogs. Recently, the DI has been shown to correlate with development of DJD in a group of cats,[1, 2] and research as to the DI's usefulness as a selection criterion for breeding is ongoing.

Until the heritability of FHD is calculated based on the hip-extended radiographic view or stress radiography, the genetic significance or impact of applying either test as a guide for a breeding program is speculative. This is not to discourage radiographing stud toms and queens, but rather is a word of caution, based on our current understanding of FHD. Whichever means of evaluating the hip joints of breeding cats is used, cats should receive yearly radiographic evaluation of their hips to ascertain maintenance of normal hip-joint conformation. Recently, the authors evaluated a stud tom that was scored by OFA as "Good" at 3 years of age, and "Moderate HD" with DJD when evaluated at 7 years of age. This cat, scored first as "normal," has been passing genes for poor hip-joint conformation to subsequent generations. Currently, heritability studies on passive hip laxity in cats, as measured by stress radiography, are ongoing. From these studies, we will be able to determine the most effective means for evaluating the hip joints at an early age. Longitudinal evaluation of cats also is being conducted to determine the youngest practical age of evaluation, and to establish normal laxity profiles for the various breeds of cats.

REFERENCES

1. Langenbach A, Green P, Giger U, et al: Relationship of degenerative joint disease and laxity in the coxofemoral joint by use of distraction index and Norberg angle measurement in a group of cats. J Am Vet Med Assoc 213:1439–1443, 1998.
2. Murphy TP, Biery DN, Smith GK: Hip dysplasia in a group of 82 Maine coon cats (Abstract). 6th Annual Conference of European Association of Veterinary Diagnostic Imaging, Vienna, Austria, 1999, p. 87.
3. Hedhammer A, Olsson SE, Anderson SA, et al: Canine hip dysplasia: Study of heritability in 401 litters of German shepherd dogs. J Am Vet Med Assoc 174:1012–1018, 1979.
4. Leighton EA: Genetics of canine hip dysplasia. J Am Vet Med Assoc 210:1474–1479, 1997.
5. Henricson B, Norberg J, Olsson SE: On the etiology and pathogenesis of hip dysplasia: A comparative review. J Small Anim Pract 7:673–687, 1966.
6. Riser WH: The dog as a model for the study of hip dysplasia: Growth, form, and development of the normal and dysplastic hip joint. Vet Pathol 12:224–234, 1975.
7. Riser WH: Canine hip dysplasia. In Bojrab MJ (ed): Disease Mechanisms in Small Animal Surgery, 2nd ed. Philadelphia, Lea & Febiger, 1993, pp. 793–803.
8. Lust G, Geary JC, Sheffy BE: Development of hip dysplasia in dogs. Am J Vet Res 34:87–91, 1973.
9. Kealy RD, Olsson SE, Monti KL, et al: Effects of limited food consumption on the incidence of hip dysplasia in growing dogs. J Am Vet Med Assoc 201:857–863, 1992.
10. Kealy RD, Lawler DF, Ballam JM, et al: Five-year longitudinal study on limited food consumption and development of osteoarthritis in coxofemoral joints of dogs. J Am Vet Med Assoc 210:222–225, 1997.
11. Kealy RD, Lawler DF, Monti KL, et al: Effects of dietary electrolyte balance on subluxation of femoral heads in growing dogs. Am J Vet Res 54:555–562, 1993.
12. Cardinet GH, Kass PH, Wallace LJ, et al: Association between pelvic muscle mass and canine hip dysplasia. J Am Vet Med Assoc 210:1466–1473, 1997.
13. Lust G, Williams AJ, Burton-Wurster N, et al: Effects of intramuscular administration of glycosaminoglycan polysulfates on signs of incipient hip dysplasia in growing pups. Am J Vet Res 53:1836–1843, 1992.
14. Riser WH, Cohen D, Lindquist S, et al: Influence of early rapid growth and weight gain on hip dysplasia in the German shepherd dog. J Am Vet Med Assoc 145:661–668, 1964.
15. Priester WA, Mulvihill JJ. Canine hip dysplasia: Relative risk by sex, size, and breed and comparative aspects. J Am Vet Med Assoc 160:735–739, 1972.
16. Hedhammer A, Wu FM, Krook L, et al: Overnutrition and skeletal disease: An experiment in growing Great Dane dogs. Cornell Vet 64(Suppl 5):1–157, 1974.
17. Kasstrom H: Nutrition, weight gain and the development of hip dysplasia. Acta Radiol Suppl (Stockh) 344:135–179, 1975.
18. Jessen CR, Spurrell FA: Heritability of canine hip dysplasia. In Proceedings: Canine Hip Dysplasia Symposium, October 19–20, 1972, St. Louis, 1973, pp. 53–61.
19. Riser WH: Diseases of the locomotor system. In Catcott EJ (ed): Feline Medicine and Surgery, 1st ed. Santa Barbara, CA, American Veterinary Publishing, 1964, pp. 296–297.
20. Holt E: Hip dysplasia in a cat. J Small Anim Pract 19:273–276, 1978.
21. Kolde DL: Pectineus tenectomy for treatment of hip dysplasia in a domestic cat: A case report. J Am Anim Hosp Assoc 10:239, 1975.
22. Hayes MH, Wilson GP, Burt JK: Feline hip dysplasia. J Am Anim Hosp Assoc 15:447–448, 1979.
23. Keoppel E, Ebner J: Die Hueftgelenksdysplasie der Katze. Kleintierpraxis 35:281–298, 1990.
24. Rabin KL, Haan JJ, Ackerman N: Hip dysplasia in a litter of domestic shorthair cats. Fel Pract 22:15–19, 1994.
25. Patsikas MN, Papazoglou LG, Komninou A, et al: Hip dysplasia in the cat: A report of three cases. J Small Anim Pract 39:290–294, 1998.
26. Corley EA, Keller GG: Hip dysplasia: A Guide for Dog Breeders and Owners, 2nd ed. Columbia, MO: Orthopedic Foundation for Animals, 1989, pp. 1–27.
27. Lust G, Beilman WT, Dueland DJ, et al: Intra-articular volume and hip joint instability in dogs with hip dysplasia. J Bone Joint Surg 62A:576–582, 1980.
28. Wright PJ, Mason TA: The usefulness of palpation of joint laxity in puppies as a predictor of hip dysplasia in a guide dog breeding program. J Small Anim Pract 18:513–522, 1977.
29. Morgan SJ: The pathology of canine hip dysplasia. Vet Clin North Am Small Anim Pract 22:541–550, 1992.
30. Smith GK, Biery DN, Gregor TP: New concepts of coxofemoral joint stability and the development of a clinical stress-radiographic method for quantitating hip joint laxity in the dog. J Am Vet Med Assoc 196:59–70, 1990.
31. Smith GK, Gregor TP, Rhodes WH, et al: Coxofemoral joint laxity from distraction radiography and its contemporaneous and prospective correlation with laxity, subjective score, and evidence of degenerative joint disease from conventional hip-extended radiography in dogs. Am J Vet Res 7:1021–1042, 1993.
32. Smith GK, Popovitch CA, Gregor TP, et al: Evaluation of risk factors for degenerative joint disease associated with hip dysplasia in dogs. J Am Vet Med Assoc 206:642–646, 1995.
33. Smith GK, Langenbach A, Green PA, et al: Evaluation of the association between medial patellar luxation and hip dysplasia in cats. J Am Vet Med Assoc 215:40–45, 1999.
34. Olsewski JM, Lust G, Rendano VT, Summers BA: Degenerative joint disease: Multiple joint involvement in young and mature dogs. Am J Vet Res 44:1300–1308, 1983.
35. Lust G, Beilman WT, Rendano VT: A relationship between degree of laxity and synovial fluid volume in coxofemoral joints of dogs predisposed for hip dysplasia. J Am Vet Med Assoc 41:55–60, 1980.
36. Schrader SC, Sherding RG: Disorders of the skeletal system. In Sherding RG (ed): The Cat: Diseases and Clinical Management, 1st ed, vol. 2. New York, Churchill Livingstone, 1989, pp. 1247–1292.
37. McManus JL, Nimmons GB: Ruptured anterior cruciate ligament in a cat. Can Vet J 7:264, 1967.
38. Scavelli TD, Schrader SC: Nonsurgical management of rupture of the cranial cruciate ligament in 18 cats. J Am Anim Hosp Assoc 23:337, 1987.
39. Zaki FA, Hurvitz AI: Spontaneous neoplasms of the central nervous system of the cat. J Small Anim Pract 17:773–782, 1976.
40. Gilmore DR: Feline pelvic limb paresis/paralysis. Compend Contin Educ Pract Vet 5:408–412, 1983.
41. Lane SB, Kornegay JN, Duncan JR, et al: Feline spinal lymphosarcoma: A retrospective evaluation of 23 cats. J Vet Intern Med 8:99–104, 1994.
42. Spodnick GJ, Berg J, Moore FM, et al: Spinal lymphoma in cats: 21 cases (1976–1989). J Am Vet Med Assoc 200:373–376, 1990.
43. Levy MS, Mauldin G, Kapatkin AS, et al: Nonlymphoid vertebral canal tumors in cats: 11 cases (1987–1995). J Am Vet Med Assoc 210:663–664, 1997.
44. Ducote JM, Dewey CW, Coates JR: Clinical forms of acquired myasthenia gravis in cats. Compend Contin Educ Pract Vet 21:440–448, 1999.
45. Breton L, Guerin P, Morin M: A case of mucopolysaccharidosis VI in a cat. J Am Anim Hosp Assoc 19:891–896, 1983.
46. Konde LJ, Thrall MA, Gasper P, et al: Radiographically visualized skeletal changes associated with mucopolysaccharidosis VI in cats. Vet Radiol 28:223–228, 1987.
47. AVMA Council on Veterinary Services: Report of panel on canine hip dysplasia. J Am Vet Med Assoc 139:791–798, 1961.
48. Lust G: Hip dysplasia in dogs. In Slatter D (ed): Textbook of Small Animal Surgery, 2nd ed, vol. 2. Philadelphia, WB Saunders, 1993, pp. 1938–1944.
49. Barr ARS, Denny HR, Gibbs C: Clinical hip dysplasia in growing dogs: The long-term results of conservative management. J Small Anim Pract 28:243–252, 1987.

50. Smith GK, Fordyce HH, Gregor TP: Non-surgical management of severe hip dysplasia: Long-term results. Proceedings, 26th Annual Meeting of Veterinary Orthopedic Society, Sun Valley, ID, February 27–March 6, 1999, p. 12.

51. Boothe DM: Controlling inflammation with non-steroidal anti-inflammatory drugs. Vet Med 84:875–883, 1989.

52. Mankin HJ, Conger KA: The acute effects of intra-articular hydrocortisone on articular cartilage in rabbits. J Bone Joint Surg Am 48:1383–1388, 1966.

53. Behrens F, Shepard N, Mitchell N: Alterations of rabbit artic-ular cartilage by intra-articular injection of glucocorticoids. J Bone Joint Surg Am 57:70–76, 1975.

54. Johnston SA, Fox SM: Mechanisms of action of anti-inflammatory medications used for the treatment of osteoarthritis. J Am Vet Med Assoc 210:1486–1492, 1997.

55. Falconer DS: Introduction to Quantitative Genetics, 3rd ed. New York, John Wiley & Sons, 1989, pp. 163–186.

56. Smith GK, LaFond E, Heyman SJ: Biomechanical characterization of passive laxity of the hip joint in dogs. Am J Vet Res 58:2078–2082, 1997.

76

◆ Understanding the Feline Genome

Leslie A. Lyons

Genomics is the analysis of DNA and the structure and function of genes. Genome initiatives, some highly organized and some cottage industries, exist today for many species. This chapter focuses on the genome initiative for the domestic cat, how genetic issues have affected cat breeds, and how comparative genetics will assist new research. Veterinarians who understand how to use this knowledge effectively will be better able to exert significant influence on feline breeding and health, and simultaneously add a measure of diversity to their practices.

◆ BACKGROUND

History of Genetics

During the mid-1800s, Gregor Mendel, the father of genetics, tested laws of inheritance with pea plant characteristics. These visible characteristics, flower color or pea shape, are called *phenotypes*. Mendel proved that phenotypes can be inherited dominantly, recessively, or codominantly. By knowing the inheritance model, the phenotypes of offspring, and the frequency of their appearance, can be predicted from the phenotypes of mated parents. About the same time, Charles Darwin was documenting the phenotypic diversity of plants and animals throughout the world. Darwin hypothesized that natural selection played a role in altering the frequency of phenotypic characteristics, resulting in population diversity, genetic isolation, and finally, in speciation. Chromosomes were discovered nearly a half-century later, and DNA finally was discovered a full century after Mendel's studies.

One Gene, One Protein

Chromosomes carry genes that consist of sequences of DNA. Cats have 19 pairs of chromosomes, inheriting 1 member of each pair from the dam and the other from the sire. Each chromosome is a very long DNA string; therefore, cats have 38 strings of DNA (19 pairs) in every cell, except for the egg and sperm, which carry 1 copy of each chromosome, combining at fertilization to again yield the full cellular DNA complement. DNA is a long string of 4 chemical bases called *nucleotides* (adenine, guanine, cytosine, and thymine). An average gene contains approximately 1 million bases, repeated over and over in different orders and combinations. With 50,000 to 100,000 genes in an individual's DNA complement,

human beings (or cats) have nearly 3 billion bases making up their DNA.

Any gene appears only once, in 2 copies, in a normal individual. Genes code for synthesis of proteins, which in turn control phenotypic characteristics. A phenotype can be produced by 1 protein or by an interaction of several proteins. When the DNA base sequence of a specific gene varies slightly, the protein coded may vary slightly as well. For example, tyrosinase is a protein that is involved in melanin production. Melanin is responsible for the color (phenotype) seen in the cat's coat. The gene (base sequence) for tyrosinase may be slightly different among individuals in a population, meaning that tyrosinase has different alleles. The alleles for tyrosinase in the cat are termed *full color, burmese, siamese,* and *albino.* Changing 1 of the bases in a specific area of the gene may cause no significant color difference. Alternatively, it may cause a slight, nonpathologic change in the tyrosinase protein, perhaps just enough to cause tyrosinase to function differently. The change may cause a phenotypic variation, making full-color black coats lighter, or burmese. Or the result of the base change may be more striking, causing a black cat to be albino. Other changes may affect the protein much more seriously, so that a disease or malformation results. If changes in both members of the gene pair are required for the dysfunction to cause a disease, then the disease is caused by a recessive mutation. If the consequences of the alteration are more severe, and only 1 copy can cause a disease, then that disease is caused by a dominant mutation.

When 2 or more alleles for a gene are present in a population, the gene is called *polymorphic* (many "morphs" or types). Homozygous (*homo-* meaning same) implies that the same allele is present on both chromosomes. Heterozygous (*heter-* meaning different) implies that the alleles are different, and the individual is polymorphic. Tonkinese cats are heterozygous for tyrosinase alleles; therefore, they are polymorphic at the tyrosinase locus.

Every time a new cell is formed, all DNA has to be copied. During this copying process, 1 in 1 million nucleotides is copied incorrectly. Such a spontaneous change occurs at random; this is the source of natural variation. When a kitten suddenly appears with color that cannot be explained by the parents' colors (phenotypes), proper identification of paternity may not be the issue. Mutations are natural, and no 2 cats are the same. Thus, genetic differences can be inherited from parents, or they can be created naturally by mutations.

The molecular study of genes is an exploding area of scientific research. Each living organism, from the smallest microbe to the largest blue whale, has a set of genes in DNA or RNA form, governing its survival and reproduction. Emergence of life on our planet, and evolution from single-cell to multicelled and higher organisms, can be traced in our genes. Thus, examination of the genetics of 1 species aids understanding of the genetics of another species. This field of science, called *comparative genetics*, has facilitated development of genome initiatives in species other than human beings and mice.

Inheritance Versus Environment

Although Mendel introduced the science of genetics over 150 years ago, geneticists still must establish inheritance patterns for important phenotypes. Phenotypes can be influenced by outside, nongenetic (generally meaning noninherited) factors, which at times makes understanding them a very complex problem. Diseases like epilepsy, asthma, and hip dysplasia have complex inheritance patterns and significant environmental components. Nongenetic influences, such as drugs, toxins, infections, metabolic disorders, sporadic damage or other alterations of DNA, and environmental factors, such as diet, exercise, and social surroundings, can produce a phenotype that looks just like an inherited characteristic or disease. This is called a *phenocopy*. Oxalate crystals can be produced by ethylene glycol intoxication or by a single-gene inherited defect. Some diseases may present differently in different tissues. These are termed *pleotrophic effects* of the same gene. For example, some completely white cats can be just white, whereas others also may be odd-eyed or have blue eyes, and may be deaf. The first task of the geneticist is to segregate environmental from nonenvironmental (genetic) effects on the phenotype.

Simple genetic investigations have become commonplace, and therefore exploration of more complex phenotypes has become the new frontier. Geneticists must team up with clinicians, epidemiologists, and breeders to accomplish this new research. The geneticist may not be trained for clinical diagnosis and therapy, whereas the clinician may not be trained to identify problems with genetic components, or to conduct evaluations that may be necessary to differentiate potentially genetic problems that have similar presentations. For both, however, the first task is to recognize a genetic problem correctly.

◆ POPULATION CHARACTERISTICS OF GENETIC DISEASES

Phenotypes can be described as diseases, traits, or types that can be desirable (except, of course, for most diseases) or undesirable. Phenotypes can result from actions of single genes, from interactions among several genes, from accumulation of environmental exposures, or from combinations of these effects. The clinician can help to define the status of study subjects, and segregate individuals that probably have genetic disorders. The geneticist would like to identify and evaluate individuals with phenotypes that primarily are genetic. Breeders would like to know if a phenotype has a large genetic component, and how to alter husbandry to increase or reduce the frequency of appearance. Hopefully, geneticists will be able to identify markers to the phenotype, or even the exact mutation, so that breeders can design very specific breeding practices to either eliminate or maintain the phenotype. A veterinarian may choose a different route of clinical management, or make a different prognosis, if a phenotype is known to be genetic. If the same condition is found in other species, veterinarians may have opportunities to try novel approaches for health care. Several characteristics that are common to genetic diseases can help separate sporadic, nongenetic occurrences from inherited diseases.

Six characteristics of inherited diseases are

1. Early age of onset
2. Bilateral and/or multiple presentation
3. Found in a closed population
4. Indication of inbreeding
5. Age of parents
6. Uniformity in presentation

Two examples of diseases that present with sporadic and inherited forms are polycystic kidney disease (PKD) and lymphosarcoma. The 6 listed characteristics of genetic diseases facilitate isolating individuals that carry genetic factors controlling these diseases. Only 1 characteristic, age of parents, has not been shown to have an effect in cats with genetic diseases.

Kidney cysts may occur in many cats, but inherited PKD occurs as early as 6 to 8 weeks of age. Both kidneys are affected, and multiple cysts generally are found. The cysts are of nonuniform size, but of course have common etiology. PKD is common in Persian cats, and thus may be present in related breeds, such as exotics and Himalayans. PKD is a dominant disease that technically could be eliminated by breeding practices alone. PKD may not compromise health until advanced age, when chronic health problems are accepted more readily as normal events. Dissemination throughout the Persian breed has been facilitated because breeding and show performance are events that occur earlier in life, when affected cats usually have not yet developed clinical signs.

Lymphosarcoma also occurs frequently in cats, but usually it is found in older cats, and in cats that have been infected with, and test positive for, feline leukemia virus (FeLV). However, a very high rate of lymphosarcoma has been identified in silver Oriental shorthairs that are FeLV-negative. Related breeds, such as Siamese, color-point shorthairs, and long-haired Siamese, also should be suspected. Affected cats generally develop a mediastinal tumor, but not universally. Age of onset is 1 to 2 years, and the tumors respond well to chemotherapy. Thus, this disease is found in a closed, probably inbred population, and has early onset and fairly uniform presentation. Although it is recessive, implying that breeding practices alone will not eliminate it, the early onset compromises breeding and showing, and thus it is disseminated less widely than PKD. Detecting carriers is the primary difficulty, and test breedings are cumbersome, inaccurate, and costly.

A genetic problem that occurs with high frequency can be found in nearly every breed, and therefore no one breed can be considered to be more healthy than others. However, the breed itself does not cause the problem. Husbandry practices of breeders and rules of cat fancy registries tend to be more problematic in this respect. Detrimental genes are found in random-bred cats also. The important difference is that, with recessive or dominant diseases that do not cause early clinical signs, breeders can be completely unaware that they are propagating a deleterious gene. Such is the case for PKD, and for amyloidosis that is found in Abyssinians. Breeds with no obvious health problems still may have low genetic diversity, which could predispose to decimation of varying but significant proportions of the entire breed. A classic example is the loss of a large portion of a captive cheetah colony to feline infectious peritonitis (FIP). Low genetic diversity is considered to be a major factor in the death of 33 per cent of a colony of cheetahs that were exposed to coronavirus. Apparently healthy, adult cheetahs did not have sufficient immune competence to overcome the infection, as do most cats. Because this particular group had little diversity, the pathogenic strain of coronavirus that caused FIP was able to affect many cats. This probably is the reason that particular lines of other types of cats may be either more or less susceptible to FIP.

Health problems, genetic and nongenetic, also may occur because of the conformation or "type" desired for the breed. Shortened skull structures and nasal canals cause Persians to have weeping eyes and increased susceptibility to upper respiratory tract diseases. The fine, elegant skeletal structures of Abyssinians and Siamese seem to facilitate patellar luxation. The largest breed of domestic cats, the Maine coon, is under investigation for hip dysplasia (HD), a very common problem in large dog breeds (see Chapter 75, Hip Dysplasia). Certainly, these problems have a genetic component, but determining the number and effects of involved genes will be difficult. Complex diseases also are under intense scrutiny in the genome projects of other species. The role of the geneticist and the veterinarian is not to place blame, but to assist with development of corrective husbandry practices by providing genetic counseling to breeders and the cat fancy

organizations, and to help place required study materials in the hands of the appropriate researchers.

◆ CAT BREED POPULATION DYNAMICS

The "Gold Standard"

Random-bred cats should be the most healthy feline population, genetically speaking. They are exposed to infectious diseases, poor nutrition, the outside environment, territorial disputes, and less health care, when compared with fancy-bred cats. These naturally selective forces act to reduce the frequency of detrimental genes that compromise migration, survival, and propagation. Isolated populations of cats also may have a characteristic defect, like taillessness on the Isle of Man. If the trait generally does not affect propagation, it becomes disseminated. Fancy-bred cats usually are the groups that have higher frequency of inherited diseases. The same defects can occur in random-bred populations, but fancy-bred cats are highly influenced by their human companions.

Founder Effects

Over 40 different cat breeds are recognized throughout the world. The number and nomenclature of the breeds differ according to the cat fanciers' organizations, but approximately 30 breeds are standard. Of these breeds, approximately 20 were recognized before the establishment of the cat fancy in the late 1800s. Folklore often obscures the true origins and identity of breeds, but the breeds listed in Table 76–1 are considered to be foundation breeds because of the early time of recognition and the isolated areas in which they apparently were developed. The breeds listed in Table 76–2 were developed from other breeds, or at least from populations that have a gene pool that is likely to be found in other breeds. Such are the Cornish and Devon rexes. These two breeds are approximately 50 years old, and were developed from random-bred cats in the United Kingdom. Random-bred cats and British shorthairs are likely to have the same genetic composition as these breeds.

The foundation cat breeds found in Table 76–1 should have the most genetic diversity. They are very old breeds, generally established from random-bred cats of the region. (Darwin noted that Asian cats looked different from British cats, although he did not apply a breed label at the time.) Thus, the foundation stock for these cats probably was broad at the time that they were "formally" developed into a breed. These breeds can be considered to have a small founder effect. A founder effect implies that only a few cats were used to develop a breed, and whatever genetic diversity was present in the founders represents the diversity available for the

Table 76–1. Founder Populations for Cat Breeds

Breed	Location of Origin	Date Established	Related Breeds
Abyssinian	Ethiopia	1868	Somali
American shorthair	United States	1966	
Birman	Burma	Founder	Snowshoe
British shorthair	England	1870s	
Burmese	Burma	1350–1767	Bombay, Tiffany, Malayan
Chartreux	France	1300	
Egyptian Mau	Egypt	1953	Bengal
European shorthair	Italy	1982	
Japanese bobtail	Japan	500–1100	
Korat	Thailand	1350–1767	
Maine coon	United States	1860s	
Manx	Isle of Man	Founder	Cymric
Norwegian forest cat	Norway	Founder	
Persian	Persia	Founder	Exotic, Kashmir, Himalayan, Sterling
Russian blue	Russia	Founder	Nebelung
Siamese	Thailand	1350–1767	Color-point, Javanese, Balinese, Oriental
Siberian	Russia	Founder	
Singapura	Singapore	1971	
Sokoke forest	Africa	1977	
Turkish angora	Ankara	1400	
Turkish Van	Van Lake	Founder	

breed. If the founders have excellent traits, then the breed is more likely to be generally healthy. If the founders have detrimental (usually recessive) traits, then the breed may experience more frequent problems that result from low genetic diversity.

Reduced Migration

Migration also contributes to genetic diversity. Migration in this sense is not necessarily movement of cats around the world, but rather indicates mating of different cat populations, or breeds, thereby facilitating "migration" of different genes into a breed's gene pool. The nature of breed development and breed registries reduces migration. A closed studbook implies no migration. A group of cats are considered to be a breed when they "breed true"; that is, mating produces cats like themselves, perhaps in different colors that would be predictable. To achieve this effect, a defined breeding program that uses cats with particular characteristics must be established. The more rigid these initial characteristics are, the less gene flow occurs from other populations. The result is reduced migration, which leads in turn to reduced genetic diversity. Both Abyssini-

Table 76–2. More Recently Developed Cat Breeds

Breed	Origin	Foundation Stock	Date	Location
American bobtail	Mutation	Random bred	1960s	United States
American curl	Mutation	Random bred	1981	United States
American wirehair	Mutation	Random bred	1966	United States
Australian mist	Crossbreed	Several breeds	1976	Australia
Bengal	Hybrid	*Felis bengalensis* × *Felis catus*	1963	United States
Burmilla	Crossbreed	Persian × Burmese	1981	England
California spangled	Crossbreed	Several breeds	1971	United States
Cornish rex	Mutation	Random bred	1950	England
Coupari	Mutation	Scottish fold	1980s	England
Devon rex	Mutation	Random bred	1960	England
Havana brown	Crossbreed	Orientals	1952	Great Britain
LaPerm	Mutation	Random bred	1986	United States
Munchkin	Mutation	Random bred	1991	United States
Ocicat	Crossbreed	Siamese × Abyssinian	1964	United States
Ojo azules	Mutation	Random bred	1984	United States
Pixiebob	Crossbreed	Random bred	1990s	United States
Ragamuffin	Crossbreed	Persian × Birman	1994	United States
Ragdoll	Crossbreed	Persian × Birman	1960s	United States
Safari	Hybrid	*O. geoffroyi* × *F. catus*	1970s	United States
Savannah	Hybrid	*Felis serval* × *F. catus*	1990s	United States
Scottish fold	Mutation	Random bred	1961	Scotland
Selkirk rex	Mutation	Random bred	1987	United States
Serengeti	Hybrid	*Felis chaus* × *F. catus*	1990s	United States
Sphynx	Mutation	Random bred	1966	Canada

ans and Persians are very old breeds. A variety of coat colors is recognized for Persians, whereas Abyssinians are more restricted. Therefore, even though both breeds should have diverse foundations, more genetic diversity can be expected in the Persian breed, because cats of many different colors were used to produce the recognized varieties (i.e., more genetic variation has been maintained in the population). When new breeds are being established and are considered provisional, outcrossing is allowed. This implies that migration of new genes into the breed is not yet limited. The longer such outcrosses are allowed, the more genetic diversity can enter. However, 1 result of this procedure is that it is more difficult to get cats to "breed true."

Inbreeding

Inbreeding quickly reduces genetic variation and increases the frequency of recessive genes. Recessive genes can be desirable (points on a Siamese), or they can be undesirable (progressive retinal atrophy [PRA]). Inbreeding occurs in different degrees. A sibling-parent cross can be much closer, or inbred, than sibling crosses, or a sibling-grandparent cross. Each parent provides half of its genetic complement to the offspring. Parents and offspring always are 50 per cent genetically identical, although the distribution is random. Thus, any 2 siblings can be completely different, 50 per cent alike, or even 100 per cent alike. On average, siblings are 50 per cent alike, but parents and offspring are exactly 50 per cent alike genetically. The more inbred a group of cats becomes, the less the genetic variation, and the higher the likelihood that they will be inheriting the same set of genes. If any detrimental genes exist in the population, these also become more frequent. Line breeding is a form of inbreeding. Developing a line is the first step toward developing a new breed. The line has specific founders and reduced migration, and is becoming inbred. The strength of the inbreeding depends on the other population dynamics, the foundation size, and the degree of migration.

Population Bottlenecks

Population bottlenecks occur frequently in the cat fancy. The term is not recognized universally, but the practice is extremely common. A bottleneck occurs when only specific individuals of a population contribute to the next generation. This can occur as a result of many individuals dying, such as the lions in the Ngorongoro Crater because of the biting fly epidemic, or because someone prevents cats from breeding. Cat fanciers have competitions. The "best" cat wins, based on the adherence to an established breed standard. Because of subsequent high breeding demand, the genes of this cat can be disseminated quickly and widely in the breed, particularly if the cat is male. A popular stud can reduce the contributions of other males, creating a manufactured population bottleneck. Bottlenecks constantly occur to varying degrees, influenced by gender, cooperativeness among breeders, mating success, litter size, and kitten viability. A good example of a population bottleneck can be found in Burmese cats in the United States. In the early 1970s, a winning cat became very popular and helped found a new variety, the contemporary Burmese. Several years after development of this new variety, an autosomal recessive head defect began to appear. The defect was confined to the contemporary variety and can be traced to 1 or 2 cats at the foundation of the group. This congenital defect is a result of a population bottleneck.

Genetic diversity generally implies improved health for the individual and the population. The development of breeds is contradictory to maintaining genetic diversity, but awareness of the population dynamics that influence diversity can help breeding programs remain effective. A good breeding program starts with a large, outbred population as its foundation. Open studbooks help the migration of new genes.

Recognizing many colors helps to maintain a good genetic foundation for a breed. Breeder cooperation and awareness can reduce the inbreeding and bottleneck effects. Beautiful and healthy breeds can be maintained by balancing husbandry practices with concerns about genetic diversity. Veterinarians can help breeders with husbandry counseling and reviews of good breeding practices.

◆ GENETIC DISEASE ASCERTAINMENT

The first individual to recognize an inherited problem usually is a breeder/owner or a veterinarian. The feline species has a "gold standard": random-bred, genetically diverse domestic cats. Most veterinarians are familiar with the frequency of malformations and diseases found in random-bred cats, but may need assistance with distinguishing genetic from sporadic occurrences. Geneticists and specialists can help in this regard. Breeders will accept a problem as genetic more readily if they have compared data across litters, with different matings, and if they have made comparisons with other breeders. Openly admitting the problem is another story, but this is not always the entire fault of the individual.

So this cat may have an inherited problem, now what?

Consulting specialists are approached more often by breeders to help with potentially genetic problems found in cats, and less frequently by veterinarians. The breeder has more to gain by solving the genetic riddles, from financial, social, and emotional perspectives. Consulting must be done in strictest confidence. The following questions should be asked to help elucidate the nature of the problem. Asking these questions also can make a breeder more aware of the problem, more likely to consider potential genetic influences proactively, and perhaps even motivated to assist with the genetic research.

- ◆ Have you seen this problem before?
- ◆ How frequently have you seen or heard about this problem?
- ◆ How were the affected group of cats, and their parents, related?
- ◆ Were the cats that produced this problem used in other matings, either to each other or to other cats, and what were the outcomes?

If these basic questions have informative answers, then a genetic study can be considered. To proceed, the following questions also must receive affirmative responses:

- ◆ May I have copies of the health records and pedigrees?
- ◆ May I speak to your veterinarian?
- ◆ May we approach other breeders?
- ◆ Will we be able to collect samples for clinical analysis and DNA studies?

Pedigrees are required to prove the inheritance pattern and to identify the most important cats for sampling. Many breeders want to use pedigree information to identify the cat that was the cause of the problem. This action functions only to place blame. It carries many negative connotations and should be avoided. Health records and interviews with veterinarians help researchers decipher the primary cause of the presentation and perhaps the true cause of death, where mortality has occurred. Veterinarians need to be willing to help supply tissues and DNA samples, laboratory results, and necropsy reports. A study always will require contact with more than 1 breeder, for informational assistance and to help obtain samples from related cats. One or a few breeders may start a project, but eventually it becomes accepted and even very proactive for the breed.

Veterinarians could be of great assistance to the researcher if banked samples were saved from unusual problems, and especially from cases with a potentially genetic cause. The consulting geneticist often is contacted after several occurrences may have been lost to further evaluation. Recognizing these cases early is of vital importance. Better genetic laboratory techniques now allow smaller and smaller samples to be collected for study, but one must be aware that DNA is found in nucleated cells. Therefore, red blood cells, serum, plasma, and hairs without follicles do not contain a DNA source. Whole blood can be a good source of DNA because nucleated white blood cells are present. A few milliliters of whole blood can be collected and frozen until analysis. When a study is just beginning, and the gene that codes for the disease is not known, hundreds of tests have to be run. This requires larger

DNA samples. Once a test has been established, cheek swabs often can be used for subsequent study. Hair is not the best source of DNA for cats that shed, but if hair samples with follicles are obtained, then DNA studies may be successful. Veterinarians also should remember that reproductive organs can be saved and frozen as sources of DNA. Formalin-fixed tissues are necessary for histology, but generally DNA isolation from these tissues is difficult or impossible.

◆ COMPARATIVE GENETICS

During the Paleocene Period, approximately 60 to 70 million years ago, an explosive mammalian radiation occurred, leading to the present 19 orders of mammals, representing over 4000 extant species. Gene maps currently are being explored for many species, covering such diverse orders as Primata, Rodentia, Carnivora, Artiodactyla, Perissodactyla, Lagomorpha, Metatheria, and Prototheria. Other than the map for *Homo sapiens*, which is fueled by the human genome initiative, the mouse genome has been most investigated.

A genome project first requires development of a genetic map. A genetic map defines locations of genes on chromosomes, their order of occurrence, and how far apart they are. Cats have 19 pairs of chromosomes. Human beings have 23 pairs; mice have 21. Most of the genes that occur in human beings also are found in cats, dogs, elephants, mice, pigs, bats, and so on. Given the amount of genetic conservation that occurs across species, if cats have 19 chromosomes and humans have 23, how do all the genes on 23 chromosomes for 1 species locate on only 19 for the other? This is the first task of a genome project, and it defines the field of comparative genetics. Gene mapping in a species is not limited to the 2 dimensions of its own genetic map. By looking at the third dimension of genetic structure across species, small genome projects, like the cat initiative, can be just as efficient because information found in other species can be very useful.

Markers and Maps

Gene maps generally are made with 2 different types of markers, called type I and type II. Type I markers are genes, and type II markers are interesting and very useful bits of DNA that are anonymous (that is, their functions are unknown). A type II marker can be an unknown part of a gene. Most maps have many type II markers, but the exact positions and identities of genes are less well established at this time. DNA fingerprinting is done with type II markers, not genes. Like genes, markers can have different alleles with slightly different base sequences. Type II markers categorize differently, depending on the majority of the nucleotide sequence. Markers that have many small tandem repeats, like CACA-

CACACACACACACACAC somewhere in the base sequence, are called *microsatellites*. Each microsatellite marker is different somewhere in its base sequence. Microsatellites are found all over chromosomes, tend to have many alleles, and therefore are highly polymorphic. If there are many alleles, then the chance that any 2 cats have exactly the same alleles is minimal. Identification of the alleles of an individual at many different microsatellites creates the DNA fingerprint. Microsatellites are the markers of choice for identification, parentage testing, and determining gene pool diversity.

In order to allow genomes of different species to be truly comparable, common language and standards have been established by the comparative gene mapping community. The same gene landmarks must be mapped in each species so that conservation and rearrangements across genomes can be recognized. These landmarks have been called *type I markers*. Type I markers are coding genes that generally are conserved, making identification of polymorphism inherently difficult within a species. However, type I markers are the most vital resource for tracking genome organization among species. This resource offers the prospect of interpreting the evolutionary lineage of living taxonomic groups, and facilitates genetic analyses and manipulations via candidate gene theories. Type I markers are very difficult to place on a genetic map because they have very little polymorphism, but an organized effort is taking place to establish a framework list of genes that are mapped in all species. This allows researchers to determine, for example, which chromosome in human beings matches which cat chromosome. If this can be established, then all known genetic information on human chromosomes is useful for mapping the cat.

The linkage map of the cat genome also is being expedited by using feline interspecific backcrosses. The backcrosses have been established by both natural and assisted methods for reproduction. The domestic cat has been crossed to Leopard cats (*Prionailurus bengalensis*) from Asia. The F1 males of each cross adhere to Haldane's rule and are sterile, but the F1 females have been productive and are crossed back to domestic cats. Over 70 backcross cats have been produced, which is sufficient for construction of a 10-cM genetic map. The genetic map of the cat, with framework type I markers and a plethora of type II markers, is the first tool required for hunting disease genes.

Disease Identification

The genetic map is a tool that will be used to attempt to identify candidate genes for specific diseases. For example, amyloidosis occurs frequently in Abyssinians and Siamese. The presentations are slightly different, involving more renal impairment for Abyssinians and more hepatic disease in Siamese. Amyloidosis also occurs in human beings and mice. Both have sporadic and inherited forms in different ethnic groups or strains. The presentation of amyloidosis in cats can be compared with findings in human beings and mice. This comparison is done by literature and database searches and by discussions with recognized experts. Because the genome projects for these 2 species are large, background information and clues to the causative gene(s) may be identified in these species and then tested in cats.

In this example, the first research problem is to find the human or mouse presentation that most mimics that found in cats. If this is accomplished, the genetic information known for that disease can be evaluated. Hopefully, a particular gene will have been implicated in mice or human beings, and the exact mutation identified. This gene then would become the primary focus of continued investigation through attempts to isolate it in cats, and to prove that the disease is caused by the same (homologous) gene as in the other species. The homologous feline gene then would be screened for mutations, comparing affected cats with normal cats. Of course, the same gene and/or mutation may not be found across species, but this is the best place to start the investigation. If a particular gene is not identified, researchers then would need to resort to a more complex task to find the gene, where use of the genetic map and comparative genetics would be vital.

Using Comparative Genetics

Comparative genetics allows exploitation of the gene-rich species, mice and human beings, for mapping the gene-poor species (essentially all others at this time). Locations for genes causing the same disease in 2 or more species should be readily accessible if they lie within the large blocks of chromosome homology, and not at breakpoints for genomic rearrangement. Locations of homologous disease genes are less consistent between mice and human beings because of the many disruptions of the large blocks of conservation between the 2 genomes. Disease gene locations are more likely to be near rearrangement breakpoints in mice than in cats, as each is compared with human beings. Therefore, gene mapping and disease gene localizations are more difficult using direct genome comparisons with mice than with cats. For example, Figure 76–1 shows the location for PKD type 2 that is mapped to human chromosome 4. Its location is in an area that could be located on 1 of 2 mouse chromosomes, 3 and 5. But this region is conserved as a large block in the cat genome, and so mapping efforts and gene localization techniques should be easier to accomplish in cats.

Once a disease phenotype has been identified in 2 different species, gene homology must be determined. Verification that the same gene is the causative agent of the disease phenotype in different

GENE POOR ⟶ GENE RICH

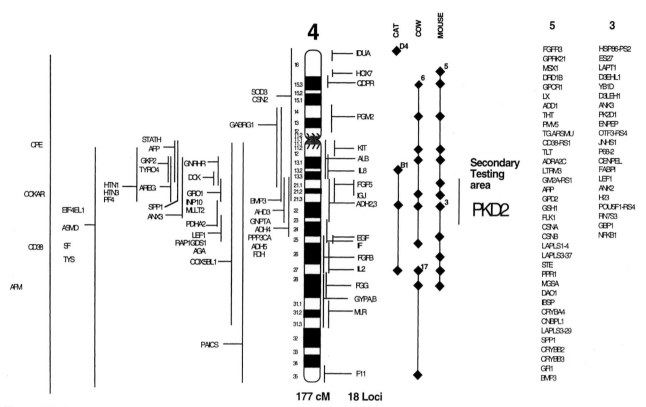

Figure 76–1. Comparative mapping: gene-rich to gene-poor. *Left,* Human genes mapping to 4q21-q23 from HGM11. *Right,* Mouse genes mapping to mouse chromosomes 5 and 3 in regions homologous to human 4q21-q23 from mouse genome database.

species may be necessary for effective development of clinical diagnostics and therapies. Diagnostic methods and drug therapies developed in 1 species can be tested for effectiveness in other species that experience the same disease. For example, the gene for PKD has been identified and mapped to human chromosome 16p (Fig. 76–2). Cats also have an autosomal dominant form of PKD, but its map location

and the gene have not been identified. The framework comparative mapping anchor loci for human 16p are HBA1, PRM1, IL4R, and PRKCB1. The feline interspecific backcross pedigree will have these 4 genes mapped, as well as linked microsatellites. Once it is shown that this region is conserved as a large block between human beings and cats, the cat microsatellites linked to the human 16p markers

Figure 76–2. Comparative mapping of polycystic kidney disease (PKD). Known feline-human homology blocks allow rapid disease homology determination. Microsatellites linked to the type I markers in the region where PKD1 is mapped can be analyzed quickly in a feline PKD family to determine homology.

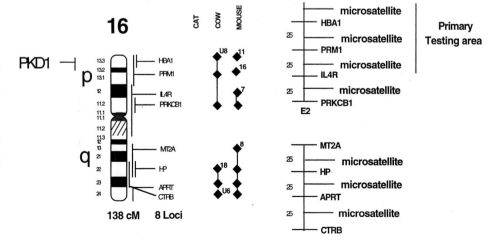

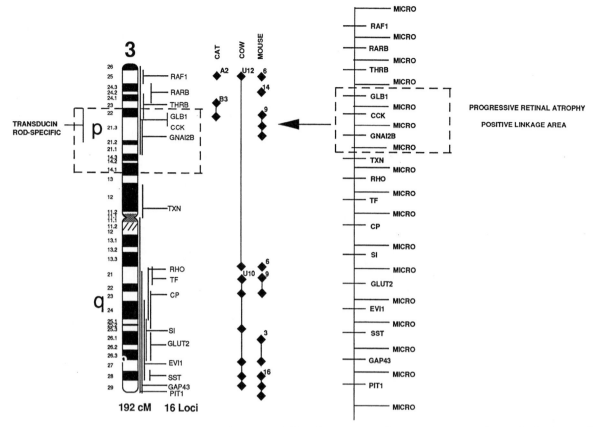

Figure 76–3. Reverse comparative genetics. Hypothetical model for the mapping of a progressive retinal atrophy in the cat. Type II markers showing linkage to the disease phenotype can be used to find the homologous regions in a gene-rich species. Type I markers linked to the type II markers allow human and/or mouse regions to be identified for candidate gene selection.

can be screened in the cat PKD pedigree for linkage to the PKD disease phenotype. Linkage would strongly suggest disease gene homology (see Fig. 76–2), but true homology cannot be determined until the exact causative mutations are discovered in each species. As shown in Figure 76–2, if feline PKD is not genetically homologous to PKD1, the region homologous to human chromosome 4 should be searched. Linkage to PKD2 has been established in human beings, but the gene has not been isolated. All the genes located in the region 4q21-q23 become possible candidates. The cat has only a few genes mapped in this region, but enough to determine the block of genome conservation. Human 4q21-q23 is maintained as a single conserved unit in the cat, and therefore investigators analyzing feline PKD may select from the plethora of human and mouse genes that are mapped to this region.

Certain lines of Abyssinian cats have an inherited form of PRA. Human beings also have PRAs, but specific genes have not been identified, and the homologous disease between human beings and cats also has not been identified. The cat disease pedigree can be screened with type II markers for linkage to feline PRA. Once linkage has been established, the neighboring type I markers can be identified. These markers then will become candidate genes. But also the homologous genomic region then can

be identified in human beings and mice. The plethora of genes in the homologous gene regions of these 2 species will provide a greater selection of possible candidate genes (Fig. 76–3). Thus, every gene does not have to be mapped in all species, but rather just enough to determine the blocks of conservation. This reverse comparative approach may identify a retina-specific gene that is mapped in either mice or human beings, and that gene would become the top candidate for the feline PRA gene.

For some diseases, linkage studies are more feasible in nonhuman species, because specific crosses and extensive pedigrees can be developed for prospective analyses. Thus, some diseases may be identified more readily in a species with a gene-poor map, but human beings may take advantage of this knowledge if the conservation blocks have been identified with type I markers.

What Will Feline Genomics Do for Breeders and Veterinarians?

Microsatellites are the markers used for parentage testing, individual identification, and forensic analyses. But the markers first must be mapped, so that investigators know that they are testing different markers that are not too close together (a very important technical issue). Finding genes and specific mutations is a difficult and time-consuming task. Often, however, type II markers may be found close to, and linked to, the gene for a trait under investigation. Pending the distance, these markers can be used to assess probability of having a recessive trait. These markers could determine whether a specific cat carries the allele that causes amyloidosis, Siamese, spasticity, wirehair, heart defect, nonagouti, cryptorchidism, and numerous other traits. Microsatellite markers can help provide data to assess whether a breed is too inbred, or the gene pool too small. This information then can be evaluated with breed history, body types, health reports, and inbreeding coefficients to facilitate development of corrective breeding measures and identification of breeds that would represent the best candidates for outcrossing. Ages of breeds, their sources, and whether they represent different domestications of cats all are questions that can be answered with reagents, techniques, and markers developed for the mapping projects.

◆ FELINE GENOME PROJECT

The cat is a model for over 20 human diseases, 80 per cent of which have no other animal model (Ta-

ble 76–3). At this time, the cat is the only animal model for human AIDS. Unlike simian immunodeficiency virus in monkeys, feline immunodeficiency virus causes disease in its host, a disease pathology that mimics that found in human beings suffering from AIDS. The cat also is ideal for evolutionary studies. Thirty-seven species of the Felidae family are extant. Cats are charismatic and attractive, and many zoos retain a number of cat species in their collections. Cooperation among zoos, reserves, and research facilities throughout the world has made the cat a good species model for many areas of this new scientific research. Unlike many canids, preservation of the feline karyotype is strong across all felid lineages. Only 1 to 2 rearrangements of the domestic cat karyotype can explain all changes in the karyotypes of small and large, and New- and Old-World feline lineages. The cat therefore should prove to be a good representative for carnivores for comparative mapping analyses.

Cats, human beings, and mice all have the same genes. The sequences are a little different, making a cat a cat, and not a human being. Overall, the genetic organization of the cat is more similar to that of human beings than it is to that of mice. The order of genes on chromosomes is more conserved between cats and human beings; human-to-mice

Table 76–3. Hereditary Human Diseases With Feline Models*

Disease	Affected Protein	Gene Symbol	Human Locus	Feline Locus
Albinism†	Tyrosinase	TYR	11q14-q12	D1
Amyloidosis†	Cystatin	CST‡	20p	
Cardiomyopathy				
Chédiak-Higashi syndrome†	(Unknown)	CHS	1q43	
Corneal dystrophy	(Unknown)	CDGG1	5q22-q33.3	
Diabetes mellitus, insulin-dependent†	Insulin	IDDM	6p21.3	
Diabetes mellitus, non–insulin-dependent†	Islet amyloid polypeptide	NIDDM	12	B4
Ehlers-Danlos syndrome	Collagen			
Ehlers-Danlos type VII	Procollagen protease			
Endocardial fibroelastosis	(Unknown)	EFE	Xq28	
Fabry's disease	Alpha-galactosidase	GLA	Xq22	X
Factor XII	Factor XII	F12	5q33-qter	
Fucosidosis	Alpha-L-fucosidase	FUCA1	1p34	C1
Globoid cell leukodystrophy†	Galactosylceraminidase	GALC	14q24.3-q32	
Glycogen storage disease type II	Alpha-1,4-glucosidase	GAA	17q23	D1
Glycogen storage disease type IV	Glycogen branching enzyme	GBE1	3p12	
GM$_1$ gangliosidosis	Beta-galactosidase	GLB1	3p21.33	B3
GM$_2$ gangliosidosis (Sandhoff's)	Beta-hexosaminidase A	HEXB	5q13	(B3)§
Hemophilia A	Factor VIII	F8C	Xq28	
Hemophilia B	Factor IX	F9	Xq27.1-q27.2	
Hyperlipoproteinemia†	Cholesterol metabolism			
Mannosidosis	Alpha-mannosidase	MANB	19cen-q12	(B3)§
Mucopolysaccharidosis type I	Alpha-L-iduronidase	IDUA	4p16.3	D4
Mucopolysaccharidosis type VI	Arylsulfatase B	ARSB	5q11-q13	
Neuronal ceroid lipofuscinosis†	(Unknown)	CLN‡		
Niemann-Pick type A	Sphingomyelin phosphodiesterase-1	SMPD1	11p15.4-p15	
Niemann-Pick type C†	(Unknown)	NPC	18q11-q12	
Ornithine aminotransferase deficiency	Ornithine aminotransferase	OAT	10q26	
Polycystic kidney disease	(Unknown)	PKD1	16p13.31-p13	
Progressive retinal atrophy				
Testicular feminization†	Androgen receptor	AR	Xq11-q12	X
Von Willebrand's disease†	Coagulation factor VIII	F8VWF	12p13.3	

*Current collaborations in **bold**.
†Diseases with murine models.
‡Several.
§HEXA-B3; MANA-B3.

gene order is very shuffled. With about 10 cuts of the scissors, a picture of cat chromosomes can be made to look like a human chromosome preparation. Much more cutting and pasting would be needed to compare human beings and mice in this fashion. If the gene that causes PKD in human beings is known, and this presentation is very similar to that found in cats, then researchers are likely to know what chromosome to search in the cat. Therefore, that gene can be isolated and analyzed faster and more efficiently.

The Human Genome Project proposes to sequence the human genome quickly, and preliminary results were announced by 2 groups in 2000. Completion of the mouse project will follow soon after. Many genes of cattle and pigs have been sequenced as part of the search for genes that influence economic traits, such as disease resistance, and quality and quantity of meat and milk production. DNA sequences are similar enough across these species that the same genes can be identified by aligning the sequences side-by-side. Also, regions that have not changed over millions of years of evolution can be identified among mice, human beings, cats, and cows. These regions of conservation help researchers identify portions of the gene that control different aspects of its function, such as replication and binding sites. If a sequence is available from an individual with a disease of interest, assays can be designed to test cats and other species for the sequence of that region.

Following is a listing and description of projects that currently fall under the Feline Genome Project.

Burmese Head Defect

A congenital head defect is found in particular lines of the contemporary Burmese. This fatal defect involves duplication of the upper maxillary region, causing 2 sets of whisker pads, 2 upper palates, and poor closure of the facial midline. Two copies of the defective gene are required for expression of this autosomal recessive defect. Cats with shorter facies may be carriers of the defective gene, but a short face does not predict a carrier with 100 per cent accuracy (neither does a longer face reliably predict a noncarrier). Face development is a complicated process involving many genes and environmental factors. Thus, the initial goals of the project were (1) to review existing data to determine whether the mode of inheritance is clear already; (2) to conduct preliminary tests of markers to determine whether the Burmese breed is sufficiently diverse to support a detailed study; and (3) to initiate research to find a genetic test to identify carriers.

No defect similar to the Burmese head defect exists in human beings or mice. Therefore, no obvious candidate gene is evident. Because many genes are known to control development of the face, markers near these genes can be evaluated to determine whether association exists. Of course, the genetic map of the cat is required to identify markers that

are near the genes of interest (the markers to test). Our laboratory at the University of California, Davis (UCD), is proceeding with identifying markers near the potential candidate genes; these genes then will be tested in the Burmese breed. If no marker around a gene of interest is found, then an entire genome scan will be performed using all the remaining genetic markers that the laboratory can produce.

Breeders have contributed to this project by supplying blood and tissue samples from normal and affected traditional and contemporary Burmese cats. As more samples are sent to our laboratory, more progress can be made toward finding a marker. When a marker is found, breeding programs will be established to eliminate this problem, while still maintaining the conformation of interest.

Havana Brown Genetic Diversity Study

The Havana brown is one of the cat breeds in the Cat Fanciers' Association (CFA) with the fewest newly registered individuals. Breeders have recognized that their gene pool is limiting, and have initiated a genetic study that should help develop a more genetically diverse breed. Any population with too few individuals can suffer from inbreeding depression that results from low genetic diversity. This has been documented in cats, the best current example being the previously described problem with FIP in the cheetah. Because this group of cheetahs had genetically similar immune systems that left them vulnerable, a particular pathogenic strain of coronavirus wiped out a third of the colony. Genetic diversity does not mean that any 1 individual may or may not have a problem. Rather, diversity ensures that an entire line, group, or population will not be decimated.

The Havana brown project includes many of the factors that influence the growth of a population or breed: present breed health concerns, the breed history, number of cats that presently are reproducing, specific cats that have been used to develop the breed to date, and the genetic diversity of the breed. We analyzed over 30 genetic markers in nearly 50 cats, and found that the genetic diversity of the Havana browns is less than that of some populations of nondomestic cats that are in critical danger of extinction, such as the Florida panther and the Gir Forest lion. All of this information will be used to help develop a breeding program for Havana browns.

The Havana brown breeding project presents many factors for consideration, as corrective measures are evaluated. Cats that can contribute to the corrective breeding population first must be identified. Not all cats need to be in the project, nor do all breeders. A balance must be achieved to maintain the type, color, and personality of the cats, while simultaneously increasing genetic diversity. Next, cats that can serve as useful outcrosses must be identified. These may include distant lines and foreign Havana browns, random-bred cats, and particular colors from other breeds. Any other varieties must be considered and minimized. The laboratory phase of this project is complete at present, and currently the number and types of outcrosses are being considered, as specifics of the long-term breeding plan are developed. The model for this project also can be used as a foundation for other breeding programs for domestic cats or for nonfeline domestic species.

Breeders can assist with this project in many ways. Particular cats and specific desired matings will be identified and sought, but the first-generation offspring of these matings may not be competitive. Enlightened breeders therefore will be accepting some sacrifice for the long-term benefit, and perhaps the long-term survival, of the Havana brown breed. It would be beneficial for the breed to grow quickly once outcrosses have been established, and breeders are the only ones who can provide for the success of this phase of the work. The project also could benefit from "surrogate" breeders. Surrogates may not necessarily want to show or produce Havana browns, but may have room in a cattery to house the expanding population until the diversity is increased and an acceptable type is produced. Still other breeders may be able to loan outcrossing candidates, again accepting some sacrifice of their own initiatives to the cause of saving the Havana brown breed. The breed council secretary or the author should be contacted by those who have interest in the Havana brown project.

Polycystic Kidney Disease

PKD is a disease that generally is not recognized unless clinical signs of kidney dysfunction and failure become evident. Many cats may be affected minimally from a clinical perspective, living well into reproducing age and beyond. In fact, this latter alternative has facilitated widespread dissemination of PKD in the Persian breed. PKD is an autosomal dominant disease that at present affects Persians at very high frequency.

PKD also exists in human beings and mice. Three genes that cause different types of cystic kidney disease have been found to date; each type is controlled by only 1 gene. The DNA sequences of each of these genes have been identified in mice, human beings, or both; 1 of them may be responsible for PKD in cats. A genetic test could be nearly 100 per cent accurate for identifying affected cats, but studies to date have been directed to finding the exact mutation that causes PKD, and not to finding a genetic marker for the disease. At present, affected cats are identified at age 6 to 8 months, using abdominal ultrasound. A genetic test could identify carriers using a cheek swab, or a very small amount of blood, from very young kittens. Breeding programs then could be established to begin slowly eliminating this disease from the Persian breed.

Progress toward elimination must be achieved slowly to avoid excessively rapid reduction of the breed gene pool, which would lead to other problems associated with diminished genetic diversity. Breeders should keep in mind, for example, that the rest of the genes in a cat with PKD are normal, and may produce a stunningly beautiful cat. No benefit accrues from discarding desirable genetic traits.

If the 3 genes of initial interest are shown not to be involved with feline PKD, then marker testing would be the next research step. Marker testing requires familial studies. Although there is an established breeding colony for this purpose, breeders could contribute samples that would improve the power of the current families. Again, the author or the breed secretary should be contacted by persons who have interest in participating in this important research.

Lymphosarcoma

Most lymphosarcoma is found in cats that are FeLV-positive. Historically, genetic susceptibility to non-FeLV lymphosarcoma has not been considered in a critical way. Recently, several cat breeders have recognized a group of Oriental shorthairs that are FeLV-negative and have an autosomal recessive form of lymphosarcoma. UCD is collaborating to help identify the gene that causes this type of lymphosarcoma. The tumors first must be characterized by cell lineage, which will facilitate comparing FeLV-negative feline lymphosarcoma with the different types found in human beings and mice. Once this is done, candidate genes could be identified, and particular genes could be screened for mutations.

Unfortunately, the affected family of Oriental shorthairs is small, and at present we are attempting to collect blood samples from as many relatives as possible. Cats have been donated to the project to extend the lymphosarcoma family in the laboratory, but many more affected cats need to be identified or bred to study this type of cancer, and to help with the genetic studies to identify markers and candidate genes.

Persian Retinal Atrophy

A recognized group of Persian cats have an autosomal recessive form of early-onset PRA. Affected cats become blind very quickly, but otherwise are very healthy and do well if their handicap is managed properly in the home environment. As part of a collaborative effort between UCD and researchers at Cornell University, the pedigrees are being evaluated, and attempts are being made to examine all available relatives. A large body of research on blindness exists for several species, including human beings, mice, and dogs. Therefore, many candidate genes might be available to study in cats, and the research plan is similar to those established for many of the other diseases (i.e., find markers to a few good candidate genes, test the markers for a correlation to the disease in the affected family, and intensively study putative responsible genes for the exact mutation). As always, the key is to have pedigrees that are large enough to establish the correlation. Because Persians are affected by this eye disease, a study colony could be developed that would maintain individuals that are useful for both the PRA and the PKD projects, which would represent a much more efficient research strategy.

Amyloidosis

Amyloidosis has been a major concern in the Abyssinian breed for years. Small studies of this problem have been initiated, but as a genetics project, amyloidosis potentially is one of the more difficult problems to investigate. The inheritance and pathophysiology are not well-understood, and the disease may be influenced strongly by genetic and environmental factors. Deposition of amyloid plaque can occur in association with various illnesses, and determining true cause-and-effect relationships therefore is challenging. Investigators in The Netherlands are studying amyloidosis in Oriental breeds, and indications are that other breeds may be involved as well. This presents the potential problem of disease heterogeneity, meaning that different genes may be causing the disease in different breeds of cats.

Diagnosis of affected cats also can be very difficult. As with PKD, many cats do not develop clinical signs until later in life, and many affected cats apparently live long, clinically normal lives. Unlike PKD, however, amyloidosis may affect different organ systems. Affected cats may present with liver failure, kidney failure, heart failure, or perhaps other problems, all secondary to organ-specific deposition of amyloid.

The plan for researching amyloidosis also is multicentric, including researchers at UCD and Ohio State University, as well as European researchers. To avoid redundancy, these various groups will work on different aspects of the amyloidosis problem. Blood samples will be collected from cats that have confirmed amyloidosis, if they have had at least 1 affected sibling, and if blood can be collected from both parents. If 200 affected cats can be collected, the project would have a good chance of producing an informative marker for amyloidosis. Any breed with amyloidosis may participate, but the breeds will be evaluated separately.

Hip Dysplasia

HD is a very common defect in many dog breeds. Despite a large volume of research, few genetic questions have been resolved. The mode of inheritance has not been determined, and several environmental effects have been documented. There exists strong suggestion that too much body weight in an adolescent dog may increase the likelihood of HD. Particular breed types clearly are more susceptible, especially the larger, working breeds (interestingly, the Maine coon cat fits this profile). Hip-joint laxity is the basic lesion of HD, although the molecular cause of the laxity is undetermined. The abnormal mechanics of affected joints can lead to severe osteoarthritis, which further compromises the affected dog.

The University of Pennsylvania and UCD are working together to initiate studies of feline HD (see Chapter 75, Hip Dysplasia). Maine coon cats are being radiographed and evaluated, using the distraction method of PennHip to establish normal and affected distraction indices for feline HD. Once baseline criteria are established, affected cats will be evaluated using blood samples and pedigree information. If sufficient baseline data can be collected, a genetic study similar to the amyloidosis investigation could be initiated.

Dwarfism

The Munchkin breed represents a type of dwarfism that is most similar to human hypochondroplasia. The gene for this type of human dwarfism is known, and the causative mutations of the gene are described. Sporadic dwarfs have been found with these exact mutations; many sporadic cases occur in human beings, and probably in cats also. Munchkin breeders have related that several different lines are available, all derived from sporadic mutations. Just as with PKD, the gene known to cause dwarfism in human beings is being investigated in cats. In collaboration with National Institutes of Health dwarfism researchers, UCD is helping to collect samples from dwarf cats, and particularly from cats of different lines. If different lines have the same (or different) mutations, breeders may be able to establish better breeding programs that would produce cats with dwarfism, but not with truly extreme conformation defects. If the human gene does not prove to be the responsible gene in cats, extensive family studies then will be conducted.

Spasticity

A muscular atrophy that affects the shoulder girdle has been reported in Devon rex cats. The mode of inheritance has not been established, and few clinical evaluations are published at present. We have collected blood samples from normal and affected cats throughout the world. The UCD muscle research laboratory will assist greatly with clinical evaluations of these cats.

◆ SUMMARY

Even though many of the current feline genetics projects focus on individual breeds, these various studies should be of interest to almost all veterinarians and cat breeders. Genetic studies should not be regarded as breed-specific, because knowledge obtained for 1 breed ultimately can have application to other breeds as well. The Feline Genome Project consists of the development of the genetic map and its use as a tool to research inherited traits, diseases, and susceptibility to disease, in domestic cats. The genetic map is being developed at the UCD School of Veterinary Medicine, and the Laboratory of Genomic Diversity at the National Cancer Institute. The cat map also can be applied to genetic interests that are not diseases, such as breed diversity issues, finding genes that control coat color, fur type, or body conformation, and breed-specific traits such as ear curl and folding, taillessness, and dwarfism. In addition, the genetic map of the cat also can help to find genes that control susceptibility and resistance to FIP, FeLV, feline immunodeficiency virus, and other infectious diseases.

77

◆ Molecular Diagnosis of Gangliosidoses: A Model for Elimination of Inherited Diseases in Pure Breeds

Henry J. Baker
Bruce F. Smith
Douglas R. Martin
Polly Foureman

◆ INHERITED DISEASES

Why should veterinary practitioners be interested in inherited diseases, especially diseases that appear as a group to be obscure and untreatable? Most veterinarians learn early in their training that inherited diseases are rare, and therefore by inference not worthy of the same attention given to infectious diseases. In fact, this "dogma" is ingrained so deeply that the words *inherited disease* are almost never spoken without the modifier *rare,* and the 3 words thus appear to be 1: *rare-inherited-disease.* If this concept is incorrect, where did it originate and why does it persist? The concept is borrowed from human medicine, where most inherited diseases indeed are rare. That is to say, in the general human population, the case incidence rate (number of affected patients in a potentially susceptible population) is very low, and with few exceptions, the carrier frequency rate (clinically normal individuals heterozygous for a trait) of recessive traits also is low. For example, the most common human gangliosidosis, Tay-Sachs disease, has a carrier frequency rate in the general population of only 1 in 300 or 0.3 per cent. However, American Jews of Eastern European origin have an ethnic predilection for this disease, and in this group the rate is 1 in 30 or 3 per cent.[1]

The basis for the overall low frequency of inherited diseases in human beings relates to religious, moral, and legal restrictions on mating between closely related individuals. Within some human families, however, the appearance of affected individuals and the carrier frequency can be very high nonetheless. The epidemiology of inherited diseases in pure breeds of cats is strikingly different from that in the human general population, and more closely resembles the pattern seen in some families. Some significant differences between affected human families and feline pure breeds are that pure breeds, depending on their popularity, are composed of thousands to tens of thousands of individuals. A popular male may mate to hundreds of females. There is no restriction on matings of closely related individuals, and in fact, this method is pre-

ferred by some breeders. Consequently, the same forces that prevent the propagation of inherited diseases in human beings are not applied to purebred animal populations, and accepted breeding practices actually encourage proliferation of inherited diseases. As a result, the carrier frequency of the gangliosidoses in some groups of pure breeds of cats and dogs has been documented to approach 20 to 40 per cent of breeding stock.

If an individual practitioner may never see an animal affected with one of the gangliosidoses, and if patients diagnosed with this disease all die within a year, how can practitioners best serve their clients? The veterinary practitioner should be the first line of defense for every animal disease, including inherited diseases. Unfortunately, pure-breed enthusiasts frequently are better informed about the inherited diseases of particular importance to their breed than most practitioners. Therefore, the goal of this chapter is to equip veterinary practitioners with the knowledge needed to fulfill their role as guardians of animal health, and to guide them to serve the pure-breed pet breeders and owners by leading the way toward detection and elimination of inherited diseases, using the feline gangliosidoses as a well-characterized example.

◆ THE GANGLIOSIDOSES

The gangliosidoses represent a class of inherited diseases known as *storage diseases,* so-called because they are characterized by the accumulation of undegraded metabolites in hypertrophied lysosomes (see Chapters 51, Neuronal Storage Disorders, and 57, Mucopolysaccharidosis). A comprehensive discussion of the feline lysosomal diseases can be found in a chapter by Wood contained in Volume 1 of this series.[2] The gangliosidoses are progressive, fatal neurologic diseases of cats, human beings, and other animals. Gangliosides accumulate principally in neuronal lysosomes,[2, 3] and are designated according to their chemical structure as G_{M1} or G_{M2}. Therefore, the diseases are identified as either G_{M1} or G_{M2} gangliosidosis, depending on which ganglioside degradative pathway is blocked. These diseases are caused by inherited defects in the genes encoding lysosomal enzymes that degrade gangliosides. G_{M1} gangliosidosis results from a mutation of the β-galactosidase gene (*GLB1*) with malfunction of the lysosomal enzyme β-galactosidase (β-gal). G_{M2} gangliosidosis results from a mutation of the hexosaminidase gene (*HEXB*) and malfunction of the β-hexosaminidase enzyme (β-hex). It is important to understand that whereas these 2 diseases involve a common biochemical pathway and induce similar clinical diseases, they actually are 2 distinct inherited diseases resulting from mutations of completely different genes (Table 77–1).

Diagnosis of affected kittens is key to recognizing that these diseases exist in a family or breed, because they are inherited as recessive traits, and "carriers" that are heterozygous for the mutation are completely normal in physical appearance. Therefore, some attention to initial diagnosis of affected cats is appropriate, even though the major emphasis of this chapter is on detection of the carrier state. Diagnosis of a kitten showing clinical signs can be accomplished by neurologic examination, histopathology, ganglioside biochemistry, and enzyme activity assays. As always, the clinician must have a high degree of suspicion and take the proper steps to achieve a correct diagnosis, usually with the assistance of centers having expertise in the pathology and biochemistry methods that are needed for definitive diagnosis. The gangliosidoses often are misdiagnosed as cerebellar hypoplasia caused by fetal infection with panleukopenia virus. The key distinguishing features are: (1) the age of onset of clinical signs in the gangliosidoses is 4 months of age or older, whereas ataxia due to cerebellar hypoplasia is present at birth, and (2) neurologic signs of the gangliosidoses are progressive, whereas those of cerebellar hypoplasia remain static or actually improve with age. The earliest signs of the gangliosidoses are fine tremors of the head and hind limbs. Owners rarely note these early signs or become concerned enough to seek professional assistance at that point. Signs progress to unsteady gait, wide stance, and inappropriate falling. Even at this stage, some owners will attribute these well-developed signs to a clumsy kitten. Therefore, when presented for diagnosis, many affected cats have advanced cerebellar signs of dysmetria to hind-limb paresis. The onset and rate of progression of clinical signs vary somewhat with the specific type of mutation. G_{M1} gangliosidosis typically becomes obvious by 4 to 6 months, is less severe, and progresses slowly over 12 to 14 months. G_{M2} gangliosidosis is apparent by 3 to 4 months, is more severe, and progresses more rapidly. Late signs include paraplegia of the hind limbs, raspy vocalization, blindness, exaggerated startle response, and grand mal seizures.

The second step in defining a potential case of feline gangliosidosis is histopathology of brain, which demonstrates accumulation of high-molecular-weight glycolipids in neurons with lesions characteristic of storage diseases. However, histopathology cannot confirm that the storage material is a ganglioside, or identify the chemical type. Definitive diagnosis can be made only by chemical identification of accumulated ganglioside in brain, and biochemical detection of reduced activity of the appropriate enzyme: β-galactosidase for G_{M1} gangliosidosis, and β-hexosaminidase for G_{M2} gangliosidosis. These assays are too specialized for most laboratories, and should be referred to a qualified diagnostic or research laboratory. Enzyme assays on tissue homogenates of affected cats are reliable for diagnosis because enzyme activity normally is high in liver and brain, and affected cats have essentially no enzyme activity. This differs distinctly from using enzyme activity to detect the carrier state, because blood has low enzyme activity normally, and results are too variable for clear prediction of genotype in many individuals.

Inheritance of the Gangliosidoses

The gangliosidoses are inherited as simple autosomal recessive traits. That is, 3 genotypes exist: (1) *normal*, meaning that both alleles are normal and the cat is normal in clinical appearance; (2) *carrier* or *heterozygote,* where 1 member of the gene pair is normal, the second is mutant (single dose of the mutation), and the individual is normal in clinical appearance; and (3) *affected* or *recessive,* where both members of the gene pair are mutant (double dose of the mutation), and the individual is affected clinically. The affected genotype is important only inasmuch as it shows that the gangliosidoses exist in the family or breed. For this reason, accurate and timely diagnosis is very important. However, affected cats represent only the tip of a potentially very large iceberg. Carriers are the most important genotype because they give no physical clues to the existence of the diseases, but transmit the mutation to half of all their progeny. In addition, the frequency of carriers in a population far exceeds the frequency of affected individuals. For example, a disease that affects just 1 per cent of the population has an estimated carrier frequency of 18 per cent! Therefore, the carrier state makes recessive diseases the most dangerous of all patterns of inheritance;

Table 77–1. The Gangliosidoses

Disease	Breeds Affected	Enzyme	Gene	Mutation
G_{M1} gangliosidosis	Siamese Korat	β-gal	*GLB1*	*CGT → CCT*
G_{M2} gangliosidosis	Korat	β-hex	*HEXB*	fHEXB Korat[a] Cytosine deletion
	DLH	β-hex	*HEXB*	fHEXB Baker[b] 25-base inversion

Abbreviation: DLH, domestic longhair, non-purebred cats.
[a]Designation of the feline HEXB mutation in Korats to distinguish from that given in note b.
[b]The feline HEXB mutation in the non-purebred cats maintained by Dr. Baker.

this is true for families, but is of overwhelming importance in pure breeds.

Typically, a recessive trait is not suspected until an individual shows clinical signs and is diagnosed accurately. If a champion tom is heterozygous for a disease trait, he will pass this trait to half of his progeny, and they in turn will pass the trait to half of their progeny. The same pattern occurs if the "founder" of the trait is a queen, but the process of dissemination in the breed is slower. Unless 2 carriers mate and have an affected kitten, the dissemination process proceeds silently, involving an ever-expanding number of cats in more and more family lines. Even if an affected kitten is born, delay of definitive diagnosis can be very long if the inherited disease is not well known to practitioners, or if laboratory assistance needed to confirm the disease is not available.

When an accurate diagnosis is made, unless there is a method that can be applied readily for detecting the carrier state, no progress can be made in understanding the breadth of the problem or working toward eliminating carriers. For example, the existence of G_{M2} gangliosidosis in Korats was demonstrated in 1985.[4] At that time, the only diagnostic procedure available was enzyme assay of peripheral blood leukocytes. This procedure was not adaptable for successful carrier screening because enzyme activity is very labile. Even when samples were processed properly, values for normals and carriers overlapped, and an unambiguous assignment of genotype could not be made consistently. An attempt was made to eliminate carriers using this method in spite of these limitations, but the effort was narrow in scope and of questionable benefit.

Molecular Characterization of Mutations in the Gangliosidoses

Before molecular characterization of a mutation, the gene responsible for an inherited disease must be determined, and the DNA of the normal gene must be sequenced. Fortunately, the lysosomal enzymes that catabolize the gangliosides have been characterized for the human diseases. More recently, the genes encoding these enzymes were sequenced for human beings and mice, providing some basis to sequence the cat genes. Hexosaminidase consists of 2 subunits, α and β, which dimerize to form different isoforms of the enzyme: Hex A (αβ) and Hex B (ββ). Each subunit of this enzyme is encoded by a different gene. Deleterious mutations in the gene encoding the β subunit of hexosaminidase (*HEXB*) affect both Hex A and Hex B enzymes, producing G_{M2} gangliosidosis variant 0 to indicate loss of both isozymes. In 1978, we described feline G_{M2} gangliosidosis, variant 0 of shorthair domestic, non-purebred cats (fG_{M2}Baker).[5] In 1985, a similar clinical disease was described in Korat cats (fG_{M2}Korat).[4] A partial sequence for the normal feline hexosaminidase gene (*HEXB*) was first reported in 1994.[6] This information was used to discover the mutation site in fG_{M2} Korats, which results from a single base deletion and frame shift that introduces a premature stop codon early in the coding sequence.[6] Based on this report, we investigated the mutation responsible for fG_{M2}Baker, sequencing the *HEXB* cDNA from fG_{M2}Baker mutants to determine if it differed from the Korat mutation. The data showed that the Baker mutation is different from the Korat mutation, and consists of a 25-base-pair inversion at the extreme 3' end of the coding sequence, which should introduce 3 amino acid substitutions at the carboxyl terminus of the β subunit and a translational stop that is 8 amino acids premature (see Table 77–1).[7] In contrast to these 2 mutations discovered to date in cats, human G_{M2} gangliosidosis, variant 0 (Sandhoff's disease) results from at least 18 different *HEXB* mutations.[1]

In 1971, we described G_{M1} gangliosidosis in Siamese cats, and similar diseases subsequently were described in non-purebred cats.[8–11] In 1998, G_{M1} gangliosidosis was described in Korats, providing the first evidence of the unexpected occurrence of both gangliosidoses in a single breed.[12] In all cases, the activity of β-galactosidase (β-gal) was absent or reduced to less than 10 per cent of normal, and G_{M1} ganglioside was the predominant storage material in brain. Although the sequence and sites of mutations have been reported for the human structural β-galactosidase gene, this information was lacking for cats. Therefore, we sequenced the full-length feline *GLB1* cDNA from normal cat brain, liver, and skin fibroblasts. Based on this normal feline *GLB1* sequence, we amplified *GLB1* from tissues of Siamese G_{M1} gangliosidosis mutants and obligate carriers. We identified a single G to C substitution (CGT→CCT) at base 1486, resulting in a change of an amino acid from Arg to Pro and loss of hydrolytic activity. This mutation does not correspond to any of the 23 mutations of the *GLB1* known to cause human G_{M1} gangliosidosis. In collaboration with DeMaria and colleagues,[12] we sequenced the *GLB1* gene from tissues of Korats with G_{M1} gangliosidosis, and found unexpectedly that this mutation was the same as that responsible for the disease in Siamese cats (see Table 77–1).[7] Because a given inherited disease in a pure breed usually results from a genetic "error" in a single individual, commonly called the *founder effect*, it can be assumed that the mutation would be unique to that breed. Even if the same syndrome is recognized in a second breed, the assumption would be that the mutations would be different, such as that observed in feline G_{M2} gangliosidosis. Finding the identical mutation in both Korats and Siamese might contradict this principle, except that both breeds originated from Siam (Thailand), and use of Siamese breeding stock was permitted in the development of the Korat breed in the West. Therefore, it is likely that the mutation of the *GLB1* gene originated in Siamese cats and was transmitted to the Korat breed decades ago.

Molecular Test for Carriers of the Gangliosidoses in Korats

Characterization of the feline *HEXB* and *GLB1* genes and the mutations responsible for the gangliosidoses of Korats allowed organization of a Korat gangliosidosis screening program that offered molecular detection of carriers of both G_{M1} and G_{M2} gangliosidosis. The advantages of a molecular test include: (1) unambiguous assignment of genotype, (2) use of a small volume (0.5 ml) of uncoagulated blood sample, (3) no requirement for processing outside of the molecular testing laboratory, (4) stability of DNA, which allows for shipping without refrigeration, and for long transit times (up to 7 to 10 days at ambient temperature), and (5) ability to store samples in the laboratory for months to years at $-70°C$.

The first samples were received for testing in March 1998, and as of May 1999 a total of 227 samples have been evaluated, which translates to 454 separate tests, because each sample is tested for both G_{M1} and G_{M2} gangliosidosis. Samples have been received from 80 Korat breeders in 11 countries: Australia, Belgium, Canada, Denmark, Finland, Great Britain, Germany, Italy, Norway, Sweden, and the United States. This high level of participation is quite remarkable for a program that is barely a year old, and makes this a truly international program.

From 227 Korats tested as of May 1999, 38 G_{M1} carriers and 14 G_{M2} carriers have been detected. Therefore, the total carrier frequency for both mutations in Korats is approximately 23 per cent. As shown in Table 77–2, there are some variations in the number of carriers detected and the distribution of G_{M1} versus G_{M2} carriers. Only 1 country (United Kingdom) appears to be unaffected to date, and Australia has no G_{M1} carriers and only 1 G_{M2} carrier. This low frequency may result from the strict quarantine of animals entering these 2 countries, which restricts entrance of new breeding animals from other countries. Except for these 2 island nations, all other countries have G_{M1} carriers. Four European countries and Canada have no G_{M2} carriers. Norway and the United States appear to have a disproportionately high frequency of G_{M2} carriers. The possibility that as many as 1 in every 5 breeding Korats is a carrier of one of the gangliosidoses is staggering! In addition to the very high carrier frequency for these mutations, these results provided additional surprises. First, G_{M2} gangliosidosis has been known as an inherited disease of Korats since at least 1985, although until now the actual magnitude of the problem had not been determined. Second, G_{M1} gangliosidosis was not known to exist in Korats until 1998, but it is clear from our sampling to date that G_{M1} appears by far to be the more important of the 2 mutations, in terms of the breadth of family lines affected. Thus far, we have not found a single Korat that carries both mutations, which is very good news, because such "compound heterozygotes" would add materially to the complexity of the problem, and could slow elimination of these diseases.

What are the keys to the early success of a screening program such as this one? First and foremost, the strong leadership of the few breeders who took the initiative to start this program has been the foundation from which progress has been built. The Korat breed is relatively small, and enthusiasts communicate easily, facilitating the exchange of information about the program and testing results. The example provided by the organizers leads directly to the remarkably high rate of participation experienced. Continued success of this program must be attributed to the 80 breeders who comprehend the gravity of this problem for the Korat breed, and who make the effort to determine which cats are affected, so that the continuing spread of these dangerous mutations can be stopped. Support of a program that defines the presence of inherited diseases is not embraced universally by breeders, and indeed there is not complete support for the Korat Gangliosidosis Screening Program. Some skepticism probably derives from the earlier limitations of the Korat G_{M2} testing program, based on enzyme activity that was not reliable for unambiguous detection of carriers. It also is clear that the rapid success and international impact that this program has enjoyed would not have been possible without the Internet and nearly universal use of e-mail. Additionally, strong leadership was provided by breed associations and registries that emphasized the importance of testing and organized sample submissions. Plans are being developed by some breed associations to require confirmation of the gangliosidosis genotype of any Korat registered.

When the Korat Gangliosidosis Screening Program first began, whole-blood samples were submitted by American and Canadian participants, and were found to be stable at ambient temperature for the usual 2 to 3 days in transit. However, DNA extraction was performed before shipment on many samples coming from other continents where speed of shipment was a concern, because purified DNA is very stable at ambient temperature. DNA extraction from cat blood is sufficiently different from other

Table 77–2. Distribution of Gangliosidosis Carriers in Korats by Nation

Country	Korats Tested (n)	G_{M1} Carriers (n)	G_{M2} Carriers (n)
Australia	19	—	1
Belgium	4	1	—
Canada	13	1	—
Denmark	9	6	—
Finland	16	3	—
Germany	21	5	2
Italy	10	7	1
Norway	12	2	3
Sweden	5	1	—
United Kingdom	49	—	—
United States	69	12	7
Totals	227	38 (16.7%)	14 (6.2%)
		52 (22.9%)	

species that most laboratories are not uniformly successful with the extraction process. As a result, we spent much time and effort trying to use some of these samples without success. It is clear now that overnight delivery service provided by most carriers, and relatively easy compliance with U.S. Department of Agriculture import requirements for cat blood (USDA Guidelines for Importing #1102), make it unnecessary to do any processing outside of our laboratory. Whole blood may be submitted from any of the participating countries, even if transit time is 5 to 7 days. We continue to use direct genetic sequence analysis for detecting carriers. This method is laborious, time-consuming, and expensive. Therefore, we are developing other methods that can be adapted more easily to high throughput processing, thus reducing processing time and expense.

In consultation with several Korat breeders who helped launch this program, we developed an official certificate that verifies test results. Results are reported by e-mail, so that owners will have access to this information as soon as possible, but the certificate is recognized as the formal document for verifying the gangliosidosis status of any Korat. To facilitate processing official certificates of test results, a sample submission form accompanies new samples. This sample submission form and instructions for submitting samples to screen Korats for the gangliosidoses are provided at the Scott-Ritchey Research Center web site at http://www.vetmed .auburn.edu/srrc.

◆ GENETIC COUNSELING OF BREEDERS

How should a clinician advise a Korat owner who learns that his or her line carries the gangliosidosis disease traits? In the past, the recommendation not to breed carriers was the standard, if not completely satisfying advice. It is clear that in Korats, the very high carrier frequency, coupled with the limited gene pool of this small breed, will not allow simple removal of all carriers from the breeding pool because of the genetic bottleneck that could result. Consequently, breeders who wish to preserve the best phenotype of champion Korats should be offered assistance in developing controlled-breeding programs. If an otherwise healthy, phenotypically superior carrier is selected for breeding, only genotypically normal cats should be selected as mates, and all kittens produced should be tested. As many as 50 per cent of kittens from these matings will be normal and available to perpetuate the best characteristics of that family line, whereas carriers should be neutered and placed as pets. The firm restrictions of this strategy are: (1) a known carrier must be mated only to a known normal to ensure that no diseased kittens are born, (2) all resulting kittens must be tested, and only normals can be returned to the gene pool as breeders, and (3) all carriers must

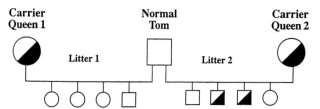

Figure 77–1. Pedigree of intentional mating of a known normal Korat tom to 2 known carrier Korat queens.

be neutered. This option probably would not be available without the unambiguous determination of genotype that the molecular test provides. This strategy is being adopted by a few breeders, and although our experience to date is limited, it appears to be working well. Figure 77–1 illustrates an actual pedigree resulting from a planned mating between 2 Korat queens known to be carriers of G_{M1} gangliosidosis and a Korat tom, known to be normal for both G_{M1} and G_{M2} gangliosidosis. In this case, the breeder had tested the breeding stock and wished to preserve the championship phenotype of the queens that tested positive as G_{M1} carriers. Of the 8 kittens produced in these 2 litters, 6 were normal genotypically and may serve as replacement breeders. These results clearly demonstrate the benefits of molecular testing in selection of breeding stock and in identification of phenotypically normal progeny, preserving a diverse and healthy gene pool for future generations of Korats. In this particular instance, litter number 2 had the expected number (50 per cent) of normals and carriers, but litter number 1 had no carriers. In addition, all of the carriers are male. This apparent disagreement with the expected distribution for an autosomal recessive trait most likely is the result of a small sample size. Without molecular testing, this powerful strategy and resulting benefits could not be offered to a breed with a small gene pool.

With pedigree analysis, testing even a relatively small number of Korats is likely to have a significant impact on identification of carriers and ultimately on elimination of the gangliosidoses from the breed. Using molecular test results, pedigree analysis serves as a powerful tool to identify the carrier status of parents, grandparents, and siblings. This is particularly applicable to the Korat breed, which requires pedigrees for all registered cats, tracing each individual back to an ancestor in their country of origin, Thailand. As the number of family lines being tested increases, pedigree analysis will become an even more powerful tool for expanding the genotypic data base.

◆ THE FUTURE OF MOLECULAR TESTING

What does the future hold? The Korat Gangliosidosis Screening Program is a historical event. Never before in veterinary medicine has molecular diagnosis been applied successfully world wide, in an attempt to eliminate an inherited disease from a pure breed. If this program ultimately is successful, it will be the first time that inherited diseases have been controlled systematically or eliminated from a pure breed through an organized testing program. Based on the enthusiastic participation experienced to date, and the self-imposed, organized restrictions placed on breeding Korats for whom the gangliosidosis status is not known, it is possible to reduce the carrier frequency substantially or even eliminate these diseases from the Korat breed entirely. This historic "experiment" will be imitated many times in the decades ahead, and may become the standard procedure to control inherited diseases, in much the same way that vaccination now is the standard for controlling infectious diseases.

REFERENCES

1. Suzuki Y, Sakuraba H, Oshima A: Beta-galactosidase deficiency (beta galatosidosis): G_{M1} gangliosidosis and Morquio B disease. *In* Scriver CR, Beaudet AL, Sly WS, Valle D (eds): The Metabolic and Molecular Bases of Inherited Disease, 7th ed. New York, McGraw-Hill, 1995, pp. 2785–2823.

2. Wood PA: Lysosomal storage diseases. *In* August JR (ed): Consultations in Feline Internal Medicine, vol. 1. Philadelphia, WB Saunders, 1991, pp. 497–501.

3. Baker HJ, Reynolds GD, Walkley SU, et al: The gangliosidoses: Comparative features and research applications. Vet Pathol 16:635–649, 1979.

4. Neuwelt EA, Johnson WG, Blank NK, et al: Characterization of a new model of G_{M2} gangliosidosis in Korat cats. J Clin Invest 76:482–490, 1985.

5. Cork LC, Munnell JF, Lorenz MD, et al: G_{M2} ganglioside lysosomal storage disease in cats with beta-hexosaminidase deficiency. Science 196:1014–1017, 1978.

6. Muldoon LL, Page MA, Neuwelt EA, Weiss DL: Characterization of the molecular defect in a feline model for type II G_{M2} gangliosidosis. Am J Pathol 144:1109–1118, 1994.

7. Baker HJ, Smith BF, Martin DR, et al: The molecular bases of feline G_{M1} and G_{M2} gangliosidoses. Feline Pract Suppl 1999, p. 11.

8. Baker HJ, Lindsey JR, Mckhann GM, Farrell DF: Neuronal G_{M1} gangliosidosis in a Siamese cat with beta galactosidase deficiency. Science 174:838–839, 1971.

9. Handa S, Yamakawa T: Biochemical studies in a cat and human gangliosidosis. J Neurochem 18:1275–1280, 1971.

10. Blakemore WF: G_{M1} gangliosidosis in a cat. J Comp Pathol 82:179–185, 1972.

11. Barker CG, Blakemore WF, Dell A, et al: G_{M1} gangliosidosis (type 1) in a cat. Biochem J 235:151–158, 1986.

12. DeMaria R, Divari S, Bo S, et al: Beta-galactosidase deficiency in a Korat cat: A new form of feline G_{M1} gangliosidosis. Acta Neuropathol 96:307–314, 1998.

78

◆ Quality of Life in Long-Term Confinement

Gary J. Patronek
Elizabeth Sperry*

Historically, owing to the numbers of animals received by animal control agencies and humane societies, animals in shelters typically were either adopted or euthanized within a fairly short time (days to weeks). Consequently, their duration of confinement in an institutional setting was relatively short. The efforts of animal protection and rescue groups, responsible breeders, veterinarians, and countless shelter workers and volunteers have finally curbed the overbreeding of companion animals. As a result, shelter intakes decreased substantially. Although the problem of "pet overpopulation" is by no means solved, many shelters today are able to house animals for much longer periods of time (sometimes weeks to months). Another development that has increased the number of companion animals living in institutional settings is an increase in the number of limited-admission or "no-kill" shelters. Limited-admission shelters, in contrast to traditional open-admission shelters, have a range of policies aimed at avoiding euthanasia. Some will euthanize only animals that are deemed unadoptable, whereas others will never euthanize a healthy animal. Therefore, most limited-admission shelters usually will not accept new animals unless there is cage space available. Although some of these shelters do attempt to adopt all of the animals they receive, animals that are not adoptable owing to age or temperament conceivably could live from months to years in the shelter. In other cases, the shelter may operate as a lifetime sanctuary, with little or no expectation that the animals ever will be adopted into new homes.

This limited-admission philosophy is becoming more widespread. In 1991, a directory of no-kill shelters listed 60 organizations, whereas the 1998 version of the same directory contained over 700 entries.[1] Although it is likely that there are now, and probably have been, many more local, community-based no-kill shelters than the number registered with the national directory, this comparison does serve as a barometer for growth of an emerging movement in animal care. Growing societal concern about euthanasia, an unavoidable consequence of irresponsible pet ownership that is borne primarily by large municipal animal control shelters, is one factor driving this shift in attitudes toward compan-

ion-animal sheltering and associated practices. Consequently, it seems inevitable that the number of animals living in long-term confinement in institutional settings will increase consistently for the foreseeable future.

Retirement homes for pets whose owners are deceased present another situation in which animals may spend the duration of their natural lives in an institutional setting. The prevalence of this type of shelter is unknown, but currently is believed to be low owing to the substantial financial endowments typically required to ensure lifetime care for a pet.

◆ CONCERNS RELEVANT TO SHELTERS

Continuing success in reducing shelter intakes and the need for euthanasia suggest that no-kill shelters eventually will become the predominant type of shelter. Many shelters in existence today were built to serve animal-control functions at a time when short-term confinement was the rule, and cats sometimes were not even considered when physical facilities were designed. An increasing number of cats likely will be housed in institutional settings that were designed primarily for dogs, and that in fact never were designed for providing long-term care for any species. Of additional concern is that limited-admission shelters tend to be smaller, local, grass-roots efforts that frequently operate with minimum resources and often rely heavily on volunteers. Cats in particular may be affected by this trend, because their small size, among other characteristics, makes them more amenable to sheltering on a small budget.

Quality of life (QOL) for animals in shelters could be compromised for several reasons. Experimental work has shown that disruption of normal social bonds is a source of great stress in a variety of animal species.[2] In addition, there is ample research demonstrating that novelty can produce considerable stress. Fear, a major problem for animals in intensive farming, is recognized as a powerful and damaging stressor that can compromise an animal's welfare seriously.[3] Inability to control or predict the environment has been shown to result in a wide variety of pathologic changes in laboratory animals.[2] Social disruption, novelty, lack of control, and both acute and chronic fear certainly have the potential to exist in the shelter environment. Animals enter-

---
*Ms. Sperry, a third-year veterinary student, was supported by a grant from the Bide-A-Wee Home Association, New York, New York.

ing a shelter have lost the important comfort cues of home (sounds, smells, routines, relationships), and the freedom to flee or hide from threats.[4] Furthermore, natural coping strategies for many species are not adapted to manufactured environments.[5] Given this situation, it should not be surprising that increased stress levels have been demonstrated for cats entering animal shelters,[6–8] boarding catteries,[5] and quarantine facilities.[9, 10] Adjustment to a shelter, as measured by reduction in stress levels, can take at least 2 to 5 weeks.[6] In 1 study of cats in boarding catteries, 4 per cent of cats never made a satisfactory adjustment.[5] The adverse effects of institutionalization and intensive confinement systems on the psychological well-being of people and farm animals, respectively, are well-recognized. The field of psychoneuroimmunology is now well-established, and has provided plausible biochemical mechanisms that have helped dismiss some of the skepticism linking mental states with somatic health.[2, 9] Therefore, it seems that trends developing in animal sheltering, and in QOL issues for animals, are timely topics for discussion.

An animal's QOL is determined in great measure by what it perceives from its unique vantage point in the world.[11] Perhaps the most salient examples of our failure to consider this seemingly obvious point are found in zoos, such as exhibits with trees painted on flat walls or concrete painted white to simulate natural environments (jungles and ice fields) for big cats and polar bears, respectively. Although these devices may serve to distract the public from the unnatural situation, animals are unlikely to be comforted by such contrivances. Yet, the animals may be as close as many captive animals come to an environment that suits their nature. Although it may not be appropriate to use the wild as a benchmark for determining characteristics of a natural environment for a domestic cat, it is fair to say that for many cats, the shelter environment remains equally artificial and therefore potentially stressful.

According to Ms. Kit Jenkins, author of a guide for recognizing stress in shelter animals, human beings fail to perceive the shelter environment from the point of view of the animal, resulting in a lack of appreciation for the degree of stress that the animals experience.[4] Sources of stress in shelters include the auditory, visual, and olfactory stimuli that are part of normal shelter activities, and the cumulative stress from all of these stimuli could be greater than the sum of stress from individual components.[4] It is important to recognize that shelter animals can suffer from understimulation or overstimulation.[4] Understimulation, or deprivation, involves denial of sometimes less obvious but no less vital psychological needs.[12] The detrimental effect of understimulation increases in importance with the duration of confinement. Long-term, low-level aversive stimuli may be more difficult to recognize than acute distress in confined cats, but may result just as inevitably in a state of distress. The result could be bore-

dom, loneliness, discomfort, anxiety, uncertainty, frustration, irritation, aggression, conflict, and distress.[12] Learned helplessness is a phenomenon seen broadly across the animal kingdom in confined animals,[2, 13] and it is an issue of concern in many human extended-care settings, such as nursing homes.[14] This condition or behavior has been induced experimentally in laboratory animals, often as a model for human depression, through repetitive electric shock or aversive stimuli from which the animal cannot escape. However, the factors that predispose to learned helplessness (e.g., no escape from a stressful situation and the inability to control or predict environmental stressors) probably are equally common in a shelter environment. Choices, as well as avenues of escape, are minimum to nonexistent for cats confined to small cages.

One final common pathway for various forms of stress is the development of stereotypies. There is debate about whether stereotypies inevitably indicate reduced welfare or whether in some cases they may represent a positive adaptation to an inadequate environment,[15, 16] and thus one way to compensate for low sensory input in a deprived environment.[17] Regardless, they are all too familiar in zoo exhibits, in which captive wild animals circle and pace incessantly or engage in self-mutilation behavior. It certainly is plausible that domestic cats confined in shelters could suffer in a similar manner, although documentation of a similar spectrum of obvious stereotypies currently is lacking. Overgrooming has been suggested as one marker of chronic stress in cats.[18, 19] Of particular concern is that some cats with high stress levels may be inconspicuous in shelters because they withdraw and show little activity, leading to the mistaken conclusion that the cat is not stressed.[5] Closer examination indicates that highly stressed cats inhibit normal behaviors such as urination, defecation, and eating.[7] In 1 study, cats that were described as inactive responders to stress actually had higher stress levels than cats that responded to stress in more identifiable ways.[7]

◆ CURRENT OVERSIGHT

Extrainstitutional public oversight to ensure the welfare of companion animals that are used in research laboratories is codified in law through the Animal Welfare Act (AWA), its amendments, and associated regulatory decisions.[12] A key feature of these amendments is that regulated research institutions must have an Institutional Animal Care and Use Committee to oversee animal care. One member of this committee must be unaffiliated with the institution, and represent community interest in proper animal care. The need for such oversight seems obvious, given that the welfare of animals used in research has the potential to be compromised owing to the nature of the experimental protocols as well as the animals' extended confinement in a research setting. However, the 1985 amendments to the AWA and subsequent regulatory decisions (e.g., those requiring researchers to provide for exercise for dogs and improve the psychological well-being of primates) indicate that community interest has expanded beyond the standards necessary to ensure the proper housing, nutrition, and veterinary care of laboratory animals.

Despite these limited protections for companion animals confined in research settings, there is no similar public process to promote QOL for animals kept for equally long, or longer, periods in other institutional settings such as animal shelters or pet retirement homes. These facilities are not covered by the AWA. Although there are exemplary shelters that excel programmatically as well as in the physical plant, there also are reports of shelters that represent the opposite end of the spectrum.[20] State and local oversight for day-to-day operations of nonprofit animal rescue and sheltering groups typically is minimum to nonexistent, and shelters in large part are self-regulated. Excuses (e.g., doing the best under the circumstances, insufficient funds, volunteer effort) for borderline animal care that would be rejected for a regulated research facility may be accepted by the public, media, and animal-protection groups when shelters are involved. It seems paradoxical that an industry whose mission is to enhance animal welfare (e.g., shelters) is not held to some developed national standard, and that resident animals have few protections beyond the good intentions of their caregivers.

Anticruelty laws in every state provide guidance for defining mistreatment and improper care of cats and other animals, prohibit certain acts and omissions, and may prescribe minimum standards for provision of food, water, and shelter. Much less information exists to characterize the opposite end of the spectrum—a state of well-being. The 1965 Brambell Report established 5 freedoms believed necessary for farm animal well-being.[21] These include the freedom to lie down, turn around, stand up, stretch, and groom. A more recent version of the Brambell recommendations has been developed. It includes freedom from thirst, hunger, and malnutrition; freedom from pain, injury, and disease; freedom from discomfort; freedom to express normal behavior; and freedom from fear and distress.[12, 22] These freedoms are accepted as essential to animal welfare by Great Britain's Farm Animal Welfare Council, the European Commission, and the World Veterinary Association.[22] No similar list of freedoms has been proposed for domestic cats, although it seems reasonable that the standards developed from Brambell might be a useful reference initially.

The greatest contributions to our scientific understanding of animal well-being, or lack thereof, come from farm animal scientists.[12] Relatively few empirical studies have addressed psychological well-being of laboratory animals,[12] and those that have been published deal mainly with primates.[23] The issue of assessing QOL for companion animals in institu-

tional settings other than laboratories has received even less attention in veterinary literature. Preference testing, which may be the best way of gauging what animals feel,[24] has not been used widely for cats.

With more and more companion animals entering a life of extended confinement, it may not be correct to assume that the good intentions underlying most sheltering efforts necessarily translate into acceptable QOL for animals. Another relevant pitfall to be aware of is that both researchers and animal protectionists concerned about laboratory animals often take for granted that caregivers know what is desirable or aversive.[12] Divergence in perceptions resulting from differences in values is a problem that has impeded consensus on how best to evaluate human QOL. Given that much of the change in animal sheltering is driven primarily by fundamental differences in the way people value prevention of animal suffering versus preservation of animal life, a common ground for discussion is needed urgently. At one extreme, there are ample reports in the popular press about large numbers of animals discovered living in homes of so-called hoarders. Typically, conditions are so terrible that they would result in immediate and severe sanctions if they were found in a research setting.[25] One justification offered by many hoarders is that the animals are being rescued or sheltered. Even under the best and most professional sheltering circumstances, when the presumption of a good QOL is reasonable, there may be a need for additional assessment criteria when an animal becomes aged or disabled, and waiting for natural death to occur could be inhumane. For similar reasons, guidelines to assess QOL systematically are needed in retirement homes. Standardized survey instruments have been developed for assessing cat stress (Table 78–1),[5, 7] socialization to other cats (Table 78–2)[6] and people (Table 78–3),[6] temperament (Table 78–4),[26] and post-treatment assessment after radiation therapy.[27] These could serve as models for development of a comprehensive instrument to assess the full spectrum of dimensions of QOL in cats.

◆ ASSESSMENT ISSUES—LESSONS FROM HUMAN MEDICINE

In contrast to the dearth of information on QOL for cats and other companion animals, considerable scholarly effort by ethicists, attorneys, insurers, clergy, physicians, and other health care professionals has been devoted to the subject of QOL for human beings. Factors stimulating work in this area include development of sophisticated medical technology that sometimes prolongs death more than it extends life, an aging human population increasingly affected by chronic diseases requiring longer and more extensive institutional care, and a society and medical establishment that are uncomfortable

Table 78–1. Seven-Level Cat-Stress Score

Score	Body	Belly	Legs	Tail	Head
1 Fully relaxed	*i:* Laid out on side or on back *a:* Not applicable	Exposed, slow ventilation	*i:* Fully extended *a:* Not applicable	*i:* Extended or loosely wrapped *a:* Not applicable	Laid on the surface with chin upward or on the surface
2 Weakly relaxed	*i:* Laid ventrally or half on side or sitting *a:* Standing or moving, back horizontal	Exposed or not exposed, slow or normal ventilation	*i:* Bent, hind legs may be laid out *a:* When standing, extended	*i:* Extended or loosely wrapped *a:* Tail up or loosely downward	Laid on the surface or over the body, some movement
3 Weakly tense	*i:* Laid ventrally or sitting *a:* Standing or moving, back horizontal	Not exposed, normal ventilation	*i:* Bent *a:* When standing, extended	*i:* On the body or curved backwards, may be twitching *a:* Up or tense downward, may be twitching	Over the body, some movement
4 Very tense	*i:* Laid ventral, rolled or sitting *a:* Standing or moving, body behind lower than in front	Not exposed, normal ventilation	*i:* Bent *a:* When standing, hind legs bent, in front extended	*i:* Close to the body *a:* Tense downward or curled forward, may be twitching	Over the body or pressed to body, little or no movement
5 Fearful, stiff	*i:* Laid ventrally or sitting *a:* Standing or moving, body behind lower than in front	Not exposed, normal or fast ventilation	*i:* Bent *a:* Bent near to surface	*i:* Close to the body *a:* Curled forward close to the body	On the plane of the body, less or no movement
6 Very fearful	*i:* Laid ventrally or crouched directly on top of all paws, may be shaking *a:* Whole body near to ground, crawling, may be shaking	Not exposed, fast ventilation	*i:* Bent *a:* Bent near to surface	*i:* Close to the body *a:* Curled forward close to the body	Near to surface, motionless
7 Terrorized	*i:* Crouched directly on top of all fours, shaking *a:* Not applicable	Not exposed, fast ventilation	*i:* Bent *a:* Not applicable	*i:* Close to the body *a:* Not applicable	Lower than the body, motionless

Abbreviations: i, cat inactive; *a,* cat active.
From Kessler MR, Turner DC: Stress and adaptation of cats *(Felis sylvestris catus)* housed singly, in pairs, and in groups in boarding catteries. Anim Welfare 6:243–254, 1997.

with viewing death as a natural part of life. Social progress toward greater human rights, holism, social welfare, and normalization of disabilities also has spurred dialogue and research into assessing QOL.[28] Consequently, a vast amount of literature on this topic has been generated for a variety of patient populations, along with a multitude of proposed determinants, conceptual models, and measurement scales for assessment of QOL.[29, 30]

The initial discussions of human QOL often were reductionist and quantitative in nature, focusing on easily measurable physical or biologic attributes of patients, and assessment of severity of medical conditions, functional abilities, or disabilities.[28–31] Determinants of QOL that have been used to evaluate individual patients and guide care include physical well-being, mental health, personal safety, fitness, mobility, ability to perform activities of daily living, valuation of handicap, size of social networks, life stress, degree of community integration, material well-being, incidence of falls, duration of sickness, number of medicines, and living space.[29, 32, 33] One reason for the predominance of quantitative evaluation was that qualitative methods were slow to emerge and become accepted.[31] There have been arguments that "hard" data are more valid. The determinants that were measured also reflected the choices and biases of the researcher, which often favored objective clinical measures of health. Although good health is one universal indicator of QOL, QOL is a broader concept than health alone, encompassing psychological as well as biologic components.[28] QOL is greater than the objective circumstances under which people live.[31] As early as 1948, the World Health Organization defined QOL as a state of complete physical, mental, and social well-being, and not as merely the absence of disease.[28, 29] In his discussions of the Great Society in

Eyes	Pupils	Ears	Whiskers	Vocalization	Activity
Closed or half opened, may be blinking slowly	Normal	Half back (normal)	Lateral (normal)	None	Sleeping or resting
Closed, half opened, or normal opened	Normal	Half back (normal) or erected to front	Lateral (normal) or forward (normal)	None	Sleeping, resting, alert or active, may be playing
Normal opened	Normal	Half back (normal) or erected to front or back and forward on head	Lateral (normal) or forward	Meow or quiet	Resting, awake or actively exploring
Widely opened or pressed together	Normal or partially dilated	Erected to front or back, or back and forward on head	Lateral (normal) or forward	Meow, plaintive meow or quiet	Cramped sleeping, resting or alert, may be actively exploring, trying to escape
Widely opened	Dilated	Partially flattened	Lateral (normal), forward or back	Plaintive meow, yowling, growling, or quiet	Alert, may be actively trying to escape
Fully opened	Fully dilated	Fully flattened	Back	Plaintive meow, yowling, growling, or quiet	Motionless alert or actively prowling
Fully opened	Fully dilated	Fully flattened back on head	Back	Plaintive meow, yowling, growling, or quiet	Motionless alert

Table 78–2. Cat Approach Test for Assessing Socialization Toward Cats*

Score	Behavior
1	Reacts in an extremely friendly way toward cats
2	Reacts in a friendly way toward cats
3	Turns toward cats
4	Moves away from or avoids any form of contact with cats
5	Reacts in an unfriendly way toward cats
6	Reacts in an extremely unfriendly way toward cats

*A calm, neutered 4-year-old male cat socialized toward cats was used in this test. The test was performed placing this cat in a portable carrier constructed of metal bars and covered with a cloth. This was placed 1 m from the back of the single cage housing the cat to be tested. After 4 min, the cover was removed from the front half of the portable carrier, and the cats were allowed visual contact for 1 min. Cats were defined as *socialized toward cats* if the mean score of 8 tests resulted in a score below 3. Cats were defined as *nonsocialized toward cats* when the mean score was greater than 4.

Adapted from Kessler MR, Turner DC: Socialization and stress in cats *(Felis sylvestris catus)* housed singly and in groups in animal shelters. Anim Welfare 8:15–26, 1999.

Table 78–3. Human Approach Test for Assessing Socialization Toward People*

Score	Behavior
1	Reacts in an extremely friendly way toward people
2	Reacts in a friendly way toward people
3	Turns toward people
4	Moves away from or avoids any form of contact with people
5	Reacts in an unfriendly way toward people
6	Reacts in an extremely unfriendly way toward people

*The test was performed by having the observer approach the front of the cage and greet the cat, touching the grate for 1 min. After 1 min, the observer opened the door of the cage for a few seconds before closing it. The test was repeated twice a day for 4 days. Cats were defined as *socialized toward people* if the mean score of 8 tests resulted in a score below 3. Cats were defined as *nonsocialized toward people* when the mean score was greater than 4.

Adapted from Kessler MR, Turner DC: Socialization and stress in cats *(Felis sylvestris catus)* housed singly and in groups in animal shelters. Anim Welfare 8:15–26, 1999.

Table 78–4. Cat Temperament Scale

Score	Behavior
5	Friendly, approaches front of cage when door is opened; may vocalize; purrs, rubs, may lie down; easy, relaxed attitude; tail raised, may knead
4	Friendly, may approach front of cage when door is opened; slightly cautious in interaction with observer; may warm to observer with time
3	Confident but not friendly; walks in cage; will return to back of cage if handled but does not show aggression; sits sternally or lies laterally, may try to escape
2	Mildly aggressive; does not approach but will allow observer to handle; may purr or growl; flicks tail
1	Outwardly aggressive; does not approach unless to strike; sits sternally in back of cage; may growl, hiss, or bite; pupils dilated; cannot be handled without protection

Adapted from Carroll GL, Howe LB, Slater MR, et al: Evaluation of analgesia provided by postoperative administration of butorphanol to cats undergoing onychectomy. J Am Vet Med Assoc 213:246–249, 1998.

the 1960s, President Lyndon Johnson emphasized his concern not with how much life, but with "how good" life is.[31]

Primacy of the patient is one area of this debate in which there seems to be consensus.[30] Unfortunately, several studies have shown that physicians and professional caretakers do not always predict patient satisfaction or preferences accurately,[30] and that divergence in perceptions probably is the norm rather than the exception.[33] In a medical setting, physical condition and severity of pain or symptoms clearly are important, but pain alone is not the only determinant of an intolerable QOL. Psychological components are so important that patients' self-reported QOL may not correspond to objective measures (e.g., medical status or level of disability) made by caregivers. It is essential to evaluate dimensions of personal meaning for patients, such as life satisfaction, happiness, and well-being, that are much more subjective. Although there is no universal agreement on the number or importance of specific determinants for evaluating QOL, the consensus is that a holistic approach is needed, in which the emphasis is on the whole person in interaction with his or her environment.[28] It also is important to include a qualitative component to supplement any quantitative measure.[33] It has been recognized that the effect of any determinant is not pure, and that it can be modified substantially by interacting factors.[34] For example, high levels of social support can improve well-being in otherwise negative situations.

In human medicine, the main subjective dimensions of QOL include self-reported health status and life satisfaction. In many situations, these measures can be obtained simply by asking the patient. However, when disability or mental status make communication of wants, needs, and satisfaction imprecise or unclear, it is difficult to obtain information in this manner. Major ethical issues arise when patients are unable to communicate their own desires, and there is a need to make decisions about medical treatment and potentially life-sustaining care that are based on subjective assessment by third parties. Persons with severe intellectual impairment, infants, persons at the end of life, and persons with multiple disabilities often are not able to communicate their subjective feelings directly about well-being and life satisfaction, yet these may be the very populations for whom accurate assessment of QOL is most important for determining the scope and nature of care.

◆ EVALUATING QUALITY OF LIFE FOR SHELTER ANIMALS

Assessing QOL for unwanted pets in shelters is not straightforward, particularly in light of the fact that assessing the state of well-being of any animal involves the controversial problem of surmising an ultimately unknowable subjective experience. Conceptual models and measurement scales published for human beings may be a useful starting point to increase our understanding of QOL issues, but their relevance for cats in shelters is questionable. The desire to apply rigorous scientific principles to this problem has produced extensive and often circuitous debates over definitions of terms such as well-being, welfare, anxiety, fear, stress, distress, and suffering. Although the colloquial meanings of many of these terms are understood, general agreement about their precise definitions is lacking.[35] The relevance of serum, urine, or fecal cortisol and other physiologic measures, the meaning of animal preference testing, the role of human values, and subjectivity in evaluating welfare also have been debated.[11, 12, 16, 36] Because the vast majority of animals in shelters are former pets accustomed to living in homes, providing a suitable QOL may pose some unique problems. Breed-specific differences and the number of geriatric and disabled animals that could be involved also raise special concerns.

In addition to these controversies, the bulk of published literature pertinent to QOL for animals deals primarily with animals in laboratory, farm, and zoo settings. The limited number of reports relevant to QOL issues for companion animals outside of laboratory settings involves dogs with disabilities such as blindness[37] and paraplegia,[38] the owner's perceptions of their pets' QOL after amputation,[39–41] or QOL after cancer treatment.[42] Two approaches used when faced with the challenge of deciding how best to assess QOL in human patients whose ability to communicate is severely compromised seem relevant for animals in shelter settings. They are the use of proxy respondents, such as caregivers, and direct observation of subjects' expressions of satisfaction or dissatisfaction by neutral third parties.[43] The following general criteria for determinants being considered objective indicators of human QOL seem equally relevant for evaluating determinants proposed for shelter animals[33]:

- QOL can be measured by observers using a common yardstick.
- The measures developed and applied have equal meaning and appropriateness for most subjects.
- Measurements can be made accurately.
- The commonalities among subjects are more important than their differences.

Criteria that seem at least superficially consistent with these assumptions and that lend themselves to assessment by proxy respondents (e.g., staff and/ or veterinarians) in animal shelters include body weight, mobility, activity level, appetite, coat condition and grooming, attitude, fearfulness or approachability, interest in surroundings, general health, results of physical examinations, and serum biochemistry values. The presence of grossly abnormal behaviors or stereotypies, as well as expression of natural behavior, also could be included in the category of objectively observable phenomena. Owing to differences in interpretation of even objective criteria for human beings, it has been suggested that it is important to have more than 1 proxy to obtain convergent views on QOL being assessed.[43] Such a precaution seems equally appropriate for animals. In vulnerable human populations (infants, mentally impaired patients, or persons unable to communicate in standard ways), it is considered critical to include a qualitative component that allows people to tell their own story in ways that are meaningful to them.[33] Although most animals cannot communicate their feelings and wants directly, the field of ethology offers important tools for enabling animals to "tell their own stories." In a shelter environment, where it is possible to observe animals closely for a prolonged period, caretakers often develop significant intuition about the well-being of animals in their care, and can detect changes in mood through observation of subtle changes in body posture, tenseness, eye contact, or response to voice.[4] The services of an academically trained animal behaviorist could be extremely helpful in evaluating shelter cats and interpreting the observations of caregivers. One method that may prove useful for neutral third parties or proxies in understanding what may be meaningful to a cat's QOL is to attempt to appreciate the shelter environment as the animal might experience it. The merit of this approach has been documented in livestock handling and slaughter facilities,[44] where observations have led to modifications in physical plants and programs that have greatly alleviated animal stress during movement and slaughter.

When evaluating the situation of any nonhuman animal, it is tempting to default to our own perceptions of comfort, stress, and distress.[12] However, even a cursory examination of this premise should illustrate the potential pitfalls in judging animal welfare based solely on what is appealing to human beings. Scientists as well as animal protectionists have been guilty of uncritical anthropomorphism.[12] In the 1960s and 1970s, achieving a high level of sanitation was a cornerstone of the movement to professionalize animal shelters, control disease, and maintain an adequate level of physical health. However, recent mandates for attention to the psychological well-being of primates and exercise for dogs indicate that rows of clean cages are believed necessary, but not sufficient, to ensure an adequate QOL for laboratory animals.

It has been argued that our criteria for animal welfare should reflect, through critical anthropomorphism, a complete range of factors that may compromise an animal's welfare.[12] *Critical anthropomorphism* has been defined as empathy tempered by objective knowledge of the species and the individual's history, behavior, and physiology.[12, 35] The starting point for any such assessment for shelter animals should begin with recognizing relevant differences owing to species and breed. Ultimately, any attempt to evaluate an animal's subjective experience also should be considered in light of the animal's age, history, and individual temperament. Geriatric and very young animals may experience the same situation very differently, as may animals with different temperaments or backgrounds. A systematic practical guide that, in essence, applies the principles of critical anthropomorphism in animal shelters, involves consideration of a variety of factors to be evaluated carefully in light of an animal's species, age, breed, and history, in order to better appreciate sources of stress and poor QOL.[4] Critical factors include:

Degree of Stimulation

One way of gauging the overall stress of the environment is to consider whether the environment is one of high or low stimulation.[4] It is important to evaluate intensity, duration, acute versus chronic, and predictability of the stimulating factors. For example, high-stimulation cages are more likely to be in high-traffic or work areas.[4] Known preferences and/ or history may provide clues as to how a particular animal is likely to react in a given situation. Whether an animal prefers a high- or low-stimulation environment also could change over time. Behavioral markers of acute stress in cats include increased rates of autogrooming, oral behavior, scratching, and head shaking.[19] A 7-level cat stress score (see Table 78–1) may be useful in gauging stress imposed by the environment.[5, 7]

Line of Vision. The cat's view from its cage may be quite different from what a human perceives in the same general location.[4] Careful consideration of what the animal can or cannot see from its vantage point may reveal sources of stress, including animal and human traffic, other animals in cages, strangers, and shelter staff members.

Sounds. Sounds from cleaning equipment, radios, ventilation, and slamming doors or gates; human sounds such as voices, paging systems, and telephones; and animal sounds such as barking, whining, and sounds of aggression or fear could be sources of stress.[4]

Smells. Animals receive much of the information about their environment through smell.[4] Therefore, olfactory stimulation from chemicals such as cleaning materials and disinfectants, other animals, food, and visitors should be considered.

People. Cats may respond differently to men and women,[4] as well as unfamiliar and familiar people.[45] Also, the stress level of caretakers in the workplace may influence the degree of animal stress directly. A pleasant work environment for people may improve animal welfare indirectly but significantly. For human beings in situations of high dependence on caregivers, QOL and quality of care become inseparable.[43] Given the dependence of animals on human caregivers, it seems that the training and supervision of these individuals must be at the highest possible level to ensure adequate welfare.

Environmental Comfort. Factors that influence environmental stress include temperature, humidity, ventilation rate, method, intensity and duration of illumination, natural versus artificial light, population density, concentration of airborne particulates and gaseous contaminants, and the nature of structural materials in cages or kennels.[46]

Primary Enclosure Size, Space, Territory

Factors to consider are whether an animal has freedom of movement, whether the caging or kenneling provides for suitable postural and locomotive expression, and whether the animal can establish a reasonable amount of personal space or territory. The ability to hide away from other animals, the public, and caretakers should be evaluated.[4, 7] For all types of laboratory animals, there has been great debate about whether improving animal welfare can be achieved best through engineering standards (e.g., specifying cage sizes or quantity of space) or performance standards (e.g., specifying a goal or functional outcome to be achieved).[47] The AWA prescribes cages with 3 square feet of floor space for cats weighing 8.8 lb or less and 4 square feet for cats weighing more than 8.8 lb. All cages must be at least 24 inches high, and all must have an elevated resting surface impervious to moisture.[48] However, it has been recognized that welfare also encompasses more than that which can be provided by adhering to engineering standards, and that engineering standards can be influenced by other factors. For example, if a dog is housed individually in a research facility, it must have more space for its primary enclosure. If this condition is not met, the dog must exercise at least 30 minutes per day.[49] There is great debate among animal welfare advocates and within the research community about the relative merits of performance versus engineering standards. It is recognized that engineering standards may promote, but certainly do not ensure, a particular desired outcome. Much of the controversy exists not because of the lack of merit of performance standards, but because of distrust and suspicion that the existence of "softer" measures would provide researchers with a means of circumventing the intent of the regulations. Above a critical minimum, improving the quality may be more important than the quantity of cage space.[50, 51]

Exercise

The necessity of mandatory exercise for confined animals has been questioned on the premise that in nature, animals that are fed, warm, and not afraid of predators or not sexually frustrated do not exercise. They either play with one another or just sleep.[52] There are additional disagreements because studies have not documented consistently significant improvements in physical, psychological, or physiologic parameters for dogs kept in cages of different sizes.[53] There are no regulations for cat exercise, nor are any anticipated. For dogs, it is considered particularly important to provide exercise if there is no visual or physical contact with other dogs.[49] This seems to suggest that the socialization that may accompany exercise is a more overriding need than exercise per se. This reasoning may be applied to cats as well.

Socialization

It is believed that domestic cats prefer a solitary existence despite numerous studies of free-ranging cats that indicate a range of social structures from completely solitary to close association centered around a food source.[23, 54] This belief, along with substantial capital investment in single cages and physical-plant limitations in shelters, may explain why single caging for cats probably is the rule, rather than the exception. Solitary confinement has been described as one of the greatest stressors that can be bestowed on most social species, as well as most individual animals.[53] For laboratory dogs, it is recognized that socialization is very important, and therefore it is recommended that dogs be maintained in compatible groups. In 1991, the U.S. Department of Agriculture expanded regulations requiring exercise of laboratory dogs to include socialization. Socialization may be one of the most important tools for helping dogs cope with the stress of confinement, and an issue such as cage size can be relatively unimportant if these other concerns are addressed adequately.[55] No such directive for socialization exists for laboratory cats, although anecdotal reports suggest that some research institutions have voluntary initiatives to provide group housing and socialization. It probably is as true in shelters as it is in laboratory settings that "hardware" (money) for facilities and cages is easier to justify than time spent in socialization.[53]

People can be a source of rich stimulation for confined cats. In 1 study, urinary cortisol was increased in cats when petting was withheld.[56] There are numerous opportunities for human social interaction during routine activities such as feeding and cleaning, and even radio voices may help timid cats adjust.[50, 51] However, for cats inadequately socialized as kittens, timid cats, aged cats, cats with restricted experience, and cats already stressed by caging, socialization may be an additional source of stress. Therefore, socialization must be individualized. For cats with gender-specific fear of people, particular attention should be paid to the gender of caretakers. The detrimental effect of fear on the well-being of other species is well-established, and fear should be avoided or at least minimized in the shelter environment.

Although some authors have argued that single caging is the most barren environment possible for cats,[51] studies of different types of housing (group, single, pair) have produced inconsistent results. During a 2-week stay in a boarding cattery, there was no difference in cat stress levels whether housed singly, in pairs, or in groups.[5] In another study, contact with other cats seemed to increase stress for short stays, and diminish stress during longer stays.[8] Cats not socialized to people seemed to have higher stress levels regardless of the type of housing, whereas cats not socialized to other cats had increased stress only in group housing.[6] Other investigators have found that cats in groups spend most of their time alone, and maintain that solitary housing may not be particularly detrimental if cats have daily human contact as well as a view of other cats and opportunities for play.[45]

Although the process of introduction to a group situation must be individualized, even cats unsocialized to human beings can be maintained successfully in group housing. One of the largest animal sanctuaries (Best Friends Animal Sanctuary, Kanab, UT) houses approximately 1500 animals, including over 700 cats, most in group housing in catteries of 15 to 20 cats each. The indoor portion of each cattery is filled with donated cat beds and hand-built platforms that are staggered around the walls to provide ample space for jumping, resting, and time away from other cats. The catteries all open onto large, covered, screened-in areas with an outdoor view. This area contains natural logs for climbing and claw sharpening as well as additional feline furniture for lounging. There also is a spacious outdoor enclosure for feral cats that were rescued from unsafe living conditions and that are not accustomed to contact with people.

Good Physical Health

Good physical health clearly is an important component of QOL. The evaluation of physical health in cats is a topic that has been addressed thoroughly by standard veterinary texts and is not reviewed here. Special concerns for geriatric animals do merit discussion because of their relevance for shelters and retirement homes (see Geriatric Cats section).

Recognition of Pain and Pain Control

The American College of Veterinary Anesthesiologists has issued a position paper stating that animal pain and suffering are clinically important conditions that adversely affect an animal's QOL.[57] Until recently, recognition and control of animal pain received little attention in veterinary literature and clinical practice,[58, 59] even though animals frequently were used in research to study pain. Denial that children were in pain, plus unwarranted fear of addiction to opioids, are some of the barriers that have compromised good pain control in human patients.[59] Similar attitudinal problems, knowledge deficits, and veterinarians' inability to recognize animal pain have been identified as barriers to better pain control in cats and other animals.[58, 59] The few pain scales that have been published refer to dogs, not cats, and tend to emphasize postsurgical pain rather than chronic pain.[59-62] In addition to increases in physiologic signs of stress such as sweating or salivation, oculonasal discharge, teeth grinding, increased heart and respiratory rates and body temperature, detection of animal pain relies in large part on recognizing subtle departures from normal behavior. These can include changes in personality, attitude, posture, activity level, appetite, facial expression, coat condition, bowel movements, and urination.[57] Adequate recognition of subtle signs of chronic pain may be one of the most pressing issues for those caring for geriatric cats.

Sanitation

As a result of efforts to professionalize the animal-shelter community and upgrade conditions generally in shelters, great emphasis has been placed on sanitation. Sanitation is 1 objective indicator of a well-run shelter. Good sanitation is important for prevention of disease as well as to provide for the comfort of the animal. However, animals communicate with each other through a variety of marking and scent-related behaviors. It is possible that maximizing sanitation, particularly if this involves the use of strong chemicals, could interfere with important cues about territory and social structure.[4]

The tendency to rely exclusively on human notions of a comfortable level of cleanliness may need to be tempered when attempting to optimize QOL for animals in institutional settings, particularly if normal intraspecies communication, ability to hide from view of caretakers or the public, socialization, and ability to perform natural behaviors are sacrificed as a result.

◆ ANIMAL BEHAVIOR AS A TOOL TO ASSESS QUALITY OF LIFE

Animal well-being has important behavioral components, and expression of normal species-specific behavior generally is considered to reflect psychological well-being in confined animals, whether in laboratory, farm, or zoo settings. Inability to express normal behaviors in these circumstances is considered by many to be a major welfare problem. The opportunity to express normal behavior is viewed as so essential to well-being that several European countries have enacted legislation to reduce or eliminate intensive agricultural rearing practices that greatly limit the behavioral repertoire of animals.[22] Because the intention of sheltering is to improve animal welfare, it seems reasonable to expect that opportunities to express normal ranges of behavior in a shelter should at least meet, if not exceed, those for animals being raised for utilitarian purposes. Similarly, every attempt should be made to minimize expression of abnormal behaviors.

When evaluating behavior in companion animals, it is important to consider how an animal of a given age, breed, species, and gender would be expected to behave, and to modify these expectations as necessary from an intake history that includes the animal's normal daily routine. Abnormal behaviors in confined dogs are well-described, and include spinning and circling, pacing, pouncing, bounding and rebounding off kennel walls or doors, leaping up and down in a repetitive manner, excessive licking with formation of granulomas, flank sucking, and wearing of toenails from pacing, chewing, or digging. Studies of stereotypic behavior in captive wild cats are limited, and even less information is available regarding stereotypic behaviors in domestic cats. It is possible that this is due simply to lack of reporting, that confined domestic cats exhibit a different range or more subtle abnormal behaviors than captive wild cats, or that perhaps domestic cats tolerate confinement better. However, 1 report identifies the following problems in confined domestic cats: boredom, aggression, fear, withdrawal, escape behavior, anorexia and weight loss, tail-chasing, and self-mutilation.[51] In 1 large shelter with a formal program to monitor resident cats for abnormal behavior, caretakers are alert for the following characteristics as indicators of the need for evaluation by a behaviorist: increased sensitivity to touch, changes in eating pattern, lethargy, boredom, and

aggression (E. Sperry, personal observation during site visit, July 1998, San Francisco SPCA, San Francisco, CA). In any shelter, systematic observation by caregivers and recording of data over time are important for detecting abnormal behavior as well as subtle changes in expression of normal behavior. If for no other reason, formal monitoring should be done to ensure that cats become more, rather than less, habituated to shelters over time.[7] However, use of standardized instruments (see Table 78–1) to facilitate such observations in shelter cats has not been implemented widely.

◆ ENVIRONMENTAL ENRICHMENT

It has been proposed that general characteristics of an animal with a good QOL include[63]:

- ◆ Ability to cope effectively with day-to-day changes in social environment, with reference to meeting its own needs
- ◆ Ability to engage in beneficial species-typical activities
- ◆ Absence of maladaptive or pathologic behavior (e.g., stereotypies) that results in self-injury or other undesirable consequences
- ◆ Presence of balanced temperament (appropriate balance of passivity and aggression), and absence of chronic signs of distress as indexed by the presence of affiliative versus distress vocalizations, facial expressions, posture, and physiologic responses

The extent to which these characteristics are achieved depends on whether the animal's environment is enriched or deprived. An enriched environment provides an animal with the means to exhibit a range of behaviors that are found in the unconfined state, as well as choices about time and place.[50] This should help decrease the frequency of undesirable or harmful behaviors.[23] Any environment can be made more stimulating and less predictable through environmental and social enrichment, which can be achieved by maximizing the complexity of whatever habitat is present.[50, 51] The lack of studies on enrichment strategies for laboratory cats has been noted.[23] Five characteristics of cat ecology and ethology that are relevant to enriching the feline environment have been identified[50, 51]:

- ◆ Their relative inactivity most of the day
- ◆ The complexity of their natural environment
- ◆ Their predatory lifestyle and playfulness, which persist into adulthood
- ◆ Their sociability
- ◆ Given time, their remarkable adaptability

Shelves and climbing opportunities can extend the available cage space and increase vertical complexity.[50, 51] If structures such as shelves are movable, they provide the opportunity to introduce novelty into the environment. Hiding places and elevated vantage points are particularly important at times of stress.[6, 7, 50, 51] Cortisol levels and stereotypic behaviors in captive wild cats have been shown to decrease in cages with hiding places and enrichment devices.[56] Even when group housing is provided, some cats remain relatively solitary. When integrating a cat into a colony, a variety of retreats and resting places are essential to provide choices in degree of seclusion.[6, 7, 50, 51] Resting places such as corners or edges enable a cat to watch other cats without fear of being approached from behind.[51] Introducing a variety of textures can enrich the environment of confined cats. For example, certain substrates, such as cardboard and rush matting, may encourage scratching.[50, 51] Cages with perches and a view of the outdoors or other areas of activity can be a source of enrichment. Characteristics of environmentally enriched housing for cats have been proposed.[64] These criteria include:

- A more domestic or homelike ambience
- Avoidance of long corridors and rows of animals in "cells"
- Avoidance of cages and bars
- A feeling of light and space
- Access to the outdoors in all weather where and/or appropriate
- Environmentally enriched living accommodations
- Access for visitors

The goals include housing cats in social groups in conservatories with ample light. The facilities provide cats with a choice of environment, height, temperature, and natural, variable light. Shelves, ladders, and climbing poles are used to help cats have a choice of location, views of gardens, access to other cats, and areas of human activity. It has been recommended that providing opportunities for confined cats to exhibit behavior associated with the natural predatory sequence may be an additional way to enhance QOL.[65] This could be accomplished through introduction of novel foods or novel ways of presentation, as well as by extending the stages of feeding (detection, capture, and handling). In 1 study of small cats confined in zoos, multiple feedings helped to decrease the frequency of stereotypic pacing.[66] Hiding food or using food puzzles and making the cat work for at least part of its food has a similar effect.[51] Toys that mimic prey characteristics also are successful in promoting play, but their play value decreases quickly, so toys should be rotated.

◆ ANIMALS WITH DISABILITIES OR CHRONIC ILLNESSES

When reviewing the human disability literature, it is clear that a deficiency or handicapping condition by itself does not necessarily indicate reduced QOL. To imply that disabled individuals have a poorer QOL than able-bodied persons has been described as a reinforcement of stereotypes that underlie discriminatory practices.[30] QOL for persons with disabilities is composed of the same factors as for those without disabilities.[33] Human beings with chronic illnesses have shown remarkable adaptive ability, and often report better QOL than healthy individuals asked to imagine themselves with a specific disease or condition.[67]

Studies of companion animals with disabilities are limited, as is information about management of disabled animals in a shelter environment. One study of quadriplegic pet dogs in homes indicated that these dogs enjoyed good QOL when fitted with a cart and provided with appropriate medical management.[38] Although animals with disabilities or chronic illnesses may require a different level of care, there is no reason to believe that the factors that constitute good QOL are any different from those for nonhandicapped animals. Given the current trends in animal sheltering, there is every reason to believe that the numbers of handicapped animals and sheltered animals living with chronic diseases will increase.

The number of shelters that have specific programs to accommodate the special needs of disabled animals is unknown, but it probably is small at present. One sanctuary contains a separate state-of-the-art building that houses approximately 100 disabled cats (Best Friends Animal Sanctuary, Kanab, UT). This includes cats with chronic medical problems such as renal failure or feline leukemia virus infection, as well as neurologic disorders. The catteries contain ramps for cats that are unable to climb, and have furniture carefully placed for cats with visual impairments. Incontinent cats, most of which are partially paralyzed from car accidents or an abusive past, also have a separate cattery. The immediate reaction to this room of cats may be one of surprise and even shock. However, time spent with these cats by one of the authors (ES) during a site visit indicated that this was a successful housing situation. The cats were maintained well, and were provided with appropriate washable bedding. Resting places were accessible easily from the ground because many of these cats cannot jump. Shelter included indoor and outdoor spaces, and there was routine bathing and bladder expression. The cats sought out human contact, purred when given attention, played with toys, and enjoyed the basic pleasures that a physically healthy cat is able to enjoy. However, it is important to emphasize that this is not a typical shelter environment. Owing to the expert and constant care required to attend properly to a cat with such a disability, it should not be attempted without appropriate facilities, highly trained support staff, and excellent medical care. It is clear from this example that significant advances are possible.

◆ GERIATRIC CATS

During the last third of their lives, cats may undergo physical and metabolic changes that could cause them discomfort and change their behavior. When caring for older cats, shelter staff need to be sensitive to changes in behavior that may indicate loss of vision or hearing; these changes could add stress to a previously tolerable daily routine.[4] Older animals often are more resistant or sensitive to changes in routine, and this should be considered in a shelter environment.[4] More warning may be needed when approaching senior cats. Social problems also may develop if cats become unable to maintain their position in the group hierarchy.[4] Osteoarthritis may produce pain and difficult ambulation. Softer resting places to accommodate cats with decreased muscle mass and nonskid surfaces to prevent slipping are additional strategies that can make an institutional setting more suited to geriatric animals.

To date, much of geriatric medicine has focused on prevention, recognition, and treatment of organ dysfunction associated with aging. One recent development that is particularly relevant for animals in sanctuaries and retirement homes is recognition of cognitive dysfunction syndrome (CDS) in cats and dogs[68] (see Chapter 74, Cognitive Dysfunction in Geriatric Cats). CDS is defined as age-related deterioration of cognitive abilities characterized by behavioral changes that cannot be attributed entirely to medical factors. CDS has been described as similar to Alzheimer's disease in human beings, and is likewise a diagnosis of exclusion. Clinical signs suggestive of canine CDS include decreased activity, energy, playfulness and enthusiasm, and interaction with caregivers; changes in sleep/wake cycle; loss of established housetraining habits; disorientation in familiar surroundings; and compulsive behavior. Until recently, it commonly was believed that cognitive decline was an inevitable consequence of aging. However, L-deprenyl (Anipryl) has been effective in alleviating these clinical signs in older dogs.[68] Similar data have not been reported for cats, and the clinical signs of CDS in cats seem less well-described. It has been noted that owners of senior dogs tend to underreport the occurrence of signs compatible with CDS unless specifically queried, and it seems likely that the same would be true of cat owners or caretakers. A behavior history form has been developed to facilitate early identification of geriatric behavior problems for dogs (Senior dog behavior history form. Cognitive dysfunction syndrome diagnostic aid. Developed for Pfizer, Inc., 1998, by Ilana Reisner, D.V.M., Ph.D., D.A.C.V.B. A similar instrument for cats is included in Chapter 74, Cognitive Dysfunction in Geriatric Cats).

◆ EUTHANASIA

Both limited-admission shelters and pet retirement facilities still may be faced with situations in which euthanasia truly is the most humane decision for an animal believed to be suffering owing to old age or untreatable chronic medical problems. Such a decision may be particularly difficult when natural

death directly as a result of disease may not be imminent, but the animal is believed to be in a poor state of well-being. Occasionally, a healthy animal may never make a satisfactory adjustment from a home setting to an institutional environment, and may be in a constant state of distress. In these cases, observations and opinions of the animal's immediate caretakers must be considered carefully. Stress on caregivers for dependent human beings is a valuable indicator of human QOL, and it is likely that evaluating stress on animal caretakers would be equally relevant.

There are several reasons why the decision to euthanize or continue to maintain an animal with reduced QOL should not be at the discretion of any single individual or constituency. Owing to their attachment to the animal, caretakers may not be objective. No one with a financial interest in the outcome (e.g., the administration of a pet retirement facility) should have sole discretion in such matters. Therefore, in order for the public to have confidence in the process, and to alleviate some of the stress on staff and caregivers, formal external review is desirable. Such oversight undoubtedly will increase in importance as the status of animals in society increases. In human medicine, decisions often must be made regarding life-prolonging medical treatments for individuals who cannot communicate their feelings directly. Approval for such decisions often resides within an institutional review board. Typically, such a board could include physicians, nurses, other caregivers, ethicists, attorneys, and lay persons, as well as an individual designated as a patient advocate. There is little precedent in the animal-sheltering community for guidance in these matters. Even at well-established no-kill shelters, where euthanasia is performed only when an animal reaches a state in which suffering is unavoidable, anecdotal reports suggest that although euthanasia is performed only after careful evaluation, the review process itself tends to be ad hoc. A review board similar to that used in human health care settings should be constituted to advise an animal shelter or retirement home on QOL issues and euthanasia decisions. Likely members would include an attorney, a cat breeder, a veterinary technician, an animal behaviorist, a member of an animal-protection group, staff members of the shelter, and an ethicist or university faculty member. The judgment of a veterinarian not having a primary financial interest in the facility should have substantial influence.

◆ CONCLUSIONS AND RECOMMENDATIONS

With more and more animals projected to live in institutional settings for longer periods of time, it is vital that commendable efforts directed at avoiding death do not result in a compensatory increase in animal suffering because issues of QOL are not addressed adequately. Research on human QOL has identified 1 pitfall that may be particularly relevant to the animal-shelter environment. In 1 study, socially devalued people were more likely to report satisfaction under conditions that other people would describe as adverse.[32] This has been attributed to lower aspirations and levels of dissatisfaction in the absence of hope. The facts that many shelters are underfunded and struggling to provide the bare minimum of care, and that many animals remain unadopted are evidence that the potential for a similar situation clearly exists for animals. Any tendency to accept a lower QOL for shelter residents than for an animal in a home or laboratory environment, simply because they are unwanted and society is providing the best it can under the circumstances, should be resisted. Careful thought is needed concerning permissible concessions, and the extent to which standards can be permitted to deviate from those considered acceptable for owned pets or even laboratory animals, simply to avoid euthanasia.

Validating the subjective experiences of animals incontrovertibly with objective data will be a difficult and perhaps impossible standard by which to initiate meaningful improvements in QOL for cats in shelters. Biologic markers of stress such as fecal cortisol, as well as other objective health and behavioral parameters, can provide some useful information, but are unlikely to provide unambiguous guidance. Agreement on determinants believed to be most important for evaluating feline QOL, reproducible measurement tools, and appropriate and feasible biologic indicators clearly are needed. In the interim, a practical working assumption is that it is possible to evaluate the subjective experience, or QOL, of animals in long-term confinement by drawing on expert opinion and experience, by using accepted principles of clinical ethology, by implementing and/or modifying existing measurement tools, and by supporting clinical observations with biologic data. Existing temperament[26] and stress[6, 7] scales may be useful for evaluating new cats, their suitability for group versus single housing, and changes in stress. Increased use of formal evaluation and standardized data collection would be valuable for monitoring both increases and decreases in cats' well-being over time, which is essential in establishing husbandry and environmental enrichment procedures to maximize QOL for cats living in institutional settings.

REFERENCES

1. Dowling JM, Stitely C: Killing ourselves over the euthanasia debate. Anim Sheltering Sept-Oct 1997, pp. 4–15.
2. McMillan FD: Influence of mental states on somatic health in animals. J Am Vet Med Assoc 214:1221–1225, 1999.
3. Jones RB: Fear and distress. In Appleby MC, Hughes BO (eds): Animal Welfare. Cambridge, UK, CAB International University Press, 1997, pp. 75–87.
4. Jenkins K: Recognizing and reducing stress in shelter ani-
mals. 1997 Elisabeth Lewyt Humane Recognition Award. Denver, Denver Dumb Friends League, 1997.
5. Kessler MR, Turner DC: Stress and adaptation of cats (Felis sylvestris catus) housed singly, in pairs, and in groups in boarding catteries. Anim Welfare 6:243–254, 1997.
6. Kessler MR, Turner DC: Socialization and stress in cats (Felis sylvestris catus) housed singly and in groups in animal shelters. Anim Welfare 8:15–26, 1999.
7. McCune S: Caged cats: Avoiding problems and possible solutions. Companion Animal Behaviour Therapy Study Group Newsletter 7:33–40, 1994.
8. Smith DFE, Durman KJ, Roy DB, Bradshaw JWS: Behavioural aspects of the welfare of rescued cats. J Feline Advis Bur 31:25–28, 39, 1994.
9. Rochlitz I, Podberscek AL, Broom DM: Effects of quarantine on cats and their owners. Vet Rec 143:181–185, 1998.
10. Rochlitz I, Podberscek AL, Broom DM: Welfare of cats in a quarantine cattery. Vet Rec 143:35–39, 1998.
11. Clark JD, Rager DR, Calpin JP: Animal well-being II. Stress and distress. Lab Anim Sci 47:571–579, 1997.
12. Clark JD, Rager DR, Calpin JP: Animal well-being I. General considerations. Lab Anim Sci 47:564–570, 1997.
13. Eisenstein EM, Carlson AD: A comparative approach to learned helplessness. Behav Brain Res 86:149–160, 1997.
14. Foy SS, Mitchell MM: Factors contributing to learned helplessness in the institutionalized aged: A literature review. Phys Occup Ther Geriatr 9:1–23, 1990.
15. Mench JA, Mason GJ: Behaviour. In Appleby MC, Hughes BO (eds): Animal Welfare. Cambridge, UK, CAB International University Press, 1997, pp. 127–141.
16. Clark JD, Rager DR, Calpin JP: Animal well-being III. An overview of assessment. Lab Anim Sci 47:580–585, 1997.
17. Fox MW: Canine behavior. In Mench J, Krulisch L (eds): Canine Research Environment. Conference Proceedings, June 22, 1989. Bethesda, MD, Scientists Center for Animal Welfare, 1989, pp. 21–28.
18. Willemse T, Spruijt BM: Preliminary evidence for dopaminergic involvement in stress-induced excessive grooming in cats. Neurosci Res Commun 17:203–208, 1995.
19. Van den Bos R: Post-conflict stress-response in confined group living cats (Felis sylvestris catus). Appl Anim Behav Sci 59:323–330, 1997.
20. Rifkin M: A lesson in patience: Baltimore County Animal Control still needs work. Our Animal Wards, Spring 1999, pp. 5–9.
21. Ryder RD: Animal revolution: Changing attitudes towards speciesism. Cambridge, MA, Basil Blackwell, 1989, p. 271.
22. Crook AD, Heider LE: The veterinarian's role in farm animal welfare: Directions in production and practice. J Am Vet Med Assoc 204:388–395, 1994.
23. De Monte M, Le Pape G: Behavioural effects of cage enrichment in single-caged adult cats. Anim Welfare 6:53–66, 1997.
24. Duncan IJH: Practices of concern. J Am Vet Med Assoc 204:379–383, 1994.
25. Patronek GJ: Hoarding of animals: An under-recognized public health problem in a difficult-to-study population. Public Health Rep 114:81–87, 1999.
26. Carroll GL, Howe LB, Slater MR, et al: Evaluation of analgesia provided by postoperative administration of butorphanol to cats undergoing onychectomy. J Am Vet Med Assoc 213:246–249, 1998.
27. Burk RL, Maudlin N: Use of a performance scale in small animal radiation therapy. Vet Radiol 33:388–391, 1992.
28. Brown I, Renwick R, Nagler M: The centrality of quality of life in health promotion and rehabilitation. In Renwick R, Brown I, Nagler M (eds): Quality of Life in Health Promotion and Rehabilitation. Conceptual Approaches, Issues, and Applications. London, Sage, 1996, pp. 3–13.
29. Testa MA, Simonson DC: Assessment of quality of life outcomes. N Engl J Med 334:835–840, 1996.
30. Leplege A, Hunt S: The problem of quality of life in medicine. JAMA 278:47–50, 1997.
31. Day H, Jankey SG: Lessons from the literature: Toward a holistic model of quality of life. In Renwick R, Brown I, Nagler M (eds): Quality of Life in Health Promotion and

Rehabilitation. Conceptual Approaches, Issues, and Applications. London, Sage, 1996, pp. 39–50.

32. Felce D, Perry J: Exploring current conceptions of quality of life. *In* Renwick R, Brown I, Nagler M (eds): Quality of Life in Health Promotion and Rehabilitation. Conceptual Approaches, Issues, and Applications. London, Sage, 1996, pp. 51–62.

33. Raphael D: Defining quality of life. Eleven debates concerning its measurement. *In* Renwick R, Brown I, Nagler M (eds): Quality of Life in Health Promotion and Rehabilitation. Conceptual Approaches, Issues, and Applications. London, Sage, 1996, pp. 146–165.

34. Raeburn JM, Rootman I: Quality of life and health promotion. *In* Renwick R, Brown I, Nagler M (eds): Quality of Life in Health Promotion and Rehabilitation. Conceptual Approaches, Issues, and Applications. London, Sage, 1996, pp. 15–25.

35. Morton DB, Burghardt GM, Smith JA: Section III Critical anthropomorphism, animal suffering, and the ecological context. Hastings Center Rep (Suppl) May/June 1990, pp. 13–19.

36. Clark JD, Rager DR, Calpin JP: Animal well-being IV. Specific assessment criteria. Lab Anim Sci 47:586–595, 1997.

37. Chester Z, Clark WT: Coping with blindness: A survey of 50 blind dogs. Vet Rec 123:668–671, 1988.

38. Bauer M, Glickman N, Glickman L, et al: Follow-up study of owner attitudes toward home care of paraplegic dogs. J Am Vet Med Assoc 200:1809–1816, 1992.

39. Carberry CA, Harvey HJ: Owner satisfaction with limb amputation in dogs and cats. J Am Anim Hosp Assoc 23:227–232, 1987.

40. Fox LE, Geoghegan SL, Davis LH, et al: Owner satisfaction with partial mandibulectomy or maxillectomy for treatment of oral tumors in 27 dogs. J Am Anim Hosp Assoc 33:25–31, 1997.

41. Withrow SJ, Hirsch VM: Owner response to amputation of a pet's leg. Vet Med Small Anim Clin 74:332, 1979.

42. Slater MR, Barton CL, Rogers KS, et al: Factors affecting treatment decisions and satisfaction of owners of cats with cancer. J Am Vet Med Assoc 208:1248–1252, 1996.

43. Oullette-Kuntz H, McCreary B: Quality of life assessment for persons with severe developmental disabilities. *In* Renwick R, Brown I, Nagler M (eds): Quality of Life in Health Promotion and Rehabilitation. Conceptual Approaches, Issues, and Applications. London, Sage, 1996, pp. 268–278.

44. Grandin T: Factors that impede animal movement at slaughter plants. J Am Vet Med Assoc 209:757–759, 1996.

45. Podberscek AL, Blackshaw JK, Beattie AW: The behaviour of laboratory colony cats and their reactions to a familiar and unfamiliar person. Appl Anim Behav Sci 31:119–130, 1991.

46. Besch EL: Environmental variables and animal care. *In* Mench J, Krulisch L (eds): Canine Research Environment. Conference Proceedings, June 22, 1989. Bethesda, MD, Scientists Center for Animal Welfare, 1989, pp. 53–57.

47. Scientists Center for Animal Welfare. *In* Gonder JC, Krulisch L (eds): Performance Standards and Animal Welfare: Definition, Application and Assessment. Part 1. Greenbelt, MD, November 1997.

48. Animal Welfare Act 9. CFR section 3.6.

49. Schwindaman D: Regulatory requirements for exercise in dogs. *In* Mench J, Krulisch L (eds): Canine Research Environment. Conference Proceedings, June 22, 1989. Bethesda, MD, Scientists Center for Animal Welfare, 1989, pp. 3–8.

50. McCune S, Hawthorne A: Environmental enrichment for confined cats. Waltham Focus 7:28–31, 1997.

51. McCune S: Enriching the environment of the laboratory cat—A review. *In* Holst B (ed): Proceedings of the Second International Conference on Environmental Enrichment, August 21–25, 1995. Copenhagen, 1995, pp. 103–116.

52. Hughes HC, Campbell S: Effects of primary enclosure size and human contact. *In* Mench J, Krulisch L (eds): Canine Research Environment. Conference Proceedings, June 22, 1989. Bethesda, MD, Scientists Center for Animal Welfare, 1989, pp. 66–73.

53. Wolfe TL: Policy, program and people: The three P's to well-being. *In* Mench J, Krulisch L (eds): Canine Research Environment. Conference Proceedings, June 22, 1989. Bethesda, MD, Scientists Center for Animal Welfare, 1989, pp. 41–47.

54. Liberg O, Sandell M: Spatial organization and reproductive tactics in the domestic cat and other felids. *In* Turner DC, Bateson P (eds): The Domestic Cat: The Biology of Its Behaviour. Cambridge University Press, Cambridge, UK, 1988, pp. 83–98.

55. Roswell HC: Regulations for canine well-being in Canada. *In* Mench J, Krulisch L (eds): Canine Research Environment. Conference Proceedings, June 22, 1989. Bethesda, MD, Scientists Center for Animal Welfare, 1989, pp. 11–18.

56. Carlstead K, Brown JL, Monfort SL, et al: Urinary monitoring of adrenal responses to psychological stressors in domestic and non-domestic felids. Zoo Biol 11:165–176, 1992.

57. American College of Veterinary Anesthesiologists' position paper on the treatment of pain in animals. J Am Vet Med Assoc 213:628–630, 1998.

58. Hansen B, Hardie E: Prescription use of analgesics in dogs and cats in a veterinary teaching hospital: 258 cases (1983–1989). J Am Vet Med Assoc 202:1485–1494, 1993.

59. Hellyer PW, Frederick C, Lacy M, et al: Attitudes of veterinary medical students, house officers, clinical faculty, and staff toward pain management in animals. J Am Vet Med Assoc 214:238–244, 1999.

60. Conzemius MG, Hill CM, Sammarco JL, Perkowski SZ: Correlation between subjective and objective measures used to determine severity of postoperative pain in dogs. J Am Vet Med Assoc 210:1619–1622, 1997.

61. Pibarot P, Dupuis J, Grisneaux E, et al: Comparison of ketoprofen, oxymorphone hydrochloride, and butorphanol in the treatment of postoperative pain in dogs. J Am Vet Med Assoc 211:438–444, 1997.

62. Firth A, Haldane SL: Development of a scale to evaluate postoperative pain in dogs. J Am Vet Med Assoc 214:651–659, 1999.

63. Anonymous: Nonhuman primates. SCAW Scientists Center for Animal Welfare Newsl 20:13, 16, 1998.

64. Loveridge GG: Provision of environmentally enriched housing for cats. Anim Technol 45:69–87, 1994.

65. Anonymous. Environmental enrichment for confined cats. Waltham Researcher, May 1997, pp. 14–17.

66. Shepherdson DJ, Carlstead K, Mellen J, Seidensticker J: The influence of food presentation on the behavior of small cats in confined environments. Zoo Biol 12:203–216, 1993.

67. Adang EMM: Quality of life ratings in patients with chronic illnesses (Letter). JAMA 277:1038, 1997.

68. Leveque NW: Cognitive dysfunction in dogs, cats: An Alzheimer's like disease. J Am Vet Med Assoc 212:1351, 1998.

◆ Index

Note: Page numbers in *italics* refer to illustrations; page numbers followed by the letter t refer to tables.

A blood type, feline, 461
AB blood type, feline, 461
Abandoned cats, 563. See also *Feral cat population(s).*
Abdomen, imaging studies of, for lymphosarcoma, 500
for splenectomy, *442,* 443, *443*
in cancer patients, 549–550, 552–554, *552–555*
in patients with chronic diarrhea, 132t, 133
strengths and weaknesses of, 548t
Abyssinian cats, amyloidosis in, 612
Acarbose, for non–insulin-dependent diabetes mellitus, 170–171, 171t
Acemannan therapy, for vaccine-associated feline sarcomas, 546
Acepromazine, for aortic thromboembolism, 302
for high blood pressure, following renal transplantation, 324
Acetazolamide, for hydrocephalus, 416
Acetylcholine (ACh) receptors, at neuromuscular junction, 374, *375*
Acetylsalicylic acid, for upper respiratory tract infection, 510
Acidifying diets, in prevention of calcium oxalate urolithiasis, 361–362
Acidosis, metabolic, in chronic renal failure, sodium bicarbonate for, 345t
treatment of, 331
Acitretin, for pre–squamous cell carcinoma, 193
Acne, ectopic feline, 205
Acquired immunodeficiency syndrome (AIDS). See *Feline immunodeficiency virus (FIV) infection; Human immunodeficiency virus (HIV) infection.*
Acromegaly, in insulin-resistant diabetes, 516
ACTH (adrenocorticotropic hormone), endogenous, 165
measurement of, 167
ACTH stimulation test, 165
results of, interpretation of, 165–166
Actinic keratosis, 193
vs. Bowen's disease, 210
Acute monocytic/monoblastic leukemia, 491, 491t
Acute myelogenous leukemia, 491, *491,* 491t
Acute myelomonocytic leukemia, 491, 491t
Acute undifferentiated leukemia, 492
Acyclovir, for chronic rhinitis, 59
for FHV-1 infection, 58, 286
Addison's disease (hypoadrenocorticism), 163–165
clinicopathologic findings in, 163–164, 164t
treatment of, 164–165
Adenocarcinoma, nasal. See also *Intranasal tumor(s).*
CT scan of, 531, *531*
thyroid, scintigraphic imaging of, *558*

Adenomatous hyperplasia, of thyroid, scintigraphic imaging of, *557*
Adenosine triphosphate (ATP), inadequate, in neural infarction, 405
Adhesions, induced, in management of chylothorax, 275
Adoption, of unclaimed cats, 573–574
Adrenal function tests, 165
interpretation of, 165–167
normal values for, 166t
Adrenal tumor(s), 159
treatment of, 161
Adrenalectomy, for adrenal tumor, 161
for pheochromocytoma, 182
for pituitary-dependent hyperadrenocorticism, 161
α_2-Adrenergic antagonists, classification of, 110t
β-Adrenergic blocking agents, for hyperthyroidism, 154
Adrenocortical disease(s), 159–167. See also specific disease, e.g., *Hyperadrenocorticism.*
Adrenocorticotropic hormone (ACTH), endogenous, 165
measurement of, 167
Adulticide therapy, for heartworm disease, 257–258
Advanced glycation end products (AGEs), role of, in pathogenesis of diabetic neuropathy, 139–140
Aerosolized bronchodilators, 288
Afferents, gut, in emesis, 109
Agenesis, of corpus callosum, 419
AGEs (advanced glycation end products), role of, in pathogenesis of diabetic neuropathy, 139–140
Aggression, increased, in geriatric cats, 584
Agyria, 419
AIDS (acquired immunodeficiency syndrome). See *Feline immunodeficiency virus (FIV) infection; Human immunodeficiency virus (HIV) infection.*
AIGR (amended insulin:glucose ratio), 183
Airway, bacteria isolated from, 283, 283t
Albendazole, thrombocytopenia associated with, 475
Alder-Reilly bodies, 454
Aldosterone, measurement of, 165, 167
Allergen(s), cat, 233–234
food, chemistry of, 114
Allergic conjunctivitis, 234
Allergic rhinitis, 234
Allergy(ies), alopecia associated with, 196–197
food, 114–116, 114t
to pets, 233–240. See also *Cat allergy.*
Alopecia, in photodermatitis, 191, *191*
paraneoplastic, 196–201
clinical features of, 196, *197*
diagnosis of, 199–200, *200*
differential diagnosis of, allergic disorders in, 196–197

Alopecia *(Continued)*
drug-induced disorders in, 199
endocrine disorders in, 198
immune-mediated disorders in, 198
infectious disorders in, 197–198
neoplastic disorders in, 199
parasitic disorders in, 198
etiopathogenesis of, 196
treatment of, 200–201
psychogenic, 199
Alopecia areata, 198
Alpha blockers, for hypertension, 370
Alpha-L-iduronidase deficiency (mucopolysaccharidosis I), 452–453
Alpha-mannosidosis, 400–401
Amended insulin:glucose ratio (AIGR), 183
Amikacin, for respiratory infections, 285t
Amitriptyline, for aggression in geriatric cats, 584
for feline interstitial cystitis, 316–317
Amlodipine, for hypertension, 281, 370, 408
in chronic renal failure, 334
Amoxicillin, for *Helicobacter* infection, 95
Amoxicillin-clavulanate, postoperative, for renal transplant recipient, 323
Amoxicillin-clavulanic acid, for respiratory infections, 285t
Amphotericin B, for cryptococcosis, 45
Ampicillin, for respiratory infections, 285t
Amputation, rear-leg, for vaccine-associated sarcomas, 5
Amyloid plaque deposition, in geriatric cats, 585
Amyloidosis, hepatic, 90
in Abyssinian cats, 612
Anagen defluxion, 199
Anaphylactoid reactions, to food, 116
Anemia, feline infectious, 12–16. See also *Hemobartonellosis.*
in chronic renal failure, prevention and treatment of, 331–332, 332t
therapeutic agents for, 345t
in lymphoma, 507
Anencephaly, 418
Anesthesia, for examination and sterilization of feral cats, 568
for renal transplantation, 321–322
Angiography, nonselective, in heartworm disease, 255–256, *256,* 256t
Angiotensin-converting enzyme (ACE) inhibitors, for hypertension, 281
in chronic renal failure, 334
Animal behavior, in assessment of shelter animals, 630
Animal shelter. See *Feline animal shelter(s).*
Animal Welfare Act, 622
Anorexia, associated with chemotherapy, 523–524
intradialytic, 347
Antibiotics, for mycobacterial panniculitis, 226–227

Antibiotics *(Continued)*
 for respiratory disease, 283–284, 285t
 postoperative, for renal transplant recipient, 323
Antibody(ies), detection of, in hemobartonellosis, 15
 insulin, 177
Anticoagulants, for aortic thromboembolism, 410–411
Anticruelty laws, maltreatment defined by, 623
Antiemetic therapy, 107–111
 classification of, 109–110, 110t
 for chemotherapy patients, 111
 for delayed gastric emptying, 111
 for dysautonomia, 383
 for motion sickness, 110
 for uremia, 110–111
 irrational use of, in undiagnosed patient, 111
 rational use of, in diagnosed patient, 110–111
  in undiagnosed patient, 111, *111*
Antifungal therapy, for respiratory disease, 284, 286
Antigens, in immunocontraception, delivery of, 579
 oocyte, 578–579
 sperm, 578
Antihistamines, for mosquito-bite hypersensitivity, 188–189, 188t
Antihypertensive therapy, *369*, 369–370
Anti-inflammatory therapy, for respiratory disease, 286–287
Antimicrobial susceptibility testing, 225–226
Antirejection therapy, for renal transplant recipient, 324–325
Antithyroid agents, thrombocytopenia associated with, 475
Antivenin, coral snake, 378–379
Antiviral therapy, for FHV-1 infection, 57–58
 for respiratory disease, 287
Anxiety, in geriatric cats, 584
Aortic thromboembolism, 299–305
 clinical features of, 301, 409–410
 diagnosis of, 301–302, 410, *410*
 epidemiology of, 299–300
 etiology of, 299
 hypertrophic cardiomyopathy as risk factor in, 299
 pathogenesis of, 300–301
 prevention of, 303–305
 prognosis associated with, 411
 treatment of, 302–303, 410–411
Aortic valve insufficiency, echocardiographic imaging of, 250–251
Aortic valve stenosis, echocardiographic imaging of, 251
Aortotomy, 303
Apolipoprotein(s), 214
Appetite, decreased, in chronic renal failure, 332–333, 333t
Appetite stimulants, 345t
APUDoma, 181
Arnold-Chiari malformation, 420
Arteriolar response, to hypertension, 278
Arylsulfatase B deficiency (mucopolysaccharidosis VI), 451, *452–453*
 pathologic findings in, 452, *454–455*
 radiographic findings in, 451–452, *454*
Aspiration, fine-needle. See *Fine-needle aspiration.*

Aspirin, for aortic thromboembolism, 302
 for hip dysplasia, 596
 prophylactic, for aortic thromboembolism, 303, 411
 for saddle thrombus, 265
Asthma, definition of, 234
Atenolol, for hypertension, 281, 370
 for hypertrophic cardiomyopathy, 265
Atopy, definition of, 234
ATP (adenosine triphosphate), inadequate, in neural infarction, 405
Atrial septal defects, echocardiographic imaging of, 252
Atrioventricular valve dysplasia, echocardiographic imaging of, 252
Atrium, echocardiographic imaging of, 248, *249–250*
Atropine, for organophosphate and carbamate toxicity, 379
 for sedation during blood collection, 463
 premedication with, for renal transplantation, 322
Autoimmune disease(s), vs. mosquito-bite hypersensitivity, 188
Azalides, for respiratory infections, 284
Azathioprine, for inflammatory bowel disease, 503–504
Azithromycin, for cryptosporidiosis, 36
 for *Helicobacter* infection, 95
 for respiratory infections, 284
Azotemia, in chronic renal failure, 328
 minimizing, 329–330

B blood type, feline, 461, 461t
Bacteria, isolated from airway, 283, 283t
Bacterial diarrhea, 129t
Bacterial infection, of respiratory tract, treatment of, 283–284, 285t
Balloon dilatation therapy, esophageal, *104*
 principles of, 103t
Barium meal, 73
Barium paste, 73, *74–75*
Barium sulfate suspension, used in upper gastrointestinal series, of small intestines, 79, *80*
 of stomach, 75, 76, *77*
Bartonella species, detection of, PCR assay in, 481–482
Bartonellosis (cat-scratch disease), 23–24, 565
Basal cell carcinoma, 193
Basophilic leukemia, 492
Benazepril, for hypertension, 281, 370
 in chronic renal failure, 334
Beta blockers, for hypertension, 370
 for hyperthyroidism, 154
 for hypertrophic cardiomyopathy, 265
Beta-glucuronidase deficiency (mucopolysaccharidosis VII), 453, *455*
Bethanechol, for dysautonomia, 383
Bile-duct carcinoma, paraneoplastic alopecia associated with, 196
Biliary cystadenoma, cytology of, 123, *123*
 diagnostic imaging of, *552, 554*
Bilirubin, conjugated (direct), 87–88
 unconjugated (indirect), 87
Biopsy, CT-guided, of meningioma, 389
 fine-needle aspiration. See *Fine-needle aspiration.*
 mucosal, in inflammatory bowel disease, 500–501, *501*
 muscle, in diabetic neuropathy, 142–143

Biopsy *(Continued)*
 peripheral nerve, in diabetic neuropathy, 142
Bismuth, for *Helicobacter* infection, 95
Bites, mosquito, hypersensitivity to. See *Hypersensitivity, mosquito-bite.*
 zoonotic disease associated with, 23–24
Blastomycosis, antifungal therapy for, 286
Bleeding time, in thrombocytopenic disorders, 470
Blood banks, veterinary, 462t
Blood collection, feline, 463–465, *464*
 sedation in, 463
Blood pressure, Doppler monitoring of, in renal transplant recipient, 324
 high. See *Hypertension.*
 measurement of, 280
  cuff factors in, 367
  environmental factors in, 368
  equipment choice in, 366–367
  protocol in, 366t
Blood substitutes, transfusion of, 466–467
Blood test, for *Helicobacter* infection, 95
Blood transfusion, 461–467
 administration of, 465
 adverse reactions to, 465–466
 collection of blood for, 463–465, *464*
  sedation in, 463
 crossmatching and blood-typing for, 462–463, *463*, 463t
 donor sedation for, 463
 donor selection for, 462, 462t
 prior to renal transplantation, 321
 synthetic colloids and blood substitutes in, 466–467
  advantages of, 467
Blood types, feline, 461–462, 461t
Blood typing, for transfusions, 462–463, *463*
Blood urea nitrogen (BUN), in chronic renal failure, 329
BMT. See *Bone marrow transplantation (BMT).*
Bobcats, cytauxzoonosis in, 436
Bone marrow, evaluation of, in thrombocytopenic disorders, 470
Bone marrow transplantation (BMT), for mucopolysaccharidosis, *455,* 456
 thrombocytopenia associated with, 473–474
Bordetella bronchiseptica, vaccination recommendations for, 8
Bordetellosis, 24
Borison-Wang model, for vomiting, 107
Borna disease, 65–68
 clinical and pathologic findings in, 66–68, *67*
 epizootiology of, 65–66
 etiopathogenesis of, 66
 vs. spongiform encephalopathy, 63t
 zoonotic risk in, 68
Botulism, 379
Bovine spongiform encephalopathy (BSE), 62. See also *Encephalopathy, spongiform.*
Bowen's disease, 208–212
 clinical signs of, 208, *208–209*
 differential diagnosis of, 209–210, 211t
 etiology of, 210–211
 histopathology of, 208–209, *210*
 treatment of, 211–212
Brain. See also *Forebrain; Hindbrain.*
 CT-guided biopsy of, meningioma in, 389
 herniation of, following excision of meningioma, 390, 390t

Brain *(Continued)*
    tumors of, in geriatric cats, 585
Breed population dynamics, bottlenecks
    in, 604
    founder effects in, 602–603, 603t
    "gold standard" in, 602
    inbreeding in, 604
    reduced migration in, 603–604
Breeders, genetic counseling of, 619, *619*
Bronchodilator therapy, 287–288, 288t
BSE (bovine spongiform encephalopathy),
    62. See also *Encephalopathy,*
    spongiform.
BUN (blood urea nitrogen), in chronic
    renal failure, 329
BUN:creatinine ratio, in chronic renal
    failure, 330
Burmese cats, craniofacial malformations
    in, 419
    head defect in, 610
Buspirone, for victim of aggression, 584
Butorphanol, for aortic thromboembolism,
    411
    with pain, 302

Calcitriol synthesis, decreased, in chronic
    renal failure, 331
Calcium, supplemental, following
    thyroidectomy, 156
Calcium and phosphorus balance, in
    chronic renal failure, maintenance of,
    330–331
Calcium channel blockers, for
    hypertension, 281, 370
    for hypertrophic cardiomyopathy, 265
Calcium gluconate, for hypocalcemia, 156
Calcium ipodate, for hyperthyroidism,
    153
Calcium oxalate crystallization, *356–358*
    altered inhibitors and promoters of, 355
    in urolith formation, 354–355
Calcium oxalate urolithiasis. See
    Urolithiasis, calcium oxalate.
Calicivirus infection, vaccination
    recommendations for, 8
Caloric supplementation, postoperative,
    for renal transplant recipient, 323
Calvarium, dome-shaped, in
    hydrocephalus, 416, *416*
Campylobacteriosis, 18
Cancer. See also at anatomic site, e.g.,
    Esophagus, cancer of; specific
    neoplasm, e.g., *Lymphoma.*
    chemotherapy for. See *Chemotherapy.*
    diagnostic imaging of, 548–558
        abdominal radiography in, 549–550,
            552, *552–554*
        computed tomography in, 555–557,
            556–557
        magnetic resonance imaging in, 555–
            557, *556*
        scintigraphy in, 557–558, *557–558*
        thoracic radiography in, 548–549,
            549–552
        ultrasonography in, 552–555, *554–555*
    hematologic abnormalities associated
        with, 473
    paraneoplastic alopecia associated with,
        196
    second, concurrent with lymphoma,
        516–517
Carbamate toxicity, 379
Carbenicillin, for respiratory infections,
    285t

Carboplatin, 522–523
    dosage of, 522
    for vaccine-associated feline sarcomas,
        546
    tumors responding to, 522t
Carcinoid, metastatic, radiographic
    imaging of, *551*
Carcinoma. See *Cancer;* specific type, e.g.,
    Squamous cell carcinoma.
Carcinoma in situ, cutaneous, 192
    multicentric squamous cell. See *Bow-*
        en's disease.
Cardiac abnormality(ies), associated with
    hypertension, 278
Cardiac shunt (shunting),
    echocardiographic imaging of,
    251–252
Cardiomyopathy(ies), dilated,
    echocardiographic features of, 249t
    hypertrophic, 261–266
        as risk factor in aortic thromboembo-
            lism, 299
        clinical signs of, 262
        differential diagnosis of, 264–265
        echocardiographic features of, 249t
        echocardiographic imaging of, 248,
            248–249
        electrocardiograms of, 262, 264, *264*
        etiology of, 261
        pathology of, 261
        pathophysiology of, 261–262
        prognosis associated with, 265–266
        radiographic studies of, 262, *263*
        thromboembolic episodes in, 265
        treatment of, 265
    in geriatric cats, 585
    restrictive, echocardiographic features
        of, 249t
Cardiovascular instability, as
    complication of hemodialysis, 344,
    346
Cat allergy, 233–240
    clinical symptoms of, 234
    diagnosis of, 234–235
    Fel d 1 allergen in, 233–234
        key points concerning, 236
    management of, 235
        strategy(ies) for, 236–240
            bedroom modification as, 239–240
            change home furnishings as, 238–
                239
            change home ventilation as, 239
            clean clothes and laundry as, 239
            cleaning procedures as, 240
            make cat less allergic as, 238
            minimize exposure to allergen as,
                237
            restricting cat habitats as, 237–238
    removal of pet in, comments regarding,
        235–236
Cat approach test, for assessment of
    socialization toward cats, 625t
Cat breeds, 603t. See also *Breed*
    population dynamics.
Cat temperature scale, 626t
Cat-scratch disease (bartonellosis), 23–24,
    565
Cat-stress score, 624t–625t
CBC (complete blood count), for chronic
    diarrhea, 130, 131t
Cefazolin, postoperative, for renal
    transplant recipient, 323
Cefoxitin, for respiratory infections, 285t
Ceftiofur, for respiratory infections, 285t
Central nervous system (CNS), disorders
    of. See specific disorder, e.g.,
    Encephalopathy, spongiform.

Central nervous system (CNS) *(Continued)*
    inflammatory, 425–433. See also *Infec-*
        tious disease(s), involving central
        nervous system.
Cephalexin, for respiratory infections,
    285t
Cerebellum, cortical atrophy of,
    hereditary, 422
    degeneration of, parvoviral-induced,
        420–421, *421*
Cerebral edema, in inflammatory CNS
    diseases, 429
Cerebrospinal fluid (CSF), analysis of, for
    meningioma, 388
    in CNS inflammatory disease, 427–
        428
    in cryptococcosis, 431
    in feline infectious peritonitis, 429
    in toxoplasmosis, 433
    increased, in hydrocephalus, 415–416
Cerebrovascular disease, 405–409
    intracranial hemorrhage as, 406–409,
        407–408, 407t
    ischemic encephalopathy as, 405–406,
        406
Ceroid lipofuscinosis, neuronal, 401–402
Cetirizine, for mosquito-bite
    hypersensitivity, 188t
Challenge testing, for allergies, 234–235
Chemical restraint, of sheltered animals,
    571–572
Chemoreceptor trigger zone (CRTZ),
    activation of, 108
    vomiting through, 107, *108*
Chemotherapy, 521–524. See also specific
    agent, e.g., *Doxorubicin.*
    antiemetics with, 111
    causing thrombocytopenia, 475–476
    client-related issues in, 524
    commonly used drugs in, updates on,
        521
    for lymphoma, adverse effects of, 508
        mediastinal, 539
        renal, 514
    for vaccine-associated feline sarcomas,
        6, 545–546
    myelosuppression secondary to, 517
    new agents in, 523
    nutritional support with, 523–524
Chiari malformation(s), 420
Chlamydia psittaci, 509. See also
    Respiratory tract infection.
    vaccination recommendations for, 8
Chlamydiosis, 24
    vs. FHV-1 infection, 55, 55t
Chlorambucil, for inflammatory bowel
    disease, 504
    for lymphosarcoma, 504t
Chloramphenicol, for hemobartonellosis,
    16
    for respiratory infections, 285t
    thrombocytopenia associated with, 475
Chlorpheniramine, for mosquito-bite
    hypersensitivity, 188t
Cholangiocarcinoma, cytology of, 121,
    123, *123*
Cholangiocellular carcinoma,
    paraneoplastic alopecia associated
    with, 196, 200–201
Cholangiohepatitis, 89–90
Cholestasis, hepatic, cytology of, 124,
    125, 126
Cholesterol, 214
M_1-Cholinergic antagonists, classification
    of, 110t
Chromium picolinate, for non–insulin-
    dependent diabetes mellitus, 171t,
    172

Chromosomes, feline, 600
Chronic illness, quality of life issues associated with, 631
Chronic myelogenous leukemia, 492
Chyle, 267, *267–268*
Chylothorax, 267–275
  clinical signs of, 269
  diagnosis of, *269–270*, 269–271
  etiology of, 271, 271t
  idiopathic, 271
  management of, medical, 271–272, 272t
    surgical, 272–275
      pericardiectomy in, 273
      pleurodesis in, 274–275
      pleuroperitoneal shunting in, 273–274, *274*
      thoracic duct ligation with mesenteric lymphangiography in, 272–273, *273*
Chylous effusions, 267–269. See also *Chylothorax.*
  characteristics of, 268t
  cytologic appearance of, 267, *268*
Cimetidine, for esophagitis, 106
  for splenomegaly, 444
Ciprofloxacin, for mycobacterial panniculitis, 226, 227
Circulatory overload, as reaction to transfusion, 466
Cirrhosis, 90
Cisapride, for esophagitis, 106
Cisplatin, stealth liposome-encapsulated, 523
Citrate, in prevention of calcium oxalate crystals, 362
Clarithromycin, for *Helicobacter* infection, 95
  for leprosy-like disease, 228
Cleft palate, 419
Clindamycin, for respiratory infections, 285t
  for toxoplasmosis, 433
Clofazimine, for leprosy-like disease, 228
Clostridium botulinum toxin, 379
Clotting factors, vitamin K–dependent, warfarin inhibition of, 304
Cloxacillin, for respiratory infections, 285t
CNS (central nervous system), disorders of. See specific disorder, e.g., *Encephalopathy, spongiform.*
  inflammatory, 425–433. See also *Infectious disease(s), involving central nervous system.*
Cobalt irradiation, for pituitary-dependent hyperadrenocorticism, 161
Cognitive dysfunction syndrome, in geriatric cats, 632
Colloid(s), synthetic, transfusion of, 466
Colon, contrast radiographic studies of, 80–81, *82–83*
  normal anatomy in, 79–80, *81*
  peritoneography in, 81, *83*
  pneumocolon in, 80–81, *82*
Coma, nonketotic hyperosmolar, 178
Complete blood count (CBC), for chronic diarrhea, 130, 131t
Computed tomography (CT), diagnostic, in cancer patients, 555–557, *556–557*
  of hydrocephalus, *415*
  of intracranial hemorrhage, 407, *407*
  of intranasal tumor, *529, 530, 531*
  of mediastinal tumor, 537
  of meningioma, 388, *389*
  of vaccine-associated feline sarcomas, 543, *544–545*

Computed tomography (CT) *(Continued)*
  strengths and weaknesses of, 548t
Confinement, long-term, quality of life in, 621–633. See also *Quality of life, in long-term confinement.*
Confinement status of cats, 563
Conjunctivitis, allergic, 234
  in FHV-1 infection, 53, 54
Conn's syndrome (hyperaldosteronism), 162–163
Constipation, in chronic renal failure, 333
  in geriatric cats, 583
Contrast agent(s). See also named agent, e.g., *Barium* entries.
  iodinated, for hyperthyroidism, 153
  water-soluble, in peritoneography, 81
Contrast echocardiography, 247
Contrast radiography, in evaluation of gastrointestinal tract, 73–85
Coral snake envenomation, 378–379
Corneal clouding, associated with mucopolysaccharidosis, 451, *452*
Corneal sequestration, associated with FHV-1 infection, 54, *54*
Corpus callosum, agenesis of, 419
Corticosteroids, for alimentary lymphosarcoma, 504
  for bronchial inflammatory disease, 286
  for hydrocephalus, 416
  for inflammatory bowel disease, 504
  for inflammatory CNS diseases, 428–429
Cortisol, 165
Cortisol:creatinine ratio, urinary, 165
  measurement of, 167
Coxiella burnetii infection, 31–32
Coxofemoral joint, laxity of, evaluation of, 593
Cranial and intracranial malformation(s), congenital, 413–422
  classification of, 413t
  differential diagnosis of, 415
  embryology of, 414–415
  etiology of, 413–414, 414t
  involving forebrain, 415–420. See also specific malformation, e.g., *Hydrocephalus.*
  involving hindbrain, 420–422. See also specific malformation, e.g., *Cerebellum, degeneration of, parvoviral-induced.*
  teratogenic agents causing, 414t
Craniofacial malformations, in Burmese cats, 419
Craniorachischisis, 418
Crossmatching, for blood transfusions, 462–463, 463t
CRTZ (chemoreceptor trigger zone), activation of, 108
  vomiting through, 107, *108*
Cryosurgery, for squamous cell carcinoma, 193–194
Cryptococcosis, 39–49, 431–432
  antifungal therapy for, 284
  diagnosis of, 43–44, *44*
  etiopathogenesis of, 39–43, *40–42*
  prognosis associated with, 48
  public health concerns associated with, 48
  treatment of, 44–48
    in cats with meningoencephalitis, 46–48, *47*
    in cats without CNS involvement, 45–46
    medical, 45, 432
    surgical, 45

Cryptococcus neoformans, 39, 431
Cryptococcus neoformans var gattii, 39
Cryptosporidiosis, 18, 20
  clinical reports of, 35, 35t
  diagnosis of, 35–36, *36*
  etiology of, 34
  pathogenesis of, 34–35
  prevention of, 37
  treatment of, 36–37
  zoonotic aspects of, 37
Cryptosporidium parvum, 18, 34
  oocysts of, *36*
Cryptosporidium species, life cycle of, 34
Crystallization, calcium oxalate, *356–358*
  altered inhibitors and promoters of, 355
  in urolith formation, 354–355
CSF. See *Cerebrospinal fluid (CSF).*
CT. See *Computed tomography (CT).*
Culture (culturing), of *Cryptococcus neoformans* organisms, 43–44, *44*
  of *Haemobartonella felis* organisms, 15
Cushing's syndrome, 159. See also *Hyperadrenocorticism.*
  treatment of, 160–161
Cutaneous xanthoma. See *Xanthoma(s), cutaneous.*
Cuterebra larva migration, in ischemic encephalopathy, 405–406, *406*
Cuterebra larval myiasis, 430–431
Cyclophosphamide, for lymphosarcoma, 504t
  myelosuppression secondary to, 517
Cyclosporine, for bronchial inflammatory disease, 286
  for renal transplant recipient, 324
Cyclosporine challenge, prior to renal transplantation, 320–321
Cyproheptadine, as appetite stimulant, 524
  for bronchial inflammatory disease, 286
  for mosquito-bite hypersensitivity, 188t
Cyst(s), mediastinal, 534
Cystadenoma, biliary, cytology of, 123, *123*
  diagnostic imaging of, *552, 554*
Cystitis, interstitial. See *Feline interstitial cystitis (FIC).*
Cytauxzoon felis, 436, *436–437*
  detection of, PCR assay in, 482
  thrombocytopenia associated with, 474
Cytauxzoonosis, clinical findings in, 437
  etiology and epidemiology of, 436, *436–437*
  implications of, for practitioner, 438
  survival of, 437–438
Cytosine arabinoside, for acute myeloid leukemias, 493t
  for lymphosarcoma, 504t

Dalteparin, prophylactic effect of, thromboembolism and, 305
DAMNITT scheme approach, to thrombocytopenia, 471t, 473–476
Dandy-Walker syndrome, 420
Day-tripper cats, 571
Defecation, outside litter box, 583
Degenerative disease(s), in geriatric cats, 584
  of joint, 592–597. See also *Hip dysplasia.*
Delayed gastric emptying, disorders of, antiemetics for, 111
Deoxyribonucleic acid. See *DNA* entries.

L-Deprenyl, for cognitive dysfunction, in geriatric cats, 586
Dermatitis, associated with *Malassezia*, 204
    facial, 205
    solar, 191–195. See also *Photodermatitis.*
Dermatophytosis, concurrent with lymphoma, 512–513
    in feral cat populations, 565
Dermatosis, sun-induced, vs. mosquito-bite hypersensitivity, 188
Desoxycorticosterone pivalate, for hypoadrenocorticism, 164
Devon rex cats, spasticity in, 612
Dexamethasone, for *Cuterebra* larval myiasis, 431
    for hypoadrenocorticism, 164
    for inflammatory bowel disease, 504
    for ischemic encephalopathy, 406
Dexamethasone suppression test, 165
    results of, interpretation of, 166
Dextrans, transfusion of, 466
DI (distraction index), in measurement of hip-joint laxity, 593, 595–596, *596*
Diabetes mellitus, concurrent with lymphoma, 515–516
    insulin-dependent, 169
        insulin therapy for, 175–178
            complications of, 178
            monitoring of, 176–178, 176t
            owner/client factors in, 175
            pharmacokinetic factors in, 175–176
    non–insulin-dependent, 169
        diet and exercise therapy for, 169–170
        oral hypoglycemic therapy for, *170,* 170–172, 171t
            agents improving peripheral insulin sensitivity in, 171t, 172
            agents inhibiting hepatic glucose output in, 171–172, 171t
            agents inhibiting intestinal glucose absorption in, 170–171, 171t
            agents promoting pancreatic release of insulin in, 171, 171t
            insulin with, 172
Diabetic ketoacidosis, 178
Diabetic neuropathy, 139–143
    clinical signs of, 140, *141–142*
    diagnosis of, electrophysiology in, 142, *143*
        peripheral nerve and muscle biopsy in, 142–143
    differential diagnosis of, 140, 142
    etiology and pathogenesis of, current theories on, 139–140
    plantigrade stance secondary to, 178
    prevention of, 143
    treatment of, 143
Dialysate, composition of, 343
Dialysis, peritoneal, 337. See also *Hemodialysis.*
    for lily nephrotoxicity, 309
Dialysis catheter, transcutaneous double-lumen, 339, *340–341*
    transcutaneous single-lumen, 339, *342*
Dialysis dysequilibrium syndrome, 346
Diarrhea, acute, 127
    chronic, 127–134
        causes of, 127–128, 128t, 129t
        diagnostic studies for, 129–130, 131t–132t, 133
        disorders associated with, 129t
        history of, 128, 130t

Diarrhea *(Continued)*
        physical findings in, 128–129
        treatment of, 133–134
    definition of, 127
Diazepam, for ischemic encephalopathy, 406
    for post-hemorrhage seizures, 408
    for sedation during blood collection, 463
Diet, for non–insulin-dependent diabetes mellitus, 169–170
    high-fiber, for chronic diarrhea, 134
    Hill's Prescription, for hypercalcemia, 313
    in chronic renal failure, management of, 334–335
    in prevention of calcium oxalate urolithiasis, 361–362, 363t
    low-fat, for chylothorax, 272t
    modification of, for feline interstitial cystitis, 316
Diethylcarbamazine, prophylactic, for heartworm disease, 259
Diffusion, principles of, in hemodialysis, 338, *339*
Dilated pupil syndrome. See *Dysautonomia.*
Diltiazem, for hypertrophic cardiomyopathy, 265
Diminazene aceturate, for cytauxzoonosis, 437
Diphenhydramine, for *Cuterebra* larval myiasis, 431
    for ischemic encephalopathy, 406
    for organophosphate and carbamate toxicity, 379
    for splenomegaly, 444
Diphenylhydantoin, causing congenital cranial malformations, 414t
Dirofilaria immitis, in heartworm disease, 253, 259
Dirty face syndrome, 205
Disabilities, quality of life issues associated with, 631
Disorientation, in geriatric cats, 585
Disseminated mycobacterial disease, with lymph node or organ involvement, 229–230, *230*
Distraction index (DI), in measurement of hip-joint laxity, 593, 595–596, *596*
Dithiazanine, for heartworm disease, 258
Diuretics, for hypertension, 281
    thiazide, for hypertension, 370
        in prevention of calcium oxalate urolithiasis, 362–363
DNA fingerprinting, 605, 606
DNA sequence, amplification of, PCR assay and, 479, *480*
    microsatellites in, 606
    of genes, 600–601
Donor(s), blood, sedation of, 463
    selection of, 462, 462t
Donor kidney, 321. See also *Renal transplantation.*
    acute rejection of, 325–326
D2-Dopaminergic antagonists, classification of, 110t
Doppler echocardiography, 247
Doxil, for vaccine-associated feline sarcomas, 545
Doxorubicin, dosages of, 521
    for renal lymphoma, 514
    myelosuppression secondary to, 517
    for vaccine-associated feline sarcomas, 545
    stealth liposome-encapsulated, 523

Doxycycline, for ehrlichiosis, 31
    for hemobartonellosis, 16
    for mycobacterial panniculitis, 227
    for respiratory infections, 285t
Drug(s). See also named drug or drug group.
    alopecia caused by, 199
    cancer. See *Chemotherapy.*
    for cognitive dysfunction, in geriatric cats, 585–586
    interaction of, with warfarin, 304
Dwarfism, in Munchkin breed, 612
Dysautonomia, clinical signs of, 381, 382t
    diagnosis of, 381–383, *382*
    pathologic findings in, 381
    treatment of, 383
Dysplasia, hip, 592–597, 612. See also *Hip dysplasia.*
Dyspnea, associated with chylothorax, 269
    intradialytic, 347

Ear-tipping, of spayed or neutered feral cats, 568–569
Echocardiography, 245–252
    contrast, 247
    diagnostic, in acquired heart disease, *248–250,* 248–251, 249t
        in congenital heart disease, 251–252
    Doppler, 247
    feline, normal values in, 246t
    imaging planes in, *247,* 247–248
        from right hemithorax, 247–248, *248*
    in heartworm disease, 248, *248–249,* 251
    in hypertrophic cardiomyopathy, 248, *248–249*
    M-mode, 245–247, *246,* 246t
    two-dimensional, 245
Ectopic feline acne, 205
Edema, cerebral, in inflammatory CNS diseases, 429
    peritumoral, associated with meningioma, 386–387
    pulmonary, in dialysis patient, 346, *347*
Efferents, gut, in emesis, 109
Effusion(s), chylous, 267–269. See also *Chylothorax.*
    characteristics of, 268t
    cytologic appearance of, 267, *268*
    pleural, associated with thymoma, 535
        in dialysis patient, 346, *347*
Ehrlichia species, 28, *28*
    detection of, PCR assay in, 482
Ehrlichiosis, 24, 28–31
    clinical signs of, 29, 30t
    diagnosis of, 29, 31
    etiologic agent in, 28, *28*
    laboratory abnormalities associated with, 29
    pathogenesis of, 28
    public health aspects of, 31
    transmission of, 28–29
    treatment of, 31
Eicosapentaenoic acid, for mosquito-bite hypersensitivity, 189
Electrocardiography. See also *Holter monitoring.*
    in hypertrophic cardiomyopathy, 262, 264, *264*
Electrophysiologic studies, of diabetic neuropathy, 142, *143*
ELISA (enzyme-linked immunosorbent assay), for cryptosporidiosis, 36

ELISA (enzyme-linked immunosorbent assay) *(Continued)*
for heartworm disease, 254–255
Embolism, aortic, 409–411, *410.* See also *Aortic thromboembolism.*
definition of, 405
fibrocartilaginous, 409
Emesis, as reaction to transfusion, 466
in chronic renal failure, 332–333
intradialytic, 347
mechanisms of, 107–108, *108*
neurotransmitters and receptors in, 108–109
vs. regurgitation, 99
Emetic center, regulation of vomiting at, 108
Employee relations, in animal shelters, 574–575
Enalapril, for hypertension, 281, 370
for hypertrophic cardiomyopathy, 265
Encephalocele, 418–419
Encephalopathy, ischemic, 405–406, *406*
spongiform, 62–65
clinical and pathologic findings in, 64, *65*
epizootiology of, 62–64, *63*
etiopathogenesis of, 64
vs. borna disease, 63t
zoonotic risk in, 64–65
uremic, in dialysis patient, 346
Enclosure size, in evaluating life of shelter animal, 628
Endocrine disorder(s). See also specific disorder, e.g., *Hyperadrenocorticism.*
alopecia associated with, 198
Endoscopy, for chronic diarrhea, 132t, 133
in removal of esophageal foreign bodies, 101, *102*
Endothelin 1 (ET-1), RAAS activation of, 277
Enemas, saline, in colonic studies, 76
Enrofloxacin, for ischemic encephalopathy, 406
for mycobacterial panniculitis, 227
for respiratory infections, 285t
Envenomation, coral snake, 378–379
Environmental comfort, in evaluating life of shelter animal, 628
Environmental enrichment, for shelter animals, 630–631
Environmental modifications, for geriatric cat, 586
Environmental toxins, causing thrombocytopenia, 476
Enzyme-linked immunosorbent assay (ELISA), for cryptosporidiosis, 36
for heartworm disease, 254–255
Eosinophilic granuloma complex, 187
Eosinophilic keratitis, associated with FHV-1 infection, 54–55, *55*
Eosinophilic leukemia, 492
Erythema, necrolytic migratory, 199
solar-induced, 191, *191*
Erythremic myelosis, 491
Erythrocyte(s), 484–485
hereditary disorder(s) of, 484–489
diagnostic approach to, 486–487
glycolytic erythroenzymopathies in, 485, 485t
heme defects in, 485, 485t
increased osmotic fragility in, 485t, *486,* 488
membrane defects in, 485, 485t
methemoglobin reductase deficiency as, 485t, 487–488

Erythrocyte(s) *(Continued)*
porphyria as, 485t, 487
pyruvate kinase deficiency as, 485t, 488–489
Erythroenzymopathy(ies), glycolytic, 485, 485t
Erythroleukemia, 491, *492*
Erythromycin, for respiratory infections, 285t
Esophageal balloon dilatation therapy, *104*
principles of, 103t
Esophagitis, 105–106, *106*
Esophagoscopy, of esophageal disease, 100–101
Esophagostomy tube, nutritional support via, 524
Esophagram, barium, 73–74, *74–75*
Esophagus, cancer of, 103, *105*
contrast radiographic studies of, 73–74, *74–75*
normal anatomy in, 73, *74*
disorders of, 99–106. See also specific disorder, e.g., *Megaesophagus.*
classification of, 99, *100*
clinical findings in, 99
diagnosis of, 99–101
esophagoscopy in, 100–101
radiography in, 99–100, *100*
obstruction of, 101–103
foreign bodies causing, 101, 101t, *102*
strictures causing, 102, *102–103*
treatment of, 102–103, 103t, *104*
ET-1 (endothelin 1), RAAS activation of, 277
Ethanol injection(s), ultrasound-guided percutaneous, for hyperthyroidism, 157
Etretinate, for pre–squamous cell carcinoma, 193
Euthanasia, in long-term confinement shelters, 632
of feral cats, 561
criteria for, 568
of unredeemed cats, 574
Euthanasia program, responsible, 574
Excision, of meningioma, 389–390
recurrence following, 390–391
Excrement, feline, zoonotic disease in human beings associated with, 19t
Exencephaly, 418
Exercise, for non–insulin-dependent diabetes mellitus, 169–170
for shelter animals, 628
Exudative diarrhea, 128

Facial dermatitis, idiopathic, 205
Facial structures, development of, 414–415
Fading kitten syndrome, 413
Family house pets, 571
Farm cat, 563
FCV (feline calicivirus infection), vaccination recommendations for, 8
Fear, in geriatric cats, 584
in shelter animals, 621
Febrile nonhemolytic reactions, to transfusions, 465
Fecal smears, for chronic diarrhea, 130, 131t, 133
Fel d 1 allergen, 233–234. See also *Cat allergy.*
key points concerning, 236
Feline acne, ectopic, 205

Feline animal shelter(s), 571–575
control and prevention of disease in, 573
employee relations in, 574–575
housing, feeding, and follow-up care in, 572–573
impoundment procedures in, 572
limited-admission (no-kill), 621
open-admission, 621
population control in, 575
quality of life in. See *Quality of life, in long-term confinement.*
restraint of cats in, 571–572
unclaimed cats in, adoption of, 573–574
euthanasia of, 574
veterinarian in, 575
Feline calicivirus (FCV) infection, vaccination recommendations for, 8
Feline excrement, zoonotic disease in human beings associated with, 19t
Feline genome project, as model for human disease, 609–613, 609t
Feline herpesvirus-1 (FHV-1) infection, 51–60
clinical signs of, 52–55
diagnosis of, 56–57
differential diagnosis of, major pathogens in, 55, 55t
minor pathogens in, 55–56
etiology and epidemiology of, 51
pathogenesis of, 51–52, *52–53*
primary, 53, *53*
recrudescent or persistent, 53–54
syndromes associated with, 54–55, *54–55*
treatment of, adjunctive, 58–59
antiviral agents in, 57–58, 286
supportive, 57
vaccination in, 59–60, 59t
recommendations for, 7–8
Feline immunodeficiency virus (FIV) infection, *C. neoformans var gattii* in, *41*
concurrent with lymphoma, 509
Feline infectious anemia (FIA), 12–16. See also *Hemobartonellosis.*
Feline infectious peritonitis (FIP), 429–430
vaccination recommendations for, 9
Feline interstitial cystitis (FIC), course of disease in, 315
treatment of, 315–317
amitriptyline in, 316–317
diet in, 316
glycosaminoglycans in, 317
stress management in, 315–316
Feline leprosy–like disease, 227–229, *228–229*
Feline leukemia virus (FeLV) infection, and coinfection with *Haemobartonella felis,* 14, 15
concurrent with lymphoma, 508–509
vaccination recommendations for, 8–9
Feline lifestyle, categories of, 571
parameters defining, 562–563
Feline population control, 575
Feline socialization, human approach test in, 625t
in assessment of shelter animal, 628–629
Feline viral rhinotracheitis, calicivirus, and panleukopenia (FVRCP) vaccine, 541
Feline welfare, of feral populations, 566
FeLV infection. See *Feline leukemia virus (FeLV) infection.*

Fenbendazole, for *Giardia* infection causing chronic diarrhea, 134
for hookworm and roundworm infections, 25
Feral cat box, 567
Feral cat population(s), 561–569
control of, grass-roots efforts in, 563–564
immunocontraception in, 577–581. See also *Immunocontraception.*
resource and teaching providers in, 564
service providers in, 564
definitions of, 562–563
extent of problem of, 561–562, 562t
in practice setting, 567–569, 567t, *568*
issue(s) involving, 564–566
feline welfare as, 566
impact on wildlife as, 565–566
nuisance complaints as, 566
public health as, 564–565
role of veterinarian in, 566–567
trap, neuter, and return (TNR) programs for, 561, 562t
Feral cats, true, 571
Ferrous sulfate, for iron deficiency, 332
FHV-1 infection. See *Feline herpesvirus-1 (FHV-1) infection.*
FIA (feline infectious anemia), 12–16. See also *Hemobartonellosis.*
Fiber, dietary, in prevention of calcium oxalate urolithiasis, 362, 363t
Fibrocartilaginous embolism, 409
Fibrosarcoma, CT imaging of, *556–557*
injectable products causing, 542. See also *Vaccine-associated feline sarcoma (VAFS).*
Fibrosing pleuritis, associated with chylothorax, *270,* 270–271
FIC. See *Feline interstitial cystitis (FIC).*
Fine-needle aspiration, of liver, 118–126
cholestasis in, 124, *125,* 126
inflammatory disease cytology in, 120–121, *120–121*
lipidosis cytology in, 121, *121–122*
neoplasia cytology in, 121, 123–124, *123–125*
normal hepatic cytology in, 119–120
retrospective study of, 119
technique of, 118–119
of mediastinal mass, 537–538
of spleen, cytology in, 443–444, *443–444*
FIP. See *Feline infectious peritonitis (FIP).*
FIP (feline infectious peritonitis), 429–430
vaccination recommendations for, 9
FIV (feline immunodeficiency virus) infection, *C. neoformans var gattii* in, *41*
concurrent with lymphoma, 509
Flares, in feline interstitial cystitis, 315
Flea-bite hypersensitivity, vs. mosquito-bite hypersensitivity, 187
Fluconazole, for cryptococcosis, 45, 432
for respiratory infections, 284, 286
Flucytosine, for cryptococcosis, 45
Fludrocortisone, for hypoadrenocorticism, 164
Fluid therapy, for lily nephrotoxicity, 309
postoperative, for renal transplant recipient, 323
"Foam cells," in cutaneous xanthomas, 216, *217*
Food, adverse reactions to, 113–114
metabolic, 116

Food *(Continued)*
terminology used in, 114t
anaphylactoid reactions to, 116
pharmacologic reactions to, 116
Food allergens, 114
Food allergy, 114–116, 114t
Food hypersensitivity, 114–116
Food idiosyncrasy, 114t, 116
Food intolerance, 114t, 116–117
Food poisoning, 114t, 116–117
Food sensitivity, 113–114, 114t
Footpad lesions, in mosquito-bite hypersensitivity, 187, *187*
Forceps, grasping, for surgical removal of heartworm, 258, *258*
Forebrain, malformation(s) of, 415–420
agenesis of corpus callosum as, 419
holoprosencephaly as, 419
hydranencephaly/porencephaly as, 417–418
hydrocephalus as, 415–417, *415–418,* 416t
neural tube defects as, 418–419
neuronal migration disorders as, 419–420
Foreign bodies, in esophagus, 101, 101t, *102*
Francisella tularensis, 449
thrombocytopenia associated with, 474
Furazolidone, for *Giardia* infection causing chronic diarrhea, 134
Furosemide, for cerebral edema, 428
for hydrocephalus, 416
FVRCP (feline viral rhinotracheitis, calicivirus, and panleukopenia) vaccine, 541

GAGs. See *Glycosaminoglycans (GAGs).*
Gallbladder, contrast radiographic studies of, 82–83, *84*
Gamma-linolenic acid, for mosquito-bite hypersensitivity, 189
Gangliosidosis, 615–619
carriers of, in molecular test for, 618–619, 618t
GM$_1$, 394–395, *395,* 615–616, 616t
GM$_2$, 395–396, 615–616, 616t
inheritance of, 616–617
mutations in, molecular characterization of, 617
signs of, 616
Gastric emptying, delayed, antiemetics for, 111
Gastric function, naturally acquired infection and, 93
Gastric inflammation, *Helicobacter* infection and, 93–94
Gastrinoma, 183–184
Gastritis, uremic, in chronic renal failure, 333
Gastroesophageal reflux, 73–74
Gastrogram, double-contrast, 76
Gastrointestinal tract. See also specific part, e.g., *Esophagus.*
afferents and efferents of, emesis involving, 109
and adverse reactions to food, 113–117, 114t
complications of, in chronic renal failure, 332–333
contrast radiographic studies of, 73–85
ancillary structures in, 81–85
Gastrostomy tube, nutritional support via, 524

Gene(s), 600–601
pleiotropic effects of, 601
Gene mapping, comparative, 606, *607*
of polycystic kidney disease, *607,* 607–608
of progressive retinal atrophy, 608, *608*
markers in, 605–606
used in disease identification, 606
Gene markers, types I and II, 605–606
Genetic counseling, of breeders, 619, *619*
Genetic diseases, inherited problems in, 604–605
population characteristics of, 601–602
Genetics, comparative, 601, 605–609
disease identification in, 606
markers and maps in, 605–606
use of, 606–608, *607–608*
history of, 600
patterns of inheritance in, 600
environment and, 601
Genital tract zoonoses, feline and canine, 20t
Genome project, feline, as model for human disease, 609–613, 609t
Genomics, use of, for breeders and veterinarians, 608–609
Gentamicin, for mycobacterial panniculitis, 226
for respiratory infections, 285t
Geriatric cat, 583–590
behavior history in, 587–590
case studies of, 586–587
dysfunction in, cognitive, 585
differential diagnosis of, 584–585
drug treatment for, 585–586
signs of, 583–584
environmental modifications for, 586
shelters for, 631–632
GFR (glomerular filtration rate), augmented, in chronic renal failure, 333
Giardia lamblia, 20
Giardiasis, 20–21
diarrhea associated with, treatment of, 134
vaccination recommendations for, 9
GLB$_1$ gene, sequencing of, in Korat cats, 617
Glimepiride, for non–insulin-dependent diabetes mellitus, 171t
Glipizide, for non–insulin-dependent diabetes mellitus, 171, 171t
Globoid cell leukodystrophy (Krabbe's disease), 402–403
Glomerular filtration rate (GFR), augmented, in chronic renal failure, 333
Glucocorticoids, for hemobartonellosis, 16
for insulinoma, 183
for mosquito-bite hypersensitivity, 188
Glucose absorption, intestinal, hypoglycemic agents inhibiting, 170–171, 171t
Glucose output, hepatic, hypoglycemic agents inhibiting, 171–172, 171t
Glycogen storage disease, 401
Glycolytic erythroenzymopathies, 485, 485t
Glycosaminoglycans (GAGs), for feline interstitial cystitis, 317
in mucopolysaccharidosis, pathologic findings of, 452, *454–455*
storage of, 450, 451, 451t
in urine, detection of, 455–456, *455–456*

GM₁ gangliosidosis, 394–395, *395*, 615–616, 616t
GM₂ gangliosidosis, 395–396, 615–616, 616t
Granuloma, cryptococcal, *42*
Grasping forceps, for surgical removal of heartworm, 258, *258*
Grass-roots efforts, in feral cat control, 563–564
Griseofulvin, causing congenital cranial malformations, 414t
    for dermatophytosis, 513

Haemobartonella bodies, on erythrocytes, 14
Haemobartonella canis, transmission of, 12–13
Haemobartonella felis, 12, *12*
    detection of, PCR assay in, 480–481, 481t
    Hfsm and Hflg variants of, 12, 13, 15–16
    infection with. See *Hemobartonellosis.*
Hair loss. See *Alopecia.*
Havana brown cat, genetic diversity study of, 610–611
HDL (high density lipoprotein), 215
Head defect, in Burmese cats, 610
Head development, 414t–415
Heart disease, acquired, diagnostic echocardiography in, *248–250*, 248–251, 249t
    congenital, diagnostic echocardiography in, 251–252
Heart rate and rhythm, variations of, Holter monitoring of, 295–297, *298*
Heartworm(s), surgical removal of, 258, *258*
Heartworm disease, 253–259
    angiography of, 255–256, *256*, 256t
    clinical pathology/serology of, *254*, 254–255, 254t
    diagnosis of, 253–254
    differential diagnosis of, 256–257
    Dirofilaria immitis in, 253, 259
    echocardiographic imaging of, 248, *248–249*, 251
    epidemiology of, 253
    prevention of, 258–259
    radiographic imaging of, 255, *255*
    routine testing for, 259
    treatment of, 257–258
Helicobacter felis, 91
Helicobacter heilmanni, 91
Helicobacter pametensis, 91
Helicobacter pylori, 91
Helicobacteriosis, 21, 91–96
    diagnosis of, invasive tests in, 94
        noninvasive tests in, 94–95
        urea breath and blood tests in, 95
    experimental studies of, 93–94
    naturally-acquired, 93
    of stomach, 91, *92*
    pathogenicity of, 93
    prevalence of, 91–92, 91t
    public health concerns associated with, 93
    transmission of, 92
    treatment of, 95–96
Hematologic complications, of hemodialysis, 347
Hematoma, intracranial, surgical removal of, 408–409
Heme defects, in hereditary erythrocyte disorders, 485, 485t

Hemerocallis species, nephrotoxicity caused by, 308
Hemithorax, right, echocardiographic images from, 247–248, *248*
Hemobartonellosis, 12–16, 33. See also *Haemobartonella* entries.
    clinical, 13–14
    diagnosis of, 15–16
    epidemiology of, 12–13
    etiology of, 12, *12*
    pathogenesis and immunity of, 13
    pathology of, 14–15
    prevention and treatment of, 16
Hemodialysis, 337–350
    and concurrent medical therapy, 343–344, *344*, 345t
    complication(s) of, 344, 346–349, 346t
        anorexia, nausea, and vomiting as, 347
        cardiovascular instability as, 344, 346
        hematologic, 347
        infectious, 348–349
        neurologic, 346
        respiratory, 346–347, *347*
        technical, 347
        thrombosis as, 348, *348–349*
        vascular access as, 347–348, *348*
    efficacy of, 349, *350*
    equipment for, 339–343, 339t, *340–342*
    indications for, 337t
    objective of, 337
    outcome of, 349–350, *350*
    principles of, 338, *338–339*
    regional referral centers for, 350t
Hemodialysis delivery system, 338, *338*
Hemodialysis prescription, 343, 343t, 344t
Hemodialyzers, classification of, 340–341, *341–342*
Hemoglobin, unstable, 485t
Hemolysis, 89
Hemolytic reaction(s), to transfusions, acute, 465
    nonimmunologic, 465–466
Hemoparasites, detection of, use of polymerase chain reactions in, 479–482
Hemorrhage, as complication of anticoagulation therapy, 410
    intracranial, 406–409, *407–408*, 407t
Hemostasis, 468
Heparin, for aortic thromboembolism, 302, 410–411
    for saddle thrombus, 265
    low-molecular-weight, 304–305
Hepatic. See also *Liver.*
Hepatic amyloidosis, 90
Hepatic cholestasis, cytology of, 124, *125*, 126
Hepatic glucose output, hypoglycemic agents inhibiting, 171–172, 171t
Hepatic lipidosis, 89
    cytology of, 121, *121–122*
Hepatic lymphoma, cytology of, 123–124, *124–125*
Hepatic neoplasia, cytology of, 121, 123–124, *123–125*
Hepatic sarcoma, metastatic, cytology of, 124, *125*
Hepatitis, portal lymphocytic, 89
Hepatocellular carcinoma, cytology of, 123, *124*
Hepatocytes, normal, 119
Hereditary cerebellar cortical atrophy, 422
Hereditary erythrocyte disorder(s), 484–489. See also *Erythrocyte(s).*
Hereditary seborrhea oleosa, primary, in Persian cats, 202, *203–204*. See also *Seborrhea.*

Herniation, brain, following excision of meningioma, 390, *390t*
Herpesvirus-1 infection. See *Feline herpesvirus-1 (FHV-1) infection.*
Hetastarch, transfusion of, 466
High density lipoprotein (HDL), 215
High-fiber diet, for chronic diarrhea, 134
Hill's Prescription Diet, for hypercalcemia, 313
Hindbrain, malformation(s) of, Chiari, 420
    Dandy-Walker syndrome as, 420
    hereditary cerebellar cortical atrophy as, 422
    parvoviral-induced cerebellar degeneration as, 420–421, *421*
Hip dysplasia, 592–597, 612
    clinical signs of, 594
    control and prevention of, 597
    diagnosis of, 594–596, *595–596*
    differential diagnosis of, 594
    epidemiology of, 593
    etiology of, 592–593
    pathogenesis of, 593–594
    treatment of, conservative, 596–597
        surgical, 597
H₁-Histaminergic antagonists, classification of, 110t
Histoplasma capsulatum, thrombocytopenia associated with, 474
Histoplasmosis, antifungal therapy for, 286
HIV infection. See *Human immunodeficiency virus (HIV) infection.*
Holoprosencephaly, 419
Holter monitor attachments, 291–294
    supplies used for, 292t
Holter monitoring, 291–297
    attachment of monitor during, self-adhesive elastic wrap in, 293, *294*
    electrodes in, 291
        attachment of, 292–293, *293–294*
    equipment for, 291
    hook-up procedure in, 292, *292*, 292t
    lead wires in, 292, *293*
    of heart rate and rhythm variations, 295–297, *298*
    recording leads in, 292
    report from, 294–295, *295*
    request form and disclosure printout for, 293–294, *295*
Hormones, in immunocontraception, 578
House cat, 563
House soiling, by geriatric cats, 583
Housing, in animal shelters, 573
5-HT₃-serotonergic antagonists, classification of, 110t
5-HT₄-serotonergic antagonists, classification of, 110t
Human familial hyperlipoproteinemia, classification of, 215t
    syndromes resembling, 215
Human immunodeficiency virus (HIV) infection, cryptosporidiosis associated with, 35
Humoral pathway, for emesis, 107–108, *108*
Hydralazine, for high blood pressure, following renal transplantation, 324
Hydranencephaly, 417–418
Hydration status, in chronic renal failure, maintenance of, 333–334
Hydrocephalus, cause of, 415
    clinical signs of, 416, *416*
    pathogenesis of, *415*, 415–416

Hydrocephalus *(Continued)*
   prognosis associated with, 417
   treatment of, 416–417, *417–418*
Hydrochlorothiazide, for hypertension, 370
   in prevention of calcium oxalate uro-lithiasis, 363
Hydroxyurea, causing congenital cranial malformations, 414t
   for chronic myeloid leukemias, 493t
Hydroxyzine, for mosquito-bite hypersensitivity, 188t
Hyperadrenocorticism, 159–161
   abdominal imaging for, 160
   adrenal function tests for, 165
      interpretation of, 165–167
      normal values for, 166t
   alopecia associated with, 198
   clinical findings in, 159, 160t
   clinicopathologic results of, 159–160, 160t
   in insulin-resistant diabetes, 516
   pituitary-dependent, 159
      cobalt irradiation for, 161
   treatment of, 160–161
Hyperaldosteronism (Conn's syndrome), 162–163
Hyperbilirubinemia. See also *Icterus.*
   pathophysiology of, 87–88
Hypercalcemia, clinical signs of, 311–312
   diagnosis of, laboratory findings in, 312
   differential diagnosis of, 312–313
   pathogenesis of, 311
   treatment of, 313
Hypercalciuria, 354–355
Hyperchylomicronemia, familial, 1–2
Hypercortisolism. See *Hyperadrenocorticism.*
Hyperlipidemia, primary, pathogenesis of, 214–215
   secondary, pathogenesis of, 216
Hyperlipoproteinemia, human familial, classification of, 215t
   syndromes resembling, 215
Hyperoxaluria, 355
Hyperphosphatemia, in chronic renal failure, aluminum hydroxide for, 345t
Hyperprogesteronism, 161–162
Hypersensitivity, flea-bite, vs. mosquito-bite hypersensitivity, 187
   mosquito-bite, 186–189
      clinical signs of, 186–187, *186–187*
      differential diagnosis of, 187–188
      pathogenesis of, 186
      prevention of, 189
      treatment of, 188–189, 188t
      vs. flea-bite hypersensitivity, 187
Hypertension, 277–282, 365–370
   arteriolar response to, 278
   causing intracranial hemorrhage, 408
   clinical signs of, 278, 365–366
   control of, 281
   diagnosis of, 279–280, 366–368, 366t, *368*
   differential diagnosis of, 279, 279t
   epidemiology of, 365, 365t
   etiology of, 277–278
   in chronic renal failure, management of, 334
      therapeutic agents for, 345t
   management of, 280–281, 368–370
      antihypertensive therapy in, *369,* 369–370
   pathogenesis of, 277–278, 365
   pathologic findings associated with, 281–282

Hypertension *(Continued)*
   prevention of, 281
   secondary to hyperthyroidism, 278
   secondary to renal failure, 277
Hyperthyroidism, 145–149
   alopecia associated with, 198
   basal free thyroid hormone determinations in, 147, *147*
   concurrent with lymphoma, 514–515
   echocardiographic features of, 251t
   hypertension secondary to, 278
   preexisting renal disease with, 151
   resting serum thyroid hormone concentrations in, 145–147, *146*
   thyroid hormone suppression test for, 147–148, *148*
   treatment of, 151–157
      beta-adrenergic blocking agents in, 154
      iodinated contrast agents in, 153
      monitoring following, 151–152
      permanent options in, 154–157
      radioiodine therapy in, 154–155
      reversible options in, 152–153
      stable iodine preparations in, 154
      surgical, 155–157
      thioureylene drugs in, 152–153
      ultrasound-guided percutaneous ethanol injection in, 157
   TRH stimulation test for, 148–149, *149*
Hypertrophic cardiomyopathy. See *Cardiomyopathy(ies), hypertrophic.*
Hypervolemia, clinical manifestations of, 344t
Hypoadrenocorticism (Addison's disease), 163–165
   clinicopathologic findings in, 163–164, 164t
   treatment of, 164–165
Hypocalcemia, postsurgical, treatment of, 156
Hypoglycemia, insulin overdose causing, 177–178
Hypoglycemic therapy, for non–insulin-dependent diabetes mellitus, *170,* 170–172, 171t
   agents improving peripheral insulin sensitivity in, 171t, 172
   agents inhibiting hepatic glucose output in, 171–172, 171t
   agents inhibiting intestinal glucose absorption in, 170–171, 171t
   agents promoting pancreatic release of insulin in, 171, 171t
   insulin with, 172
Hypokalemia, in chronic renal failure, potassium gluconate for, 345t
Hypothyroidism, alopecia associated with, 198

IBD. See *Inflammatory bowel disease (IBD).*
I-cell disease (mucolipidosis II), 398
   vs. mucopolysaccharidosis, 453–454
Icterus, detection of, 87
   diagnostic tests for, 88–89
   differential diagnosis of, 89–90
   hemolytic causes of, 89
   hepatic causes of, 89–90
   physical examination and laboratory testing for, 88
   posthepatic, 90
   prehepatic causes of, 89
Icterus index, 88

Idarubicin, dosage of, 523
IDDM. See *Insulin-dependent diabetes mellitus (IDDM).*
IER (illness energy requirement), calculation of, 320
IFA (immunofluorescent assay), for cryptosporidiosis, 36
   for FHV-1 infection, 56
IGFs (insulin-like growth factors), role of, in pathogenesis of diabetic neuropathy, 139
IgG (immunoglobulin G), in hemobartonellosis, 13
Illness, chronic, quality of life issues associated with, 631
Illness energy requirement (IER), calculation of, 320
Imaging modality(ies), diagnostic, 548–558. See also specific type, e.g., *Computed tomography (CT).*
   strengths and weaknesses of, 548t
Imidazoles, for respiratory infections, 284
Imidocarb dipropionate, for cytauxzoonosis, 437
Immiticide, for heartworm disease, 257
Immune disorder(s), alopecia associated with, 198
   thrombocytopenia associated with, 475
Immune response, humoral and cell-mediated, against *H. felis,* 13
   in immunocontraception, 577–578
   to *Salmonella*/ZP, 580, *580*
Immunization. See *Vaccine (vaccination).*
Immunocompetent host, localized mycobacterial disease in, *230,* 230–231
Immunocontraception, to control feral cat population, 577–581
   delivery of antigens in, 579
   future developments in, 581
   hormones in, 578
   immune responses in, 577–578
   oocyte antigens in, 578–579
   Salmonella strain and zona pellucida type in, *578–579, 579*–581
   sperm antigens in, 578
Immunofluorescent assay (IFA), for cryptosporidiosis, 36
   for FHV-1 infection, 56
Immunoglobulin G (IgG), in hemobartonellosis, 13
Immunosuppressed people, zoonotic transfer of infection in, 18, 19t, 20–25, 20t. See also specific infection, e.g., *Toxoplasmosis.*
Immunosuppression therapy, for acquired myasthenia gravis, 377
Immunotherapy, for cat allergies, 235
   for vaccine-associated feline sarcomas, 546
Inbreeding, in population dynamics, 604
INF (interferon), for FHV-1 infection, 58
Infarction, neural, pathophysiology of, 405
Infectious disease(s). See also *Feline infectious* entries; specific infection, e.g., *Ehrlichiosis.*
   alopecia associated with, 197–198
   as complication of hemodialysis, 348–349
   causing thrombocytopenia, 474
   concurrent with lymphoma, 508–513
   control and prevention of, in animal shelters, 573
   involving central nervous system, 425–433. See also specific infection, e.g., *Cryptococcosis.*

Infectious disease(s) (Continued)
    clinical signs of, 426
    diagnosis of, 426–428
    differential diagnosis of, 426, 427t
    etiology and epidemiology of, 425
    pathogenesis of, 425–426
    pathology of, 429
    treatment of, 428–429
Inflammation, definition of, 425
    gastric, Helicobacter infection and,
        93–94
    in development of vaccine-associated fe-
        line sarcomas, 542
Inflammatory bowel disease (IBD),
        499–504
    clinical signs of, 499–500
    diagnosis of, 500–501
    etiopathogenesis of, 499
    histopathology of, 502, 502–503
    treatment of, 503–504
    vs. alimentary lymphosarcoma, 503
Inflammatory liver disease, cytology of,
        definition of, 120–121, 120–121
Inherited disease(s), 615. See also specific
        disease, e.g., Gangliosidosis.
    elimination of, in pure breeds, 615–620
    human, with feline models, 609t
Insulin absorption, poor, 176
Insulin antibodies, 177
Insulin formulations, 175–176
Insulin overdose, causing hypoglycemia,
        177–178
Insulin release, pancreatic, hypoglycemic
        agents promoting, 171, 171t
Insulin resistance, 177
    diagnosis and treatment of, 177t
    in diabetic cat with lymphoma, 516
Insulin sensitivity, peripheral,
        hypoglycemic agents improving, 171t,
        172
Insulin storage, 175
Insulin therapy, 175–178, 176t
    combining oral hypoglycemic therapy
        with, 172
Insulin-dependent diabetes mellitus
        (IDDM), 169. See also Diabetes
        mellitus.
    insulin therapy for, 175–178
    complications of, 178
    monitoring of, 176–178, 176t
    owner/client factors in, 175
    pharmacokinetic factors in, 175–176
Insulin:glucose ratio, amended, 183
Insulin-like growth factors (IGFs), role of,
        in pathogenesis of diabetic
        neuropathy, 139
Insulinoma, 182–183
Interferon (INF), for FHV-1 infection, 58
Intestinal glucose absorption,
        hypoglycemic agents inhibiting,
        170–171, 171t
Intracranial hemorrhage, 406–409
    diagnosis of, 407–408, 407–408, 407t
    of epidural or subdural origin, 406
    treatment of, 408–409
Intranasal tumor(s), clinical signs of, 529,
        530t
    diagnosis of, 529–530, 530
    epithelial, CT imaging of, 557
    etiology and epidemiology of, 529
    pathophysiology of, 529, 529
    prognosis associated with, 531
    treatment of, 530–531, 531
Iodinated contrast agents, for
        hyperthyroidism, 153
Iodine preparations, stable, for
        hyperthyroidism, 154

Iohexol, used in upper gastrointestinal
        series, of small intestines, 79
    of stomach, 75
Ipodate, for hyperthyroidism, 153
Iron dextran, for iron deficiency, 332
Ischemia, neural, pathophysiology of, 405
    peripheral nerve, 409–411
Ischemic encephalopathy, 405–406, 406
Isotretinoin, for pre–squamous cell
        carcinoma, 193
    for primary hereditary seborrhea oleosa,
        206
Itraconazole, for cryptococcosis, 45, 432
    for dermatophytosis, 513
    for respiratory infections, 284, 286
Ivermectin, for Cuterebra larval myiasis,
        431
    for ischemic encephalopathy, 406
    prophylactic, for heartworm disease,
        258–259

Jaundice, 87. See also Icterus.
Joint disease, degenerative, 592–597. See
        also Hip dysplasia.
Joint laxity, 593, 594, 595–596

Keratitis, eosinophilic, associated with
        FHV-1 infection, 54–55, 55
Keratosis, actinic, 193
    vs. Bowen's disease, 210
Ketamine, for sedation during blood
        collection, 463
Ketoacidosis, diabetic, 178
Ketoconazole, for cryptococcosis, 45
    for Cushing's syndrome, 160
    for respiratory infections, 284
Key-Gaskell syndrome. See
        Dysautonomia.
Kidney(s). See also Renal entries.
    donor, 321
        acute rejection of, 325–326
    polycystic. See Polycystic kidney dis-
        ease (PKD).
Korat cats, carriers of gangliosidosis in,
        molecular testing for, 618–619,
        618t
    future of, 619–620
    GLB₁ gene in, sequencing of, 617
Krabbe's disease (globoid cell
        leukodystrophy), 402–403
Kupffer cells, 455

Laparotomy, exploratory, for chronic
        diarrhea, 132t, 133
    for splenomegaly, 444
Large-intestinal diarrhea, vs. small-
        intestinal diarrhea, 128t
Laser surgery, for Bowen's disease, 211,
        212
    for squamous cell carcinoma, 194
LDL (low density lipoprotein), 214
Leprosy-like disease, 227–229
    clinical features of, 228, 228
    diagnosis of, 228, 229
    treatment of, 228–229
Leukemia(s), 490–494. See also Feline
        leukemia virus (FeLV) infection.
    acute, 491–492, 491–492
    chronic, 492–493
    clinical signs of, 490

Leukemia(s) (Continued)
    cytochemical staining characteristics of,
        491t
    diagnosis of, 490–491
    mast cell, 493–494, 494
    myeloid, classification of, 490t
    treatment of, 493t
Levamisole, for heartworm disease, 258
Lifestyle, feline, categories of, 571
    parameters defining, 562–563
Lilium species, nephrotoxicity caused by,
        308
Lipid(s), dietary, in renal disease, 335
Lipidosis, hepatic, 89
    cytology of, 121, 121–122
Lipofuscinosis, neuronal ceroid, 401–402
Lipoprotein(s), capillary leakage of. See
        Xanthoma(s).
    high density, 215
    low density, 214
    metabolism of, 214
    very low density, 215
Lipoprotein lipase, 214, 215
Liposome-encapsulated chemotherapy
        agents, 523. See also Chemotherapy.
Lisinopril, for hypertension, 281
Lissencephaly, 419–420
Liver. See also Hepatic; Hepato- entries.
    contrast radiographic studies of, 81–82
        portography in, 82, 84
    fine-needle aspiration biopsy of, 118–
        126
        cholestasis in, 124, 125, 126
        inflammatory disease cytology in,
            120–121, 120–121
        lipidosis cytology in, 121, 121–122
        neoplasia cytology in, 121, 123–124,
            123–125
        normal hepatic cytology in, 119–120
        retrospective study of, 119
        technique in, 118–119
LMWH (low-molecular-weight heparin),
        304–305
Location descriptions, of cats, 563
Loratadine, for mosquito-bite
        hypersensitivity, 188t
Low density lipoprotein (LDL), 214
Low-fat diet, for chylothorax, 272t
Low-molecular-weight heparin (LMWH),
        304–305
Low-protein diet, for chronic renal
        failure, 335
Lufenuron injections, causing
        fibrosarcomas, 542. See also Vaccine-
        associated feline sarcoma (VAFS).
Lung cancer, metastatic, radiographic
        imaging of, 549–551
Lymph node(s), enlargement of. See
        Lymphadenopathy.
    function of, 445
    involvement of, in disseminated nontu-
        berculous mycobacterial disease,
        229–230, 230
    peripheral, hyperplasia of, 447–448
    plague and tularemia affecting, 449
    plexiform vascularization of, 448–449
Lymphadenomegaly, mandibular,
        cryptococcal, 42
Lymphadenopathy, 445–449
    clinical approach to, 445, 446
    diagnostic approach to, 447
    diseases causing, 447–449, 448t
    physical examination in, 445, 447
    resembling lymphoma, 448
Lymphangiography, mesenteric, thoracic
        duct ligation with, in management of
        chylothorax, 272–273, 273

Lymphoma, diagnostic imaging of, *552–555*
  disease concurrent with, 506–517
    chronic renal failure as, 513–514
    clinical presentation of, 506
    dermatophytosis as, 512–513
    diabetes mellitus as, 515–516
    diagnostic tests for, 506–507
    hyperthyroidism as, 514–515
    management of, complications during, 507–508
    retroviral infection as, 508–509
    salmonellosis as, 511–512
    second cancer as, 516–517
    staging of, 506–507, 507t
    upper respiratory tract infection as, 509–511
  hepatic, cytology of, 123–124, *124–125*
  lymphadenopathy resembling, 448
  mediastinal, 534
    cytologic evaluation of, 537
    treatment of, 539
  nasal, treatment and prognosis of, 531
  T-cell, alopecia associated with, 199
Lymphosarcoma, 611
  alimentary, 499–504
    clinical signs of, 499–500
    diagnosis of, 500–501
    etiopathogenesis of, 499
    histopathology of, *502*, 502–503
    treatment of, 503, 504t
    vs. inflammatory bowel disease, 503
  sporadic and inherited forms of, 601–602
Lysine, oral, for FHV-1 infection, 287

Magnesium, dietary, in prevention of calcium oxalate urolithiasis, 361, 363t
Magnetic resonance imaging (MRI), diagnostic, in cancer patients, 555–557, *556*
  of *Cuterebra* larva migration, *406*
  of intracranial hemorrhage, 407, *408*
    at medium field strength, 407t
  of mediastinal tumor, 537
  of meningioma, 388, *389*
  of oral rhabdomyosarcoma, 526, *527*
  strengths and weaknesses of, 548t
Malassezia, dermatitis associated with, 204
Mandibular lymphadenomegaly, cryptococcal, *42*
Mannitol, for cerebral edema, 428
  for intracranial hemorrhage, 408
Manual restraint, of sheltered animals, 571–572
Marbofloxacin, for respiratory infections, 283
Mast cell leukemia, 493–494, *494*
Mediastinal cyst(s), 534
Mediastinal tumor(s), 533–539
  clinical signs of, 533, *534*
  diagnosis of, advanced imaging in, 537, *537*
    cytology in, 537–538
    histopathology in, 538
    radiography in, 535, *536, 552*
    thyroid scintigraphy in, 538
    ultrasonography in, 535, 537, *552*
  differential diagnosis of, 533–535
  treatment of, 538–539
Medical therapy, concurrent with hemodialysis, 343–344, *344*, 345t
Megaesophagus, 103, 105

Megaesophagus *(Continued)*
  congenital, radiographic imaging of, *100*
Megakaryocytic/megakaryoblastic leukemia, 492
Megaplatelets, 470
Megestrol acetate, as appetite stimulant, 524
Melanin, 190
Melanoma, 193
Membrane defects, in hereditary erythrocyte disorders, 485, 485t
MEN (multiple endocrine neoplasia), 184
Meningioma, 385–391
  clinical findings in, 386–387, 387t
  diagnosis of, 387–389
    cerebrospinal fluid analysis in, 388
    CT and MR imaging in, 388, *389, 556*
    CT-guided brain biopsy in, 389
    skull radiographs in, 387–388
  etiology of, 386
  incidence of, 385
  location of, 385
  pathologic findings in, 386
  recurrence of, 390–391
  treatment of, goals in, 389
    radiation therapy in, 391
    surgical, 389–390
    survival data following, 390t
Meningitis, cryptococcal, *41*
Meningocele, 418–419
Meningoencephalomyelitis, nonsuppurative, 430
Meowing behavior problems, in geriatric cats, 583–584
Mesenchymal tumor(s), of oral cavity, 528
Metabolic acidosis, in chronic renal failure, sodium bicarbonate for, 345t
  treatment of, 331
Metabolic diseases, in geriatric cats, 585
Metabolism, lipoprotein, 214
Metformin, for non–insulin-dependent diabetes mellitus, 171–172, 171t
Methemoglobin reductase deficiency, 485t, 487–488
Methemoglobinemia, 485t
Methicillin, for respiratory infections, 285t
Methimazole, for hyperthyroidism, 152–153, 515
  side effects of, 153
Methotrexate, for lymphosarcoma, 504t
N-Methyl D-aspartate receptors, role of, in pathogenesis of diabetic neuropathy, 140
Methylmercury, causing congenital cranial malformations, 414t
Methylprednisolone, for hypoadrenocorticism, 164
  for toxoplasmosis, 22
Metoclopramide, for dysautonomia, 383
  for esophagitis, 106
Metronidazole, for *Giardia* infection causing chronic diarrhea, 134
  for *Helicobacter* infection, 95
  for inflammatory bowel disease, 503
  for respiratory infections, 285t
Metyrapone, for Cushing's syndrome, 161
Microsatellites, in DNA sequencing, 606
Microscopy, of *Haemobartonella felis* organisms, 15
Microsporum canis infection, vaccination recommendations for, 9
Microsporum gypseum, 512. See also *Dermatophytosis.*
MICs (minimum inhibitory concentrations), for antibiotics, 225–226

Migration, reduced, in breed population dynamics, 603–604
Milbemycin oxime, prophylactic, for heartworm disease, 259
Minimum inhibitory concentrations (MICs), for antibiotics, 225–226
Mitotane, for hyperadrenocorticism, 160
Mitoxantrone, dosage of, 522
  for acute myeloid leukemias, 493t
Mitral valve insufficiency, echocardiographic imaging of, 249–250
M-mode echocardiography, 245–247, *246, 246t*
Molecular testing, for carriers of gangliosidosis, in Korat cats, 618–619, 618t
  future of, 619–620
Mosquito bites, hypersensitivity to. See *Hypersensitivity, mosquito-bite.*
Motility disorders, diarrhea associated with, 128
  esophageal, evaluation of, 73–74
Motion sickness, antiemetics for, 110
MRI. See *Magnetic resonance imaging (MRI).*
Mucolipidosis II (I-cell disease), 398
  vs. mucopolysaccharidosis, 453–454
Mucopolysaccharidosis, 398–400, 450–456
  feline, 451
    classification of, 451t
    clinical and laboratory features of, 451t
    diagnosis of, 455–456, *455–456*
    differential diagnosis of, 453–455
    I (alpha-L-iduronidase deficiency), 452–453
    prevention of, 456
    treatment of, 456
    VI (arylsulfatase B deficiency), 451, *452–453*
      pathologic findings in, 452, *454–455*
      radiographic findings in, 451–452, *454*
    VII (beta-glucuronidase deficiency), 453, *455*
    vs. mucolipidosis II, 453–454
  in children, 450, *450*
Multicentric squamous cell carcinoma in situ. See *Bowen's disease.*
Multiple endocrine neoplasia (MEN), 184
Munchkin breed, dwarfism in, 612
Muscle biopsy, in diabetic neuropathy, 142–143
Myasthenia gravis, acquired, clinical signs of, 375–376, *376*, 376t
  diagnosis of, 376–377
  pathophysiology of, 374–375
  prognosis associated with, 378
  treatment of, 377–378
Mycobacterial disease(s), nontuberculous, 221–231
  agents causing, 221–222
  diagnosis of, molecular method of, 222–223
  disseminated, with lymph node or organ involvement, 229–230, *230*
  feline leprosy–like disease as, 227–229, *228–229*
  inflammatory response in, 222
  localized, in immunocompetent host, *230*, 230–231
  panniculitis as, 223–227. See also *Panniculitis, mycobacterial.*

Mycobacterial disease(s) *(Continued)*
  public health significance of, 231
Mycobacterium fortuitum, 223. See also
    Panniculitis, mycobacterial.
  identification of, 225
Mycobacterium lepraemurium, 227. See
    also *Leprosy-like disease.*
Mycobacterium smegmatis, 223. See also
    Panniculitis, mycobacterial.
  identification of, 225
Mycotic diarrhea, 129t
Myelodysplasia, 490
Myelodysplastic syndrome, 493
Myeloproliferative disorders. See also
    Leukemia(s).
  classification of, 490, 490t
  clinical signs of, 490
  diagnosis of, 490–491
  treatment of, 493t
Myelosis, erythremic, 491
Myelosuppression, secondary to
    chemotherapy drugs, 517
Myiasis, *Cuterebra* larval, 430–431
Myocardial disease, echocardiographic
    imaging of, 248–249, *248–250,* 249t

NA (Norberg angle), in measurement of
    hip-joint laxity, 593, 595
Nasal discharge, chronic, differential
    diagnosis of, 530t
Nasal oxygen therapy, for chronic rhinitis,
    289
Nasal tumor(s). See *Intranasal tumor(s).*
Nausea. See also *Emesis.*
  intradialytic, 347
Necrolytic migratory erythema (NME),
    199
Needle thoracentesis, to relieve dyspnea,
    269–270
Neighborhood cat, 563
Nephroliths, 359
Nephrotoxicity, lily, clinical signs of, 308,
    308t
    etiology and epidemiology of, 308
    pathology of, 308–309
    treatment of, 309
Neural crest cells, in embryogenesis, 415
Neural infarction, pathophysiology of, 405
Neural ischemia, pathophysiology of, 405
Neural pathway, for emesis, 107–108, *108*
Neural tube, defects of, 418–419
  embryogenesis of, 414
Neurologic complications, associated with
    hypertension, 278
  in renal transplant recipient, 324
  of hemodialysis, 346
Neuromuscular junction, anatomy and
    physiology of, 374, *375*
  disorders of, 374–379. See also specific
    disorder, e.g., *Myasthenia gravis.*
Neuronal ceroid lipofuscinosis, 401–402
Neuronal migration, disorders of, 419–420
Neuronal storage disorder(s), 393–403
  alpha-mannosidosis as, 400–401
  diagnosis of, 393
  gangliosidosis as, 394–396, *395.* See
    also *Gangliosidosis.*
  globoid cell leukodystrophy (Krabbe's
    disease) as, 402–403
  glycogen storage disease as, 401
  mucolipidosis II (I-cell disease) as, 398
  mucopolysaccharidosis as, 398–400
  neuronal ceroid lipofuscinosis as, 401–
    402

Neuronal storage disorder(s) *(Continued)*
  sphingomyelinosis (Niemann-Pick dis-
    ease) as, 396–398, *397*
Neuropathy, diabetic. See *Diabetic
    neuropathy.*
Neurotransmitter-receptor systems,
    associated with vomiting, 108–109
Neutering services, provided by
    veterinary hospitals, 564
Neutraceuticals, for hip dysplasia, 597
Nicergoline, for cognitive dysfunction, in
    geriatric cats, 586
NIDDM. See *Non–insulin-dependent
    diabetes mellitus (NIDDM).*
Niemann-Pick disease
    (sphingomyelinosis), 396–398, *397*
NME (necrolytic migratory erythema), 199
N-methyl D-aspartate receptors, role of, in
    pathogenesis of diabetic neuropathy,
    140
Nodule(s), inflammatory, after
    vaccination, 542. See also *Vaccine-
    associated feline sarcoma (VAFS).*
Non–insulin-dependent diabetes mellitus
    (NIDDM), 169. See also *Diabetes
    mellitus.*
  diet and exercise therapy for, 169–170
  oral hypoglycemic therapy for, *170,*
    170–172, 171t
    agents improving peripheral insulin
      sensitivity in, 171t, 172
    agents inhibiting hepatic glucose out-
      put in, 171–172, 171t
    agents inhibiting intestinal glucose ab-
      sorption in, 170–171, 171t
    agents promoting pancreatic release
      of insulin in, 171, 171t
    insulin with, 172
Nonketotic hyperosmolar coma, 178
Nonsteroidal anti-inflammatory drugs
    (NSAIDs), for hip dysplasia, 592, 596
Norberg angle (NA), in measurement of
    hip-joint laxity, 593, 595
NSAIDs (nonsteroidal anti-inflammatory
    drugs), for hip dysplasia, 592, 596
Nuclear medicine imaging. See
    Scintigraphy.
Nucleotides, 600
Nuisance complaints, regarding feral cat
    populations, 566
Nutrition program, in animal shelters,
    572–573
Nutritional disorders, in geriatric cats,
    585
Nutritional support, concurrent with
    hemodialysis, 344, *344,* 345t
  for acquired myasthenia gravis, 378
  for chemotherapy patients, 523–524
  thrombocytopenia associated with, 473

Obstruction. See at anatomic site, e.g.,
    Esophagus, obstruction of.
Ocular secretions, feline, zoonotic disease
    in human beings associated with, 20t
Odontogenic tumor(s), 528
Omeprazole, for esophagitis, 106
Oocyte antigens, in
    immunocontraception, 578–579
Ophthalmic conditions, associated with
    hypertension, 278
Optic neuritis, cryptococcal, *41*
Oral tumor(s), 526–528
  clinical presentation of, 526
  diagnosis and staging of, 526–527, *527*

Oral tumor(s) *(Continued)*
  treatment of, 527–528
Organ system(s), dysfunction of,
    thrombocytopenia associated with,
    476
Organophosphate toxicity, 379
Osmotic diarrhea, 127
Osmotic fragility, increased, in hereditary
    erythrocyte disorders, 485t, *486,* 488
Osteodystrophy, renal, calcitriol for, 345t
Overattachment, in geriatric cats, 584
Overresponsiveness, in geriatric cats, 584
Ownership, of cats, 563
Oxalic acid, 355
Oxidative stress, role of, in pathogenesis
    of diabetic neuropathy, 140
Oxygen therapy, nasal, for chronic
    rhinitis, 289
Oxyglobin, transfusion of, 466–467
Oxymorphone, premedication with, for
    renal transplantation, 322
Oxytetracycline, for hemobartonellosis, 16

p53 gene, role of, in vaccine-associated
    feline sarcomas, 4, 542
Pachygyria, 419
Pain/pain control, recognition of, in
    evaluating shelter animals, 629
Palate, cleft, 419
Pancreas, cancer of, paraneoplastic
    alopecia associated with, 196, 201
  contrast radiographic studies of, 83, 85,
    85
Pancreatic release, of insulin,
    hypoglycemic agents promoting, 171,
    171t
Panleukopenia, vaccination
    recommendations for, 7
Panniculitis, mycobacterial, 223–227
  agents causing, 223
  clinical features of, 223–224, *224*
  diagnosis of, antimicrobial suscepti-
      bility testing in, 225–226
    bacteriology in, 225
    cytology in, 224–225, *225*
    strain identification in, 225
  treatment of, 226–227
Papules, in mosquito-bite
    hypersensitivity, 187, *187*
Paralysis, tick, 378
Paraneoplastic disorder(s). See also
    Alopecia, paraneoplastic.
  definition of, 196
Parasitic diarrhea, 129t
Parasitic disorders, alopecia associated
    with, 198
Paromomycin, for cryptosporidiosis, 36
Paroxetine, for aggression in geriatric cats,
    584
Parvoviral-induced cerebellar
    degeneration, 420–421, *421*
Patent ductus arteriosus,
    echocardiographic imaging of, 252
PCR assay. See *Polymerase chain reaction
    (PCR) assay.*
People, familiar and unfamiliar, shelter
    animal's response to, 628
Pericardial disease, echocardiographic
    imaging of, 251
Pericardiectomy, in management of
    chylothorax, 273
Periodontal tumor(s), 528
Peripheral nerve biopsy, in diabetic
    neuropathy, 142

Peripheral nerve ischemia, 409–411
Peritoneal dialysis, 337. See also
    Hemodialysis.
  for lily nephrotoxicity, 309
Peritonitis, infectious, vaccination
    recommendations for, 9
Peritumoral edema, associated with
    meningioma, 386–387
Persian cats, idiopathic facial dermatitis
    in, 205
  primary hereditary seborrhea oleosa in,
    202, *203–204.* See also *Seborrhea.*
  retinal atrophy in, 611–612
Phenobarbital, for ischemic
    encephalopathy, 406
  for post-hemorrhage seizures, 408
Phenocopy, 601
Phenotypes, 600
  desirable vs. undesirable, 601
Phenoxybenzamine, for hypertension, 281
Pheochromocytoma, 181–182
Phosphorus, dietary, in prevention of
    calcium oxalate urolithiasis, 361, 363t
Photoallergy, 190
Photodermatitis, clinical signs of, 191,
    191–192
  diagnosis of, 191–192
  pathogenesis of, 190–191
  prognosis associated with, 192–193
  treatment of, 193–195, *194–195*
Photodynamic therapy, for Bowen's
    disease, 211–212
  for squamous cell carcinoma, 195
Photosensitivity, 190
Phototoxicity, 190
PHSO (primary hereditary seborrhea
    oleosa), in Persian cats, 202, *203–204.*
    See also *Seborrhea.*
Physical health, of shelter animals, 629
Pilocarpine, for dysautonomia, 383
Pinnectomy, for squamous cell carcinoma,
    194, *194*
PKD (polycystic kidney disease), 611
  comparative gene mapping of, *607,*
    607–608
  sporadic and inherited forms of, 601
Plague, 449
  in feral cat populations, 565
Plantigrade stance, secondary to diabetic
    neuropathy, 178
Platelet(s), in thrombocytopenic disorders,
    decreased production of, 471
  destruction of, 472
    excessive utilization/consumption of,
    472–473
  sequestration of, 472
Platelet count, in thrombocytopenic
    disorders, 469–470
Pleural effusion, associated with
    thymoma, 535
  in dialysis patient, 346, *347*
Pleuritis, fibrosing, associated with
    chylothorax, *270,* 270–271
Pleurodesis, induced, in management of
    chylothorax, 274–275
Pleuroperitoneal shunting, in
    management of chylothorax, 273–274,
    274
Pneumogastrogram, modified, 74–75, *76*
Pneumonitis, uremic, in dialysis patient,
    347
Poikilocytosis, 485, 485t, *486*
Poisoning, food, 114t, 116–117
Polycystic kidney disease (PKD), 611
  comparative gene mapping of, *607,*
    607–608

Polycystic kidney disease (PKD)
    (Continued)
  sporadic and inherited forms of, 601
Polycythemia rubra vera, 492–493
Polymerase chain reaction (PCR) assay,
    advantages of, 479
  and amplification of DNA sequence,
    479, *480*
  for CNS inflammatory disease, 428
  for feline infectious peritonitis, 430
  for FHV-1 infection, 56–57
  in detection of *Bartonella henselae,*
    481–482
  in detection of *Cytauxzoon felis,* 482
  in detection of *Ehrlichia* species, 482
  in detection of *Haemobartonella felis,*
    15–16, 480–481, 481t
  in detection of *Trypanosoma* species,
    482
  limitations of, 479
Population bottlenecks, in breed
    dynamics, 604
Porencephaly, 417–418
Porphyria, 485t, 487
Portal hepatitis, lymphocytic, 89
Portography, 82, *84*
Potassium, total-body, maintenance of, in
    chronic renal failure, 330
Pralidoxime chloride, for
    organophosphate and carbamate
    toxicity, 379
Prausnitz-Küstner test, for mosquito-bite
    hypersensitivity, 186
Prazolin, for hypertension, 370
Prednisolone, for bronchial inflammatory
    disease, 286
  for heartworm disease, 257
  for hemobartonellosis, 16
  for hydrocephalus, 416
  for hypoadrenocorticism, 164
  for inflammatory bowel disease, 503
  for insulinoma, 183
  for lymphosarcoma, 503, 504t
  for mosquito-bite hypersensitivity, 188
  for renal transplant recipient, 324
  for toxoplasmosis, 22
  prior to renal transplantation, 321
Prednisone, for hypercalcemia, 313
  for hypoadrenocorticism, 164, 165
Pre–squamous cell carcinoma lesions,
    treatment of, 193
Primary hereditary seborrhea oleosa
    (PHSO), in Persian cats, 202,
    203–204. See also *Seborrhea.*
Prion-protein (PrP), in spongiform
    encephalopathy, 64
Prochlorperazine, for dysautonomia, 383
Promethazine, for mosquito-bite
    hypersensitivity, 188t
Propentofylline, for cognitive dysfunction,
    in geriatric cats, 586
Propranolol, for hypertension, 281
  for hyperthyroidism, 153
  for hypertrophic cardiomyopathy, 265
  for renal transplant recipient, 324
Protein(s), dietary, in prevention of
    calcium oxalate urolithiasis, 361, 363t
Protein formulations, commercial feline
    modified, 345t
Prothrombin time (PT), measurement of,
    in anticoagulation for aortic
    thromboembolism, 410
Protozoal diarrhea, 129t
PrP (prion-protein), in spongiform
    encephalopathy, 64
Psychogenic alopecia, 199

PT (prothrombin time), measurement of,
    in anticoagulation for aortic
    thromboembolism, 410
Public health issues, of feral cat
    populations, 564–565
Pulmonary edema, in dialysis patient,
    346, *347*
Purkinje cells, in Niemann-Pick disease,
    396, *397*
Purpura, definition of, 469
Pyridostigmine bromide, for acquired
    myasthenia gravis, 377
Pyruvate kinase deficiency, 485t, 488–489

Quality of life, assessment issues in,
    623–624, 626
  in long-term confinement, 621–633. See
    also *Feline animal shelter(s).*
  animal disabilities and chronic ill-
    nesses and, 631
  assessment of, animal behavior as
    tool in, 630
  concerns relevant to, 621–622
  environmental enrichment and, 630–
    631
  euthanasia and, 632
  evaluation of, 626–630
    degree of stimulation in, 627–628
    enclosure size, space, and territory
    in, 628
    necessity of exercise in, 628
    pain and pain control in, 629
    physical health in, 629
    sanitation in, 629–630
    socialization in, 628–629
  of geriatric cats, 631–632
  promotion of, current oversight in,
    622–623, 624t–625t, 626t
  WHO definition of, 624

RAAS (renin-angiotensin-aldosterone
    system), in hypertension, 277
Rabies, in feral cat populations, 564–565
  vaccination recommendations for, 9
Radiation, solar, skin changes due to, 190.
    See also *Photodermatitis.*
Radiation therapy, for intranasal tumors,
    531
  for mediastinal lymphoma, 539
  for meningioma, 391
  for pituitary-dependent hyperadrenocor-
    ticism, 161
  for vaccine-associated feline sarcomas,
    6, 544, 545
Radiography, 548–552
  abdominal, for cancer patients, 549–
    550, 552, *552–554*
    for patient with chronic diarrhea,
    132t, 133
    for splenectomy, *442,* 443
    of lymphosarcoma, 500
  contrast, of gastrointestinal tract, 73–85
  indications for, 548
  of calcium oxalate uroliths, *356–357,*
    357–359
  of chylothorax, 269–270, *269–270*
  of esophageal disease, 99–100, *100*
  of heartworm disease, 255, *255*
  of hip dysplasia, 594–595, *595–596*
  of hypertrophic cardiomyopathy, 262,
    263
  of mediastinal tumors, 535, *536*

Radiography *(Continued)*
of mucopolysaccharidosis VI, 451–452, *454*
of vaccine-associated feline sarcomas, 543, *544*
skull, of meningioma, 387–388
strengths and weaknesses of, 548t
thoracic, for cancer patients, 548–549, *549–552*
Radioiodine therapy, for hyperthyroidism, 154–155
Ranitidine, for esophagitis, 106
for *Helicobacter* infection, 95
Recombinant human erythropoietin (rHuEPO), for anemia, 332
Red blood cell(s). See *Erythrocyte(s).*
Reflux, gastroesophageal, 73–74
Regional hemodialysis referral centers, 350t
Regurgitation, defined, 99
Renal. See also *Kidney(s).*
Renal disease, preexisting, with hyperthyroidism, 151
role of dietary lipids in, 335
Renal failure, chronic, 328–335
anemia in, prevention and treatment of, 331–332, 332t
arterial hypertension in, management of, 334
azotemia in, minimizing, 329–330
calcium and phosphorus balance in, maintenance of, 330–331
client education in, 329t
concurrent with lymphoma, 513–514
constipation in, 333
decreased appetite in, 332–333, 333t
decreased calcitriol synthesis in, 331
definition of, 513
dietary management in, 334–335
hemodialysis for, 337–350. See also *Hemodialysis.*
hydration status in, maintenance of, 333–334
kidney transplant for, 319–326. See also *Renal transplantation.*
metabolic acidosis in, treatment of, 331
monitoring of, 328–329
selected diagnostic considerations for, 328
therapeutic agents used in, 345t
total-body potassium in, maintenance of, 330
uremic gastritis in, 333
urinary tract infection in, 335
vomiting in, 332–333
secondary to hypertension, 277
Renal osteodystrophy, calcitriol for, 345t
Renal transplantation, 319–326
active feline programs for, in United States, 319
costs incurred in, 320
donor in, 321
recipient in, 319–321
anesthetic management of, 321–322
long-term care of, 325–326
postoperative management of, 323–325
preoperative management of, 321
results of, 326
surgical procedure in, 322–323, *323*
thrombocytopenia associated with, 473
Renin-angiotensin-aldosterone system (RAAS), in hypertension, 277
Resection, for squamous cell carcinoma, 194, *194*

Resource and teaching providers, in feral cat control, 564
Respiratory complications, of hemodialysis, 346–347, *347*
Respiratory disease, antibiotics for, 283–284, 285t
antifungal therapy for, 284, 286
anti-inflammatory therapy for, 286–287
antiviral therapy for, 287
bronchodilator therapy for, 287–288, 288t
isolated bacteria in, 283, 283t
supportive care for, 289
vaccines for, 288–289
Respiratory secretions, feline, zoonotic disease in human beings associated with, 20t
Respiratory tract infection, upper, concurrent with lymphoma, 509–511
diagnosis of, 509–510
management of, 510
role of vaccination in, 510–511
Restraint, manual or chemical, of sheltered animals, 571–572
Retinal atrophy, in Persian cats, 611–612
progressive, comparative gene mapping of, 608, *608*
Retinoids, for primary hereditary seborrhea oleosa, 206
for squamous cell carcinoma, 194–195
Retirement home, for pets, 621
Retroviral infections, concurrent with lymphoma, 508–509
Rhabdomyosarcoma, of oral cavity, MR imaging of, 526, *527*
Rhinitis, allergic, 234
chronic, nasal oxygen therapy for, 289
treatment of, 59
cryptococcal, 40, *40, 41*
Rhinosinusitis, role of FHV-1 in, 59
rHuEPO (recombinant human erythropoietin), for anemia, 332
Rickettsia felis, in zoonotic disease, 24
Rickettsia felis infection, 32–33
Rickettsial disease(s), 28–33. See also specific disease, e.g., *Ehrlichiosis.*
Rifampicin, for leprosy-like disease, 228
16S rRNA gene, sequence information from, in PCR assay, 480, 481

Saddle thrombus, treatment of, 265
Saline enema, in colonic studies, 76
Salmonella typhimurium, 511
Salmonella vaccine strain, choice of, in immunocontraception, 579–581
genetic engineering of, 579–580, *579–580*
Salmonellosis, 21
combined with lymphoma, 511–512
Sanitation, in evaluating life of shelter animal, 629–630
Sarcoma(s), hepatic, metastatic, cytology of, 124, *125*
vaccine-associated, 3–6, *4–5*, 541–546. See also *Vaccine-associated feline sarcoma (VAFS).*
Scaling, in photodermatitis, 191, *191*
Sciatic-tibial nerve, motor conduction of, in cat with diabetic neuropathy, *143*
Scintigraphy, strengths and weaknesses of, 548t
thyroid, 538
of cancer patients, 557–558, *557–558*

Scratches, zoonotic disease associated with, 23–24
Seborrhea, 202–207
classification of, 204t
clinical signs of, 202–203, *203–204*
definition of, 202
diagnosis of, 205
etiology and pathogenesis of, 202
management of, 205–206
prevention of, 206–207
primary, 203–204
secondary, 204–205
Secretory diarrhea, 127–128
Seizure(s), associated with hypertension, 278
in inflammatory CNS disease, 428
postoperative, as complication of renal transplantation, 324
Selamectin, prophylactic, for heartworm disease, 259
Semiferal cats, 571
Sepsis, as reaction to transfusion, 466
Septicemia, gram-negative and gram-positive, icterus associated with, 90
5-HT3-Serotonergic antagonists, classification of, 110t
5-HT4-Serotonergic antagonists, classification of, 110t
Service providers, in feral cat control, 564
Shelter(s). See *Feline animal shelter(s).*
Shift platelets, 470
Shunt (shunting), cardiac, echocardiographic imaging of, 251–252
for hydrocephalus, 417, *417*
pleuroperitoneal, in management of chylothorax, 273–274, *274*
Siamese cats, facial dysmorphia in, 451, *453*
Skin, cancer of, 192–195. See also specific type, e.g., *Squamous cell carcinoma.*
in patient with paraneoplastic alopecia, 200, *200*
Skin fragility syndrome, acquired, 199
Skull radiographs, of meningioma, 387–388
Small intestine, contrast radiographic studies of, 78–79, 79t, *80*
normal anatomy in, 76t, 77–78, *78–79*
Small-intestinal diarrhea, vs. large-intestinal diarrhea, 128t
Smells, in evaluating life of shelter animal, 628
Snake envenomation, 378–379
Sociability spectrum, of cats, 563
Socialization, feline, human approach test in, 625t
in assessment of shelter animal, 628–629
Sodium, restriction of, in prevention of calcium oxalate urolithiasis, 361
Solar radiation, skin changes due to, 190. See also *Photodermatitis.*
Sorbitol accumulation hypothesis, of pathogenesis of diabetic neuropathy, 139
Sounds, sheltered animal's response to, 628
Space, in evaluating life of shelter animal, 628
Spasticity, in Devon rex cats, 612
Spaying services, provided by veterinary hospitals, 564
Sperm antigens, in immunocontraception, 578
Sphingomyelinosis (Niemann-Pick disease), 396–398, *397*

Spina bifida, 418
Spironolactone, for hypertension, 370
Spleen, anatomy of, 439, *439*
   fine-needle aspiration of, cytology in,
      443–444, *443–444*
Splenectomy, for mast cell leukemia, 494
   for splenomegaly, 444
   hemobartonellosis exacerbated by, 13
Splenomegaly, 439–445
   diagnostic approach to, 439–444
      clinical history in, 440
      physical examination in, 440, *440*
      tests in, 440–441, *441–444, 443–444*
   diseases resulting in, 440t
   treatment of, 444–445
Spongiform encephalopathy. See
   Encephalopathy, spongiform.
Squamous cell carcinoma, histopathologic
      changes in, 192
   of oral cavity, 527–528
   prognosis associated with, 193
   treatment of, medical, 194–195, *195*
      surgical, 193–194, *194*
Squeeze cages, used in feral cat
      population, 567, *568*
"Staggering disease." See *Borna disease.*
Stance, plantigrade, secondary to diabetic
      neuropathy, 178
Stenosis, aortic, echocardiographic
      imaging of, 251
Sterilization, of feral cat, 568
Stimulants, appetite, 345t
Stimulation, degree of, in evaluating
      shelter animals, 627–628
Stomach. See also *Gastric; Gastro-*
      entries.
   contrast radiographic studies of, 74–77
      modified pneumogastrogram in, 74–
         75, *76*
      normal anatomy in, 74, *75*
   Helicobacter species infecting, 91, *92.*
      See also *Helicobacteriosis.*
Storage disorder(s), lysosomal, 450–456.
      See also specific disease, e.g.,
      Mucopolysaccharidosis.
   neuronal, 393–403. See also *Neuronal*
      storage disorder(s).
Strabismus, vertical, in hydrocephalus,
      416, *416*
Stray cats, 561–562, 563. See also *Feral*
      cat population(s).
Stress, in shelter animals, 622
   management of, in feline interstitial cys-
      titis, 315–316
Stress platelets, 470
Stricture, esophageal, diagnostic tests for,
      102, *102–103*
   treatment of, 102–103, 103t, *104*
Sulfasalazine, for inflammatory colitis,
      134
Sunburn, 192–193
Sun-induced dermatosis. See also
   Photodermatitis.
   vs. mosquito-bite hypersensitivity, 188
Supportive care, for respiratory disease,
      289
Surgery. See specific procedure, e.g.,
   Adrenalectomy.
Symblepharon, in FHV-1 infection, 52, *52*
Synthetic colloids, transfusion of, 466
Systemic lupus erythematosus, alopecia
      associated with, 198

T_3. See *Triiodothyronine (T_3)* entries.
T_4. See *Thyroxine (T_4).*

Tay-Sachs disease, 395
T-cell lymphoma, alopecia associated
      with, 199
Technical complications, of hemodialysis,
      347
Telogen defluxion, 199
Teratogenic agent(s), causing congenital
      cranial malformations, 414t
Terbutaline, for lung disease, 288
Territory, in evaluating life of shelter
      animal, 628
Tetracycline, for hemobartonellosis, 16
   for respiratory infections, 285t
Tetralogy of Fallot, echocardiographic
      imaging of, 252
Theophylline, drug interactions with,
      288t
   for heartworm disease, 257
   sustained-release, for lung disease, 288
Thiacetarsamide, for heartworm disease,
      257
   for hemobartonellosis, 16
Thiazide diuretics, for hypertension, 370
   in prevention of calcium oxalate uro-
      lithiasis, 362–363
Thioureylene agents, for hyperthyroidism,
      152–153
   prior to surgery, 156
Thoracentesis, needle, to relieve dyspnea,
      269–270
Thoracic duct ligation, with mesenteric
      lymphangiography, in management of
      chylothorax, 272–273, *273*
Thorax, radiographic studies of, in cancer
      patients, 548–549, *549–552*
   strengths and weaknesses of, 548t
Thrombocythemia, essential, 493
Thrombocytopenia, 468–477
   clinical approach to, 471–476
      basic mechanisms in, 471–473, 471t
      DAMNITT scheme in, 471t, 473–476
   diagnostic approach to, 468–470
   management of, 476–477
Thromboembolism, aortic. See *Aortic*
   thromboembolism.
   associated with adulticide therapy, 257–
      258
Thrombosis, as complication of
      hemodialysis, 348, *348–349*
Thrombotic thrombocytopenic purpura
      (TTP), 472–473
Thrombus, definition of, 405
   saddle, treatment of, 265
Thymoma, 534–535, *536*
   alopecia associated with, 199
   cytologic evaluation of, 538
   treatment of, 539
Thyroid adenocarcinoma, scintigraphic
      imaging of, *558*
Thyroid hormone(s), basal free, in
      hyperthyroidism, 147, *147*
   resting serum, in hyperthyroidism, 145–
      147, *146*
Thyroid hyperplasia, adenomatous,
      scintigraphic imaging of, *557*
Thyroid scintigraphy, 538
   diagnostic, in cancer patients, 557–558,
      557–558
   strengths and weaknesses of, 548t
Thyroidectomy, for hyperthyroidism,
      156–157
Thyroid-stimulating hormone (TSH)
      secretion, inhibition of, 147
Thyrotropin-releasing hormone (TRH)
      stimulation test, for hyperthyroidism,
      148–149, *149*

Thyroxine (T_4), concentration of, before
      and after administration of
      liothyronine, 148, *148*
   before and after TRH stimulation,
      148–149, *149*
   resting serum, 145–147, *146*
   decreased levels of, 151–152
   following thyroidectomy, 157
   free, 147, *147*
Tick(s), *Cytauxzoon* transmission by, 436
   Ehrlichia transmission by, 28–29
Tick paralysis, 378
Toxicity, organophosphate and carbamate,
      379
Toxin(s), environmental, causing
      thrombocytopenia, 476
Toxoplasma gondii, 21, 432, 565
Toxoplasma gondii titers, prior to renal
      transplantation, 320, 321
Toxoplasmosis, 21–23, 432–433
   in feral cat populations, 565
Transfusion. See *Blood transfusion.*
Transmissible spongiform
      encephalopathies (TSEs), 62. See also
      Encephalopathy, spongiform.
Transplantation, bone marrow. See *Bone*
   marrow transplantation (BMT).
   renal. See *Renal transplantation.*
Trap, neuter, and return (TNR) programs,
      for feral cat populations, 561, 562t
Trap, sterilize, vaccinate, and release
      programs, in animal shelters, 575
Traumatic injuries, in geriatric cats, 585
Tricuspid valve insufficiency,
      echocardiographic imaging of,
      249–250
Trifluridine, for herpesvirus-1 (FHV-1)
      infection, 58
Triglycerides, 214
Triiodothyronine (T_3), decreased levels of,
      151–152
   free, 147
   resting serum concentrations of, 145–
      147, *146*
Triiodothyronine (T_3) suppression test,
      147–148
Trimethoprim/sulfonamide, for respiratory
      infections, 285t
Troglitazone, for non–insulin-dependent
      diabetes mellitus, 171t, 172
Trypanosoma species, detection of, PCR
      assay in, 482
TSEs (transmissible spongiform
      encephalopathies), 62. See also
      Encephalopathy, spongiform.
TTP (thrombotic thrombocytopenic
      purpura), 472–473
Tularemia, 449
Tumor(s). See at anatomic site, e.g., *Oral*
      tumor(s); specific tumor, e.g.,
      Meningioma.
Tumor suppressor genes, role of, in
      vaccine-associated feline sarcomas, 4,
      542
Two-dimensional echocardiography, 245
Tylosin, for clostridial colitis, 134
   for cryptosporidiosis, 36

Ulceration, of conjunctiva, in FHV-1
      infection, 53, *53*
   of ear-tip, solar-induced, 191, *191*
   of muzzle, in mosquito-bite hypersensi-
      tivity, 187, *187*
Ultrafiltration, principles of, in
      hemodialysis, 338, *339*

Ultrasonography, abdominal, of lymphosarcoma, 500
of pancreatic adenocarcinoma, in patient with paraneoplastic alopecia, 200, *200*
of patient with chronic diarrhea, 132t, 133
of spleen, 443, *443*
diagnostic, in cancer patients, 552–555, *554–555*
strengths and weaknesses of, 548t
of lymphoma with concurrent disease, 507
of mediastinal tumors, 535, 537
of patient with acquired heart disease, *248–250*, 248–251, 249t
Ultraviolet-A (UVA), 190
Ultraviolet-B (UVB), 190
Underresponsiveness, in geriatric cats, 584
Upper gastrointestinal series, of small intestine, 78–79, 79t, *80*
of stomach, 75–77, *77*
Urea breath test, *for Helicobacter* infection, 95
Uremia, antiemetics for, 110–111
Uremic encephalopathy, in dialysis patient, 346
Uremic gastritis, in chronic renal failure, 333
Uremic pneumonitis, in dialysis patient, 347
Ureteroliths, 359
Urethroliths, 359
Urinalysis, in diagnosis of calcium oxalate uroliths, 356, *356*
Urinary cortisol:creatinine ratio, 165 measurement of, 167
Urinary tract infection, in chronic renal failure, 335
Urinary tract zoonoses, feline and canine, 20t
Urination, outside litter box, 583
Urine, chemical analysis of, 357–358
glycosaminoglycans in, detection of, 455–456, *455–456*
saturation of, calcium oxalate crystallization in, 354–355
concept of, 352–354, *353–354*
tests for, 358
Urobilinogen, 88
Urocystoliths, 359
Urolith(s), formation of, calcium oxalate crystallization in, 354–355
mechanism of, 352–354, *353–354*
radiographic imaging of, 356–357, *357–359*
voided or retrieved, analysis of, 358–359
Urolithiasis, calcium oxalate, 352–363
clinical signs of, 355
diagnosis of, analysis of retrieved uroliths in, 358–359
endocrine testing in, 357
imaging characteristics in, 356–357, *357–359*
patient signalment in, 356
serum biochemical analysis in, 356
urinalysis in, 356, *356*
urine chemistry analysis in, 357–358
urine saturation in, 358
differential diagnosis of, 355–356
epidemiology of, 352
etiopathogenesis of, 352–355, *353–354*

Urolithiasis *(Continued)*
hypercalcemia associated with, 311
prevention of, 359, *360*, 361–363
dietary considerations in, 361–362, 363t
pharmacologic therapy in, 362–363
treatment of, 359
UVA (ultraviolet-A), 190
UVB (ultraviolet-B), 190
Uveitis, idiopathic, associated with FHV-1 infection, 55

Vaccine (vaccination), feline, in shelter medicine, 572
recommendations regarding, 546t
for *Bordetella bronchiseptica*, 8
for *Chlamydia psittaci*, 8
for feline calicivirus, 8
for feline herpesvirus-1, 7–8, 59–60, 59t
for feline infectious peritonitis, 9
for feline leukemia virus, 8–9
for feline viral rhinotracheitis, calicivirus, and panleukopenia, 541
for *Giardia* species, 9
for *Microsporum canis*, 9
for panleukopenia, 7
for rabies, 9
for respiratory disease, 288–289
recommendations for, current, 6–7
sarcomas at site of. See *Vaccine-associated feline sarcoma (VAFS)*.
Vaccine Associated Feline Sarcoma Task Force (VAFSTF), 541
guidelines by, 543t
Vaccine-associated feline sarcoma (VAFS), 3–6, *4–5*, 541–546
clinical signs of, 542, 543t, *544*
diagnosis of, 543, *544–545*
epidemiology of, 3, 542
etiology of, 541–542
pathogenesis of, 4–5, 542
prevention of, 5, 546, 546t
treatment of, 5–6, 543–546, 543t
chemotherapy in, 545–546
immunotherapy in, 546
radiation therapy in, 545
surgical, 544–545
vs. non-vaccine site sarcoma, 3
VAFS. See *Vaccine-associated feline sarcoma (VAFS)*.
VAFSTF (Vaccine Associated Feline Sarcoma Task Force), 541
guidelines by, 543t
Valvular insufficiency, echocardiographic imaging of, 249–251
Vanadium, for non–insulin-dependent diabetes mellitus, 171t, 172
Vascular access, complications of, in hemodialysis, 347–348, *348*
Ventricular outflow obstruction, echocardiographic imaging of, 251
Very low density lipoprotein (VLDL), 215
Veterinarian, in animal shelter medicine, 575
role of, in feral cat solution, 566–567
Veterinary blood banks, 462t
Veterinary practice, feral cats in, 567–569, 567t, *568*
Vidarabine, for herpesvirus-1 (FHV-1) infection, 58
Vincristine, 521–522
dosage of, 522
for lymphosarcoma, 504t

Viral-associated diarrhea, 129t
Virus(es), isolation of, in FHV-1 infection, 56
role of, in vaccine-associated feline sarcomas, 4, 542
Vision, line of, of caged animal, 627–628
Vitamin B_6, in prevention of calcium oxalate urolithiasis, 362
Vitamin C, restriction of, in prevention of calcium oxalate urolithiasis, 362
Vitamin D, restriction of, in prevention of calcium oxalate urolithiasis, 362
supplemental, following thyroidectomy, 156–157
Vitamin K antagonists, bleeding associated with, 476
Vitamin K_1, for reversal of effects of warfarin, 411
Vitamin K–dependent clotting factors, warfarin inhibition of, 304
VLDL (very low density lipoprotein), 215
Vocalization, in geriatric cats, 583–584
Vomiting. See *Emesis*.

Warfarin, drug interactions with, 304
for aortic thromboembolism, 410
prophylactic, 303–304
Water, in prevention of calcium oxalate urolithiasis, 362, 363t
Welfare, of feral cats, 566
Wildlife, impact of feral cat populations on, 565–566
World Health organization (WHO) definition, of quality of life, 624

Xanthoma(s), cutaneous, 214–218
clinical signs of, 216, *216–217*
diagnosis of, 216–218, *217*
treatment of, 218

Yersinia pestis, 449, 565

Zolazepam, chemical restraint with, 572
Zollinger-Ellison syndrome, 183
Zona pellucida, type of, in immunocontraception, 579–581
Zoonotic disease, 18–25
associated with feline and canine urinary and genital tracts, 20t
associated with feline excrement, 19t
associated with feline respiratory or ocular secretions, 20t
avoidance of, recommendations for, 24–25, 25t
bite and scratch–associated, 23–24. See also specific disease, e.g., *Bartonellosis (cat-scratch disease)*.
emerging, 24. See also specific disease, e.g., *Ehrlichiosis*.
enteric, 18, 20–23. See also specific disease, e.g., *Cryptosporidiosis*.
transmission of, by feral cat populations, 564–565
treatment of, 25
ZP4 gene, expression of, 579–580, *579–581*